Voigt's Pharmaceutical Technology

Voigt's Pharmaceutical Technology

Prof. Dr. Alfred Fahr

Institute of Pharmaceutical Technology
Friedrich - Schiller University of Jena, Germany

Translated by Prof. Dr. Gerrit Scherphof

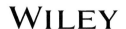

Registered Office(s)
John Wiley & Sons, Inc., 111 River Street, Hoboken, NJ 07030, USA
John Wiley & Sons Ltd, The Atrium, Southern Gate, Chichester, West Sussex,
PO19 8SQ, UK

Editorial Office
The Atrium, Southern Gate, Chichester, West Sussex, PO19 8SQ, UK

For details of our global editorial offices, customer services, and more information about Wiley products visit us at www.wiley.com.

Wiley also publishes its books in a variety of electronic formats and by print-on-demand. Some content that appears in standard print versions of this book may not be available in other formats.

Library of Congress Cataloging-in-Publication Data

Names: Fahr, Alfred, author.
Title: Voigt's pharmaceutical technology / by Alfred Fahr; translated by Gerrit Scherphof.
Other titles: Voigt Pharmazeutische Technologie. English | Pharmaceutical technology
Description: Hoboken, NJ: Wiley, 2018. | Includes bibliographical references and index. |
Identifiers: LCCN 2017031789 (print) | LCCN 2017033911 (ebook) | ISBN 9781118972434 (pdf) |
    ISBN 9781118972441 (epub) | ISBN 9781118972625 (cloth)
Subjects: | MESH: Technology, Pharmaceutical
Classification: LCC RS380 (ebook) | LCC RS380 (print) | NLM QV 778 | DDC 615.1/9–dc23
LC record available at https://lccn.loc.gov/2017031789

Cover image: © Lightspring/Shutterstock
Cover design by Wiley

Set in 9/12pt JoannaMtStd by Aptara Inc., New Delhi, India.
Printed and bound in Singapore by Markono Print Media Pte Ltd

10 9 8 7 6 5 4 3 2 1

Contents

Note: Online supplementary material for the book can be found at http://booksupport.wiley.com

Contributors

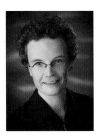

Prof. Dr. Heike Bunjes
Institut für Pharmazeutische
Technologie
Technische Universität Braunschweig
Braunschweig, Germany

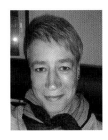

Prof. Dr. Judith Kuntsche
Department of Physics, Chemistry
and Pharmacy
University of Southern Denmark
Odense, Denmark

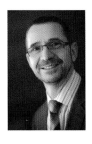

Prof. Dr. Rolf Daniels
Institute for Pharmacy
Pharmaceutical Technology
Eberhard Karls University Tübingen
Tübingen, Germany

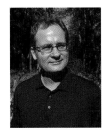

Prof. Dr. Sylvio May
Department of Physics
North Dakota State University
Fargo ND, USA

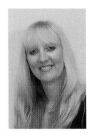

Prof. Dr. Dagmar Fischer
Institute for Pharmacy
Department of Pharmaceutical
Technology
Friedrich-Schiller University of Jena
Jena, Germany

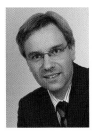

PD Dr. habil. Stefan Scheler
Novartis Technical Operations
Biologics Technical Development &
Manufacturing
Sandoz GmbH
Langkampfen, Austria

Foreword

During my studies in Oxford, I had to follow a class in electrochemistry, and in the Bodleian library I found an excellent textbook on this topic. Comfortably stretched out on the perfectly trimmed lawn of my college, I started to read it. To my surprise, I quickly discovered that I was able to easily grasp the meaning of all the statements and formulas, which had given me so much trouble years before in Germany when I was following a similar class using a German textbook. I considered that, rather than due to my increased wisdom, this was due to the difference in style of textbook writing between German and Anglo-Saxon countries. In other words, "A German author likes to emphasize the complexity of matters that only he understands."

At the end of my studies, I decided that, whenever I would have the opportunity to write my own textbook, I would bring into practice the ideas and recommendations that famous writers and philosophers have provided us with over the centuries. For example, Voltaire left us the consideration that "The secret of being a bore... is to tell everything."

The chance to write a textbook came when Rudolf Voigt, the founder of the original German version of this textbook half a century ago, asked me to continue his life's work, 20 years ago. Over the following German editions, while basically sticking to Voigt's original intentions, I tried to follow the early philosophers as much as scientific restrictions would allow. Obviously, by doing so it was unavoidable to accept compromises, some of which I have specified below.

Teaching the complex subject of *pharmaceutical technology* is approached differently in different areas of the world. In some countries, pharmacy students are just taught to make an ointment and become acquainted to various extents with other technologies by means of demonstrations or videos. In Europe, on the other hand, pharmaceutical technology is taught to pharmacy students in extensive and comprehensive courses, including several practical courses concluded by highly demanding exams. In Germany, each individual student prepares ALL conceivable formulations in the lab so that he or she is familiar with each relevant detail of each product sold in a pharmacy and also gains a solid background for a career in pharmaceutical industry.

Students do not invariably undergo this learning process with great pleasure and enthusiasm. This makes teachers aware of specific difficulties that students experience in thoroughly understanding the scientific background of the various technologies. At the same time, it will hopefully teach them to effectively and elegantly handle situations arising from the lack of understanding of students. The educational experience, thus gathered over the past decades, has been gradually integrated into this book. Thus, we have tried to visualize the manifold principles of the different technologies and their applications, both by means of text and technical illustrations.

We are aware that for many students, it is a nightmare to discover that understanding pharmaceutical technology is based on a solid background in fields such as chemistry, physics, biology, material science, medicine, and (worst of all!) mathematics (statistics).

The reader will find these topics in the first few chapters, including, for example, statistics. In Germany, statistics is not taught at the required level in the regular pharmacy curriculum. Therefore, the statistics chapter was added with the idea in mind that the combination of any rudimentary exposure to stats with thorough reading of this chapter should enable the reader to build a sufficient level of comprehension to serve as a solid base in statistics for a professional career in pharmacy.

As the reader may have guessed, this is one of the compromises I mentioned above. I do believe it is worthwhile.

The other compromise the reader will encounter is in Chapter 5, in which we deal with all known excipients. A large number of German readers (students and professionals alike) were in favor of this idea. A potential drawback of this decision is that it may occasionally require the reader to browse through this chapter for detailed information on certain excipients described in the context of pharmaceutical formulations in other chapters (but that is why the index register was created!).

Other features which may be helpful to the reader are the boxes explaining details and text boxes derived from paragraphs of the Ph. Eur., which may serve to give insight in the way scientific observations find their way into regulatory texts. In the English edition, we added in these text boxes the corresponding texts from USP and the Japanese Pharmacopeia in a comparative way. The Annex section was improved similarly. Here the reader can find descriptions of representative pharmaceutical formulations taking into consideration the differences with respect to preparation methods and tests between the three main pharmacopeias for the dosage forms chosen. We trust this will be helpful not only for the pharmacy student to guide her or him on the way to become a pharmacist and beyond, but will be appreciated by the established professional pharmacist as well.

About the English edition: The mission of all of us was to compose a textbook that was both comprehensive and comprehensible. It was meant to offer relatively easy but scientifically sound reading to an audience of students and professionals, much like the latest German edition. When Wiley suggested that publication of an English version of the book might be worth considering, we set out to find someone knowledgeable enough in the field to grasp at least the scientific backgrounds of the immense field involved and at the same time possessing enough passive knowledge of the German language to understand the German texts and active knowledge of English to produce an acceptable first draft of an English text, although not necessarily being a native speaker. Such a person was found, and his initial English texts were edited by us for scientific and terminological correctness. The resulting texts were subsequently edited by five motivated British PhD students of pharmacy. In addition to language editing they also provided useful suggestions for missing content.

Together with the contributors, I monitored all these processes.

Meanwhile—this process alone took over one year—I also consulted a number of highly competent colleagues from industry and academia about novel trends, devices, and processes. It was highly gratifying to observe how generously all these experts were willing to provide me with relevant information. The names of all these individuals can be found below. Thus, this first English edition has become much more than a mere translation of our 12th German edition. I already have started thinking about translating the English edition into our next 13th German edition.

We anticipate that Wiley's decision to produce a multicolored edition will substantially add to its readability and thus to the digestion by the reader. Prof. Dr. Judith Kuntsche, who created the modern graphics in the latest German editions, appropriately transformed those and produced new ones to offer a new dimension in visualisation.

My special thanks go to Rebecca Stubbs and Sarah Keegan at Wiley in the UK for their constant support and unconventional assistance all through the translating part of the project. I thank Cheryl Ferguson in the USA for the very interactive time during her copy editing work and her teaching of good (American) English. The final production process of the book including composing and the almost never-ending story of proofreading and—changing was done on another continent for this international book by Audrey Koh in Singapore and Shalini Sharma in India, two very lenient and patient ladies. Surely there were many other people at Wiley involved whom I want to say "Thank You" for accompanying me on this long journey.

I would also thank my family for their understanding for the last years. This goes especially to my kids Sophie and Fabian, that on many days an unshaved man appeared to finish off his breakfast or dinner in the upper rooms of the house, rapidly disappearing again in his hades back to his computers and books. *Was this daddy?*—Yes! my loving wife would have answered. Thanks for understanding my interpretation of the word "retired", dear Sabine!

We all hope that you will appreciate our efforts. We do not have the illusion that this book will be different from other textbooks by being flawless (particularly as being the 1st edition). Therefore, we are soliciting your alertness for typos and—yes, we will be prepared to face it—blatant errors and other mistakes like untranslated German words.

Please email me when you have found one or more of those in this book. I will collect all errors found by the users of the book and every half year I will draw one of the reporters for a prize. For the German edition, I have awarded thus far bottles of wine from my hometown on Lake Constance as a token of our appreciation. For the international book, I might have to think of a less fragile item.

The elimination of any bugs and additional information about new trends in pharmaceutics and more profound and detailed insights into technologies you might find on my website www.alfred-fahr.com. Please email me (alfred.fahr@uni-jena.de) for any suggestions.

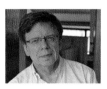

Prof. Dr. Alfred Fahr
Professor Emeritus
Institute of Pharmacy
Friedrich-Schiller University of Jena
Jena, Germany

Acknowledgements

We would like to thank the translator, Gerrit Scherphof, for his translation of the German text. He has also pinpointed many unclear wordings and offered his continuous support on addressing difficult translation problems and changing my Denglish to decent English.

We would also like to thank the five British PhD students who read the translated text for comprehensibility and checked the pharmaceutics wording. They also gave useful hints for making difficult items more understandable: Carla Roces-Rodriguez, Mandeep Marwah, Thomas Dennison, Jasdip Koner, and Swapnil Khadke.

I am very thankful to many experts in industry and academia, who spent a lot of time for and with me showing and demonstrating new devices and methods we know—if at all—only from literature. I am also indebted for many drawings and photographs I was permitted to use in the updated chapters. Among these gentle persons are: Dr. Karlheinz Seyfang (Harro Höfliger); PD Dr. Martin Tegtmeier (Schaper & Brümmer), Dr. Ruth Leu-Marseiler (Novartis), Dr. Tereza Pereira de Souza (Harvard University), Dr. Hanns-Christian Mahler (Lonza); Prof. Sven Stegemann (Capsugel); Prof. Dr. Karl Wagner (University of Bonn); Marten Klukkert (Fette); Dr. Brigitte Skalsky (Evonik); Lilian Schmalenstroer (GEA); Anita Meister and Alexander Muskat (Groninger); Dr. Norbert Pöllinger (Glatt); Mark W. Ayles (Pall); Petra Silbereisen (Sotax); Peter Keller (Filtrox); Bärbel Kroll (Uhlmann); and Jarrett Mallory (Frain).

I also thank Trevor Rigby, Jasmine Weidenbach, and Jennifer Benson in Marburg for many discussions and help on British and American English.

Finally, I would like to thank Kalpa Nagarsenker and Mukul Ashtikar, for their proofreading and contributions in providing explanations at the proper places to make this book even more readable.

List of Abbreviations

A

AE	anion exchanger
AAS	Atomic absorption spectrometry
ACTH	adrenocorticotropic hormone
ADME	absorption, distribution, metabolism, elimination
AFM	Atomic Force Microscopy
AIO	all in one
ANM	amylum non mucilaginosum
API	active pharmaceutical ingredient
ASTM	American Society for Testing and Materials
AUC	Area under the curve

B

BA	bioavailability
BBB	blood brain barrier
BE	bioequivalence
BET	bacterial endotoxin test
BET theory	Brunauer-Emmett-Teller theory
BFS	blow fill seal
BHA	butylhydroxyanisole
BHT	butylhydroxytoluene
BODI	Bioadhesive ophthalmic drug inserts
BSE	Bovine Spongiform Encephalopathy

C

CAP	cellulose acetate phthalate
CCS	container closure system
CE	cation exchanger
CEN	Comité Européen de Normalisation (European Committee for Standardization)
CFR	Code of Federal Regulations
CFU	colony forming unit
CMC	critical micelle concentration (the concentration of surfactants above which micelles are spontaneously formed)
CMV	cytomegalovirus
COC	certificat of conformity
COMOD	continuous mono dose
CQAs	critical quality attributes
CTD	common technological document

D

d	day
DAB	Deutsches Arzneibuch (German Pharmacopeia)
DAC	Deutscher Arzneimittel-Codex (German Drug Codex)
DB	double blind
DCJI	disposable-cartridge jet injector
DER	Drug-Extract-Relation
DIN	Deutsche Industrienorm (German Industrial Standard)
DIN	German Institute for Normalization

DLVO theory	named after Boris Derjaguin, Lev Landau, Evert Verwey and Theodor Overbeek
DOE	design of experiments
DPI	Dry powder inhaler
DSC	differential scanning calorimetry
DVS	Dynamic Vapor Sorption

E

EDTA	ethylenediaminetetraacetate
ELISA	enzyme-linked immunosorbent assay

F

FDA	Food and Drug Administration (federal agency of the United States Department of Health and Human Services)
FIP	Fédération Internationale Pharmaceutique (International Pharmaceutical Federation)
FTIR	Fourier transform infrared spectroscopy

G

GACP	Good Agricultural and Collection Practice
GCP	Good Clinical Practice
GIT	gastrointestinal tract
GLP	Good Laboratory Practice
GMP	Good Manufacturing Practice
GRAS	generally recognized as safe

H

HAB	Homöopathisches Arzneibuch (Homeopathic Pharmacopeia)
HDPE	high density polyethylene
HEC	hydroxyethylcellulose
HEMA	hydroxyethylmethacrylate
HEPA filter	high-efficiency particulate air filter
HES	hydroxyethyl starch
HFA	hydrofluoroalkane
HFC	partially fluorinated hydrocarbon
HIV	human immunodeficiency virus
HLB	hydrophilic–lipophilic balance
HPC	hydroxypropylcellulose
HPMC	hydroxypropylmethylcellulose
HPMCP	hydroxypropylmethylcellulose phthalate

I

ICH	International Council for Harmonisation of Technical Requirements for Pharmaceuticals for Human Use
IUPAC	International Union of Pure and Applied Chemistry

J

JP	Japanese Pharmacopeia

L

LADME	liberation, absorption, distribution, metabolism, excretion
LAF	laminar air flow
LAL	Limulus Amebocyte Lysate (test)
LDPE	low density polyethylene (see also PE-LD)
lg	logarithm with base 10
LOD	limit of detection
LVP	large-volume parenterals

M

MA	methacrylic acid
MAT	monocyte activation test
MC	methylcellulose
MCC	microcrystalline cellulose
MCT	medium chain triglyceride
MDI	metered dose inhaler
MEC	minimal effective concentration
MEMS	micro-electromechanical
MFG	modified fluid gelatin
MMA	methyl methacrylate
MR	modified release
MRT	mean residence time
MVD	maximum valid dilution

N

Na-CMC	sodium carboxymethyl cellulose
NEMS	nano-electromechanical
NF	National Formulary (Excipient monographs in the USP-NF)
NMR	nuclear magnetic resonance
NODS	new ophthalmic delivery system
NVP	N-vinylpyrrolidone

O

OPC	one-point-cut (-ampoule)

P

PAT	Process Analytical Technology
PCS	photon correlation spectroscopy
PE	polyethylene
PEG	polyethylene glycol or poly(ethylene glycol)
PE-LD	low density polyethylene (soft polyethylene)
PEO	polyethylene oxide
PETP	polyethylene terephthalate
PFC	fully fluorinated hydrocarbons
Ph. Eur.	European Pharmacopeia
PIC	Pharmaceutical Inspection Convention
PIT	phase inversion temperature
PLGA	poly(lactic-co-glycolic acid)
pMDI	pressurized metered dose inhaler
PMMA	polymethylmethacrylate
PTFE	polytetrafluorethylene
pull point	time point of sample withdrawal
PVA	polyvinyl alcohol
PVC	polyvinyl chloride
PVDC	polyvinylidene chloride
PVDF	polyvinylidenefluoride
PVP	polyvinylpyrrolidone

Q

Quats	quaternary ammonium cations

R

RH	relative humidity
RIA	radio immuno assay
RMM	rapid microbiological methods

RMS	root mean square
RNS	rigid needle shield
RRSB	Rosin, Rammler, Sperling, Bennet (distribution)
RSE	reference standard endotoxin

S

SAL	sterility assurance level
SLN	solid lipid nanoparticles
SODI	Soluble ophthalmic drug inserts
SOP	standard operating procedure
SVP	small-volume parenterals

T

TAMC	total aerobic microbial count
TOC	total organic carbon
TPN	total parenteral nutrition
TS	therapeutic system
TTS	transdermal therapeutic system

U

UAP	Ultraamylopectin®
USP	United States Pharmacopeia (contains the monographs for drug substances, dosage forms, and compounded preparations)

W

WFI	water for injections
WHO	World Health Organization

Index of Pharmacopeia Boxes

Dosage Forms

Despite all available protocols, rules and regulations, the development of a new formulation is still an exciting endeavor. And often even, this endeavor turns out to be an open-ended adventure, because numerous poorly understood factors engaged in ill-defined interactions with each other, may turn out to play an essential part in the process. George Wald described this sensation in his Nobel lecture (1967) with the words, "I have often had cause to feel that my hands are cleverer than my head." This notion is also quite commonly experienced by pharmaceutical scientists, who in many cases have to rely on the phenomenon of "serendipity" (keyword: "chance favors only the prepared mind"). It may be comforting to the reader that this book, even though not helpful in affecting chance, may do so by preparing the reader's mind.

Drug Formulations as Application System—Science and Legal Provisions

1.1 General Principles

The main objective to formulate a drug is to deliver it in a reproducible, reliable, safe, and optimally effective manner, thus allowing it to exert its proper therapeutic effect under quality-controlled conditions. Only in rare cases will it be possible to administer a drug without any formulation, such as a single, measured dose (e.g., a single-dose powder only containing the active ingredient itself). In most cases, however, the active agent(s) will have to be transformed into a medication (i.e., a drug formulation) by means of appropriate pharmaceutical techniques employing one or more preferably inert substances, while taking into consideration therapeutical and biopharmaceutical requirements, as well as machinability, stability, and appearance.

Thus, a drug product consists of active and inactive substances, as shown in Fig. 1-1.

The definition of the term *pharmaceutics* varies with the legislature of individual countries. Often, it includes active substances as well as drug products. But it may also refer to individual prescriptions, bulk formulations, or large-scale supplies of ready-to-use products. Pharmaceuticals are distinguished from medical devices (*for an elaborate definition, see chapter 5.1*) by their principal mechanism of action (metabolic, immunological, or pharmacological for the former, and physical or physicochemical for the latter, even if they serve therapeutic or diagnostic purposes).

The inactive substances, known as *excipients*, play an important role in the formulation of drugs (see chapter 5). Not only are they responsible for the characteristic appearance of a formulation, but most of all they ensure the drug's biological availability and therapeutic action as well as its controlled and economically accountable production.

It is only after an active agent has been transferred into a suitable formulation that a certain kind of application becomes possible. For example, for peroral administration, drugs are most often formulated as tablets or capsules, but liquid preparations such as solutions, suspensions, or emulsions may also serve as vehicles. For the treatment of skin conditions, ointments, pastes, and liniments are often applied (chapter 15). Suppositories or rectal capsules are suitable for rectal applications, while for application into the blood stream therapeutic agents are formulated as solutions or suspensions for injection or infusion (chapter 21).

Aerosols are most suitable for the treatment of bronchial or pulmonary epithelia (chapter 23). Particle dimensions of novel drug formulations tend to reach the micro- or nanometer range—for example, microparticles or nanoparticles such as liposomes (chapter 20.2). The turbulent development of molecular and gene technology requires multifunctional, "intelligent," and conductible (i.e., site-directed) formulations to allow effective delivery of medicines with limited water solubility, low-membrane permeability, or insufficient stability, such as peptides, proteins, DNA, RNA, or strongly lipophilic substances.

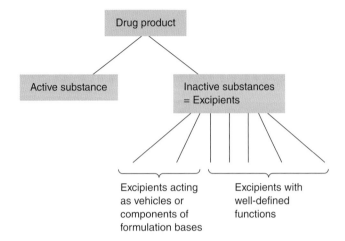

Fig. 1-1 Components of a drug product.

Definition of Active Pharmaceutical Ingredient (API) (or Drug Substance or Active substance) by the FDA (U.S.A.): "Any substance or mixture of substances intended to be used in the manufacture of a drug (medicinal) product and that, when used in the production of a drug, becomes an active ingredient of the drug product. Such substances are intended to furnish pharmacological activity or other direct effect in the diagnosis, cure, mitigation, treatment, or prevention of disease or to affect the structure and function of the body." Also the expression AI (active ingredient) or pharmacon is used.

In contrast, the active ingredient in plant material is called *active constituent*.

These are only a few examples, but they clearly illustrate the many available possibilities to design appropriate formulations to administer pharmaceutically active agents in or on the human and animal body. The choice of formulation will depend on the site to be treated and the site of action, the type of disease, the patient population (i.e. adults or children), and the desired effect. Nowadays, such formulations are often referred to as *drug delivery systems*, meant to allow tailored deployment of a pharmaceutical agent for a defined and exclusive therapeutic goal (targeted delivery). So-called therapeutic systems release the active drug at the site of action in a controlled way with a well-defined premeditated constant release rate for a fixed time period. Examples of such systems are the Transdermal Therapeutic Systems (TTS) (see chapter 16) or the Oral Osmotic Systems (OROS) (see chapter 12.6.3).

It is important to note that the formulation has, by no means, only a carrier function. The basic ingredients and excipients, as well as the manufacturing technology, strongly influence the ultimate effect of the drug. The onset, duration, and intensity of the drug action depend on the way it is formulated. Therefore, the formulation plays a substantial role in the ultimate efficacy of the drug. It represents a complex system whose individual components (active substance(s) and excipients (see Fig. 1-1)) should not just be regarded as isolated entities, but rather, in combination with the numerous possible interactions of the individual components. It is important to stay aware that the manufacturing technology may act on each of them in many different ways (see Fig. 1-2).

Accurate dosing of the drug formulation is important for the patient not to experience harmful side effects as a result of dose deviations. This implies that weight and drug content of single-dose medication, e.g. individual tablet, is controlled in a narrow range.

A further requirement of the formulation concerns sufficient stability of the active ingredient, but also all excipients. Often, the proper choice of packaging may already diminish or prevent stability loss.

Drug formulations should as well have an appealing appearance. Most pharmacopeias, therefore, allow the use of pigments (water-soluble, fat-soluble, or insoluble coloring substances; see section 5.4.1). For the sake of making the product more appealing, for better recognition (to prevent mixing up different medicines) or psychological aspects. This is, in particular, used for (coated) tablets, capsules, and suppositories. Coloring of medicines does not always come without problems. Under certain conditions, dyes may be oncogenic, embryotoxic, or teratogenic. Therefore, only formally approved dyes have to be used. Initiatives are underway to establish their safety by scientific data as a prerequisite for permanent listing. Depending on the physicochemical properties of the dyes, undesirable changes in the drug system, including interactions or incompatibilities between active ingredient and excipients, cannot be rigorously excluded. Apart from that, the sustainability of a medicine also applies to the stability of the applied pigments (check by means of color charts or colorimetry).

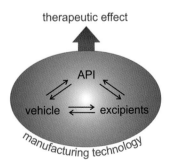

Fig. 1-2 The drug formulation as a system.

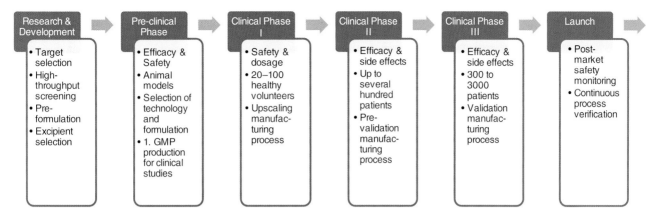

Fig. 1-3 Drug development process.

Furthermore, in the case of orally administered medicines, it is advisable to conceal bad flavor or odor with suitable excipients.

The development of a drug formulation is a complex process that, grossly simplified, is characterized by the following stages (see Fig. 1-3):

- In the pre-formulation stage, the physicochemical properties of the active ingredient (e.g., solubility, stability, distribution coefficient, acid-base characteristics, particle size, salt selection, polymorphism, etc.) is intensively investigated. This is meant to serve as the basis for the selection of a suitable formulation, to predict the behavior of the new drug form and to facilitate planning of the developing process by identification of critical parameters at this stage.

- Furthermore, investigations are conducted with the aim to select suitable excipients for the formulation of a medicine—for instance, with respect to possible interactions with the active ingredient. While earlier these processes were predominantly depending on a trial-and-error approach, nowadays a more rational strategy, based on statistically supported research planning is prevailing.

- Based on the results of these investigations formulation development takes place under laboratory conditions. Using different excipients and technologies a suitable formulation for first human studies is developed and assessed for stability.

- The selected formulation is produced under GMP conditions in order to supply the first clinical study

- After successful completion of a series of first clinical studies (so-called phase I, conducted on healthy volunteers to determine patient tolerance, the distribution in the body, single ascending dose and multiple ascending dose) upscaling follows (verification in the pilot facility).

- If the clinical phase II study (activity and dose finding in several hundreds of patients) turns out to be successful as well, the project will finally be transferred to the production department of the pharmaceutical industry.

- This transfer to mass production, also described as upscaling, may cause problems in the adjustment of methodology, especially in case of complex novel drug formulations. Efforts spent in the developing process are decisive for the technical feasibility and, in connection to that, the economic feasibility of the project, precipitating in the production costs.

The leading principle is most certainly the implementation of the regulations concerning quality certification of the entire production process. Pioneering work in this connection was performed by the approval authorities of the United States, who brought together a number of already-existing guidelines, drawn up in 1962, under the concept of Good Manufacturing Practice (GMP). Several other countries also adopted these efforts. Global guidelines were worked out by the *International Council for Harmonisation of Technical Requirements for Pharmaceuticals for Human Use* (ICH) and should, at least for Europe, the United States, and Japan, form the basis for approval. The WHO-GMP guidelines are, however, directional in more than 100 (predominantly developing) countries.

1.2   Good Manufacturing Practice (GMP)

Since the late 1960s, recurring incidents with medicines such as switching incidents (mix-ups of medications), cross contaminations, (bacterial) contaminations, and the discovery of serious shortcomings during test procedures have gradually led to the introduction of stringent measures *vis-à-vis* quality security of active ingredients, excipients, and drug product. Since then, solid proof of safety, efficacy and quality of the drug as well as drug products for the entire shelf life is requested.

Fulfillment of these essential requirements must be undisputable before approval will be obtained. They are laid down in drug laws that regulate the development, approval, and commercialization of medicines. The approval of medicines is granted at the national level, such as a request of approval in a given country is submitted to the qualified authorities in that country (e.g., USA: FDA; Germany: BfArM; Japan: MHLW). Within the European Union, centralized and decentralized procedures can be distinguished. In case of a centralized procedure, the request is filed at the European Medicines Agency for all EU countries alike. In case of decentralized procedures (DCP), there is an additional distinction as compared to the Mutual Recognition Procedures (MRP). For a MRP, an approval request is first submitted to only one country, and after obtaining approval a procedure is started to obtain mutual approval in other EU countries. In the DCP, approval requests are filed simultaneously in several countries and one of them is selected as a reference country. The other countries carry out an evaluation of the submission in a coordinated mutual approval process.

The World Health Organization (WHO) drafted in 1968 a document called "Draft Requirements for Good Manufacturing Practice in the Manufacture and Quality Control of Drugs and Pharmaceutical Specialties" as an instrument for the introduction of quality criteria, suggested for use in all member states, to accomplish a harmonized standard of production and quality control.

This document, which in its current version is called "WHO Good Manufacturing Practices: Main Principles for Pharmaceutical Products," has repeatedly been supplemented and revised over the years. Nowadays its key message is worldwide known as Good Manufacturing Practice (GMP).

As a further completion of the original *WHO-GMP Guidelines,* (mainly European) authorities in charge of its surveillance on their turn launched a frequently up-dated agreement on the mutual recognition of inspections of pharmaceutical industries (PIC—Pharmaceutical Inspection Convention) in 1970.

In this agreement, furthermore, the basic rules and regulations for GMP-compatible manufacturing of pharmaceutical products are laid down (PIC-GMP rules). The document stipulates in particular the guidelines for the manufacturing of sterile products, the handling of raw materials, and the packaging of pharmaceutical products.

In the early 1990s, the EU established its own GMP rules (EU-GMP-regulations) that were basically adopted from PIC. Today, the EU-GMP regulations consist of two parts, the mandatory guidelines and the nonmandatory but highly recommended manual.

The current, revised and expanded WHO-GMP set of rules encompasses and goes beyond all principles, standards, and procedures contained in the *PIC-GMP-guidelines*. For example, in the WHO documents, the requirements for in-process control procedures are more precise.

That means that as a rule, a WHO-conformed quality control will be in line with PIC requirements; reversely, however, PIC-conform quality control systems may not necessarily be fully in accordance with the WHO guidelines. That refers also to the EU-GMP guidelines, as this set of GMP rules, except for minor differences (e.g., in educational requirements), is identical to the PIC-GMP guidelines.

Earlier, the GMP rules were not covered by legal jurisdiction in the context of national legislature, but were to be interpreted as strong recommendations on how to achieve pursued quality goals and to fulfill basic quality requirements.

Today, the GMP set of rules forms, together with GLP (Good Laboratory Practice) and GCP (Good Clinical Practice), constitutes an integral part of a complex quality assurance system and requires comprehensive surveillance and quality control in each phase of the manufacturing process, adjusted to state of the art of science and technology. Compliance with the GMP rules is a strict precondition to obtain approval of the product.

Also, the requirements of the quality management system according to ISO 9000 series of standards (established in 1994 and revised in 2005, *describing fundamentals of quality management systems*) are fully covered by the extensive legislative provisions on medicines as well as the current framework of GMP rules.

The essential requirements of the WHO-GMP guidelines (extended form) are:

– Extreme care during all production phases by well-trained quality-aware and responsible personnel.
– Availability of appropriate spatial arrangements providing separate spaces for manufacturing, packaging, labeling, and testing of the medicines.
– Erroneous switching incidents and cross-contamination should be avoided by appropriate spatial separation of different production and packaging processes, as well as unambiguous labeling of the contents of all containers and pieces of equipment used in the different steps of production.
– To avoid contamination, production hygiene should be meticulous, ascertained by regular cleaning of all working spaces and equipment as well as by regular health checks of the personnel and environmental monitoring.
– In order to fulfill the requirements of microbial purity, hygienic measures are particularly mandatory in the production of medicines, which are not subjected to sterilization.
– Active ingredients with exceptionally high bioactivity must be processed in separate spaces provided with an adequate ventilation system in order to avoid cross contamination.
– High quality of all materials involved in the production of the medicine must be guaranteed; the guidelines were expanded with additional paragraphs concerning reagents, culture media, reference standards, and waste materials.
– Further recommendations concern the quality control system and the handling and documentation of complaints as well as reports of unwanted (side) effects.
– In-process controls: Quality should be produced and should be reproducible! The controls should support and confirm the GMP-conform production of a medicine as an auxiliary measure, and apply to all critical parameters during the production process

  • These control procedures make it possible to improve quality assurance as well as continuous monitoring/correction/optimization of the running production processes (e.g., control of tablet mass, disintegration time, homogeneity of mixtures, filling volume of ampoules).

– Control of raw materials as well as of final products including packaging material
– Registration of each individual production step that might affect the quality of the final product
– Control of stability of the medicine
– Control of the batch protocols
– Throughout the product lifecycle, all processes are monitored and evaluated. This additional knowledge is utilized for adjustment of processes as part of the continual improvement of the drug product.
– Guidelines for the manufacturing of sterile pharmaceutical products; for example, sterile filtration is considered to be a sterilization process.
– The requirements with respect to self-inspection and audit have to be expanded with aspects concerning the extent of self-inspection and the subsequent follow-up measures, as well as supplier control (audit). In the context of the audit, the contract provider is obliged to ascertain the competence of the supplier. The supplier is obliged to act according to GMP rules and must have the necessary equipment and personnel at his disposition.

One key aspect of the GMP idea is the "validation" principle that was introduced in the late 1970s, initially for the sterile production of parenterals and later for all other drug products. According to the EU-GMP guideline, validation is the systematic and documented proof that procedures, processes, equipment, materials, production cycles, or systems reliably, reproducibly and truly lead to the intended results, in line with the principles of good manufacturing practice. This regards the validation of processes, methods, cleaning, and installation of instruments, computers, and other equipment. In the latter cases, we speak, in a narrower sense, of qualification. All actions with respect to a validation or qualification must be planned and documented, and specified outcomes and acceptance criteria must be indicated.

As a rule, validations are performed *prospectively* (i.e., before market authorization) or, alternatively and only when supported by solid argumentation, concurrent with market authorization on minimally three consecutive batches. Nowadays, retrospective activities of already established installations by exploitation of preexisting data material (approx. 10 to 30 production cycles) hardly stand a chance to become formally recognized. The basis for all validation work is knowledge of all critical parameters in which minor changes have a significant influence on the quality of the final product, which normally involves practical determinations by experiments covering all parameter influences (according to "Design of Experiments" methodology; DoE). The determination and characterization of these parameters and their importance are collectively referred to as risk analysis.

It is generally understood that qualification of instruments, installations, and equipment implies documented proof that such systems have been constructed according to predefined specifications and function in accordance with those. This documentation must be continuously available during the entire life cycle of the system.

A permanent, verifiable, and orderly documentation is a compelling condition for the surveillance and transparency of the overall process and thus of the reliability of pharmaceutical quality. According to EU-GMP guidelines, availability of the following documents is imperative:

- *Standard operation procedures* (SOP) are defined working instructions for a process with an unequivocally documented outcome. Such instructions have to be followed most accurately in order to ascertain comparability of results and reproducible quality of the final product.
- *Specifications* define the requirements of the raw materials, in-process products, and final product.
- *Manufacturing protocols* (*Master Batch Records*) and packaging instructions determine all outcomes and procedures with respect to processing and packaging.
- *Protocols* (Executed Master Batch Records) document the complete course of events of each individual batch produced.

According to EU-GMP guidelines, extreme care should be taken to avoid any unpredicted deviation from an adopted standard. Deviations may occur during the manufacturing as well as during the testing of medicines and can be characterized as either process-dependent (e.g., inadequate optimization or design of the process) or process-independent (e.g., failure of equipment or human errors). If deviations occur, the root cause(s), the effect on product quality, and measures to solve the problem must all be identified.

In contrast to deviations, changes are defined as planned and lasting modifications of an adopted standard. Changes are introduced in the course of processes and procedures preferentially based on progress in technical developments. In a change control procedure, all actions leading to the modification, as well as their effect on the validation status and approval, have to be defined and coordinated.

The *qualified person* (QP) is responsible for the completion and testing of each individual batch, according to GMP protocols. This is anchored in the drug law.

In 2002, the FDA launched a new offensive by means of the GMP initiative "Pharmaceutical cGMPs for the Twenty-First Century—A Risk-Based Approach" with four objectives:

1. Encourage development and innovations in pharmaceutical development.
2. Exploit modern science and techniques in a more goal-oriented and efficient way.
3. Modernize pharmaceutical regulations.
4. Improve approval, surveillance, and safety procedures.

In its narrow sense, a qualified person is just responsible for the release of the batch, but this presupposes completion and testing of the batch.

In this connection, process understanding and risk management deserve reinforced significance.

Formerly, the traditional approach in the production of medicines was characterized by exploiting empirical methods with a focus on final product testing. By contrast, nowadays a system is created by means of process analytical technology (PAT) for the design, analysis, and monitoring of the production process using real-time assessments of critical parameters of quality and performance of raw materials, in-process products, and processes, thus safeguarding the quality of the final product. The thorough understanding of the overall process and the application of novel technologies—in particular, real-time assessments and real-time release—should enhance safety, shorten production time, enlarge yields, and reduce costs.

As another follow-up of the FDA initiatives, the quality by design (QbD) concept was introduced as an extension of the systematic pharmaceutical development program with its own guideline (Quality Systems Approach Guideline). QbD can be seen as a systematically structured developmental effort, starting with predefined targets particularly emphasizing process understanding and control. The initiative rests on solid scientific grounds and intensive quality-risk management.

The concept includes the following principles:

– Prospective definition of the quality characteristics of a product as a *quality target product profile* (QTPP), which exerts an essential influence on factors such as activity, quality, and safety
– Recording of critical chemical, physical, and biological quality attributes of active ingredient as well as excipients (e.g., identity, purity, content etc.), which sums up to CQA (critical quality attribute of the drug product) and CMA (critical material attributes of excipients or API)
– Selection of an appropriate production process allowing the achievement of the chosen characteristics
– Defining of a control strategy and suitable control mechanisms to monitor process performance and process quality
– Demonstrate process capability and efficiency of the control strategy
– Surveillance and monitoring of the process capability during the entire life cycle of the project

The principles for this concept are risk management, statistic calculations, and PAT.

Thus, in the last decades, the notion of quality has developed from mere quality control, in which only at the end of the process is a test performed to ascertain that the final product meets all predetermined specifications, to comprehensive quality management involving the integrated action of people, technique, and organization processes. What began in the early twentieth century as a simple final quality control (QC) of a significant percentage of the produced items has evolved as a result of increasing production rates, via quality assurance (QA) based on random sampling into statistically secured test protocols. It was recognized that workers in their interaction with technique and organization are essential to QA. This initially led to the concept of quality management (QM) and later—upon integration of company exceeding factors such as environment, client demands, security, and economics—to the notion of total quality management (TQM). This company philosophy presumes the collaboration of all actively involved individuals to achieve the ultimate goal of the system: quality.

As can already be sensed from this introductory chapter, each newly developed drug is a true challenge for pharmaceutical technology, despite the vast body of knowledge that has been accumulated over many decades and in numerous places. That holds true for all stages on the way of development, from the initial formulation design to its optimization and then onto its mass production for the market. The ever-sharpening quality requirements for the protection of the patient are not merely tested but, rather, incorporated in the process. During the development stage, that applies particularly to newly introduced excipients for a given API but also to (new) combinations of known components. Even in the late stages (e.g., the scaling-up phase) the complexity of the interactions between all components may present unexpected problems. Profound knowledge of the individual process steps, including seemingly simple procedures like mixing or granulation, and the combination of knowledge on the individual steps is necessary to prevent the pharmaceutical scientist from getting lost

The Common Technical Document (CTD) is a set of specifications for application dossier for the registration of Medicines and designed to be used across Europe, Japan and the United States. It is an internationally agreed format for the preparation of applications regarding new drugs intended to be submitted to regional regulatory authorities in participating countries. It was developed by the European Medicines Agency (EMA, Europe), the Food and Drug Administration (FDA, US) and the Ministry of Health, Labour and Welfare (MHLW, Japan). The CTD is maintained by the International Council for Harmonisation of Technical Requirements for Pharmaceuticals for Human Use (ICH). The CTD consists of five modules:

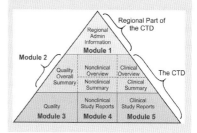

in a thicket of information. It is only then that we will be able to meet the ever-increasing demands concerning quality security of medicines, in a predictable yet scientific manner.

> Despite all available protocols, rules and regulations, the development of a new formulation is still an exciting endeavor. And often even, this endeavor turns out to be an open-ended adventure, because numerous poorly understood factors engaged in ill-defined interactions with each other, may turn out to play an essential part in the process. George Wald described this sensation in his Nobel lecture (1967) with the words, "I have often had cause to feel that my hands are cleverer than my head." This notion is also quite commonly experienced by pharmaceutical scientists, who in many cases have to rely on the phenomenon of "serendipity" (keyword: "chance favors only the prepared mind"). It may be comforting to the reader that this book, even though not helpful in affecting chance, may do so by preparing the reader's mind.

A note to the Pharmacopeia Boxes _____

As written in the foreword, these boxes help
  1. to show how scientific expertise find its way into legal context
  2. to see how tests are performed
  3. to identify the differences between three main pharmacopeias in this world

The boxes in the German version of this book were originally based on the Ph. Eur. rules. Three main pharmacopeial commissions (JP, Ph. Eur., USP) work together for harmonization of the pharmacopeias (cf. General part Ph. Eur. 5.8). Many other countries (e.g., China, India, Russian Confederation) are *observer countries* and work in harmonization groups (see, e.g., www.ich.org) on this behalf. Despite these efforts, there are still many differences between the main pharmacopeias. We compare in the pharmacopeia boxes and in the monography chapter the rules described in the three main pharmacopeias for a better understanding. If only one or two pharmacopeias are mentioned in a box, this normally means, that there is no information about the special items in those pharmacopeias. This might work as a guidance for the professional pharmacist.

USP–NF is a combination of two compendia, the United States Pharmacopeia (USP) and the National Formulary (NF). Monographs for drug substances, dosage forms, and compounded preparations are featured in the USP. Excipient monographs are in the NF.

JP is the Japanese Pharmacopeia. The basis for our comparative work is USP 38, NF 38, and JP 16. The German book was based on Ph. Eur. 7.8, which we took as reference. In this book we had adapted the relevant text from Ph. Eur. 9.1. These editions of the main pharmacopeias are also the basis of the appendix (Selected Pharmaceutical Preparations (Compared between Ph. Eur., USP, and JP). Each of the pharmacopeias contains at least one chapter on pharmaceutical dosage forms where definitions, sub-classifications and relevant tests can be found. The appendix describes the dosage forms which are listed there and compares the requirements specified in the three different pharmacopeias.

General and Technological Principles and Unit Operations

PART 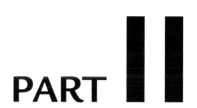 II

From craftsmanship one can rise to artistry, but never so from botchery

(Johann Wolfgang Goethe)

Unit Operations

2.1 Comminution (Particle Size Reduction)

2.1.1 General

Most active ingredients and excipients for the preparation of medicines can only be processed after suitable size reduction. The particle or grain size is a determinant for the uniformity as well as for optimal pharmaceutical activity and nonirritability of the medicine. For several pharmaceutical formulations, such as inhalation aerosols, *comminution*—that is, reduction of particle size to a certain level—is a prerequisite to reach the site of action. Also, herbal drugs have to be reduced in size in order to facilitate quantitative extraction of the relevant substances. Size reduction correlates with an increase in surface area, which, in turn, may have a strong influence on biopharmaceutical parameters such as release or absorption.

2.1.2 Mechanisms of Size Reduction

The extent of size reduction of a substance is defined by the degree of reduction:

$$Z = d_0/d_1 \qquad\qquad (2\text{-}1)$$

Z = degree of reduction
d_0 = initial grain size
d_1 = grain size after size reduction

Particle size reduction can be achieved by compression, impaction, attrition, shock, or shear forces. Which one of these forces most effectively results in the required particle size depends on the properties of the material such as hardness and elasticity. Under the impact of the fragmentation forces, the material is elastically and plastically deformed until it breaks upon exceeding a certain force level. Particles of solid substances usually possess different types of weak spots, like, for example, dislocations in the crystal lattice or cracks (see 3.2.1), where fractures preferentially occur.

The number of suitable weak spots decreases with increasing comminution so that with diminishing particle size, higher energy input will be required for a further reduction in size. Also during grinding of granules fractures always occur first at weak sites—in this case, particularly in solid bridges between individual particles formed by hardened binders and crystallized solids.

Of the total energy input, only the fraction required for the formation of new surface area is stored as surface energy in the pulverized material. The remainder is mainly dissipated as

Voigt's Pharmaceutical Technology, First Edition. Alfred Fahr.
© 2018 John Wiley & Sons Ltd. Published 2018 by John Wiley & Sons Ltd.

heat. In order to minimize the amount of required energy, the following measures should be taken:

- Enhance the chance of brittle fracture—that is, ensure minimal elastic deformation (e.g., cold grinding when applicable).
- Remove very small particles before and, when possible, during the comminution process.
- Allow higher degree of reduction by stepwise comminution and classification.
- Do not go unnecessarily beyond the smallest required particle size.

2.1.3   Comminution Techniques

In addition to the predominantly used dry grinding, comminution can also be performed under addition of a liquid (wet grinding) or at low temperatures (cold grinding).

2.1.3.1   Wet Grinding

The substance to be fragmented is mixed with a liquid in which it is not soluble and then subjected to the appropriate treatment. Liquids with high polarity, such as water and alcohols, are preferred. In some cases, addition of surface active agents may be necessary. By means of wet grinding, the grinding effect is substantially enhanced due to the better transduction of the shear forces, resulting in a further reduction of the achievable grain size. Additional advantages are the reduction of surface energy of the newly formed surfaces as a result of solute adsorption, the reduction of the aggregation tendency, the lower heat burden on the material, and reduced oxidation at the fracture faces. As a rule, the dispersion liquid has to be removed from the material after the grinding process, which, in turn, can lead to reaggregation during the drying process.

2.1.3.2   Cold Grinding

In cold grinding, comminution is performed at low temperatures. With decreasing temperature, the brittleness of the material increases such that fractures are formed more easily. Cold grinding is especially applied with substances with a low melting point or with substances that tend to form eutectic mixtures. It is important to avoid condensation of air moisture on the material to be ground.

2.1.3.3   Problems Occurring During Fragmentation

Usually, during dry grinding the material experiences a heat burden, which may, for example, lead to polymorphic transformations. A strong reduction in particle size worsens the flow characteristics of the powder as a result of an enhanced aggregation tendency. The enlarged surface area in materials with strongly reduced particle size may induce higher reactivity, which, in turn, might lead to degradation of sensitive substances.

Dry grinding of organic substances such as starch-containing products brings along the risk of dust explosions caused by electrostatic charging of the particle surfaces. In this connection, essentially important factors are particle size and fine dust concentration in the air. To avoid the risk of a dust explosion, the grinder can be electrostatically grounded. Alternatively, an inert gas may be introduced in order to diminish oxygen content of the air. In wet grinding, the risk of dust explosions is minimal because the fine particles are dispersed in the fluid.

In order to avoid contamination of the ground material by wear or abrasion of the mill, the grinding parts of the machine should be at least one Mohs degree harder than the material to be ground (see 3.2.6).

2.1.4   Comminution Equipment

At the level of prescription formulations, comminution is commonly performed by means of manual methods (e.g., a mortar and pestle types). Dry plant materials can be disintegrated in a mortar or, as long as they are not too hard, with mashing (pounding) or mincing knives or rotary cutters.

Table 2-1 Performance of Fragmentation Equipment

Equipment	Principle	Particle Size Product
cutting mill	rotating knives	20–0.25 mm
roll/jaw mill	attrition, compression	10–1 mm
hammer mill	impact, pounding	2–0.3 mm
disk mill	attrition, shear	5–0.1 mm
ball mill	attrition, compression, pounding	2–0.001 mm
pin mill	crushing, impact, pounding	500–20 µm
mortar mill	compression, attrition	100–10 µm
air-jet mill	impact, attrition	100–<1 µm
colloid mill	attrition, shear	30–<1 µm

Due to different construction options of individual grinder types and dependence of achievable fragmentation grades on the nature of the starting material, the presented particle size ranges should be taken as indications.

Disintegration of fresh or dried herbal drugs can be achieved with special herb cutting knives. For the disintegration of larger batches of material, a variety of mechanical comminution equipment such as grinders is available.

The selection of equipment in a particular case will be dictated by the amount and the physical properties (hardness, elasticity, stickiness) of the material, but also on the particle size of the starting material and the required particle size of the final product. Depending on the achievable disintegration degree equipment for, coarse, medium and fine fragmentation can be distinguished (Table 2-1).

2.1.4.1   Jaw Crusher and Roller Mill

Jaw grinders are particularly useful for hard and medium hard substances. The grinding space is usually funnel-shaped; the slit width of the product outlet can be adjusted to the desired fineness of the product. Fragmentation results predominantly from the pressure burden between a fixed and a mobile crushing arm. In the roller mill (Fig. 2-1), the material to be disintegrated is pressed between two or more counter-rotating rollers, where the surface of the rollers can be differently shaped (e.g., smooth, jagged, etc.). Disintegration results from pressure and friction (attrition) and, depending on rotation velocity, also from shear forces. For coarsely dispersed materials the surfaces will be provided with notches or teeth or the like, while for the production of smaller fragments rollers with a smooth surface are preferred (see three-roll mill, section 15.4.2).

2.1.4.2   Mortar Mills

In mortar mills (Fig. 2-2) the material is squeezed between the rough surfaces of the grinding vessel and the pestle. The motion between vessel wall and pestle is mostly achieved by rotation of the vessel. In order to keep the material within the fragmentation zone, the resulting powder that sticks to the vessel wall must be scraped off the wall perpetually. This is achieved by a scraper, which also ensures optimal mixing of the material.

2.1.4.3   Disk Mills

This type of grinder is used for disintegration of elastic or fibrous substances. Comminution occurs in the narrow space between the disks, of which one is fixed (stator) and the other rotates with high velocity (rotor). Both disks can either be smooth or covered with ripples, notches or teeth. The distance between the disks is adjustable according to the required grain size. At relatively low velocities, the disintegration process proceeds mainly by pressure and shear forces, while at higher speeds pounding comes into play as well.

2.1.4.4   Hammer (Impact) Mills, and Pin Mills

The material is hurled against the wall of the grinder by rapidly rotating beating bars, crosses or pins. The comminution is the result of a collision process. The efficiency of the grinding

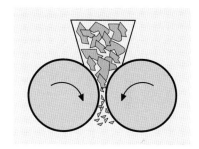

Fig. 2-1 Roller mill (roller crusher).

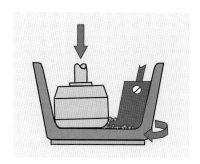

Fig. 2-2 Mortar mill (mortar grinder).

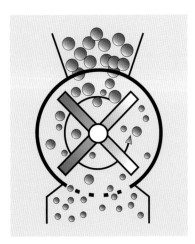

Fig. 2-3 Hammer mill.

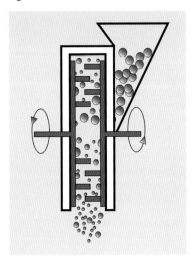

Fig. 2-4 Pin mill.

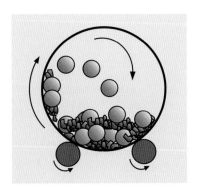

Fig. 2-5 Ball mill.

becomes higher with increasing rotation speed and density of the material. The fine material thus formed can be collected at the edges of the grinder by sieving.

Hammer mills (Fig. 2-3) are provided with hammers serving as grinding machinery; they are either freely hanging from the rotor or fixed to it. Movable hammers, which as a result of centrifugal force are swinging outward, have the advantage that they can give way in case of heavy or nongrindable material (protection against overburdening). These grinders are often provided with a sieve grid for the outlet of the fine material and determining the upper limit of the grain size of the product.

The *pin mill* (Fig. 2-4) consists of two vertically positioned metal pin bearers rotating with high velocity in opposite directions, as a result of which the material particles are hurled outward through rows of pins and disintegrate by collision and pounding. The distance between the two pin bearers is adjustable to the desired fineness of the particles and the final grain diameter.

2.1.4.5 Ball Mills

The material is disintegrated by rolling or dropping spheres in a cylindrical vessel. These spheres can be made of steel, hard porcelain, or agate. The principle of this type of grinder may be applied, for example, in a ball mill with horizontally positioned bearings (Fig. 2-5). As a result of the rotation of the grinding chamber, the spheres are carried some distance along the chamber wall until they drop back on the material due to gravity. At higher rotation speed, the dropping motion of the spheres leads to a coarser fragmentation than when grinding proceeds during the dragging of spheres occurring at lower rotation speed. For the preparation of a relatively coarse product, preferably larger, heavier spheres are employed. For more finely dispersed products, larger numbers of smaller spheres are used. Beyond a certain critical rotation velocity, the spheres stick to the vessel wall as a result of the centrifugal force, thus preventing an effective grinding process.

At the critical rotation speed n_{crit} the centrifugal force (F_c) exerted on the spheres equals the weight force F_G of the spheres:

$$F_c = m \cdot (2\pi n)^2 \cdot \frac{D}{2} \quad \text{is equal } F_{grav} = m \cdot g$$
$$\text{therefore}: \ m \cdot (2\pi n)^2 \cdot \frac{D}{2} = m \cdot g \tag{2-2}$$

By rearranging the equation to n, the critical rotation speed can be calculated:

$$n_{crit} = \frac{1}{2\pi} \cdot \sqrt{\frac{2g}{D}} \tag{2-3}$$

m = mass of one sphere [g]
n = rotation speed [rev/min]
D = internal diameter of the grinding chamber [m]
g = gravitational constant [m/s^2]

As a rule, ball mills are operated at rotation speeds of 60–75% of the critical rotation speed, which is in physical numbers about 0.5 rotations per second. The filling degree (see eq. 2-4) may vary, but a value of about 0.5–0.6 is mostly used. The spheres contribute here to about 0.4–0.5 and the material to be ground about 0.3–0.4, as the empty space between the spheres are also filled with material (the theoretical empty space between perfectly stacked spheres is 26% of the total volume). Optimal grinding involves also other factors, like the ratio of the diameter between mill drum and spheres.

$$\text{Filling degree } \varphi = \frac{\text{Bulk volume}}{\text{Grinding chamber volume}} \ (\text{Grinding media+Material to be ground}) \tag{2-4}$$

The *centrifugal ball mill* carries out a horizontal rotary motion. An eccentric bearing of the mill vessel ensures that the spheres, in addition to the rolling motion, also undergo a motion similar to the falling motion in the mill provided with a horizontal bearing. In the *planetary ball mill*, the grinding vessel undergoes, in addition to the circular motion, a rotation around

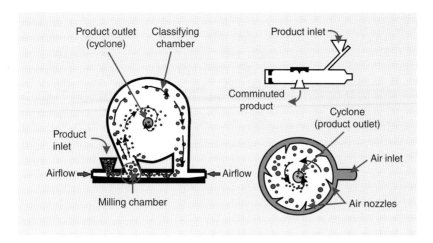

Fig. 2-6 Air jet mill (left: opposed jet mill; right: spiral jet mill in side and top view).

its own axis. In this case, not only the centrifugal motion of the circular motion but also the centrifugal force of its own rotation as well as the Coriolis force act upon the material, which causes the material to experience a higher grinding burden.

In the *vibration mill*, the spring-borne grinding vessel filled with the material and grinding spheres is subjected to vibrations. With this motion, the intended imbalance of the grinding vessel favors the fragmentation, resulting from the swinging movements of the grinding spheres and the vibration of the material.

2.1.4.6   The Air Jet Mill

This type of micronizer is employed for the production of very fine powders. There are several differently constructed grinders of this type (Fig. 2-6). The material to be disintegrated is introduced in a compressed air jet that is led into the mill with sonic or even supersonic velocity. Collisions with other particles or with the vessel wall are responsible for the grinding effect. Prefragmentation may be required. The air is exhausted by a vortex in the center of the mill, causing the powder particles to be forced into spiral paths, dependent on particle size, under strong acceleration. While the finest material leaves the mill via the central discharge channel, the coarser particles stay behind in the grinder by virtue of their inertia and will be further reduced in size until the required size has been reached. Due to these classifying effects, relatively narrow size distributions can be obtained. Particle sizes down to the lower micrometer range, partly even the nanometer range, can be obtained. Due to the cooling air jet, the heat burden on the material is low in this type of grinder. For this reason, the high energy expenditure of this method is considered acceptable in case thermo-labile drugs need to be reduced to the required degree of fineness in a gentle way. A disadvantage is the high aggregation tendency and often the poor wettability of the formed particles.

2.1.4.7   Colloid Mills

A conical rotor rotates with high velocity within a housing. The adjustable distance between rotor and housing wall amounts to not more than a few tenths of a mm (Fig. 2-7). The material to be diminished is introduced into the grinder as a suspension and further reduced in size by shear forces occurring during the forced passage through the narrow space between rotor and wall. With colloid grinders particle sizes down to below 1 μm can be attained.

2.2   Mixing

2.2.1   General

Mixing procedures serve to obtain the highest possible homogeneity in a mixture of multiple substances. Homogeneous distribution of the components is an absolute requirement for exact dosing of medicines. The overall notion "mixing" includes *stirring* (mixing of liquids

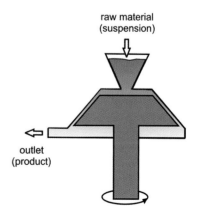

Fig. 2-7 Colloid mill.

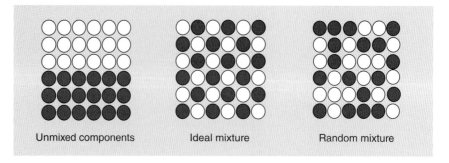

Unmixed components   Ideal mixture   Random mixture

Fig. 2-8 Ideal and stochastic homogeneity.

with liquid, solid, or gaseous substances), *kneading* (treatment of dough-like or plastic masses), and *blending* (mingling of powdery or granular substances).

During mixing, the particles of one substance accommodate themselves in between the particles of one or more other substances. Ideally, the resulting distribution is purely random (Fig. 2-8), implying that the probability that a certain particle is present at a certain position in the mixer is identical for each particle (stochastic homogeneity, uniform chance-determined mixing). Ideal, or perfect homogeneity, for which even the smallest sample of the mixture has exactly the same composition as every other sample of that size, cannot be attained by simple mixing procedures. An approach to ideal mixing is represented by *ordered mixtures*. Ordered mixtures are attained for example by adhesion of fine-powder particles to larger particles, by coating of particles with a film containing an active ingredient, or by embedding of particles in a matrix. In these instances, we are not dealing with mixing procedures.

The number of times per unit of time that the particle changes position in all three dimensions is a key parameter in the mixing effect. During mixing, three forces act on the material: pulling or pressure forces that only bring about a volume change of the material, and three-dimensional shear forces, which are ultimately responsible for the actual mixing process. A turbulent motion process is favorable in order to destroy any aggregates that might occur. To facilitate three-dimensional movement, the mixer should not be overfilled.

In essence, the material undergoes three types of motion (Fig. 2-9):

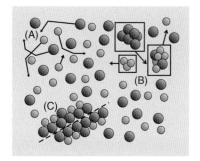

Fig. 2-9 Types of movement of the material: (A) Diffusion-like motions of single particles; (B) Convection-like motion of particle clusters; (C) Shear motion.

- Diffusion-like motion of single particles relative to one another as a result of chance
- Convection-like motion of groups of particles relative to one another
- Shear motion—shifting of particle layers by formation of shear planes

Mixing is a time-dependent process that initially proceeds rapidly and after a while no longer leads to further effectiveness. Particularly size, shape, and size distribution of the grains as well as concentration and flow characteristics affect the mixing effectiveness. Particle density only plays a role when there are substantial density differences between the individual components. Forces that favor the formation of aggregates (e.g., cohesion and adhesion forces, moisture) reduce the dispersion effect. As such surface forces increase with diminishing particle size, it is often the extremely fine powders that cause problems. Also problematic is the processing of components that are present in only very small proportions.

Depending on the properties of the material, a continuous increase in quality of the mixture may occur during the mixing process (cohesive materials) or an optimum is observed, following which demixing (i.e., segregation) may occur (especially in the case of free-flowing materials). Materials that tend to segregate should, whenever possible, be mixed immediately before preparation or further processing. Shocks, vibrations, or treatments that induce flow or free fall of particles should be avoided. In case of needle-shaped substances, the occurrence of strong segregation tendencies should be taken into account. By virtue of their space-consuming shape, these particles create holes through which finely powdered components can drop down. With equally sized spherical particles, such segregation effects do not occur.

To establish optimal mixing time and to ensure uniformity of content of the dosage forms, *mixing quality* is defined and assessed with the help of statistical parameters such as standard

Mixing and demixing can nowadays be precisely studied by image analysis of mixing processes (Daumann and Nirschl (2008)).

deviation. It is important that a sufficient number (minimally 20) of samples are taken and that sample size is adequate. Sampling occurs randomly at various positions in the mixer.

As described, mixing quality is dependent on mixing time. But also grain size, shape, and size distribution, as well as flow characteristics, moisture, density, and concentration of the individual components decisively affect mixing quality, which is, amongst others, crucial for accurate dosing. According to statistical considerations, a sufficiently large number of active agent particles have to be present in each and every tablet. Only when this condition is fulfilled will the inevitable variation of particle number per tablet not lead to unacceptably large dose variations between single tablets. Particle size plays an important role in this connection. The acceptable maximum particle size to achieve dose accuracy ($s_{rel} = 1\%$) is dose-dependent and is designated *particle size limit*. Table 2-2 presents particle size limits determined for an active ingredient with an average density of 1.25 g/mL in a tablet of 100 mg.

The requirement for content uniformity is described in more detail in the pharmacopeia box Ph. Eur. 2.9.40 (p. 364).

2.2.2 Mixing of Liquids

Stirring processes serve the purpose of mixing liquids, dissolving solids, exchanging heat during heating or cooling of a liquid mixture, as well as dispersing solids or emulsifying liquids. These procedures are mostly performed in closed vessels (Fig. 2-10). The container can be provided with a thermo-regulated jacket or with a vacuum device in order to avoid air entrapment in the liquid.

The choice of stirrer is predominantly dictated by the type of task it has to perform: dispersion or emulsifying processes require, for instance, a strong shear action of the stirrer, whereas for pure mixing procedures, a simple whirling motion suffices. Furthermore, viscosity of the liquid and, among others, also the total amount of material to be mixed is important.

The various types of stirrers deploy their mixing action in accordance with the specific processing of the material to be mixed: axial (propeller, slanting blade, coil stirrers), radial (blade, grid, crossed bars, inverted propeller, and disc stirrers), or tangential (anchor stirrers) (Fig. 2-11).

For mixing of liquids with a low viscosity propeller, impeller, flat-blade, and pitch-blade turbines are most appropriate, for medium viscous liquids cross-arm, blade and gate-blade stirrers are preferred, while high-viscosity liquids require deployment of for example an

Table 2-2 Particle Size Limit as a Function of Dose (tablet mass 100 mg)

Active Ingredient in Tablet (mg)	Particle Size Limit (μm)
0.1	25
1.0	54
5.0	95
10.0	125

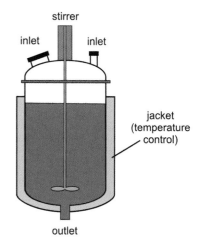

Fig. 2-10 Stirring vessel.

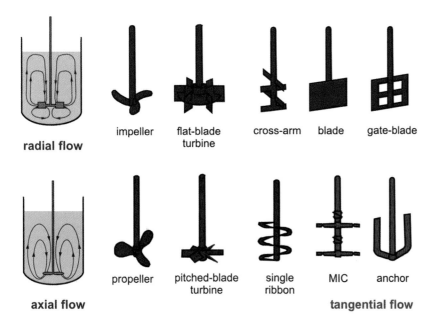

Fig. 2-11 Constructions of stirrers with corresponding flow schemes.

Tangential flow follows a circular path around the stirrer shaft (till the circumference of the vessel) and creates a vortex.

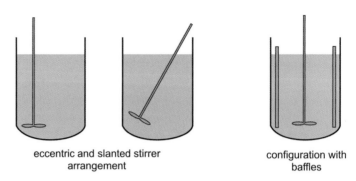

eccentric and slanted stirrer
arrangement

configuration with
baffles

Fig. 2-12　Eccentric and slanted positioning of a propeller stirrer with and without baffles.

anchor or single ribbon stirrer. Stirring elements for mixing formulations of high viscosity are usually larger, relative to the mixing container, than devices for low-viscosity liquids and are operated at lower speed.

Especially with high-viscosity material, it is advisable to ensure appropriate mass exchange near the wall of the mixing container by using mixing elements that get into close vicinity to the wall, in order to prevent the formation of highly viscous or even solid layers of material, which might affect heat exchange (e.g., during cooling) or cause heat overload. Central positioning of the stirring element may lead to mere "co-rotation" of the material and to the formation of a central whirl. This phenomenon can be counteracted by the installation of baffles—for example, metal blades positioned perpendicular to the wall. These do however, increase the force input and prolong, as a result of the occurrence of "dead zones," mixing time. With sufficiently small-sized stirrers, eccentric or slanting positioning can be helpful (Fig. 2-12).

For complex mixing problems, as occur, for example, during manufacturing of disperse systems or semi-solid preparations, it may be useful to combine the stirrers described in the foregoing with mixing elements with high dispersing potency. In this manner, an anchor stirrer may, for instance, be combined in one mixing container together with rotor-stator systems (see 15.4.5).

Currently, static mixers are increasingly applied. The static mixer is in most commercially available options composed of a smooth tube with incorporated left- and right-turning coils. The mixer leads the flowing product against the wall of the tube and back. By means of the alternatingly positioned right- and left-turning mixing elements, an inversion of the rotation and flow distribution is brought about. The advantages of the static mixer over the stirred systems lie in the continuity of the process, little loss of pressure, short and evenly distributed residence time, and assured quality of the mixing process.

2.2.3　Mixers for Solids

A large number of different types of mixers are available, which, depending on the construction, allow a variety of force impacts on the material to be mixed. The choice of mixer is dictated by properties and amount of material to be mixed. In order to achieve optimal mixing action, the following points need to be considered:

- The expansion of the powder bed is a prerequisite for the mutual permeation of the powder constituents. The loading level is accordingly adjusted to 30% to 80% of the maximal capacity of the mixing vessel, depending on mixer type.
- During the mixing process, forces from all directions in the vessel should act on the material. Particularly, turbulent movement of the particles is a favorable condition for effective mixing. In case only two-dimensional motions occur, mixing proceeds very slowly.
- The entire mass should be simultaneously in motion in order to avoid the occurrence of dead zones.

Fluid: anything that flows. This includes gases and liquids.
Gases: their volume is defined by the container.
Liquid: has a fixed volume but no shape.
Solid: has a definite volume and a definite shape without any container.

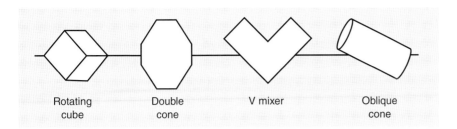

Fig. 2-13 Schematic representation of tumbling mixers.

- The mixer should exert sufficient shear forces on the material to ensure appropriate disaggregation of cohesive materials. However, higher shear forces increase the risk of damaging sensitive materials (e.g., granules).
- To prevent demixing effects, movements inducing a free fall of the particles should be avoided.

For each individual material and each individual mixer a suitable mixing time needs to be chosen.

2.2.3.1   Tumbling Mixers

This type of mixer consists of rotating drums of various size, shape, and working principle (Fig. 2-13). In a continuously operating zigzag mixer (Fig. 2-14) at one side the loading takes place and at the other side the mixed product is withdrawn. As a result of the rotation of the zigzag-shaped arm, which is bent toward the outlet, the material is mixed and moved toward the outlet.

Mixing in a tumbling mixer is accomplished by convection and shear movements without strongly burdening the mix material. Grain size remains constant, so that this apparatus is also suitable for the use of sensitive granules. By incorporating baffles, mixing efficiency can be enhanced. This type of mixer is unsuitable for extra fine or strongly cohesive materials, because in such cases the shear forces are insufficient to take apart larger aggregates.

2.2.3.2   Shaking Mixers

A special case is the Turbula shaker mixer. In this apparatus, a certain shear burden and an enhanced diffusion-like movement of the particles is achieved by means of a complex

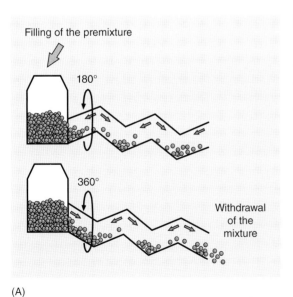

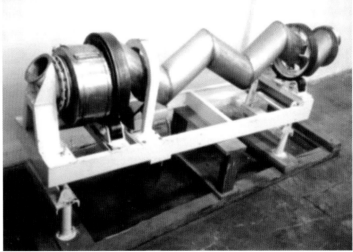

(A)   (B)

Fig. 2-14 Zigzag mixer: Scheme (slope of the mixer arm exaggerated) (A); Example (B).
Reproduced with permission from Frain Group © 2016.

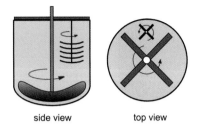

side view   top view

Fig. 2-15 High-speed mixer.

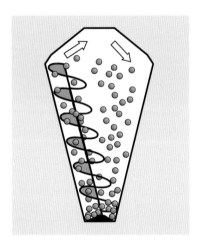

Fig. 2-16 Nauta mixer.

three-dimensional motion pattern of mixing consisting of rotation, translation, and inversion movements. However, this also brings along an enhanced challenge on the material to be mixed, in that it may, for example, lead to deterioration of granule cohesiveness.

2.2.3.3   Shear and Forced-Circulation Mixers

Blade mixers contain blades and scrapers that mostly run in opposite directions and thus accomplish the mixing process. High-speed mixers (Fig. 2-15), for example, may be deployed for high-shear granulation. Horizontally rotating wings and sidewise positioned cutters accomplish thorough mixing of the material.

Although, because of the high rotation velocity of these mixers, strong concomitant shear forces allow high mixing effectiveness and short mixing times, they are not suitable for mechanically sensitive materials. In a continuous ribbon agitator mixer, the material (analogous to the transport in a meat mincer) is blended during its transport towards the outlet by means of a horizontal axis to which a coil or a coil-shaped blade is attached. This type is less suitable for mechanically sensitive materials because of the strong friction forces that occur between the worm and the vessel wall. The Nauta mixer (Fig. 2-16) consists of an upright-positioned conically shaped container in which a coil-shaped screw rotates in a planet-like path along the wall. The material to be mixed is transported upward along the wall of the vessel and then falls back in the vessel, thus accomplishing the blending effect. The mechanical burden on the material is lower than in the continuously operating worm-drive mixer.

2.2.3.4   Compounding-Scale Production of Powder Mixtures

Mixing of smaller quantities at compounding scale most often occurs by trituration. Mixing procedures carried out with mortar and pestle are different from the mixing methods described in the foregoing paragraphs. In the former cases, mixing proceeds much less uniformly because at any moment only that fraction of the material is in motion that is in direct contact with the pestle. As the amount of material in the mortar increases, uniformity of the mixing process diminishes and the occurrence of dead zones grows. Frequent scraping of the mortar wall and pestle head is essential to achieve satisfactory mixing quality. Grain size reduction often occurs during this procedure as a result of the high pressure and shear burden. When mixing small quantities of active ingredient with excipients, geometric dilution (doubling-up) is recommended. To that end, gradually increasing amounts of the excipient are added stepwise to the ground active substance (see Fig. 2-17) and mixed thoroughly after each addition. This procedure results in high mixing quality.

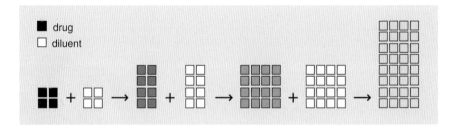

Fig. 2-17 Compounding-scale mixing by stepwise geometric dilution.

2.3   Filtration

2.3.1   General

In a filtration process, either the filter residue is collected as the main product (separation filtration) or the liquid is freed from undesired particulate matter (clarification or germ-freeing filtration). In the context of pharmaceutical-technological separation procedures we are mostly dealing with the latter option. When filtration proceeds without additional application of pressure or vacuum, we speak of a gravity filtration. The flow rate (throughput) depends on the cut-off size of the filter, the filter area, the amount, size and structure of the material to be filtered out, viscosity of the liquid and the available pressure difference. It may be enhanced by applying excess pressure (positive pressure filtration) or reduced pressure (negative pressure filtration). This is described by the Darcy equation:

$$\frac{v}{A} = \frac{\Delta p}{\eta \cdot (\beta_S \cdot h_S + \beta_K \cdot h_K)} \qquad (2\text{-}5)$$

v = filtration rate (volume/time)

A = filter area

Δp = pressure gradient

η = viscosity of the filtrate

β_i = specific resistance, fictitious pore length in the filter (S) or cake layer (K)

h_i = corresponding layer thickness

The cut-off value is defined as smallest particle size retained by the filter. It is a more accurate parameter for filter efficacy than sheer pore diameter, as particle adsorption within the filter also plays an important role and is not taken into account when only pore diameter is considered.

One speaks of *surface filtration* when, as a result of sieve action, the solid substances are retained on the surface of the filter. In case of depth filtration, the solid substances are not retained on the surface of the filter but rather, in the matrix of the filter material—that is, separated out inside the angular or winding pores. In practice, the two processes usually occur simultaneously.

Depending on flow input, static and dynamic (tangential) filtration are distinguished (Fig. 2-18). In case of *static filtration* (also called *dead-end filtration*) the feed is pressed against the filter surface. Impurities precipitate within or on the filter and the filtrate is collected. During *dynamic filtration* (also called *cross-flow* or *tangential-flow filtration*), the feed is circulated tangentially along the filter. As the pressure at the feed side is higher than on the filtrate side, part of the volume flow is pressed through the filter. This fraction is called the *permeate*. In this way, the impurities are not filtered out on or in the filter, but flow along the filter surface, thus preventing the filter from becoming clogged. The fraction enriched with impurities is designated the *retentate*.

2.3.2 Traditional Filtration Techniques

For filtration at the laboratory level, often filter paper is used. The filter equipment (funnels) is made from glass or porcelain and in some cases also from metal or synthetic polymers. For large-size filter funnels, inlays are applied to prevent ripping of the filter paper in the tip by the very weight of the liquid.

Henry Darcy (1803–1853, Dijon, France) was an engineer. He studied the flow of water through beds of sand and started with this equation the scientific field of hydrogeology.

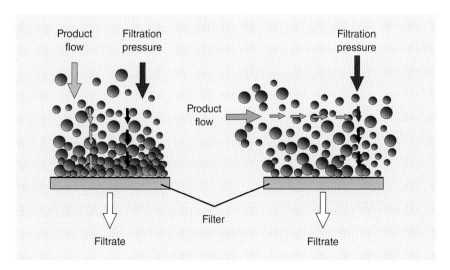

Fig. 2-18 Static (left) and dynamic (right) filtration.

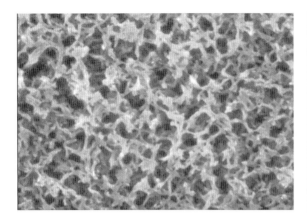 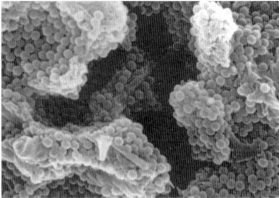

Fig. 2-19 Left: Foamed polyamide membrane (Ultipor N$_{66}$®, Pall Corp.). Right: foamed positively charged polyamide membrane with adsorbed negatively charged latex particles (Posidyne N$_{66}$®, Pall Corp.), considerable enlargement.

In many cases (e.g., for the removal of particulates from pharmaceutical solutions), regular filter paper is not suitable as it continuously releases fibers. In such cases fused-glass filters (glass funnels containing fused-in layers of filter material composed of sintered glass) can be employed. Such filters come in a variety of sizes and pore diameters and bring along numerous advantages over paper filters. They are resistant to acidic and basic agents, are reusable after cleaning, and can be sterilized by hot air or autoclaving.

2.3.2.1 Membrane Filters

Membrane filters come in a large variety and can be distinguished either by the material they are made of or the way they are produced, as well as by the type of application. *Foamed membranes* (Fig. 2-19, Table 2-3) possessing a homogeneous sponge-like structure, are manufactured by a phase inversion procedure. In this procedure, a homogeneous polymer solution is separated into a polymer-rich solid phase and a fluid phase.

As a result of evaporation of the fluid phase, pores are formed as cavities between the foam lamellae formed from the solid phase. The classical substances from which this type of membrane is manufactured include cellulose acetate and -nitrate, mixed esters and regenerated cellulose. As these substances usually require the addition of plasticizers and/or crosslinking agents, nowadays industry rather prefers polyamide, polyvinylidenefluoride or polyether sulfone. Such membranes have typical cut-off pore diameters of 20 nm to 5 μm, with a layer thickness of around 100 μm and a pore surface area of up to 80%. Often, these membranes are reinforced by incorporation of support layers.

Generally, foamed membranes are hydrophilic and are therefore the product of choice for sterile filtration of aqueous fluids.

Polyamide membranes are also available in a variety that possesses positive surface charge. As a result, additional adsorption forces are coming into play that can bind negatively charged microorganisms and bacteria-derived endotoxin (Fig. 2-19 shows latex particles as example).

Table 2-3 Examples of Foamed Membranes

Material	Manufacturer	Product Name
Polyamide	Cuno	Zeta Plus
	Pall	Ultipor N$_{66}$, N$_{66}$ Posidyne
	Sartorius	Sartolon
Polyether sulfone	Pall	Supor
	Sartorius	Sartopore
Polyvinylidene fluoride	Millipore	Durapore
	Pall	Fluorodyne
Cellulose acetate	Sartorius	Sartobran
Cellulose, mixed ester	Domnick Hunter	Asypore

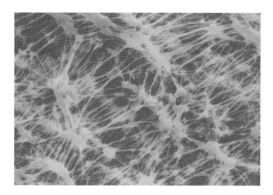

Fig. 2-20 Stretched polytetrafluorethylene membrane (Emflon®, Pall Corp.).

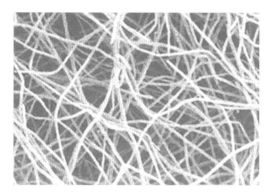

Fig. 2-21 Polypropylene microfiber membrane (HDC®, Pall Corp.).

In *stretched membranes* (Fig. 2-20, Table 2-4), the pores are formed by controlled two-dimensional stretching of polymer leaflets. Typical material for this type of membrane is polytetrafluorethylene. Typical cut-off pore-size values are 0.04 to 0.45 μm, with a layer thickness of 20 μm and a porosity of 60%. By virtue of the material from which they are made, stretched membranes are hydrophobic and are therefore mostly applied as an air or a gas filter or as an aeration filter.

Since the cut-off size of a membrane filter critically depends on the depth of the matrix, often double membrane filters are employed to enhance safety. For that purpose, either two stacked membranes of identical pore size are employed or, alternatively, two membranes of different pore size (e.g., one of 0.1 μm and another one of 0.2 μm pore size). Additionally, such double membranes guarantee further safety enhancement as the upper one may serve to cover potential "large" pores.

Asymmetric membranes consist of homogeneous material in which pore size gradually diminishes across the filter layers (e.g., from 10 to 0.1 μm), causing larger particles to sediment in the upper zone of the membrane, thus preventing smaller pores in the lower zone from becoming clogged. As a result, such filters possess highly favorable flow-through capacities.

For the manufacturing of *microfiber membranes* (Fig. 2-21) all materials can be used that allow processing in fibrous form; these comprise polymers such as polypropylene, polyamide,

Table 2-4 Stretched Membranes

Material	Manufacturer	Product Name
Polytetrafluorethylene	Cuno	Microfluor
	Domnick Hunter	Highflow Tetpor
	Millipore	Aerex
	Pall	Emflon
	Sartorius	Sartofluor

Table 2-5 Microfiber Membranes

Material	Manufacturer	Product Name
Glass fiber	Domnick Hunter	Prepor GF
	Millipore	Lifegard
	Pall	Ultipor GF plus, Preflow
	Sartorius	Sartopure GF
Polypropylene	Cuno	PolyPro, Betafine
	Domnick Hunter	Peplyn Plus
	Millipore	Polygard
	Pall	HDC, Profile Star
	Sartorius	Sartopure PP

polyvinylchloride and polyaramide, but also a large variety of organic and inorganic substances like cellulose, glass, stainless steel etc. (Table 2-5). Important is that a fully cross-linked network of microfibers is obtained as this prevents shedding of fibers and deformation of the membrane structure which in turn might lead to breakthrough of particles. This membrane type covers a wide selection of cut-off sizes, ranging from 0.5 μm to over 100 μm. The thickness of the layer varies from 200 to 300 μm, but may in rare cases also be substantially larger. The pore fraction varies from about 50% to about 80%, depending on material and fineness. Microfiber membranes are nearly exclusively deployed as pre- or particle filters.

Track-etched membranes represent a very special type of membrane filter. Thin leaflets of, for example, polycarbonate or polyester are bombarded with neutrons. Along their path (tracks), these neutrons create chemical changes in the material that can be removed by a chemical etching procedure, such that highly identical pores are formed (Fig. 2-22). Pore density (porosity) of such membranes varies around 10%. Higher densities would require denser irradiation, which might lead to multiple pores. *Track-etched filters* are genuine surface filters and are of little relevance for production at the industrial scale because of the high risk of clogging and low flow capacity. However, their exceptionally narrow pore-size distribution has widely promoted their use in particle and microbiological analysis technology.

As a rule, filtration by means of membrane filters is performed under pressure or vacuum while the filter is tightly fixed in a filter holder. For smaller samples, filter disks are employed; for larger samples, filter cartridges are preferred. In the pharmaceutical industry

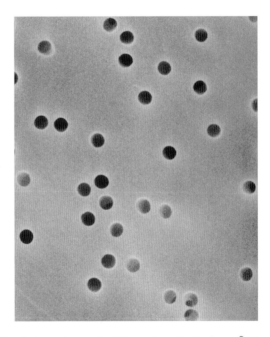

Fig. 2-22 Scanning electron micrograph of the surface of a Nuclepore® filter (Corning Costar, Bodenheim).

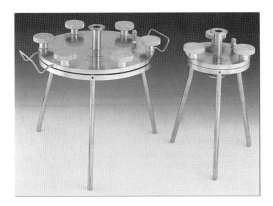

Fig. 2-23 Disk filter support.

and biotechnology, membrane filters have proven their value for liquid as well as gas filtration over a period of several decades.

The oldest form of membrane filtration requires the incorporation of filter disks in a membrane holder (Fig. 2-23). This form of membrane filtration is still customary at the extemporary formulation and compounding-scale level. Also, the syringe filter, commonly used in the laboratory setting and for formulations, relies on this principle (Fig. 2-24).

Commonly, membrane filters have a porosity of approximately 80%. Nonetheless, this high proportion of active filter surface cannot be fully exploited because generally the holes in the filter support comprise only 25% to 40% of the total surface area of the support. The smooth surface of this filter support, usually photo-etched sieve plates made from stainless steel, cover a substantial proportion of the overlying filter surface. As a result, the effective filter surface is reduced by 20% to 32% and so is the flow capacity of the filter and its capacity toward solids. Cloth backing will substantially reduce the contact surface between filter and support and thus enhance throughput.

2.3.2.2   Filter Cartridges

Nowadays, industry nearly exclusively employs filter cartridges, consisting of folded filter material. These are incorporated in a filter housing, which is commonly made of stainless steel. For special applications, filter housings made of other metals or of polymeric material are available as well.

The essential advantage of cartridges is that they allow a large filter surface to be accommodated within a relatively small space. For a standard filter cartridge of 70 mm diameter and 10 inches long (it is not uncommon to refer to diameter in cm and to length in inches) the total filter surface ranges from 0.5 to 1.6 m^2, depending on the structure of folding. This is achieved by star-shaped folding the membrane material with the help of a suitable support and drainage material (Fig. 2-25). The support material enhances the firmness of the folded structure and thus the maximally allowed pressure difference, while the drainage layers ensure full exploitation of the filter surface.

For prefiltering conditions and for particle filtration so-called depth-filter cartridges are employed in addition to folded filter cartridges, because of their higher capacity to collect residue. In this category, coiled cartridges and sintered cartridges are distinguished. In the coiled cartridge, fibers of materials such as cellulose, cotton, fiberglass, or polymers are coiled around a core. Sintered filter cartridges consist of metal, ceramic, glass, or polymer powders thermally fused together with or without additional adhesives. Depending on operational conditions, these filter cartridges allow flow capacities of several m^3/h. For even higher capacities multiple cartridges are installed together in one filter housing. In such cases, the cartridges can be aligned either side by side or on top of each other in order to achieve maximal packing density. In the pharmaceutical industry, filter housings containing 20 to 30 cartridges are not uncommon. In chemical as well as (soft) drink industries the number can even amount to over 100. In standard operation, flow direction in the cartridges is from outside to inside. In so far as the operation mode of the filter will allow it to be cleaned from solvent remains, this should be performed by rinsing in the flow direction in order to avoid

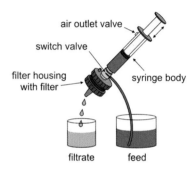

Fig. 2-24 Filtration of a small sample with a syringe filter.

air outlet valve

switch valve

filter housing with filter

syringe body

filtrate   feed

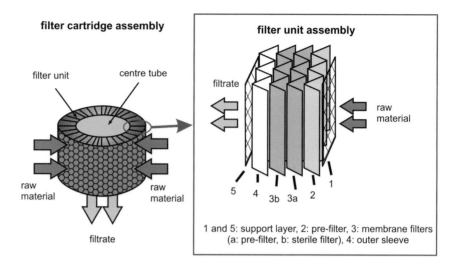

filter cartridge assembly

filter unit
centre tube
filtrate
raw material
raw material
filtrate

filter unit assembly

filtrate
raw material

5　4　3b　3a　2　1

1 and 5: support layer, 2: pre-filter, 3: membrane filters
(a: pre-filter, b: sterile filter), 4: outer sleeve

Fig. 2-25　Folded filter cartridge.

contamination on the filtrate side. Particles collected in the interior of the filter cannot, as a rule, be washed out by counterflow rinsing.

2.3.2.3　Single Use Filter Capsules

In case of single use filter capsules, cartridges and filter housing form a fixed unit. In the pharmaceutical industry, disposable filter cartridges are increasingly employed since validation of the cleaning procedure, which is required for classical cartridge filters, can be disregarded. This filter type has also proven its usefulness for the filtration of toxic substances and other critical products.

2.3.2.4　Depth Filter Sheets

Depth filter sheets are based on cellulose as a matrix material. Individual cellulose fibers stick together by means of resins in order to form a three-dimensional network. The resins also render the matrix moisture-proof and have an effect on charge. Addition of diatomaceous earth, perlite, or activated charcoal can influence specific filtration characteristics.

With respect to their structural make-up, depth filter sheets resemble a three-dimensional matrix consisting of an extremely fine maze-like meshwork with a porosity of 70% to 85%. The liquid to be filtered flows relatively slowly through these channels so that there is prolonged contact between the liquid and the filter surface. Thus, on their way through this maze, particles, microorganisms, colloids, viruses, and pyrogens are retained, while adsorption by surface charge supplements the mechanical 3-D binding.

2.3.2.5　Classical Flat Sheet Filtration with Frame Filter Press

Filter press constructions for accommodation of flat sheet are established equipment for clarification and prefiltration, dregs filtration and for the separation of bulk amounts of solids. They present discontinuously operating pressure filters with vertically or horizontally positioned filter chambers, in between which filter layers with various separation mechanisms can be installed. Their application offers the possibility to adjust filter media and filter surfaces according to changing requirements. In this way, large installations are formed of several meters in length and corresponding width and, by virtue of the commonly used steel constructions, of appreciable weight.

Frame filter presses are composed of a frame containing a variable number of vertically positioned filter chambers with alternating feed and filtrate chambers and often separated from each other by layers of filters (Fig. 2-26). After assembly, the entire construction is either manually (e.g., by means of a manual spindle press) or automatically pressed together hydraulically.

Each chamber is provided with two or more cylindrical supply openings (channel eyes). By compression of the chambers, the channel eyes, which are closed off by virtue of their close packing, form the supply and outlet channels.

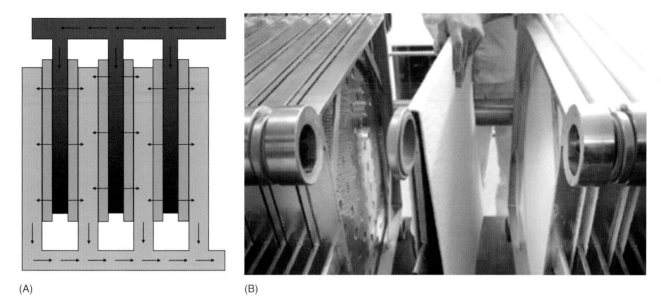

(A)   (B)

Fig. 2-26 Principle of sheet filtration (A); sheet filter in reality (B). Reproduced with permission from Filtrox AG © 2016.

The feed enters the supply channel in the inlet chamber and is filtered over the filter layer. The filtrate flows into the outlet chamber and is ultimately removed through the outlet channel.

2.3.2.6   Module Filters

State of the art depth filtration is performed by filter modules, which essentially are composed of a number of filter cells around a central tube (Fig. 2-27). The individual filter cells consist of filter layer material and a drainage system that is edge-sealed by an injection molding process. The individual filter cells are piled up on the central tube, compressed, and combined into one unit. Special adapters seal the filter modules off from the filter housing. The filter modules are installed in stainless steel housings before use or already molded into plastic capsules at the manufacturer. Thus, a complete and tightly closed filter system emerges, without losses, in contrast to the layer filter, in which, pertaining to its very design, leaky spots can occur.

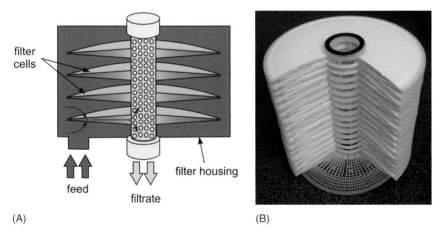

(A)   (B)

Fig. 2-27 Assembly of a module filter (A); module filter in reality. Reproduced with permission from Pall Corporation © 2016.

2.3.3   Centrifugation

In industry, separation is commonly performed by *filter centrifugation*. A filter centrifuge consists of an axially rotating sieve drum, which on the inside is coated with a filter. The dregs are

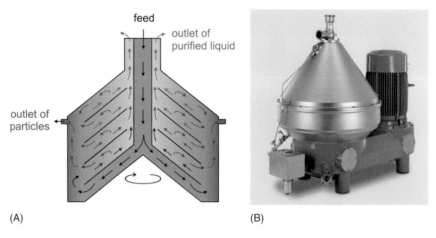

Fig. 2-28 Separator: (A) Principle; and (B) realization. Courtesy of GEA.

led into the interior of the drum and by rotation of the drum the solid fraction precipitates on the filter while the liquid passes through it.

For continuous clearance of liquids, mostly *separators* are used. Variations in construction make those suited for separation of liquids, dehydration of oils, desledging, or freeing fluids from solid material, respectively (Fig. 2-28). The whole device is rotating and the process is in dynamic equilibrium. The liquid from the intake pushes the liquid already in the device upward after it has reached the lower corners by centrifugal forces, guided by the inner elements. The heavier solid particles, experiencing a slightly stronger centrifugal force, are pushed to the wall and ultimately to the lower exit, whereas the lighter "filtrate" leaves the separator at the upper outlet.

2.4   Drying

2.4.1   General

Drying (desiccation) is the withdrawal of fluids, commonly water, by means of evaporation, vaporization or sublimation. The mostly used desiccating agent is air, which can accommodate water vapor up to saturation. As with increasing temperature, the water uptake capacity of air and thus the drying rate increase substantially, commonly hot air is used for this purpose. This also serves to compensate for the loss of heat by the evaporation process. Solid materials that need to be dried should be spread in a thin layer so as to bring about a larger surface area and a shortened diffusion path and thus an enhanced drying rate.

During a drying process, equilibrium is established between the wetness (moisture) of the substance to be dried and that of the gas phase (usually air) in contact with it. Therefore, it is in general not possible to dry a substance to such an extent that no traces of the removed liquid are left. When drying is performed at temperatures below the boiling point of the liquid and vapor pressure in the surrounding drying gas is lower than in the material to be dried, this is called *evaporation drying*. When, on the other hand, temperature and vapor pressure are close to those at the boiling point of the liquid, the drying process is rather referred to as *vaporization drying*.

In case of freeze-drying, moisture is removed directly from the solid phase of the liquid—a process called sublimation.

The supply or transfer of heat can be established by convection, radiation, or conductance. During convection drying, heat is led onto the drying substance by a gas stream (usually air). Simultaneously, the airflow provides for removal of the water vapor. In case of radiation drying the absorbed radiation (infrared radiation) is transformed into heat. That may lead to high temperatures on the surface of the drying material. In contact drying, the material to be dried is in direct contact with a heated surface; heat and water flow in the same direction from the heated surface to the surface of the drying material.

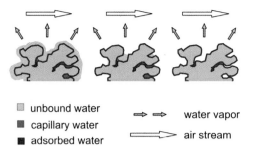

Fig. 2-29 Time course of the drying of a granule.

In most cases, drying leads to enhanced stability of the material, as in the dry state both chemical reactions and microbiological processes proceed at very low rates. That applies to chemical compounds as well as to products of vegetable and animal origin. Water removal thus represents a very effective stabilization method. When heat is applied, it is important to strive for the shortest possible heat exposure, as with increasing temperature the reaction velocity of a chemical conversion increases and physical instabilities are favored (e.g., polymorphic transitions).

2.4.2   Course of the Drying Process

Water can be bound to a solid in different ways (Fig. 2-29). The type of binding is of decisive importance for the drying process. A measure of the strength of binding is the binding heat, representing the energy required to abolish the binding:

- *Adhesive water.* This sits at the surface of the granule as well as in its larger cracks and microcapillaries (diameter >0.1 μm). It is unbound, freely movable water displaying the same vapor pressure as unbound bulk water. Adhesive water is easy to remove.
- *Capillary water.* In microcapillaries (radius <0.1 μm), vapor pressure depends on the radius of curvature of the liquid surface. In water-filled microcapillaries vapor pressure is clearly lower than in wider capillaries or compared with that of unbound water. With diminishing capillary radius, the reduction of vapor pressure becomes larger. As a result, capillary water is more difficult to remove than adhesive water.
- *Water of hydration ("swelling water").* Hydrophilic organic macromolecules such as cellulose derivatives and gelatin swell by adsorption of water. The strength of this binding is relatively low, so this swelling water can be removed by simple drying methods.
- *Adsorbed water.* At the surface of solid materials, adhesion forces are operational, which can retain water molecules. These forces are substance-specific. The surface loading begins with the formation of a monomolecular layer that displays strong binding forces. On this initial layer, additional layers of water molecules can attach with correspondingly lower binding forces. The attachment can be accomplished by interaction of water dipoles to salt ions or by the formation of hydrogen bridges to suitable functional groups (e.g., hydroxyl, carboxyl, or amino groups). Complete removal of water bound by adsorption requires intensive drying procedures.
- *Water of crystallization.* Crystalline substances can accommodate water molecules under the formation of hydrates. Water thus incorporated forms a structural element of the crystal lattice. Due to the strength by which this water is bound, it can only be removed by elevated temperatures, leading to loss of the corresponding crystal structure.

Most pharmaceutical substances are hygroscopic and bind water in small capillaries, in addition to the superficial adhesive water. During drying of hygroscopic materials, several characteristic drying stages are observed.

First, the loosely bound adhesion water is dried off with a relatively constant drying velocity. The drying air is then nearly fully saturated with water vapor. The rate at which the adhesive water is removed depends on the flow speed and the moisture of the air stream. After

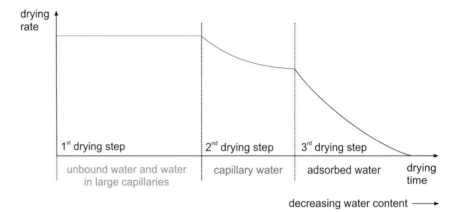

Fig. 2-30 Drying diagram.

removal of the adhesive water, the evaporation site moves deeper and deeper into the core of the granule. At that point, the drying rate is predominantly determined by the vapor diffusion rate. Removal of the water adsorbed to the granule surface requires more drastic drying measures and proceeds quite slowly.

Drying diagrams, which present the correlation between drying rate and moisture content, commonly display abrupt discontinuities, characteristic for the individual stages of the drying process (Fig. 2-30). In most cases, complete drying is not pursued, since a small amount of residual moisture may be required (e.g., for further processing of granules).

2.4.3   Drying Procedures

The choice of drying procedure depends on condition, quantity and physicochemical properties of the material to be dried (thin or thick liquid, paste-like, solid).

2.4.3.1   Cabinet or Vacuum Dryers

For drying at elevated temperatures, electrically heated drying cabinets are used. Hot air is led into the cabinet's interior and over a number of stacked trays containing the material to be dried. Modern drying cabinets are provided with fans and air circulation to create turbulence in order to establish evenly distributed temperatures inside the cabinet and appropriate flow speed, while at the same time ensuring continuous exhaustion of the water-saturated drying air. Heat-sensitive substances can be dried under reduced pressure in vacuum drying cabinets. In those cases, heat is supplied by heating the shelves on which the drying material is spread out.

2.4.3.2   Channel or Drum Dryers

In industry, drying is most often a continuous process. In *channel dryers* the spread material to be dried is transported on a conveyor belt and introduced into a channel that is heated by steam, hot water, or hot air. Blowers provide sufficient turbulence in the air stream. The dried material is then collected from the other end of the channel. The *drum dryer* consists of a slightly slanting drum mounted on roller bearings. The steadily supplied drying material is stirred by rotation of the drum and is gradually transported to the outlet due to its inclined position. The drying air can be led either in the direction of the mass movement or opposite to that. In other types of dryers (e.g., snail, blade, and trough dryers), the material to be dried is advanced by variously shaped mechanic insertions. They are heated in a similar manner and allow continuous throughput of material.

2.4.3.3   Fluidized-Bed Drying

With this drying method, the moist granular material (grain size 0.01–10 mm) is spread out on a porous bed (sieve plate) and is dried from below by a whirling stream of hot air. The high air-flow capacity allows a very rapid (up to 100 tons/h) drying process. It is to be

In physics, fluidized-bed situations occur, when a solid/fluid mixture behaves as a fluid. In our case, the granular material are fluidized in a stream of hot air.

noted that loss of ultrafine particles can occur as a result of precipitation in the filter caused by excessively high flow rates of the drying air stream.

2.4.3.4 Roller Drying

Roller dryers (Fig. 2-31) are applied for drying of fluid, pulp, and paste-like substances. They are particularly suitable for the manufacturing of larger batches of, for instance, milk powder, pigments, and the like, but occasionally also for the industrial manufacturing of larger quantities of dried pharmaceutical concentrates. The material is applied in a thin layer from a stock supply container by means of heated metal rollers. Heat transfer is accomplished directly from the roller to the drying material. With an appropriately heated roller surface, the drying process takes only a few seconds, so that the dried material can already be scraped from the roller before one full turn is made. For substances that do not even tolerate this short heat exposure, vacuum rollers can be employed.

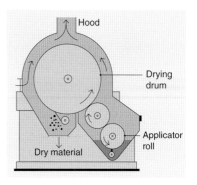

Fig. 2-31 Roller dryer.

2.4.3.5 Air Drying

A simple drying procedure, which is particularly used for the drying of (medicinal) plant material, is air drying. The material to be dried is spread on trays or shelves or in cabinets, protected from direct sunlight, and dried on the air.

2.4.3.6 Infrared Drying

Infrared (IR) radiation ($\lambda > 800$ nm) is particularly known for its heating capacity. Ideally, the amount of radiation energy applied with this method is just sufficient to penetrate the spread material onto the support construction, such that the entire layer of drying material absorbs the radiation.

2.4.3.7 Microwave Drying

During microwave drying, microwaves ($\lambda \sim 12$ cm, frequency ~ 2.45 GHz) excite predominantly the water molecules in the material to vibration. The heat thus formed causes the water to evaporate. The evaporation process can be speeded up by applying reduced pressure, which will lower the boiling point of the water. The water vapor thus formed is pumped out of the vacuum chamber.

2.4.3.8 Spray Drying

A particularly fast method to dry liquid materials can be achieved by spray towers (Fig. 2-32). By nebulization of nonviscous or moderately viscous solutions or dispersions

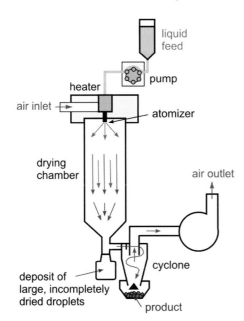

Fig. 2-32 Spray-dryer.

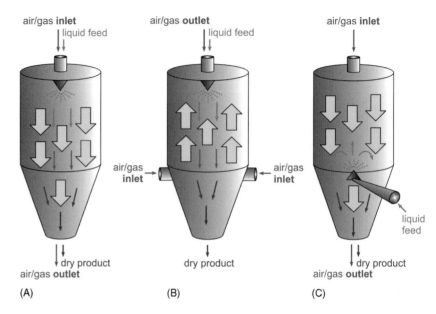

Fig. 2-33 Spray-dryer configurations: Co-current (A) and counter-current (B and C) flow.

in a hot-air stream, fine droplets are formed and, as a result of the strong surface enlargement, the material dries in fractions of a second into a fine powder. Nebulization can be achieved by means of an atomizer disk or a spray nozzle.

Different configurations of air inlets and feeds into the drying chamber are used (see Fig. 2-33). Residence time of the particles drying in the counter-current chamber types (Figs. 2-33 B and C) is long and larger particles—if desired—can be the consequence. In the co-current chamber design (Fig. 2-33 A), which nowadays is the most often used design, feed liquid is introduced from the top into the hot air zone. Here, the resulting fast evaporation caused by the atomization (for an explanation of atomization see Fig. 2-34) rapidly dissipates the heat energy. The hot air is thus cooled down before it continues its path through the chamber, which makes this configuration particularly well-suited for drying of heat-sensitive powders.

2.4.3.9   Atomizer Disk

With this equipment the liquid is introduced in the center of a rapidly rotating disk (4,000 to 50,000 rpm) (Fig. 2-34 A). The centrifugal force transports the liquid to the edge of the disk, while forming a thin film of liquid, which at the ridge of the disk is fragmented into small droplets.

2.4.3.10   Nebulization

In the *single-fluid nozzle* variant of the nebulizer the liquid is pressed under high pressure through a narrow orifice and thus forced into a spiral movement in a swirl chamber (Fig. 2-34 B). Upon exiting the nozzle, the liquid film is disrupted into small droplets. A drawback of the single-fluid nozzle equipment is that it tends to clog because of the small diameter of the orifice. It is therefore less suited for nebulization of dispersions. *Two-fluid nozzles* are constructed of two tubes sliding into one another. In the inner tube, the liquid is introduced into a centrally positioned opening. From a circular slit around this opening, a gas (commonly atmospheric air) is introduced with high velocity. This gas stream fragments the liquid upon exiting the nozzle into a fine spray mist. Two-fluid nozzles are less sensitive to clogging than the single-fluid nozzle variant.

The material to be dried is usually led into the spray tower from the top. During *direct-current drying*, the drying air is led into the spray direction. Thus, the hottest air hits the droplets containing most liquid, which are continuously cooled by the released negative heat of evaporation and thus already dried in an energy-conserving manner. The droplets stay in the airflow only relatively briefly but, by creating a spiral-shaped airflow, retention time can be prolonged. When the drying air is introduced counter-currently with respect to the fluid,

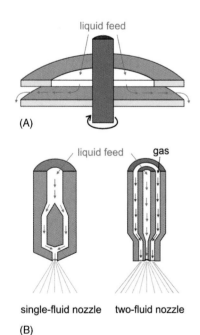

Fig. 2-34 Atomizer disk (A) and single-fluid and two-fluid nebulizers (B).

we speak of *counter-current drying*. Although in this way the droplets remain longer in the air stream, a disadvantage is that the hottest air now hits the already partly dried droplets, causing a larger heat burden on the material than the direct-current variant. Very fine droplets can be carried again upward and thus gain size by condensation, causing the granules thus obtained to display a relatively narrow size distribution.

Based on the spherical shape of the sprayed liquid droplets mostly approximately spherical particles of 20 to 200 μm are obtained. Often, hollow particles or fragments thereof are formed as a result of crust formation on the surface of the drying droplet. The dry-foam character of the particles favors their rapid dissolution. Spray-drying is also applied for the microencapsulation of essential oils and oxidation-sensitive compounds such as vitamins.

2.4.3.11 Freeze-Drying

Freeze-drying or lyophilization is a particularly gentle procedure to dry thermo-labile and hydrolysis-sensitive agents. It is applied for the drying of antibiotics, vitamins, hormones, blood plasma, sera, vaccines, proteins, sensitive herbal extracts, as well as colloidal preparations (e.g., liposome formulations).

The principle of the freeze-drying technique rests on the observation that frozen water has a significant vapor pressure and can therefore be removed by sublimation. Fig. 2-35 presents the phase diagram of water. Sublimation of frozen water is possible only when the partial vapor pressure close to the ice surface is lower than the saturation vapor pressure. In addition, the water vapor formed must be pumped off continuously and/or removed from the system as condensate.

Lyophilization systems consist of a temperature-controlled drying chamber with adjustable trays to accommodate the material to be dried, a condensation chamber for the separation of the formed water vapor, and a vacuum pump (Fig. 2-36).

During freeze-drying, three stages can be distinguished (Fig. 2-35; Fig. 2-37):

1. Freezing
2. Primary drying
3. Secondary drying

The freezing stage is accomplished under normal pressure. The applied conditions are more complex for pharmaceutical preparations than for pure water. The presence of active ingredients and excipients will lower the freezing point of the water and in the phase diagram multiple-phase areas show up (see Ch. 3.2.5). During cooling, first only pure water is separated from the solution (the size of the ice crystals formed affects not only the course of events during drying but also the subsequent redissolution of the dried material), resulting in an increase in concentration of the other components in the solution.

In case of simple eutectic behavior, the last remaining fluid domains will crystallize upon reaching the eutectic temperature of the entire system (for common pharmaceutical products,

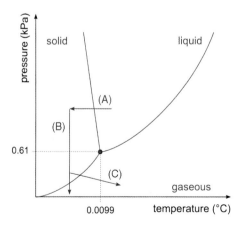

Fig. 2-35 **Phase diagram of water und stages of freeze-drying: (A) Freezing; (B) primary drying; (C) secondary drying.**

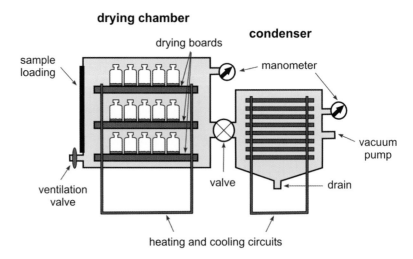

Fig. 2-36 Freeze-dryer.

this is usually between −20°C and −30°C). However, it may also occur that during the freezing process the concentrated solution solidifies in an amorphous phase, besides the ice crystals already formed. Such behavior, which may, for instance, occur in the presence of sugars, can enhance the stability of sensitive agents such as proteins suppressing harmful effects such as those caused by extremely high salt concentrations or precipitation of buffer salts (cryo-protection). In any case, the freezing conditions should be chosen such that complete solidification of the material to be dried is guaranteed.

During the primary drying stage, the frozen water is removed by sublimation under reduced pressure, as a result of which pores are formed in the product at the place of the disappearing ice crystals. The water vapor formed is trapped on a condenser with a temperature below that of the drying material. Further cooling of the sample by loss of sublimation heat is counteracted by supplying heat to the support trays. Heat supply should be controlled in such a way that the sample temperature remains below the eutectic temperature of the mixture, respectively, the glass transition temperature of the amorphous domains, in order to avoid loss of structure of the forming drying product by softening. The thickness of the layers of drying material should be minimal in order to guarantee adequate transport of the sublimating water from the deeper layers of the material.

The secondary drying serves to remove traces of remaining moisture. To that end, the product is additionally dried under vacuum at elevated temperature (e.g., 20°C).

For the manufacturing of parenteral products, the freeze-drying process must be performed under aseptic conditions. Usually, final sterilization of the end product is not possible.

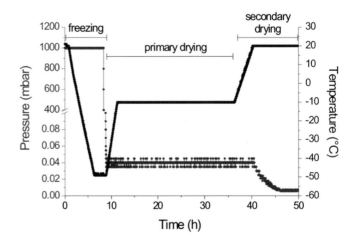

Fig. 2-37 Course of a conventional freeze-drying cycle.

Loading of the lyophilizing system should be possible from a clean room area, while the necessary technical equipment (vacuum pumps, compressors, etc.) should remain outside. After the complete drying process, the vials containing the dry material are automatically sealed inside the drying chamber.

The remaining moisture of freeze-dried product is very low (<1%). Such lyophilized materials are characterized by a fine, highly porous structure, which allows rapid dissolution because fluid can easily penetrate. Often excipient molecules with large numbers of hydroxyl groups are added (mostly sugars or sugar alcohols), which can stabilize polypeptides and proteins, facilitate dissolution of the lyophilized substance and at the same time serve to render the reconstituted preparation isotonic.

Further Reading

Chamayou, A. and Dodds, J.A. "Air jet milling." *Handbook of powder technology* 12 (2007): 421–435.

Daumann, B. and Nirschl, H. "Assessment of the mixing efficiency of solid mixtures by means of image analysis." *Powder Technol* 182(3) (2008): 415–423.

Franks, F. and Auffret, T. "Freeze-drying of Pharmaceuticals and Biopharmaceuticals." Royal Society of Chemistry Publishing, Cambridge, 2008.

Yokoyama, T. and Inoue, Y. "Selection of fine grinding mills." *Handbook of powder technology* 12 (2007): 487–508.

3

Physical and Physicochemical Principles of Drug Formulation

3.1 Drug Formulations as Disperse Systems

3.1.1 General Principles

For the characterization of drug formulations, we distinguish single-component and multi-component systems, in which each defined chemical compound is to be considered a single component that can occur as a solid, liquid, or gaseous phase.

Drug formulations generally consist of multiple components and are therefore classified as multicomponent systems. Systems consisting of at least two phases are designated as *disperse systems (dispersions)* when one of them (*dispersed phase*) is finely distributed in the other (*dispersing medium or dispersant*, also called *continuous phase*). Both the dispersed phase and the dispersing phase can be solid, liquid, or gaseous, but also *transitions* occur. Disperse systems are characterized by their *dispersion grade*, expressed, for example, by the volume-related total surface area of the dispersed phase or by particle (droplet) size.

When the dispersed particles are homogeneous in shape (e.g., spherules) we speak of monoform particles; in case of different shapes, they are called polyform particles. Systems with monoform particles of identical size are called *monodisperse* or *isodisperse*, and systems with heterogeneous particle size are *hetero-* or *polydisperse* (Fig. 3-1). According to particle size, *coarse*, *colloidal*, and molecular dispersion systems are distinguished (Table 3-1).

This classification principle is merely schematic since no step-wise changes in properties occur from one system to another. The classification is based on a scheme proposed by Hermann Staudinger (Nobel laureate, 1881–1965), who based his classification on the number of building elements, because a classification according to particle size applies, strictly speaking, only to spherical particles. The shape of the particles has a substantial influence on the properties of disperse systems.

When the dispersed particles are distributed in the dispersion agent without having contact with each other (i.e., when only the dispersion agent forms a coherent phase), we are dealing with an *incoherent system*. Examples of such systems are emulsions or suspensions. In coherent systems, the dispersed particles can interact with each other and build a three-dimensional scaffold structure such that both phases penetrate into one another (Fig. 3-2). Such conditions prevail in gels (ointment bases, bentonite gel; see section 15.3).

A classification of the multitude of disperse systems based on the aggregation state of the phases involved, as proposed by Wilhelm Ostwald (Nobel laureate, 1853–1932), provides helpful systematics. The dispersed systems presented in Table 3-2, including examples from pharmaceutical technology, are made up according to the same classification principle.

It should be noted that to some extent sliding transitions occur between the individual systems due to a lack of sharp borderlines between the states of aggregation. This, in turn,

Voigt's Pharmaceutical Technology, First Edition. Alfred Fahr.
© 2018 John Wiley & Sons Ltd. Published 2018 by John Wiley & Sons Ltd.

Table 3-1 Classification of Disperse Systems

	Coarse	Colloidal	Molecular
Number of building elements in one particle	$> 10^9$	$10^3–10^9$	$< 10^3$
Particle size	> 1 μm	1 μm (500 nm) to 1 nm	< 1 nm
Visualization of the particles	Naked eye or microscopically	Only in electron microscope	Invisible
Separation between dispersing agent and dispersed substance	Filtration with common filter paper	Filtration through nano-porous or ultrafilters	Cannot be filtered
Examples	Microparticles for injection; oral suspensions	Protein solutions, mucilages, liposomes (SUV, LUV)	NaCl solution (genuine solutions), gas- and liquid mixtures

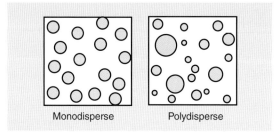

Fig. 3-1 Disperse systems.

is related to the difficulty to accurately define at any time the prevailing consistency of the phases and the disperse system.

3.1.2 Molecularly Disperse Systems

In molecularly disperse systems, the dispersed substance is genuinely dissolved in the solvent. Such mixtures are uniform and homogeneous and therefore no interfaces occur within the system. The mutual distribution of the components in the solution is molecular

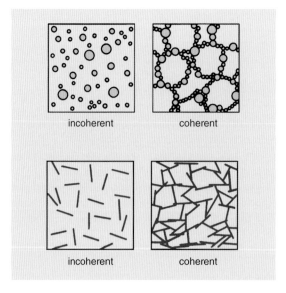

Fig. 3-2 Examples of incoherent and coherent disperse systems.

Table 3-2 Drug Formulations as Disperse Systems

Dispersed Phase	Dispersion Agent	State of the System	Designation	Examples Colloidally Dispersed	Coarsely Dispersed
Solid	Solid	Solid	"Solid suspensions"		Suspension suppositories
Liquid	Solid	Solid	"Solid (rigid) emulsions"		Emulsion suppositories
Gaseous	Solid	Solid		Activated carbon, zeolite as molecular sieve	Lyophilisate
Solid	Liquid	Liquid	Suspension	Dispersions of sun protecting pigments, polymer- and lipid nanoparticles	Shake lotions, parenteral suspensions (i.m., s.c.)
Solid	Liquid	Semi-solid		Aerosil and bentonite gel, petrolatum, triglyceride- and polyethylene glycol based ointment base	Moist granulate substance
Liquid	Liquid	Liquid	Emulsions	Parenteral lipid emulsions	Silicon oil emulsions, dermal emulsions
Liquid	Liquid	Semi-solid	Highly concentrated emulsions		
Gaseous	Liquid	Liquid/semi-solid			Medicinal foams, gas bubble dispersions as contrast agent
Solid	Gaseous	Gaseous	Smoke, aerosols		Powder aerosols; inhalation of solid particles
Liquid	Gaseous	Gaseous	Mist, nebulizer aerosols		Inhalation of liquid particles

when the particle size of the components in the solution is around 0.1 to 1 nm. The most abundant component is designated the solvent, in which the other component is (genuinely) dissolved. The ratio between the amount of solute and the amount of solvent is called *concentration*. Solutions in which both components are present in similar amounts and, in pure form under identical external conditions of temperature and pressure, both have the same aggregation state as the solution, are called *mixtures*. The term *solution* is commonly reserved for liquid or solid mixed phases.

3.1.3 Colloidally Disperse Systems

3.1.3.1 Principles

Colloidal dispersion systems take an intermediate position between molecularly dispersed and coarsely dispersed systems. *Colloids* are molecules or aggregates of molecules consisting of 10^3 to 10^9 building blocks with a particle size in at least one dimension between 1 nm and 1 μm (in some definitions, the upper size limit is taken as 500 nm) and in which the particles are distributed in a dispersing agent.

In contrast to the molecularly dispersed systems, a colloidal system is not merely defined by the thermodynamic parameters pressure, temperature, and concentration; also size, shape, and structure of the particles determine the properties of the system. The size of the colloidal particles and the degree of homogeneity of their distribution in the dispersing agent frequently give rise to the formation of interfaces (in contrast to molecularly dispersed systems) and may bring about a multitude of interfacial phenomena such as adsorption and interfacial tension.

Colloidal particles, which can be of inorganic as well as organic nature, do not possess a uniform shape or identical structure. They are predominantly characterized by their size (for polydisperse systems average size and size range). These parameters can be determined, for instance, by dynamic light scattering or electron microscopy. According to particle shape, one can distinguish sphero-colloids, which are obviously sphere-shaped (e.g., colloidal silica), platelet-like *laminar colloids* (e.g., bentonite), and fiber-like *linear colloids* (fiber-shaped macro-molecules).

3.1.3.2   Classification of Colloids

Colloidal dispersion systems can be classified as follows: single-molecule *molecular colloids, association colloids* arising from aggregation of smaller building blocks, and *dispersion colloids* formed by fragmentation of a phase.

Molecular Colloids

Molecular colloids consist of molecules that by themselves have already the dimensions of a colloidal particle. Examples are cellulose derivatives and other polymers (e.g., polyvinyl compounds). In solution some macromolecules can aggregate to even larger entities (macromolecular associates) as a result of the action of secondary valence forces. As a rule, in macromolecular solutions particles of various sizes occur. For linear colloids the average size can be estimated by viscosity measurements. Thread-like macromolecules are applied as mucilages, not only therapeutically, as for example in a laxative, but also as excipients for the stabilization of emulsions and suspensions, as binding agent for the manufacturing of granulates or for the formation of hydrogels, for example.

Association Colloids (Micellar Systems)

Association colloids can be formed from surfactants. When these are dissolved in low concentrations, molecularly disperse solutions are formed. Upon exceeding the so-called critical micelle concentration (CMC), association of the surfactant molecules results in the formation of more or less spherical aggregates called micelles. They are discussed more elaborately under 3.7.6 in connection with their significance as solubilizers for poorly water-soluble drugs.

Dispersion Colloids

All colloidal-dispersed systems that are obtained by dispersing (i.e., finely distributing) a compact phase belong to the category dispersion colloids. Depending on the physical state of the dispersed phase and of the dispersing agent, colloidal systems are formed of the type presented in Table 3-2. Dispersion colloids can be prepared by means of a variety of methods, as briefly explained in the following section:

- *Dispersion methods.* Dispersion occurs when a compact substance is disintegrated by the action of external forces (e.g., colloid mill, ultrasound, high-pressure homogenization). Also liquids can be dispersed by such methodology.
- *Condensation methods.* Starting from a molecularly disperse solution a supersaturated solution can be formed by cooling or by addition of a solvent in which the dispersed substance is insoluble (antisolvent). Alternatively, by means of a chemical reaction a poorly soluble product is formed which precipitates in the form of colloidal particles. Condensation methods aim at the aggregation of small (subcolloidal) particles such as molecules into particles of colloidal size. Measures should be taken (e.g., addition of stabilizers) to ensure that the aggregation terminates at the desired particle size and does not lead to the formation of a coarsely dispersed system.
- *Peptization.* With this method, colloidal particles that are held together merely by weak van der Waals forces are converted into a colloidal solution, or an ultra-fine dispersion (sol) by addition of electrolyte solutions. This is explained as follows: aggregated colloidal particles preferentially adsorb only one type of ion (anion or cation); as a result they all acquire similar charge, which leads to electrostatic repulsion between the particles. A transition to the sol phase occurs when repulsion forces exceed the attraction forces that caused the aggregation.

3.1.3.3   Stability and Stabilization

Molecules at the interface possess a higher free energy than molecules in the bulk phase. As the ratio between surface-oriented molecules and inner-phase molecules increases with diminishing particle size, dispersion colloids possess a large excess of free energy and thus tend to fuse together into larger aggregates to lower their free energy. The process leading to this aggregation is called coagulation. A further grouping together of particles, which ultimately will lead to the formation of one compact coherent phase, is called coalescence. The coagulation process can be prevented by taking appropriate stabilizing measures, which is discussed in more detail in chapters 18 and 19.

- *Surface charge.* Many dispersion colloids carry a surface charge by virtue of either chemical dissociation or adsorption of ions. The magnitude of the surface charge of the colloid particles (either + or −) can be chosen such that it is stronger than the van der Waals attraction forces. The kinetic energy of the particles should not allow them to approach each other so closely that coagulation can occur.
- *Solvation.* Also when, as a result of the deposition of molecules of the dispersing agent, the colloidal particles acquire a solvation layer (in case of water, hydration), free energy diminishes. Colloids with a strong solvation coating are designated *lyophilic colloids*, while those with a weakly solvated coating or no coating at all are called *lyophobic colloids*.
- Decisive for this classification is the affinity of the colloid particle to the dispersing agent. For example, starch is lyophilic toward water by virtue of the many hydrophilic groups in the molecule. Silver particles, on the other hand, prove themselves lyophobic in water because of their lack of affinity to the latter. Lyophobic colloids coagulate when electrolytes are added. The strength of the tendency to coagulate depends on the nature (in particular the charge) and the concentration of the added electrolyte.
- *Protective colloids.* As lyophobic colloids possess no or insufficient solvate coating, they are basically only protected against coagulation by their electric charge. Even tiny amounts of electrolytes, such as can be released from glass, for instance, can lead to charge neutralization and thus to coagulation. Lyophilic macromolecules added to such colloids act as a *protective colloid* (e.g., gelatin), in that they coat the lyophobic particles and form a solvation layer, thus preventing coagulation events. The protective action of protein is, for example, applied for the stabilization of silver colloids.

3.1.3.4   Properties of Colloidal Solutions

The colloidal structure of dissolved substances can be demonstrated by *dialysis*. Molecularly dissolved substances diffuse easily through semipermeable membranes (parchment paper, cellulose acetate or cellulose nitrate). Colloidally dissolved substances can only traverse through a semipermeable membrane when particle size is below the cut-off limit of the membrane. The cut-off or exclusion limit is commonly expressed as Dalton (Da), the unit for molecular weight. The dialysis procedure is quite suitable for the separation of low-molecular weight components from colloidal systems and thus for purification purposes. Colloidal systems consisting of particles with a size below the wavelength of visible light display the so-called *Tyndall effect*. When a sample of such a colloid is sideways illuminated with light, a bluish light scattering becomes visibly apparent. In particular, colloidal solutions of proteins and micellar solutions show this effect.

In an electric field, charged colloidal particles travel like ions (*electrophoresis*). The addition of electrolytes leads to decharging of the colloid particles, as these adsorb counter-charged ions (counter ions). This is called charge-neutralization coagulation. Also, the addition of other solvents can bring about disturbance of the solvation layer. At the iso-electric point, the particles no longer possess electric charge, so that as a result of the lacking repulsion forces coagulation can occur.

Of particular significance are also the rheological properties of colloidal systems. They depend on concentration, temperature, particle size, and shape, as well as on the mutual interaction between the colloidally dispersed particles and the nature of the dispersing agent.

A dilute colloidal solution is also designated as sol. Nonetheless, depending on the size of the dispersed particles, in many cases we are not dealing with a solution but rather with a suspension of colloidal particles. When in such cases, at increasing particle concentration, the forces between particles become so strong that a network of connections is formed, sols can be transformed through several steps into gels. Concomitant stepwise increased viscosities characterize these transformation steps.

3.1.4   Coarsely Dispersed Systems

As can be seen in Table 3-2, many drug formulations form coarsely dispersed systems. Occasionally, the coarse size range is further subdivided in macroscopically disperse (>0.1 mm) and microscopically disperse, according to the particle dimensions. Suspensions and emulsions are simple disperse systems, as far as they consist of one dispersed substance (e.g., oil dispersed in water). However, often we are dealing with systems that are more complex. Ointment bases may by themselves already represent a dispersed system, such as petrolatum, which consists of two phases: One phase of liquid paraffin is embedded in a phase of solid paraffin (see section 15.3.1.1). Thus, petrolatum is defined as *simple disperse system*. When zinc oxide is processed into petrolatum, a double-disperse system is formed. In emulsions, it gets even more complicated: the addition of an insoluble active ingredient forms a double-disperse system—an oil-in-water emulsion and an active-ingredient-in-water suspension. When taking into account that the active ingredient may be present not only in the water phase of the emulsion but also in suspended form in the oil droplets, even a triple-disperse system may result. When the fat phase of an emulsion consists of petrolatum rather than of liquid paraffin or a fatty oil, as is the case for many creams, even four- or five-phase disperse systems may be formed.

It is mainly due to this complexity that only in recent years have the physical or physicochemical laws and theoretical approaches that, strictly speaking, have validity only for single disperse systems, been applied to solve pharmaceutical-technological problems.

3.2   Pharmaceutical Solids

The majority of active ingredients and excipients are solids. Knowledge of the properties of solid materials is therefore indispensable for the manufacturing of medicines. Solid raw substances for pharmaceutical and preparative use can occur in various crystalline, amorphous, or partially crystalline states and affect by their very physical state the biopharmaceutical properties of the active ingredients involved.

3.2.1   Crystallinity

Table 3-3 Examples of active substances with polymorphic behavior

Acetylsalicylic acid
Ampicillin
Cefazoline
Chininhydrochloride
Cimetidine
Clotrimazole
Caffein, theophyllin
Cortisonacetate, hydrocortisone
Cyclophosphamide
Digitoxin, digoxin
Erythromycin
Estradiol, progesterone, testosterone
Glibenclamide
Griseofulvin
Indometacine
Meprobamate
Morphine
Nifedipine, nitrendipine
Nystatin
Paracetamol
Ritonavir
Spironolactone
Sulfanilamide, sulfathiazol
Tetracycline, oxytetracycline

Many solid compounds occur in a crystalline form. That is, their molecules or their constituting atoms are positioned at defined locations in a three-dimensional crystal lattice. The structure of a crystal lattice made up of organic molecules is, by virtue of the highly complex structure of its building blocks, substantially more complex than that of inorganic substances. The cohesiveness of such a molecular crystal is accounted for on the one hand by the covalent bonds within individual molecules and on the other hand by the occurrence of various intermolecular interactions.

Which shape of a crystal of a given material prevails not only depends on the internal structure of the crystal lattice but also on the question of which of the crystal planes is favored during crystallization. Thus, crystals with fully identical internal structure may take entirely different shapes when collected from different solvent systems. For the development of formulations, the shape of crystals is important in connection with their processing properties such as flow- and compression behavior.

3.2.1.1   Polymorphism

Many substances are capable of forming various crystal structures and therefore can occur in multiple structural *modifications*. This property is known as *polymorphism*. It is generally assumed that the majority of pharmaceutically active agents are capable of adopting polymorph forms (a few examples are shown in Table 3-3). The various crystal modifications are the result of the relative position of the molecules in the crystal lattice, causing the prevailing binding forces and the corresponding lattice energy to be different.

That brings along consequences for the physicochemical properties of the substances: crystal modifications vary, for example, in density, melting point, melting and dissolution heat, and solubility, as well as in mechanical behavior. Under given external conditions always only one crystal modification is stable, specifically the one with the lowest free energy or vapor pressure. Unstable modifications may convert to the stable form. However, conversion between different polymorphic crystal states is often kinetically inhibited by the limited mobility of the molecules in the crystal lattice and thus is characterized by high activation energy. This implies that thermodynamically unstable forms may very well prevail in a metastable state throughout pharmaceutically relevant periods of time.

When at different external conditions (e.g., different temperature ranges) particular modifications are stable, the conversion is reversible in case external conditions change (*enantiotropy*). Fig. 3-3a schematically presents the vapor pressure curves of a pair of enantiotropic modifications. In this example, modification II is stable at low temperatures and at temperature T_3, it is converted into modification I. Upon further heating, modification I remains stable up to its melting point T_1. On the other hand, also polymorphic substances are known of which in the given temperature range always only one modification is stable, so that the conversion into this modification proceeds irreversibly (*monotropy*). A schematic presentation of the vapor pressure curve of a pair of monotropic modifications is given in Fig. 3-3b. Modification I in this example is unstable in the entire temperature range and can only be preserved by undercooling of the molten mass up to temperature T_1. It will sooner or later transform into the more stable modification II. In this case, a conversion into the other direction is not possible because, upon heating modification II, the energy-richer modification I will not be formed at the theoretical conversion temperature T_3 but instead the substance begins to melt already at T_2.

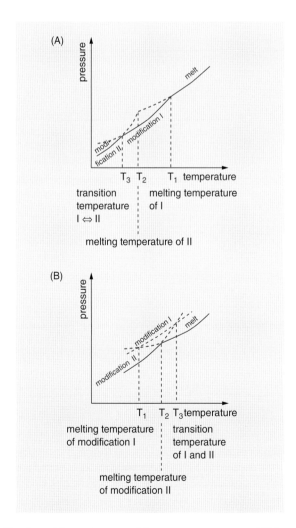

Fig. 3-3 Modifications. Schematic course of the vapor pressure curve; (A) for a pair of enantiotropic modifications, (B) for a pair of monotropic modifications.

Different modifications of a substance can be formed depending on the solvent from which it is crystallized or on the thermic treatment applied. Also factors such as pressure and temperature during processing (e.g., granulation or tableting) can lead to conversions in modification. In finished dosage forms conversion into a more stable form may take place during storage.

The different physical properties (section 25.3.1.1) of the crystal modifications can substantially affect the pharmaceutical characteristics of a drug formulation. For example, differences in crystal shape or in mechanical properties may profoundly affect tableting behavior. The difference in energy content of the various crystal forms also affects solubility and consequently the rate of dissolution (see section 3.9.3). This may have severe consequences for bioavailability, in particular for poorly water-soluble active agents, for which dissolution is the rate-limiting step in the absorption process. Also differences in stability toward chemical or enzymatic processes may occur. For example, the rate of enzymatic hydrolysis of chloramphenicol palmitate proceeds at rates, which are dependent on the nature of the prevailing modification. By the same token, light sensitivity of certain substances is modification-dependent (e.g., oxytetracyclin hydrochloride).

Ph. Eur. 5.9 Polymorphism _____

The Ph. Eur. dedicates a separate chapter to polymorphism, describing the phenomenon in general clarifying terms. In the substance monographs, the term *polymorphism* is used for polymorphism of molecular crystals, the allotropy of chemical elements, the existence of solvates or hydrates of a compound or for the occurrence of amorphous forms. The following methods are recommended for the analysis of polymorphic modifications.

- X-ray diffraction of powders
- X-ray diffraction of single crystals
- Thermal analysis (differential scanning calorimetry, thermogravimetry, thermomicroscopy)
- Microcalorimetry
- Moisture absorption analysis
- Optical and electron microscopy
- Solid-state nuclear magnetic resonance spectroscopy
- Infrared absorption spectrophotometry
- Raman spectrometry
- Measurement of solubility and intrinsic dissolution rate
- Density measurement

Investigation of solvates is preferentially done by means of differential scanning calorimetry (DSC) or thermogravimetry, combined with measurements of solubility, intrinsic dissolution rate and X-ray diffraction. In case of hydrates, sorption/desorption isotherms are determined to demonstrate the zones of relative stability.

3.2.1.2   Pseudopolymorphism

The process of crystallization of substances from solutions can give rise to inclusion of solvent molecules in the crystal structure. As a consequence, so-called solvates arise, which in case of water inclusion are designated *hydrates*. As solvates and hydrates commonly display an anomalous crystal structure this is often called *pseudopolymorphism*. From a technological point of view altered dissolution behavior and the possibility to release or incorporate solvent molecules during processing are of particular significance.

3.2.1.3   Real Crystals

Crystals produced and obtained under common conditions possess a highly ordered structure only within severely limited size ranges. For example, disturbances in the crystal structure already arise by the presence of minute quantities of an impurity. Nonetheless, also the innate lattice building blocks can adopt slight order deviations and thus cause the occurrence of *crystal defects*. Such defects may merely concern single positions in the crystal lattice (point defects, e.g. vacant sites, extraneous components at interstitial lattice sites), or alternatively stretch as edge dislocations or screw dislocations along so-called dislocation lines (line defects) or, furthermore, expand in a sheet-wise manner near grain boundaries (planar defects).

At the border of the grains the lattices of different individual crystals meet in a certain angle—for example, in aggregates of grown-together crystals, which often arise during technical processes (*polycrystallinity*). But even in single crystals so-called *domains* may commonly be encountered, with a typical size of ~1 μm, and crystal lattices that are slightly tilted toward each other. Other irregularities in crystal structures can arise, for example, when dealing with mixtures of different crystalline components or as macroscopic defects such as microcracks or pores.

3.2.2   Amorphous Solids

Particularly in the realm of polymers (e.g., lactic-acid/glycolic-acid copolymers), we may encounter substances that, as a result of their molecular structure, lack the potential to organize into a highly ordered crystal structure. Upon cooling from the melted state they solidify amorphously, that is, in a state lacking long-range order, which could be considered a *solidified liquid*. Instead of a sharply defined melting point we observe for such substances a *softening point*, which is characterized by a *glass transition temperature*.

Also for a variety of low-molecular weight substances, which normally occur in crystalline form, an amorphous phase is sometimes observed. Many sugars, for example, but also several active agents, tend to solidify in a glass-like state when they are rapidly cooled down from the molten state or dried from a solution (e.g. trehalose). Likewise, a strong mechanical challenge such as occurs during comminution, can lead to amorphousness. Since for such substances the amorphous state is instable or only metastable, recrystallization phenomena can occur during further processing or storage.

As mechanical behavior, hygroscopicity and solubility of amorphous substances may differ substantially from the properties of crystalline materials (Table 3-4), alterations of essential properties of a product may be the result. It is also conceivable that a substance simultaneously possesses amorphous and crystalline domains (semi-crystallinity). Thus, a "crystalline" polymer such as cellulose, commonly contains substantial proportions of amorphous material, while its chains assemble only locally into crystalline structures.

3.2.3   Characterization Methods

It should be kept in mind that, even though a substance may exist in different solid states, these states are nonetheless composed of chemically identical molecules. It is obvious, therefore, that these states cannot be identified by common chemical analytic procedures, the more so because in most cases it will be necessary to dissolve the substance before analysis. Therefore, physical assay methods need to be employed, which allow direct or indirect conclusions with respect to the molecular structure of the solid substance. Techniques often used for this purpose are X-ray diffraction, thermal analysis, and various spectroscopic methods (see Pharmacopeia Box Ph. Eur. 5.9 Polymorphism, page 46). Chemical methods, however, can be applied to detect the presence of solvent molecules in the crystal lattice and to determine their fraction.

Table 3-4 Different Properties of Crystalline and Amorphous Solid States

Crystalline Solid Material	Amorphous Solid Material
Highly ordered three-dimensional long-range internal structure	Unordered or short-range ordered inner structure
Defined melting point	Softening point (glass transition)
Optically anisotropic (exception: cubic crystal structure), birefringence	Optically isotropic
Mechanically anisotropic	Mechanically isotropic
Lower (apparent) solubility	Higher (apparent) solubility

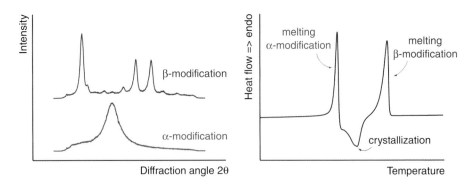

Fig. 3-4   X-ray diffraction pattern of a polymorphic substance (left) and DSC thermograph of the same substance (right).

3.2.3.1   X-ray Diffraction

The wavelengths of X-rays lie in the range of the distances between atoms in a crystal lattice. As a consequence, characteristic diffraction patterns are observed when the X-rays hit a crystal lattice. These patterns represent a function of the crystal structure and can thus be employed to determine this. Every crystalline substance has a crystal structure-determined characteristic diffraction pattern, comparable to an IR fingerprint.

In the context of drug formulation development, predominantly powder diffraction methods are employed, which allow characterization of powders of raw materials as well as of complete formulations. In this way, a distinction can be made not only between crystalline and amorphous material (the latter does not produce a sharp diffraction pattern because it lacks an ordered structure), but also between different polymorphic and pseudo-polymorphic forms, even within drug formulations such as tablets (Fig. 3-4). When properly performed, this method can also produce quantitative data, for instance with respect to the proportion of crystalline material in an otherwise amorphous sample, or concerning the mixing ratio of different modifications.

Ph. Eur. 2.9.33 Characterization of Crystalline and Partially Crystalline Solids by X-ray Powder Diffraction (XRPD) _____

USP ⟨941⟩ Characterization of Crystalline and Partially Crystalline Solids by X-ray Powder Diffraction (XRPD)

JP 2.58 X-Ray Powder Diffraction Method

X-ray powder diffraction (XRPD) is a procedure that allows determination of the qualitative as well as quantitative composition of a substance by characterizing its crystal structure, thereby distinguishing the crystalline from the amorphous phase as well as the various polymorphous modifications. This technology is based on the principle that X-rays are scattered by interaction with the electron clouds of individual atoms in the material. When the lattice planes of a crystal are positioned in a certain angle with respect to the direction of an incident monochromatic X-ray beam, the latter is scattered in defined angles by the successive superimposed lattice planes. The traveled path lengths of the rays differ from each other by an integral number of wavelengths used. In the direction of these angles, the scattered rays oscillate in phase and thus are amplified, while for in between angles the phase-shifted oscillations lead to attenuation or even extinction. These interference conditions are quantitatively described by the Bragg equation:

$$2d_{hkl}\,\sin\theta_{hkl} = n\lambda$$

d_{hkl} = distance between two consecutive lattice planes
θ_{hkl} = angle between incident beam and the deflecting lattice plane
λ = wavelength
n = integral number

Thus, for each lattice plane direction in the crystal a first-order diffraction maximum and additional higher-order maxima are observed. In case of a powder sample, a large number of statistically distributed crystals or crystallites occur within each individual powder grain. For each type of lattice plane occurring in the crystal and for each order of possible diffraction angles, such a sample contains a large number of powder grains, which are oriented by chance in such a way in the powder bed that for each case they fulfill the Bragg conditions. For such measurements nowadays mostly equipment of the Bragg-Brentano goniometer type is used. An X-ray source produces monochromatic radiation, which is paralleled by collimators. Often the Cu K_α radiation of a copper anode is used as an X-ray source.

The X-rays hit a swiveling sample holder, which rotates during the measurement, at half the angle at which the detector moves, in a circular path around the sample holder. This assures that the angle at which the deflected rays are received always complies with the angle of incidence. The sample must be positioned on the holder such that the grain particles are maximally randomly distributed and do not favor any specific direction. Particularly for needle- or disk-shaped particles comminution (not below 0.5 μm) can improve the result.

For qualitative phase analysis—that is, the identification of the phase composition of an unknown sample, it is appropriate to record the diffraction pattern in a 2θ-range from as near to 0° as possible to at least 40°. If the sample and the reference have the same crystal form the corresponding signals coincide with an error of maximally 0.2°. With hydrates and solvates, however, greater deviations can occur. When in a sample, two or more known phases occur, of which maximally one is amorphous, it is possible to obtain the quantitative composition of the sample by evaluation of the peak heights or areas of a number of selected diffraction signals or by computer-assisted analysis of the overall diffraction pattern. The sample diffraction pattern can be compared not only with the powder pattern of a reference substance but also with the XRPD pattern calculated from the crystallographic data of a particular substance. Thus, every known mono-crystal structure of a certain substance can be used for the identification of a powder sample.

3.2.3.2   Thermal Analysis

A frequently applied method for the characterization of organic solids is differential scanning calorimetry (DSC), as shown in Fig. 3-4. With this technique, the uptake or release of heat energy by the sample during a temperature program is recorded. In this way, any process that is accompanied by heat exchange, such as melting, crystallization, glass transitions, release of hydrate water or chemical conversions, can be characterized. Thus, it is, for instance, possible to discriminate between amorphous (glass transition) and crystalline (sharply defined melting temperature) material, or to identify polymorphic forms by determining melting temperatures and melting heats. Thermally induced processes, accompanied by loss or gain of mass, can be identified by means of *thermo-gravimetry*. By polarization microscopy amorphous and crystalline substances can be distinguished (except for cubic crystal structures) on the basis of their optical properties: Amorphous substances are optically isotropic; most crystals are anisotropic. Microscopic examination during a temperature program (*thermo-microscopy*) provides additional indications about polymorphous conversions or the presence of solvates.

Ph. Eur. 2.2.34 Thermal Analysis _____

USP ⟨891⟩ Thermal Analysis

JP 2.52 Thermal Analysis

Thermal analysis comprises a group of techniques in which the variation of a physical property of a substance is measured as a function of temperature. The most commonly used techniques, thermogravimetry, and differential scanning calorimetry are described in Ph. Eur. and JP. Thermomicroscopy is included in Ph. Eur. as an additional technique. In the USP the chapter has a mainly application-oriented structure:

- Transition and melting point temperatures
- Determination of transition temperature (melt onset temperature) and melting point temperature
- Thermogravimetric analysis
- Hot-stage microscopy
- Eutectic impurity analysis

Thermogravimetry (Ph. Eur., JP), Thermogravimetric Analysis (USP)

In this method, the mass of a substance is measured during the passage of a defined temperature program. It allows the recording of the mass as a function of temperature or—under isothermic conditions—of time.

Proper functioning of the balance can be verified by the weight change of reference materials (e.g., water release of calcium oxalate monohydrate) (Ph. Eur.). Calibration is performed by the use of standard weights (USP). For temperature calibration advantage is taken of the change in magnetic properties of nickel at the Curie point, which causes an apparent weight change at 385°C when the sample is placed in a magnetic field (USP).

Differential Scanning Calorimetry (Ph. Eur.), Differential Thermal Analysis, or Differential Scanning Calorimetry (JP)

Differential scanning calorimetry allows the quantitative assessment of changes in enthalpy and specific heat during heating or cooling of a substance and the estimation of the temperatures at which these changes take place. To that end, the heat released or absorbed by the sample is measured relative to a reference sample. Measurements can be done in two ways: either the amount of absorbed heat required to compensate for the temperature difference between sample and reference is recorded (DSC in the narrower sense) or the temperature differences occurring during a constant heating (or cooling) rate are recorded (often termed differential thermal analysis, DTA). In both cases, a graphic plot of energy change against temperature is obtained. The intersection of the tangent of the first inflexion point of a curve peak and the baseline identifies the start of the thermal event (onset temperature), while the top of the peak marks the end of it. The enthalpy of the thermal process is proportional to the peak area above the baseline. Calibration is performed by measuring the melting heat of a known substance (e.g., indium) under identical conditions. The DSC method allows quantitative assessment of multiple thermal processes such as melting, solidifying, evaporation, sublimation, desolvation, polymorphous, and amorphous-crystalline transitions. In addition, the purity grade of a substance can be derived from the melting point and the molar melting heat (Eutectic impurity analysis, USP).

Thermo-Microscopy (Ph. Eur.), Hot-Stage Microscopy (USP)

Thermo-microscopy serves to identify phase transitions by means of polarization-microscopic analysis of morphological changes.

3.2.3.3   Spectroscopic Methods

Although infrared spectroscopy is based on the interaction of radiation with bonds within individual molecules, these spectra, especially in the fingerprint range, also express differences in crystal structure. For the investigation of polymorphism preferentially FTIR spectra are recorded, which also allow quantitative conclusions concerning the contribution of the form of interest. Information about the environment of individual atoms or groups in different solid states can be obtained by means of solid-state NMR spectroscopy. In view of its high cost, however, this technique is not commonly employed for routine assays.

3.2.4   Crystallization

Crystallization of pharmaceutical substances is not only important during the production of active ingredients but also for their processing. Examples are the events occurring during freeze- and spray drying, the solidification of raw materials for the production of suppositories, sugar coating of tablets or the granulation process. The crystallization process from a melt or a solution of a substance includes two subsequent stages: formation of a nucleus and crystal growth. For the formation of crystals, either a melt of the substance has to be cooled down to below the melting point or a solution of the substance has to be concentrated to

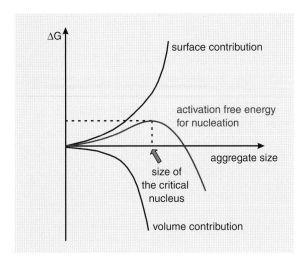

Fig. 3-5　Processes during the formation of crystal nuclei.

Recent studies employing modern methods like AFM showed that nano-sized structures are present in supersaturated solutions before nucleation occurs. This lowers the energy barrier to nucleation and consequently for crystallization. The conclusions of these results are still under debate. If this is of interest, read the paper by Habraken et al. (2013), who present, besides the experiments on nucleation of calcium phosphate, also a "compromise" between old and new theories. In any case, it is clear that these findings will change our view of crystallization mechanism in the future.

above the saturation concentration. After the temperature has dropped below the melting temperature or the concentration has increased to above the saturation concentration, crystallization will not immediately start. To begin with, the formation of a crystal nucleus is an energy-requiring process during which a sufficient number of molecules have to align together from the melt or the solution in the correct orientation (Fig. 3-5). The probability of nucleus formation increases with increasing undercooling or increasing saturation, respectively. As soon as a certain critical extent of undercooling/oversaturation has been reached, numerous crystal nuclei are spontaneously formed. Normally, no spontaneous nuclei formation is observed within the meta-stable range between melting point or saturation limit, respectively, and the range of spontaneous nuclei formation. Nonetheless, crystal growth is possible under those conditions when, for instance, seed crystals of the material in question are added. By following this procedure, it is also possible to achieve crystallization of a predetermined polymorph form.

With increasing undercooling of a melt viscosity also increases. The spontaneous alignment of the molecules to form a crystal nucleus is impeded, then, so that the rate of nucleus formation decreases again and nucleus formation comes to a halt. The high viscosity also explains why nucleus formation in amorphous solids (e.g., window glass) is often barely or even not at all possible.

During formation of crystal nuclei enhanced binding forces between the aligned molecules come into play, leading to a negative contribution to the free energy of the system (crystallization heat), and thus advancing the process (see Fig. 3-5). Nonetheless, nucleus formation is also associated with a positive enthalpy contribution, as between the mother phase and the aligned molecules an interface is formed. In the early stages of nucleus formation, this interface contribution outweighs the volume contribution resulting from the associating molecules, such that nucleus formation is not favored and the nascent crystals tend to dissolve again. Only after a critical nuclear radius is exceeded, the net amount of free energy diminishes again, thus stabilizing the nucleus and allowing it to grow. The number of molecules required for the formation of a stable nucleus decreases with increasing undercooling or oversaturation of the liquid system, causing an increasing probability of nucleus formation.

The process of crystal growth following nucleus formation has an essential influence on the shape of the formed crystals. The crystal faces onto which the molecules from the liquid preferentially arrange themselves—and where therefore the highest crystal growth rate will occur—are relatively small in the fully-grown crystal and may even disappear. On the other hand, crystal faces onto which the molecules attach slowly keep growing to large surfaces. The presence of foreign compounds (e.g., ions or surfactants) can impede the molecular association on certain surfaces and thus affect the shape of the forming crystals.

3.2.5   Solid-State Mixtures

3.2.5.1   Eutectic Behavior

Most crystalline materials do not mix in the solid state, even if they are freely miscible in the liquid state. Mixtures of such substances often display eutectic behavior (Fig. 3-6), which macroscopically becomes particularly apparent as a lowering of the melting temperature as compared to the melting points of the single components. The lowest melting

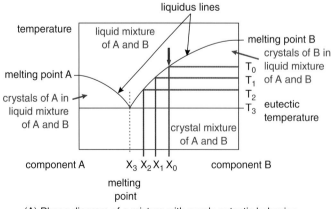

(A) Phase diagram of a mixture with purely eutectic behavior   (B) Eutectic behavior with "edge solubility"

Fig. 3-6 Eutectic behavior.

point is observed for a composition of the system, which is known as the eutectic mixture or simply eutectic, consisting in the solid state of very fine crystals of both components. The formation of very fine crystals during solidification of a eutectic mixture of a readily water-soluble substance with a poorly soluble active ingredient can provide the ultimate product with favorable solubility properties (cf. section 2.4.3.11).

In the topical anaesthetic Emla®-Cream, the employment of a liquid (at room temperature) eutectic mixture of two solid local anesthetics allows it to be processed in the liquid state. On the other hand, liquefaction occurring during processing (e.g., granulation, tableting) of mixtures of powdery components with eutectic behavior can lead to complications in the processing procedure. Eutectic behavior of an active ingredient mixed with a suppository base may result in unacceptable product properties due to a lowered melting point of the base. To counteract this effect, a suitably higher melting base may then be added. Also during lyophilization of complex mixtures eutectic behavior may play an important role.

When two solid substances display eutectic behavior, the melting point of their mixture lies below that of either one of the two components. In the liquid state the two substances mix indefinitely in the range above the two liquidus lines in the phase diagram. Below either one of the liquidus lines (e.g., for the mixture with composition X_0 in diagram A at temperature T_0) crystalline material of one of the pure components (in the example component B) separates out so that a mixture emerges consisting of solid pure substance and a liquid mixture of both components. The composition of the liquid mixture corresponds then with the position on the liquidus line at the corresponding temperature. Upon continued cooling of the mixture, evermore pure component crystallizes out of the mixture, thus depleting the liquid mixture of this component, causing it to approach the eutectic composition (via X_1 and X_2 to X_3). Below the eutectic temperature, the entire system solidifies while the two pure components crystallize separately. Only at the composition of the system corresponding to that of the eutectic mixture (also known as the eutecticum), the system can completely solidify immediately upon cooling. The eutectic mixture exhibits the lowest possible melting point of the two-component system. Mixtures differing from this composition melt in a temperature range of varying width. As a rule, in real systems displaying eutectic behavior the two components are to some extent mutually soluble in the solid state. In the phase diagram, this is expressed in areas of "limited solubility" (Fig. 3-6B). As a result, the pure components do not crystallize there but, rather, the prevailing solid solutions. In some mixtures, the position of the "eutectic" mixture has fully shifted in favor of one of the two components. In such cases, we speak of a monotecticum.

EMLA® (**e**utectic **m**ixture of **l**ocal **a**nesthetics) from Astra Zeneca: Prilocaine and lidocaine form an eutectic at a mixture of 50:50, which is then an oil. This can be formulated as an O/W emulsion at much higher concentrations than the respective substances dissolved in oil.

3.2.5.2 Solid Crystalline Solutions

In these situations, the two components of a system crystallize together in mixed crystals. Most often, the miscibility at the edges of the phase diagram is limited, but occasionally also in the crystalline state complete miscibility is observed (Fig. 3-7). In such cases, molecules of one component are replaced by molecules of the other in the crystal lattice, or small molecules nestle between the lattice elements of the "solvent." The latter behavior is for

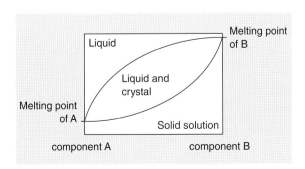

Fig. 3-7 Phase diagram of a continuous crystalline solid solution.

instance observed with solutions in solid macromolecules (e.g., hydrocortisone acetate in polyethylene glycol 6000).

3.2.5.3 Mixtures with Amorphous Components

A substance may dissolve in an amorphous solid, like it would in a liquid, or be suspended in crystalline form. Such amorphous matrices can be formed for example by citric acid, urea, sugar, polyvinyl-pyrrolidone or polyethylene glycol. Also precipitation of an amorphous active substance in a crystalline matrix is possible.

3.2.6   Mechanical Behavior of Solids

Mechanical properties of solid materials under stress play a role in pharmaceutical technology, particularly in relation to comminution and deformation processes (tableting, for example). Mechanical behavior of a solid material can be categorized with respect to several characteristic aspects, depending on the applied stress (ideal or disproportional elastic behavior, flow plasticity, fracture) (Fig. 3-8).

In contrast to crystalline solids, solid amorphous substances are mechanically isotropic upon deformation (i.e., their mechanical properties are independent of the direction of the applied deformation). Crystalline substances, on the other hand, may display clearly anisotropic behavior under these conditions. Deformation then follows privileged slide planes, along which the crystal building blocks can be readily displaced. Irregularities in the crystal lattice play an important role in the mechanical behavior of crystalline substances. In connection with plastic deformation edge dislocations are important. They may move relatively easily through the crystal and thus contribute to satisfactory deformability. Various types of crystal defects, also at the macroscopic level, are preferred weak points for fractures to occur in crystals because at such sites a fracture requires much less energy than disruption of an intact crystal lattice.

The mechanical characteristics of a solid under strain stress may be described by means of a stress-strain diagram shown in Fig. 3-8.

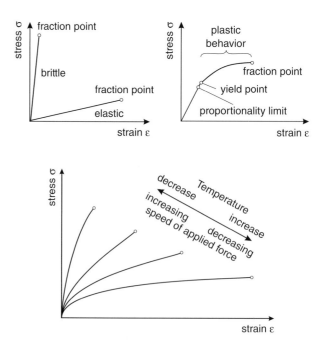

Fig. 3-8 Stress-strain diagram in tension.
Top left diagram: materials with ideally elastic behavior, top right diagram: material with plastic behavior, bottom diagram: dependence of plasticity on temperature and rate of force application.

At relatively low mechanical stress challenge a solid body will respond ideally elastic, i.e. deformation is linearly proportional to the applied stress. This is described by Hooke's law:

$$\frac{F}{A} = E \cdot \frac{\Delta l}{l_0} \quad \text{with} \quad \frac{F}{A} = \sigma \text{ and } \frac{\Delta l}{l_0} = \varepsilon$$

σ stress: pulling force F per area A
ε relative change of length l with regard to the initial position l_0
E elasticity modulus

The more easily the material stretches, the smaller is the elasticity modulus. In the range of ideal elastic deformation behavior, the material adopts its original length upon release of the strain force. This still applies in the range of supra-proportional elasticity, which follows the Hooke range, whereas no linear proportionality is observed between strain and extension. When an even higher strain is applied, the material starts to deform plastically, in other words it begins to flow. Upon releasing the strain force in this range, resilience is observed only as far as it is in accordance with the earlier applied elastic deformation; however, the flow process is irreversible. A further increase of the strain force will eventually lead to fracture of the material. Although the different ranges described here in a general fashion may in principle be observed in all materials, their individual relevance may vary distinctly (e.g., brittle vs. plastically deformable materials). In addition, mechanical behavior often depends on temperature ("low-temperature brittleness") as well as on the rate of force application (rapid processes may lead to suppression of the plastic deformation, see bottom diagram in Fig. 3-8).

The hardness of solid materials is particularly important for the choice of milling equipment. It is expressed by the resistance of the material against the penetration of a foreign object and can be assayed in different ways. A very simple way to classify hardness of materials is the Mohs hardness scale (Table 3-5), in which materials are ranked according to their susceptibility to being scratched by the next material on the scale. As a rule, active substance crystals display low hardness. Grinding equipment should always be selected such that the material it is made of takes a clearly higher position on the hardness scale than the material to be ground in order to prevent abrasion of the grinder.

Table 3-5 Scratching Hardness According to Mohs

Substance	Hardness
Talcum	1
Gypsum	2
Calcite	3
Fluorite	4
Apatite	5
Potassium feldspar	6
Quartz	7
Topaz	8
Corund	9
Diamond	10

3.3   Particle Size

Particle size correlates tightly to pharmaceutically relevant physicochemical characteristics of materials such as dissolution rate, adsorption capacity, adhesive power, and rheological properties. Particularly for poorly soluble drugs, small particle size is a prerequisite to achieve sufficient dissolution rates and thus drug absorption. The grain size spectrum that is relevant in pharmaceutical technology ranges from the nm size to several mm. As a result, there is no common technology for size measurement available that covers the entire size range of relevant particles (Table 3-6). For the selection of the assay method, size range and physical characteristics (powder, suspension, emulsion, etc.) must be taken into consideration. Requirements with respect to accuracy and speediness of the method are decisive for pharmaceutical industry in order to ascertain quality during the production process. Whenever particle size of a sample is given, the applied assay method must be revealed, because measured particle size may vary with the assay technique (see section 3.4).

3.3.1   Grain Size and Grain Size Distribution

As a rule, assemblies of particles such as powders are heterogeneous; they consist of particles varying in size within a broader or narrower range. Only for an ideally spherical particle its size is accurately defined by means of a given diameter. Particles used in pharmaceutical technology commonly possess a more or less anisometric nonspherical shape. Depending on the assay method, particle sizes are given by different statistical diameters and equivalent diameter which may yield different values.

Table 3-6 Overview of Most Important Size Measurement Techniques

Technique	Approximate Size Range	Application Examples
Sieve analysis	5 μm to 125 mm	Powders, granules
Microscopy		
light microscopy	0.5 to 250 μm	Powders, suspensions, emulsions
electron microscopy	1 nm to 10 μm	Colloidal suspensions and emulsions
Light scattering		
Laser scattering	1 to 2000 μm	Powder, suspensions, emulsions, aerosols
with submicron equipment	< 50 nm to 2000 μm	Suspensions and emulsions
Photon correlation spectroscopy	5 nm to 1 μm	
Sedimentation		
Pipette analysis	1 to 100 μm	Suspensions, emulsions
Sedimentation balance	1 to 100 μm	Suspensions, emulsions
Sedimentation in centrifugal field	50 nm to 5 μm	Suspensions, emulsions
Electrozone sensing (Coulter counter)	0.4 to 1200 μm	Suspensions, emulsions
Filtration		
Gravity air classification	5 mm to several mm	Powders, granules
Centrifugal air classification	2 to 80 μm	Powders
Light obscuration (light blockage)	1 to 2500 μm	Emulsions, suspensions, powders

3.3.1.1   Statistical Diameter

In microscopic particle size analysis two statistical diameter definitions are common: the diameter according to Martin (d_M) and the diameter according to Feret (d_{Fer}). The d_M is defined as the length of the line, which—in the direction of measurement—cuts the projection area of the particle in two equal parts. The d_{Fer} is defined as the distance between the two tangents to the particle projection perpendicular to the direction of measurement. From Fig. 3-9, it is clear that the two different methods yield different values for the diameter of the same anisotropic particle. By measuring the sizes of a statistically significant number of particles, arranged randomly on the microscopic slide, the average size of the particle assembly is obtained.

3.3.1.2   Equivalent Diameter

Examples of common equivalent diameters are:

- *Stokes diameter* (diameter of a sphere with the same sedimentation properties as the particle in question).
- *Sieve diameter* (maximal diameter of a sphere still passing through a sieve with a pore size allowing the passage of the particle in question).
- *Volume equivalent diameter* (diameter of a sphere with the same volume as the particle in question).

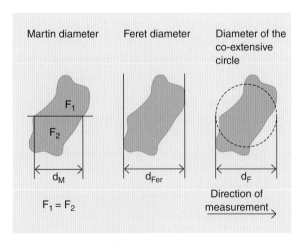

Fig. 3-9 Characterization of particle diameter by microscopy.

From the microscopically measured surface area of the particle projection, the equivalent diameter of the surface-equivalent circle can be determined (Fig. 3-9).

Ph. Eur. 2.9.37 Optical Microscopy _____

USP ⟨776⟩ Optical Microscopy
JP 3.04 Particle Size Determination, Method 1. Optical Microscopy
Under the heading "Optical Microscopy," the Ph. Eur. presents detailed information on the design and handling of a light microscope as well as on sample preparation. This section also describes light microscopy as a method to analyze size and shape of particles and their visual appearance, to determine the presence of particular contaminants and to characterize their crystalline nature (polarization microscopy). Light microscopy is a suitable characterization technique, in particular for nonspherical particles, and may also be seen as a basis for the development of more rapid routine methods.

3.3.2 Graphic Representation

In general, an average value for the fineness of a particle assembly does not suffice to accurately describe it. It is important to also know the frequency of a certain particle size in the sample and the width of the size distribution. Most simply, grain size distributions may be presented in the form of a table, but these are most often not highly illustrative. Therefore, size distributions are commonly presented graphically, with the independent variable (grain size, degree of fineness) depicted on the abscissa and the dependent variable (e.g., mass or number of particles) on the ordinate.

3.3.2.1 Histograms
The simplest graphic representation is the histogram or column diagram. The size range is divided in individual particle size classes (in case of sieve analysis, the width of the classes is determined by the mesh size of the applied sieve). On the abscissa, the grain size parameters of the individual fractions are plotted, on the ordinate the mass or number of particles belonging to each individual grain class, the relative frequency or the density distribution (Fig. 3-10).

3.3.2.2 Density Distribution Curve
When for each class the relative frequency is divided by the width of the class, a discrete density distribution is obtained with a total surface area of 100%, or 1. By applying certain assumptions concerning the distribution model (e.g., Gaussian distribution) a continuous density distribution curve is obtained (Fig. 3-10).

3.3.2.3 Cumulative Distribution Curve
When on the ordinate the sum of the masses or of the number of particles per class is plotted, a cumulative distribution curve is obtained. Usually, two curves, one for the undersize cumulative distribution (i.e., passing fraction distribution curve) and one representing the cumulative distribution of the sieve residues are plotted (Fig. 3-11).

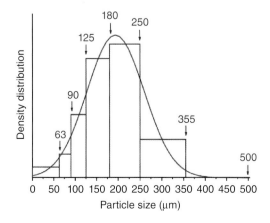

Fig. 3-10 Histogram and density distribution curve of a sieve analysis (the numbers in the histogram signify the mesh sizes of the applied sieves).

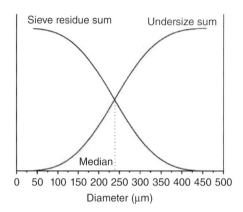

Fig. 3-11   Cumulative distribution curves.

3.3.2.4   Mass and Number Distribution

Depending on the applied method, either the mass (or volume) contribution (in this case to be considered equivalent) or the number of particles in the corresponding grain size class is determined. As large particles have a greater impact on the mass and volume distribution than on the number distribution, obvious differences are observed between the two distributions (Fig. 3-12). In most methods applied in pharmaceutical technology, a mass distribution is obtained—for instance, with sieve analysis, sedimentation analysis or light scattering. Electrozone sensing and microscopy methods, on the other hand, are examples of methods with which number distributions can be obtained. Under certain assumptions (e.g., identical particle shape and density), the two distribution types can be converted into one another by calculation.

3.3.2.5   Location and Dispersion Parameters

The *location parameter* is a measure for the average fineness of a sample. In practice, different location parameters are used: the *median* (D_{50}) is the particle size at 50% permeation or retention, respectively, in the undersize distribution. The median divides the density distribution curve in two exactly identical surface areas. The *mode* designates the most frequently occurring particle size in the sample; it corresponds to the maximal density distribution (density average). The *mean* is defined as the arithmetic average of all measured particle sizes. For a Gaussian normal distribution, the three condition parameters have identical values.

The *dispersion parameter* is a measure of the width of a distribution. For a Gaussian distribution, it corresponds to the standard deviation.

3.3.2.6   Model Distributions

The determination of location and dispersion parameters, the dealing with measured particle size distributions as well as the comparison of different assays or samples will become significantly easier when the measured distribution can be modeled by a mathematical function. However, as generally applicable rules are lacking, this will in most cases only be possible by

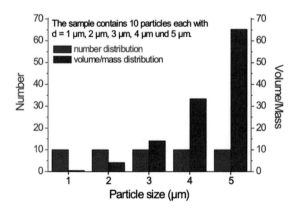

Fig. 3-12   Mass and number distributions.

using appropriate approximations. For many grain size distributions in pharmaceutical systems, at least approximate linearization is possible by presenting the undersize distribution in a special, non-linear coordinate system. In practice, it is useful to present the results of a grain size analysis graphically in different linearized diagrams and determine location and dispersion parameters from these diagrams by means of the best fitting straight line.

The simplest model distribution is the normal Gaussian distribution. Other often-applied model distributions are the logarithmic normal distribution and the RRSB (Rosin, Rammler, Sperling, Bennett) distribution (Fig. 3-13). All specified model distributions assume a mono-modal distribution with only one maximum in the density distribution curve. The mathematical description of bi- and multi-modal distributions (two or more maxima) requires more complex evaluation procedures.

3.3.2.7 Normal Distribution

The sizes of particles formed during a natural growth process, such as for instance starch grains, frequently display a normal distribution. The distribution maximum corresponds to the arithmetic average and serves as location parameter, dividing the total area under the curve in two identical halves (Modal value = Average value = Median value). The standard deviation serves as dispersion parameter. By plotting the data in a probability diagram (see section 6.2) the undersize distribution can be linearized.

3.3.2.8 Logarithmic Normal Distribution

This model deals with asymmetric, mono-modal distributions with a maximum that is shifted to smaller particle sizes. By a logarithmic presentation of the abscissa a symmetric bell-shaped curve is obtained, which can be analyzed like a normal distribution. The most frequent grain size (modal value) does not equal the central grain size (median) and this does not equal the arithmetic average; an average diameter value as a location parameter must therefore by necessity be specified. By presenting the data in a logarithmic probability plot the undersize distribution can be linearized and a dispersion parameter can be determined. Particles produced by means of a rapid and disturbed random process often follow this model distribution. Examples of such production processes are spray drying, high-pressure homogenization and powder production by precipitation.

3.3.2.9 RRSB Distribution

Many materials, in particular those that are produced by means of grinding processes, cannot be described by the distributions discussed above. For these substances often a good approximation can be obtained by plotting in a Rosin, Rammler, Sperling, Bennett plot (RRSB distribution), in which the abscissa has a logarithmic and the ordinate a double-logarithmic scale (Fig. 3-13). This distribution is described by the following empirical approximation equation:

$$1 - D = R = 100 \cdot e^{-\left(\frac{d}{d'}\right)^n}$$

D = undersize sum (%)
R = sieve residue sum (%)
d = grain diameter (μm)
d' = grain size parameter (μm)
n = uniformity number

By plotting in a RRSB grain size grid in which undersize or sieve residue is presented, a straight line is obtained if the sample follows a RRSB distribution. The location parameter corresponds to the characteristic grain size d' for a retention of 36.8%, i.e. a permeation of 63.2%.

$$\text{for } d = d' \text{ applies: } R = 100 \cdot e^{-\left(\frac{d'}{d'}\right)^n}$$
$$= 100 \cdot e^{-1} = \frac{100}{e} = 36,8\%$$
(3-2)

The width of the distribution (dispersion parameter) is described by the slope of the straight line. In earlier times, special RRSB grid paper was used to calculate the RRBS parameter like the volume-related surface S_V (see section 3.5) or the uniformity number n. The smaller

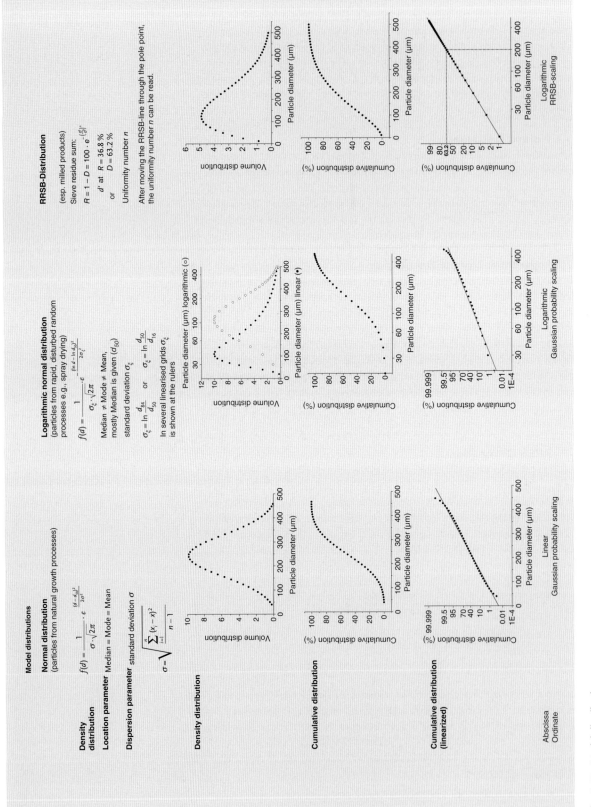

Fig. 3-13 Model distributions.

the value of *n*, the broader the particle size distribution of the sample will be. However, nowadays a simple computer program serves this purpose without the necessity of complex grid paper.

3.4 Particle Size Assay Methods

Preceding any particle size analysis, a representative sample must be taken from the large amount of material usually at hand. It is crucial to avoid the occurrence of "demixing," as either fine or coarse material may selectively be sampled from a material that has undergone segregation. By careful sampling, this systematic error can be minimized. In case of very large amounts of material multiple samples should be taken, while the sites of sampling should be selected according to a premeditated sampling plan.

The following sections discuss the various methods that can be used to assess particle size.

3.4.1 Sieve Analysis

Sifting is a classical procedure for materials consisting of particles with different grain sizes, which are to be separated either for preparative or analytical purposes. It is the separation of coarse from fine material using a meshed or perforated surface. In ancient Egypt, this was done for sizing grains. The sieves in those days were made of woven reeds and grass. Today, sieve analysis is one of the standard methods for analyzing distributions of granular material. If done correctly, it is not only a cheap but also reliable and quick method.

For this procedure, metal or textile fabrics are used or occasionally also perforated disks with holes of uniform mesh or pore size. The sieves are either manually or mechanically agitated either in horizontal circles or swung vertically. To intensify the motion of the material auxiliary devices such as rubber balls or brushes can be used. While during preparative sieving a further comminution may occur as a desirable side effect, in case of analytical sifting any change in particle size should by all means be avoided.

The effectiveness of the sieve process depends on size and shape of the holes, their total surface in relation to the total sieve surface as well as on the mode of agitation applied. The presence of moisture, unfavorable crystal forms, and electric charge of the particles reduce the sieve performance and may falsify the result.

The two fractions obtained with one single sieve are designated passing fraction or *undersize* (fine powder) and *residue* (coarse powder). The maximal grain size passing the sieve is called *grain* limit. Pharmacopeias describe sieves with defined mesh sizes characterized by numbers that can be referred to when describing the comminution grade of a powder (Ph. Eur. 2.1.4 and 2.9.12).

For fractionation in more than two grain classes, multiple sieves are arranged below each other in decreasing mesh size (sieve set or sieve tower). In this way, the particle size distribution of a crude mixture of particle sizes can be determined.

Grain sizes fractionated by an analytical sieve range from approximately 5 μm to 125 mm:
- Manual sieve or sieve tower: 40 μm to 125 mm
- Air jet sieve: ~10 to 500 μm
- Wet sifting with micro-precision sieves ~5 to 50 μm

An example of the evaluation of a sieve analysis is presented in Fig. 3-14. With a common vibration or shaking sieve, with or without application of auxiliary means, separations of grain sizes down to 40 μm can be achieved. In most cases, smaller particles obstruct the permeability of the sieve as a result of aggregation.

3.4.1.1 Wet Sieving

By means of wet sieving, bulk phases with particle sizes down to 5 μm can be classified. To that end the material is suspended in a neutral liquid, which causes a strong reduction of the aggregation tendency of the particles. The sieves are brought into a vibrational or shaking motion and simultaneously flushed with liquid.

Class i	Lower Limit of Class x_{il} (μm)	Upper Limit of Class x_{iu} (μm)	Class Width Δx_i (μm)	Mean Class Value x_m (μm)	Partial Mass ΔM_i (g)	Sum of Partial Masses $\Sigma \Delta M_i$ (g)	Relative Frequency h_i (%)	Cumulative Frequency Q_{3i} (%)	Distribution Density q_{3i} (%/μm)
	Sieve with smaller mesh size	Sieve with larger mesh size	$\Delta x_i = x_{iu} - x_{il}$	$x_m = \dfrac{(x_{iu}+x_{il})}{2}$	Weighed masses on the Sieve Representation in histogram (A)	Sum of weighed masses	$h_i = \dfrac{\Delta M_i}{M_{tot}} \cdot 100$ Representation in histogram (A)	$Q_{3i} = \sum \dfrac{\Delta M_i}{M_{tot}} \cdot 100$ Representation in sum curve (B) Undersize sum	$q_{3i} = \dfrac{h_i}{\Delta x_i}$ Representation in histogram or density distribution curve (C)
1	0	63	63	31.5	4.25	4.25	2.8	2.8	$4.44 \cdot 10^{-2}$
2	63	90	27	76.5	4.04	8.29	2.7	5.5	$1.00 \cdot 10^{-1}$
3	90	125	35	107.5	14.08	22.37	9.4	14.9	$2.69 \cdot 10^{-1}$
4	125	180	55	152.5	41.94	64.31	28.0	42.9	$5.09 \cdot 10^{-1}$
5	180	250	70	215	59.84	124.15	39.9	82.8	$5.70 \cdot 10^{-1}$
6	250	355	105	302.5	25.67	149.82	17.1	99.9	$1.63 \cdot 10^{-1}$
7	355	500	145	427.5	0.11	14.93	0.07	99.97	$4.83 \cdot 10^{-4}$
8	500	700	200	600	0.5	149.98	0.03	100.0	$1.50 \cdot 10^{-4}$

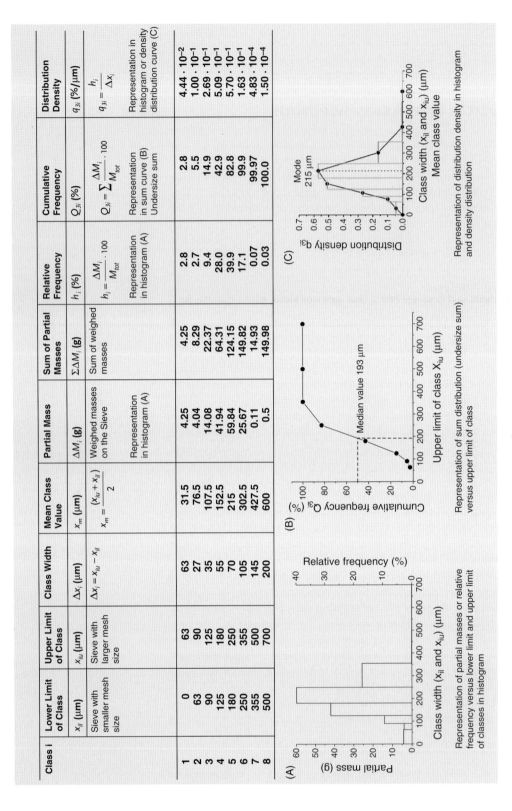

(A) Representation of partial masses or relative frequency versus lower limit and upper limit of classes in histogram

(B) Representation of sum distribution (undersize sum) versus upper limit of class

(C) Representation of distribution density in histogram and density distribution

Fig. 3-14   Evaluation of a sieve analysis of calcium phosphate (Emcompress®).

3.4.1.2   Manual Sieving

During manual sieving, the powder is first deposited on the finest sieve in order to eliminate fine dust, which may cause aggregation, clogging of the sieve pores, and adhesion to larger particles. The residue is then placed on the sieve with the largest pore diameter. The passing fraction is subsequently fractionated on a stack of sieves with decreasing mesh size. Such a procedure is obviously very time-consuming but offers the advantage that the process can be monitored and problems that might occur during the process, such as aggregation and grain comminution, can be dealt with.

Ph. Eur. 2.1.4 Sieves, Table 2.1.4.-1 _____

Ph. Eur. 2.9.38 Particle Size Distribution Estimation by Analytical Sieving, Table 2.9.38.-1

USP ⟨786⟩ Particle Size Distribution Estimation by Analytical Sieving, Table 1. Sizes of Standard Sieve Series in Range of Interest

JP 3.04 Particle Size Determination, Method 2. Analytical Sieving Method, Table 3.04-1. Sizes of Standard Sieve Series in Range of Interest

The sieve sizes described in Ph. Eur., USP, and JP are based on ISO 3310-1: Test Sieves—Technical Requirements and Testing—Part 1: Test Sieves of Metal Wire Cloth. Ph. Eur. sieve numbers refer to the nominal dimension of the apertures. The use of these values is also recommended by the USP, although the latter additionally includes U.S. sieve no., defined by the U.S. standard mesh series (number of openings per inch). Also, Japanese sieve numbers are based on the mesh standard, however, showing some slight differences with respect to the U.S. mesh series.

ISO Nominal Aperture	U.S. Sieve No.	Recommended USP Sieves (μm)	European Sieve No.	Japanese Sieve No.
11.20 mm[1,2]			11200	
8.00 mm[1,2]			8000[3]	
5.60 mm[1,2]			5600	3.5
4.75 mm[2]				4
4.00 mm[1,2]	5	4000	4000	4.7
3.35 mm[2]	6			5.5
2.80 mm[1,2]	7	2800	2800	6.5
2.36 mm[2]	8			7.5
2.00 mm[1,2]	10	2000	2000	8.6
1.70 mm[2]	12			10
1.40 mm[1,2]	14	1400	1400	12
1.18 mm[2]	16			14
1.00 mm[1,2]	18	1000	1000	16
850 μm[2]	20			18
710 μm[1,2]	25	710	710	22
600 μm[2]	30			26
500 μm[1,2]	35	500	500	30
425 μm[2]	40			36
355 μm[1,2]	45	355	355	42
300 μm[2]	50			50
250 μm[1,2]	60	250	250	60
212 μm[2]	70			70
180 μm[1,2]	80	180	180	83
150 μm[2]	100			100
125 μm[1,2]	120	125	125	119
106 μm[2]	140			140
90 μm[1,2]	170	90	90	166
75 μm[2]	200			200
63 μm[1,2]	230	63	63	235
53 μm[2]	270			282
45 μm[1,2]	325	45	45	330
38 μm[2]			38[4]	391

[1] Principal sizes (R 20/3)
[2] Supplementary sizes (R 40/3)
[3] Only in Table 2.1.4.-1 of Ph. Eur. 2.1.4 but not in Table 2.9.38.-1 of Ph. Eur. 2.9.38
[4] Only in Table 2.9.38.-1 of Ph. Eur. 2.9.38 but not included in Table 2.1.4.-1 of Ph. Eur. 2.1.4

In the United States, sieves are characterized by mesh per inch.

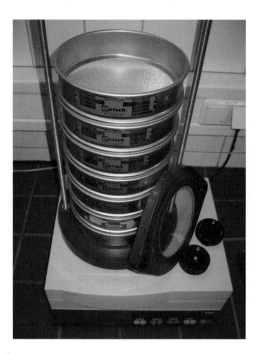

Fig. 3-15 Sieve tower.

3.4.1.3 Mechanical Sifting with a Sieve Tower

The sample is sifted from top to bottom through a set of 5 to 10 sieves with decreasing pore diameter. Below the sieve with the smallest mesh size, a collecting dish is placed (Fig. 3-15). The material to be fractionated is introduced in the top sieve and the sieve tower is closed off with a cover. The tower is then agitated by vibration and the amount of material in each fraction is determined by weighing the residues on each sieve. Sieve time varies from 10 to 20 minutes but depends on the properties of the material (e.g., particle size and density, aggregation tendency). When equipped with a special device, the sieve tower also allows wet sieving.

3.4.1.4 Air Jet Sieving

Dry material consisting of very fine powders can be fractionated by means of *air jet sieving*. The material is placed on the sieve mesh. Powerful pressurized rotating air jets break up aggregates and clean clogged sieve pores (Fig. 3-16). The sieve mesh is then flushed with an

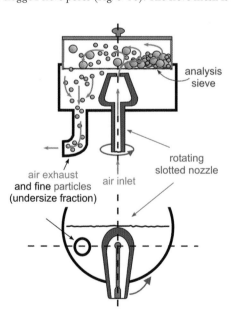

Fig. 3-16 Air jet sieve (top: cross section; bottom: top view).

upward-directed air stream coming from a slit-shaped nozzle rotating closely below the mesh. The air stream constantly agitates the material. At other sites of the sieve, the direction of the airstream is reversed. The air carries the particles smaller than the mesh size down through the sieve openings and is extracted together with the undersize particles. Air jet sieving allows the use of micro-sieves with mesh widths down to 10 μm. The sieve procedure starts with the smallest mesh width and the residue on the sieve is weighed. Also, the undersize, if recovered and collected, can be weighed. When applicable, further classification with additional sieves of increasing mesh width may be performed.

Ph. Eur. 2.9.38 Particle-Size Distribution Estimation by Analytical Sieving _____

USP ⟨786⟩ Particle Size Distribution Estimation by Analytical Sieving

JP 3.04 Particle Size Determination, Method 2. Analytical Sieving Method

Commonly, sieving is the method of choice for classification of coarse powders or granules. The majority of the particles should be larger than 75 μm. An analytical sieve tower consists of a set of stacked sieves with, from top to bottom, decreasing mesh sizes (usually with a factor of about $\sqrt{2}$). Most widely used are sieves of 200 mm or 76 mm in diameter. Before the analysis, the tare weight of each individual sieve is determined with an accuracy of 0.1 gram. Depending on the density of the material, 25 to 100 g of the substance to be analyzed is placed on the top sieve (diameter 200 mm). One-seventh that amount is applied in case of 76-mm sieves. Since oversized samples will lead to incomplete sifting, the appropriate sample quantity should be determined in a pilot experiment. Substances that easily absorb or release water should be analyzed at appropriate humidity. Electric charge acquisition can be minimized by addition of 0.5% colloidal silicon dioxide and/or aluminum oxide. The sieve tower is brought into a vertical, horizontal, or circular motion. The procedure is interrupted at intervals of 5 minutes and each sieve is weighed. The process is terminated when none of the sieves has changed weight by more than 5% or 10% for 200-mm and 76-mm sieves, respectively, within a 5-minute interval. For a conclusive and reproducible analysis, it has to be ascertained that the residue on each individual sieve contains only single particles and no aggregates. When more than 50% of the entire sample has accumulated on one individual sieve, the procedure is repeated, placing an additional sieve with an intermediate mesh size right above the sieve in question. After weighing the residue on each individual sieve, the result is usually presented in the form of a cumulative mass distribution.

Particularly, for samples consisting of small particles, the air jet or sonic sieving method may be deployed, instead of vibration. Air jet sieving cannot be achieved in one single step with a sieve tower. It requires sequential analyses on individual sieves, starting with the finest sieve to obtain a particle size distribution.

3.4.1.5 Problems and Failures with Sieve Analysis

Sample size and sifting time are both important when considering sieve analysis. The size of the sample to be analyzed can significantly affect the analysis. On the one hand, the amount of material should just be sufficient to cover the sieve surface with a thin layer of aggregate-free material. On the other hand, the amount of material on the sieve should be sufficient to allow accurate weighing.

Optimal sifting time is strongly dependent on the powder characteristics and should be empirically determined for each individual bulk phase to be analyzed. Periodical monitoring of the mass changes on the individual sieves will indicate whether the sifting procedure can be terminated.

Not all materials are suitable for characterization by sieve analysis. Particularly, the following properties can lead to problems or errors during the sifting analysis:

- Strong aggregation tendency and adhesion to the sieve (solution: wet sieving; adding a small amount of colloidal silica; sieve auxiliaries)
- Electrostatic charge of the powder during the sieving process (solution: wet sieving)
- Abrasion-susceptible materials such as granules (solution: manual sieving)
- Strongly anisometric, needle-shaped particles

Ph. Eur. 2.9.12 Sieve Test _____

The degree of fineness of a powder may be expressed by reference to sieves—that is, in relation to one or two sieve numbers. The weight fraction (m/m) of the material that passes the sieve(s) is determined. In case of two sieves, the sieve with number A allows the passage of $\geq 95\%$ of the sample and the sieve with number B the passage of $\leq 40\%$. Based on these numbers, the Ph. Eur. defines four terms, describing the degree of fineness:

Degree of Fineness	Sieve Number A	Sieve Number B
Coarse powder	1400	355
Moderately fine powder	355	180
Fine powder	180	125
Very fine powder	125	90

When the degree of fineness of a powder is expressed by one sieve number only, 97% of the material passes the sieve of that number.

3.4.2   Microscopy

Microscopic methods provide information on particle size and shape, but also allow evaluation of aggregate formation. It should be kept in mind, however, that microscopic images only present a two-dimensional representation of a small number of the particle population. During sample preparation particles tend to arrange themselves in a way that is mainly dictated by their shape. For example, they usually settle with their flattest side on the microscope slide. Particularly when comparing particle sizes with those obtained by a procedure in which particle size is independent of particle orientation, deviations may occur. It is therefore important to specify which method was used to determine particle size. In order to determine the average particle size (statistic diameter) a sufficient number of particles should be analyzed. The introduction of computer-assisted image analysis techniques has allowed the determination of number distributions and the conversion into volume distributions within a reasonable time frame.

3.4.2.1   Light Microscopy

The resolution of a microscope is determined by the wavelength of visible light and the numeric aperture of the microscope objective, allowing for a maximal resolution of approximately 0.5 μm. Objects of this size and even smaller can be observed in the light microscope but they cannot be measured in this way. As a rule, particles smaller than the resolution maximum appear larger than they really are. With a suitable illumination method (dark field), also smaller light-scattering particles are visible. This method, which is used to count small particles in a light microscope, is called ultra-microscopy. Upon transfer of dispersions to the microscope slide, a certain degree of particle classification may occur, as smaller particles may be carried preferentially to the edge of the cover slip while the sample droplet flows out.

Direct manual measurement of particle sizes has been replaced almost entirely by computer-assisted procedures. It is only still in use to obtain a quick impression of particle size and shape. Special auxiliary tools such as specialized ocular insets, have greatly facilitated size classification and particle counting. Modern computation techniques, combined with high-resolution video chips, allow analysis of microscopic images with respect to particle shape and number. Number distribution can thus be completed with shape factor and particle surface distribution and, derived from those, volume distribution.

3.4.2.2   Electron Microscopy

The application limits of the electron microscope lie between 1 nm and 10 μm. For the purpose of particle size analysis, images are taken that can be enlarged later. Image evaluation is performed analogous to light microscopic images. Sample preparation is comparatively expensive and time consuming.

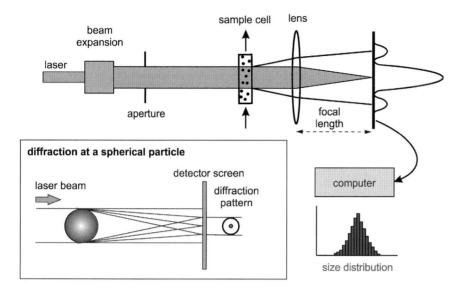

Fig. 3-17 Laser beam diffraction by a spherical particle.

3.4.3 Light-Scattering Procedures

In all light-scattering techniques, a laser serves as a light source emitting monochromatic coherent and linearly polarized light of high intensity. In this connection, scattering represents any change in light direction caused by physical deflection, diffraction or reflection.

3.4.3.1 Laser Diffraction

In drug formulation, nowadays often laser diffraction devices (Fig. 3-17) are used for quality control of powders, emulsions, and suspensions. The method is based on the interaction of laser light with the particles present in the laser beam. For many pharmaceutically relevant preparations, the observed phenomena can be described according to the Fraunhofer diffraction principle. In a homogeneous medium, the light waves initially propagate as a straight line. When a spherical particle is hit by the light beam, the two edges of the particle form two separate light waves. In the particle's shade the two waves undergo interference as they coincide with respect to wavelength and vibrational phase. Thus, a typical pattern of diffraction rings is formed (Fig. 3-17).

Smaller particles scatter the light more strongly than larger particles. The diffraction pattern of larger particles produces small diffraction rings with high intensity, whereas that of smaller particles displays large rings with lower intensity. Special detector geometries compensate for this difference in intensity so that, independent of the particle size distribution in the sample, equal particle volumes produce approximately identical signals (intensities), allowing calculation of the particle size distribution from the diffraction pattern of a collection of particles.

The diffraction theory according to Fraunhofer is, strictly speaking, only valid for particles with a diameter significantly larger than that of the applied laser light. For smaller particles, the Mie theory rather applies. This theory is much more complex, however, and requires additional information on the physical properties of the particles such as refractive index and absorption properties.

> **Ph. Eur. 2.9.31 Particle Size Analysis by Laser Light Diffraction** _____
>
> **USP ⟨429⟩ Light Diffraction Measurement of Particle Size**
> **JP G2 Solid-State Properties, Laser Diffraction Measurement of Particle Size**
> Based on the ISO standards 13320-1 and 9276-1, the Ph. Eur. describes laser diffraction as a routine method for particle size analysis in the size range of 0.1 to 3000 μm (newer instruments are capable of exceeding this range). The method is based on measurement

Gustav Mie (1868–1957) was professor at the university of Freiburg (Germany) from 1924–1935. He played an active role in the university opposition against Nazism during the Nazi dictatorship. He tried to develop a "universal function" and was thereby a competitor of Albert Einstein (both failed on this project). It is hard to understand today how he could develop his extensive theory at that time (Mie 1908) without the help of computers. The Mie theory covers – as we know today – the light scattering events caused by particles over a large size range: from colloids up to planets. Tributes to his achievements and personality were published by Pedro Lilienfeld (1991) and by Helmuth Horvath (2009).

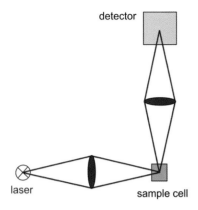

Fig. 3-18 Schematic representation of a PCS instrument.

of diffraction patterns of dispersed particles and their evaluation by means of a theoretical model, usually the Fraunhofer or Mie theory. The former is a suitable and relatively easily manageable model for larger particles (above 1–2 μm). No information on refractive indices is required for application of the Fraunhofer model. For small or transparent particles, the Mie theory provides less-biased size distributions. To apply this method, the refractive index of the particles with its real and imaginary part as well as the real part of the refractive index of the medium must be known, at least approximately. To obtain an acceptable signal-to-noise ratio and at the same time to avoid multiple scattering, the suitable particle concentration must be determined beforehand. Operational qualification as well as periodical performance qualifications and calibrations of the instrument are preferably performed with spherical test particles of defined size. The calibration requirements are met if the measured median particle size (d_{50}) deviates not more than 3% from the certified diameter of the reference material (for d < 10 μm not more than 6%).

The diffraction patterns of particles with diameters in the nm range do not vary significantly, which hampers their evaluation. For the analysis of such particles differences in polarized light scattering can be used instead (polarization intensity differential scattering (PIDS)^{TM}). The intensity of the scattered light depends on the plane of polarization, wavelength of the incident light, particle size and angle between incident and scattered beam. This dependence can be determined in addition to the "normal" diffraction data. In this way, the entire measurable size range can be extended down to below 50 nm.

3.4.3.2   Dynamic Light Scattering—Photon Correlation Spectroscopy (PCS)

Scattered light by particles in a colloidal dispersion is measured, for example, at an angle of 90° with respect to the incident laser beam (Fig. 3-18). Variations in intensity of the scattered light are monitored over time by an electronic evaluation system connected to the detector. These variations are caused by the motion of the particles in the sample. The diffusion coefficient and thus the diffusion rate are dependent on particle size and with those the time-dependent variations in the scattered light as well. The smaller the particles, the faster they move and the higher the frequency of variations in scattered-light intensity. With suitable evaluation algorithms and with knowledge of further parameters (e.g., viscosity of the medium) particle size can be calculated involving the well-known Stokes-Einstein equation (Tscharnuter 2000). This procedure is applicable to sizes from the lower nm range up to about 1 μm.

3.4.3.3   Nanoparticle Tracking Analysis (NTA)

NTA is a rather new method that tracks particles by a combination of laser light-scattering microscopy and a camera. The software identifies single particles and relates the diffusional path length during a defined time directly via the Stokes-Einstein equation to particle size. This method has a better peak resolution than the PCS method, which only allows detection of peaks which differ in size at least by a factor of 3 (Filipe et al. 2010).

The Stokes-Einstein equation *hydrodynamic diameter* $= \frac{kT}{3\pi\eta D}$ is easily applicable for the NTA case, as D (diffusion coefficient) can be easily determined as the speed of the single particle.

3.4.3.4   Light Blockage (Light Obscuration, Particle Optical Sensing)

With this procedure, single particles can be counted and their size estimated down to a size of approx. 0.5 μm. The sample is passed through a capillary tube that is evenly irradiated by a laser beam (Fig. 3-19). During their passage through the tube the particles attenuate the intensity of the laser beam to an extent that is dependent on the size of the particle. The intensity drop of the beam is measured by a detector and converted into corresponding pulses. Modern equipment can measure up to 10,000 particles per second so that the particle

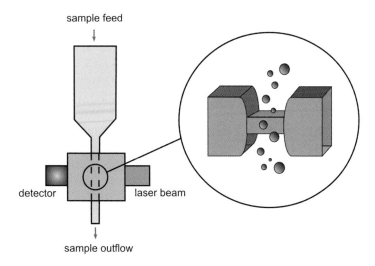

Fig. 3-19 Schematic representation of a light blockade instrument (AccuSizer®).

size distribution in a sample can be obtained in a few minutes. Because individual particles are evaluated, optimal resolution rates can be obtained. This procedure can also be applied for quality control of parenteral solutions in order to determine particulate contamination (see section 21.20.2).

3.4.4   Sedimentation Methods

Also, the dependence of sedimentation rate on particle size can be exploited for particle size analysis. However, because nowadays more precise, faster and less error-prone methods are available for the analysis of particles in the size range accessible to sedimentation methods the latter are hardly used anymore in pharmaceutical practice.

3.4.5   Pulse Procedures (Electrical Zone Sensing)

This procedure was originally developed by the Coulter Company for the counting of blood cells. Although nowadays equipment from other manufacturers is also on the market, this procedure is often still called the Coulter-counter method. The method is basically a counting procedure (Fig. 3-20). The particles to be counted are suspended in an electrolyte solution in

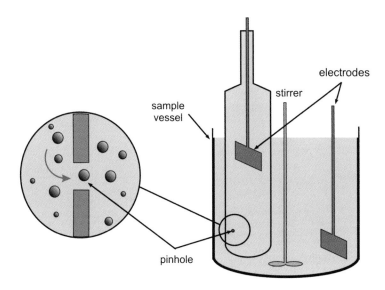

Fig. 3-20 Principle of electrical zone sensing (pulse procedure).

which the particles do not dissolve, swell, or undergo chemical changes. In the vial containing the strongly diluted sample a closed glass tube is immersed, filled with an electrolyte solution, which is connected via a microscopic hole with the solution in the sample vial. An electrode is placed in both solutions. A pump system aspirates a defined volume of the sample through the orifice, the diameter of which can be adjusted (20–2,000 μm) according to the prevailing particle size spectrum (from 3 to 50 times the particle diameter).

During the passage of a particle through the strong electric field prevailing in the orifice the electric resistance inside the orifice undergoes a transient change; this change is proportional to the volume of the particle. The advantages of this method are speediness of the analysis and the small sample size required. Disadvantages are the susceptibility of the orifice to clogging and the potential counting error when two particles pass simultaneously. In addition, many pharmaceutical preparations are not stable in the electrolyte solutions used. Also, air bubbles in the electrolyte solution during the analysis can lead to counting errors.

3.4.6   Sifting (Air Classifying)

Sifting implies that, as for sieving, the material to be probed is separated in minimally two particle size classes (coarse and fine material). Mainly, two sifting principles are applied for preparative purposes: counterflow and cross-flow sifting. Both can be applied either individually or in combination, supported by either gravitational or flow force. As a rule, no sharply defined separation limits apply because it is inevitable that a larger or smaller fraction of the particles remains within the separation range, reason why we prefer to speak of a separation limit range. This method has been used for thousands of years, as in ancient Egypt, when wheat had to be *winnowed*, or separated from chaff.

3.4.6.1   Counter-Flow Wind Sifting in a Gravitational Force Field

The separation limits range from 5 to 40 μm. The equipment consists of a perpendicular cylindrical tube that is perfused from bottom to top by a constant airflow (Fig. 3-21) and the material to be examined is introduced in the airflow. Particles with a sedimentation rate lower than the airflow velocity are carried upward by the airflow, while particles with sedimentation rates higher than the airflow velocity settle at the bottom of the tube. Particles with intermediate sedimentation velocities tend to stay floating in the airflow.

3.4.6.2   Cross-Flow Wind Sifting in a Centrifugal Force Field

The separation limits of these sifters ranges from 2 to 30 μm. The sifter consists of a cylindrical perpendicularly positioned tube, which rotates around its axis and is perfused from bottom to top with air at a constant flow velocity. Because of the rotation of the cylinder, the air in the separation zone experiences a rotation component that is maintained over the entire length of the tube. The material to be separated is introduced at the upper end of the separation zone and dispersed in the airflow. The particles are then separated along the axis

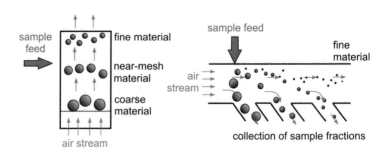

Fig. 3-21 **Sifters: Gravitational-counterflow (left) and gravitational-cross-flow (right) sifter.**

into classes with decreasing sedimentation velocity and deposited on the inside wall of the cylinder. The material can thus be separated into more than two fractions.

3.4.6.3 Cross-Flow Wind Sifting in a Gravitational Force Field

Also with this principle, the material can be separated into more than two fractions. The separation limits range from 10 μm to a few mm. The material to be separated is introduced into the separation zone of the horizontally positioned tube, perpendicular to the flow direction of the airflow (Fig. 3-21). The particles then travel downward along paths corresponding to their sedimentation velocity and spread out within the separation zone. They are deposited per sedimentation velocity class in an ordered way on the wall opposite the sample introduction site.

3.4.7 Aerodynamic Evaluation of Aerosols

The aerodynamic properties of aerosol particles can be assessed by means of a multistage impactor device. With this procedure, the aerodynamic diameter of the particle is determined as the equivalent of the diameter of a sphere of density 1 g/cm^3 displaying, under the impact of external mechanical forces in force equilibrium, the same migration velocity with respect to the dispersion agent as the examined aerosol particle. In such devices, the conditions prevailing in the respiratory tract should be mimicked as accurately as possible, allowing evaluation of the behavior of the aerosol particles intended for inhalation purposes. However, physiological conditions can be taken into account only to a limited extent, so that no firm conclusions can be drawn with respect to the particles' behavior in the respiratory tract. The procedure serves to compare different inhalation devices and is used for quality control.

The principle of the impactor device is based on the inertia-mediated deposition of particles along a curved track of a gas flow, such as air. Particles of a certain size or mass follow a track that deviates from the track of the gas due to their inertness. By increasing the flow speed of the gas and the curvature of the track, smaller and smaller particles are deposited. The individual stages of an impactor determine the separation limits. These are defined as the 50% probability that a certain particle size is deposited. The flow velocity of the gas is determined by the diameter of the orifices, the curvature of the gas track by the distance of the orifices from the impact plate (Fig. 3-22).

In a cascade impactor, an array of orifices of gradually decreasing diameter is lined up one after the other, such that the gas flow velocity increases step by step. At the same time, the distance between the orifice and the impact plate decreases, causing the curvature of the flow track to become stronger and stronger. The larger the particles, the more difficulty they will have to follow the curved flow track; they will then be deposited at a relatively low flow rate. Fine particles will be transported along with the gas flow and only deposited at higher flow velocities. Finally, the amounts of deposited material on the plates will be determined.

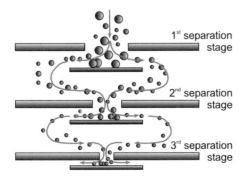

Fig. 3-22 Schematic representation of the separation principle of a cascade impactor with three separation stages.

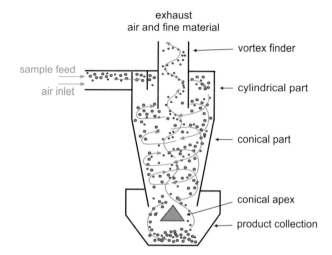

exhaust
air and fine material

← vortex finder

sample feed →
air inlet →

← cylindrical part

← conical part

← conical apex

← product collection

Fig. 3-23 Operation principle of a cyclone.

3.4.8   Gas Cyclones

Gas cyclones serve to separate fine particles. They can be installed at the end of a manufacturing process such as grain comminution in an air-stream grinder or spray drying.

The gas containing the dispersed particles flows tangentially in the cylindrical part of the cyclone (Fig. 3-23). Due to the cylindrical construction, a spiral airflow (vortex) is formed that continues down the cylinder and is ultimately carried off through a vortex finder sticking into the cylinder. Due to the centrifugal force the particles in the gas are slung outward onto the cylinder wall from where they slide downward in a spiral track (vortex). Very fine particles will follow the track of the gas flow and are carried together with the gas out of the cyclone. The size of the deposited particles is mainly determined by the dimensions of the cyclone and the flow speed of the gas.

Ph. Eur. 2.9.18 Preparations for Inhalation: Aerodynamic Assessment of Fine Particles _____

USP ⟨601⟩ Inhalation and Nasal Drug Products: Aerosols, Sprays, and Powders—Performance Quality Tests: C. Aerodynamic Size Distribution—Inhalation Aerosols, Sprays, and Powders

The particle or droplet size distribution in the plume discharged from inhalation aerosols and sprays and the particle size distribution in the cloud discharged from inhalation powders should be tested with a method, which allows determination of the aerodynamic size distribution. The aerodynamic diameter of an aerosol particle is equal to the diameter of a sphere of unit density whose gravimetric settling velocity is the same. Ph. Eur. describes four test devices to classify inhalation aerosols. Three of them are also covered by the USP together with an additional device. The underlying principle of all these methods is the fractionated inertia-dependent separation of particles. From stage to stage, the particles pass through narrowing tube openings or orifices with stepwise increased velocity. The particles are deposited on the plate below as soon as their size no longer allow them to follow the curved streamlines at the prevailing velocity. From the amount of deposited material cumulative size distributions can be calculated with all USP devices, including Ph. Eur. devices C, D, and E. In case of Ph. Eur. device A, only two fractions can be determined (single cut-point size 6.4 μm at 60 L/min). The following table shows which devices are intended for testing of powder inhalers and which for metered dose inhalers. For both applications the pharmacopeias provide detailed user instructions. In case of Ph. Eur. device A, also a test procedure for nebulizers is described. However, in Ph. Eur. 2.9.44 (Preparations for Nebulizers—Characterization) and USP chapter ⟨1601⟩ (Products for Nebulization—Characterization Tests) the Next Generation Impactor (Ph. Eur. device E, USP device 5) is specified as the test device for aerodynamic assessment of nebulized aerosols.

Device	Glass Impinger	Multistage Liquid Impinger	Andersen Cascade Impactor	Next Generation Impactor (NGI)	Marple Miller Impactor
Device in Ph. Eur.	Apparatus A	Apparatus C	Apparatus D	Apparatus E	–
Device in USP (tested dosage form)	–	Apparatus 4 (IP)	Without preseparator: Apparatus 1 (IAS) With pre-separator: Apparatus 3 (IP)	With preseparator: Apparatus 5 (IP) Without pre-separator: Apparatus 6 (IAS)	Apparatus 2 (IP)
Number of stages	2	4 + integral after-filter (Stage 5) (impaction stage 1 = pre-separator)	8 + final filter + optional preseparator	7 + microorifice collector[1], + optional pre-separator	5 + after-filter
Applicability	Pressurized inhalers, Powder inhalers, Nebulizers	Pressurized inhalers, Powder inhalers	Pressurized inhalers, Powder inhalers (for powder inhalers configuration with preseparator)	Pressurized inhalers, Powder inhalers (for powder inhalers configuration with preseparator)	Powder inhalers

IAS = Inhalation aerosols and sprays   IP = inhalation powders

[1] The microorifice collector is an impactor plate with nominally 4032 holes (70 μm). Most particles not captured on stage 7 of the impactor will be captured on the cup surface below the microorifice collector.

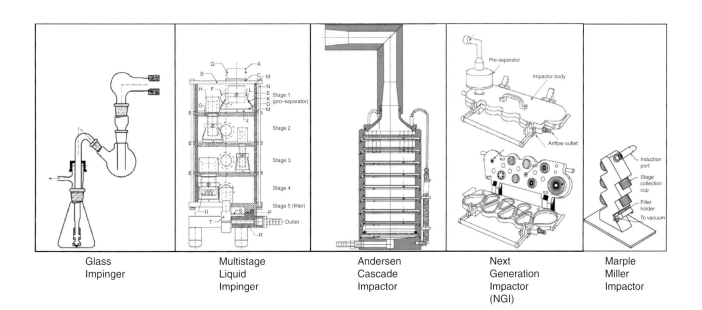

| Glass Impinger | Multistage Liquid Impinger | Andersen Cascade Impactor | Next Generation Impactor (NGI) | Marple Miller Impactor |

3.5   Surface Area Assay Methods

The surface area of a powder sample is determined by particle size as well as porosity. A distinction is made between outer and inner surfaces, the latter representing pores and capillaries. The specific surface area can be presented in relation to either volume or mass, both entities being related by the equation:

$$S_m = \frac{S_v}{Q_s \rho_s} \tag{3-3}$$

S_m = mass-related specific surface area
S_v = volume-related specific surface area
ρ_s = density of the solid

The surface area of a powder influences, for instance, the wetting and dissolution velocity of the material. In practice, the surface area is determined by indirect methods:

- From the particle size distribution: This merely yields the geometric surface without surface roughness and pores.
- Gas permeability procedures: This measures the flow resistance in a gas stream experienced by a powder sample of known size. Especially the outer surface area is determined, including surface roughness.
- Gas adsorption procedures: The amount of gas adsorbed to the powder surface is determined. In addition to the total outer surface also the accessible part of the interior surface is determined in this way.
- Entropy effect: During wetting of a powder sample a certain amount of heat is released, which is dependent on the exterior plus interior surface area.

The different physical assay methods yield different results. The method of choice will depend on the purpose of the assay and the problem to be solved.

3.5.1   Determining Specific Surface Area from Particle Size Distribution

Particle size of a sample corresponds with the outer, geometric surface area of a bulk phase, allowing calculation of the surface area from a particle size distribution. However, the distribution width and, in particular, the lack of uniformity and the anisometric shape of the particles render this method inaccurate; therefore, it produces only a rough estimate of the exterior surface area. The method can, for example, be applied to determine the amount of lubricant during tableting procedures.

For a powder sample with an RRSB distribution, the surface index number O_k can be obtained from its RRSB diagram. The specific surface area S_v can be calculated from O_k by means of the following equation:

$$S_v = \frac{O_k \cdot f}{d'} \tag{3-4}$$

S_v = volume-related specific surface area
O_k = surface index number
d' = characteristic grain size at D = 63.2% (see Ch. 3.3.1)
f = shape factor accounting for the shape of the particle

3.5.2   Determining Specific Surface Area by Means of Permeability Measurements

These methods exploit the friction of gases on the surface of the particles during the through-flow of a powder sample. The flow rate of the gas will increase as the surface of the solid diminishes. In powders with fine particles, and concomitantly larger specific surface area, relatively narrow capillaries are formed between the powder particles, allowing the gas to flow only slowly. For laminar flows through cylindrical capillaries, the law of Hagen and Poiseuille applies:

$$v = \frac{\Delta V}{\Delta t} = \frac{\Delta P \cdot \pi \cdot r^4}{8 \cdot \eta \cdot l} \tag{3-5}$$

v = average velocity of the flowing medium
V = flow-through volume
ΔP = pressure gradient between the capillary endings
r = radius of the flow cross section
η = dynamic viscosity of the flowing medium
l = capillary length

In real powder beds, the capillaries are shaped irregularly and the flow will not necessarily be laminar. This notion is taken into account by the Carman-Kozeny equation:

$$\frac{dV}{dt} = \frac{A \cdot \Delta P \cdot \varepsilon^3}{S_v^2 \cdot \eta \cdot l \cdot C \cdot (1-\varepsilon)^2} \tag{3-6}$$

dV/dt = flow velocity
A = cross section of the perfused column
ΔP = pressure gradient
ε = porosity of the powder bed
S_V = volume-specific surface area of the powder
η = dynamic viscosity of air
l = length/height of the power bed
C = capillary shape specific constant

In the Blaine apparatus (Fig. 3-24), the powder sample is condensed in a sample container with the aid of a plunger, such that porosity is adjusted to a predefined value. The required

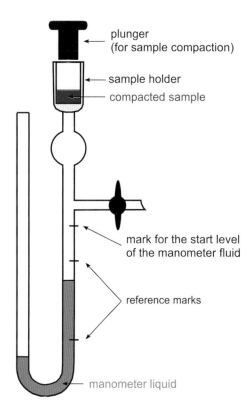

Fig. 3-24 Blaine apparatus.

amount of sample is calculated by means of the known volume of the sample holder and the porosity to be applied:

$$m = V \cdot \rho_s \cdot (1 - \varepsilon)$$
(3-7)

m = mass of the powder
V = volume of the sample holder
ρ_s = density of the solid material
ε = porosity of the powder bed

The porosity to be adjusted depends on the nature and fineness of the solid substance. It should be chosen such that, in consideration of the calculated sample size, the sample can easily be condensed. Often a porosity of 0.5 is applied. The sample container is placed on top of one of the legs of an open U-tube gauge and the plunger is removed from the sample container. Because of the lowering manometer liquid air is aspirated through the probe and the time required for the meniscus of the manometer liquid to drop from the upper to the lower mark on the tube is measured. The mass-related specific surface area can then be calculated by means of the following equation:

$$S_m = \frac{k \cdot \sqrt{\varepsilon^3} \cdot \sqrt{t}}{\rho_s \cdot (1 - \varepsilon) \cdot \sqrt{\eta}}$$
(3-8)

S_m = mass-related specific surface area
k = instrument constant
ε = porosity of the powder bed
t   = permeation time
ρ_s = density of the solid
η = dynamic viscosity of air

3.5.3   Determination of Surface Area by Means of Gas Adsorption

In this assay method, the internal surface accessible to the gas molecules is included. The following types of gas adsorption on solid material are distinguished:
- Chemisorption. The gas molecules are bound tightly to the solid surface (chemical bonding). This results in the formation of a monomolecular layer at the solid surface; the binding is only partially reversible.
- Physisorption. In this case the binding of the gas molecules is achieved by random, unspecific Van-der-Waals forces. The adsorption can be reversed by temperature increase or pressure decrease.

For the assessment of the specific surface area physisorption is applied. The assay deploys inert gases like nitrogen or krypton, which are dosed in preevacuated sample cells.

3.5.3.1   Gas Adsorption Process at Solid Surfaces

After the introduction of the probing gas, equilibrium is achieved between free and surface-bound gas molecules. Every further addition of gas will lead to an increase in pressure and more gas molecules will adsorb to the sample surface; nonetheless, not all additional gas molecules will be bound. In order to allow assessment of relative pressure, the sample is cooled to a temperature below the critical temperature of the assay gas (-147°C for N_2). The usual procedure involves the adsorption of nitrogen at its boiling point (-196°C). For powders with small specific surface area (< 1 m^2/g), the proportion of adsorbed gas is only minor. In such cases, krypton is applied as assay gas by virtue of its lower vapor pressure.

Ph. Eur. 2.9.14 Specific Surface Area by Air Permeability _____

The device described in the Ph. Eur. is similar to the Blaine apparatus according to DIN 66126 and ASTM C-204 and allows the assessment of specific surface areas in the range between 0.1 and 0.4 m^2/g. The equipment consists of a permeation cell and a U-tube gauge filled with dibutylphtalate. The weighed powder sample is introduced in the permeation cell and compacted with the piston of the apparatus. The packing must be so dense that during gas perfusion no air channels are formed and the particles do not change places with respect to one another. On the other hand, the particles should not be deformed or reduced in size by the compacting process. After suction of the manometer liquid up to the first marker level, the time required for the meniscus to travel the distance between the two marker lines is measured. The formula used to calculate specific surface area from the travel time follows from the Kozeny-Carman equation by compiling all procedure-dependent factors into an instrument constant. This instrument constant is determined during the calibration procedure by means of a reference powder with known density and specific surface area.

3.5.3.2 Theory of Brunauer, Emmett, and Teller (BET)

The BET theory (published 1938) describes the adsorption of gases on solid surfaces under the formation of multiple adsorption layers (Fig. 3-25). For adsorption isotherms of type II equation 3-9 applies:

$$\frac{1}{V_A \cdot \frac{P_0}{(P-1)}} = \frac{1}{V_M \cdot C} + \frac{(C-1)}{V_M \cdot C} \cdot \frac{P}{P_0} \qquad (3\text{-}9)$$

V_A = volume of the adsorbed gas
V_M = gas volume required to form a monolayer on the sample surface
C = substance-specific constant including the enthalpy of the gas adsorption
P = partial pressure of adsorbate in equilibrium
P_0 = saturated vapor pressure of the gas

Adsorption isotherms describe the correlation between amount of adsorbed gas and equilibrium pressure at constant temperature. IUPAC distinguishes six different types of adsorption isotherms.

In type I large quantities of gas adsorb at relatively low pressure, followed by plateau formation. The gas molecules are retained by virtue of relatively high surface energies, such as in microporous systems (pore radius < 1 μm). The type-I adsorption isotherm is furthermore typical of chemisorption. In case of type-II adsorption isotherms the amount of adsorbed gas is substantially lower. The inflection point of the curve represents the formation of a monolayer on the nonporous sample material. Subsequently, multiple additional gas layers are accommodated on top of this. This behavior is quantitatively described by the theory of Brunauer, Emmett, and Teller, which is used for the assessment of surface areas by means of gas adsorption. The type IV adsorption isotherm displays a characteristic hysteresis phenomenon, that traces back to the filling of meso-pores (pore radius between 1 and 25 nm) and macropores (pore radius > 25 nm) with the adsorbing gas. At low relative pressures type-II adsorption may be described by the BET theory. Type III, V, and VI adsorption isotherms (not shown) represent rare and complex cases.

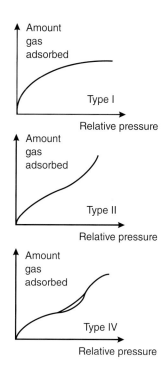

Fig. 3-25 Types of adsorption on solid surfaces.

Ph. Eur. 2.9.32 Porosity and Pore-Size Distribution of Solids by Mercury Porosimetry _____

USP ⟨267⟩ Porosimetry by Mercury Intrusion

Mercury porosimetry is based on the estimation of the volume of mercury that under pressure penetrates into the pores of a solid. The pressure under which a nonwetting liquid penetrates into a pore is proportional to the inner diameter of the pore opening. For cylindrical pores this correlation is described by the Washburn equation. For more complex pore structures, like we find in most porous materials, there is no theory by which the absolute pore size distribution can be calculated precisely from the assay data; therefore, this method is basically only meaningful for comparative measurements. The assay range varies from 3 nm to 400 μm; however, it has to be taken into consideration that the surface areas of closed pores are not included. By the same token, it is in most cases not possible to differentiate between intra-particle and inter-particle porosity.

A mercury pycnometer consists of a sample chamber with a calibrated capillary tube attached to its opening through which the sample can be evacuated and through which mercury can enter. The filling level of the mercury in the capillary is read while it is pressed into the sample by means of an overlaying hydraulic liquid. For precise measurements the expected pore volume of the sample should be between 20% and 90% of the capillary volume. After evacuation and degassing of the probe at $\leq$ 7 Pa, pressure is increased either stepwise or continuously for low-pressure measurements to 4–300 kPa and for high-pressure measurements to beyond 300 kPa.

The raw data yield the cumulative volume of mercury-filled space as a function of applied pressure. By means of the Washburn equation or by an alternative model, the latter can be converted to the pore diameter. With these data the pore volume of each pore diameter can be plotted as a histogram or a continuous density function. Because mercury porosimetry cannot be applied for absolute measurements, but only as a comparative test, the pharmacopeias do not provide instructions for calibration of the equipment. Nonetheless, they recommend to conduct performance tests on a regular basis.

The Japanese Pharmacopeia does not include a detailed description of mercury porosimetry but mentions the method in section G2 (solid-state properties) as a technique to determine particle density.

By plotting the left term in Equation 3-9 against the corresponding relative pressure (P/P_0), we obtain, in case of monomolecular adsorption in the relative pressure range of 0.05 to 0.3 kPa, a straight line, the so-called BET adsorption isotherm. From the slope of this line and the intercept with the y-axis, the volume of gas required to cover a monolayer can be calculated, and with that, the total surface area of the sample:

$$S_m = \frac{V_M}{m} \cdot \frac{N_A \cdot a}{V_{Mol}}$$

(3-10)

S_m　= mass-related specific surface area
V_M　= gas volume required to form a monolayer
m　= sample mass
N_A　= Avogadro's number ($6.023 \cdot 10^{23}$ mol^{-1})
a　= cross section of a test gas molecule (for N_2 0.162 nm^2)
V_{Mol} = mole volume of a gas

3.5.3.3　Procedure for Gas Adsorption Method

For the actual assay, the sample is degassed by evacuation in order to remove surface-bound foreign substances (e.g., solvate layers). Pressure and temperature are set in such a way that the sample surface will not undergo any changes. The subsequent assay is performed by at least three readings (multiple-point method) at various partial pressures, or by only one reading at one partial pressure (single-point method). The latter is applied when the substance-specific constant C in the BET equation is much larger than 1, and therefore the intercept with the y-axis lies close to the origin. It can also be applied when a series of similar samples are assayed for which C can be considered constant and determined only once by means of the multiple-point method.

The principle of the construction of an instrument for surface area determination by means of the multiple-point method is presented in Fig. 3-26. By introducing various defined volumes of test gas, the gas volume adsorbed to the sample at the relevant relative pressure is determined. The volume of adsorbed gas is the difference between the pressure of the defined test gas volume and the actual pressure.

With respect to instrumentation, the surface area assay by means of the single-point difference procedure according to Haul and Dümbgen (*areameter*) is essentially less complex than

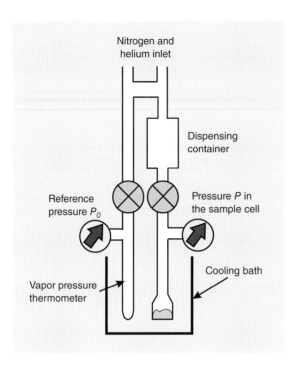

Fig. 3-26 Multiple-point method—Measuring set-up for the volumetric assay.

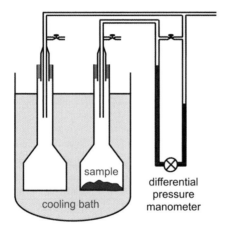

Fig. 3-27 End-point method: Schematic representation of an areameter.

the multipoint assay (Fig. 3-27). The apparatus consists of two vessels of equal volume, one of which contains the degassed sample and the other serves as a reference chamber. The two vessels are connected via a differential gauge. At the start of the measurement, nitrogen is introduced (pressure difference between the vessels is zero). After dipping the vessels in a cold bath with liquid nitrogen, the pressure in the sample vessel falls more steeply because nitrogen adsorbs at the sample surface. The specific mass-related surface area of the sample follows from the pressure difference, atmospheric pressure, and sample mass.

3.6 Density

The density ρ is a temperature-dependent matter constant for homogeneous solid, liquid, or gaseous substances. It is defined as the ratio between the mass (m) of a substance and its volume (V).

$$\rho = \frac{m}{V} \left(\frac{kg}{m^3} \right)$$

(3-11)

The temperature dependence of the density or of the volume of a substance is expressed by the expansion coefficient κ $(1/K)$, which for many substances is practically constant within a certain temperature interval and for liquids substantially larger than for solids.

The relative density is the ratio between the density of the test system and the density of a reference system under conditions that have to be defined for both systems. It is dimensionless. The relative density is mostly referred to the density of water at 20°C or 4°C. Density is an important substance characteristic that is used as proof of identity and purity of drugs and additives, particularly of liquids and wax-like substances.

Ph. Eur. 2.9.26 Specific Surface Area by Gas Adsorption _____

USP ⟨846⟩ Specific Surface Area

JP 3.02 Specific Surface Area by Gas Adsorption

The pharmacopeias describe two different methods to estimate adsorption of a test gas (N_2 or Kr) on the sample surface to be tested:

Method I: Dynamic

In this method, a mixture of test gas (in general nitrogen) and helium first flows through a thermal conductivity detector, subsequently through the sample, and then again through a thermal conductivity detector. The thermal conductivity detectors produce a signal that, after integration, is proportional to the volume of the flowing gas. Upon cooling the sample cell with liquid nitrogen, the sample adsorbs gaseous nitrogen from the test gas mixture, causing a difference signal between the two thermal conductivity detectors. During the desorption process, after removal of the cooling liquid, a coextensive but opposite difference signal can be measured. The latter signal is used for the surface calculation because it is more accurately defined than the adsorption peak. At least three measurements with different mixing ratios of N_2 and He are performed.

Method II: Volumetric Method

For the volumetric determination, the sample is cooled in a small test tube with liquid nitrogen at −196°C. After evacuating the sample cell down to the required pressure (as a rule 2–10 Pa), defined volumes of gaseous nitrogen are introduced and the corresponding pressures, after reaching adsorption equilibrium, are measured. From these values the adsorbed volumes V_a, as well as the corresponding relative pressures P/P_0 (partial vapor pressure of test gas in equilibrium with the surface / saturated pressure of adsorbate gas) can be calculated. As a rule, at least three determinations are required—that is, three value pairs of V_a and corresponding P/P_0 (multiple-point method). Under certain circumstances (e.g., comparison of similar powder samples), a single-point measurement may be acceptable.

For the analysis of samples with low specific surface area (<0.2 m^2/g), the use of krypton as the assay gas (but likewise at −196°C) is recommended as its lower vapor pressure reduces assay errors. The applied amount of sample should have a surface area of minimally 1 m^2 for an assay with nitrogen and minimally 0.5 m^2 for an assay with krypton. The quality of the measurement critically depends on effective degassing of the sample. Care should be taken that the sample surface is not altered by overheating. For regular functional verification of the equipment, reference substances such as aluminum trioxide are employed.

Ph. Eur. 2.2.5 Relative Density _____

JP 2.56 Determination of Specific Gravity and Density

The relative density d_{20}^{20} of a substance is the ratio between the mass of a certain volume of this substance at 20°C and the mass of an identical volume of water of the same temperature. Most common is the determination of d_4^{20} that relates to the mass of a volume of water at 4°C. Based on the following values for the absolute densities of water at

20°C and 4°C, the conversion formulas between relative and absolute density, expressed as g/cm^3, are:

$$\rho_{20(H_2O)} = 0.998203 \frac{g}{cm^3}$$
$$\rho_{4(H_2O)} = 0.999972 \frac{g}{cm^3}$$
$$\rho_{20} = 0.998202 \, d_{20}^{20}$$
$$d_{20}^{20} = 1.00180 \, \rho_{20}$$
$$\rho_{20} = 0.999972 \, d_4^{20}$$
$$d_4^{20} = 1.00003 \, \rho_{20}$$

Relative density and absolute density are determined by means of a density bottle (= pycnometer) (solids and liquids), a hydrostatic balance (solids), a hydrometer (fluids), or an oscillating transducer density meter (= oscillator-type density meter) (liquids and gases).

Oscillator-Type Density Meter

An oscillator-type density meter consists of an U-shaped glass tube, which is caused to oscillate as a cantilever oscillator by means of a magneto-electrical or piezo-electrical excitation system, and a sensor for measurement of the vibration frequency. After filling the tube with the liquid to be assessed, the resonance frequency is determined, which is a function of the spring constant and the mass of the system. The volume of the liquid that participates in the vibration is limited by the vibration node at the site where the end of the tube is attached and therefore is constant. The instrument is calibrated by measuring two different samples of known density (e.g., degassed water and air). A sample viscosity that deviates from the calibration media can distort the measurement. Many devices are equipped with an automatic correction for viscosity.

3.6.1   Density of Liquids

In addition to their property to serve as an identity and purity criterion, the density of liquids represents a critical parameter regarding the development of multiple-phase systems such as emulsions. Furthermore, knowledge about density is a prerequisite for certain analytical procedures, such as for viscosity assays (see 3.12) or density measurements of solid substances (see 3.6.2). It can be determined by weighing a defined volume of the liquid, by applying buoyancy phenomena or by other procedures. All measurements should take place while avoiding the formation of gas bubbles and, related to the strong temperature dependence of density, under accurately controlled temperature conditions.

3.6.1.1   Pycnometers
After establishing the mass of a liquid in a vessel with defined volume, its density can be calculated directly from these variables. For practical reasons, mass assessment is performed with the liquid pycnometer, which can be filled up to an exactly defined volume.

3.6.1.2   Buoyancy Phenomena
Also, the observation that solid objects in a liquid experience buoyancy can be applied to establish the density of a liquid. Buoyancy b represents the mass of the amount of liquid that is displaced by the object, m_{fl}, or the product of the displaced volume V and the density ρ of the liquid:

$$b = m_{fl} = \rho \cdot V \tag{3-12}$$

3.6.1.3   The Hydrometer (Areometer)
Hydrometers consist of a hollow glass body, the bulb-shaped bottom part of which is provided with a lead ballast weight. The upper part extends into a thin graduated glass column with a density scale. For the measurement, the instrument is immersed into the liquid to

be measured, such that it freely floats. From the scale marker aligned with the meniscus of the liquid, the density can be directly read. However, even when using a set of instruments, comprising various hydrometers with different measuring ranges, this method will not allow very accurate measurements.

3.6.1.4　　Hydrostatic Weighing

With this method the apparent mass m_{app} of a body with known volume V placed in a liquid is determined. The weight of the body in air (m_{air}) is reduced by its buoyancy, in other words by the mass of the displaced fluid m_{fl}:

$$m_{app} = m_{air} - m_{fl} = m_{air} - \rho \cdot V$$
$$\rho = \frac{m_{air} - m_{app}}{V}$$

(3-13)

Special constructions attached to a modern analytical balance permit simple application of this type of measurement, often allowing direct reading of the density on the display of the balance.

3.6.1.5　　The Flexural Resonator Method (Oscillator-Type Density Meter)

This is an instrumentally complex but fast and accurate method, which is also suitable for density measurements of very small volumes of liquid (<1 mL). The method exploits the observation that the natural frequency (eigenfrequency) of a mechanical oscillator depends on its mass. As an oscillator, for instance, a U-shaped capillary tube with a defined volume is used that is filled with the liquid to be measured ($m_{oscillator} = m_{capillary} + V_{capillary} - \rho_{fluid}$).

3.6.2　　Density of Solids

As compared to liquids the definition of density of solid bodies is considerably more complex (see also Ph. Eur. 2.2.42, density of solids). The true density of a solid object can be determined only when the object is available in a form which is perfectly free from pores and hollow spaces. For crystals it can be calculated from crystal structure data obtained by X-ray diffraction. For inhomogeneous solids and powders containing pores and hollow spaces density is not unambiguously defined. To describe the density of powder particles the particle density can be utilized, which implies however that any hollow spaces in the particle are included in its volume. As a consequence, particle density is always smaller than true density. Bulk and tapped density characterize the apparent density of a mass (see section 8.6.1) and do not refer to individual grains. The spaces in between individual particles are included in the volume of the mass (Ph. Eur. 2.2.42).

Ph. Eur. 2.2.42 Density of Solids _____

USP ⟨699⟩ Density of Solids

JP G2 Solid-State Properties, Solid and Particle Densities

Ph. Eur. and JP distinguish four types of density of solids: Crystal density, particle density, bulk, and tapped density.

The USP applies another classification that differentiates between true density (corresponding to crystal density), pycnometric density, and granular density (the last two being subclasses of particle density according to Ph. Eur. and JP). Beyond these main classes, the USP mentions bulk density as a separate type, as it depends not only on the powder particles but also on their packing.

Crystal Density

This comprises exclusively the solid fraction of a material, exclusive of all voids that are not a fundamental part of the molecular packing arrangement. It is also designated *true density*.

- Calculated crystal density (from crystallographic data and relative molecular mass)
- Measured crystal density (ratio of mass and volume of a single crystal)

Particle Density

This also includes the volume due to intraparticulate pores
- Pycnometric density (by means of the gas displacement method, Ph. Eur. 2.9.23, USP ⟨699⟩, JP 3.03)
- Mercury porosimeter density (= granular density, determined by mercury intrusion). Various granular densities can be obtained from one sample, as for each applied mercury intrusion pressure a density value is obtained corresponding to the pore-size limit at this pressure.

Bulk and Tapped Density

Bulk density (= apparent density) of a powder includes the contribution of interparticulate void volume as part of the volume of the powder. Therefore, bulk density depends on both the powder particle density and the spatial arrangement of particles in the power bed. Thus, while reporting bulk density, it is essential to specify how the powder bed was prepared. The pharmacopeias specify conventional methods for determination of bulk density and tapped density (Ph. Eur. 2.9.34. Bulk Density and Tapped Density of Powders, USP ⟨616⟩ Bulk Density and Tapped Density of Powders, JP 3.01 Determination of Bulk and Tapped Densities) (Practical Application see Ch. 8.6.1).
- Bulk density (determined from a loose powder bed prepared by passing a powder sample through a screen into a graduated cylinder)
- Tapped density (determined from a compacted powder bed prepared by tapping the cylinder containing the powder sample in a specified manner)

3.6.2.1   Determination of Particle Density

The challenge presented by measuring density of granular or powder-like substances lies in the determination of the particle volume (mass determination, which is also required to calculate density, is performed simply by weighing). Dependent on the method used to determine particle volume, the intraparticulate pores are included to different extents. As a result, the obtained particle density depends strongly on the applied assay method.

Gas Pycnometric Methods
Sample volume is determined by means of a pressure measurement with the aid of an inert gas such as air or helium, which can penetrate into the fine pores without being adsorbed. In this way values can be obtained that closely approach the true volume of the solid. As the test gas cannot penetrate into closed pores, the sample should be powdered to the finest possible degree.

Air Comparison Pycnometer
This pycnometer consists of two chambers (sample chamber and reference chamber) with identical defined volumes. The two chambers are connected via a differential pressure gauge. The sample is introduced in the sample chamber, as a result of which the gas volume in this chamber is reduced by the volume of the sample and in both chambers the same pressure prevails. In both chambers, the gas volume is subsequently compressed to the same pressure by a piston. Because of the smaller gas volume in the sample chamber the gas is not as strongly compressed here as in the reference chamber, which leads to a difference in the distance the pistons move. The product of this path difference and the surface area of the plunger is directly proportional to the sample volume (Fig. 3-28).

$$V_s = \frac{a \cdot A_0 \cdot V_1}{(V_1 - V_2)} \tag{3-14}$$

V_s = sample volume
V_1 = volume of the chambers before compression
V_2 = volume of the reference chamber after compression
a = path length difference of the pistons
A_0 = surface area of the pistons

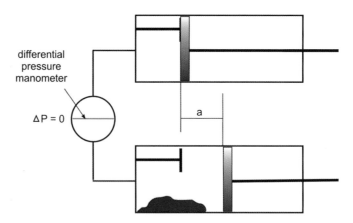

Fig. 3-28 Air comparison pycnometer.

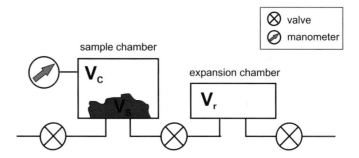

Fig. 3-29 Gas pycnometer.

Gas Pycnometer

The sample is introduced into the sample chamber, which has a defined void volume. The chamber is connected via a manometer and a valve with an expansion chamber of defined void volume. After gassing the sample with helium, the reference pressure P_r is read with open valve and, when appropriate, set to zero. The valve is then closed and the pressure in the sample chamber is enhanced by introducing the test gas and subsequently read (initial pressure P_i). Then the valve is opened, the test gas in the sample chamber expands because of the pressure disparity in the expansion chamber and the pressure in both chambers equalizes to the final pressure P_f (Fig. 3-29). The sample volume can then be calculated per the following equation:

$$V_s = V_c + \frac{V_r}{\left(1 - \frac{P_i}{P_f}\right)} \tag{3-15}$$

V_s = sample volume
V_C = volume of the sample chamber
V_r = volume of the expansion chamber
P_i = initial pressure in the sample chamber
P_f = equalized final pressure

Before the actual measurement is performed, the volumes of the two (empty) chambers are determined by means of steel spherules of defined volume.

Derivation _____

Gas Pycnometer

The basis for the calculation of the sample volume is the ideal gas law:

$$P \cdot V = n \cdot R \cdot T$$

Situation at the start of the assay:

Expansion chamber $P_r \cdot V_r = n_3 \cdot R \cdot T$
Sample chamber $P_r \cdot (Vc - Vs) = n_1 \cdot R \cdot T$

Before the actual measurement P_r can be set at zero in order to simplify evaluation. Then the valve between the two chambers is closed and the test gas (n_2 particles) is introduced into the sample chamber up to an initial pressure P_i.

Sample chamber $P_i \cdot (V_C - V_S) = (n_1 + n_2) \cdot R \cdot T$

After reading the initial pressure P_i in the sample chamber the valve is opened so that the pressure in the two chambers equalizes to the final pressure P_f.

$$P \cdot V = \text{const.}, T = \text{const.}, P_r = 0 \qquad \begin{array}{l} P_f \cdot (V_c - V_s + V_r) = (n_1 + n_2 + n_3) \cdot R \cdot T \\ P_i \cdot (V_c - V_s) = P_f \cdot (V_c - V_s + V_r) \end{array}$$

This yields the sample volume V_S as follows:

$$V_s = V_c + \frac{V_r}{\left(1 - \frac{P_i}{P_f}\right)}$$

The above equations are valid as such only when at the start of the measurement the initial pressure P_r is set at zero; if not, the actual P_r value should be included in the equations.

Symbols

V_r, V_C, V_S = volumes of the expansion chamber, the empty sample chamber and the sample
P_r = reference pressure (set at 0) before the measurement
P_i = initial pressure in the sample chamber after gassing
P_f = final pressure after equalizing pressure in sample and expansion chamber
n_1, n_2, n_3 = quantity of gas (mol) in the sample chamber before gassing; additional quantity of gas (mol) due to gassing; quantity of gas (mol) in the expansion chamber before the start of the measurement.
R = gas constant
T = absolute temperature

3.6.2.2   Determination of Densities with the Aid of Liquids

Determination of particle densities may also be done with liquid pycnometers. With these methods the mass of a powder is estimated by the amount of liquid it displaces. Via the density of the liquid the volume of the displaced liquid and thus the volume of the sample can be determined. Various liquids can be used as pycnometer liquid, provided they do not cause the powder to swell or dissolve. Mercury is the preferred liquid for this purpose, as it will not spontaneously penetrate into the pores due to its high surface tension. With increasing pressure, however, also the mercury will penetrate in increasingly narrower pores, so that, after determining the dependence of the amount of penetrating mercury on the applied pressure, the pore size distribution can be determined (mercury intrusion procedure).

3.7   Relative and Absolute Humidity

3.7.1   Mixtures of Air and Water Vapor

Assuming ideal conditions, the total pressure of a mixture of water vapor and air follows from the sum of the partial pressures of these gases. The saturated vapor pressure is the maximal partial pressure that can be attained in a water vapor-air mixture at a certain temperature; it corresponds to the vapor pressure of water at that temperature.

The *absolute air humidity* represents the water content in grams per kg dry air. It is independent of pressure and temperature. In praxis, however, the *relative air humidity* is used:

$$\varphi = \frac{P_D}{P_S} \cdot 100\% \tag{3-16}$$

φ = relative air humidity
P_D = partial pressure of water vapor
P_S = saturated water vapor

Saturated vapor pressure and thus the relative humidity are strongly temperature and pressure dependent.

3.7.2   Mollier Diagram

The correlation between relative humidity, absolute humidity, enthalpy, and temperature of a water-vapor/air mixture can be represented in a modified h-x-diagram according to Mollier (Richard Mollier, professor for applied physics, 1863–1935), Fig. 3-30. On the abscissa, absolute water content is plotted and on the ordinate the temperature. The adiabatic lines (straight lines with identical enthalpy) run diagonally towards the abscissa. As, practically speaking, only enthalpy *changes* are of interest, the enthalpy at 0°C for water-free air is set at 0. The isopsychric lines (straight lines of identical relative humidity) take a curved course. The isopsychric line with 100% relative humidity is designated the saturation or dew point curve. The presented conditions are valid only for a specific pressure, which must be stated in the diagram.

The following information can be derived from the Mollier diagram:
- Dew point of air as a function of relative humidity
- Absolute humidity of air with a specific relative humidity as a function of temperature

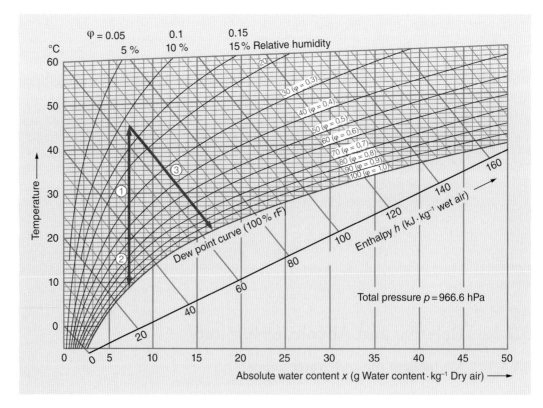

Fig. 3-30 Mollier diagram.

- Amount of heat to be added/removed for isothermal moisturizing/drying of air
- Temperature differences occurring under adiabatic conditions (i.e., without heat exchange with the environment)
- Relative humidity changes as a function of temperature

Relative humidity is particularly relevant for drying processes. In pharmaceutical production environments it varies as a rule between 30% and 50%.

Ph. Eur. 2.9.23 Pycnometric Density of Solids _____

USP ⟨699⟩ Density of Solids, Gas Pycnometry for the Measurement of Density
JP 3.03 Powder Particle Density Determination

The gas pycnometric density of a powder is determined by measuring the gas volume that under defined conditions is displaced by the powder. The applied apparatus consists of a test cell with a defined empty volume V_c, which is connected through a valve to an expansion cell with a volume V_r, a manometer and a system capable of pressurizing the test cell with a test gas (e.g., He or N_2) to a defined pressure. After the powder sample is filled into the test cell, the latter is sealed and volatile components are removed by a constant purge of gas or under vacuum. At open connection between test and reference cell the reference pressure P_r of the system is measured. After closing the connecting valve the test cell is filled with test gas up to an initial pressure P_i. Subsequently the valve is opened to allow equalization of the pressures and the resulting final pressure P_f is read. The sample weight is determined after this process because volatiles may evolve during the measurement. The sample volume V_s is calculated by the following equations:

$$V_s = V_c - \frac{V_r}{\left(\frac{P_i - P_r}{P_f - P_r}\right) - 1}$$

The powder particle density ρ results as the ratio of final mass and sample volume.

$$\rho = \frac{m}{V_s}$$

Before the measurement, the volumes of the cells are calibrated by means of polished steel balls whose volume is known to the nearest 0.001 cm^3. Measurement is performed at a temperature between 15°C and 30°C, which should vary not more than 2°C during the measurement.

3.7.3   Determination of Relative Humidity—Hygrometry

3.7.3.1   Hair Hygrometer

In this method, threads made of collagen, nylon or keratin, whose length depends on the amount of moisture, serve as sensors. The main advantage of such devices is their low cost. Disadvantages are the error range of the measurements (at least 3% of the relative humidity), the required maintenance and regeneration as well as the long adjustment time. The hair hygrometer is predominantly used for orientation measurements.

Examples

Mollier Diagram

1. Air with a relative humidity of 50% and a temperature of 20°C is heated in a closed space to 45°C. The absolute humidity of approximately 7.5 g water per kg dry air is kept constant. Phase changes proceed along the perpendicular lines (constant absolute

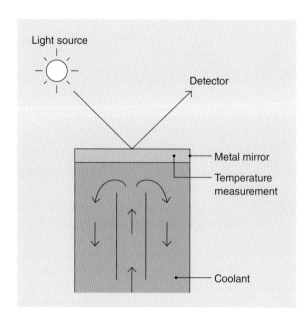

Fig. 3-31   Dew point hygrometer.

humidity) in the Mollier diagram: relative humidity drops to 12% and enthalpy of the air raises from 40 to 65 kJ/kg (Fig. 3-30, arrow 1).

2. The air of example 1 (relative humidity = 50%, temperature = 20°C) is cooled down in a closed space. Relative humidity increases until the dew point is reached at 9°C (arrow 2). Upon further cooling, the water vapor condensates and the phase change proceeds along the dew point line; the absolute water content of the air diminishes.

3. The heated air from example 1 (relative humidity 12%, temperature 45°C) is used to dry granules. The fed energy remains unchanged (enthalpy of air = 65 kJ/kg). The air absorbs water from the drying material (increase of absolute humidity from 7.5 to 17 g water per kg dry air) and, ideally, becomes saturated with water (relative humidity 100%). The temperature of the air drops from 45°C to 22°C (arrow 3). The amount of drying air required for the drying of the granules can now be estimated from the water content of the granules and the difference between the absolute humidity of the supplied air and that of the saturated drying air.

3.7.3.2   Dew Point Hygrometer

During cooling of unsaturated air, at a certain temperature the saturated state (dew point) will be reached; the water vapor is condensed on a cool surface in the form of very fine dew droplets. For this assay, polished metal mirrors are used, for which the temperature can be monitored precisely by means of a thermocouple. The backside of the mirror is slowly cooled down until the first dew deposition becomes visibly detectable (Fig. 3-31). The relative humidity is then derived from the measured dew point temperature and the original air temperature and can, for instance, be read from a Mollier diagram.

3.7.4   Psychrometer

A psychrometer consists of two thermometers, the bulb of one of them being wrapped in a moisturized fabric (wet-bulb thermometer). Air is passed along both thermometers at a certain velocity (Fig. 3-32). Dictated by the withdrawal of evaporation heat, lower temperatures prevail at the wet-bulb thermometer. The temperature difference (psychromatic difference) becomes larger as the air is drier and thus represents a measure of air humidity.

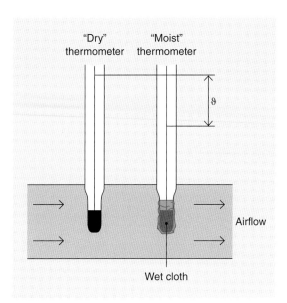

"Dry" thermometer   "Moist" thermometer

ϑ

Airflow

Wet cloth

Fig. 3-32   Psychrometer.

3.8   Water Content of Solid Substances

The estimation of absolute water content of solids is important for the manufacturing of powders, tablets, and coated tablets, as well as several other manufacturing processes. For example, the water content of powders affects the ability to flow, aggregation tendency and miscibility of bulk material. During the fabrication of tablets, the moisture content is particularly important for the granulation, compression, disintegration and fracture strength of the tablets. The terms moisture and humidity are applicable to both gases and solid materials, but it is emphasized that for solids the term water content is mostly used.

Ph. Eur. 2.9.39 Water-solid interactions: Determination of Sorption-Desorption Isotherms and Water Activity _____

USP ⟨1241⟩ Water-Solid Interactions in Pharmaceutical Systems

The Ph. Eur. and the USP describe in general terms common methods for the determination of sorption and desorption isotherms, as well as the water activity. Sorption isotherms can be determined by storage of samples in chambers at various relative humidities and measuring the mass gained or lost after the equilibration of the water content. Alternatively, the determination can be perfomed by means of automated dynamic gravimetric water sorption systems (dynamic vapor sorption = DVS). In the latter, the test sample is placed on a microbalance in an air-conditioned chamber in which at constant temperature the relative humidity is automatically stepwise changed at predefined intervals. After moving to each next environmental humidity level, another data point for the determination of the sorption isotherm is taken as soon as a sufficiently constant signal indicates that the sample has reached a new equilibrium. The advantage of the DVS method is that the time dependence of the water uptake or release can be assessed and that assay errors as a result of a change in water content during weighing of the sample outside the chamber can also be excluded. As a rule, the water content is given in mass percentage and plotted against relative humidity. When water uptake proceeds predominantly by adsorption, it is more informative to determine additionally the specific surface of the substance and to express the water content per unit area of the solid surface.

   The water activity of a substance is determined by placing a sample in an airtight, accurately temperature-controlled chamber with an integrated hygrometer or moisture sensor until the relative humidity above the sample has reached equilibrium. The equilibrium humidity above the sample corresponds to the water activity of the substance. The water activity is a function of the temperature and should therefore always be measured together with the temperature during the assay. In order to avoid the sorption state of the sample changing during the measurement, it is important to ensure a sufficient filling degree of the assay chamber (i.e., the volume of air above the sample must be small in relation to the sample volume).

3.8.1   Hygroscopicity

Water can be bound to solids in several ways. The strength of the binding depends on the nature of the binding. This, in turn, is determined by the specific properties of the material (see Ch. 2.4.2). We distinguish between hygroscopic and nonhygroscopic substances. *Nonhygroscopic* substances bind water only weakly at their surface; the vapor pressure corresponds to the saturated vapor pressure of water. It mostly concerns poorly soluble substances with coarse pores. Such substances can be completely dried without rigorous drying procedures. *Hygroscopic* substances display a decrease in vapor pressure below a certain amount of water content because of their stronger water binding. Above this critical water content, they behave like nonhygroscopic substances. Often, hygroscopic substances cannot be dried to completion. It is emphasized that most substances that are processed in pharmaceutical technology are hygroscopic. When the material is exposed to the environment an equilibrium state will be reached between the water content of the substance and the relative air humidity. This equilibrium depends on temperature, nature and properties of the material. By plotting the water content of a sample against increasing relative humidity (adsorption isotherm) or decreasing relative humidity, respectively (desorption isotherm), the water vapor sorption isotherm is obtained. For hygroscopic materials, the desorption isotherm will display higher water contents than the adsorption isotherm (hysteresis).

3.8.2   Determination of Water Content of Solid Materials

3.8.2.1   Gravimetry (Assessment of Weight Loss on Drying)

These gravimetric procedures are based on differential weight determinations; in the simplest case, the material to be dried (powder, tablets, granules) is weighed before and after the drying process and water content presented as percent difference (loss of mass). This procedure is not applicable when the material to be dried contains volatile components. More up-to-date procedures employ an infrared moisture balance or a device with which absolute water content can be determined (Ph. Eur. 2.2.32).

Ph. Eur. 2.2.32 Loss on Drying _____

USP ⟨731⟩ Loss on Drying

JP 2.41 Loss on Drying Test

Loss on drying is a method to measure the loss in mass of the sample, when dried under specified conditions. USP and JP indicate only the framework conditions of the test in the method chapters ⟨731⟩ and 2.41, respectively and refer to the monographs for further specifications. By contrast, the Ph. Eur. lists five different drying methods and gives a short description for each of them:

- "In a desiccator" (over P_2O_5 at atmospheric pressure and room temperature)
- "In vacuo" (over P_2O_5 at 1.5 to 2.5 kPa and room temperature)
- "In vacuo within a specified temperature range" (over P_2O_5 at 1.5 to 2.5 kPa and the indicated temperature)
- "In an oven within a specified temperature range"
- "Under high vacuum" (over P_2O_5 at ≤ 0.1 kPa and the specified temperature)

When "dry to constant weight" is specified in a monograph or when the duration of the drying process is not indicated, drying should be continued until two consecutive weight determinations do not differ by more than 0.50 mg per g of substance taken, the second weighing following an additional hour of drying (Ph. Eur. 1.2 Definitions, USP ⟨731⟩).

3.8.2.2   Karl-Fischer Titration

This method is based on the reduction of iodine by sulfur dioxide, which proceeds only in the presence of water (Ph. Eur. 2.5.12). The endpoint of this titration can be determined visually or electrochemically, the latter method yielding more accurate values.

Ph. Eur. 2.5.12 Water: Semi-Micro Determination ⎯⎯⎯⎯⎯⎯⎯⎯⎯⎯⎯⎯⎯⎯⎯⎯

USP ⟨921⟩ Water Determination

JP 2.48 Water Determination (Karl-Fischer Method)

The Karl-Fischer method for the titration of water is based on the quantitative reaction of water with sulfur dioxide and iodine in a suitable anhydrous medium in the presence of a base, which shifts the equilibrium towards the side of the reaction products. The endpoint is determined biamperometrically or bivoltametrically.

Ph. Eur. describes only a volumetric titration method whereas USP and JP additionally include a coulometric method. In case of the volumetric titration, a iodine-containing standard solution is added until no more iodine is consumed by the reaction and an excess of I_2 signals the endpoint (Ph. Eur. A, USP Ia, JP 1.4.1). Alternatively, a back titration with a water-containing standard solution can be performed after addition of an excess amount of iodine (Ph. Eur. B, USP Ib, JP 1.4.2).

In case of the coulometric method (USP Ic, JP 2), iodine is not added as a titrant but rather is electrochemically produced from iodide at a second pair of electrodes. The water content is calculated from the quantity of electricity (Electric current × Time) required for the production of iodine during the titration.

3.8.2.3   Azeotropic Distillation

The material to be assessed is distilled with a solvent, which is not miscible with water but forms an azeotropic mixture with it (e.g., toluene or chloroform). By separating off the water in a graduated measuring tube, the water content of the sample can be determined. The method is less suitable for substances with low water content.

3.8.2.4   Assessment of Hygroscopic Moisture Equilibrium

The relative air humidity above the material is measured. With the aid of the sorption isotherm, the approximate water content of the sample can be established.

3.9   Solubility

3.9.1   General Introduction

Solutions are considered to be homogeneous mixtures of different substances in which as a rule the dissolved components form the smaller fraction of the mixture while the solvent represents the larger part. In addition to fluid solutions of gases, liquids, and solids, also solid solutions are known—for example, glass, alloys and mixed crystal formations. The dissolved component is often molecularly dispersed (see Ch. 3.1.2) in the solvent (true solutions). In some cases, however, a solution may contain finely distributed larger entities (colloidal solutions).

During the formation of a solution, the dissolved components often lose their properties while the characteristics of the whole system are determined by the solvent. Nonetheless, solutions usually display properties that differ from those of the pure solvent, such as with regard to their osmotic and thermal behavior (freezing point depression, boiling point elevation), their density, refractive index, and conductivity (electrolyte solutions). Solutions of solid substances in liquids are relevant in the manufacturing of drug formulations and for the study of biopharmaceutical behavior. Therefore, in the following section particularly such systems will be discussed.

3.9.2   Concentration Units

Concentrations of dissolved substances in a solvent are usually expressed by one of the following units:

- Mass percent (mass % or %): gram substance in 100 g solution
- Volume percent (vol.%): milliliter substance in 100 mL solution
- Molarity (mol · l^{-1}): mol substance in 1000 mL solution
- Molality (mol · kg^{-1}): mol substance in 1000 g solvent (elimination of volume variability)

For special cases, also other units are used, such as International Units (I.U.) for sera and antibiotic solutions. In the pharmacopeia, the applied indicators for solubility of substances can be found under the heading "solubility" (Ph. Eur. 1.3).

3.9.3   Elementary Processes during Dissolution

The solubility of a substance is defined as its saturation concentration in a given solvent at a defined temperature and atmospheric pressure. The amount of a substance that can be dissolved in a solvent depends on the chemical nature of both components. As a rule of thumb, a particular solute dissolves in a solvent of similar nature (*similia similibus solvuntur*), that is, substances with polar groups dissolve best in polar media and nonpolar substances preferentially in nonpolar media. Thus, non-electrolytes capable of forming hydrogen bonds can dissolve in water, but are practically insoluble in non-polar solvents such as petroleum ether. As solubility of (pharmaceutically) active ingredients is of utmost importance for the development of drug formulations, numerous attempts have been made to predict these parameters from the chemical structure of the compounds involved. Although up to now no general valid theory has been put forward that would permit such a prediction with great precision, some conclusions with respect to solubility can be drawn from the knowledge of certain parameters, so that at least comparative considerations are possible.

By mixing two substances between whose molecules perfectly identical interactions occur (*ideal mixtures / solutions*), an increase in entropy occurs. Thus, the mixture is favored over the nonmixed situation. The complete miscibility of gaseous substances, between whose molecules only very little interaction occurs, is based on the same consideration. Such a situation, however, does not occur in this form in real systems. In these situations, the mutual interactions between molecules of the solute will at least to some extent differ from those between the molecules of the solute and those of the solvent. For that reason, introduction of the solute into the solvent will be accompanied by a heat transfer. This transfer formally can be considered as the heat transfers of three elementary processes that are depicted in Fig. 3-33.

1. In order to pass over into the solution, a molecule of the solute first has to leave the organization of the solid material. To that end, work (W_{22}) has to be performed in order to overcome the attractive forces between the molecules of the solid. The spent energy W_{22} corresponds to the evaporation heat of this molecule. The "hole" that is left behind by the escaped molecule can be filled up by rearrangement of neighboring molecules.

2. In order for the molecule to be accommodated in the solution, a corresponding space must be created in the solvent; for that purpose, an amount of energy (W_{11}) must be spent that suffices to overcome the attractive force between the solvent molecules.

3. After the solid-substance molecule has passed over in the "empty space" created in the solvent, attractive forces between the molecule and the neighboring molecules of the solvent become operational. The molecule is *solvated* (or, in case water is the solvent, it is *hydrated*). As a result, an amount of energy $2W_{12}$ is released, which corresponds to the strength of the interactions that thus arise. The total amount of energy of these three processes is commonly expressed as the sum of two identical quantities of energy,

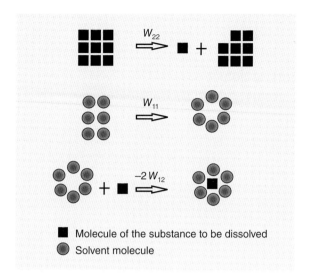

Fig. 3-33   **Elementary processes during dissolution.**

because two surfaces—that of the solid molecule and the empty-space surface—are involved, which interact with each other.

The total amount of work spent is therefore:

$$W_{tot} = W_{22} + W_{11} - 2W_{12} \qquad\qquad (3\text{-}17)$$

When the sum of the energy of the first two processes is smaller than the amount that is released in the third (solvation heat), the dissolution process is exothermic (solution warms up). Alternatively, when $W_{22} + W_{11}$ is larger than $2W_{12}$, we are dealing with an endotherm dissolution process (solution cools down).

From the above considerations, it becomes clear that in theoretic reflections with regard to solubility, additional considerations play a role: In particular, potential interactions between the dissolved molecules and the molecules of the solvent should be taken into consideration, as well as intermolecular bonds within the solid substance to be dissolved and within the solvent. In this connection, the latter will be less important than the former.

Ph. Eur. 1.3 Solubility _____

USP General Notices and Requirements 5.30. Description and Solubility
JP General Notices 29

The data on solubility that can be found in the pharmacopeia monographs have the following meaning:

Descriptive term	Parts of solvent required for 1 part of solute (Ph. Eur.: mL per g of solute, USP: part per part of solute, JP: (Ph. Eur.: mL per g of solute or mL per mL of solute)		
Very soluble	less than	1	
Freely soluble	from	1	to	10
Soluble	from	10	to	30
Sparingly soluble	from	30	to	100
Slightly soluble	from	100	to	1,000
Very slightly soluble	from	1,000	to	10,000
Practically insoluble	more than	10,000	

The strength of the bonds within the solute depends among other things on the structure of the solid. It is, for example, weaker in the amorphous state than in the corresponding crystalline form. The melting and evaporation heat as well as the approximate melting and boiling points roughly reflect the binding forces. Often, substances with high melting point and high melting heat display poor solubility in any solvent.

3.9.4   Interactions between Dissolved Substances and Solvent—Solubility Parameter

Estimating the contribution of solute and solvent to the dissolution process is a highly complex venture. The contribution of the polar groups on the surface of the dissolved molecules plays a pronounced role in its interaction with water. Substituents on the molecular skeleton can be distinguished in hydrophobic (e.g., alkyl groups, halogens), slightly hydrophilic (e.g., methoxy, nitro and carboxyl groups), hydrophilic (e.g., primary amino and aldehyde groups), and strongly hydrophilic (e.g., hydroxyl, ammonium and carboxylate groups). The possibilities of the substituents to engage in interactions with water not only depend on the nature and number of these groups, but also on their position on the molecular skeleton.

There are numerous methods to quantitatively approach the solubility of one substance in another or the mutual miscibility of two substances. One of the most widely used methods is based on the application of the *Hildebrand solubility parameters*, named after Joel Henry Hildebrand, 1881–1983. These describe the cohesion between identical molecules in a liquid. In order to separate such molecules from one another during the dissolution process, the same forces have to be overcome as those occurring during evaporation of compound; as a consequence, the cohesive energy is directly related to the heat of evaporation. The cohesive energy related to the molar volume is called cohesive energy density (CED). It can be derived from the molar heat of evaporation ΔH_v and the molar volume V_m:

$$CED = \frac{\Delta H_v - RT}{V_m} \tag{3-18}$$

In 1924 Joel Henry Hildebrand wrote a monograph on the solubility of non-electrolytes, which served as a widely accepted reference for half a century. He won all important science prizes except the Nobel Prize. He was the manager of the US Olympic ski team at the Olympic Winter Games in Germany in 1936. His entire academic life he worked at Berkeley where he retired in 1952, but he remained active as professor emeritus till 1983, when he died at the age of 101.

R and T are the gas constant and absolute temperature, respectively. The square root of the CED represents the *Hildebrand solubility parameter* δ of the substance concerned:

$$\delta = \sqrt{CED} = \sqrt{\frac{\Delta H_v - RT}{V_m}} \tag{3-19}$$

The smaller the difference between the solubility parameters of two substances, the better they mix. That may be explained as follows:

Two substances (dissolved component (solute) and solvent) together form an ideal solution when the cohesive forces between the molecules of one substance are identical to the forces between the molecules of the other. In real-life solutions, the cohesive forces are not identical and the molecules of the individual components are not ordered and statistically distributed, causing solubility of the dissolved components in the solvent (expressed as the mole fraction X_2) to differ by a factor γ_2 (the rational activity coefficient) from the ideal solubility X_2^i:

$$X_2 = X_2^i / \gamma_2 \tag{3-20}$$

$$-\ln X_2 = -\ln X_2^i + \ln \gamma_2 \tag{3-21}$$

The logarithm of the ideal solubility is a function of the heat of fusion ΔH_f and the melting temperature T_f of the dissolved substance as well as of the temperature T of the solution. On the other hand, the rational activity coefficient includes the energy that is spent or released during the dissolution process. In equation 3-22 W_{11} and W_{22} represent the energies per volume that are required to release the solvent and solute molecules, respectively, from their bonds with identical neighboring molecules. W_{12}, on the other hand, is the energy released during the formation of new interactions between molecules of the solute and the solvent (cf. equation 3-17).

$$-\ln X_2 = -\ln X_2^i + \ln \gamma_2 = \frac{\Delta H_f}{RT} \left(\frac{T_f - T}{T_f} \right)$$
$$+ (W_{11} + W_{22} - 2W_{12}) \frac{V_2 \Phi_1^2}{RT} \tag{3-22}$$

V_2 is the molar volume of the solute and Φ_1 is the volume fraction of the solvent. When W_{12} is described as the geometric average of W_{11} and W_{22}, that is, as $(W_{11} \cdot W_{22})^{1/2}$, which in case of regular solutions is approximately correct, equation 3-22 can be converted as follows:

$$
\begin{aligned}
-\ln X_2 = -\ln X_2^i + \ln \gamma_2 &= \frac{\Delta H_f}{RT} \left(\frac{T_f - T}{T_f} \right) \\
&+ \left(\sqrt{W_{11}} - \sqrt{W_{22}} \right)^2 \frac{V_2 \Phi_1^2}{RT}
\end{aligned}
\tag{3-23}
$$

As W_{11} and W_{22} represent cohesive energy densities, their square roots represent the solubility parameters of the two substances, in accordance with the definition above:

$$
\begin{aligned}
-\ln X_2 = -\ln X_2^i + \ln \gamma_2 &= \frac{\Delta H_f}{RT} \left(\frac{T_f - T}{T_f} \right) \\
&+ (\delta_1 + \delta_2)^2 \frac{V_2 \Phi_1^2}{RT}
\end{aligned}
\tag{3-24}
$$

Equation 3-24 shows that, the smaller the difference between the solubility parameters, the closer the solubility approaches the ideal solubility X_2^i and, because of that, the higher the solubility of the substance in the solvent. This correlation renders the solubility parameter a meaningful aid in the prediction of solubility, particularly in cases where direct measurement is impossible.

For many substances, solubility parameters are reported in literature. However, they may also be calculated quite easily when heat of vaporization and molar volume of the substance are known (equation 3-19). In addition, with the help of the group contribution method, they can be approximated from the structural formulas of the molecules by summation of every structural element and every functional group in the molecule.

As shown in the derivation, a major disadvantage of the Hildebrand solubility parameters is that they are limited to regular solutions. This disregards possible associations of molecules, via polar bonds or hydrogen bonds. In order to take into account such interactions and to broaden the application range of this method, multidimensional solubility parameters (partial solubility parameters) have been developed. The most frequently used among those is the concept of Hansen's solubility parameter (named after Ch. M. Hansen, 1938). In this approach, a substance is characterized by three separate parameters, δ_d, δ_p, and δ_h, which describe the contributions to the cohesive energy accounted for by dispersive (van der Waals), polar and hydrogen bond interactions, respectively. These three-dimensional parameters can be visualized in a three-dimensional coordinate system. The distance Ra between them, signifying a measure of the mutual miscibility of two substances (the closer they are the better the miscibility), is described by the Euclidean distance (the dispersive component being weighed with a factor of four):

$$
Ra = \sqrt{4(\delta_{d2} - \delta_{d1})^2 + (\delta_{p2} - \delta_{p1})^2 + (\delta_{h2} - \delta_{h1})^2}
\tag{3-25}
$$

Also, Hansen's solubility parameters can be found in literature for numerous substances. These parameters can be determined experimentally or, likewise, calculated by group contribution methods from the molecular structure.

Solubility parameters may be considered as universal aids to estimate and evaluate variation in solubility and affinity between different substances. Starting with their original applications in the plastics and paint industry, solubility parameters are increasingly applied to resolve a large variety of problems in the field of pharmacy. Besides classic issues concerning selection of solvents, this also relates to interactions between components of active ingredients, between active substance and excipient as well as to interactions with packaging materials or the release of active substances from carrier systems. Also distribution and permeation processes in biological systems such as the skin or the intestinal mucosa can be characterized to some extent by means of solubility parameters.

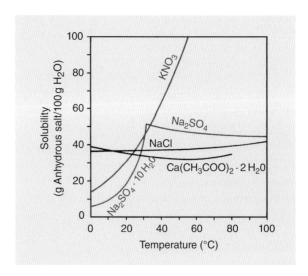

Fig. 3-34 Temperature-dependent solubility.

3.9.5   Dependence of Solubility on Temperature

As a rule, solubility is a temperature-dependent variable. A temperature increase may lead to an increase or a decrease in solubility; occasionally the temperature effect is only small (Fig. 3-34). During a dissolution process that is accompanied by heat change, Le Chatelier's principle predicts that solubility will depend on temperature in such a way that the solubility of substances that produce heat during dissolution will decrease upon increasing temperature, whereas the solubility of substances that dissolve endothermally will increase under identical conditions (Henry Le Chatelier, 1850–1936, Sorbonne). Anomalous dissolution behavior (angulate curve) may occur for salts, which can exist as hydrates (e.g., Na_2SO_4), since the solubility of hydrates differs from that of the corresponding anhydrate (see Section 3.9.7.1).

3.9.6   pH-Dependence of Solubility of Weak Electrolytes

Most active ingredients are weak bases or acids and can therefore exist in ionized and un-ionized forms, dependent on pH. Due to the large difference in polarity of the two forms, their solubility in water also differs considerably. This pH-dependent solubility is technologically, as well as from the pharmaceutical point of view, of crucial importance but can be described with the help of simple equations. In these, total solubility of the active substance (sum of the solubilities of the dissociated and the nondissociated forms) is designated C_S and solubility of the nondissociated form (also called *intrinsic solubility*) C_{S_0}. The dissociation equilibrium for a weak acid HA reads

$$HA + H_2O \leftrightarrows H_3O^+ + A^-$$

The corresponding equation for the acid constant K_a is

$$K_a = \frac{[H_3O^+]\,[A^-]}{[HA]}$$

Substituting C_{S_0} for HA yields

$$K_a = \frac{[H_3O^+]\,[A^-]}{c_{S_0}}$$

After conversions:

$$\frac{K_a}{[H_3O^+]} = \frac{[A^-]}{C_{S_0}}$$

By substituting $C_S - C_{S_0}$ for $[A^-]$ we obtain

$$\frac{K_a}{[H_3O^+]} = \frac{c_S - c_{S_0}}{c_{S_0}}$$

By taking the logarithm we obtain

$$\log K_a - \log[H_3O^+] = \log\left(\frac{c_S - c_{S_0}}{c_{S_0}}\right)$$

or

$$pH - pK_a = \log\left(\frac{c_S - c_{S_0}}{c_{S_0}}\right)$$

For a weak base B, the dissociation equilibrium, using the corresponding acid constant K_a, reads

$$K_a = \frac{[H_3O^+][B]}{[BH^+]}$$

Now the concentration of the poorly soluble nondissociated form is in the numerator, so that after substitution by C_S and C_{S_0}, respectively, the following equation appears:

$$\frac{K_a}{[H_3O^+]} = \frac{c_{S_0}}{c_S - c_{S_0}}$$

By analogy to the conversions described above, this yields

$$pH - pK_a = \log\left(\frac{c_{S_0}}{c_S - c_{S_0}}\right)$$

In so far as the solubility of the nondissociated form and pK_a are known, the solubility of the weak electrolyte can be calculated for any pH value. It should be noted that the equations assume an infinitely high solubility for the ionized form. Practically speaking, this will obviously be limited when the solubility product of the salt is exceeded due to the presence of counter ions.

3.9.7 Dependence of Solubility on Physical State and Particle Size

3.9.7.1 Dependence on Physical State

Metastable crystal modifications and amorphous substances display higher solubility than thermodynamically more stable crystal forms because the internal binding forces are weaker. Independent of the solvent, at moderate concentrations relative solubility of polymorphous forms and their vapor pressure (as an expression of thermodynamic stability) correlate as follows:

$$\frac{c_{S_1}}{c_{S_2}} = \frac{p_1}{p_2} \tag{3-26}$$

$c_{S_{1,2}}$ = solubility (saturation concentration) of modification 1 and 2, respectively

$p_{1,2}$ = vapor pressure of modification 1 and 2, respectively

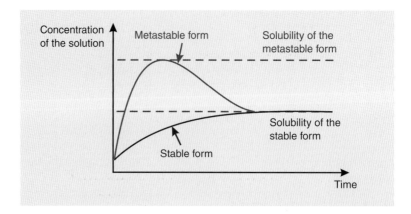

Fig. 3-35 Supersaturated solutions.

Solutions made from the metastable forms are supersaturated as compared to the stable crystalline modification, leading to a separation of crystalline material as soon as one crystal of the stable modification is formed in the system (Fig. 3-35). As a result, the concentration of the solution will drop over time to the saturation concentration of the stable form. Therefore, the solubility of the metastable form is commonly called *apparent equilibrium solubility*. Consequently, these metastable forms cannot serve to produce stable solutions with concentrations higher than the saturation concentration of the stable form. In cases where storage stability of the forming solution is not required or the saturation concentration is not even reached during the dissolution process, the enhanced dissolution velocity may nonetheless have pharmaceutical relevance. Specifically, it can be exploited to enhance the dissolution rate of poorly soluble active ingredients in the gastrointestinal tract (see 3.10.4.1). The resulting differences in biological activity between crystalline and amorphous active substances can be quite considerable for poorly water-soluble substances. For example, the antibiotic Novobiocin is only biologically active when administered in the amorphous form.

Also pseudo-polymorphous forms of active agents (solvates, hydrates) exhibit solubility characteristics that deviate from those of the solvate-free crystal. Likewise, this can be relevant for the dissolution behavior after administration. In general, active ingredients without hydrate-water dissolve better than the corresponding hydrates. For example, the solubility of water-free theophylline at room temperature is twice as high as that of the hydrate. By contrast, solvate-containing crystals often dissolve better in organic solvents than solvate-free crystals. This has been demonstrated, for example, for hydrocortisone esters (in ethanol) and succinyl-sulfathiazole (in n-pentanol). Table 3-7 presents examples of solubilities of various forms of solids.

Table 3-7 Examples of Active Substances with Different Solubilities of the Different Solid Forms

Active Substance (Temperature)	Better Soluble/Less Soluble Form	Solubility Ratio
Glibenclamide (37°C)	modification II / modification I	1.6
Mebendazole (25°C)	modification B / modification A	7.2
Meprobamate (25°C)	modification II / modification I	1.9
Ampicillin (20°C)	anhydrate/hydrate	2.2
Erythromycin (30°C)	anhydrate/dihydrate	2.2
Theophylline (25°C)	anhydrate/monohydrate	2.0
Caffeine (25°C)	amorphous/crystalline	6.5
Theophylline (17°C)	amorphous/crystalline	58
Morphine (20°C)	amorphous/crystalline	268

3.9.7.2 Dependence on Particle Size

According to the Ostwald-Freundlich correlation, solubility also depends on particle size.

$$\ln\frac{c_S}{c_{S_0}} = \frac{2\gamma \cdot V}{r \cdot R \cdot T} \tag{3-27}$$

c_S = solubility (saturation concentration) of fine particles with radius r
c_{S_0} = solubility (saturation concentration) of relatively coarse powder particles
V = mol volume
R = ideal gas constant
T = absolute temperature
γ = surface tension

Small particles have higher solubility than larger ones. Nonetheless, this size dependence is only relevant for ultra-fine particles. Only for powders with colloidal particle size, which, however, can't be easily manufactured or manipulated, practically relevant improvement of solubility can be attained.

The correlation between particle size and solubility is responsible for the *Ostwald ripening* phenomenon observed in drug formulations containing finely disperse active substance particles (e.g., suspensions and suspension ointments). Due to the different solubilities of smaller and larger particles, the latter may become larger in time at the expense of the smaller particles. As a result, an undesired shift in particle size distribution may occur.

3.9.8 Solvent Properties of Water

The most important solvent in the manufacturing of medicines, water, has exceptional properties. Physical parameters of water, such as density, evaporation heat, surface tension, heat conductance, and solubilizing properties, deviate from those that would be expected from the values within the homologous series. Of special importance for the anomalous behavior of water—as for all liquids forming hydrogen bonds—are the exceptionally strong and highly directional intermolecular forces. This exceptional position is determined by the structure of the water molecule. It is the only molecule that, from a single-atom center, can form hydrogen bonds in the direction of all four corners of a tetrahedron via its two hydrogen atoms and the two solitary electron pairs.

In the strictly symmetric structure of the lattice of ice, the water molecules are arranged in such a way that each oxygen atom is surrounded in a tetrahedral manner by four hydrogen atoms. Upon melting, the ice lattice collapses, but a considerable fraction of the hydrogen bonds is preserved. The proportion of free, unbound OH groups amounts to a mere 10% at 0°C and still only about 21% at 100°C. In many structural theories of liquid water, it is proposed that conglomerates of water molecules form small short-range domains consisting of a three-dimensional network with a tetrahedral structure (cluster model), from which continuously single molecules are split off and attached again at another site of the cluster (Fig. 3-36). A number of the anomalies of water (but by no means all of them) can be explained with this clustered-structure model.

Various compounds can influence the structure of water. For example, upon a temperature increase, the proportion of hydrogen bonds diminishes. During dissolution of numerous salts (e.g., NaCl, KNO_3), the number of hydrogen bonds is reduced and the state or ordering of the water diminishes. The increase in hydrogen bond defects, causes the water to become more "hydrophilic," as a result of which solvent properties for polar substances increase. Such ions are designated as *structure breakers*. Urea, for example, has such an effect. Oppositely, other substances (e.g., Na_2CO_3, $MgSO_4$) lead to an enhanced proportion of hydrogen bonds, analogous to the effect occurring during cooling of pure water, which causes the water to become more hydrophobic and the dissolving capacity to diminish. Such compounds are designated as *structure makers*.

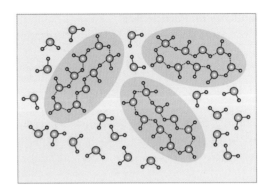

Fig. 3-36 Cluster structure of water.

3.9.9   Measures to Enhance Solubility

For the processing of active substances, solubility in water is of eminent importance. While in case of drug formulations for topical or oral use solvents other than water might be considered, for the preparation of solutions for injection, particularly in case of large-volumes for intravenous administration, most often only water will qualify as an acceptable carrier medium. Water solubility also plays a central role in the administration of solid drug formulations, as active ingredients will only be absorbed when dissolved in water.

The solubility of active substances can be enhanced by chemical and technological means (Table 3-8). An increase in solubility can be achieved by means of alterations of the drug molecule (salt formation or dissociation after changing pH of the solution, introduction of hydrophilic groups), as well as by the addition of dissolution mediators (complex formers; co-solvents, surfactants). The latter excipients should be perfectly safe and not display any incompatibility with the active ingredient. A special form of dissolution facilitation is achieved with surfactants as micelle formers. It is known as *solubilization* and the applied surfactants as *solubilizers*. Especially the manufacturing of injection fluids often depends on the addition of dissolution enhancers to obtain sufficiently high drug concentrations.

Table 3-8 Measures to Improve Dissolution Behavior

Measure to Enhance Solubility	Examples
Modification of the Active Ingredient	
• Salt formation, changing pH	Alkaloid salts
• Introduction of hydrophilic groups	
Addition of Dissolution Enhancers	
• Complex formation	Cyclodextrin inclusion compounds
• Application of co-solvents	Addition of ethanol, propylene glycol
• Solubilization in micelles	Addition of polysorbate, Cremophor EL

Measures to Enhance Dissolution Rate

Enhancement of solubility/saturation concentration: all above-mentioned measures, plus:
- Reducing particle size
- Application of metastable modifications, amorphous substances, solvates

Increasing the Surface Area Available for the Dissolution Process
- Reducing particle size
- Crystallization from a surfactant-containing solution
- Spray and freeze drying
- Spray embedding
- Melt extrusion, co-evaporates

Table 3-9 Examples of Achievable Increase in Water Solubility by Salt Formation (Parts substance + Parts solvent)

	Counter Ion	Acidic or Alkaline Form	Salt Form
Phenobarbital	Na^+	1+5 000	1+1.5
Phenoxymethylpenicillin	Ca^{2+}	1+1 700	1+120
	K^+		1+1.5
Papaverine	Cl^-	1+50 000	1+40
Procaine	Cl^-	1+770	1+1
Acetylsalicylic acid	Ca^{2+}	1+300	1+4

3.9.9.1   Choice of pH Value of Solutions

The exponential correlation between pH value and solubility of weak acids and bases, as presented in 3.7.4, demonstrates that considerable improvement of solubility can be achieved by the proper choice of pH value. When applying this approach, certain aspects of physiological tolerance and chemical stability as well as possible effects on biopharmaceutical behavior should be taken into consideration. Furthermore, it should be taken into account that dilution of nonbuffered solutions may cause a pH change during administration and, as a consequence, alter solubility of the active agent (under certain conditions even leading to precipitation of the agent). This effect can be suppressed by deployment of an appropriate buffer provided the latter is tolerated.

3.9.9.2   Formation of Water-Soluble Salts

This method, which can lead to considerable solubility improvements (Table 3-9), is widely applied for poorly soluble basic drugs such as alkaloids (e.g., pilocarpine hydrochloride, morphine hydrochloride and acid derivatives of drugs (e.g., sodium benzoate). The solubility of the drug strongly depends on the nature of the applied counter ions.

3.9.9.3   Introduction of Polar Groups in the Molecule

Polar groups such as carboxyl, hydroxyl, hydroxylalkyl, polyoxyethylene, sulfate, and amino groups can be introduced in the molecule to make it more hydrophilic. Nonetheless, the options to improve solubility by chemical measures are limited, because structural alterations often change pharmacological properties, enhance toxicity or reduce stability.

3.9.9.4   Complex Formation

In this connection, complexes are to be understood as compounds that may arise, by hydrogen bonding or dipole-dipole interactions, or by hydrophobic interactions, between different drugs as well as between drugs and specific additives. Complex formation is often connected with a change in drug properties such as durability, absorption, and tolerance; this implies that in each individual case, meticulous testing is indispensable. The conjunction of caffeine and procaine is an example of improvement of water solubility by complex formation between low-molecular-weight substances.

Substantial solubility improvement can be attained by deployment of inclusion compounds (see also section 5.3.3.5). Cyclodextrins are cyclic oligosaccharides composed of 6 to 8 glucose units interconnected so as to build a hollow cylinder and resulting in correspondingly different ring diameters (Fig. 3-37). Per ring size they are designated as α- (6 glucose units), β- (7 units) or γ-cyclodextrin (8 units). The external surface of the cylinder is hydrophilic while the inner surface has hydrophobic properties and thus can engage in nonpolar interactions with drug molecules. As the ring-shaped hollow space has a limited volume (ring diameters varying from 0.45 to 0.9 nm) only drug molecules with corresponding structure and molecular size can be enclosed. Commonly, 1:1 complexes are formed, sometimes enclosing only parts of the host molecule. The different cyclodextrins display different water solubility. Solubility can be improved by formation of derivatives, which is particularly important in case of β-cyclodextrins (e.g., hydroxypropyl-β-cyclodextrin and sulfobutyl ether β-cyclodextrin). For numerous poorly soluble active substances, significant enhancement of solubility and dissolution rates can be achieved (Table 3-10). In addition, enclosure of sensitive agents can lead

Water solubility of cyclodextrins

β-CD: 1.85 g/100 mL
α-CD: 14.5 g/100 mL
γ-CD: 23.2 g/100 mL
all at room temperature.

The solubility of CDs increases strongly with increasing temperature.

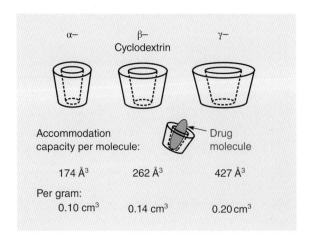

Fig. 3-37 Cyclodextrins.

to improvement of stability. In dried form, cyclodextrin inclusion complexes can be readily processed into tablets and capsules.

Formation of complexes or associations may not only lead to enhancement of solubility, but in some instances can also bring along retardation of the rate of dissolution or release.

3.9.9.5   Application of Co-solvents

Co-solvents are water-miscible or partly water-miscible organic solvents such as ethanol, propylene glycol, polyethylene glycol, glycerol and dimethyl-acetamide, which can form hydrogen bonds but also possess hydrocarbon domains. By mixing with water, the interaction options between the water molecules diminish and the potential to dissolve nonpolar substances is enhanced. The solvent properties of the resulting mixture lie between those of the pure organic solvent and those of water, leading to the following approximate correlation for solutions of nonpolar substances (Fig. 3-38):

$$\log c_{s_{mix}} = \log c_{s_w} + m \cdot f_c \tag{3-28}$$

$c_{s_{mix}}$ = solubility in co-solvent system
c_{s_w} = solubility in water
m = constant
f_c = volume fraction of the co-solvent

If, on the other hand, the polarity of the solute lies between that of water and that of the chosen co-solvent, we can expect a maximum in the solubility curve, as the highest solubility is reached only then when the polarity of the solvent mixture coincides with that of the solute.

The employment of co-solvents is a commonly used procedure to enhance solubility of organic substances in aqueous media (Table 3.11), taking into consideration the compatibility of the solvent mixtures under consideration. For example, the co-solvent ethanol, which is often used in oral formulations, is considered unfavorable for children. Likewise, ethanol is not employed for ophthalmological formulations because of its irritating action. Glycerol and propylene glycol can cause hemolysis and thrombophlebitis when applied intravenously

Table 3-10 Examples of Medicines Exploiting Solubility Enhancement by Cyclodextrins

Active Agent	Cyclodextrin	Commercial Product	Application
Alprostadil	α-Cyclodextrin	Prostavasin®	Solution for infusion
Itraconazole	Hydroxypropyl-β-cyclodextrin	Sempera® Liquid	Solution for oral administration
Voriconazole	Sulfobutyl ether β-cyclodextrin	VFend®	Solution for infusion
Ziprasidone mesylate	Sulfobutyl ether β-cyclodextrin	Zeldox®	Solution for injection

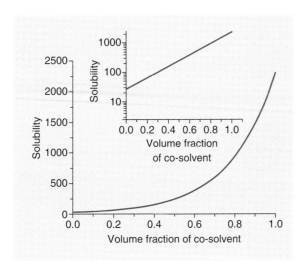

Fig. 3-38 Typical solubility curve of a nonpolar substance in a co-solvent system (Insert: logarithmic presentation).

in high concentrations. Furthermore, intramuscular application of co-solvents may cause tissue irritation. Occasionally it may be possible to keep the proportion of particular co-solvents within the required limits by a combination of multiple substances. Analogous to the employment of different pH values, application of co-solvents may lead to precipitation of the solute upon dilution or administration. This should be taken into consideration, particularly in view of the logarithmic correlation between solubility and co-solvent concentration.

3.9.9.6   Formation and Properties of Micelles

Micelles are associations of surfactant molecules with particle sizes in the lower nm range which can be determined, for example, by means of dynamic light scattering (e.g., ca. 3 nm for micelles of sodium lauryl sulfate or 10 nm for micelles of poly-oxy ethylated castor oil). They form in aqueous solutions of surface-active substances above the so-called *critical micelle concentration* (CMC). The potential to form micelles is based on the specific chemical structure of surfactants, which is characterized by the presence of a hydrophilic (either ionic or non-ionic) and a hydrophobic moiety (see section 5.3.6 and 18.4). While the hydrophilic part of the molecule can interact intensively with water molecules, this is impossible for the

Table 3-11 Examples of finished medicinal products based on Co-Solvent Systems

Active Agent	Product	Formulation	Co-solvent
Carmustin	Carmubris® powder and solvent for preparation of solution for infusion	i.v.-infusion after dilution	ethanol
Nifedipine	Adalat® pro infusione	solution for infusion	ethanol, macrogol 400
Nimodipine	Nimotop® S solution for infusion	solution for infusion	ethanol, macrogol 400
Glycerol-trinitrate	Perlinganit® solution	solution for infusion	propylene glycol
Esmolol-HCl	Brevibloc®	concentrate for solution for infusion; for dilution	ethanol, propylene glycol
Piroxicam	Clinit®	solution for injection	ethanol, propylene glycol
Prednisolone acetate	Ultracortenol®	eye drops	macrogol 400
Digitoxin	Digimerck®	solution for injection	propylene glycol, ethanol
Digoxin	Lanicor® Lenoxin® Liquidum	solution for injection solution for oral administration	propylene glycol, ethanol

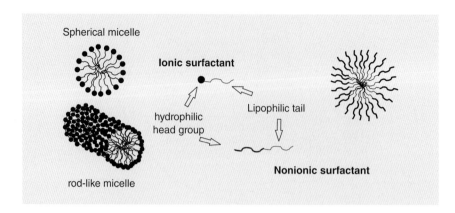

Fig. 3-39   Forms of micelles.

hydrophobic moiety. Thus, it is energetically advantageous for the system to arrange itself above the CMC in such a way that the individual surfactant molecules group together into micelles. In that situation, the hydrophobic parts of the surfactant molecules turn toward each other and build a fluid core that is shielded from the surrounding water by the polar head groups (Fig. 3-39). The fluid character of the micelles offers the possibility to incorporate hydrophobic and amphiphilic foreign molecules (solubilization).

Depending on the surfactant and its concentration, micelles can be composed of relatively few molecules (e.g., approx. 60–80 for sodium lauryl sulfate micelles). They can, however, also consist of hundreds to even thousands of individual molecules. Furthermore, micelles come in different shapes. Immediately after exceeding the CMC, they commonly adopt a spherical shape; upon a further increase in concentration, often formation of rod-shaped or sometimes discoid associations occurs. Finally, at even higher concentrations liquid crystalline structures can be formed (section 15.3.5).

Not all surfactants will form micelles in water. Some are capable of forming micelles in organic solvents or lipidic media; we speak of *reverse micelles* in such cases. The hydrophilic groups of the surfactant will then concentrate in the core of the micelle; the hydrophobic residues, present on the outside, are responsible for the solubility of the association complex in the solvent under consideration.

The formation of micelles upon increasing detergent concentration occurs in a narrow concentration range, the CMC (Fig. 3-40). Below the CMC, individual surfactant molecules are present in a molecularly dispersed solution, or sometimes are grouped together in associations of very few molecules. The surfactant molecules display a strong tendency to adsorb at the surface of the solution (air-water interface), which leads in this concentration range up to the CMC, to a gradual decrease in surface tension. The surfactant molecules in the solution and those at the surface are in equilibrium with each other. Upon reaching the CMC, suddenly micelles are formed. Micelle formation occurs spontaneously; the essential driving force is an entropy increase in the system, the cause of which is not yet fully understood. An essential contribution is given by the *hydrophobic effect*. When individual surfactant molecules are present in the solution, ordered water structures arise in the areas of contact between the hydrophobic chains of the surfactant and the water molecules. By the repositioning of the hydrophobic chains in the core of the micelles, this ordering is abolished again, resulting in an entropy increase. Possibly, a conformation change in the lipophilic chains upon transfer into the micelles contributes to the entropy increase. Thus, the micellar system formed is thermodynamically stable and in an equilibrated state, allowing active exchange of surfactant molecules between the micelles and the solution. The concentration of the surfactant monomers barely increases above the CMC, so that from then on, essentially no further change in surface tension will occur.

Whether or not, at a certain surfactant concentration, individual surfactant molecules, associations of a few molecules or micelles are present, is determined predominantly by the nature of the surfactant, in addition to a number of external parameters (e.g., temperature, solvent, electrolyte concentration). Surfactants with a relatively large lipophilic moiety already

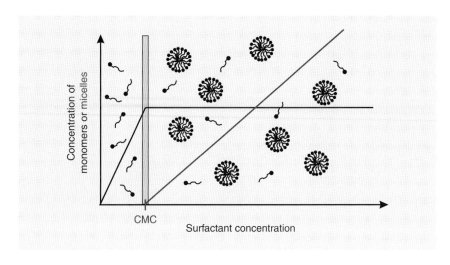

Fig. 3-40 Micelle formation as a function of surfactant concentration.

arrange into micelles at substantially lower concentrations (low CMC) than comparable more hydrophilic surfactants (high CMC). For ionic surfactants, the CMC is again higher than that of comparable nonionic surfactants, because prior to the accommodation of such surfactants into a micelle the electrostatic repulsion of the head groups will have to be overcome. Micelle formation can only start when the solubility of the surfactant is sufficiently high to reach the CMC.

Particularly surfactants with relatively long lipophilic chains dissolve only poorly in water at a given temperature (e.g., sodium cetyl stearyl sulfate). No micelles will be formed unless the temperature reaches a value at which the solubility of the surfactant reaches the CMC (*Krafft point*). For many nonionic surfactants, in particular those that contain polyoxyethylene groups, an upper critical temperature limit is defined, which by virtue of the formation of a cloudy turbidity in the solution is designated *cloud point*. At this temperature, hydration of the polyoxyethylene groups is strongly reduced, inducing the onset of fusion of micelles and the formation of a separate surfactant-rich phase. This phenomenon can be observed, for instance, during autoclaving of such surfactant solutions. By contrast, the dissolution behavior of ionic surfactants is barely temperature-dependent.

The structural change that takes place at concentrations in the CMC range comes to expression as a jump in the physicochemical properties of the solution, including surface tension, equivalent conductivity, osmotic pressure, freezing point depression, viscosity, refractive index, and spectroscopic characteristics (Fig. 3-41). All these parameters may be

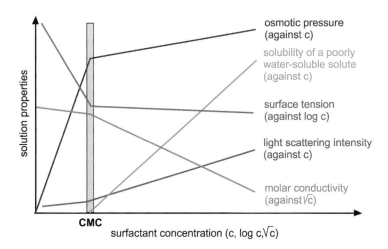

Fig. 3-41 Changes of the physical properties of surfactant solutions at concentrations around the CMC.

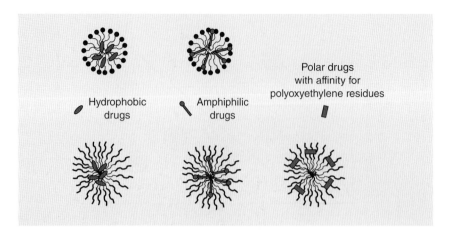

Fig. 3-42 Localization of active agents in micelles.

used to determine the CMC. Simple methods specifically exploit surface tension, equivalent conductivity (for ionic surfactants), light scattering, or the capacity of micelles to solubilize lipophilic dyes. The latter approach exploits the change in the absorption spectrum of the dye that occurs upon micelle formation and/or causes a color change in the solution.

3.9.9.7 Solubilization

Solubilization is commonly understood as an improvement of solubility by means of surface-active compounds. Such so-called *surfactants* are capable of conveying poorly soluble or insoluble pharmaceutical agents into clear, or at most opalescent, aqueous solutions without causing changes in the chemical structure of the agent. The solubilizing potency of surfactants is based on the formation of micelles. In addition to micelles, other colloidal structures, such as liposomes or emulsion droplets, can be exploited to solubilize very poorly water-soluble substances.

Poorly soluble substances can be incorporated into micelles; their localization in the micelle depends on their chemical properties, in particular polarity (Fig. 3-42). Highly non-polar substances are accommodated in the hydrophobic core of the micelle whereas more polar molecules may also be found in the more polar peripheral areas of the micelle. In micelles composed of a surfactant with polyoxyethylene groups, association of molecules of appropriate affinity with the "polyoxyethylene shell" is possible. The accommodation of foreign substances in the core of the micelle leads to a size increase because the core swells, whereby additional surfactant molecules are accommodated in order to shield the increased nonpolar area from the water.

Micellar solutions of active agents are thermodynamically stable systems. Nonetheless, also for these colloidal systems certain stability issues must be taken into consideration. Micelles can, for instance, become supersaturated with solubilized substances. Upon prolonged storage of such preparations, there is an increasing risk that the solubilized drug is separated in crystalline form from the solution or that aggregates are formed. Super-saturation may also occur upon dilution of micellar solutions, as the equilibrium between molecularly dispersed and micelle-associated surfactant has to be reinstalled by dissociation of surfactant molecules from the micelles.

Addition of surfactant can affect chemical stability of a solubilized active agent either in a positive or in a negative way. For example, some substances turn out to be highly susceptible to oxidation when incorporated in micelles. On the other hand, the hydrolysis rate of esters often diminishes at concentrations above the CMC. Also, the applied surfactants themselves may be susceptible to chemical alterations (e.g., polysorbates and fatty alcohol ethers of polyoxyethylene are liable to autooxidation).

In pharmaceutical technology, particularly nonionic surfactants (section 5.4.4) are used as solubilizers which are largely inert toward purely chemical influences (Table 3-12). Often lipophilic vitamins (A, D, E, K), steroids and cytostatics are converted into aqueous solubilized preparations for oral or parenteral administration. Essential oils and their components can be turned into water-clear solutions by means of solubilization (aromatic waters). Addition of

Table 3-12 Examples of Surfactants as Solubilizers

Active Agent	Product	Formulation	Surfactant (+ Co-solvent)
Prednisolone acetate	Inflanefran®	eye drops	Polysorbate 80
Dexamethasone	Isopto-Dex®	eye drops	Polysorbate 80
Diclofenac-sodium	Voltaren® ophta	eye drops	Macrogol ricinoleate
Tocopherol acetate	E-Vicotrat®	solution for infusion	Polysorbate 80
e.g., Vitamins Λ, D, E	Multibionta®-drops	solution for oral intake	Macrogol-1500-glycerol triricinoleate
Phytomenadione	Konakion® MM	solution or oral intake	Lecithin, Glycocholic acid
e.g., Vitamins A, D, E	Cernevit®	lyophilizate for preparation of solution for infusion	Phospholipids, Glycocholic acid
Travoprost	Travatan®	eye drops	Macrogol glycerol-hydroxystearate
Etoposid	Vepesid®	concentrate for preparation of solution for infusion	Macrogol 300 Polysorbate 80 30% Ethanol
Paclitaxel	Taxol®	concentrate for preparation of solution for infusion	Macrogol-1500-glycerol triricinoleate Ethanol
Teniposid	VM 26-Bristol®	concentrate for preparation of solution for infusion	Macrogol-1500-glycerol triricinoleate, Ethanol Dimethyl-acetamide
Tacrolimus	Prograf®	concentrate for preparation of solution for infusion	Macrogol ricinoleate 60, Ethanol

surfactants also greatly improves extraction of essential oils and other natural substances from herbal drugs.

Mixed micelles composed of phospholipids and bile salts are often used for parenteral administration of drugs, such as for solubilization of menadione in Konakion® MM. Dissolution in lipophilic solvents (inverted micelles) is rather facilitated by means of the more lipophilic sorbitane esters or by polysorbates. Mixed micelles are also formed naturally in the gut, when lipases cleave triglycerides into monoglycerides and fatty acids. Together with bile salts these formed mixed micelles are able to host lipophilic drugs. These mixed micelles are prone to break down at the epithelial cell membranes releasing the drug there, which can then readily diffuse through the epithelial cells into the systemic circulation.

When using solubilizers, it is important to keep in mind that surfactants may have a physiological activity by themselves, so that toxic reactions cannot be excluded. Particularly in case of deployment of solubilizers for manufacturing solutions for injection or infusion, extensive pharmacological and toxicological testing should be performed. It is known, for instance, that many surface-active compounds possess hemolytic activity. Also, anaphylactic reactions have been described in connection with the administration of surfactant-containing infusion liquids (e.g., with Cremophor EL® (Macrogol-1500-glycerol-triricinoleate)). Surfactants often also cause eye irritation. For oral use, one should keep in mind that surfactants, because of their unpleasant taste, cannot always be used, unless in combination with taste maskers.

The activity of medicines is not always enhanced by surfactants; it may also be attenuated. Weakening of activity has, for instance, been observed for anesthetics and antibiotics. Occasionally, preservatives will not fully develop their growth-inhibiting action in presence of surfactants (see section 26.2). Anionic micelle formers can form poorly soluble complexes with nitrogen-containing drug substances and thus reduce their therapeutic effect.

3.10   Dissolution Rate

3.10.1   General Principles

From the dissolution rate the information on the time course of the dissolution process may be derived. This parameter is particularly important in the formulation of medicines because for many poorly soluble drugs it represents the rate-limiting step in the absorption process. This applies particularly when the dissolution rate of a substance is lower than the absorption rate. By increasing the dissolution rate, the conditions for rapid absorption can be improved (section 7.6.2).

3.10.2   Physical Laws

The fundamental physical laws governing dissolution rates were formulated in 1879 by Noyes and Whitney:

$$\frac{dc}{dt} = C \cdot (c_S - c_t) \tag{3-29}$$

dc/dt = dissolution rate (change in concentration per time unit)
c_S = solubility (saturation concentration of the solute in the solvent)
c_t = solute concentration at time t
C = constant, referring to diffusion coefficient, the volume of the saturated
             solution and the thickness of the diffusion layer

The equation states that the dissolution rate is dependent on the concentration gradient between the saturation concentration and the concentration at time point t. During the dissolution process of a solid substance, a thin layer of saturated solution is formed on the surface of the solid material; from there the substance diffuses into the bulk of the surrounding solution (Fig. 3-43).

By taking into account diffusion retardation, the Noyes and Whitney equation can be formulated more precisely: by employing the first diffusion law of Fick, the relation derived by Nernst and Brunner results:

$$\frac{dc}{dt} = \frac{D \cdot A}{h \cdot V} \cdot (c_s - c_t) \tag{3-30}$$

dc/dt = dissolution rate (concentration change per time unit)
D = diffusion coefficient of the drug in the solvent in question (in the
            diffusion layer)
A = particle surface area of the nondissolved drug
h = thickness of the diffusion layer around a drug particle
V = volume of the solvent
c_S = saturation concentration (solubility)
c_t = drug concentration at time t

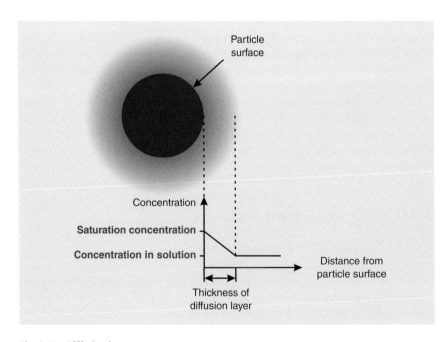

Fig. 3-43 Diffusion layer.

According to this equation, the dissolution rate is directly proportional to the total surface area of the solid drug particles, the diffusion coefficient of its molecules in the solvent as well as to the concentration gradient built up around the particle at time t. It is inversely proportional to the thickness of this diffusion layer. For poorly soluble substances, the concentration gradient $(c_s - c_t)$ will become so low that the total surface area of the particles practically speaking becomes the limiting factor determining the dissolution rate.

From equation 3-30 it follows that the dissolution rate can be enhanced substantially by a large surface increase (e.g., micronization). When applying the Nernst & Brunner equation it should be kept in mind that the total particle surface changes with time during the dissolution process, leading to a reduction in dissolution rate.

3.10.3 The Cube Root Law

The cube root law of *Hixson and Crowell* (published in 1938) also considers, in addition to the transport through the diffusion layer, the decrease in particle size and thus the decrease of the available surface area during the dissolution process. This law assumes uniform particle size or the dissolution of a single particle, respectively:

$$\sqrt[3]{m_0} - \sqrt[3]{m} = k \cdot t \quad \text{with} \quad k = \frac{\sqrt[3]{m_0}}{d} \cdot \frac{2D \cdot c_s}{h \cdot \rho} \tag{3-31}$$

m_0 = total mass of solid material at time 0
k = dissolution rate constant for the cube root law
d = particle diameter
D = diffusion coefficient
h = thickness of the diffusion layer
c_S = solubility, saturation concentration
ρ = density of the solid material

Although these laws illustrate the basic principles of the process, their strict applicability assumes rigorously standardized conditions, which in the reality of drugs and formulations (different particle sizes and shapes) do not prevail. In addition, the geometric conditions of the test equipment and the flow conditions in the solution must be precisely defined in order to obtain reliable results. The reality of practice is therefore better served by dissolution tests (see section 9.9.1).

3.10.4 Measures to Enhance Dissolution Rate

Potential measures to enhance the dissolution rate can be derived from the Noyes-Whitney or the Nernst-Brunner equation (equation 3-30), respectively. Particular parameters that can be influenced technologically are the saturation concentration c_s (see section 3.9.7) and total surface area A available for dissolution of the nondissolved drug. The surface area can be enlarged by mechanical comminution (micronization) or by applying excipients and processes that, in addition to other possible effects, lead to smaller particle size of the active agent (spray drying, spray or melt embedding, formation of solid dispersions).

3.10.4.1 Increase of Saturation Concentration

Of the variety of measures used to increase the saturation concentration, as shown in Table 3-8, particularly the changes in molecular properties (salt formation, introduction of hydrophilic groups) are relevant, especially in connection with the enhancement of the dissolution rate of solid drugs in the gastrointestinal tract. The properties of the prevailing "solvent" (gastrointestinal fluid) are barely susceptible to manipulation. Besides, also here the influence of the physical state, as discussed in section 3.9.7, can be exploited (application of suitable polymorph forms or amorphous substances, use of very small particles), because stability of the saturated solution is not required to increase dissolution rate in the intestinal tract. In case of very poorly soluble substances, for which the dissolution process represents the rate-determining step in the absorption process, the saturation concentration will not be reached at all, since the drug will have been carried off before that could occur.

Ph. Eur. 2.9.29 Intrinsic Dissolution _____

USP ⟨1087⟩ Intrinsic Dissolution

The intrinsic dissolution rate is defined as the dissolution rate of a pure solid under conditions of constant surface area of the solid and constant temperature, pH value, composition, ionic strength, and stirring velocity of the solvent. In order to keep the surface area between the material to be tested and the dissolution medium at a constant level, a cylindrically compacted sample is produced that, after compression, remains in the die and is exposed there to the solvent solution only at its free, circular surface (diameter 0.1–1 cm). The opposite opening of the die is closed off with a threaded shoulder screw attached to a laboratory stirring device. Commonly, the assembly of a type 1 or 2 dissolution apparatus is used for this purpose. Instead of a basket or a stirring blade, a holder containing the die is mounted to its shaft. The free sample surface is pointing downward and is positioned 3.8 cm above the bottom of the vessel, which is filled with a suitable volume of the dissolution medium. While the sample is rotating, the concentration of the dissolved substance in the medium is measured at certain time intervals. The intrinsic dissolution rate is expressed in terms of dissolved mass per unit of time and per exposed area ($mg \cdot min^{-1} \cdot cm^{-2}$). Its value is affected by all properties of the solid, including crystal form, crystallinity, amorphism, polymorphism, particle size, and specific surface area. The intrinsic dissolution rate is used to evaluate dissolution behavior of medicinal substances under biopharmaceutical aspects as well as to compare different drug and excipient batches for reasons of quality control. In case of pharmaceutical substances with an intrinsic dissolution rate below 0.1 to 1 $mg \cdot min^{-1} \cdot cm^{-2}$, the dissolution rate will significantly limit bioavailability.

3.10.4.2   Comminution

Decreasing particle size is one of the most important measures one can take to enhance dissolution rate. While the effect of small particle size on *solubility* is commonly relatively small (see Ch. 3.7.5), the increase in specific surface area that goes along with it often leads to a substantial boost in *dissolution rate*. This is important above all for poorly soluble substances, which may have an absolute requirement for micronization. In addition to enlargement of the specific surface area, this process may cause parts of the processed material to become amorphous, which in turn may further accelerate dissolution. A well-known example of enhanced effectiveness of a drug as a result of micronization is griseofulvin, a practically insoluble antimycotic drug (see section 7.6.2.1). Recent years have seen a boost in the development of procedures allowing the manufacturing of particles in the nm size range (nanonization) in order to further optimize dissolution rate (see section 20.6). In this case the increase in solubility may become relevant as well. Oppositely, an increase in particle size may serve to delay dissolution and drug release, allowing the establishment of a depot effect. By combining large and small crystals or a mixture of different crystal forms, it is often possible to achieve a prolonged drug effect.

3.10.4.3   Recrystallization from a Surfactant-Containing Solution

In case of distinctly hydrophobic pharmaceutical substances (e.g., propyphenazone), particle comminution may result in deterioration rather than improvement of dissolution properties. This finds its cause in that the resulting increase in surface area is accompanied by a larger, nonwettable interface. Because wetting by the solvent is a prerequisite for the dissolution process, the latter is strongly inhibited in this case. When such problems occur, the dissolution rate can be enhanced by recrystallization of the substance from a surfactant-containing solution (e.g., 0.5% polysorbate). Traces of the surfactant that accumulate during recrystallization at the particle surface apparently facilitate wetting and thus the dissolution process.

3.10.4.4 Spray and Freeze Drying

During spray-drying (section 2.4.3.8) from fluid solutions mostly hollow spherically shaped particles are formed (ca. 20–200 μm) with a dry-foam character. As a result of the accompanying surface area increase, dissolution will be accelerated compared to that of the crystalline powder. In addition, active agents, commonly present in crystalline form, can be transformed partly or completely into the amorphous state by spray drying. As a result, an increase in solubility and dissolution rate occurs. Also products obtained by means of freeze-drying (*lyophilization*, section 2.4.3.11) display increased dissolution rates due to their highly porous structure and the formation of hydrophilic (easily wettable) surfaces.

3.10.4.5 Solid Dispersions

The dissolution rate of poorly soluble pharmaceutical substances can furthermore be enhanced by processing with a highly water-soluble carrier substance (e.g., polyvinyl pyrrolidone, polyethylene glycol, cellulose derivatives, sugars, sugar alcohols, urea). This proceeds by jointly melting the drug and the carrier followed by rapid solidification of the melt (melt embedding, melt extrusion) or by dissolving the active ingredient and the carrier together in an organic solvent (when appropriate, also super-critical carbon dioxide may be used), followed by evaporation of the solvent (*co-precipitation*) and subsequent grinding. Alternatively, solid dispersions can be prepared by spraying a melt into a cold environment (*spray congealing, spray embedding*) or by *spray- and freeze-drying* of the mostly aqueous solution of both components. Thus, the products formed may represent eutectic mixtures, solid solutions, solutions, or suspensions in a glass-like carrier, amorphous precipitates in a crystalline carrier substance, composite, or complexed compounds. They contain the active ingredient in finely dispersed form in an inert, likewise solid carrier substance. After rapid dissolution of the hydrophilic matrix, an enormous surface area (even culminating to that of individual active drug molecules) becomes available for transfer into the solvent. These improved dissolution conditions thus rely on the finely disperse distribution, and occasionally also on the interactions between drug and polymer carrier (e.g., solubilizing properties of the carrier material). Most notably, however, they may find their cause in the conversion of a crystalline substance into an amorphous state.

During preparation of solid dispersions containing metastable (e.g., amorphous) material, care should be taken that product properties do not alter in time due to transition to a more stable state.

3.11 Interfacial Phenomena

An interface is the contact area between two different phases of either identical or different chemical and/or physical nature (e.g., water/oil or ice/water). Interfaces can therefore exist as solid/solid, solid/liquid, solid/gas systems (solid interfaces) but also as liquid/liquid and liquid/gas systems (liquid interfaces). In case one of the phases is a gas, the corresponding interface is called a *surface*. At interfaces physicochemical properties change abruptly, sometimes leading to quite complex interfacial phenomena that may also be relevant with respect to the manufacturing of medicines.

Solid/solid interfaces arise, for example, during the preparation of solid dispersions or of suspension suppositories. Processes at solid/liquid interfaces are highly significant during dissolution processes (see section 3.9 and 3.10) and in the stabilization of suspensions (see section 19.3, 19.4). Solid surfaces can serve for instance as a target surface for adsorption processes from the gas phase, such as those occurring during adsorption of water vapor or during the assessment of the specific surface area of powdered substances by means of gas adsorption. Processes at the liquid/liquid interface are crucial during the formation and stabilization of emulsions (see section 18.3, 18.4), while the properties of liquid surfaces are for instance relevant with respect to the process of droplet formation (e.g., during spray drying).

Several interfacial processes involve not just two, but rather three phases. This relates for instance to *wetting processes* at solid or fluid interfaces by a liquid. Such processes occur, for example, during processing of powdery substances with liquids, the distribution of fluid coating formulations on tablet surfaces or the emptying of injection vials.

Surfactants play a special role in connection with interfacial phenomena (see section 5.4 and 18.4) because of their tendency to accumulate at interfaces (*interfacial activity*).

Specific problems regarding individual interfacial phenomena will be dealt with in the corresponding chapters. In the following section, merely the basic principles of interfacial tension and wetting will be discussed, as well as the pertaining assay procedures.

Ph. Eur. 2.9.45 Wettability of Porous Solids Including Powders _____

Wettability of solid surfaces is characterized by the contact angle. That is the angle formed by the edge of a cross-sectional representation of a fluid droplet on a solid surface with that surface. The European Pharmacopeia describes a direct and an indirect method to determine this angle.

Sessile Drop Method

The direct method deploys a goniometer with which a liquid droplet can be sized in lateral view. The droplet is formed upon deposition of a defined volume of fluid on the surface to be investigated (e.g., a tablet or a film coating) by means of a microliter pipette. For the examination of a powder a flat smooth surface is produced by compacting a powder sample. Wetting properties may, however, be altered by this procedure since, due to a change in crystalline structure, the free surface energy may increase. Porous surfaces, into which the fluid may quickly penetrate, are hard to characterize by means of this method. For this purpose, the Washburn method is more suitable.

The Washburn Method

The Washburn method (*Edward W. Washburn, 1881–1934*) is an indirect procedure to determine the contact angle of porous substances in the range of 0° to 90°. It involves the measurement of the rate at which a liquid penetrates a compacted powder bed. The sample holder may be either a small glass cylinder which at the bottom side is closed off with a glass frit, or an aluminum cylinder with holes in the bottom plate.

After covering the bottom of the tube with a filter disk and filling the sample holder by approximately two-thirds its volume with the material to be examined, the surface of the powder bed is covered with a filter disk and the stamp of the device is put in place to compress the powder. Compaction can be achieved by means of a tapped density tester or by centrifugation (*A tapped density tester consists of a graduated cylinder located vertically in a fixture which is slidingly mounted on a snail cam. As the cam rotates, the cylinder is repeatedly raised and allowed to drop under its own weight a specific distance*). The loaded sample holder is attached to the load cell of the instrument, which is constructed like the assembly of a ring tensiometer. Similar to the latter, it possesses a height-adjustable liquid-filled vessel, which is pulled up to a height just allowing the liquid surface to touch the powder bed. While the fluid penetrates into the powder bed, the mass increase is recorded as a function of time. The ratio of the square of the mass of liquid m soaked up and the time t required for this is part of a material constant, which includes, among others, the cosinus of the contact angle θ. Solved for cos θ results in the following relation:

$$\cos\theta = \frac{m^2}{t} \cdot \frac{\eta}{c \cdot \rho^2 \cdot \gamma}$$

in which η represents the viscosity of the liquid, ρ its density, γ its surface tension and c the material constant, which depends on the pore structure of the powder. The material constant is determined by performing the measurement in liquids like n-heptane, or hexamethyl disiloxane for which a contact angle of 0° (cos 0° = 1) can be assumed. After substitution of cos 0° and the other parameters of the applied liquid into the equation it is solved for c. When the material constant is known, the contact angle can be calculated from the measured data for other liquids.

3.11.1 Interfacial Tension and Surface Tension

The intermolecular interactions at the interface of two phases are clearly different from those in the pure phase and result in the phenomenon of *interfacial tension* γ or, as a special case, *surface tension* σ. The surface tension of a liquid originates from the mutual attraction of the liquid molecules. As each molecule in the bulk liquid is equally affected by all its surrounding molecules, the mutual attraction forces fully compensate each other (Fig. 3-44). At the surface, however, not all these forces can be compensated, as the interactions with the molecules of the gas phase (in most cases air) are only weak. The resulting inward-directed force, perpendicular to the liquid surface, causes the surface tension. The molecules at the surface will yield to the inward pull, until the surface area has reached a minimal value. As long as gravitation or other forces do not disturb the system, the liquid phase under consideration will adopt a spherical shape (e.g., droplets in an emulsion or in free fall), because the geometric body with the smallest surface-to-volume ratio is a sphere. Often, however, additional forces are involved. For example, a water droplet on a nonwettable solid surface will spread out (and thus be deformed) to some extent by gravity.

Enlargement of a liquid surface area requires energy (Fig. 3-45). This is called *free surface energy* and is equal to the product of surface tension σ and surface area increase. The surface or interfacial tension σ (γ) is thus defined as the amount of mechanical work that is required to enlarge a surface or interface under isothermal and isobaric conditions by one surface area unit:

$$\sigma = \frac{\Delta W}{\Delta A} \left(\frac{J}{m^2} = \frac{N}{m} \right) \tag{3-32}$$

ΔW = mechanical work /energy to be spent

ΔA = increase of surface or interfacial area

The functioning of surface tension can be elegantly illustrated by means of a lamella of liquid stretched out in a wireframe, one of the sides of which can be moved to vary the surface area of the lamella (see figure).

The area increase $\Delta A = 2 \cdot l \cdot \Delta s$. Mind that the liquid lamella has two surfaces thus explaining the factor 2. In order to enlarge the surface area, the action of a force F along the distance Δs is required to produce an amount of (surface) work $\Delta W = F \cdot \Delta s$. Taking into consideration the definition of surface tension (equation 3-32), the surface tension σ can now be calculated as follows:

$$\sigma = \Delta W / \Delta A = F \Delta s / 2 \cdot l \cdot \Delta s = F / 2 \cdot l$$

Considering the situation at the wireframe, we may conclude that the surface tension may also be expressed as force per unit of length. Accordingly, the force F_σ acting along a contact line of length l (in this case the length of the movable side) results from the surface tension as follows:

$$F_\sigma = \sigma \cdot l$$

This consideration is applied to describe the conditions in several methods used to determine surface or interfacial tension. Also the wireframe method can be used to assess surface tension by means of a suitable experimental set up (wireframe method according to Lenard) but is not commonly employed.

The values of the interfacial tensions prevailing in the pharmaceutical field for liquid interfaces vary from 0 to 80 mN/m. The surface tension of water at 20°C, for example, amounts

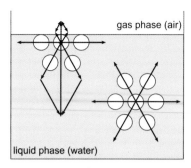

Fig. 3-44 Force impact on a molecule at the surface and in the bulk of a liquid.

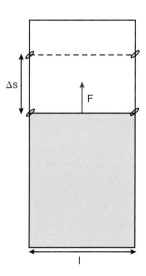

Fig. 3-45 Example of surface tension action.

Table 3-13 Examples of Surface or Interfacial Tension at 20°C.

Substance	Surface Tension (mN/m)	Interfacial Tension versus Water (mN/m)
Water	72.8	–
Glycerol	63	–
Ethanol	22	–
Chloroform	27	33
Olive oil	36	23
Mercury	476	375

Table 3-14 Development of Surface Parameters during Fragmentation of a Water Droplet of 1 cm Diameter into Smaller Fragments

Droplet Diameter	Number of Droplets	Total Surface Area of All Droplets	Volume-Specific Surface	Surface Energy of Entire System
1 cm	1	3.14 cm^2	6 cm^{-1}	0.02287 mJ
1 mm	10^3	31.4 cm^2	60 cm^{-1}	0.2287 mJ
100 μm	10^6	314 cm^2	600 cm^{-1}	2.287 mJ
10 μm	10^9	$3,140 \text{ cm}^2$	$6,000 \text{ cm}^{-1}$	22.87 mJ
1 μm	10^{12}	$31,400 \text{ cm}^2$	$60,000 \text{ cm}^{-1}$	228.7 mJ
100 nm	10^{15}	$314,000 \text{ cm}^2$	$600,000 \text{ cm}^{-1}$	$2,287 \text{ mJ}$

to 72.8 mN/m (table 3-13). That means that $72.8 \cdot 10^{-7}$ J is required to enlarge the area of a water surface by 1 cm^2. The value of the interfacial or surface tension is determined by the differences between the potential molecular interactions in the bulk of the phase under consideration (cohesion forces) as compared to those between the molecules of the two phases involved across the interface (adhesion forces).

The larger these differences are, the higher the interfacial or surface tension. That is why the surface tension of a solid body is higher than that of the liquid form. Due to its hydrogen bonds, water has an exceptionally high surface tension when compared to other solvents. Interfacial tensions between two liquid phases commonly have values in between the surface tensions of the individual liquids. In case of exceptional interaction possibilities between the phases involved, values below the surface tensions of either liquid are sometimes observed.

During fragmentation of a phase into smaller volume units, surface area increases strongly, causing energy to be stored in the newly formed surface area (Table 3-14). Due to the increasing ratio between surface area and volume of the material during the fragmentation, surface phenomena gradually play an increasingly important role. The system will try to counteract the increase in surface energy by diminishing its surface area. This is the very driving force of the destabilization of emulsions (see section 18.3).

The interfacial tension not only depends on the nature of the participating phases but may also be influenced by other factors. From a technological point of view, the most important influential factor is the addition of surface-active substances (surfactants), which reduce the surface tension and thus facilitate emulsifying and dispersion procedures. But also other dissolved components can change the surface tension of liquids. In addition, surface tension is temperature-dependent, which should be taken into consideration as well when performing assays of interfacial or surface tension.

3.11.2 Wetting

Wetting is a phenomenon that occurs notably at interfaces between solid bodies and liquids, such as in systems consisting of solid material, liquid, and gas. It is defined as the potential of a liquid to spread over the surface of a solid body. For pharmaceutical products, wettability of solids plays an important role, for instance during disintegration of tablets, in dissolution processes, and in dispersion and aggregation of solid materials. In addition, wetting is relevant for various methods by which surface tension is determined.

One measure of wettability is the *contact angle* (wetting angle) θ, which is formed at the contact line between a solid body and a liquid (Fig. 3-46). The degree of wettability depends on the ratio between the interfacial tensions solid/liquid ($\gamma_{s/l}$), solid/gas (air) ($\sigma_{s/g}$) and liquid/air ($\sigma_{l/g}$). At the droplet, between these interfacial tensions a state of equilibrium exists to which the Young equation applies (note that the vectors representing the interfacial tensions point parallel to or in the interface):

$$\sigma_{s/g} = \gamma_{s/l} + \sigma_{l/g} \cdot \cos \theta \tag{3-33}$$

The term $\sigma_{l/g} \cdot \cos \theta$ equals the perpendicular projection of the vector representing the liquid's surface tension. Thus, $\cos \theta$ describes the interactions between the three interfacial

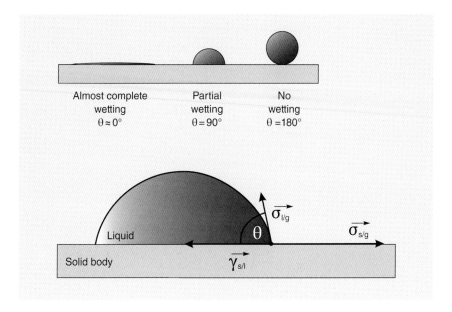

Fig. 3-46 Wetting of a solid surface by a liquid.

tensions. Several manifestations of the wetting state are conceivable (Fig. 3-46): when the contact angle equals 0°, we speak of complete wetting, while a contact angle of 180° signifies complete nonwettability.

Wetting conditions can also be expressed by comparison of adhesion and cohesion energy. The adhesion energy W_{adh} is the energy required to separate the system along the solid/liquid interface (or the energy that is released during the formation of the interface). It expresses therefore the interaction potential between liquid and solid. During separation of the system new solid/gas and liquid/gas interfaces are formed, while the solid/liquid interface disappears. In accordance with this the following equation applies:

$$W_{adh.}/A = \sigma_{s/g} + \sigma_{l/g} - \gamma_{s/l} \qquad (3\text{-}34)$$

The cohesion energy W_{coh} is a measure of the mutual interaction of the liquid molecules among each other. It can be expressed as the energy required to divide a certain volume of liquid in such a way that two new liquid/gas interfaces are formed:

$$W_{coh.}/A = 2\sigma_{l/g} \qquad (3\text{-}35)$$

When the adhesion energy is larger than the cohesion energy, the solid will be wetted by the liquid, while in the opposite case poor wetting will occur.

The equilibrium described by the Young equation (*Thomas Young*, 1773–1829) is time and temperature dependent. In practice, we distinguish the so-called advancing angle (wetting of the dry solid body) and the receding angle (starting from an already wetted solid surface). Conditions similar to those occurring during the wetting of solid surfaces are observed at liquid surfaces. Commonly, in such cases formation of a liquid lens is observed in the equilibrium state.

3.11.3 Methods to Investigate Interfacial Phenomena

For the measurement of interfacial and surface tensions of liquids, a wide variety of methods is available. Not all of them, though, are suitable for the measurement of both interfacial and surface tension. They can be distinguished in those where the size of the interface under consideration remains constant (static methods) and those in which the area of the interface changes (dynamic methods). With methods allowing control of area changes during

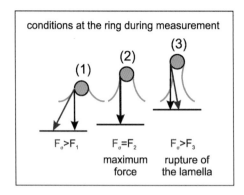

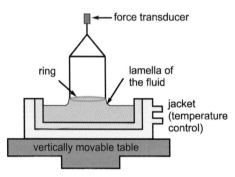

Fig. 3-47   Ring tensiometer.

measurement, kinetic processes can be investigated, such as the diffusion rate of surfactant molecules at newly formed interfaces.

All methods discussed in the following exploit a typical property of liquids, that is, their deformability. As a consequence, such methods are unsuited for determining interfacial tensions of solid bodies. As a rule, the latter are only amenable to indirect assay methods.

3.11.3.1   Ring Tensiometer Method According to du Noüy

This commonly used method (Fig. 3-47) is similar to the wireframe method described above (Fig. 3-45). A horizontally suspended ring of defined dimensions, commonly consisting of platinum/iridium wire, serves as a measuring bob. The material of the ring should be maximally wettable by the liquid to be investigated. The ring is immersed into the liquid and then brought in contact with its surface. Subsequently, the ring is pulled from the liquid (alternatively, the level of the liquid is lowered), causing the formation of an adhering lamella of liquid below the ring. The ring experiences now a downward force composed of the weight force F_w of the lamella of liquid below the ring (for which the measured value has to be corrected later) and a surface-tension-derived force F_σ acting on the ring along the wetted length.

$$F_\sigma = \sigma \cdot 2\pi (r_i + r_0) \cdot \cos\theta$$
$$\sigma = \frac{F_\sigma}{2\pi \cdot (r_i + r_0) \cdot \cos\theta} \tag{3-36}$$

σ = surface tension of the liquid

r_i, r_0 = inner resp. outer radius of the ring ($2\pi \cdot (r_i + r_0)$: wetted length l of the ring)

θ = contact angle (at complete wetting (ideal case) $\theta = 0$)

Principle of the Ring Method

The force that pulls the ring downward will be maximal when the force vector acting on the ring as a result of the surface tension is exactly perpendicular to the liquid's surface, or the plane of the ring (Fig. 3-47). When, after reaching the maximal force, the ring is pulled further out of the liquid, the liquid lamella will tear.

The maximal force measured immediately before the liquid lamella breaks is taken as the outcome value. For the determination of the interfacial tension this value needs to be corrected for the weight of the liquid lamella hanging from the ring (in practice, a correction factor is commonly applied for that purpose; in modern equipment the force is determined by means of a digital balance system, which also allows to measure the force just before the lamella breaks):

$$\sigma = \frac{F_{max} - F_W}{2\pi \cdot (r_i + r_0) \cdot \cos\theta} \qquad (3\text{-}37)$$

F_{max} = total force acting on the ring immediately before the lamella breaks
F_W = weight force resulting from the liquid lamella
r_i, r_0 = radii of the ring
θ = wetting angle

The ring method also allows for the determination of interfacial tensions; for that purpose the ring is placed at the interface between two liquid phases instead of at a liquid surface.

3.11.3.2   Wilhelmy Plate Method

In this method, instrumental arrangement and force assessment correspond to those of the ring method. Instead of the ring, however, a thin roughened platinum plate (Wilhelmy plate) of defined dimensions is used (Fig. 3-48).

For the measurement, the plate is dipped briefly into the liquid to ascertain that it is maximally wetted. When using a roughened platinum platelet, wetting is usually complete—that is, the contact angle θ equals 0. Subsequently, the plate is pulled up from the liquid until the lower side is at the level of the meniscus. Due to the surface tension, a downward force F_σ now acts on the plate along the wetted length, which can be assessed by means of the balance system.

$$F_\sigma = \sigma \cdot l \cdot \cos\theta \text{ respectively } \sigma = \frac{F_\sigma}{l \cdot \cos\theta} \qquad (3\text{-}38)$$

l = wetted length (circumference) of the plate

With the Wilhelmy plate method no new surface area is formed during the assessment, so here we are dealing with a static procedure. Therefore, it is possible to assess time-dependent changes in surface tension with this method. Concomitantly, it also allows assessment of interfacial tensions. However, in this case, the buoyancy of the plate in the upper phase must be taken into account. Instruments of this kind also allow the assessment of wetting angles

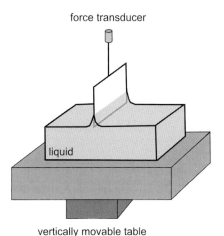

force transducer

liquid

vertically movable table

Fig. 3-48 Principle of the plate method.

($<90°$) when a liquid of known surface tension and, instead of the platinum plate, a sample of the solid under consideration are used.

The contact angle is calculated from the following equation:

$$\cos \theta = \frac{F_\sigma}{\sigma \cdot l} \tag{3-39}$$

3.11.3.3 Drop Volume Method and Drop Weight Method

With this dynamic method both surface tension and interfacial tension can be determined. To that end, a defined volume or mass of a test liquid is allowed to drip from a capillary tube with defined outflow tip surface area and the number of drops formed from this amount of liquid is determined. The size of the droplets formed (i.e., their number per sample volume) depends on the surface or interfacial tension of the liquid with respect to its surrounding medium. The drop formed at the tip of the capillary grows until the weight force F_w acting on it outweighs the force F_σ caused by the surface or interfacial tension and thus the drop falls off.

The conditions at the site of drop formation are often difficult to define physically accurately. Therefore, in practice, often relative measurements are performed using calibration liquids (e.g., water).

For that purpose, a *stalagmometer according to Traube* is often used, a calibrated glass capillary with a horizontal surface-ground narrow end extension to facilitate drop formation. The method exploits the proportionality between interfacial tension on one hand and mass, volume, or number of droplets formed, on the other hand. The larger the size of the droplets (i.e., the smaller the number of droplets per volume of fluid), the higher is the surface tension. From the number of droplets Z_x formed from a given volume of test liquid and that formed from of the calibration fluid Z_C, the surface tension σ_x of the test liquid can be calculated:

$$\frac{\sigma_x}{\sigma_c} = \frac{m_x}{m_c} = \frac{V_x \cdot \rho_x}{V_c \cdot \rho_c} = \frac{z_c}{z_x} \cdot \frac{\rho_x}{\rho_c}$$

$$\sigma_x = \frac{Z_c}{Z_x} \cdot \frac{\rho_x}{\rho_c} \cdot \sigma_c \tag{3-40}$$

σ_x, σ_c = surface tension of test and calibration liquid, respectively

m_x, m_c = droplet mass of test and calibration liquid, respectively

V_x, V_c = droplet volume of test and calibration liquid, respectively

ρ_x, ρ_c = density of test and calibration liquid, respectively

z_x, z_c = number of droplets formed from a given volume of test and calibration liquid, respectively

In this procedure, it is assumed that wetting conditions at the outlet of the capillary are not significantly different for test and calibration liquid, respectively. However, this often does not apply to aqueous surfactant solutions. In addition, because of the rapid drop formation in the stalagmometer, the adsorption equilibrium of the surfactant on the newly formed surface area is often not reached quickly enough. As a consequence, the stalagmometer is mainly suited for the assessment of surface tensions of pure liquids.

The conditions described for the stalagmometer also apply to the droppers, described in the pharmacopeias for dosing liquids (e.g., essential oils or stock solutions). Also, in this case, the size of the droplets depends on density and surface tension of the liquid to be dosed, necessitating calibration of the apparatus for each individual liquid used.

Ph. Eur. 2.1.1 Droppers _____

USP $\langle 1101 \rangle$ Medicine Dropper

In magistral preparations small volumes of liquid are often dosed dropwise. Since droplet mass depends, among others, on shape and size of the drop outlet, exact dosing is only possible with a standardized dropper. The droppers described in Ph. Eur. and USP consist of a glass tube (USP also allows other transparent material) which is constricted at the delivery end to a circular opening with an external diameter of about 3 mm. While this is the only dimensional requirement specified by the USP, the Ph. Eur. includes a detailed drawing with further specifications for shape and dimensions. The droppers of both pharmacopeias are designed to provide water droplets with a weight of 50 mg. According to USP the volume error should not exceed 15%, the Ph. Eur. requests an accuracy of even ±5%. Most medicinal liquids do not have the same surface tension and viscosity characteristics as water, and therefore drop size will vary from one preparation to another. In the German Drug Codex (DAC), a table can be found with the drop masses of important liquids applied in drug formulations.

3.11.3.4 Bubble Pressure Method

The bubble pressure method is based on measurement of the pressure in a capillary from which an air bubble is blown into a liquid (Fig. 3-49). The method exploits the dependence of the pressure in the bubble on its radius (*curvature pressure, Laplace pressure*). This phenomenon is described by the Gauss-Laplace equation:

$$P_c = \frac{2\sigma}{r} \tag{3-41}$$

P_C = curvature pressure of the bubble
r = radius of curvature of the bubble

The curvature pressure of the bubble and the hydrostatic pressure (depending on the immersion depth) acting on it are in equilibrium with the mechanical counter pressure that is coming along with bubble formation. During bubble formation, the radius of curvature diminishes continuously so that curvature pressure gradually increases. It will be maximal when the radius of the bubble reaches that of the capillary. From the measured maximal pressure, the surface tension of the liquid can be calculated:

$$p_m = p_c + p_h = \frac{2\sigma}{r} + \rho \cdot g \cdot h \text{ respectively}$$
$$\sigma = \frac{r}{2} \cdot (p_m - \rho \cdot g \cdot h) \tag{3-42}$$

p_m = mechanical counter pressure
p_h = hydrostatic pressure
ρ = density of the fluid
h = immersion depth
g = gravity

The bubble pressure method can also be applied for the measurement of the interfacial tension between two liquids. Instead of an air bubble, a drop of the "foreign" liquid is then forced into the measurement liquid.

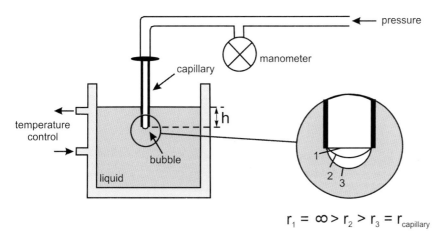

$$r_1 = \infty > r_2 > r_3 = r_{capillary}$$

Fig. 3-49 Bubble pressure method.

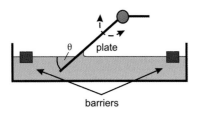

Fig. 3-50 Method of the tilted plate.

3.11.4   Measurement of Contact Angles

3.11.4.1   Sessile Drop Method

A defined amount of liquid is placed on the solid surface. Subsequently, contact angle measurements can be performed by means of microscopic observation, projection of an enlarged image of the drop on a screen, by photography or by reflection of a light beam at the edge of the droplet, while at the point of contact between liquid and solid a tangent is constructed (Fig. 3-46). By increasing or decreasing the size of the droplet (e.g., by means of a syringe), the advancing and receding angles can be determined.

3.11.4.2   Method of the Tilted Plate

In this method a slab or sheet ("plate") of the material to be assayed or coated with it (e.g., an object slide coated with ointment) is put on one side in the temperature-controlled fluid (e.g., water). The position of the plate with respect to the liquid surface is altered in such a way that the liquid surface shows no curvature up to the contact line with the plate. The angle of the slope of the plate, which can be read by means of a goniometer, corresponds to the contact angle. By successive rotation of the holder as represented in Fig. 3-50, the advancing as well as the receding angle can be determined. The advancing contact angle is determined by immersion of the part of the plate that has not yet been in contact with the liquid, while the receding contact angle is determined at the part of the surface that has just been lifted from the liquid. When applying this method, any contaminations of the liquid surface with surface-active substances can be eliminated by just pushing them aside with a barrier placed on the surface.

3.11.4.3   The Washburn Method

In case of wetting systems (contact angle $<90°$), the wetting angle can also be determined on powdered substances. For this purpose, the Washburn method employs the capillary action of a powder bed that has been compacted under controlled conditions. From the infiltration rate of the fluid the wetting angle can be calculated when viscosity, density, and surface tension are known. A prerequisite for this assay is, however, the prior determination of a material constant of the powder bed with the aid of perfectly wetting fluids.

3.12   Rheology

Rheology describes the flow properties of substances and systems prepared thereof. It comprises the physical laws concerning flow and deformation of liquids, semi-solid systems, and in a broader sense also of solid bodies (see section 3.2.6). As such, it plays a major role in every possible step in the development of pharmaceutical products.

3.12.1   Viscous Flow

In order to make substances flow, the interactions between the constituting molecules (internal friction) have to be overcome. The resistance that counteracts the flow of a substance is characterized by the *viscosity* η.

3.12.1.1   Ideal Viscous Flow

To visualize the events during the flow of a substance one can envisage the liquid as a stack of parallel sheets (Fig. 3-51). When a force F acts on the upper sheet of liquid with an area A, the sheet will be shifted with a certain velocity v in the direction of the force. The sheets underneath will also move but, because of the frictional resistance, for each consecutive sheet with decreasing velocity. The lowest sheet of liquid will ultimately remain in place. In order to move the upper sheet with a certain velocity with respect to the lower sheet a force is

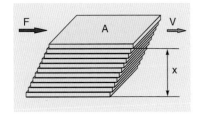

Fig. 3-51 Stack of cards model.

therefore required to overcome the frictional resistance. The latter results from Newton's law as follows:

$$\frac{F}{A} = \eta \frac{dv}{dx} \qquad (3\text{-}43)$$

F = force acting on the fluid (N)
A = surface area of the fluid sheet (m^2)
η = dynamic viscosity of the fluid (Pa · s)
v = velocity of the fluid sheet (m/s)
x = distance between the sheet under consideration and the lowest, stationary sheet (m)

The ratio F/A is designated the *shear stress* τ, the differential quotient dv/dx is known as the *shear rate* or *velocity gradient* D. Equation 3-43 can thus be simplified to:

$$\tau = \eta \cdot D \text{ respectively } \eta = \frac{\tau}{D} \qquad (3\text{-}44)$$

τ = shear stress (N/m^2)
D = shear rate (s^{-1})

The proportionality factor between shear stress and shear rate represents the *dynamic viscosity* η (unit: Pa · s or mPa · s). Dividing the dynamic viscosity by the density of the test liquid yields the so-called kinematic viscosity v (m^2/s). Liquids with a flow behavior obeying Newton's law are called *ideally viscous liquids* or *Newtonian liquids*. In such cases, viscosity is a constant. Ideal flow behavior like this is observed, for example, in pharmaceutically used solvents such as water, ethanol, glycerol, and fatty oils, as well as their molecularly dispersed solutions (e.g., salt, sugar and active agent solutions (Table 3-15)). Also systems that exhibit plastic flow at room temperature, such as fats and petrolatum, can display ideally viscous behavior in molten form.

When plotting shear stress τ against shear rate D for ideally viscous fluids, a straight line through the origin is obtained with a slope that is a measure of the dynamic viscosity (Fig. 3-52). Plotting η against τ or D yields a horizontal straight line, allowing estimation of η by one single measurement.

Also systems consisting of an ideally viscous liquid containing finely dispersed isometric particles may display Newtonian flow in case the volume contribution of the dispersed phase is relatively small (<1%). In this case an increase in viscosity is observed with respect to that of the solvent (η_0). According to Einstein, this increase depends on the volume contribution Φ of the dispersed phase:

$$\eta = \eta_0 (1 + 2.5\Phi) \qquad (3\text{-}45)$$

η = dynamic viscosity of the dispersion (mPa · s)
η_0 = dynamic viscosity of the solvent (mPa · s)

Table 3-15 Viscosities of Different Liquids

Substance	Viscosity (mPa · s) at 20°C
chloroform	0.56
water	1.00
ethanol	1.19
blood	4–15 (at 37°C!)*
medium-chain triglycerides	~ 30
light liquid paraffine	25–80
liquid paraffin	110–230
olive oil	~ 100
castor oil	~ 1000

*The value for blood is given for the sake of comparison although blood is not an ideally viscous fluid

More concentrated dispersions or dispersions with anisometric particles (which can be formed, for example, by deformation of emulsion droplets) display, on the other hand, a flow behavior that is dependent on the shearing load.

The viscosity of liquids barely depends on pressure, but is strongly dependent on temperature. In contrast to gases, viscosity of liquids diminishes with increasing temperature, because the interaction forces between the individual molecules decrease. The temperature-dependent viscosity change follows the relation

$$\mathrm{Log}\,\eta \sim \frac{1}{T} \quad (T\colon \text{ absolute temperature (K)}).$$

3.12.1.2   Non-Newtonian Flow

In many systems, viscosity depends on the applied shear stress, or, when applicable, on the prevailing velocity gradient. Shear stress and velocity gradient are not linearly proportional to one another. A comprehensive characterization of the flow behavior of such non-Newtonian bodies requires recording of a complete flow curve. To each point of this curve a viscosity value can be assigned, the *apparent viscosity*. Essentially three idealized shear load-dependent flow types can be distinguished: pseudo-plastic (shear-thinning), dilatant (shear-thickening) and plastic flow (Fig. 3-52).

3.12.1.3   Pseudo-Plastic (Shear-Thinning) Flow

Like Newtonian fluids, *pseudo-plastic systems flow* already at the lowest possible shear stress (origin of the flow curve in point zero). Their viscosity decreases, however, with increasing shear challenge and the system will become more fluid (shear thinning). Typical representatives of this group are solutions with linearly shaped macro molecules (e.g., fluid preparations of cellulose derivatives and natural gums) and suspensions of anisometric particles.

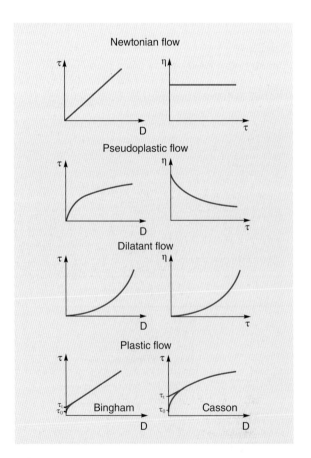

Fig. 3-52 Flow behavior.

Upon increasing shear challenge, the initially nonordered molecules or structural elements in these systems orient themselves in the flow direction so that the internal resistance against the flow diminishes, in other words viscosity decreases. Referring to Newton's law, this can be approximated with $\tau = k_1 \cdot D^n$ ($n < 1$), where the value of n characterizes deviation from ideally viscous (Newtonian) flow. The parameter k_1 represents the flow coefficient.

From the moment when the orientation process has finished, viscosity remains constant, meaning that the flow curve transforms into a straight line (*infinite shear viscosity*). Also at low shear challenge, when movement of the molecules or structural elements is still fast enough to counteract the orientation effect, a Newtonian viscosity value is observed (*zero shear viscosity*).

Also emulsions or liquids containing aggregated particles may display pseudo-plastic flow. In that case increasing fluidity can be explained by deformation of the emulsion droplets or by a dis-aggregation process: the dispersion liquid contained within the aggregates will be partially set free and become available for the flow process.

3.12.1.4 Dilatant (Shear-Thickening) Flow

Dilatant systems are characterized by the condition that their viscosity increases with shear challenge, bringing along increased resistance against flow. Dilatency can thus be seen as the opposite of pseudo-plastic behavior. This phenomenon is rather rarely observed in pharmaceutical preparations; it is displayed by dispersions with an extremely high (typically >50%) proportion of solid material (e.g., highly concentrated starch suspensions and pastes). Under shear challenge the particles in highly concentrated dispersions start to engage in a rotating motion, which in case of anisometric particles causes a demand for more space. As a result, the volume of available free dispersion liquid diminishes and flow-hampering interactions between individual particles occur. At higher shear load, the coating of the particles with dispersion liquid, which acts as a lubricating film, may be lost, which additionally increases viscosity. In extreme cases, a total lack of flow may occur, causing the system to behave like an elastic solid body (e.g., wet sand). Dilatant behavior should therefore be taken into consideration, for example, during mixing processes in order to prevent overstressing of the equipment.

3.12.1.5 Plastic Flow

Plastic bodies have a yield value. Therefore, a minimal shear stress must act on the system in order to initiate a flow process. At lower shear stresses the plastic body behaves as a solid but elastic substance. This behavior can be explained by the presence of a coherent structure in the system (e.g., as a result of interparticulate or intermolecular interactions). This structure first has to be broken down to allow initiation of a flow process. Such flow behavior is of pharmaceutical interest, for example, in case of formulations for dermal application. These systems should form a soft strand upon being squeezed from a tube but subsequently allow distribution on the skin upon application of appropriate mechanical force.

Below the practical yield value, τ_0 bodies with plastic flow behavior behave like a solid body. After exceeding the yield value, they can display different types of behavior. When, shortly after onset, flow proceeds like for a Newtonian fluid (entirely straight "curve"), we are dealing with a *Bingham* or *ideally plastic body*. In this case, the system can be characterized unequivocally by providing the yield value and the viscosity value calculated from the slope of the straight part of the curve (plastic viscosity according to Bingham, η_B, a constant). Because direct assessment of the practical yield value is difficult, commonly shear stress is rather used. This can be obtained by extrapolation of the straight part of the curve to the τ axis and is then called the *theoretical yield value*.

When, by contrast, the sample displays a curved τ/D relation, we are dealing with a *Casson* or *non-ideally plastic body*. In this case, viscosity values (plastic viscosity according to Casson, η_C) calculated from the slopes of the corresponding curves will depend on the prevailing shear conditions.

After an initially structure-related viscous behavior, also Casson bodies ultimately display mostly ideally viscous behavior upon a further increase of the shear stress. Extrapolation of the straight part of the τ/D plot to the τ axis will yield a theoretical yield value τ_t which, like the practical yield value, is used to characterize such plastic systems.

Genuine Bingham bodies occur rarely and do not play a significant role in pharmaceutics. In contrast, many semi-solid pharmaceutical preparations (ointments, creams, gels, and most pastes) are Casson bodies.

3.12.2   Thixotropy and Other Time-Dependent Effects

The often-observed decrease in viscosity occurring upon the application of shear stress finds its basis in a disruption of internal structures in the system under consideration. Such structures are often not immediately reestablished when the shear stress is reduced, but regenerate only slowly. This time-dependent reconstruction of texture under isothermal conditions, which can be observed in systems with plastic and pseudo-plastic flow behavior, is known as thixotropy. Viscosity of thixotropic systems not only depends on the intensity of the applied shear challenge (e.g., the applied shear stress) but also on its duration (Fig. 3-53). When, for example, an ointment sample is continuously challenged mechanically for a certain amount of time, viscosity will drop to a certain final value, as a result of the destruction of the internal network. When the stressed system is subsequently left to stand, the initial viscosity will be restored after some time (*regeneration time*), as the internal structure is gradually rebuilt. In many cases, such as with bentonite gels, shear may lead to complete destruction of the internal structure (fluidization), which nonetheless is reversible (gel-sol-gel conversion). Irreversible shear-induced destruction of the network, as is observed, for instance, in gelatin gels, is called *rheo-destruction*.

Thixotropic and rheo-destructive behavior are reflected in a rheogram in the sense that the ascending and descending τ/D curves (obtained by continuously increasing respectively decreasing shear load) do not coincide. At identical shear stress, the descending curve shows a steeper slope due to the diminished viscosity, leading to a hysteresis effect (Fig. 3-53).

Under appropriately normalized assay conditions and under exclusion of rheo-destruction the hysteresis area between the two curves may serve as a simple measure of the degree of thixotropy. Flow behavior of all systems with time-dependent rheological behavior strongly

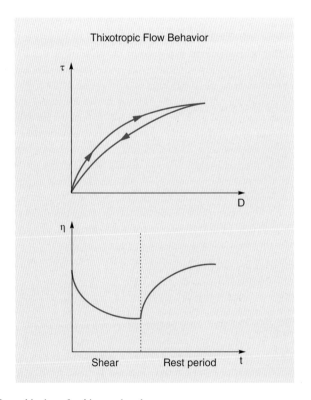

Fig. 3-53 Shear thinning of a thixotropic substance.

depends on the rheological pretreatment. Reproducible results of rheological investigations can therefore be obtained only under strictly identical conditions (including sample preparation).

Ointments are among the substances possessing a less or more pronounced rheo-destructive and partially thixotropic behavior. For the stability of fluid dispersions (e.g., suspensions for oral administration), pronounced thixotropy can be of great benefit. Ideally, such systems, when in rest, show a very high viscosity or yield value, in order to suppress sedimentation of the dispersed particles and thus secure homogeneity during prolonged storage. When they are shaken they change into a fluid state for a length of time sufficient to allow taking a sample from the container and application. Subsequently, the system remaining in the container gradually regains its (highly viscous) resting state appearance.

In addition to thixotropy, other time-dependent rheological phenomena are known, which however are rarely encountered in pharmaceutical systems. An example is rheopexy, the phenomenon that with increasing shear time a reversible structure building occurs.

3.12.3 Measuring Instruments

Because an ideally viscous liquid possesses a viscosity that is independent of the applied shear load or velocity gradient, it is not absolutely necessary to construct a rheogram in order to characterize its flow properties; rather, a single-point measurement will suffice. The comprehensive characterization of systems with a viscosity that depends on the prevailing shear load does require, however, construction of a complete flow curve. The presentation of one single viscosity value without specifying the measuring conditions is meaningless for such systems.

Precise and reproducible assessment of viscosity requires a laminar flow of the system to be investigated, because when turbulence occurs (Fig. 3-54), that is, when the critical Reynolds number is exceeded (see below), disturbing influences of unmanageable dimensions come into play. Under correct assay conditions, the most common instruments will allow production of a laminar flow. For all rheological studies precise temperature control is mandatory. Samples with time-dependent rheological behavior also require reproducible pretreatment (preshearing, resting time), particularly during filling of the assay system. Systems with temperature-sensitive structure (many ointment bases), require monitoring and recording of the thermic history of the sample (preparation temperature, storage conditions), because also thermally disrupted internal structures will only slowly regain their initial state.

The flow of liquids and gases can be laminar or turbulent (Fig. 3-54). While in case of laminar flow a liquid moves along ordered and approximately parallel streamlines, turbulent flow is characterized by formation of eddies (swirls). Turbulent flow is connected with increased energy input, which has to be taken into consideration, for example, in the transport of liquids through pipelines. It is difficult to predict when laminar flow changes into turbulent flow. Influential factors in this connection are particularly the dimensions and geometry of the system involved, as well as flow rate and viscosity of the flowing liquid. Low flow rate and high viscosity favor a laminar flow process. To estimate the situation of the transition between laminar and turbulent flow, commonly the dimensionless Reynold's number is applied:

$$\mathrm{Re} = v \cdot d \cdot \rho / \eta$$

v = average flow rate of the fluid
d = characteristic factor determined by flow-relevant dimensions of the system (e.g., diameter of the pipe through which or the sphere around which the liquid flows)
ρ = density of the liquid
η = dynamic viscosity of the liquid

For values below a critical Reynold's number, stable laminar flow may be expected. At higher values of Re, turbulence may come into play. Occasionally, also above the critical Reynold's number laminar flow may still be observed. This flow is, however, no longer stable and may,

laminar flow   turbulent flow

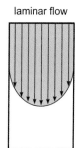 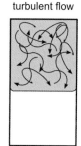

Fig. 3-54 Laminar and turbulent flow.

even at the tiniest disturbance, transform into turbulent flow. The Reynold's number is therefore suited to estimate up to what limit values in rheological measurement systems laminar flow may be expected to occur. The value of the critical Re value depends on the system under consideration. For flow in a smooth cylindrical pipe, the critical Re value amounts to approximately 2,300; for flow around a sphere, it is lower than 1.

3.12.4   Single-Point Assay Methods

3.12.4.1   Capillary Viscometer

In capillary viscometers, flow time of a defined volume of test liquid through a normalized capillary is measured. According to Hagen-Poiseuille's law, describing the velocity of the laminar flow of liquids in cylindrical tubes, flow time is directly proportional to viscosity:

$$\frac{V}{t} = \frac{\Delta p \cdot \pi \cdot r^4}{8 \cdot \eta \cdot l} \text{ respectively } \eta = \frac{\Delta p \cdot \pi \cdot r^4 \cdot t}{8 \cdot l \cdot V} \tag{3-46}$$

V = volume of liquid (m^3), flowing through the capillary in time t (s)

l = length of capillary (m)

r = radius of capillary (m)

Δp = pressure gradient between capillary ends (Pa)

The most common type of capillary viscometer is the Ubbelohde type with a vertically oriented capillary (Fig. 3-55). The attachment of a widening with an air inlet immediately below the capillary allows the outflow of the liquid against a constant pressure, the external air pressure. Therefore, the apparatus should not be filled with too large volumes of fluid. The hydrostatic pressure p at the upper end of the capillary follows from the height h of the liquid column above it, the density of the liquid ρ and the gravitational acceleration g: p = $\rho \cdot h \cdot g$. Because the height of the liquid column drops during the measurement, the average value h_m of initial and final height is introduced in the calculation.

This results in the following format of Hagen-Poiseuille's law:

$$\eta = \frac{\rho \cdot h_m \cdot g \cdot \pi \cdot r^4 \cdot t}{8 \cdot l \cdot V} \tag{3-47}$$

The instrument-specific parameters are usually combined in the instrument constant k.

$$k = \frac{h_m \cdot g \cdot \pi \cdot r^4}{8 \cdot l \cdot V} \tag{3-48}$$

k = instrument constant

h_m = average column height (m)

Viscosity can then be calculated by means of: $k \cdot t = v$ (kinematic viscosity) or $\rho \cdot k \cdot t = \rho \cdot v = \eta$ (dynamic viscosity). Determination of kinematic viscosity v is therefore possible by measuring outflow time without the need to involve other measured parameters, whereas for the determination of dynamic viscosity also the density of the liquid must be taken into account.

For different ranges of viscosity, viscometers with different capillary sizes are available, so that, by choosing a suitable viscometer, both laminar flow and sufficiently long measuring time can be ensured. Capillary viscometers allow very precise measurements of the viscosity of Newtonian liquids with relatively small sample sizes.

3.12.4.2   Falling Sphere Viscometer

In a falling sphere (or ball) viscometer, such as the common viscometer according to Höppler (Fig. 3-56), the dropping time of a ball in a liquid serves as the read out parameter. The fall of

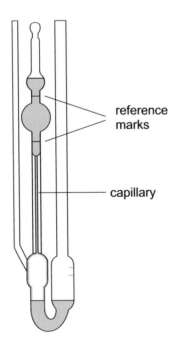

reference marks

capillary

Fig. 3-55 Capillary viscometer Ubbelohde type.

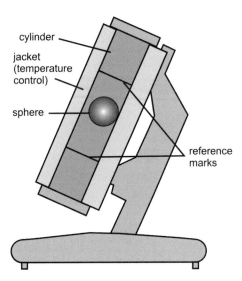

Fig. 3-56 Falling sphere viscometer according to Höppler.

a sphere with a smooth finish in a vertically positioned, infinitely wide tube, after reaching a constant falling velocity v, is described by Stokes' sedimentation law (*George Stokes* 1819–1903):

$$v = \frac{h}{t} = \frac{2}{9}\frac{(\rho_s - \rho_f) \cdot r^2 \cdot g}{\eta}$$
$$\eta = \frac{2}{9}\frac{(\rho_s - \rho_f) \cdot r^2 \cdot g \cdot t}{h}$$

(3-49)

v = velocity of the falling sphere (m/s)
h = height fallen (m) per unit of falling time t (s)
ρ_s = density of the sphere (kg/m^3)
ρ_f = density of the liquid (kg/m^3)
r = radius of the sphere (m)
g = gravitational acceleration (m/s^2)
η = dynamic viscosity of the liquid (mPa s)

Thus, dropping time of the sphere is proportional to the viscosity of the liquid. In the falling sphere viscometer after Höppler, Stokes' sedimentation law cannot, however, be rigorously applied, as the requirement that the sphere diameter should be very small relative to the tube diameter is not fulfilled (the sphere diameter is only slightly smaller than that of the tube).

In addition, the tube is positioned in a slanted way in order to ascertain stable movement of the sphere, implying that we are not dealing here with a free fall phenomenon. The deviations from Stokes' law resulting from this are taken into account by means of a sphere-dependent constant c, which also includes the instrument-specific constant parameters and h. With the help of these constants, which are determined by the manufacturer by calibration with standard oils, dynamic viscosity η can be obtained from the time t required for the sphere to travel the distance h according to the following equation:

$$\eta = c \cdot (\rho_s - \rho_f) \cdot t$$

(3-50)

This formula assumes, however, that the density of the test liquid is known; the density of the sphere will be given by the manufacturer. To allow for measurements on liquids in a wider viscosity range, spheres with different densities are available which may be selected in accordance with the properties of the liquid to be measured. Care should be taken that the sphere, before passing the first mark on the tube, has travelled the entire available distance from the upper end of the tube, in order to ascertain that at the start of the assay it has attained a constant velocity.

A disadvantage of the falling sphere viscometer is the usually quite large volume of liquid required.

3.12.5 Assay Systems for the Recording of Flow Curves

To recording a flow curve, the system has to be assayed under different shear stress conditions. This can be accomplished with a rotational viscometer in which the sample can be stressed either in an annular gap between two concentric cylinders (*cylinder method*, Fig. 3-57) or between a flat cone and a plate (*cone-plate method*, Fig. 3-58). Either the shear forces resulting from predetermined shear velocities are measured (*controlled rate*), or the shear velocities resulting from predetermined shear stress values are recorded (*controlled stress*).

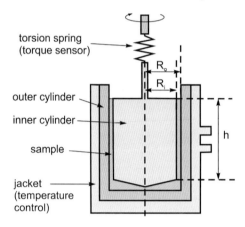

Fig. 3-57 **Rotating viscometer (concentric cylinder method).**

3.12.5.1 Rotating Viscometer (Rotational Viscometer)

Concentric Cylinders Method

Shearing occurs in an annular gap between a hollow cylinder (outer cylinder) and a solid cylinder placed inside it (inner cylinder), either one of which can be rotated, depending on the specific construction. In case the outer cylinder rotates at a predetermined velocity and torque is determined as a measure of the shear stress, we speak of a *Couette procedure*. However, in the instruments most commonly used nowadays, the sample is sheared by rotation of the inner cylinder, the torque of which is measured at the same time (*Searle principle*).

As a result of the rotation, a cylindrical laminar flow profile arises in the annular gap, leading to maximal velocity of the test substance at the surface of the rotating cylinder, while the velocity at the stationary cylinder equals 0. In contrast to the situation in the stack-of-cards model, the shear velocity in these instruments is not constant over the entire width of the gap, but diminishes in the Searle construction, for instance, from inside to outside. By using systems with the narrowest gap possible this complication can be reduced to a negligible level.

For determination of rheological properties only the conditions in the gap are relevant, while other influences on the acting torque should be maximally suppressed. Particularly, interactions of the bottom surface of the inner cylinder with the test material are important in this connection. They can be substantially reduced by inserting an expanded air bubble in the specially made bottom of the inner cylinder or they may be dealt with by correction factors.

Computational assessment of viscosity is carried out by means of the following equation. The instrument constant c is determined via the radii of the two cylinders (R_o and R_i, Fig. 3-57) and the cylinder height h.

$$\eta = \frac{c \cdot M}{\omega} \tag{3-51}$$

η = dynamic viscosity
ω = angular velocity
c = instrument constant
M = torque

Concentric cylinder systems are particularly suited to examine low or moderately viscous samples. Highly viscous samples or samples with a high yield value are difficult to introduce into the system in a homogeneous and reproducible manner. Samples of low-viscosity liquids need the employment of a special measurement body with maximized surface area (e.g., double gap), in order to achieve sufficient sensitivity. As a rule, measurements with the concentric-cylinder method require relatively large amounts of sample.

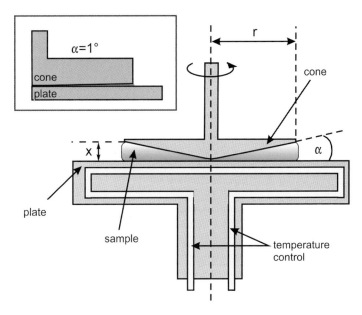

Fig. 3-58 Rotating viscometer (cone-plate method); note that the angle α is strongly exaggerated (see insert for realistic proportions).

Cone-Plate Method

Characterization of flow behavior of highly viscous and plastic systems usually requires the deployment of the cone-plate method (Fig. 3-58). A movable and very flat cone with truncated tip rotates on a stationary temperature-controlled and horizontally positioned plate. The cone can have variable radii and opening angles (e.g., $1°$–$4°$). In some cases, a second plate is used instead of the cone (*plate-plate method*). The cone is positioned so far down toward the plate that its (virtual) tip just touches it. The arising ring-shaped wedge is filled completely with the sample. Depending on the measuring mode the core rotates at a predetermined angular velocity and the torque M is determined. Alternatively, a torque M is applied and the resulting velocity measured. The shear stress then follows from the following relation:

$$\tau = \frac{3 \cdot M}{2 \cdot \pi \cdot r^3} \tag{3-52}$$

For the shear velocity applies, at each desired radius r_y:

$$D = \frac{\Delta v_y}{\Delta x_y} \text{ with } \Delta v_y = \omega \cdot r_y \text{ and } \Delta x_y = r_y \cdot \tan \alpha \tag{3-53}$$

v_y = orbital velocity of the cone at radius r_y
x_y = distance between cone and plate at radius r_y

This results in:

$$D = \frac{\omega}{\tan \alpha} \approx \frac{\omega}{\alpha} \tag{3-54}$$

The approximate numerical equality between tan α and α applies only for very small opening angles, which, in fact, are commonly used in this method.

Because increased orbital velocity for a larger cone radius is compensated by a larger height of the gap, the shear rate is constant over the entire gap space in a cone-plate instrument, but this does not apply for a plate-plate instrument. In addition to these better-defined measuring conditions, also the lower sample-size requirement and amount of work are clear advantages over the concentric cylinders method. For samples containing particulate constituents, the cone-plate method can be used only as long as particle size is considerably smaller than the gap at its narrowest site.

3.12.5.2   Assessment of Visco-Elastic Properties with the Oscillation Rheometer

During deformation, particularly semi-solid dosage forms display characteristics of viscous (liquid-like) as well as of elastic (solid-like) properties (*visco-elasticity*). Viscometers with a steadily rotating measurement body are only suitable for the investigation of viscous properties. Due to the forced flow movement, they are not capable of assessing any elastic properties that manifest themselves as resilience—for example, after removal of shear stress. However, investigation of visco-elastic properties is possible when the measurement body performs small sinusoidal rotational movements. In that case, the deflection is sufficiently low to ensure retention of the internal structure of the sample during shear.

To obtain information on the internal structure of the intact system, the time-dependent response of the system to an imposed oscillation is investigated. For example, in this way the time course of occurring shear stress as a function of deformation of the system may be determined.

Upon sinusoidal deformation, the relaxation behavior of the elastic body is reflected in a phase shift between stress and deformation. For purely elastic systems, which follow deformation without delay, the phase shift equals 0, while for purely viscous systems it is 90°. By means of elaborate analysis of the response curve, the contributions that are in phase with the applied oscillation or are shifted by 90°, respectively, are determined and from this a so-called *storage modulus* and a *loss modulus* are obtained**.** The storage modulus is an expression of the elasticity contribution of the properties of the system, while the loss modulus reflects its viscous properties.

Ph. Eur. 2.2.8–2.2.10, 2.2.49 Viscosity _____

USP ⟨911⟩, ⟨912⟩, ⟨913⟩ Viscosity

JP2.53 Viscosity Determination

In Ph. Eur. Chapter 2.2.8, "Viscosity," a number of general principles for viscosity determination are presented.

Capillary viscosimetry is described in Ph. Eur. 2.2.9 (Capillary Viscometer Method), USP ⟨911⟩ (Viscosity—Capillary Methods) and JP 2.53 (Viscosity Determination). While Ph. Eur. and JP only include suspended-level viscometers (= Ubbelohde-type viscometers), the USP describes application of this viscometer type only for method I and a simple U-tube viscometer (= Ostwald-type) for method II. The USP does not specify which capillary diameter should be chosen for a certain viscosity range. By contrast, Ph. Eur. lists 9 and JP lists 14 different viscometer sizes (with different instrument constants) each of them covering a specified viscosity range within the total range from 3.5 to 100,000 mm^2/s (Ph. Eur.) or from 1 to 100,000 mm^2/s (JP). A detailed description of the test procedure (e.g., temperature control, minimal passage time, time measurement) is provided by all pharmacopeias.

The falling sphere viscometer is only included in Ph. Eur. (2.2.49 Falling Ball Viscometer Method) and USP ⟨913⟩ Viscosity—(Rolling Ball Methods). These chapters contain a brief description of the instruments as well as detailed instructions for the assay procedure and evaluation.

Rotational viscosimetry is used for assessment of non-Newtonian systems. Information is provided in Ph. Eur. 2.2.10 (Rotating Viscometer Method), USP ⟨912⟩ (Viscosity -

Rotational methods) and JP 2.53 (Viscosity determination). All pharmacopeias include three types of rotational viscometers: Concentric cylinders viscometers (= USP method II), cone-plate viscometers (= USP method III), and spindle viscometers (= single cylinder-type rotational viscometers = Brookfield type viscometers, USP method I). The relevant details for the measurement, like viscometer type, angular velocity, or shear gradient to be applied, are specified in the relevant monographs referring to the method.

3.13 Physicochemical Characterization of Biologics

According to existing guidelines (cf. ICH Q6B, cf. Berkowitz et al. 2012), physicochemical characterization of biologics such as proteins or DNA demands, besides structural analysis, also investigation of aggregation phenomena. This is a major concern in producing biologics (especially proteins); aggregates can range from dimers to a size containing several billions of monomers. This can be analyzed by several methods already described in section 3.4. A useful overview on the application of these (and other) methods on biologics is available in Mahler et al. 2009 (see Fig. 3-59 for a graphical summary on detection methods for aggregation of biologics). The analysis of subvisible particulate matter in therapeutic protein injections by light obscuration and by microscopy is described in USP ⟨787⟩.

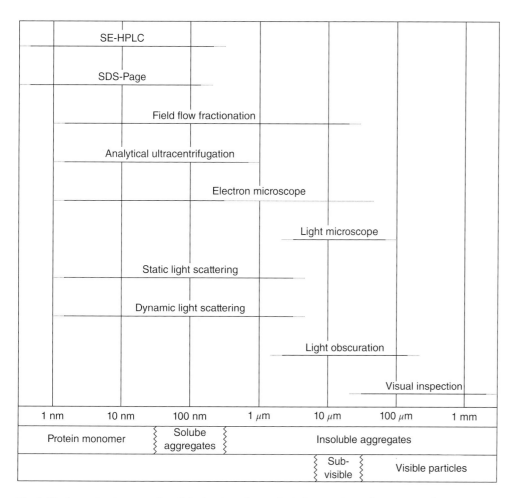

Fig. 3-59 Approximate range of particle size detection methods for proteins and aggregates of proteins. Reprinted from Mahler et al. 2009, © 2009 with permission from Elsevier; see end of chapter for reference.

Further Reading

Berkowitz, S. A., Engen, J. R., Mazzeo, J. R., and Jones, G. B. "Analytical Tools for Characterizing Biopharmaceuticals and the Implications for Biosimilars." *Nature Reviews Drug Discovery* 11(7) (2012): 527–540.

Brunauer, S., Emmett, P., and Teller, E. "Adsorption of gases in multimolecular layers." *J Am Chem Soc* 60 (1938): 309–319.

Byrn, S., Pfeiffer, R., Ganey, M., Hoiberg, C., and Poochikian, G. "Pharmaceutical solids: a strategic approach to regulatory considerations." *Pharmaceutical Research* 12(7) (1995): 945–954.

Filipe, V., Hawe, A., and Jiskoot, W. "Critical Evaluation of Nanoparticle Tracking Analysis (NTA) by NanoSight for the Measurement of Nanoparticles and Protein Aggregates." *Pharmaceutical Research* 27(5) (2010): 796–810.

Habraken, W. J., et al. "Ion-association complexes unite classical and non-classical theories for the biomimetic nucleation of calcium phosphate." *Nat Commun* 4 (2013): 1507.

Hildebrand, J. H. "Solubility." American Chemical Society. Monograph Series, New York: Chemical Catalog Company, 1924.

Horvath, H. "Gustav Mie and the scattering and absorption of light by particles: Historic developments and basics." *J Quant Spectrosc Radiat Transfer* 110(11) (2009): 787–799.

Lilienfeld, P. "Gustav Mie: the person." *Appl Opt* 30(33) (1991): 4696–4698.

Mahler, H. C., Friess, W., Grauschopf, U., and Kiese, S. "Protein aggregation: pathways, induction factors and analysis." *Journal of Pharmaceutical Sciences* 98(9) (2009): 2909–2934.

Mie, G. "Beiträge zur Optik trüber Medien, speziell kolloidaler Metallösungen[Contributions to the optics of turbid media, particularly of colloidal metal solutions)." *Annalen der Physik* 330(3) (1908): 377–445.

Tscharnuter, W. "Photon Correlation Spectroscopy in Particle Sizing." *Encyclopedia of Analytical Chemistry.* Chichester U.K.: John Wiley & Sons, 2000, 5469–5485.

Florence, A. F., and Attwood, D. *Physicochemical Principles of Pharmacy, In Manufacture, Formulations and Clinical Use,* 6th edition. London: Pharmaceutical Press, 2016.

Sterilization of Drug Formulations: Procedures to Reduce Microbial Count

4

4.1 General Introduction

Drug formulations that are not administered via the gastro-intestinal tract are often required to be sterile, that is, free of microorganisms. This holds true in particular in case of preparations for injection or infusion, but also for other drug formulations sterility may be required under specific conditions, for instance for solutions intended for bladder irrigation, eye drops, ointments and powders. Furthermore, sterility is required for syringes, cannulas, many bandage materials, clothes, and so on. Finally, vials or other containers for sterile drug formulations need to be sterile as well.

A large variety of microorganisms can cause diseases and therefore their presence in drug formulations is undesirable. But also nonpathogenic microorganisms can be detrimental to the activity of a drug product, for instance, by releasing metabolic or lysis products. Growth and multiplication of microorganisms require certain environmental conditions such as the availability of nutrients, temperature, pH, osmotic pressure, oxygen supply, humidity and light. When the required conditions are lacking the organism will not multiply and eventually die. A number of microorganisms (aerobic Bacillus strains, anaerobic Clostridiae) have the ability to form spores. Spores are highly durable forms of life that are able to withstand extreme conditions and to evolve again under favorable conditions into viable bacterial cells which can reproduce by growth and division.

The resistance of microorganisms toward deleterious influences varies substantially. For the complete inactivation of microorganisms, various procedures are in use. The most common are those in which high temperature is involved. Effective methods include dry heat as well as, and even predominantly so, hot water vapor.

The microbicidal effect of high temperatures was discovered in the late 1800s by Lazarro Spallanzani (1729–1799, University of Pavia in Italy, scientist and Jesuit). His discovery, however, did not lead to a practical application because at that time it was not yet known that microorganisms were the cause of infectious disease. It was Louis Pasteur (1822–1895, Institut Pasteur, Paris), who in 1860 for the first time accomplished dry heat sterilization. Koch and Wolffhügel of the University of Göttingen (Germany) were the first to conduct systematic experiments on the killing of spores in 1881. Koch also recognized that for sterilization a stream of steam has a clear advantage over dry quiescent hot air, which requires a longer exposition time. The application of dry heat in surgical practice followed in 1884 by the Frenchman Terrilon, while his compatriot Redard (Paris) deployed pressurized saturated steam in 1887. The following definitions delimit the various methods to inactivate, remove and keep away microorganisms or prevent microbial infections.

Voigt's Pharmaceutical Technology, First Edition. Alfred Fahr.
© 2018 John Wiley & Sons Ltd. Published 2018 by John Wiley & Sons Ltd.

Sterilization implies the elimination by killing or removal of viable forms of microorganisms occurring in raw materials, preparations and objects. These entities only then can be considered sterile when they are free from viable forms of microorganisms whose presence could be confirmed under the culture conditions applicable to a sterility assay. In most pharmacopeias this definition is further specified to the extent that procedures and measures should lead to a probability of nonsterility (sterility assurance level, SAL) of $\leq 10^{-6}$. That means that in a batch of 1 million units (e.g., infusion bottles) maximally 1 vial may be contaminated. This internationally accepted high level of safety is the basis for the calculation and evaluation of sterilization procedures.

Disinfection includes procedures that can convert viable as well as nonviable material to a condition in which it can no longer cause an infection. In contrast to sterilization, disinfection is a measure to prevent infection by pathogenic microorganisms. This definition does not include the inactivation of spores. Disinfection measures in the context of pharmaceutical preparation methods serve to inactivate not only pathogenic germs but rather, all of them. In this context, the term *sanitization* is also used, which seems to be more appropriate.

> Cleaning: process of removing material from surfaces
>
> Sanitizing: process of reducing the number of microorganisms
>
> Disinfecting: reducing the number of microorganisms beyond the level of sanitizing to a harmless level of microorganisms
>
> Sterilizing: removal of all microorganisms

In the selection of the disinfection or sanitization method, the effectiveness, particularly the activity against problematic germs (pseudomonas, salmonellae, and staphylococci), the required exposition time, but also the compatibility with materials and the environmental burden are parameters to be considered. In order to prevent the selection of resistant germs, the disinfection method should be changed monthly.

Hand disinfection is preferably performed with agents based on aliphatic alcohols (ethanol, propanol). For disinfection of surfaces and equipment, phenolic compounds, peracetic acid preparations, and aldehydes in combination with quaternary ammonium compounds are commonly used. In case of minor contamination, the time- and labor-saving simultaneous cleaning/disinfection may be justified. For the disinfection of rooms with gaseous or volatile agents, hydrogen peroxide is now preferred to formaldehyde.

Antiseptic agents are disinfecting agents that can kill microorganisms occurring on mucosal tissue and wounds, while *aseptic* procedures include a whole spectrum of measures aiming at keeping away microorganisms from living tissue and thus are suitable to prevent microbial infections. Aseptic handling is for doctors (use of sterile instruments, rubber gloves, bandage materials, surgical clothing, mouth cover, decontamination of air, operation theaters) equally important as for pharmaceutical workers (aseptic preparation of formulations).

Disinfestation implies the eradication of any insects (e.g., lice, flees, bedbugs, flies, mosquitos) and small animals such as mice and rats, that are often acting as transmitters of disease. In pharmaceutical processes disinfestation is mainly relevant in the production of herbal medicines (see chapter 24).

Sterilization is predominantly achieved by heat. At higher temperatures, microorganisms are killed due to protein denaturation. Of crucial importance in this connection are the duration of the exposition to heat, the nature, age and density of the bacterial culture, the pH of the medium, the presence of chemicals, blood, and pus (the latter may coat the organisms, thereby changing their heat resistance). Moist heat (steam) is superior to dry heat with respect to sterilization effectiveness. That is explained by the notion that water is an excellent heat conductor and contains, by virtue of the stored heat of evaporation, substantially more energy than dry air. This energy can be effectively transmitted onto the material to be sterilized, which in moist conditions adopts the surrounding temperature substantially faster than under dry conditions. Dry hot air requires a comparatively considerably longer time to penetrate into the object than moist hot air. In addition, protein coagulation proceeds much faster in a humid environment. In general, microorganisms display a higher tolerance toward detrimental impact, especially heat, under dry conditions. The capacity of microorganisms to resist moist heat is characterized by four stages (Table 4-1).

When noxious physical or chemical influences act upon microorganisms, not all of these are momentarily killed. Biological rules, characterized by a certain order of destruction, dictate the killing process. This order depends on the nature (e.g., heat, radiation), intensity of the impact and the duration of the treatment as well as on the resistance of the various types and forms of microorganism.

Table 4-1 Resistance of Microorganisms to Sterilization Conditions

Resistance Stage	Resistance Capacity	Microorganism
1	Instantaneous killing in streaming water vapor (100°C)	Nonspore forming bacteria, vegetative forms of spore formers
2	Killing within 20 min in streaming water vapor (100°C)	Anthrax spores
		Culture spores of nonpathogenic spore formers (Hoffmann spores)
3	No killing within 20 min in streaming water vapor, but killing after 5 min in pressurized saturated steam at 121°C	Soil spores (native and genuine spores)
4	Killing in streaming water vapor (100°C) practically impossible and in pressurized, saturated steam at 134°C only after about 30 min	Highly resistant native spores of thermophilic spore formers

4.2   Procedures

4.2.1   General Introduction

The pharmacopeias describe various methods to make a material germ-free. Generally, two approaches have to be distinguished: those that comprise terminal sterilization in the final container and those to decontaminate materials that do not allow or tolerate terminal sterilization.

Sterilization for pharmaceutical or medical purposes commonly involves the following methods:

- Steam sterilization: treatment with pressurized saturated steam in an autoclave at a temperature of at least 121°C for 15 minutes (standard procedure) or at another suitable combination of time and temperature.
- Dry heat sterilization: heat treatment at 160°C, 170°C or 180°C for 120, 60, or 30 minutes, respectively, or at another suitable time-temperature combination. The standard procedure according to the Ph. Eur. is a treatment of minimally 2 hours at minimally 160°C. Some materials can be heated till glowing red (approximately 500°C); this is a simple and secure method for the sterilization of inoculation loops, spatulas etc., although such conditions are obviously demanding on the material. Treatment of spatulas, tweezers, simple glassware or ceramic material by slow and repeated movement through an open flame (flaming) does not represent an effective way to kill germs and is therefore to be discouraged.
- Sterilization with microbicidal gas: treatment with ethylene oxide, formaldehyde, or hydrogen peroxide in a gas sterilization chamber.
- Radiation: treatment with γ-rays or an electron beam.

Procedures that must be applied when terminal sterilization cannot be applied, because the respective material does not tolerate the treatment especially because of insufficient thermostability, should always be part of an aseptic protocol. They do not provide the high reliability of a sterilization procedure and are rather to be considered as a second-best substitute that cannot be renounced because of the lack of a better procedure.

These procedures include:

- Germ removal by filtration: use of bacteria-retaining filters under aseptic working conditions.
- Aseptic manufacturing: application of a complex set of measures that prevent the introduction of germs during a manufacturing process.
- Thermal substitute procedures: thermal methods operating at lower temperatures than in thermal sterilization procedures, which lead to a pronounced but often selective killing of microorganisms. During *pasteurization*, which is mainly used to preserve

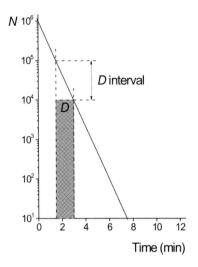

Fig. 4-1 Definition of the *D*-value exemplified by the killing curve of *Geobacillus stearothermophilus* in saturated steam under pressure at 121°C.

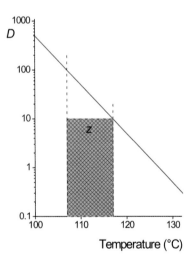

Fig. 4-2 Definition of the *z*-value exemplified by the killing curve of *Geobacillus stearothermophilus* in saturated steam under pressure.

foodstuffs, the material is exposed for a short period to temperatures between 60°C and 90°C. Thus, prolonged heating (30 minutes, 62°–65°C), brief heating (15–30 seconds, 72°–75°C) and high-temperature heating (4–10 seconds, 85°C) are distinguished. During ultra-high temperature treatment, the material is heated for 2 to 3 seconds at 135°C to 150°C and immediately cooled again to 4°C to 5°C.

A further method, known as tyndallization (fractionated sterilization), can only be used as additional measure under rare circumstances in the pharmaceutical field. The procedure includes the repeated heating of the material to be decontaminated to approximately 100°C on minimally four consecutive days, while keeping it in between at room temperature. This assures that possibly present spores germinate or swell to such an extent that they will be killed at the next heat treatment. In case of chemothermic treatment, used for disinfection of solutions containing a preservative, the preparation is exposed to a boiling water bath or a stream of steam for about 30 minutes. The increase in temperature causes a significant enhancement of the preservative activity.

- Disinfection with microbicidal fluids: treatment of objects and equipment with solutions of microbicidal agents such as peracetic acid, formaldehyde or glutaraldehyde.

4.2.2 Calculation and Assessment of the Effectiveness of a Sterilization Procedure

The killing of microorganisms at a certain temperature follows the kinetics of a first order reaction (see section 25.2.2). That implies a linear relationship between the logarithm of the number of germs N and time (Fig. 4-1). The rate of the killing process is represented by the D-value, the decimal reduction value. This is the time required to decrease the number of germs by one log. In case of sterilization by means of radiation the absorbed radiation dose serves as the D-value, under otherwise analogously defined conditions. The D-value is germ and procedure specific and is meaningful only as long as the experimental conditions are accurately defined.

Likewise, to describe the temperature dependence of the killing process of a population of microorganisms, the germ- and procedure-specific z-value (temperature coefficient) is defined. The z-value represents the temperature difference in K (Kelvin), which is required for a tenfold change in the D-value (Fig. 4-2). Table 4-2 presents the D- and z-values for a number of spore-forming bacteria in case of steam sterilization at 115° and 121°C. The two values allow the calculation of the effectiveness (lethality) of the (thermic) sterilization procedure as an F-value, in which N_0 is the initial number of germs, N the number of germs at the end of the germ-killing treatment and n the total number of logs of the reduction of N.

$$F = (\log N_0 - \log N) \cdot D = \log \frac{N_0}{N} \cdot D = n \cdot D \tag{4-1}$$

As for the sterilization procedure a safety factor of 10^6 is required (i.e., $N = 10^{-6}$), equation 4-1 can be converted to equation 4-2:

$$F = (\log N_0 - \log 10^{-6}) \cdot D \tag{4-2}$$

Table 4-2 D- and z-values for some bacteria spores upon treatment with pressurized saturated steam

Type of Bacteria (Spores)	D-value (min)		z-value (K)
	at 115°C	at 121°C	
Geobacillus stearothermophilus	10–24	1.5–4.0	6–7
Bacillus atrophaeus	2.2	0.4–0.7	8–13
Clostridium sporogenes	2.8–3.6	0.8–1.4	13
Clostridium botulinum		0.2	10

For steam sterilization the F-value can be calculated, at a D-value of 1 minute and under a bioburden in the material to be sterilized, of 10^6 germs per container, as follows:

$$F = (\log 10^6 - \log 10^{-6}) \cdot 1.0 \text{ min} = (6 - 6) \cdot 1.0 \text{ min} = 12 \text{ min}. \qquad (4\text{-}3)$$

As can be seen, the required sterilization time amounts to 12 minutes. Sterilization procedures, which, at a prevailing D-value of 1 min, achieve a reduction of the number of germs by at least 12 logs ($n = 12$) are internationally considered overkill procedures. In line with this view, the standard and reference steam sterilization process at 121°C for 15 minutes, as favored by most pharmacopeias, represents such an overkill procedure. According to experience, in the pharmaceutical field the presence of mesophilic germs with a D-value of <1 minutes is to be expected, implying that the standard procedure and equivalent procedures operational at other temperature-time combinations, but with the same effectiveness as the standard procedure, ensure a high degree of safety.

For equivalent procedures the F-value (F_T-value) representing the required sterilization time under the chosen conditions can be calculated as

$$F_T = \frac{F_{121}}{10^{\frac{T-121}{z}}} \qquad (4\text{-}4)$$

Alternative procedures, which must be deployed when limited heat stability of the treated material does not allow treatment at the temperature of the standard or equivalent procedure, show a lower effectiveness at an identical sterilization safety of 10^6. The deployment of alternative procedures requires that the microbiological burden of the material to be sterilized has to be determined taking into account nature, quantity and temperature sensitivity of the germs, which will bring along high labor cost.

4.2.3 Validation and Control of Sterilization Procedures

The success of sterilization procedures critically depends on the starting germ count. GMP approved design of the overall manufacturing process should guarantee that the microbial contamination of raw materials (active ingredients as well as excipients), the manufacturing equipment and all other materials applied, is as low as possible. Besides, microbiologically controlled operating conditions should be organized in such a way that introduction and multiplication of germs is avoided. Special attention should be paid to raw materials that are to be regarded as particularly at risk toward microbiological contamination. In the pharmacopeia the reader can find special purity requirements for some raw materials used for parenteral formulations (Table 4-3).

Table 4-3 Examples of active ingredients and excipients for the preparation of parenteral drug formulations with microbial purity requirements according to the Ph. Eur. [TAMC: total aerobic microbial count; CFU: colony-forming units]

	Acceptance Criterion TAMC max. CFU/g Substance
Calcium gluconate for injection	10^2
Dextrans for injection	10^2
Hydroxyethyl starches	10^2
Hydroxypropylbetadex intended for use in the manufacture of parenteral preparations	10^2
Erythritol	10^2
Mannitol	10^2
Paclitaxel	10^2
Sorbitol intended for use in the manufacture of parenteral preparations	10^2

Every sterilization procedure should be validated taking into account the nature of the product under consideration. That means that evidence should be procured by means of appropriate methods that the applied de-germination procedure is suited for the intended purpose and that compliant with the established methodological/instrumental conditions it will ensure sterility.

The validation of the procedure includes (as qualification) proof of the technical functionality of the sterilizer, including the calibration of the measuring and control devices.

The validation should be repeated periodically, with a frequency to be specified depending on the nature of the product and the sterilization procedure (revalidation). Revalidation is required when essential changes are made concerning the composition or the manufacturing of the product, the sterilization mode (e.g., degree of loading of the sterilizer), or repair work on the sterilizer, in particular the measuring and control devices.

The validity of a sterilization process is first of all evidenced by providing proof that the critical physical parameters (e.g., temperature, pressure, radiation dose) were adhered to. In addition, biological indicators are deployed in order to prove the efficiency of the sterilization procedure. However, these should by no means be considered as acceptable replacement of the physical validation measures. Biological indicators are spores of microorganisms with a high resistance against the respective biocidal agent. In most cases biological indicator preparations contain, on a suitable carrier (paper, glass or metal sheets), a defined number of preferably nonpathogenic microorganisms (Table 4-4).

These indicators, which should be labeled in a clearly recognizable manner in order to avoid mix-up with the material to be sterilized, must be placed at such locations in the sterilizer load that, according to experience, cannot easily be reached by the sterilizing agent.

After termination of the sterilization process the carriers are transferred to a culture medium and incubated. The availability of biological indicators in the forms of test ampoules that already contain a culture medium presents an important reduction of the workload involved.

The validation of each individual sterilization procedure is, however, based on physical assessment methods, which can also be used for process control. For thermal sterilization, preferentially thermo-sensors are applied, positioned at the thermally critical places, to assess the temperature distribution within the useable volume of the sterilizer or to localize the "cold spot" of the load. For procedure as well as in-process control of radiation sterilization, dosimeters are preferred that allow the measurement of the absorbed radiation dose in the immediate vicinity or even at the very site of the goods to be sterilized.

In contrast to biological indicators, chemical indicators (e.g., temperature- or gas-sensitive indicator labels with an irreversible color switch) merely indicate that the product has been

Table 4-4 Biological Indicators for Assessing the Effectiveness of Sterilization Methods (Ph. Eur. 5.1.2 "Biological Indicators of Sterilization"; corresponding information can also be found in JP G4 "Microorganisms—Terminal Sterilization and Sterilization Indicators")

Method	Microorganism (Spores)	Number of Viable Spores per Carrier	D-value	Requirements for Proof of Sterilization Effectiveness
Steam sterilization	*Geobacillus stearothermophilus*	$>5 \cdot 10^5$	≥ 1.5 min (121°C)	Growth after 6 min treatment (121±1°C), No growth after 15 min treatment
Dry-heat sterilization	*Bacillus Atrophaeus* In case of dry heat sterilization/ depyrogenization at >220°C: heat-resistant bacterial endotoxin preparation	$>1 \cdot 10^6$	≥ 2.5 min (160°C)	No growth after the spores have been subjected to the sterilization procedure to be tested In case of dry heat sterilization/depyrogenization at temperatures >220°C demonstration of a 3 log reduction in bacterial endotoxin can be used as replacement for biological indicators.
Ionizing radiation sterilization	*Bacillus pumilus*	$>1 \cdot 10^7$	≥ 1.9 kGy	No growth after treatment with 25 kGy (minimally absorbed dose)
Gas sterilization	*Bacillus atrophaeus* (for gas sterilization with ethylene oxide)	$>1 \cdot 10^6$	≥ 2.5 min at 54°C and 60% rel. humidity for 1 test cycle with 0.6 g/L	No growth after 1 test cycle for 25 min; Growth after 1 test cycle for 50 min at 30°C

subjected to the sterilization procedure. They are deployed in order to prevent mixing up of sterilized and nonsterilized material.

4.2.4 Steam Sterilization

4.2.4.1 General Introduction

Steam sterilization utilizes pressurized saturated steam and is performed in steam sterilizers (sterilization autoclaves). The method is based on the following physical principles: as is generally known, the boiling point of water depends on the prevailing pressure; water, for example, boils in an open container at a pressure of 0.1 MPa (760 mm Hg) at 100°C thereby transforming into the gas phase. The situation changes when water is heated in a closed vessel. Then the temperature of water and vapor increases to above 100°C while simultaneously pressure increases. In this situation we are dealing with *pressurized* (water) *vapor*. While the vapor of the boiling water (*streaming vapor*) features a pressure of 0.1 MPa (1 bar), pressurized air-free vapor of 121°C exhibits a pressure of 0.2 MPA (2 bar). We speak of *saturated steam* when water vapor and fluid water are in equilibrium. As long as there is fluid water available, pressure will rise with increasing temperature. Unsaturated steam prevails when a volume, saturated with steam but no longer containing fluid water, is increased, because saturated steam now fills up the additional space thereby turning into unsaturated steam with a pressure that no longer represents the vapor pressure of water at the given temperature.

Overheated steam is formed when additional heat is supplied to a given space in which no more fluid is present. Unsaturated and, in particular, overheated steam is insufficiently microbicidal. When during cooling part of the saturated vapor condenses on the walls of the sterilization chamber we are dealing with *wet steam*.

Sterilization is performed with pressurized saturated steam that is retained in a simple laboratory autoclave in the following way:

- during the initial heating the steam valve of the autoclave remains open so that the air can escape from the sterilization chamber,
- when a strong steam jet exits through the valve the latter is kept open for another 5 minutes so that remaining air will be expelled from the chamber,
- the valve is closed, upon which pressure and temperature will increase till pressure has raised to 2 bar and temperature to 121°C.

Only air-free steam will really reach this pressure/temperature combination. In case there still is air in the sterilization chamber, the total pressure (i.e., air pressure plus vapor pressure of the water) is higher than can be expected for pressurized water vapor at the prevailing temperature. It should furthermore be ensured that the autoclave contains a sufficient water supply, so that equilibrium can be established between liquid and gaseous water. When still air is present in the sterilization chamber the sterilization effect is diminished.

The vapor phase and the liquid phase are in condensation-evaporation equilibrium with each other. The heat that is released during the condensation of water on the treated material supplies the energy required to kill the microorganisms.

Because, at a given temperature, mixtures of air and water vapor possess a higher pressure than air-free vapor, it is possible to obtain information about the amount of air in the pressurized vapor, by simultaneous assessment of pressure and temperature. Too-high-pressure values relative to temperature indicate incomplete removal of air.

Steam sterilization is preferentially applied for bandaging material, cellulose (pulp), paper, linen goods, work clothes, instruments, and empty glassware (surface sterilization), water, and aqueous solutions of heat-stable solutes (sterilization in closed containers).

4.2.4.2 Equipment

Simple, small steam sterilizers are single-walled (Fig. 4-3). The water in the lower part is separated from the sterilization chamber by a sieve plate, which at the same time functions as the support plate for the material to be sterilized. Similar to the procedure customary for larger sterilizers, heating is usually achieved by means of electricity. The vapor/air mixture that is formed penetrates through the chamber from below and is released via a valve in the

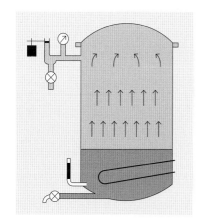

Fig. 4-3 Single-walled autoclave.

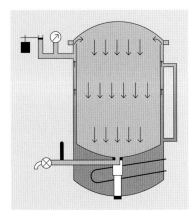

Fig. 4-4 Double-walled autoclave.

upper part of the chamber until for about 5 minutes a strong steam jet has escaped. Then it can safely be assumed that extensive displacement of air has taken place. Only then the valve is closed, causing temperature and pressure to rise.

Double-walled steam sterilizers are of much higher practical relevance (Fig. 4-4). In these devices, the feed water for the steam formation is contained in the lower part of the jacketed vessel. A glass window in the vessel serves to check that the autoclave contains a sufficient amount of water. The steam flows from the top into the sterilization chamber, thus ensuring the expulsion of the relatively heavy cold air which accumulates in the lower part of the chamber, where an exhaust stopcock allows the release of the air/vapor mixture (*gravity air displacement*).

Additional elements of the autoclave are a manometer, which can be mounted at various sites (most commonly on the lid or the exhaust nozzle) and serves to control the pressure, a thermometer and a safety valve.

In more sophisticated autoclaves temperature sensors and control mechanisms ensure automated energy supply. The expulsion of air is facilitated by air separators, which are provided for in some constructions (Fig. 4-5). They consist of a cooling coil through which the vapor is channeled before it leaves the autoclave via the air- and steam-release stopcock. Here, the steam condenses, thus causing a volume reduction, which, in turn, yields a suction drawing the air out of the sterilization chamber. In such equipment, the valve is closed as soon as steam starts escaping. The air in the autoclave chamber can also be removed by applying a vacuum before steam is introduced (*pre-vacuum procedure, dynamic air removal*). Alternatively, steam injection alternating with air suction is deployed (*fractionated pre-vacuum procedure*). This procedure is particularly suited for porous sterilization material, from which the air cannot readily be expelled.

To dry the sterilized material, larger autoclaves have devices to exhaust the vapor in the cooling phase and to perfuse the chamber with hot, sterile air. A general problem connected with autoclaves is the long time they require to cool off; this can amount up to several hours. Therefore, the entire sterilization process is quite time consuming and therefore immediate reuse after termination of a sterilization process is not possible. In addition, active ingredients are exposed to prolonged thermal stress, which can cause disintegration. Larger autoclaves are thus often provided with cooling and pressure release devices. Cooling can be achieved

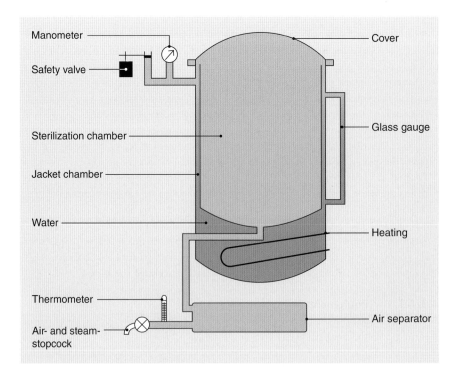

Fig. 4-5 Autoclave with air separator.

by means of transfusion of cold water through a pipe system incorporated in the wall of the instrument. Without additional measures this principle is, however, only applicable for surface sterilization. During sterilization of solutions for injection the rapid pressure release in the chamber may lead to cracking of the (glass) container if not simultaneously compressed air provides compensation. If the material to be sterilized permits, constructions are preferred which are provided with a special device allowing water jets to be sprayed on the injection vials. Also in this case it may be useful (at least until the temperature in the vessel reaches 100°C) to blow in compressed air in order to account for the slower pressure drop in the containers compared to that in the chamber.

It will not be possible to sterilize solutions in plastic containers under the conditions described in the foregoing, as with increasing temperature the increasing pressure in the containers is likely to lead to their rupture. In the rototherm procedure, an appropriate counter pressure is achieved by circulating the heating or cooling medium in a pressure-resistant chamber by means of strong ventilators. Cooling is achieved by means of filter-sterilized compressed air.

In pharmaceutical companies, centralized sterilization departments and hospital pharmacies automated steam sterilizers are the standard sterilization device of choice. Especially convenient with regard to workflow are types constructed in a pass-through design and incorporated as such into a wall. The autoclave is loaded in one room, and in the other room the sterilized material is taken out. The procedure can be programmed.

Large-volume autoclaves are equipped with temperature and pressure assessment devices, which ascertain an uninterrupted assessment and registration of these important process parameters.

Instead of pressurized saturated steam, steam-air or steam-air-water mixtures can be used as media to transfer thermal energy to the items to be sterilized. With these, an evenly distributed temperature is achieved in the sterilization chamber by means of a recycling distribution system (circulation blowers or pumps), additionally bringing along a substantially shortened cooling time.

Spraying the load with hot water in the steam-air-water procedure comes along with a high-precision temperature control. For the sterilization of preparations in foil bags or other thin-walled vessels, the techniques using vapor/air mixtures are well suited (*support pressure procedure*). In a sealed container a total pressure is developed according to Dalton's law, which equals the sum of the vapor pressure of the water and the pressure of the air above it and is therefore higher than the pressure in an autoclave chamber filled with air-free water vapor only. By applying a vapor/air mixture, a higher "support pressure" can be built up outside the vessel, which may help to prevent it from bursting.

4.2.4.3 Practical Implementation

For the practical implementation of the sterilization procedure, knowledge of some conceptual terms that characterize the operating procedure are helpful. The time required for an entire sterilization cycle (i.e., the time period from the start of the sterilization procedure until its termination) is composed of the following elements:

- Come-up time: the time from the start of the continuous heat supply until the required sterilization temperature at the site of the thermometer device has been reached.
- Equilibrium time: time required to reach the required temperature at all sites of the material to be sterilized.
- Exposure time (sterilization time): the time for which the material to be sterilized is exposed to the sterilization temperature. The sterilization time begins only after termination of the equilibrium time and represents the time required for a particular procedure, as prescribed by the Pharmacopeia. Traditionally, the sterilization time is the time required for complete germ killing plus a supplement, most commonly of 50%.
- Cool-down time: the time span between terminating the energy supply and withdrawing the sterilized material from the device.

Special attention deserves the equilibrium time, which varies depending on the nature of the material to be sterilized, the degree of loading and the texture of the cargo. It should

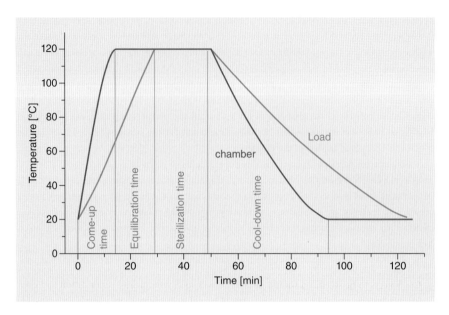

Fig. 4-6 Temperature-time diagram of the time course of a heat sterilization (schematically).

be determined by means of temperature sensors positioned in reference containers. Fig. 4-6 presents a temperature-time diagram for a steam sterilization process. The equilibrium time for an autoclave with a usable volume of 12 liters, loaded with two 500 mL infusion flasks, is 8 minutes. For thin-walled glass vessels with a volume of 10 mL approximately 3 to 5 minutes and for thick-walled glass vessels with a volume of 1000 mL approximately 18 to 20 minutes should be taken into consideration as equilibrium time.

After termination of the sterilization time and interruption of the energy supply, one should allow the system to cool down, while the valve is still closed, until the temperature in the chamber indicates 95°C. Then the valve is opened and the system is allowed to cool further down. Fig. 4-6 demonstrates that the temperature drop in the chamber occurs considerably faster than in the load. Obviously, smaller ampoules or surface material can be taken out rather soon, whereas for large volume solutions this is only allowed when the temperature in the chamber has dropped to about 50°C.

Incidents taken from daily practice call for special emphasis on the need to open the autoclave and take out material not before the required cooling time has passed. Because solutions for infusion in bottles still can have a higher temperature than the thermometer in the chamber indicates, they are under elevated pressure. When, upon opening the autoclave, breakage of a glass container occurs, it is not unlikely that this will involve not only one but rather more containers culminating in a chain reaction of exploding vessels involving several or even all vessels in the autoclave. Apart from the obvious material damage that may occur, literature also reports on the occurrence of serious injuries (including death, loss of eye sight, etc.), which can be ascribed to explosion accidents caused by failing to observe the required waiting time before taking out the sterilized material.

Particularly long waiting times are required in case of sterilized infusions, which have an additional CO_2 pressure—for instance, sodium bicarbonate solutions. They need to be cooled down, therefore, to room temperature, and even then it is required to wait for another two hours before opening the autoclave.

Table 4-5 presents the pressure conditions that must be taken into account with aqueous solutions in sealed containers. The internal pressure that develops during heating is adding up to the partial pressure of the water vapor, the air and the pressure increase caused by the expanding liquid. When a container is filled to a level of >95%, the pressure approaches an "infinite" value. Up to a filling level of 90%, the pressure difference with that in the chamber will not lead to breakage of the glass container, provided it has no material flaws.

For sterilization of surface material (e.g., surgical instruments), this should be wrapped in material that is permeable to steam but impermeable to germs in order to prevent

Table 4-5 Internal pressure and pressure difference in a sealed container with respect to the chamber during sterilization in an autoclave at 120°C and 2 bar in dependence of the degree of filling

Filling of the Vessel (%)	Internal Pressure at 120°C (MPa)	Pressure Difference with the Chamber (MPa)
50	0,34	0,14
68	0,35	0,15
85	0,4	0,2
90	0,48	0,28
>95	→∞	→∞

contamination after the sterilization process. For this purpose, compact paper as well as polyester-PET foil can be used. The pores in sterilization paper become narrower during the sterilization process, turning it into an effective bacteria filter. For that reason, pure textile wrappings are not recommended for this purpose.

The objects to be sterilized should be double-wrapped when using paper or foil and even quadruple when using pure textile. Also, stainless steel sterilization containers with a closable perforated lid have proven their practical usefulness.

Process control (e.g., regarding vapor permeation) is performed by means of temperature sensor measurements in at least two containers or with biological indicators. For that purpose also thermo-indicators, such as the four-field color indicator (Fig. 4-7), are well suited. Those provide information about the duration of the effect of the sterilization temperature by means of a color change of the individual fields (*Bowie-Dick test*).

4.2.4.4 Continuous Sterilization

Steam sterilization can also be performed in a continuous process. The construction of a continuous sterilizer is based on a hydrostatic principle. The pressure of the saturated steam in the internal space is in equilibrium with the height of adjacent water columns. By selecting the height of the water columns and the desired percolation rate through the sterilization zone, an optimal treatment can be achieved for each individual product.

The process occurs in long vertical towers. The containers to be sterilized pass through several temperature zones accompanied by water, steam or air as a medium, by means of a transport belt (paternoster type). During this passage, pre-heating, sterilization, and eventually cooling ensue. The sterilization temperature can be set at values between 105°C and 130°C. By manipulating the height of the water columns pressure and thereby the temperature can be modulated. The water columns also serve to preheat and cool the containers. By changing the velocity of the transport belt, the exposure time of the container in the sterilization zone can be controlled. Hydrostatic sterilizers are mostly used in food technology (e.g., for the manufacturing of canned food) but can occasionally also be encountered in pharmaceutical industry.

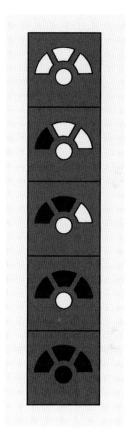

Fig. 4-7 Four-field color indicator.

4.2.5 Dry Heat Sterilization

4.2.5.1 Instruments

Conventional dry heat sterilizers are cabinet-shaped devices with a round or rectangular chamber and equipped with a thermometer for temperature control. Heating is mostly achieved by electric means. The larger dry heat sterilizers are equipped with measuring and control amenities that, by means of temperature sensors, ascertain continuous monitoring and documentation of the process. The sterilizers need to be provided with ventilation devices that ensure an even heat distribution within the material to be sterilized by means of active convection. The mechanical stirring of the air is achieved either by fans installed on the outside of the sterilization chamber or by rotors in the upper part of the chamber. Smaller devices, particularly those of older design, usually not possessing such features, are not suited for pharmaceutical applications. As a result of the merely thermally induced air convection, the good to be sterilized heats up only slowly and unevenly, which often causes the formation of "islands" of cold air with a temperature as much as up to 30°C lower than the thermometer indicates.

Dry heat sterilizers provided with laminar airflow technology ensure proper sterilization and depyrogenation while simultaneously protecting the goods to be sterilized against particulate contamination. In most cases double chamber sterilizers are deployed, consisting of a laminarly aerated heating and cooling chamber.

4.2.5.2   Practical Implementation

The process flow is characterized by the same phases as described for steam sterilization (see 4.2.4.3). Special attention deserves the equilibrium time, which can be quite considerable due to the poor heat transfer, dependent on the nature of the substance to be sterilized and on the loading of the chamber. For powders, fats and fatty oils it may correspond to a multitude of the sterilization time. In order to shorten the equilibrium time for such substances they should be warmed up before introducing them in the sterilizer. That applies in particular to powders, which in addition should be spread out in as thin a layer as possible (e.g., in a Petri dish). Oils should be dehydrated prior to the sterilization procedure by heating at approximately 120°C. When loading the chamber it is important to pack the material as loosely as possible and to avoid overloading. Sterilization of instruments (tweezers, cannulas, syringes, pipettes) is performed in metal containers, which prevent re-contamination after the sterilization process. With respect to the process control, which should be performed with the help of biological indicators or temperature sensors (at two sites minimally), it should be taken into account that the biological indicator prescribed by the Pharmacopeia (spores of *B. atropheus*) is only suited for temperatures up to 180°C maximally. Above this temperature, the D-value, due to its low value, can no longer be estimated accurately. In such cases, the assessment of the effect on endotoxins is considered more favorable; this allows at the same time an assertion concerning the effectiveness of depyrogenization. The preferred application range of dry heat sterilization procedures includes the sterilization of empty glassware (ampoules, injection vials and infusion flasks), tools and instruments (syringes, surgical tools and glass, porcelain or metal objects), thermo-stable powders, fats, oils, paraffins, waxes (e.g., also ointment bases). Rubber and plastic material, clothes, medicinal cotton and gauze as well as most pharmaceutical products cannot be sterilized by dry heat due to the high temperature burden.

4.2.5.3   Drying and Sterilization Tunnel

Continuously operating drying and sterilization tunnels have proven their usefulness in pharmaceutical industry for the purpose of sterilization and depyrogenation of empty containers for parenteral formulations. Fig. 4-8 shows the construction of a *dry heat sterilizing tunnel*. The loading of this device with the containers to be sterilized (ampoules, injection and infusion flasks) occurs either continuously by means of an upstream-located cleaning device or manually into the introduction zone to the transport belt.

In the heating and sterilization zone, the containers are dried and exposed to a 3-minute heat treatment at ≥300°C which will lead to a guaranteed killing of all germs and destruction of endotoxins. Rod-shaped infrared quartz glass radiators, installed perpendicular to the transport direction, serve as a heat source. To amplify their radiation and heat action they are coated on the backside with reflecting surfaces. Subsequently the containers travel through the cooling zone where they are cooled to the temperature required for their further processing; ultimately, they end up at the filling machine via a turning table.

Both the infeed and the cooling zone are provided with laminar flow devices. As a result of this laminar aeration and the transport through the HEPA filter preconditioned (section 4.2.8.1) air from the cooling zone in the direction of the introduction zone (counter flow), extremely particle-poor conditions are created in the entire tunnel area.

Measuring and recording devices, which are installed in a separate switch cabinet, guarantee continuous process surveillance by detection and regulation of the temperature in the heating and sterilization zone and the assessment of the laminar flow velocity in the cooling zone. It is also possible to incorporate an in-process particle assessment device, consisting of air exhaust pipes connected to a separate laser particle counter. The maximal capacity for small-sized vessels is approximately 36,000 units per hour.

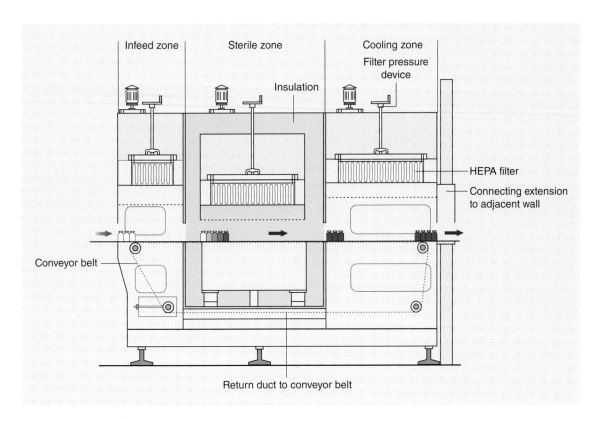

Fig. 4-8 Dry heat sterilization tunnel.

Likewise, for continuous sterilization and de-pyrogenation of empty glass containers pharmaceutical industry employs the hot air tunnel (laminar flow hot air tunnel). This device distinguishes itself from the sterilization tunnel in that the heat transfer is achieved by HEPA filter degerminated hot air of 250°C to 350°C, which is led through the sterilization zone in a down-draught flow of low turbulence at a velocity of ca. 0.7 m/s.

4.2.6 Sterilization by Radiation

Ionizing radiation includes corpuscular (α and β rays) and electromagnetic (γ and X rays) radiation. For sterilization purposes predominantly γ radiation and to a lesser degree β rays are employed. This is related to a higher penetration potential of γ rays. While β rays with 1 MeV energy do not penetrate deeper than 5 mm in water, γ rays of identical energy lose only 50% of their energy when penetrating a water layer of 30 cm thickness. Both radiation types possess similar germ-killing activity toward bacteria, molds and viruses, of which the latter, with D-values of up to 4 kGy (encephalitis virus), and spore forming bacteria with D-values up to 3 kGy (*B. atrophaeus*), display high radiation resistance. Radiation is quantified as energy dose. This is a measure of the amount of energy absorbed by the material. It cannot be determined directly in living tissue. 1 Gray (Gy) of radiation signifies that 1 kg of material has absorbed 1 Joule of energy. The amount of absorbed energy can be determined calorimetrically by measuring the heat uptake of the radiated material. The germ-killing effect depends on the dose and a number of other factors. The most important of these are germ type and age, germ density, oxygen concentration (in presence of oxygen the germs are two to three times more sensitive), and humidity.

The required radiation dose should be estimated while taking into account the characteristics of the product and the process. In addition, the bioburden of the material to be sterilized should be kept to a minimal level in order to guarantee a sterility assurance level of 10^{-6} at the most common radiation dose of 25 Gy.

For the practical execution of the sterilization procedure the material to be made germ-free is passed by the radiation source by means of a conveyer belt. The production of electron (β)

rays is achieved by a Van de Graaff accelerator, while γ rays are almost exclusively produced by means of the radio nuclide ^{60}Co. During the sterilization process, the absorbed radiation dose is monitored at or in the material to be sterilized by means of a dosimeter.

Radiation mediated sterilization is particularly suited for the treatment of thermo-labile products and is also applied for surgical suture and bandage material, transplants, implants and the like. Furthermore, certain thermolabile active ingredients (benzyl penicillin, streptomycin, polymyxin, atropine), either in powder form or processed in an ointment base, can be sterilized this way. An advantage is that the sterilization can be performed while the product is in the final container. Even so, it should be taken into account that radiation can lead to material damage and radiolytic conversions, often manifested as discoloration. For example, at the most common radiation dose of 25 Gy, glass and certain synthetic polymers such as polypropylene (PP) and polyvinylidene chloride (PVDC) display discoloration and may become brittle. Other polymers, including epoxy resins and polysterol are not susceptible to such radiation induced depreciation.

Radiation mediated sterilization of pharmaceutical products is allowed only when no other suitable methods are available.

4.2.7   Sterilization with Microbicidal Gases and Vapors

4.2.7.1   Ethylene Oxide

Gas sterilization is most commonly performed with ethylene oxide (oxirane); frequently used alternatives are for example chlorodioxide or formaldehyde. Ethylene oxide is a colorless and odorless highly reactive gas, which in concentrations from 3% to 80% forms an explosive mixture with air.

The compound is oncogenic, causes skin and mucosal irritation already at very low concentrations, leads to nausea, headache and vomiting. The lethal dose for humans is 100–200 mg/L air.

Ethylene oxide is active against vegetative bacterial spores as well as against fungi and viruses. The effectiveness depends on the gas concentration, the pressure (with increasing pressure the microbicidal effect becomes stronger), temperature and the humidity of the material to be sterilized (at least 55% relative humidity). In most cases, the humidity of the material has to be conditioned before the start of the sterilization process as otherwise the germ-killing effect may become questionable.

For sterilization purposes mostly ethylene oxide/carbon dioxide mixtures are used, for example a mixture of 90% (*V/V*) ethylene oxide and 10% (*V/V*) carbon dioxide. The treatment takes place in a closed, cabinet-like, explosion-proof device that can be operated at normal, under-, or overpressure. Overpressure is essential when operating under low-concentration conditions of ethylene oxide. In the framework of validation measures the effectiveness of the procedure has to be verified for each batch by means of biological indicators. Besides, Pharmacopeias and guidelines require that the process parameters are assessed and recorded.

Special attention needs to be paid to removal of the ethylene oxide from the sterilized material. By applying a sufficiently long desorption time, residues of ethylene oxide and ethylene oxide related products, in particular ethylene chlorhydrin, can be removed to the extent that the product can be used harmlessly. The European Medicines Agency (EMA) specifies a limit for the residual content of ethylene oxide of usually 1 ppm, for chlorinated ethylenehydrines of 50 ppm. The necessary desorption times are dependent on the material and can amount to 70 hours for rubber and polymers. This time can be shortened considerably by desorption under reduced pressure.

Ethylene oxide is suited for the sterilization of medical equipment, surgical instruments, infusion sets, bacteria-retaining filters, as well as containers or closure materials made of polymers. It is less well suited for sterilization of active ingredients because, due to the reactivity of the gas, chemical detorioration can often occur (e.g., alkylation reactions). An important application of ethylene oxide is the treatment of products that are packed in gas- and water-vapor-permeable foil. Soft polyethylene (PE-LD) foils of ca. 100 μm thickness are particularly suited for this purpose.

The Ph. Eur. prescribes that gas sterilization can only then be employed when no alternative sterilization procedure is available.

4.2.7.2   Sterilization with H₂O₂ Vapor and Plasma

Because the operation of conventional gas sterilizers comes with considerable legal constraints due to the risk of residues, there is great interest in procedures for the sterilization of thermo-labile instruments based on agents that decompose residue-free.

Liquid hydrogen peroxide has long been in use as a disinfectant agent. Only much later was it recognized that gaseous H_2O_2 already at very low concentrations (<5 mg/L) kills microorganisms and even their spores. Since then, methods that apply evaporated H_2O_2 for the sterilization of medical instruments, either as such or in the plasma phase, have become increasingly important. Meanwhile these methods are very often applied for the decontamination of aseptic working spaces, e.g., isolators (see 4.3.2).

One such procedure is the low-temperature plasma sterilization (Sterrad® procedure, Johnson & Johnson). The method involves evaporation of 58% hydrogen peroxide followed by injection of the vapor at 45°C in the evacuated sterilization chamber (injection phase). Subsequently, the vapor thoroughly perfuses all surfaces and hollow spaces of the material to be sterilized (diffusion phase). Then a high-frequency field is applied for 45 to 80 minutes, according to the selected program, which causes the hydrogen peroxide to change over in a plasma phase. A plasma is an ionized gas consisting of ions and electrons. It is often distinguished from the liquid, solid and gaseous states of matter as a fourth physical state. In this state the hydrogen peroxide decomposes into highly reactive radicals. The plasma phase is the actual sterilization phase. It is followed by an aeration phase in which any remaining H_2O_2 is removed followed by rapid decomposition into water and oxygen in the moist environment of the atmosphere. The advantage of this method is the absence of toxic side effects such as occur with the gas sterilization and the fact that, after the sterilization procedure, the sterilized material can be taken out and used immediately. A disadvantage is that the method is not suited for cellulose containing materials, textiles, covers used during surgical procedures and clothing, nor for material containing dead-end pores.

A newer method is the VHP® procedure (Steris Corporation) that similarly operates with H_2O_2 vapor but without transfer into the plasma phase. With this method, temperatures between 30°C and 40°C can be used. The entire process takes two hours.

Another low-temperature gas plasma procedure (AbTox system) utilizes an evaporated mixture of peracetic acid and hydrogen peroxide, which subsequently is carried off by means of an oxygen-hydrogen-argon mixture.

4.2.8   Filtration

4.2.8.1   General Introduction

Elimination of microorganisms by filtration, also known as *filtration through bacteria-retaining filters* or *sterile filtration*, comes into demand in case of solutions of active ingredients that do not tolerate heat sterilization due to thermo-instability of (one of) the solutes. For solutions for injection and infusion, which will undergo a final sterilization procedure, the method is used to reduce the initial number of germs in order to avoid the formation of pyrogens and to enhance the security of the final sterilization.

The separation of the microorganisms is accomplished by a mechanical sieve effect and/or by means of adsorption. Most viruses, as well as microorganisms lacking a cell wall (such as mycoplasmas), will not be retained by the filter. The separation of bacterial endotoxins with pyrogenic action is possible with filters possessing sorptive activity. Filtration methods are suited for the decontamination of true solutions of low viscosity. Filtration of colloidal and highly viscous solutions can be problematic.

A special situation prevails in case of filtration of air. While for microbiological decontamination of process gases or aeration of tanks mostly membrane filters made of hydrophobic polytetrafluorethylene (PTFE) or polyvinylidenefluoride (PVDF) are deployed, sterile filtration of larger volumes of air, such as required for ventilation of aseptic working places and for laminar flow devices (section 4.3.4) is accomplished by means of depth filtration. For that purpose, high-efficiency particulate air (HEPA) filters are deployed, which are made of pleated glass fiber fleece with a high retention capacity (particles ≥0.5 μm diameter are retained by 99.99%). This extraordinarily high-separation efficiency is based on a combination of sieve effects (particles >1 μm), inertia (particles of 0.2-1 μm), and diffusion effects (particles <0.2 μm) (see section 23.1.3).

4.2.8.2   Instruments

For the purpose of sterile filtration, the equipment already described in section 2.3 is deployed. The choice of equipment type is determined by the nature and volume of the solution to be filtered. For small-scale operations glass or metal (e.g., stainless steel) devices are in use, for industrial-scale applications mostly multi-layer filters (module filters). For routine operations, such as for the filtration of large volumes of infusions, devices allowing continuous filtration (filter equipment from Sartorius, Millipore and others) are used, enabling at the same time filtration directly into the receptacle. Decanting is thus not required and the danger of contamination is reduced. Pressure filtration is usually preferred to avoid contamination on the filtrate side of the device.

The gas commonly used to drive the process is compressed air or, for filtration of solutions containing oxidation-prone active ingredients, nitrogen or carbon dioxide. Pressure filtration is also suitable for volatile liquids such as ethers and alcohols, foam-forming solutions and highly viscous media. The filtration rate diminishes gradually with prolonged use of the filter. In this connection it is recommended to apply relatively low initial pressures of 0.12 to 0.15 MPa and not to increase the pressure above 0.25 to 0.30 MPa.

All filtration devices, including the filters, must be sterilized before use. The appropriate sterilization conditions and the procedure can be found in the documentation provided with the equipment. In most cases, autoclaving the appropriately paper-wrapped device that is provided with the filters at 120°C suffices. Filters and devices used for filtration of oily solutions can be sterilized by means of dry heat. In industry, presterilized disposable units are increasingly used.

4.2.8.3   Filter Materials

For the sterile filtration of dosage forms exclusively membrane filters are used, as they possess a defined pore structure. Membrane filters used to produce bacteria-free solutions should have a pore diameter of maximally 0.20 to 0.22 μm. When evaluating the germ retention potential of a filter it should be taken into account that the pore diameters provided by the manufacturer are calculated values obtained under idealized conditions. As a result of the filter production process, all filters also contain pores that are larger than the indicated size and therefore may allow passage of small-sized germs, as was demonstrated for membrane filters with a nominal pore diameter of 0.2 μm, by means of the test germ *Brevundimonas diminuta* or polystyrol calibration particles with a diameter of 0.23 μm. Consequently, more and more often the FDA requires the use of 0.1-μm filters.

Double-layered filters, that is, a combination of two filters with different pore sizes, for example one with 0.2 μm diameter combined with one of 0.45 or 0.60 μm, guarantee a practically complete separation of bacteria, due to the partial coverage of the larger pores. Layered filters or filter cartridges (e.g., Sartobran® II) manufactured according to this principle additionally display a high flow and loading capacity because the upper membrane with larger pores acts as a prefilter. Cellulose nitrate and cellulose acetate filters are incompatible with several organic solvents such as ethers, ketones, and esters. In such cases, filters made of regenerated cellulose, polytetrafluorethylene or polyamide are used. Sterilization of the filters within the filtration device is achieved by autoclaving at 121°C for 20 minutes. In order to avoid premature clogging of the sterile filter, it is recommended to apply a prefilter (pore size of about 10–12 μm) in case of strongly contaminated solutions.

Asymmetric filters consist of one layer of homogeneous material in which the pore size decreases throughout across the layer from, for instance, 10 down to 0.1 μm. The upper layers thus act as prefilters, and as a result, these filters offer a high retention capacity and good flow capacities.

Zeta-plus filters, which have a positively charged filter matrix, combine a mechanical sieving effect at the surface with an adsorption effect of the negatively charged microorganisms and bacterial endotoxins within the filter matrix.

Cellulose-diatomite filters (Seitz® EK-1) are deployed instead of filters containing asbestos. They feature a similar retention capacity for germs and pyrogenic bacterial endotoxins. These filter materials can be sterilized by steam.

4.2.8.4 Testing of Filters and Filtration Systems

Testing of bacteria-retaining filters for proper quality is done with the *bubble point test*. The bubble point corresponds to the pressure required to blow air through the liquid-filled pores of the filter to the extent that a clear flow of bubbles is detectable. This pressure depends on the surface tension of the liquid, the pore diameter, and the contact angle liquid/filter material.

$$p = \frac{4c\sigma \cdot \cos\theta}{d} \qquad (4\text{-}5)$$

p = bubble point pressure
c = shape correction factor
σ = surface tension
θ = contact angle
d = pore diameter

The bubble point represents for each filter type a characteristic parameter, which depends on the filter material and the manufacturing technology (Table 4-6). It provides an indication of the diameter of the "largest pore."

As in-process control, physical integrity of the filtration device (sterilized filter holder or housing with integrated filter) is assessed preferentially by means of the *pressure hold test*, which can be performed before as well as after the filtration process. In this procedure, the wet filter is exposed from the nonsterile side for 3 to 5 minutes to a pressure of about 60% of the bubble point pressure. In case the filtration system does not perform according to the requirements (e.g., leakage across defect or slipped gaskets, mechanical damage of the filter, defective glue joints of cartridge filters), a clear pressure drop is observed.

A further possibility to test the integrity of the filtration system is offered by the *diffusive flow test*. In this method, a test pressure of approximately 80% of the bubble point pressure is acting on the wet filter. The read-out parameter in this case is the rate at which the air diffuses through the filter pores. Because for the assessment of the gas-flow rate the air volume after passage through the filter needs to be measured at the sterile side and, in addition, reliable values can only be obtained for filters with a large surface area, this technique is less well suited than the pressure hold test.

Automatically recording instruments are available (e.g., Sartocheck®) for a rational implementation of the abovementioned tests.

Of the microbiological methods for the assessment of the effectiveness of sterile filters, the *bacteria challenge test* is most common. This test determines, by means of microorganisms of appropriate size, by how many logs the original germ number is reduced as a result of the filtration process. The FDA requires that, for the most commonly used sterile filter of pore size 0.2 μm, the filtration of an amount of liquid containing 10^7 colony forming units (CFU) per cm² filter surface area of the test germ *Brevundimonas diminuta* yields a germ-free product.

Table 4-6 Bubble Point Values for Membrane Filters

Nominal-Pore Width (μm)	Filter Material	Bubble Point (Bar)
0.1	Cellulose acetate	4.2
	Cellulose nitrate	9.0
	Polycarbonate	>7.0
0.2	Cellulose acetate	3.4
	Cellulose nitrate	4.8
	Polycarbonate	4.2
0.45	Cellulose acetate	>2.0
	Cellulose nitrate	3.1
	Polyamide	2.3

4.3 Aseptic Preparation

4.3.1 General Introduction

When the thermo-lability of an active ingredient does not allow heat sterilization, it will be necessary to work under strict exclusion of germs.

Aseptic manufacturing of drug formulations implies that, as far as possible, the required components (active ingredients as well as excipients) are sterilized before use and that their processing occurs with sterilized equipment and filling proceeds into sterile containers. All these individual processes need to be carried out in an environment of clean room grade A (CFU $<1/m^3$ of air) in order to bridge any aseptic gaps that may occur and are hard to completely avoid during the manufacturing process, with as little risk of contamination as possible. Thus, all aseptic measures are aimed at the diminution or exclusion of the risk of contaminations that might be brought along by the potential germ sources (nonsterilizable active ingredients, manipulation by personnel and production area). This brings along strict requirements with respect to the equipment in terms of production areas and instruments as well as to planning the process and process implementation. The validation of an aseptic manufacturing process by means of media fill generally assumes a limitation of the contamination risk to $<10^{-3}$, that is, less than 1 out of 1000 fillings is allowed to be nonsterile. For terminally sterilized preparations a sterility assurance level of 10^{-6} is required. Nonetheless, drug formulations may only be designated "sterile" when proof of sterility is presented.

4.3.2 Prerequisites Concerning Rooms and Equipment

The requirements with respect to the limitations in particles and germs during the preparation and filling of formulations are stipulated in standards and guidelines. According to the EU guidelines to Good Manufacturing Practice (GMP) (Annex 1: Preparation of Sterile Medicinal Products) four grades of cleanrooms as environment for the preparation of sterile products are distinguished (Table 4-7).

For small-scale operations, clean benches (laminar flow boxes; see 4.3.4) or isolators (glove boxes) of various dimensions and construction design are well suited. Isolators are cabinets made of (light) metal or polymers, equipped with large glass or Perspex® walls. They ensure an airtight sealing so that no microorganisms can access the cabinet from the lab space. On the front side, two or more openings are present to which rubber gloves are germ-tight attached. The gloves allow (aseptic) operations to be carried out inside the chamber compartment. By double-door airlocks, sterilized preparative instruments (balances, mortars, funnels, spoons, etc.) can be introduced, in addition to the active ingredients and excipients that need to be processed, after the chamber has been treated by spraying a disinfection agent or with hydrogen peroxide. A UV lamp can be installed in the chamber of the cabinet as an additional germ-reduction measure.

Aseptic manufacturing zones in pharmaceutical production units and hospital pharmacies have, in addition to the aseptic production rooms (clean room class A/B) preparatory spaces (class D) at their disposition, in which, among others, all containers, instruments and materials that are required for the aseptic manufacturing of drug formulations are cleaned. Such units should be designed in such a way that cleanliness can be easily maintained.

The constructional design of a room in the aseptic working area is subjected to the following principal requirements:

- Walls, ceiling, and floors as well as the working benches should have smooth surfaces, which are easy to clean and disinfect.

Table 4-7 Classification of Clean Rooms According to the EU Guidelines for GMP (Annex 1: Preparation of Sterile Medicinal Products)

		Operating Procedures in the Various Clean Room Classes				
		Max. Particle Number/m³ at Rest		Max. Germ Number/m³	Examples of Operations	
Grade	Ventilation	≥0.5 μm	≥5 μm		Terminally sterilized products	Not terminally sterilized products
A	Laminar airflow HEPA-filter	3,520	20	<1	Filling of products, when unusually at risk	Aseptic preparation and filling
B	Turbulent dilution flow HEPA-Filter	3,520	29	10	Background environment for the grade A zone	Background environment for the grade A zone
C	Turbulent dilution flow HEPA-filter	352,000	2,900	100	Preparation of products when unusually at risk, filling of products with normal contamination risk	Preparation of solutions to be filtered
D	Turbulent dilution flow	3,520,000	29,000	200	Preparation of solutions and components for subsequent filling	Handling of components after washing

- Windows and doors should allow tight closing and should be kept closed during the production process.
- The aseptic area should be accessible only via double airlocks consisting of a primary airlock (gray zone) where street clothes are taken off and a second one (white zone), where hand and forearms are thoroughly washed and disinfected and sterilized working clothes consisting of fabric nonshedding fibers are put on.
- The doors to the primary airlock and the aseptic space should be forcibly bolted.
- Ventilation should be achieved with germ-free filtered and temperature-conditioned air while the air supply should be regulated in such a way that in the production room a slight over-pressure prevails (15 Pa at least) in order to minimalize access of germ-containing air.
- Transport of materials into and out of the area should take place via separate airlocks.

The *hygienic measures* should be laid down in operating procedures that take account of company-specific matters. In general, it is mandatory that floors and working surfaces are thoroughly wet-cleaned and disinfected at least daily and walls, doors and lamps about monthly to three times monthly.

Bacteria are commonly 500 nm to 1 μm in size, *Bacillus* species up to 5 μm. The germs can be located in the air attached to dust particles. Airborne solid or liquid particles have diameters of 20 nm to 100 μm. There is, however, no correlation between germ number and the concentration of airborne particles.

The assessment of the number of particles in the air is achieved by means of laser particle counters. The microbial status of the air is assessed by the following methods:

- During filtration, air is drawn through a filter and subsequently the filter is incubated (cf. 4.4.3). This procedure allows quantitative assessment of the germ number and is frequently applied.
- Germ-containing particles are precipitated by means of impactors (see section 3.4.7) on agar plates or gelatin membrane filters, which are subsequently incubated. The Reuter-Centrifugal-Sampler blows the air, sucked in by a turbine wheel, radially against an agar strip lying flat against the cylindrical inner wall of the turbine housing. Based on a cascade-like deposition of the particles, the Andersen-impactor can provide information on the distribution of the germs in dependence on particle size.
- The Slit-Sampler sucks air through a narrow slit and the germs are slung onto a slowly rotating agar plate. Germ-number limits of <1 CFU/m^3 can be determined this way.
- The settling procedure applies agar plates onto which the germs precipitate by sedimentation. After incubation of the plates, evaluation follows—however, without allowing a quantitative assessment of the germ number in the air because the precipitation of the germs depends on the size of the precipitating particle. Only germs or dust particles larger than ca. 1 μm will precipitate by sedimentation. Smaller particles or bacteria are not susceptible to sedimentation. According to experience, with this method only 30 to 40 percent of the germs are captured.

There are no official directions indicating how often the germ number of the air should be assessed. This is left to the responsibility of the pharmaceutical manufacturer. As a rule of thumb, biweekly assessments are reasonable.

4.3.3   Personnel Hygiene

The most important source of contamination in the aseptic domain is men, who provides excellent living conditions for a large number of different microorganisms and continuously releases those into the environment (Table 4-8).

As a consequence, a series of measures is required to minimize the risk of contamination. Primarily, this concerns the education of workers with respect to proper production behavior and a high awareness of hygiene, as well as careful planning of all production steps warranting an expeditious workflow.

Table 4-8 Germ Release and Germ Content of Humans

	Number of Germs
Fingertip	20–100/cm^2
Hand	1000–6000
Saliva	10^6–10^8/mL
Nasal secretion	10^6–10^7/mL
1 x sneezing	10^4–10^6

Compliance to the following measures is required in particular:

- Wash and disinfect hands and forearms before starting work and after work interruptions.
- Wear special sterilized clean-room garments (clean room gown) including hood and face mask; the latter should cover mouth and nose and should be replaced every two hours, minimally.
- Use sterilized disposable towels and handkerchiefs, to be discarded after use in closable garbage containers.
- Avoid sneezing, coughing, and unnecessary speaking.
- Do not wear jewelry or watches on hands and forearms.

4.3.4   Laminar Flow Principle

A revolutionary step forward in aseptic technology was made in 1960 by the development and practical introduction of the laminar airflow (LAF) system. This technology makes it possible to create a sterile working place in a nonsterile environment.

It involves the uniform movement of a laminar flow of air, made particle- and microorganism-free by a high efficiency particulate (HEPA) filter, through a closed off compartment (Fig. 4-9). The flow velocity should amount to about 0.45 m/s, corresponding to an approximately 170-200-fold air exchange rate per hour, without producing a noticeable draft. By contrast, with a turbulent airflow, such as applied for the ventilation of conventional clean rooms, already a 20-fold air exchange per h is experienced as uncomfortable. The laminar airflow continuously carries off emitted particles within seconds and prevents their entrance from outside. The extraordinary performance of this process is illustrated by the following. The ambient air in cities contains, depending on season and location, about 50 to 200 million particles of size class ≥ 0.5 μm per m^3, while the concentration of animate particles (i.e., microorganisms) amounts to 100 to 500/m^3. In closed spaces, on the other hand, a germ number of 500 to 2000/m^3 air can be expected, depending on the number of people present. In conventional clean rooms, ventilated with turbulent airflow, the number of ≥ 0.5 μm

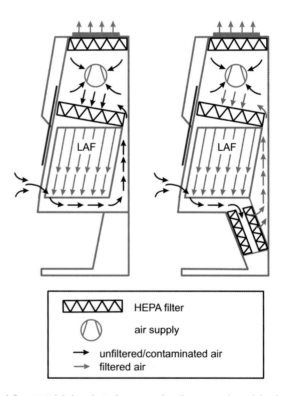

Fig. 4-9 Vertical-flow LAF lab bench. Left: conventional construction; right: bench with additional filter for processing of toxic substances.

particles may be as high as $3.520.000/m^3$ and the germ number up to $200/m^3$ (clean room grade D). With laminar flow facilities it is possible to reduce the $\geq 0.5\,\mu m$ particle count in the air to $<3520/m^3$ and the germ number to $<1/m^3$.

The laminar airflow can be carried either vertically (i.e., it flows from ceiling to floor, down flow), or horizontally (i.e., the air flows from one wall to the opposite one, cross flow). In addition, the airflow can be actively drawn off, or it leaves the aseptic space passively. The former system, provided with an installed special exhaust filter, should be applied in case one is working with toxic or infectious material.

Depending on the intended purpose, laminar airflow devices can be constructed in different ways. Portable systems, which can be transported relatively easily to microbially hazardous zones such as ampoule filling sites, can locally provide for an aseptic working space. For the aseptic manufacturing of drug formulations at a subindustrial scale (ophthalmic preparations, parenteral dosage forms) and sterility tests LAF benches (clean benches) can be used (Fig. 4-9).

For the aseptic manufacturing of drug formulations as well as for sterility tests, the equipment must be installed in a grade B clean room environment. Horizontal- and vertical-flow LAF benches, which only guarantee product protection, are distinguished from class-2 safety benches that protect the product against contamination from the ambient air but also the working individual and the environment from aerosols and microorganisms originating from the product. These safety benches are equipped with exhaust slits at the front and back edge of the working area. Since the exhaust capacity is higher than the supply rate of filtered air, at the front side not only air from the internal space of the bench is sucked in but also ambient air. As a result, an air curtain is formed at the manipulation openings, which prevents both the entrance and exit of suspended particles. Approximately 70% of the air drawn off is guided back to the inner space after sterile filtration, the remaining 30% leaves the bench via an exhaust filter. The processing of cytotoxic substances (e.g., cytostatics) requires the application of benches equipped with prefilters, which prevent contamination of the air channels in the internal parts of the device. It is important to note that heat-producing equipment (e.g., Bunsen burners) can produce air turbulence. In addition, the LAF box should only contain indispensable equipment and instruments in order to prevent disturbance of the laminar airflow, which may lead to suboptimal removal of germs. Obviously, also other principles of aseptic handling should be strictly obeyed, including hand disinfection, sterilization of equipment, materials and vessels to be used, as well as regular wet cleaning and disinfection of the working surfaces and walls of the bench.

For the surveillance of the functionality of these devices, it is necessary to assess the airflow velocity with anemometers (vane, or better even, hot-wire anemometer), the parallelism of the airflow with a suitable aerosol generator and the microbial status of the air with membrane filter devices (or, second best, a settle plates).

4.4 Sterility Tests and Microbial Contamination

4.4.1 General Introduction

Sterile drug formulations have to be free from viable microorganisms, that is, they must comply with the test for sterility. However, also for nonsterile preparations, the Pharmacopeia has established microbial quality requirements (see section 25.5.2). These vary with the nature of the application (for inhalation formulations for instance, more rigorous requirements apply than for rectal preparations) but also take into account the origin of the raw materials (special requirements for example for herbal products). Acceptability criteria with respect to microbial quality are also defined for a multitude of raw materials. Evaluation criteria include, as a rule, the total number of aerobic microorganisms (TAMC, total aerobic microbial count) and that of yeasts and molds (TYMC, total combined yeasts/molds count). Besides, often tests for specified microorganisms (e.g., *Pseudomonas aeruginosa*, *Staphylococcus aureus* and *Escherichia coli* are carried out, as an indicator of fecal contamination.

4.4.2   Test for Sterility

4.4.2.1   General Introduction

Substances, preparations, or objects may be designated sterile only then when upon a test for sterility no growth of microorganisms is observed. The test is performed on random samples selected in accordance with the Pharmacopeia. A predefined amount of the correspondingly prepared formulation is incubated in a specified culture medium. The Ph. Eur. recommends for that purpose a soya-bean casein digest medium (to detect aerobic bacteria and fungi) and a fluid thioglycollate medium (for the detection of anaerobic microorganisms). Because certain active ingredients (antibiotics, cytostatics), preservatives, but also heavy metal traces that are present in the formulation may have an inhibitory effect on the growth of microorganisms, the presence of such substances should be identified by special tests and, when applicable, they need to be removed or inactivated. The ultimate evaluation of the test is based on macroscopic evidence of microbial growth (see Ph. Eur. 2.6.1).

In order to prevent false positive results from the test procedure, this must be carried out under strict maintenance of aseptic conditions. This can be realized by using a clean bench (clean room grade A) in a clean room grade B, or an isolator. The instruments and media used in the test should be pre-sterilized as far as possible. It is, however, also important that the samples to be investigated are stored and treated in such a way that any microorganisms present in the samples will not be damaged, in order to prevent underestimation of any contamination.

Ph. Eur. 2.6.1 Sterility _____

Ph. Eur. 5.1.9. Guidelines for Using the Test for Sterility
USP ⟨71⟩ Sterility Tests
JP 4.06 Sterility Test

The test for sterility is carried out under aseptic conditions. Either the membrane filtration method or the direct inoculation method can be applied.

The membrane filtration method is applicable for liquid (aqueous and oily) and semi-solid substances or preparations as well as for soluble solids (according to Ph. Eur.). In the USP the applicability is extended to prefilled syringes, sterile aerosol products and devices with pathways labeled sterile. The test volume, which is specified in the pharmacopeias as a function of the quantity per container, is filtered through a sterile membrane filter with pore size 0.45 μm. If necessary, it may be diluted with an appropriate sterile diluent before filtration (e.g., neutral meat or casein peptone solution). Solids are dissolved in a suitable solvent. After filtration the membrane may be washed with a sterile diluent, if necessary, for example if the product has antimicrobial properties. Subsequently the filter membrane is transferred into a suitable culture medium or overlaid with this in the filtration device and incubated for at least 14 days at 30°C to 35°C (fluid thioglycollate medium) or between 20°C and 25°C (soya-bean casein digest medium). In order to apply both media the membrane can be cut aseptically into two equal parts, and one half is transferred to each of the two media.

The direct inoculation method can be used for all products for which also the membrane filtration method is applicable. In addition, the Ph. Eur. allows this method also for testing of surgical sutures for veterinary use. In the USP, the applicability is extended to solids, purified cotton, gauze, surgical dressings, and related articles, as well as sterile devices. The amount of the preparation specified in the pharmacopeias is transferred directly into the culture medium and incubated for at least 14 days at the indicated temperature. The volume of the product should not exceed 10% of the volume of the medium. If needed, the sample can be diluted with a sterile dilution medium (e.g., meat or casein peptone), or a suitable emulsifier (e.g., polysorbate 80) or inactivating agent can be added to inactivate any antimicrobially acting substance present in the sample. The inoculated media are incubated for not less than 14 days at the abovementioned temperatures.

At intervals during the incubation period and at its conclusion, the media are examined macroscopically for evidence of microbial growth. When microbial growth occurs in one or more test samples, it is considered for the whole batch that proof of sterility has failed.

The pharmacopeias recommend fluid thioglycollate medium for anaerobic as well as aerobic bacteria, in addition to soya-bean casein digest medium for bacteria and fungi. As a negative control the sterility of the used media needs to be ascertained (growth of microorganisms must not occur when portions of the media are incubated for 14 days). Furthermore, it needs to be ensured that the used media allow microbial growth, both in presence (method suitability test) and absence (growth promotion test) of the product to be tested. For that purpose, the pure and the product containing media or the filter membrane after filtration of the product are inoculated with a small number (<100 CFU) of the following test organisms: *Staphylococcus aureus, Bacillus subtilis, Pseudomonas aeruginosa, Clostridium sporogenes, Candida albicans, Aspergillus brasiliensis*. Within 5 days of incubation (or even 3 days for bacteria in case of the growth promotion test) visually observable growth should be clearly apparent. The minimal number of items that have to be tested is determined by the type of the product and the batch size. Precise instructions are presented as a table in Ph. Eur. 2.6.1, USP ⟨71⟩, JP 4.06. Additional directions concerning the test for sterility can be found in Ph. Eur. 5.1.9 (Guidelines for using the test for sterility).

The test for sterility implies testing of random samples. A negative result then merely means the absence of microbial contamination in the tested units. Simple extrapolation of this outcome to the entire batch would be based on the assumption that each container of the batch would have yielded the same test result. In case of only a minor contamination of the batch, most probably, the very few contaminated units will remain undetected and, thus, there is a high risk for false negative results.

However, the test also brings along a significant risk of false positive results. In such cases a repetition of the test is allowed only when at least one of the following conditions applies:

- Data of the microbiological monitoring of the sterility testing facility show a fault.
- A clear fault in the test procedure can be demonstrated.
- Microbial growth is found in the negative controls.
- By means of nucleic-acid homologies (RNA/DNA-sequence homology), it can be unequivocally demonstrated that the microorganisms in the contaminated sample originate from the test materials and/or from the testing environment and can be isolated from there.

4.4.2.2 Membrane Filtration Method

With this method, the preparation is filtered through a membrane filter (pore width ≤0.45 μm), leaving the microorganisms to be determined behind on the filter. The method is suitable for aqueous solutions, soluble powders, oils, and oily solutions and, when applicable, also ointments and creams that can be diluted into liquid systems (e.g., with isopropyl myristate). After the filtration through the sterile membrane filter, the latter is transferred to a liquid culture medium or overlaid with that. In order to allow a testing with both specified culture media, the filter can be cut into pieces under aseptic conditions before the testing. When the macroscopic examination during and after the termination of the incubation time (≥14 d) shows no growth of microorganisms, the sample may be considered sterile. As a rule, filters are used with a pore width larger than that applied for the sterile filtration during manufacturing processes, because in this way less stress is applied on possibly present microorganisms. In addition to the enrichment of the microorganisms on the filter, this method has the advantage that antimicrobial components that are potentially present in the preparation can be removed by rinsing with sterile dilution liquid. That is the reason why, whenever possible, this variant of the sterility test is preferred. In order to facilitate the aseptic execution of the test, nowadays prefabricated sterile disposable filtration units are commonly used, allowing overlaying the filter with the respective culture medium after the filtration. These units often also allow the partitioning of the product stream on two filters so that the contamination-prone cutting of the filter can be avoided.

4.4.2.3　Direct Inoculation Method

This method is applied to test preparations that cannot be filtered, for example certain oily liquids or semi-solid preparations. These are transferred directly into the culture medium. In the testing of oily liquids, the culture medium is supplemented with an emulsifier (e.g., polysorbate 80). In this case, validation studies are required to demonstrate that the emulsifier does not exhibit antimicrobial activity. Ointments and creams are mixed with a suitable emulsifier in an aqueous dilution solution prior to transfer into the culture medium. If the product is anti-microbially active, it is diluted with culture medium to such an extent that no more antimicrobial properties can be detected in the preparation or, alternatively, inactivating agents are added. Subsequently, the mixture is cultured for at least 14 days, upon which no germ growth should be observable.

Limits of the method. The sterility test only allows a strongly limited conclusion concerning the actual microbiological quality condition of a batch. Because for the test a limited number of randomly selected samples can be used (in most cases n = 20), extrapolation of the test result to the entire batch is problematic and is allowed only then when each unit of the batch in all stages of the manufacturing and handling is exposed to the same measures. Statistically, the probability that a batch that, upon one random sampling of n = 20, displays a contamination level of as high as 2%, is actually recognized as nonsterile and consequently rejected, is only 33%.

The sterility test may thus have an important meaning as a reference method, it is however not suitable as the only criterion for approval of a batch. The release of a batch of a sterile product therefore always occurs only in combination with the assessment of the physical characteristics of the sterilization process or of the validated processes in case of an aseptic manufacturing procedure, respectively. The recorded physical parameters of a validated sterilization process are of a much higher significance in connection to the sterility of a batch than the actual results of a sterility test. For that reason, the responsible authorities can allow to release a final product that has been terminally sterilized by means of a fully validated process exclusively on the basis of these physical parameters (i.e., waiving the necessity of the test for sterility) (*parametric release*). Until now, this procedure is not possible for aseptically manufactured products, so that the sterility test for these products is of special significance.

4.4.3　Microbiological Examination of Nonsterile Products

4.4.3.1　Microbial Enumeration Tests

The number of microorganisms is a criterion for the microbiological purity of substances, preparations or objects. For all drug formulations for which sterility is not mandatory, a limit of the number of microorganism and the absence of specified microorganisms is required.

The assessment of the number of microorganisms concerns the total number of viable and aerobic germs. This can be performed by membrane filtration or counting on agar plates and in exceptional cases also by means of dilution series (*most probable number method*). The membrane filtration method has the highest sensitivity with the additional possibility to exclude disturbing influences. The assay must be performed under aseptic conditions in order to prevent import of microorganisms. At the same time, any germs present in the samples should not be damaged.

Sample preparation. The preparation of the sample depends on the nature of the product to be tested. The latter is aseptically diluted by dissolution, suspension, or emulsification. The dispersion of water-insoluble products can be facilitated by addition of suitable surface-active agents such as polysorbate 80 and in case of fatty substances by slight warming. For aerosols and transdermal patches special preparation methods are described in the Pharmacopeia.

- **Membrane filtration**. The appropriately prepared product is filtered over a membrane filter with maximally 0.45 μm pore width. Subsequently, the filter is placed on the

Table 4-9 Most Probable Number of Microorganisms (Ph. Eur. 2.6.12 / USP <61> / JP 4.05)

Number of Tubes with Microbial Growth			Most Probable Number of Microorganisms per g or mL
0.1 g/mL per tube	0.01 g/mL per tube	0.001 mg/mL per tube	
3	3	3	>1100
3	3	2	1100
3	3	1	460
3	3	0	240
3	2	3	290
3	2	2	210
3	2	1	150
3	2	0	93
3	1	3	160
3	1	2	120
3	1	1	75
3	1	0	43
3	0	2	64
3	0	1	38
3	0	0	23

agar medium and after incubation the number of colonies is determined. Two tests should be performed, one for bacteria (TAMC) and one for fungi (TYMC), with the corresponding media and incubation conditions.

- **Plate-count methods**. Likewise, two parallel tests have to be performed, for bacteria and fungi, respectively. The test can be carried out according to either the pour-plate method or the surface-spread method. In the former case, the diluted product is mixed with slightly warmed fluid medium and then poured out. The dilution should be done in such a way that an as high as possible, but <250 (TAMC) or <50 (TYMC), number of colonies is produced on each individual plate. The number of microorganisms is taken to be the number of CFUs formed under test conditions from 1 mL or, when applicable, 1 g of the test substance. Alternatively, the samples can also be spread on prefabricated agar plates.

- **Counting by means of serial dilution (most probable number, MPN)**. This method is less reliable than the aforementioned procedures and should therefore only be applied if other methods are not applicable. Because it is not suitable for the determination of fungi, it is only carried out in soya-bean casein digest medium. The product is diluted stepwise to 1:10, 1:100 and 1:1000 dilutions (and, if need be, to further 1:10 step dilutions). For each dilution, three samples are transferred to a culture tube (thereby being diluted a further 1:10-step). After the prescribed incubation time, the most probable number of microorganisms can be estimated by evaluation of the number of turbid tubes (see Table 4-9 for the principle).

The method is based on the application of the Poisson distribution, through which the average number of microorganisms per mL of the relevant dilution step correlates with the frequency of growth-negative tubes.

4.4.3.2 Test for the Absence of Specified Microorganisms

In addition to a limitation of the number of microorganism in nonsterile products, also the absence of certain specified germs is required, which by virtue of their pathogenicity should by no means be present in a drug formulation:

- Bile salt-tolerant gram-negative bacteria (in particular enterobacteria)
- *Escherichia coli*
- Salmonellae
- *Pseudomonas aeruginosa*

- *Staphylococcus aureus*
- *Clostridiae*
- *Candida albicans*

When necessary, the test substance is dissolved, emulsified or suspended, like for the assessment of the number of microorganisms, and assayed using selective culture media. Both purposes require that any inhibitory action of the test conditions on the growth of the microorganisms be experimentally excluded and that the culture media are pre-tested for their suitability.

Ph. Eur. 2.6.12 Microbiological Examination of Nonsterile Products—Microbial Enumeration Tests

USP ⟨61⟩ Microbial Examination of Nonsterile Products—Microbial Enumeration Tests

JP 4.05 Microbial Limit Test, I. Microbial Examination of Nonsterile Products: Total Viable Aerobic Count

This test allows the quantitative enumeration of aerobic mesophilic bacteria (bacteria that grow best in a temperature range of 25-40°C). Three methods are described in the pharmacopeias: the membrane filtration method, the plate-count method, and the most probable number (MPN) method.

When applying the **membrane filtration method**, the appropriate amount of the liquid or dissolved sample or, in case of transdermal patches, the extracted solution, is filtered through each of two membrane filters with 0.45 μm nominal pore width. Both filters are rinsed with an adequate volume of a suitable fluid (e.g., a buffered NaCl-peptone solution pH 7.0). One of the membranes is transferred to a casein soya bean digest agar plate for the assessment of aerobic microorganisms (total aerobic microbial count = TAMC) and incubated for 3 to 5 days at 30°C to 35°C. The other membrane is transferred to a Sabouraud-dextrose agar plate for the assessment of yeasts and fungi (total combined yeasts/molds count = TYMC) and incubated for 5 to 7 days at 20°C to 25°C. From the number of colonies, the number of microorganisms is determined as CFU per g or per mL of the product.

The **plate-count method** can be performed either as pour-plate or as surface-spread method. In the pour-plate method, 1-mL aliquots of adequate dilutions of the test solution are mixed with 15-20 mL casein soya bean digest agar or Sabouraud-dextrose agar at a temperature of maximally 45°C (as little as possible above the gelling temperature of 42°C) in a Petri dish of 9 cm diameter and, after cooling, incubated under the above-mentioned time and temperature conditions. Per dilution at least two plates are inoculated. Of each dilution, only the plates with the highest CFU value are evaluated, provided that this value is below 250 CFU for TAMC and below 50 CFU for TYMC.

The **surface-spread method** is distinguished from the pour-plate method in that at least 0.1 mL of adequate dilutions of the test solution is evenly spread on 15 to 20 mL prefabricated agar culture plates (at least two Petri dishes for each medium and each level of dilution).

The **most-probable-number-method** is only applied for counting bacteria in certain product groups with a very low bioburden, where it may be the most appropriate method. The precision and accuracy is less than that of the membrane filtration method or the plate-count method. Unreliable results are particularly obtained for the enumeration of molds. Three culture tubes, each containing 9 to 10 mL of casein soya bean digest broth, are inoculated with 1 mL or 1 g aliquots of each dilution step of three consecutive 1:10 dilutions of the test sample. The nine inoculated tubes are incubated for 3 to 5 days at 30°C to 35°C. Based on the number of turbid tubes (i.e., those exhibiting microbial growth) in each of the three dilution steps the most probable number of microorganisms in the original solution is read out from a statistical table.

Ph. Eur. 2.6.13 Microbiological Examination of Nonsterile Products: Test for Specified Microorganisms _____

USP ⟨62⟩ Microbiological Examination of Nonsterile Products—Tests for Specified Microorganisms

JP 4.05 Microbial Limit Test, II. Microbial Examination of Nonsterile Products: Test for Specified Microorganisms _____

For the quantitative assessment of the bacteria listed below, the pharmacopeias describe methods that are based on the application of selective culture media:

- *Escherichia coli*
- *Salmonella*
- *Pseudomonas aeruginosa*
- *Staphylococcus aureus*
- *Clostridia*
- *Candida albicans*

Excipients for Drug Formulation

5

5.1   General Introduction, Requirements

The use of excipients to transform pharmacologically active substances into a suitable dosage form for application is as old as the production of medicines themselves. In combination with pharmaceutical substances, excipients may alter the pharmacological profile of the drug. On the other hand, based on merely physical effects, pure ointment bases for dermatological applications may display therapeutic effects even in the absence of any active ingredient. Pharmaceutical preparations whose activity is based on purely physical effects are referred to as "medical devices" (see box).

Excipients are substances by which pharmaceutically active ingredients can be transformed into a suitable drug formulation, with the possibility of altering the properties of the active agent. Thus, they fulfill various requirements, such as the following:

- They transform a pharmaceutically active substance into an appropriate form that can be utilized safely.
- The release of active ingredients can be modulated or targeted to the desired site of action.
- They provide sufficient stability of the active ingredient, as well as of the whole formulation.
- In the case of dermatology, cosmetic and skin care intrinsic effects may be assigned to the excipient(s).

Apart from the exceptions previously discussed, excipients should not display pharmacological activity by themselves. Therefore, they should be as inert as possible and physiologically fully inactive. The latter requirement may not always be fulfilled.

It is not always easy to make a precise distinction between excipients and active ingredients. Depending on the application, the dosage, as well as the site and method of administration, many substances can fulfill a function either as an excipient or as an active substance (Table 5-1).

When utilized as an excipient, the substance under consideration should not display either toxic or irritating activity at the applied concentration and dose, nor should it be allergenic. That is the reason why the number of approved excipients has been reduced further and further in recent years and the application of new excipients has come under more stringent regulation.

Further requirements that must be applied to excipients concern microbial contamination, compatibility, and stability.

- Many natural products that are put to use as excipients are contaminated with microorganisms. Pharmacopeias, therefore, have set limits to the count of bacteria and fungi. In addition, these materials are to be tested for the presence of various specific pathogenic

Voigt's Pharmaceutical Technology, First Edition. Alfred Fahr.
© 2018 John Wiley & Sons Ltd. Published 2018 by John Wiley & Sons Ltd.

Definitions:

United States Pharmacopeia:
USP ⟨1151⟩: Excipient: An ingredient of a dosage form other than a drug substance. The term "excipient" is synonymous with inactive ingredient.
US Code of Federal Regulations:
21CFR210.3 (8): Inactive ingredient means any component other than an active ingredient.

Table 5-1 Examples of Substances That Can Act as Active Ingredient as Well as an Excipient

Substance	Active Ingredient Function	Excipient Function
benzalkonium chloride	local antiseptic	preservative
α-Tocopherol	vitamin	antioxidant
glucose	therapy of diabetogenic coma, parenteral nutrition	tonicity agent
lactose	laxative	filler

organisms. Excipients for the preparation of parenteral or ophthalmologic formulations have to meet special requirements. For excipients where the production involves material from animal species known to be potential transmitters of transmittable spongiform encephalopathy, a risk assessment is required.

- Undesired interactions with active ingredients as well as with container and closure material should be avoided by proper selection of the excipient.
- Excipients should be sufficiently stable. Furthermore, the substances used should on the one hand maintain their function for the entire shelf life of the formulation, while on the other hand potential degradation products should not be toxic nor change the relevant properties of the formulation to any unacceptable extent.

In the documentation that has to be submitted if an application for marketing authorization is filed, excipients are treated in virtually the same way as active ingredients. The EU guideline CPMP/QWP/419/03 ("Note for guidance on excipients, antioxidants and antimicrobial preservatives in the dossier for application for marketing authorization of a medicinal product") stipulates the following:

- Type and quantity of all excipients must be specified.
- The inclusion of each individual excipient must be justified
- Specifications must be defined and justified for all excipients that are not described in any pharmacopeia monograph.
- The methods used to test the specifications must be described and validated.
- For new excipients, stability data must be determined.

In contrast to active ingredients, for most excipients it is generally not required to include qualitative or quantitative analyses in the control procedures for batch release. However, this does not apply to antioxidants and preservatives, nor, in particular cases, for other stability-relevant ingredients.

Most excipients can serve several, often very different, purposes. It is therefore difficult to list them according to application purpose. In the following, a chemical classification according to structure is presented. Only dyes, preservatives, and antioxidants, which originate from very different classes of chemical compounds, are systematically listed according to their application purpose.

Medical Devices

Medical device means any instrument, apparatus, appliance, software, material or other article to be used for human beings for diagnosis, prevention or therapy of diseases or for the investigation or modification of physiological function. It does not achieve its principal intended action in or on the human body by pharmacological, immunological or metabolic means, but might be assisted in their function by such means. (according to 93/42/EEC, abridged). In EU and USA, the legal framework for medical devices is determined by the following regulations: EU: 90/385/EEC, 93/42/EEC, 98/79/EC, 2007/47/EC, USA: 21 CFR Part 860. Combinations of medical devices with pharmaceutical agents are considered as medical devices only when the pharmaceutical agent has a merely supportive function in relation to the physical primary action (e.g., antibiotic-containing bone cement, heparin-coated catheters). When the function of the medical device is merely to deliver the pharmaceutical agent (e.g., drug-containing patches, prefilled syringes) the whole product is classified as a medicinal product according to EU regulations (formal authorization rather than CE marking). By contrast, in the USA any product composed of a combination of a drug and a device is denoted as a combination product (21 CFR 3.2(e): definition; 21 CFR part 4: regulation of combination products).

While placing a new medical product on the market requires approval by the government or a governmental agency, in EU the latter has only an indirect surveillance function when it concerns medical devices. A precondition for the initial market introduction of a medical device is that the device has undergone a conformity validation procedure (in EU: acceptance of a CE qualification), which, in the case of devices of the lowest risk class, is conducted by the manufacturer, while for higher risk classes an officially accredited authority must be involved. In the EU medical devices are categorized in the risk classes I, Is (sterile), Im (with measuring function), Ia, Ib and III. The table below presents examples of medical devices with pharmaceutical-technological relevance:

Class I	nonsterile dressing material
Class Is	sterile wound dressings, swabs, and gauze compresses
Class IIa	dental material, disinfectants for instruments and equipment
Class IIb	contact lens solutions, wound irrigation solutions
Class III	implants (also those containing active agents), sterile NaCl solutions for rinsing of catheters

A similar risk based classification also applies to medical devices according to US legislation (class I: low to moderate risk, class II: moderate to high risk, class III: high risk). Whereas most class I devices are exempt from premarket notification, most class II devices require premarket notification and most class III devices need a premarket approval.

5.2 Inorganic Excipients

5.2.1 Water

Water is undoubtedly the most important excipient; it is required not only for liquid formulations but also for the manufacturing of numerous solid dosage forms (e.g., for wet granulation). However, even if water is removed through drying after the manufacturing process, it can act as a source for chemical or microbiological contaminations that might remain in the final product. For this reason, in addition the quality of those excipients, which are only transiently in contact with the pharmaceutical product or its precursors, must not be ignored.

5.2.1.1 Water Qualities in the Pharmacopeias

The pharmacopeias distinguish different water qualities for use in medical devices or for drug formulations (regarding requirements and test procedures, see Table 5-2):

- Purified water (aqua purificata), Ph. Eur., USP, JP (Ph. Eur. submonographs: Purified water in bulk, Purified water in containers)
- Purified water in containers, JP
- Sterile purified water, USP
- Sterile purified water in containers, JP
- Water for the preparation of extracts (Aqua ad extractas praeparandas), Ph. Eur.
- Sterile water for inhalation, USP
- Sterile water for irrigation, USP
- Highly purified water (Aqua valde purificata), Ph. Eur.
- Water for injections (Aqua ad injectabilia, WFI), Ph. Eur. (submonographs: Water for injections in bulk, Sterilized water for injections)

Table 5-2 Water Qualities According to the Pharmacopeias (Requirements and Tests)

	Water for Preparation of Extracts (Ph. Eur.)	Purified Water in Bulk (Ph. Eur.)	Purified Water in Containers (Ph. Eur.)	Purified Water (USP)	Sterile Purified Water (USP)	Sterile Water for Inhalation (USP)	Water for Irrigation (Ph. Eur.) Sterile Water for Irrigation (USP)	Highly Purified Water (Ph. Eur.)
Preparation	Drinking water according to 98/83 EC or purified water	Preparation from drinking water by means of distillation, ion exchange, reverse osmosis or other suitable methods	Preparation from drinking water by means of distillation, ion exchange, reverse osmosis or other suitable methods	Preparation from drinking water by means of suitable methods	Preparation from drinking water by means of suitable methods, sterilization	Preparation from "Water for injection" that is sterilized and suitably packaged	Ph. Eur.: see Water for injections USP: Preparation from "Water for injection" that is sterilized and suitably packaged	Preparation from drinking water by means of double pass reverse osmosis in connection with other suitable techniques such as ultrafiltration or deionization
Microbial contamination	Action limit: 100 CFU/mL	Action limit: 100 CFU/mL	Acceptance criterion: TAMC: 10^2 CFU/mL	No limit specified. Where used for sterile dosage forms it has to meet the requirements of the sterility test <71>	Meets the requirements of the sterility test <71>	Meets the requirements of the sterility test <71>	Ph. Eur.: Compliant with sterility test USP: Meets the requirements of the sterility test <71>	Action limit: 10 CFU/100 mL
Bacterial endotoxins	No limit specified.	No limit specified. <0.25 IU/mL, when applied for the preparation of dialysis solutions	No limit specified. <0.25 IU/mL, when applied for the preparation of dialysis solutions	No limit specified.	No limit specified.	<0.5 IU/mL	Ph. Eur.: <0.5 IU/mL USP: <0.25 IU/mL	<0.25 IU/mL
Total organic carbon (TOC)	No test on TOC	≤0.5 mg/L alternatively: Test on oxidizable substances	Instead of TOC: Test on oxidizable substances (same limit as for Purified water in bulk)	≤0.5 mg/L	≤8.0 mg/L alternatively: Test on oxidizable substances	≤8.0 mg/L alternatively: Test on oxidizable substances	Ph. Eur.: ≤0.5 mg/L USP: ≤8.0 mg/L alternatively: Test on oxidizable substances	≤0.5 mg/L
Conductivity	≤2500 µS·cm^{-1} (20°C)	≤4.3 µS·cm^{-1} (20°C)	No test on conductivity	≤1.1 µS·cm^{-1} (20°C) for stage 1 of the test (higher values apply if the test has to be continued to stages 2 or 3)	Container vol. ≤10 mL: ≤25 µS·cm^{-1} (25°C) Container vol. >10 mL: ≤5 µS·cm^{-1} (25°C)	Container vol. ≤10 mL: ≤25 µS·cm^{-1} (25°C) Container vol. >10 mL: ≤5 µS·cm^{-1} (25°C)	Ph. Eur.: ≤1.1 µS·cm^{-1} (≥20°C, <25°C) USP: Container vol. ≤10 mL: ≤25 µS·cm^{-1} (25°C) Container vol. >10 mL: ≤5 µS·cm^{-1} (25°C)	≤1.1 µS·cm^{-1} (>20°C, ≤25°C) for stage 1 of the test (higher values apply if the test has to be continued to stages 2 or 3)
Other tests	Nitrates	Nitrates, Aluminum, Heavy metals	Nitrates, Aluminum, Heavy metals, Acidity/ Alkalinity, Chlorides, Sulfates, Ammonium, Calcium and magnesium, Residue upon drying	None[1]	Oxidizable substances as an alternative method for TOC[1]	Oxidizable substances as an alternative method for TOC[1]	Ph. Eur.: Pyrogens USP: Oxidizable substances as an alternative method for TOC[1]	Nitrates, Aluminum

[1] The USP does not specify the chemical quality of water by a series of chemistry tests for various specific and nonspecific attributes but substituted them by TOC and conductivity measurements without tightening the quality requirements. The TOC test replaced the test for oxidizable substances and a multistaged conductivity test replaced all of the tests for inorganic ions with the exception of the test for heavy metals. The latter was considered unnecessary because the source water specifications (drinking water standards) for individual heavy metals are tighter than the approximate limit of detection of the former heavy metal test and contemporary water system construction materials do not leach heavy metals contaminants. The pH test was dropped as a separate attribute test, as it was considered redundant to the conductivity test, which includes the aspect of pH dependent molecule dissociation in its test stage 3.

Water for Injections in Bulk (Ph. Eur.) Water for Injection (USP)	Sterilized Water for Injections (Ph. Eur.) Sterile Water for Injection (USP)	Water for Diluting Concentrated Hemodialysis Solutions (Ph. Eur.) Water for Hemodialysis (USP)	Purified Water (JP)	Purified Water in Containers (JP)	Sterile Purified Water in Containers (JP)	Water for Injection (JP)	Sterile Water for Injection in Containers (JP)
Ph. Eur./USP: Preparation from drinking water or purified water by means of distillation or by a purification process that is equivalent or superior to distillation (such as reverse osmosis, coupled with appropriate techniques)	Ph. Eur.: Preparation from Water for injections in bulk by distribution into suitable containers and sterilization by heat USP: Preparation from water for injection that is sterilized and suitably packaged	Preparation from drinking water by suitable methods Ph. Eur.: Preparation e.g., by distillation, ion exchange, reverse osmosis. Under certain circumstances also without further treatment	Preparation from drinking water by means of ion exchange, distillation, reverse osmosis, ultrafiltration or by a combination of these processes	Preparation from purified water by introducing it in a tight container	Preparation from purified water by introducing it into a hermetic container and subsequent sterilization or by aseptic filling of sterile purified water in a sterile, hermetic container	Preparation by distillation or by reverse osmosis and/or ultrafiltration, either from pretreated water (e.g., ion-exchange or reverse osmosis), or from purified water	Preparation from water for injection by introducing it into a hermetic container and subsequent sterilization or by aseptic filling of sterile water for injection in a sterile, hermetic container
Ph. Eur.: Action limit: 10 CFU/ 100 mL USP: No explicit limit specified	Ph. Eur.: Compliant with sterility test (2.6.1) USP: Meets the requirements of the sterility test <71>	Ph. Eur.: Acceptance criterion: TAMC: 10^7 CFU/g USP: TAMC ≤100 CFU/mL, Absence of Pseudomonas aeruginosa	No limit specified	Acceptance criterion: TAMC: 10^2 CFU/mL	Meets the requirements of the sterility test 4.06	No limit specified	Meets the requirements of the sterility test 4.06
<0.25 IU/mL	<0.25 IU/mL	Ph. Eur.: <0.25 IU/mL USP: <1 IU/mL	No limit specified	No limit specified	No limit specified	<0.25 IU/mL	<0.25 IU/mL
≤0.5 mg/L	Ph. Eur.: Instead of TOC: Test on oxidizable substances (limit 2× (if vol. ≥50 mL) or 4× (if vol. <50 mL) that for Purified water) USP: ≤8.0 mg/L alternatively: Test on oxidizable substances	Ph. Eur: Instead of TOC: Test on oxidizable substances (same limit as for purified water) USP: ≤0.5 mg/L	≤0.5 mg/L	No limit specified, instead limit for potassium permanganate-reducing substances	No limit specified, instead limit for potassium permanganate-reducing substances	≤0.5 mg/L	No limit specified, instead limit for potassium permanganate-reducing substances
≤1.1 µS·cm⁻¹ (≥20°C, <25°C) for stage 1 of the test (higher values apply if the test has to be continued to stages 2 or 3)	Container vol. ≤10 mL: ≤25 µS·cm⁻¹ (25°C) Container vol. >10 mL: ≤5 µS·cm⁻¹ (25°C)	Ph. Eur.: No test on conductivity USP: ≤1.1 µS·cm⁻¹ (20°C) for stage 1 of the test (higher values apply if the test has to be continued to stages 2 or 3)	≤2.1 µS·cm⁻¹ (25°C)	Container vol. ≤10 mL: ≤25 µS·cm⁻¹ (25°C) Container vol. >10 mL: ≤5 µS·cm⁻¹ (25°C)	Container vol. ≤10 mL: ≤25 µS·cm⁻¹ (25°C) Container vol. >10 mL: ≤5 µS·cm⁻¹ (25°C)	≤2.1 µS·cm⁻¹ (25°C)	Container vol. ≤10 mL: ≤25 µS·cm⁻¹ (25°C) Container vol. >10 mL: ≤5 µS·cm⁻¹ (25°C)
Ph. Eur.: Nitrates, Aluminum USP: None[1]	Ph. Eur.: Acidity/alkalinity, Oxidizable substances, Chlorides, Nitrates, Sulfates, Aluminum, Ammonium, Calcium and Magnesium, Residue upon drying, Particulate contaminations: non-visible particles. USP: Particulate matter in injections Oxidizable substances as an alternative method for TOC[1]	Ph. Eur.: Acidity/alkalinity, Total available chlorine, Chlorides, Fluorides, Nitrates, Sulfates, Aluminum, Ammonium, Calcium, Magnesium, Mercury, Potassium, Sodium, Zinc, Heavy metals USP: Maximum allowable chemical levels are listed in <1230>. Monitoring of these components is recommended.	None	Potassium permanganate-reducing substances	Potassium permanganate-reducing substances	None	Potassium permanganate-reducing substances, Foreign insoluble matter <6.06>, Insoluble particulate matter 6.07

- Water for injection, USP, JP
- Sterile water for injection, USP
- Sterile water for injection in containers, JP
- Water for the dilution of concentrated hemodialysis solutions (Aqua ad dilutionem solutionium concentratarum ad haemodialysim), Ph. Eur.
- Water for hemodialysis, USP

In the Ph. Eur., "Water for Irrigation" is included in the monograph "Preparations for Irrigation." It designates a water quality, intended for direct use in humans or animals by irrigation of body cavities, wounds, and surfaces, such as during surgical procedures. This water differs from "Water for Injections" only with respect to the specified type of the container closure system.

For analytical purposes more water qualities are described with special purity requirements, including "Water for BET" and "TOC water":

- Water for BET (Water for bacterial endotoxins test) (Ph. Eur., USP)
- Ph. Eur.: TOC-water (for the determination of total organic carbon) (TOC level ≤ 0.10 mg/L), USP: "Reagent water" for testing bulk water or sterile water on total organic carbon (TOC level ≤ 0.10 mg/L or ≤ 0.50 mg/L, dependent whether it is used for analysis of bulk or sterile water)

Water for pharmaceutical purposes must meet particularly high requirements with respect to its physicochemical biological and physiological properties. By contrast, water from natural sources contains dissolved substances, gases, microorganisms, pyrogens, and particulate contaminations, which must be removed to acceptable residual levels, depending on the specific purpose of use.

5.2.1.2   Water Hardness

The presence of calcium and magnesium salts determines the hardness of water. Depending on the behavior during boiling, transient hardness can be distinguished from permanent hardness. Transient hardness is caused by bicarbonates of calcium and magnesium. During boiling the dissolved carbon dioxide is expelled and the bicarbonates precipitate as carbonates (scale)

$$[Ca(HCO_3)_2 \rightarrow CaCO_3\downarrow + H_2O + CO_2\uparrow].$$

The permanent hardness (noncarbonate hardness, residual hardness) is caused by alkaline-earth chlorides, sulfates and silicates and cannot be eliminated by boiling. Water hardness is expressed as the concentration of alkaline-earth ions in mmol/L or mol/m^3.

In practice, also a variety of nationally defined hardness degrees are in use—for example, German hardness degrees (unit: °dH), American degrees (unit: ppm = mg/L CaCO$_3$), English degrees (unit: °e = °Clark) or French degrees (unit: °fH = °F) (Conversion into mmol/L: 1°dH = 0.1783 mmol/L, 1 ppm = 0.009991 mmol/L, 1 °e = 0.1424 mmol/L, 1 °fH = 0.09991 mmol/L). Nowadays, however, the only official measuring unit is mmol/L. Water hardness can be determined by complexometric titration with ethylenediaminetetraacetate (EDTA) using suitable indicators or by means of atomic absorption spectrometry (AAS).

Standard procedures to determine water hardness can be found in ASTM (American Society for Testing and Materials) and ISO (International Organization for Standardization) standards: ASTM D 1126 (Standard Test Method for Hardness in Water), ISO 7980 (Water Quality: Determination of Calcium and Magnesium—Atomic Absorption Spectrometric Method), ISO 6059 (Water Quality: Determination of the Sum of Calcium and Magnesium—EDTA Titrimetric Method).

Reduction of water hardness is desirable for many reasons. If Ca and Mg carbonates (scale) and other minerals precipitate on the walls of hot water systems, such as a kettle, they do not only reduce heat exchange and thus increase energy consumption, they are also often the cause of accidents, since the sudden pressure increase that may occur upon the chipping of such coatings (boiling delay), may cause explosion of the kettle.

In drug formulations, divalent calcium and magnesium ions may cause the complexation or flocculation of many, in particular macromolecular, anionic active and inactive ingredients. Multivalent ions may also reduce the stability of suspensions and emulsions as a result of a decrease in the zeta potential. Therefore, in the manufacturing of medicines, mostly purified water is used or even, when required, water of a higher pharmaceutical quality. Purified water in containers (Ph. Eur.) contains at most 0.05 mmol/L (Ca^{2+} + Mg^{2+}) ions.

5.2.2 Pharmaceutical Water Qualities, Preparation

Purified water is prepared from drinking water by means of ion exchange, reverse osmosis, electrodeionization, or distillation. Based on the requirement of the pharmacopeias that only drinking water must be used for the preparation of purified water, the quality of the source material is also precisely defined by the legal limits for drinking water. For the production of water for injection only distillation or purification processes equivalent to distillation, such as reverse osmosis coupled with appropriate techniques, are allowed.

5.2.2.1 Distillation

The production of pure water by means of distillation requires the use of high heat energy. Heating 1 L of water from 20°C to 100°C consumes 335.2 kJ (80 kcal) and to turn this into vapor another 2262 kJ (540 kcal) is required. During condensation of the water vapor, the vapor-generating energy is set free again and transferred to the cooling water. In older equipment, this heat is withdrawn from the system and thus distillation is much more energy consuming than ion exchange or reverse osmosis.

Equipment

Because water for injections (WFI) has the capacity to dissolve ions from materials with which it comes into contact, it may to a certain extent act corrosively. Therefore, equipment for the production of WFI has to be made of largely inert materials. Although the Ph. Eur. also allows neutral or quartz glass as a material for WFI stills, in modern installations only high-alloyed chrome-nickel-molybdenum steel is applied. The surfaces are electropolished and possess, as a rule, an average surface roughness (R_a) of ≤ 0.2 μm in order to avoid the adhesion of particles and microorganisms in the depressions of the surface structure. Because of GMP requirements for equipment qualification and process validation, simple laboratory devices, including those for the production of double-distilled water (aqua bidest), are unsuitable for the preparation of WFI. Also for small-scale WFI production, exclusively, automatically operating column distillation plants are used. The smallest versions are single effect stills with a capacity of up to 50 L/h. If even smaller amounts are required, for instance, for the prescription-wise production of parenterals in the pharmacy, it is recommended to refer to commercially available WFI in bottles or polymer ampoules. For laboratory use (e.g., in the framework of preclinical development), in most cases the use of reverse-osmosis water suffices; this can be easily prepared by means of fully automatized and user-friendly tabletop devices.

5.2.2.2 Distillation Equipment for Large-Scale Production

The development of all modern distillation equipment is characterized by the intention to utilize the required energy as economically as possible, to reduce the use of cooling water (the ratio distillate to cooling water varies from 1:10 to 1:20), and to automatize the installation.

The most frequently used distillation procedures in industry are as follows:

- The single-step or double-step pressure column procedure
- The thermo-compression procedure
- The Zyclodest®-procedure
- The thermojet-procedure

The procedures operate either as a boiling procedure, that is, by evaporation from a stationary water supply (pool) or as a dropping-film distillation in which water, while running

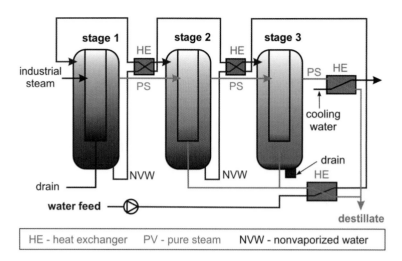

Fig. 5-1 Multistage distillation plant.

downward along the wall of a heated pipe, evaporates. All these procedures exploit the energy released during the condensation to preheat the feed water.

Multieffect Distillation Plants

In this type of equipment (Fig. 5-1), the cold feed water and the hot distillate are led counter-current-wise through the heat exchanger of the three- to eight-stage plant. As a result, the feeding water has almost attained its evaporation temperature already upon entering the first column. Only a small additional quantity of evaporation energy has to be supplied by external heating. The ultrapure vapor from each individual column is used to evaporate the feed water of the following column, while the distillate condenses and is further cooled down in heat exchangers. The impure distillate collecting at the bottom of each column acts as the feed water for the next one. In this way the water is boiled down in up to eight consecutive steps, before it leaves the last column as a concentrate of impurities dissolved in the residual volume.

Up to a demand of 50 L ultrapure water per hour, a single stage device suffices, while for demands ≥100 L/h, multieffect plants are needed. Finn-Aqua stills (Santasolo-Sohlberg Corp., Helsinki) with one to six pressure columns produce, for example, 100–26,000 L ultrapure water per hour. In this type of column, the vapor is guided upward in a spiral movement, leading to a separation of unevaporated water droplets driven by centrifugal forces.

The rational way of heat recycling, particularly in the multieffect distillation plants, allows a drastic conservation of heating energy and cooling water, as compared to classic distillation procedures.

Thermo-Compression Devices

Even more economic is the thermo-compression method, although it is quite maintenance-intensive because of its movable mechanical parts. In the thermo-compression device, the feed water is preheated and subsequently evaporated in a heat exchange tube at 105°C. The vapor arrives via special grids made from stainless steel (demister), which serve to separate droplets and particles, in the housing dome where it is condensed by a compressor. During this process the vapor is overheated to about 140°C. At this temperature it flows through the heat exchanger, where it is condensed to a distillate, while the feed water evaporates. Additional heating (by vapor or electricity) serves to make up for heat losses and to start up the system (Fig. 5-2).

Zyclodest® Procedure

A further development is the Zyclodest® procedure, which is characterized by two separate circuits, with the heat compression system (secondary circuit) having no direct contact to the distillate circuit (primary circuit). The feed water, preheated in a heat exchanger by the down-flowing distillate, is evaporated during a heating step at 135°C and corresponding

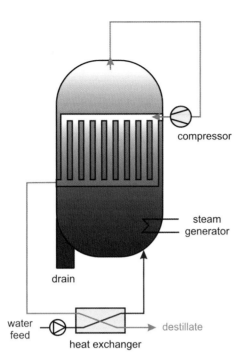

Fig. 5-2 Thermo-compression device.

over-pressure. When exiting the vaporization chamber the vapor passes a cyclone in which water droplets with sizes up to 0.5 μm are centrifuged off at about 500 times gravity. Smaller droplets are also carried along with them due to the coagulation effects. The ultrapure vapor produced is separated as a distillate in a condenser. The heat released in this process evaporates the water in the secondary circuit. The steam, is transformed by compression into a superheated state that provides the energy for the evaporation of the feed water in the heating stage. This procedure does not require any cooling water (Fig. 5-3).

The Thermojet Procedure

In the Thermojet procedure, water is heated in a feed-heating stage to about 180°C, during which a vapor pressure of 10 bar is reached. The unevaporated fluid fraction serves to preheat the feed water just before entering the heating stage. The pressure of the produced water vapor is expanded and the vapor condenses into a distillate by the cooled water from the heating step.

A comparison of the energy and cooling water requirements of various distillation procedures can be found in Table 5-3.

5.2.2.3 Ion Exchange

Exchange Materials

Ion exchangers are insoluble materials that are capable of reversibly exchanging part of the electrostatically bound ions on their surface by other ions. One finds substances possessing ion exchange activity in a variety of different chemical classes, including inorganic materials such as aluminum silicates (Zeolite) or polymers of natural or synthetic origin. The currently used exchange materials for desalting of water are synthetic polymer resins cross-linked in a three-dimensional network featuring an insoluble, swellable hydrocarbon skeleton bearing exchange-active groups. Ion-exchange resins can be synthesized by poly-condensation or by polymerization. Polycondensate resins from simply substituted phenols (phenol sulfonic acids, phenol carboxylic acids) and aldehydes (specifically formaldehyde) were the first synthetically produced ion exchange resins. Currently, used exchange resins are almost exclusively polymers based on polystyrene or polyacrylates. Polystyrene resins are obtained by polymerization of derivatives of vinylbenzenes with divinylbenzene serving as a cross-linker. Polyacrylate resins can be synthesized by copolymerization of divinylbenzene with acrylic

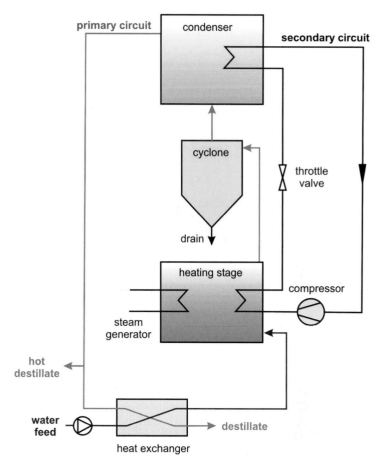

Fig. 5-3 Zyclodest® procedure.

acids. The polymer skeleton can be either swellable, but free from discrete pores (exchange resins of the gel type), or it can represent a structure interspersed with pore channels (macroporous exchange resins).

The former possess higher exchange capacity, but are active only in fluids that are capable of causing the polymer to swell. The latter are independent on the type of fluid and also facilitate the exchange of larger ions. Depending on whether the ions are bound to acidic or alkaline groups in the exchanger molecules, cation and anion exchangers are distinguished.

In cation exchangers, mainly sulfonic acid groups ($-SO_3H$), phenolic hydroxylgroups ($-OH$), and carboxyl groups ($-COOH$) are responsible for the acidic properties. The Ph. Eur.

Table 5-3 Energy and Cooling Water Requirement of Various Distillation Procedures for the Production of 100 L Distillate

	Electrical Power Input (kW)	Steam Consumption (kg)	Cooling Water Consumption (L)	Distillate Temp. (°C)
Conventional distillation	65	110	1000	30
Multieffect stills (4 columns)	18	37	84	90
Thermo-compression procedure	3.7 +1.6 (for doubling the energy by the compressor)	3.4	–	30
Zyclodest® procedure	3.0		–	cold
	11.0		–	70
Thermojet procedure	11.0		–	90

lists in the chapter "Reagents" several cation exchangers—among others, "Cation exchanger R" and "Cation exchanger, strongly acidic R." These contain sulfonic acid groups that are connected to a polystyrene skeleton, which in case of "cation exchanger R1" is cross-linked with 4% divinylbenzene. Cation exchanger weakly acidic R is a weakly acidic poly(methacrylic acid) resin with carboxylic groups. The cation exchangers are available either in protonated form or as a sodium or calcium salt.

In anion exchangers, mainly quaternary ammonium groups as well as primary, secondary or tertiary amino groups act as carriers of the alkaline properties. The Ph. Eur. lists under the heading "Reagents" a series of anion exchangers, among them the types described in the following:

"Anion exchanger R" contains quaternary ammonium groups in the chloride form, connected to a skeleton cross-linked with 2% divinylbenzene. "Anion exchanger, strongly basic R" contains quaternary ammonium groups with hydroxyl counterions, which are coupled to a polystyrene skeleton cross-linked with 8% divinylbenzene. By contrast, "Anion exchanger, weak R" possesses diethylaminoethyl groups. Other types are based on poly(methyl methacrylate), poly(ethylvinylbenzene-divinylbenzene) or polyether skeletons. Similar ion exchangers are also described by reagent monographs in the USP and JP.

Under the trademarks Lewatit®, Permutit®, Dowex®, Amberlite® and others, numerous ion exchanger types are commercially available.

A sodium chloride solution is deionized as follows:

Cation exchanger (CE): $R-SO_3H + NaCl \rightarrow R-SO_3Na + HCl$
Anion exchanger (AE): $R-NR_3'^{\oplus}OH^{\ominus} + HCl \rightarrow R-NR_3'^{\oplus}Cl^{\ominus} + H_2O$
R: exchanger skeleton
$-NR_3'^{\oplus}$:   quaternary ammonium group

Deionized (demineralized) water can be produced according to two different procedures: deionization by separated cation and anion exchangers or by mixed-bed deionization.

The latter one is nowadays the most common procedure (Fig. 5-4) and is achieved in a column in which a mixture of the cation and the anion exchange resins is packed. The water obtained by this procedure is practically neutral and of high purity.

Testing Exchanger Activity

The capacity of exchanger devices is characterized by the amount of ions that can be bound per gram of dry resin or per liters of wet resin. It is usually quoted as eq/kg (meq/g) or eq/L. One equivalent (eq) is the amount of ions that carries 1 mol of unit charge, independent of the sign of the charge.

When continuously fresh electrolyte-containing water flows through the exchange column, gradually all exchangeable ions are being replaced by ions from the water, slowly exhausting the capacity of the exchanger. Ultimately, this results in a "salt break-through" (appearance of cations and/or anions in the outflow), which can be detected by means of an electric conductivity test. Virtually all customary ion-exchange systems are equipped with conductivity meters.

Chemically pure water has a specific conductivity of 0.055 μS (Microsiemens) per cm, by virtue of its dissociation into oxonium and hydroxyl ions. Already, very small quantities of salts or carbon dioxide increase the electric conductivity, which thus represents a reliable indicator for the purity of water and for the functionality of deionization devices. Mixed-bed devices produce water with a conductivity of approximately 0.1–1 μS/cm. The conductivity limits requested by the pharmacopeias for different water qualities are listed in Table 5-2.

Regeneration

As a rule, cation exchangers are regenerated with hydrochloric acid (3%–5%) and anionic exchangers with alkali (4%). For the regeneration of mixed-bed exchange columns, it is necessary to first separate the two types of resin. This can be achieved by taking advantage of the density difference between cation and anion exchange resins. After both components are regenerated by type-specific treatments, they are remixed and are ready for further use.

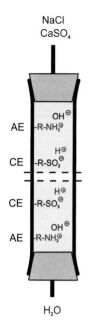

Fig. 5-4 Schematic representation of an ion-exchange column.

Though the units eq/kg and eq/L are still commonly used in application-oriented literature, the scientific correct units are mol_c/kg or mol_c/L (mol_c = moles of charge). 1 eq = 1 mol_c.

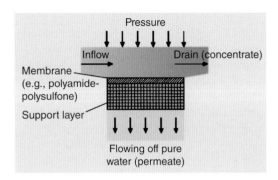

Fig. 5-5 Reverse osmosis.

Automatically operating systems are available that carry out all these regeneration steps directly on-site.

For small-scale applications, however, cartridge-based devices are commonly used that contain the resins in exchangeable polymer containers. These modules are returned to the manufacturer for regeneration.

Types of Equipment

The capacity of ion exchange devices may vary greatly. Small devices produce 50 L/h, while larger ones may produce about 400 L/h. Multiple-tank systems with arrangements of several mixed-bed columns have a capacity of about 5,000 L/h for water.

High-quality resins, when properly used, produce odorless water with a neutral taste and without any organic residues. The Ph. Eur. explicitly permits demineralization by means of ion exchange for the production of purified water and water for the dilution of concentrated hemodialysis solutions, as an alternative to distillation.

The advantage of demineralized water is that the production is far more economical than distilled water. The cost savings can amount to as much as 80% because the energy-intensive evaporation process is eliminated. Demineralization by ion exchangers is also often combined with distillation. A cation exchanger for softening of the water (removal of calcium and magnesium) is usually installed upstream to a distillation unit in order to prevent the still from scale deposit.

Because of potential microbial contamination, the pharmacopeias do not permit the use of demineralized water for the preparation of injection and infusion solutions. The organic matrix and the high surface area of the resins promote bacterial colonization.

However, at high perfusion rates, short down times and by using high-quality resins demineralization is able to produce water with a low microbial count and endotoxin concentration. By additional measures such as UV irradiation and bacteria-retaining filters the microbial count and pyrogen content can be further reduced.

5.2.2.4 Reverse Osmosis

Reverse osmosis, an established method for the desalting of seawater, has also gained widespread use in the pharmaceutical field. It is the standard procedure for the production of purified water and has also become an alternative to distillation for production of water for injections. Ultrapure water may be obtained, for instance, by double reverse osmosis, often coupled to prior treatment with an ion exchange procedure.

While during osmosis water diffuses through a semipermeable membrane, following a concentration gradient from high to low concentration, in reverse osmosis the solvent flows, under an externally applied pressure, in the opposite direction (Fig. 5-5). Reverse osmosis membranes display a selective permeability by virtue of molecular interactions between dissolved low-molecular weight substances (salts, acids), and the membrane surface. The extent of desalting can reach 98% and for multistep devices up to 99.9%. Also microbial contaminations are kept to a minimum with a bioburden reduction amounting to values of 95% to 99%. The installations are constructed for capacities of 20–2,000 l/h and operate at pressures of 1,400–2,800 kPa (14–28 bar).

Although reverse osmosis membranes are often reported to have a pore size of 0.1 nm, it is still a point of debate whether these layers are really porous or rather represent homogeneous structures without any pores running the entire width of the membrane layer, but instead have free volume spaces owing to the static or dynamic disorder of the polymer structure.

Prior to subjecting water to a reverse osmosis procedure, the feed water is pretreated by ion exchange for the removal of iron and silicate ions, which may damage the membranes. Subsequently it is introduced into the polyamide (or cellulose acetate) module where the membrane processes take place. The modules can be constructed in various ways such as: *hollow-fiber modules* consisting of thousands of very thin, tube-wise arranged bundled fibers. The prepurified water permeates the fibrous membranes and is drained off as ultrapure water via the internal space of the fibers; *Spiral modules* are filter bodies, which are spirally reeled around a core. They consist of two membranes, separated from each other by a sieve layer, and glued together at the edges, thus forming a sac. The water flows from outside inward. It is recommended that the module be cleaned by regular rinsing and disinfection. Reverse osmosis devices are relative inexpensive, but maintainance efforts, necessary to guarantee impeccable ultrapure water, are very high.

5.2.2.5　Nanofiltration

Nanofiltration is a membrane filtration technique by which (according to IUPAC definition) particles and dissolved molecules larger than 2 nm are rejected. Its cut-off size is between that of ultrafiltration (0.1 μm to 2 nm, commonly indicated as molecular weight cut-off = MWCO: 1,000,000 − 5,000 Da) and reverse osmosis (0.1 nm). Nanofiltration membranes are permeable to monovalent ions and therefore not applicable for complete demineralization of water. However, besides small organic molecules, they retain high proportions of divalent ions like calcium and magnesium, which renders nanofiltration an effective method for water softening. An advantage over cation exchange is that no additional sodium ions are added to the water in exchange for calcium and magnesium. Nanofiltration is operated at a lower pressure (5−15 bar) than reverse osmosis, resulting in lower energy consumption.

5.2.2.6　Electrodeionization

Electrodeionization (EDI) can be described as a combination of ion exchange and dialysis. The water flows through an ion exchange resin, which is regenerated in an electric field. For that purpose, multiple layers of exchange resin are placed between two electrodes, with each layer separated from the concentrate channels lying in between by ion-selective membranes. On one side the anion-permeable membranes are positioned, on the other the cation-permeable membranes. The applied voltage makes the anions move in the direction of the anode and the cations in the direction of the cathode. By virtue of the ion-selectivity of the membranes the ions can reach the neighboring concentrate channel, but from there they cannot travel further into the next resin layer. Without the exchange resin (electro-dialysis principle), the water could have been desalted down to a specific conductivity (conductance of 200 μS/cm), since unacceptably high voltages would be required to maintain the ion travel at increasing purity. This problem is solved in the EDI technology by employment of ion exchange resins. These form a conductive "flow path" by allowing the ions to move step-wise from one binding site to the next. This accounts for a virtually complete deionization of the water (Fig. 5-6). Often electrodeionization is coupled downstream of a reverse osmosis procedure.

5.2.3　Salts of Inorganic Acids

5.2.3.1　Calcium Carbonate (Calcium Carbonicum, Calcii carbonas, $CaCO_3$)

Calcium carbonate (Ph. Eur., NF; Precipitated calcium carbonate, JP) is a tasteless white powder and is practically insoluble in water. It occurs in two crystalline modifications, the hexagonal-rhombohedral calcite and the rhombic aragonite. Commercial calcium carbonate of pharmacopeia quality is produced by precipitation from calcium hydroxide with carbon dioxide. The precipitation temperature determines the modification formed.

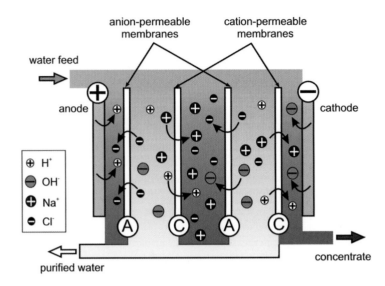

Fig. 5-6 Electrodeionization.

Application: tablet or capsule filler substance, white pigment, polishing agent for dental care.

5.2.3.2   Calcium Hydrogen Phosphate (Dicalcium Phosphate, Dibasic Calcium Phosphate, Secondary Calcium Phosphate, Calcii hydrogenophosphas, $CaHPO_4 \cdot 2H_2O$)

Calcium hydrogen phosphate (Ph. Eur.; Dibasic calcium phosphate, NF, JP) is a white, crystalline, odorless powder. It is practically insoluble in water, but soluble in acid. It crystallizes into a crystal water-containing (dihydrate) and a water-free form. Upon heating above $100°C$, the dihydrate loses its crystal water and is converted into the water-free salt. The release of crystal water can proceed slowly at temperatures from $36°C$. During storage of tablets containing calcium hydrogen phosphate, structural changes can therefore occur, with possible effects on the stability and the release of the active ingredient. Active substances, which are susceptible to hydrolysis, may be damaged by the released crystal water.

Application: calcium hydrogen phosphate is a widely used filler and dry binding agent for tablet production, in particular for direct tablet compression. Earlier efforts to replace lactose, because of potential incompatibilities (e.g., lactose intolerance), in its function as a filler, have led to an increased application of calcium hydrogen phosphate as an excipient in tablets. For tablets with sustained release properties it is suited only under certain conditions, because of its solubility in acidic media. During tableting, a powder bed of calcium hydrogen phosphate is densified almost exclusively by brittle fragmentation of the crystals with little or no plastic or elastic deformation. Thus, upon compression the substance forms numerous new uncoated fracture planes, which cause cohesion of the powder particles by mutual interaction. Due to this mechanism, and in contrast to many fillers and binders with high plasticity, even an intensive coating and hydrophobization of the particle surface by prolonged mixing with magnesium stearate, hardly affects the strength of the resulting tablets. Calcium hydrogenphosphate containing powder mixtures for tableting are therefore largely insensitive to addition of hydrophobic lubricants.

Calcium hydrogen phosphate is also applied as a polishing agent in toothpastes and it is a component of calcium phosphate cement that is used in surgery for filling up bone defects.

5.2.3.3   Sodium Hydrogen Carbonate (Sodium Bicarbonate, Natrii hydrogen carbonas, $NaHCO_3$)

Sodium hydrogencarbonate (Ph. Eur.; Sodium bicarbonate, NF, JP) is a white, crystalline and water-soluble powder. It is produced by introducing CO_2 into a solution of sodium carbonate

(Na_2CO_3). The reverse reaction occurs when sodium hydrogencarbonate solutions are heated whilst splitting off CO_2 causes the pH of the solutions to increase. This thermal decarboxylation should be taken into account when applying $NaHCO_3$ as a buffer substance for injection or infusion solutions that are to be heat-sterilized in the final container. In order to avoid a pressure increase during sterilization due to CO_2 release, the equilibrium of the reaction should be shifted toward the $NaHCO_3$ by gassing the headspace with CO_2.

Application: Apart from its function as a buffer substance, sodium hydrogencarbonate is a key ingredient for most effervescent tablets, where it acts as the source of carbon dioxide. This application benefits from the low hygroscopicity of the substance, which prevents premature release of CO_2 during storage.

5.2.4   Oxides

5.2.4.1   Titanium Dioxide (Titanium Oxide, Titanii dioxidum, TiO_2)

Titanium dioxide (Ph. Eur., NF; Titanium oxide, JP) is a white, odorless and chemically inert powder that is soluble neither in water nor in alkali or acid, except sulfuric acid and fluoric acid. Therefore, aqueous suspensions of TiO_2 react neutral. It is produced either by precipitation from sulfuric acid digestion mixtures of Ilmenite ($FeTiO_3$) or by combustion of titanium tetrachloride, which is also obtained from Ilmenite. Titanium dioxide occurs in three different crystal forms, two of which (anatase and rutile) are used as white pigments by virtue of their high refractive indices (2.55 for anatase and 2.70 for rutile), which are responsible for their high light-scattering potential. The substance is characterized by an extraordinary opacity. The intensity of the scattered light depends on its wavelength and on the particle size of the material and reaches optimal values for particles ≤ 1 μm. TiO_2 micropigments (15-20 nm), which scatter UV radiation but not visible light, can be processed into transparent sun protection preparations.

Applications: white pigment in oral dosage forms and dermatological preparations, coloring of sugar-coated and film-coated tablets, opaque pigmentation of gelatin capsules.

5.2.4.2   Zinc Oxide (Zinci oxidum, ZnO)

Zinc oxide (Ph. Eur., USP, JP) is a white, amorphous, light and odorless powder. It is insoluble in water but readily soluble in diluted mineral acids. It is produced either by the combustion of zinc vapor in air or by annealing of precipitated zinc carbonate. Common commercial qualities come in particle sizes between 0.1 and 5 μm, with the pyrogenic production method yielding a more homogeneous product. Zinc oxide has a good adsorption capacity, for water as well as for oil. Its flow properties are satisfactory, but is has practically no adhesiveness. It acts as a mild disinfectant and weak astringent. By reaction with wound and skin secretions soluble zinc salts are formed which represent the active principle for this effect. It is able to neutralize bad-smelling organic acids on the skin. However upon application on large areas of damaged skin, toxic quantities may be resorbed.

Applications: additive in dermatic preparations, if used as a mere excipient, any pharmacological action is not desirable.

5.2.4.3   Magnesium Oxide (Magnesii oxidum, MgO)

Magnesium oxide (Ph. Eur., USP, JP) is a white, fine, and odorless powder. It is practically insoluble in water, but very small proportions do dissolve under formation of $Mg(OH_2)$, causing aqueous suspensions of it to display pH values of about 10.3. MgO is soluble in dilute acids. Pharmaceutically used forms are produced by annealing magnesium carbonate. The Ph. Eur. describes two forms with different bulk volumes: *light MgO* (magnesia oxidum leve) with 150 mL/15 g and *heavy MgO* (magnesia oxidum ponderosum) with 30 mL/15 g. Magnesium oxide has good adhesion and water uptake capacity, but very poor flow properties.

Application: excipient in (make-up) powders and toothpastes.

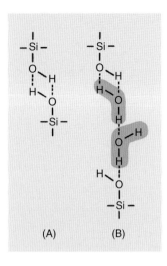

Fig. 5-7 Linking of neighboring Aerosil® particles by hydrogen bridges: (A) without water; (B) via water molecule.

5.2.5   Silicates

5.2.5.1   Colloidal Silicon Dioxide (Colloidal Anhydrous Silica, Aerosil®, Silica colloidalis anhydrica, SiO_2)

Colloidal silicon dioxide (NF; Silica colloidal anhydrous, Ph. Eur.; Light anhydrous silicic acid, JP) is a bluish white, fine, light and flaky, amorphous powder with a primary particle size distribution of 3 to 40 nm. Sticking together of the primary particles causes the formation of agglomerates or aggregates with diameters of 1 to 100 µm. The small particle size results in a BET surface of about 50–380 m^2/g. Concomitantly, the bulk volume is extremely low with 50 g/L. The production of colloidal silicon dioxide involves the flame hydrolysis of silicon tetrachloride: a homogeneous mixture of $SiCl_4$ vapor, hydrogen and air is chemically converted in the gas phase during joint combustion in a flame ($2 H_2 + O_2 \rightarrow 2H_2O$, $SiCl_4 + 2 H_2O \rightarrow SiO_2 + 4 HCl$, total: $2 H_2 + O_2 + SiCl_4 \rightarrow SiO_2 + 4 HCl$). The substance is practically insoluble in water and mineral acids, except hydrofluoric acid.

Colloidal silicon dioxide is not a pigment, because it does not have a sufficiently high refractive index (1.45) and is, thus, not applicable for light protective or opaque coatings. Because of its amorphous structure, it does not cause silicosis in the lungs. The silanol groups on the particle surface allow the formation of hydrogen bonds with neighboring particles as a result of which three-dimensional networks are formed (Fig. 5-7). In turn, this causes a substantial viscosity increase particularly in non-polar systems (e.g., paraffin, isopropyl myristate). At a proportion of 5% to 6% SiO_2, a thixotropic gel is formed. The formation of hydrogen bonds with polar substances such as water or alcohols explains the excellent adsorption capacity. Colloidal silicon dioxide can adsorb up to 40% moisture without losing its dry-powder structure.

Applications: flow regulation agent for solid dosage forms, adsorbent, hydrophilization agent for the improvement of tablet stability, suspension stabilizer, network-forming compound and gelling agent.

By chemical conversion of highly dispersed silicon dioxide with dimethyl dichlorosilan **hydrophobic colloidal silica** (Ph. Eur., NF; Silica hydrophobica colloidalis) is obtained. The primary particles of this product are surrounded by a hydrophobic layer of methyl residues, which is created by linking the –OH functions at the particle surface with >$Si(CH_3)_2$ groups and renders the surface unwettable by water. This hydrophobic silicon dioxide is predominantly used as a flow regulation agent for powders with hygroscopic properties. At the surface of the powder particles the hydrophobic silicon dioxide particles form a layer that slows down the water uptake and keeps the adhesion forces low, also at high air humidity. When applied in tablets, it delays their disintegration, diminishes their hardness, and enhances friability by virtue of its hydrophobic properties.

5.2.5.2   Precipitated Silicas

Precipitated silicas and silica gels are prepared by wet chemistry through acidification of silicate solutions. The Ph. Eur. and the NF describe two products, **colloidal hydrated silica** (Silica colloidalis hydrica, Ph. Eur.; **silicon dioxide**, NF) and **dental type silica** (Silica ad usum dentalem Ph. Eur.; NF). In the German Pharmacopeia (DAB) a monograph on **precipitated silicon dioxide** (Silicii dioxidum praecipitatum) can be found. These three products distinguish themselves by their specific surfaces (250–1,000 m^2/g) and by some other specification limits. Precipitated silicon oxide types are used as adsorption agents, as carrier materials, desiccants and abrasive cleaning agents in toothpastes as well as for the adjustment of viscosity.

5.2.5.3   Talc

Talc (Ph. Eur., NF, JP) is a pulverized hydrated magnesium silicate of natural origin, which may contain various amounts of other minerals. For pharmaceutical purposes, talc is obtained from deposits with a proven absence of asbestos. Talc belongs to the triple-layer silicates. In these structures, layers composed of two tetrahedrally coordinated silicate sublayers, with a layer of octahedrically coordinated magnesium hydroxide in between, are periodically arranged (molecular formula $Mg_{12}(OH)_8Si_6O_{40}$). Adjacent silicate layers are connected to each other only by weak Van der Waals forces, explaining the excellent fissility of this

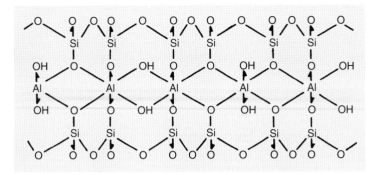

Fig. 5-8 Triple-layer structure of bentonite (schematic representation).

material and its suitability as a lubricant. Because the silicate layers are electrostatically neutral, talc cannot be used as a cation exchanger, nor is it able to take up crystal water. However, because of its lipophilic properties, it can accommodate substantial quantities of oil in between its layers. Talc is insoluble in water, acids, alkali, and organic solvents. As a pigment in film coatings, talc can enhance the moisture-insulating effect of the film. Its hydrophobic surface properties and the flaky appearance of the talcum particles, which allows a roof-tile-like arrangement in the polymer film, reduce the permeability of the film.

Applications: lubricant in tablet production, powder base, pigment for film coatings.

5.2.5.4   Kaolin (Kaolinum ponderosum, China Clay, Bolus alba)

Kaolin (NF, JP; Heavy kaolin, Ph. Eur.) is a purified naturally occurring water-containing aluminum silicate with kaolinite as the main mineral. This double-layer silicate can be described as a condensation product of tetrahedrically coordinated silicic acid layers in a periodical arrangement with octahedrically coordinated aluminum hydroxide layers. Chemical formula: $Al_2Si_2O_5(OH)_4$. Kaolin displays pronounced hydrophilic properties and has a high capacity to adsorb water. As Kaolin belongs to the non-swellable clay minerals, the water is bound exclusively on the exterior surface of the primary particles. Its high adsorption capacity is based in part on its high density of exchangeable cations on the particle surface. 1 g of kaolin can bind 1.4 mL of water.

Applications: diluent in tablet and capsule formulations, adsorbent, powder base, dispersing agent for suspensions.

5.2.5.5   Bentonite (Bentonitum)

Bentonites (Bentonite, Ph. Eur., JP; Bentonite/Purified Bentonite/Bentonite Magma, NF) are swelling clays named after the site where the mineral was first found, near Fort Benton (USA). They consist mainly of clay minerals from the smectite group (montmorillonites), that is, aluminum silicates with the chemical formula $Al_2[(OH)_2/Si_4O_{10}] \cdot n\,H_2O$. Montmorillonites have a triple-layered structure. One single-layer unit (Fig. 5-8) consists of a layer of aluminum hydroxide octahedrons, limited by two layers of silicic acid tetrahedrons. The individual layers are spaced by about 1.0 to 1.4 nm. The partly isomorph replacement of Si^{4+} tetrahedrons by Al^{3+} ions, or of the Al^{3+} ions in the octahedron layer by Mg^{2+} or Fe^{2+} ions causes a charge difference that is compensated by cations, predominantly Na^+ and Ca^{2+} ions. As these ions are easily exchangeable and since the peripheral silicic acid and aluminum hydroxide groups will dissociate depending on the pH, bentonites are cation exchangers.

The distinct tendency of bentonites to swell is based on the incompletely saturated oxygen functions of the Si-O groups at the surface of the layers. It is here that hydrogen bridges are formed (Fig. 5-9). In this way, the accumulation of water and other polar fluids (e.g., glycols and glycerol) not only occurs at the particle surface but also at the surfaces of the inner layers. This intra-crystalline swelling leads to a significant widening of the layers. Bentonite is a submicrocrystalline powder, of which the platelet-shaped crystals (thickness 5–10 nm, length 0.1–2 μm) are constructed by multiples of the layer packages described above.

For pharmaceutical purposes iron-free types should be used, which show a whitish to yellow-brown appearance. The swelling capacity of the bentonites varies with their origin

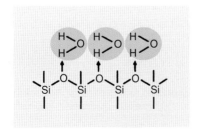

Fig. 5-9 Hydrogen bridges at the bentonite surface.

and the way they are processed. As a rule, 2 g of bentonite swells up to 24 mL in excess water. For the production of spreadable gels, concentrations of 8% to 15% are required. By mixing with small quantities of phosphate (1.5% to 2%), gel formation is facilitated.

Applications: hydrogel former, thickening agent, emulsifier for O/W emulsions, suspension stabilizer, cation exchanger.

5.3   Organic Excipients

5.3.1   Organic Solvents

5.3.1.1   Ethanol (Ethyl Alcohol, Aethanolum)

Ethanol (Ph. Eur., USP, JP) is a clear, volatile, highly flammable liquid. Ethanol for pharmaceutical purposes is produced only from agricultural sources. Like water, it is a protic, polar solvent, of which the molecules associate via hydrogen bonds. It is infinitely miscible with common organic solvents. With water it forms an azeotropic mixture of 95.57% ethanol and 4.43% water, which boils at 78.15°C. Upon mixing with water a volume contraction occurs. In the European Union, according to the Excipients-Guideline CPMP/463/00 ("Excipients in the label and package leaflet of medicinal products for human use"), ethanol-containing oral and parenteral products must be provided with a warning instruction. In connection with the ethanol concentration, this warning should call attention to specific risks for certain categories of individuals (e.g., alcoholics, pregnant women, children), potential interactions with other medication or driving capability. A similar guideline in the United States, covering the labeling and the maximum allowable ethanol concentration of oral over-the-counter (OTC) drug products, is 21 CFR Ch. I Part 28 ("Over-the-Counter Drug Products Intended for Oral Ingestion That Contain Alcohol"). In most countries, commercial ethanol is subject to taxation, with the exception of denatured alcohol, which has been made unfit for consumption by additives such as camphor, thymol, or toluene. The latter ethanol preparations are used for the manufacturing of medical products for exterior use.

Applications: solvent, co-solvent, extraction fluid, (skin) penetration enhancer, disinfection agent.

5.3.1.2   Isopropanol (Isopropyl Alcohol, 2-Propanol, Alcohol isopropylicus)

Isopropanol (JP; Isopropyl alcohol, Ph. Eur., NF) is a colorless, somewhat sharp-aromatically smelling liquid. It largely equals ethanol in chemical and physical properties. It is not any less toxic than ethanol, but has better disinfection potential.

Applications: solvent, co-solvent, extraction fluid, penetration enhancer, disinfectant.

5.3.1.3   Glycerol (Glycerin, Glycerolum)

Glycerol (Ph. Eur.; Glycerin, NF, JP) is a nearly colorless, syrupy, fatty to the touch, sweet tasting, strongly hygroscopic liquid. It is commercially available either as water-free glycerol or as glycerol 85%. It is infinitely miscible with water and ethanol, whereas it is practically insoluble in ether as well as in fats and etheric oils. It is thermally stable up to 180°C. Above that temperature a slow decomposition sets on. Water-free glycerol can be hot-air sterilized at 160°C or 180°C. Water-containing glycerol boils already at 130°C to 135°C.

Autoclaving requires special conditions according to the German dispensing formulary NRF (Neues Rezeptur-Formularium), which provides the following instructions for the sterilization of glycerol: For effective sterilization with saturated pressurized water vapor, the glycerol should contain at least 20% water. Glycerol 85% cannot be autoclaved under standard conditions. After appropriate validation, steam sterilization for 60 minutes at 130°C or for 45 minutes at 140°C can be performed. Sterilization of water-containing glycerol with dry heat is not possible in an open container without changes in composition. In a closed container, it is prohibited because of severe explosion risks. Only water-free glycerol may be sterilized by dry heat.

Applications: solvent, co-solvent, preservative, viscosity enhancer, humectant, plasticizer in soft capsules, and film formulations.

5.3.1.4 Propylene Glycol (1,2-Propylene Glycol, Propylenglycolum)

Propylene glycol is a clear, colorless, viscous, sweet but sharp-tasting, hygroscopic liquid. It is miscible with water, lower mono- and multivalent alcohols, acetone, chloroform, and etheric oils. It is insoluble in petrol and fatty oils. At concentrations higher than 15% to 20%, it has preservative activity. Exterior application of undiluted propylene glycol may lead to local irritation of skin and mucosal tissue.

Applications: solvent, co-solvent, preservative, viscosity enhancer, humectant, plasticizer in film formulations.

5.3.2 Organic Acids and Bases and Their Salts

5.3.2.1 Stearic Acid (Acidum stearicum)

Stearic acid (Ph. Eur., NF, JP) of quality according to the pharmacopeias is not a pure compound, but rather a mixture of saturated fatty acids, which, in addition to stearic acid, also contains palmitic acid, therefore, the product is also known as stearo-palmitic acid. It is a white, fatty to the touch, solid substance.

Applications: lubricant for tablet manufacturing, structure builder in creams.

Ph. Eur./NF Monograph Stearic Acid _____

The Ph. Eur and the NF distinguish three stearic acid qualities. The designation indicates the nominal content of stearic acid:

Stearic acid 50 contains 40% to 60% stearic acid and minimally 90% stearic + palmitic acid

Stearic acid 70 contains 60% to 80% stearic acid and minimally 90% stearic + palmitic acid

Stearic acid 95 contains minimally 90% stearic acid and minimally 96% stearic + palmitic acid

---

5.3.2.2 Magnesium Stearate (Magnesii stearas)

Magnesium stearate (Ph. Eur., NF, JP) contains, in addition to the magnesium salt of stearic acid (~40 to 65%), the magnesium salt of palmitic acid (~25% to 50%) and of oleic acid (max. 4%). It is a white, very fine, nearly odorless, fatty to the touch powder that is neither soluble in water nor in water-free ethanol or ether. Its suitability as a lubricant is on one hand based on its lamellar crystal structure and on the other hand on its small particle size of 3 to 15 μm.

Magnesium stearate occurs in multiple pseudopolymorphic forms. One distinguishes needle-shaped crystals containing 3 mol of water, the second a sheet-like form containing 2 mol of water and a third dried substance with only 1 mol of water. The properties of the material change with decreasing water content, which is based on the conversion of a monocline or orthorhombic into a hexagonal lattice, which brings along the abolishment of the lamellar structure. During storage, magnesium stearate can catalyze the degradation of hydrolysis-sensitive active ingredients (e.g., acetyl salicylic acid). Fine-particulate qualities display a higher catalytic activity by virtue of their larger total surface area.

Applications: Magnesium stearate is the most frequently used lubricant and mold release agent for the manufacture of tablets. The magnesium stearate particles organize themselves on the surfaces of other solid material particles in the tableting mixture and thus reduce the friction resistance when these are pressed against each other or against the die wall during the compression. When the added amounts are too high and/or the mixing time is too long, a continuous film is formed on the particle surface that unfavorably affects the binding force and the wettability of the tablet material. As a consequence, tablets with reduced hardness are obtained, leading to a slow release of the active ingredient.

Further application: lubricant for capsule production, in powders to improve lubricity and coating capacity.

5.3.2.3   Sodium Stearyl Fumarate (Natrii stearylis fumaras)

Sodium stearyl fumarate (Ph. Eur., NF) is the mono-sodium salt of fumaric acid monostearyl ester. The white poorly water-soluble powder is used as a lubricant in tablets and capsules (~0.5%–2%); its lubricating effect is as good as that of magnesium stearate.

5.3.3   Sugars and Sugar Alcohols

Sugars (saccharides) are broadly defined as multivalent alcohols with an active carbonyl function that can either be an aldehyde or a keto group, from which hydroxy aldehydes (aldoses) or hydroxy ketones (ketoses) are derived. The carbonyl group is usually present as (hemi)acetal or (hemi)ketal. Intramolecular hemiacetal or hemiketal formation leads to ring closure. Di-, tri-, tetra- (i.e., oligo-) or polysaccharides are formed by intermolecular acetal or ketal formation (glycosidic bond). Various types of sugars are widely used in drug formulation. In the Ph. Eur. and the USP/NF, monographs are devoted to the monosaccharides fructose, galactose, glucose (hexoses) and xylose (a pentose), as well as to the disaccharides lactose, lactulose, maltose (in Ph. Eur. only as reagent monograph), sucrose, and trehalose.

Sugar alcohols (alditols) are noncyclic polyols that structurally represent reduction products of saccharides. The Ph. Eur. and the USP/NF list the monosaccharide alcohols myo-inositol, **mannitol, sorbitol** (hexitols), **xylitol** (a pentitol) and **erythritol** (a tetrol), in addition to the disaccharide alcohols **maltitol** (4-O-α-D-galactopyranosyl-D-glucitol) **lactitol** (4-O-β-D-galactopyranosyl-D-glucitol), and **isomalt** (a mixture of 1-O-α-D-glucopyranosyl-D-mannitol and 6-O-α-D-glucopyranosyl-D-glucitol).

5.3.3.1   Glucose (Corn Sugar, Dextrose, α-D-glucopyranose, Glucosum, Saccharum amylaceum)

Glucose (Ph. Eur., JP; Dextrose, USP, NF) is a white, odorless, sweet-tasting powder; it is freely soluble in water (0.909 g/mL; 25°C) and very slightly soluble in ethanol. Commercially, water-free glucose and glucose monohydrate are available. By virtue of its free carbonyl group, that is, through the hydroxyl group at the anomeric carbon atom of the cyclic hemiacetal form, glucose can reduce not only Cu^{2+} ions in alkaline solution (reducing sugar), but it can also react with a host of active ingredients and excipients to cause a variety of incompatibilities.

With amines and proteins, it undergoes the Maillard reaction, a complex series of chemical steps ultimately resulting in the formation of brown-colored melanoidins. During autoclaving of aqueous glucose solutions partial degradation occurs. The degradation product is 5-hydroxy furfural, which forms yellow-brownish polymers. Simultaneously, the pH drops due to the formation of lactic acid and formic acid. For direct tablet compression starch hydrolysates such as Emdex or Celutab were developed, which consist of 90% to 92% glucose. In addition, they contain about 3% to 5% maltose and the remainder represents oligo- and monosaccharides. The Ph. Eur. describes glucose in the monographs **water-free glucose** and **glucose monohydrate**. The USP monograph "dextrose" covers both D-glucose monohydrate and anhydrous D-glucose whereas the NF monograph "dextrose" is dedicated to D-glucose monohydrate for nonparenteral use. All the aforementioned types of glucose are well distinguished from **glucose liquid** (Ph. Eur. and NF) and **glucose liquid spray-dried** (Ph. Eur.). The latter two are mixtures of glucose, di-, oligo-, and polysaccharides produced by enzymatic hydrolysis of starch. Hydrogenated glucose syrup can be found in the Ph. Eur. and NF under the name **maltitol solution**. However, this substance does not contain any glucose; during the hydrogenation a mixture of D-maltitol and D-sorbitol is formed with fractions of hydrogenated oligo- and polysaccharides.

Applications: filling substance for lozenges and vaginal tablets (in spite of the good water solubility of glucose, the dissolution rate from glucose-containing tablets is low, which is an advantage with respect to dissolution in the oral cavity), sweetener, tonicifier for parenteral formulations. Glucose syrup is used in solutions or suspensions or for pan-coating with sugar.

5.3.3.2   Lactose (Milk Sugar, 4-O-β-D-galactopyranosyl-α-D-glucopyranose, Lactosum, Saccharum lactis)

Lactose (Ph. Eur., NF, JP) is a disaccharide made up of galactose and glucose. Pharmaceutically it is predominantly utilized as the α-lactose monohydrate form and rarely as water-free lactose. The monohydrate contains 5% crystal water. It is a white, crystalline, odorless powder, which dissolves easily but slowly in water (0.189 g/mL; 25°C), while in ethanol it is practically insoluble. By virtue of its low dissolution rate the powder causes only a weak sweet-taste sensation on the tongue. The β-modification, obtained by crystallization from concentrated solutions at a temperature above 93.5°C, is more water-soluble and has a sweeter taste than α-lactose. At a temperature of 110°C to 120°C the monohydrate releases its crystal water and converts into the water-free form. Also lactose qualities with a high proportion of an amorphous nature are commercially available; they are produced by quick drying (e.g., spray drying) of aqueous lactose suspensions. The amorphous fraction contains both α- and β-lactose, at a ratio of 38:62, corresponding to the mutarotation equilibrium. As a reducing sugar, lactose can react in a Maillard reaction with amino groups of active components and excipients and thus form brown-colored melanoidins, or react with active substances containing hydrazine groups, to form poorly soluble osazones.

Lactose is a widely used filling substance for tableting processes. For the direct tablet compression process, spray-dried lactose is preferential, which is, for example, commercially available as FlowLac®. Another specialty for direct tablet compression is Tablettose, an agglomerated lactose, combining the good flow characteristics of a coarse-grained material with the optimal compressibility of a finely ground lactose. Besides particle size, the proportion of amorphous lactose is a decisive criterion for tableting capacity. Commercial products with various amorphous fractions are available: ≤2% (Tablettose 80), 7%–9% (e.g. FlowLac 100, Supertab SD11, FastFlo 315) and up to 13%–15% (FlowLac 90, Supertab SD14, FastFlo 316). With increasing proportions of amorphous lactose, tablet stability improves; this can be explained by the plastic deformability of the amorphous material. Crystallization of amorphous material during storage can, however, lead to unwanted and uncontrollable delayed hardening of the tablets. Besides the numerous commercially available lactose qualities for use as excipients in tablet manufacture, special qualities for direct tablet compression have been developed from lactose monohydrate and cellulose powder (Cellactose), microcrystalline cellulose (MicroceLac) and cornstarch (StarLac).

For deployment in powder inhalers InhaLac offers a lactose quality that distinguishes itself by a smooth crystal surface, narrow particle size distribution and absence of amorphous material. For processing with moisture-sensitive products, water-free lactose is preferable as in the crystalline state it is hardly hygroscopic. With increasing proportions of amorphous material, the hygroscopicity of lactose increases. Amorphous lactose can reach a water content of up to 11% at a relative ambient humidity of 55% before, upon further increases in humidity, crystallization starts to occur, accompanied by desorption of the bound water. The high water uptake capacity of amorphous lactose can be exploited for the stabilization of lyophilized hydrolytically sensitive active agents during storage. After lyophilization, lactose, used as filling material (cake former), is in the amorphous state and absorbs remaining moisture in the product or the stopper, thus protecting the active ingredient against small amounts of moisture that could possibly penetrate during storage.

Application: filler for tablets and capsules, base material for homeopathic triturations, cake former for lyophilization

5.3.3.3 Sucrose (Reed or Beet Sugar, β-D-fructofuranosyl-α-D-glucopyranosid, Saccharose, Saccharum)

Sucrose (Ph. Eur., NF, JP) is a disaccharide made up of glucose and fructose. It is a white, crystalline, sweet tasting, and slightly hygroscopic powder. The solubility in water is 2.1 g/mL (25°C) and in ethanol 0.0059 g/mL. The molecule has no carbonyl group and therefore no reducing properties. In acidic media sucrose can be hydrolytically cleaved into an equimolar mixture of fructose and glucose, called invert sugar. Good commercial qualities contain less than 0.015% invert sugar. Incompatibility reactions caused by free carbonyl groups can only be caused by the cleavage products. Sucrose is more hygroscopic than lactose; sucrose-containing tablets tend to display delayed hardening at elevated humidity values. The compound is therefore predominantly deployed for tablet types that should dissolve without prior disintegration.

Sucrose does not contain crystal water; nonetheless, during crystallization small quantities of mother liquor can be included in the crystals in the form of small droplets. During grinding into powdered sugar this water is released and adsorbed on the surface of the newly formed crystals; as a result, a thin film of sugar syrup is formed that causes the powder to cake during storage. In order to avoid this, the powdered sugar has to be conditioned with dry air after the grinding to remove the released moisture.

Applications: filler for lozenges and chewing tablets, sweetener, coating of sugar-coated tablets, binding agent for moist granulation, dry binding agent, thickener for syrups, lyo- and crytoprotectant and bulking agent for lyophilisates.

5.3.3.4   Trehalose (α-D-Glucopyranosyl-α-D-glucopyranoside)

Trehalose (Ph. Eur., NF, JP) is a disaccharide with two glucose molecules linked in an α,α-1,1 configuration. It is an odorless, white or almost white powder, tasting about half as sweet as sucrose. It occurs as anhydrous trehalose and (more often) as dihydrate. The substance is soluble in water (50 mg/mL). Due to the linkage at the reducing carbons of the two glucopyranose rings, trehalose is a nonreducing sugar and demonstrates exceptional hydrolytic stability. Trehalose readily forms an amorphous matrix upon drying or dehydration. This property renders it an ideal desiccation-protectant for many biomolecules. It traps the biomolecules in a glassy matix, separates them, restricts their mobility, and, thus, retards their degradation. Hydrogen bonding with the protein surface supports the stabilizing effect on protein conformation and activity. Trehalose has the highest glass transition temperature T_g of all disaccharides (110°C–120°C), which allows its use as a stabilizer in a wide range of extreme environmental conditions. As also T_g', the glass transition temperature of a maximally concentrated solution, is higher than for many other sugars and sugar alcohols, it is possible to conduct primary drying steps of freeze-drying processes at a higher temperature for trehalose-containing formulations.

Applications: Cryoprotectant in parenteral formulations, lyoprotectant and bulking agent for lyophilizates (stabilization of liposomes and proteins as well as viruses, bacteria, and tissues). Humectant in cosmetic preparations.

5.3.3.5   Cyclodextrins

Cyclodextrins are cyclic oligosaccharides consisting of six (α-cyclodextrin, **Alfadex**, Ph. Eur., NF), seven (β-cyclodextrin, **Betadex**, Ph. Eur., NF) or eight (γ-cyclodextrin, NF) glucose molecules. The ring-shaped structure of the molecule forms a hollow space with an inner diameter of 0.45, 0.7, or 0.85 nm (for α, β and γ cyclodextrin, respectively), which can accommodate molecules of appropriate size under the formation of an inclusion compound. As the hydroxyl groups of the glucose molecules are predominantly oriented outward, the hole inside is more lipophilic than the outer face of the molecule. Cyclodextrins are quite soluble in water. A further improvement of solubility can be attained by substitution with hydroxypropyl (**Hydroxypropylbetadex**, Ph. Eur, NF) or sulfobutyl groups (**Betadex sulfobutyl ether sodium**, (NF). By accommodation of a drug molecule in the cavity of a cyclodextrin molecule the solubility of the former can be improved, as well as its stability.

β-Cyclodextrin, though it is the least soluble cyclodextrin, is used most frequently, as it is cheapest. However, it can be nephrotoxic upon parenteral administration. Because of its low absorption (1%–2%) it is considered to be nontoxic if administered orally and is therefore mainly used in tablet and capsule formulations. α-Cyclodextrin has a lower toxicity upon systemic administration and therefore has its main field of application in parenteral formulations.

Applications: solubilizer, transformation of fluid substances into solid formulations, fixation of fragrances and aromas, protection against incompatibilities, improvement of storage stability.

5.3.3.6   Mannitol (Mannite, Mannitolum)

D(-)-Mannitol (Ph. Eur., USP, NF, JP) is a hexavalent alcohol (hexitol) derived from D-mannose. The white, crystalline powder is half as sweet as sucrose and exerts a cooling effect on the tongue due to its highly positive dissolution enthalpy. One part of mannitol dissolves in about 6 parts of water. It can therefore be considered freely soluble, but its solubility is considerably lower than that of sorbitol. In contrast to the latter, mannitol is not hygroscopic and can be safely stored at high air humidity values. Mannitol occurs in several polymorphic forms. If mannitol is used as bulking agent for lyophilizaton, these polymorphic forms need to be adequately monitored and controlled. Crystallization of mannitol causes expansion, possibly leading to breakage of vials during lyophilization. The polymorphic differences also have to be considered when mannitol is used as tableting excipient as the polymorphic forms display different compression characteristics. Although mannitol yields tablets of lower hardness than sorbitol, it is often preferred because of its lower hygroscopicity. It can be processed by direct compression and is often utilized, for instance, for lozenges and chewing/orally disintegrating tablets as well as for reagent tablets in diagnostic test kits. A recommended filling mixture for pharmacy-made hard capsules consists of 99.5% mannitol and 0.5% colloidal anhydrous silica to ensure proper flow characteristcs. Mannitol is not completely absorbed in the intestinal tract and leads therefore, in doses of 12 to 20 g to an osmotically induced laxative effect.

Applications: Filler for tableting, sugar substituent, dry binding agent, bulking agent for lyophilization.

5.3.3.7   Sorbitol (Sorbit, Glucitol, Sorbitolum)

D-Sorbitol (Ph. Eur., NF, JP) is a hexavalent alcohol (hexitol) derived from D-glucose. It is a white, odorless powder that is half as sweet as sucrose. Unlike mannitol, sorbitol is strongly hygroscopic and much more water-soluble (1 part sorbitol in about 0.4 parts of water). The hygroscopic property of the substance is taken as an advantage to prevent drying-out of water-containing formulations. Sorbitol exists in multiple modifications. At 121°C it can be autoclaved in neutral solutions without decomposition; in acidic media, under identical conditions, it is converted to 2,5-anhydrosorbitol by intra-molecular cyclisation and elimination of a water molecule. Under strong dehydrating conditions, this reaction leads to the formation of 1,4-sorbitan and the bicyclic sorbides (particularly isosorbide). The pharmacopeias describe several sorbitol solutions that contain either pure sorbitol ("Sorbitol liquid crystallizing", Ph. Eur.; "Sorbitol solution", USP/NF; "D-Sorbitol solution", JP) or mixtures of sorbitol, other hexitols, and hexitol anhydrides ("Sorbitol liquid non-crystallizing", Ph. Eur.), "Noncrystallizing sorbitol solution", NF, "Hydrogenated starch hydrolysate", NF). While sorbitol is derived from glucose, the noncrystallizing sorbitol solutions are obtained by catalytic hydration of starch hydrolysates. The accompanying substances in these solutions act as crystallization inhibitors. Partial acid-catalyzed dehydration results in the conversion of a sorbitol solution into a solution which contains predominantly sorbitol and 1,4-sorbitan ("Sorbitol liquid partially dehydrated", Ph. Eur., "Sorbitol sorbitan solution", NF).

Applications: sugar substituent, plasticizer for soft capsules, humectant, bases for syrups and peroral suspensions.

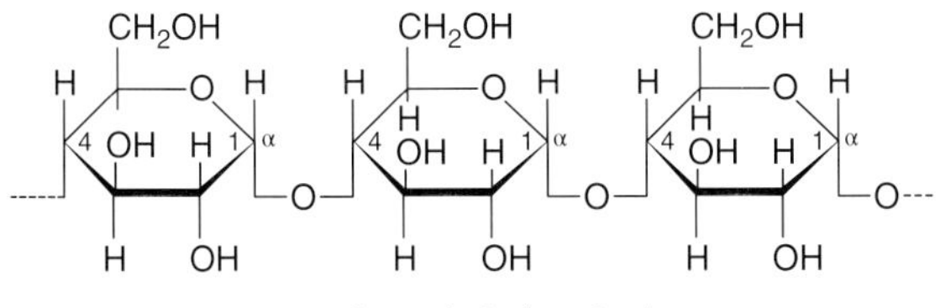

amylose chain (section)

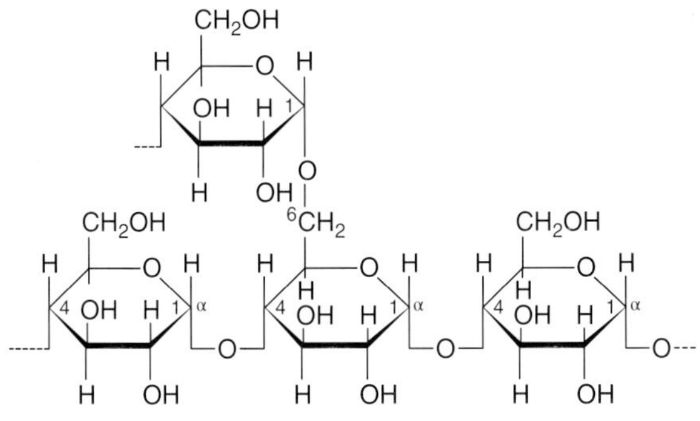

amylopectin chain (section)

5.3.4 Natural Macromolecular Excipients

5.3.4.1 Starches (Amyla)

Starches are polysaccharides built up from glucose units. The starch granules occurring in plant cells contain two types of glucose polymers: ~15% to 30% amylose and 70% to 85% amylopectin. Amylose is a linear polymeric structure formed by about 100 to 1,400 glucopyranose units linked together through 1,4-α-glycosidic bonds (M_r = 17,000 to 225,000). Unlike the β-glycosidic links in cellulose, the α-glucosidic linkages in amylose induce a coiled secondary structure in the polymer with six glucose units per winding. This channel-like form with an inner diameter of ~5 Å facilitates the formation of inclusion complexes, such as with I_3- and I_5-ions. By contrast, amylopectin, a glucose polymer consisting of 1,200 to 6,000 glucose units M_r = 200,000 to 1,000,000), is strongly branched as a result of the additional presence of polyglucoside side chains, which are linked by a 1,6-α-glucosidic bond to about every twenty-fifth glucose unit of the main chain. These side chains have a length of 15 to 25 glucose units.

All starch types are very fine, white, odorless, and tasteless powders, which produce a grinding sound, when rubbed between the fingers. They are practically insoluble in cold water and ethanol. Starch is mainly obtained from cereal grains or tubers. Starches from corn, rice, wheat, potatoes, and peas are used for pharmaceutical purposes. Size and shape of starch granules (2 to 100 μm) vary with the origin and represent a microscopically distinguishable characteristic. Starch granules are sphero-crystals, that is, aggregates made up of crystal particles arranged in concentric or excentric, alternating water-poor and water-rich layers around a growth core. Besides small amounts of proteins (0.1% to 0.15% gluten), starch granules contain 10% to 20% water that is completely released by drying at 125°C to 130°C. Due to its water content, starch may jeopardize the stability of moisture-sensitive substances.

Whereas isolated amylose is practically insoluble in cold water, because the coiled molecule, stabilized by intramolecular hydrogen bridges, becomes only poorly solvated, pure amylopectin is quite water-soluble, also in the cold. In hot water, amylose dissolves colloidally under partial decomposition. Due to its branched structure, the amylopectin fraction is able to swell in water because the molecular structure is widened by the penetrating water molecules. Hence, the amylopectin fraction is the actual gel former in starch. Gel formation with water (gelatinization of the starch) occurs only above the so-called gelatinization temperature. For the production of mucilages cereal starches such as rice, corn, and wheat starch, but above all potato starch, are used.

The gelatinization temperatures of pharmaceutically relevant starches are within the range 55°C to 77°C. In presence of glycerol and polyols a higher temperature is required. Cold swelling is possible by use of an alkali. Gelatinized starches show after some time a retrogradation, that is, the occurrence of crystalline aggregates, mostly of submicroscopic dimensions, caused by partial crystallization of the amylose fraction. This leads to an enhanced turbidity of the gel. This phenomenon is particularly pronounced in preparations from cereal starches, which contain as a rule a higher proportion of amylose than potato starch. Potato starch thus yields clearer preparations due to its generally lower content of slowly crystallizing amylose.

Spreadable preparations based on starch with glycerol are the oldest pharmaceutically applied hydrogels. Nowadays, however, they have been replaced by more suitable products. Spreadable starch gels have a sticky consistency and are prone to microbial infestation.

In tablet manufacturing, starches are exploited as fillers, binding agents, as well as disintegrants. They display a predominantly elastic compression behavior. By the partial back stretching at the end of the compression process a network of microscopic fissures is formed in the compressed material, through which water can rapidly penetrate into the matrix. Upon moisturizing, the deformed starch granules undergo uncoiling and expansion, which pushes the compressed structure apart.

For application in the direct compression tableting, modified starches have proven their usefulness: gelatinized starch is cornstarch that has been swollen for a few minutes in boiling water and subsequently dried. By this treatment the crystalline domains are widened and become amorphous, which yields a product that, upon renewed contact with water, will already swell in cold water. For direct tablet compression, a pregelatinized cornstarch is available under the name Starch 1500 (formerly: STA-RX 1500), which upon addition of a defined amount of water is pressed into briquettes, dried, and ground to powder.

The following starch types and products are listed in the pharmacopeias:

Corn starch (NF, JP), Maize starch (Ph. Eur.) (from Zea mays)

Pea starch (Ph. Eur., NF) (from Pisum sativum)

Potato starch (Ph. Eur., NF, JP) (from Solanum tuberosum)

Rice starch (Ph. Eur., NF, JP) (from Oryza sativa)

Tapioca starch (NF) (from Manihot ultissima)

Topical starch (NF) (from Zea mays; specifications differ from corn starch (NF), e.g., no limit for E. coli)

Wheat starch (Ph. Eur., NF, JP) (from Triticum aestivum)

Starch pregelatinized (Ph. Eur.) (starch that has been mechanically processed to rupture all or part of the starch granules in the presence of water and subsequently dried)

Pregelatinized starch (NF) (starch that has been chemically and/or mechanically processed to rupture all or part of the granules in the presence of water and subsequently dried)

Modified starch (NF) (starch modified by chemical means, e.g., acid-modified, bleached, oxidized, esterified, etherified, or treated enzymatically)

Pregelatinized modified starch (NF) (starch that has been chemically or mechanically processed or both, to rupture all or part of the granules to produce a product that swells in cold water)

Applications: filling substance, disintegration enhancer, lubricant, binding agent, ground substance for (cosmetic) powders, thickener.

5.3.4.2   Cellulose Powder (Cellulosi pulvis)

Cellulose is a high-molecular weight carbohydrate with the formula $(C_6H_{10}O_5)_n$, in which glucopyranose units, are linearly linked together. Depending on the origin and the way it has been processed, the products have different degrees of polymerization. While native cellulose with a molecular weight of 500,000 to 1,600,000 consists of about 3,000 to 10,000 glucose units, products that comply with the Ph. Eur. have a molecular weight of 150,000 to 200,000 and a degree of polymerization 1,000 to 1,200. The NF requests a degree of polymerization (DP) greater than 440. Cellulose types with degrees of > 200 ($M_r > 30,000$) are referred to as α-celluloses, which are distinguished from the short-chain NaOH-soluble β- (DP = 10 to 150), and γ-celluloses (DP < 10).

Powdered cellulose (Ph. Eur., NF, JP) is a fine or granular, odorless powder that is insoluble in water and organic solvents. In the polarization microscope, it is optically anisotropic and has a fibrous appearance with fiber lengths below 100 μm—in the case of fibrous cellulose, up to 350 μm. Bulk materials containing cellulose have poor flow properties, while they tend to undergo strong bridge formation.

Applications: filling substance, dry binding agent, tablet disintegration enhancer.

5.3.4.3   Microcrystalline Cellulose (Cellulosum Microcrystallosum)

Microcrystalline cellulose (Ph. Eur., NF, JP) is a white, odorless, fine, or granular powder that is practically insoluble in water and organic solvents. It is available as a spray-dried product with particle sizes of 20 to 180 μm. In the polarization microscope, it appears optically anisotropic.

Microcrystalline cellulose is obtained by partial hydrolysis of the amorphous fraction of α-cellulose with mineral acids (2.5M HCl, 105°C). This treatment reduces the DP to 200–300. Since predominantly the less ordered, amorphous molecular domains are hydrolyzed, the degree of order is enhanced, that is, the crystallization index increases (the ratio between the crystalline and the amorphous fractions). The crystallization index of α-cellulose powder varies from 0.23 to 0.34 while that of microcrystalline cellulose amounts to about 0.7.

Despite its higher crystallinity, microcrystalline cellulose is much more deformable than normal cellulose powder, due to its exceptional structure. As a result of the rapid drying during the manufacturing process, dislocations and slip planes occur, which during the tableting process can fracture and rearrange. This deformation is of plastic nature. For this reason, tableting mixtures containing microcrystalline cellulose usually yield mechanically firm tablets. Nonetheless, they possess favorable disintegration properties, since the cellulose fraction in the compressed substance causes a pronounced wick effect.

Cellulose products are not degraded in the intestinal tract (only to some degree by microbes in the colon); nonetheless, orally administered microcrystalline cellulose can be persorbed to a certain extent by the intestinal epithelium up to a particle size of 150 μm.

Applications: filling substance, dry binding agent, tablet disintegration enhancer, sedimentation delayer, ground substance for (cosmetic) powders.

5.3.4.4   Further Cellulose Products

The NF includes two monographs for carboxylated types of cellulose: Oxidized Cellulose and Oxidized Regenerated Cellulose, containing 16% to 24% and 18% to 24% of carboxyl groups, respectively. Both products have to be sterile.

Besides these pure cellulose derivatives, two mixtures of cellulose with other excipients are monographed in the pharmacopeias: Silicified Microcrystalline Cellulose (NF) is composed of intimately associated microcrystalline cellulose and colloidal silicon dioxide particles, derived from aqueous coprocessing prior to drying the material. Both, Ph. Eur. and NF, describe a compound called Microcrystalline Cellulose and Carboxymethylcellulose Sodium, which is a colloid-forming, attrited mixture of microcrystalline cellulose and carboxymethylcellulose sodium.

5.3.4.5   Gelatin (Gelatina)

Gelatin (Ph. Eur., NF, JP; Purified Gelatin, JP) is a purified protein that can be obtained by hydrolysis of collagen. Structurally, it differs substantially from conventional proteins. Like collagen, about one third of the molecule consists of glycine. Also noticeable is the high proportion of proline and the unusual protein amino acid hydroxyproline. The exceptional amino acid composition renders gelatin a protein with low nutritional value.

Like collagen, the peptide chains of gelatin have a unique helical structure, which, in terms of dimensions, is not identical to α-helices of common proteins. Three of these helices are twisted together and cross-linked by hydrogen and covalent bonds. During alkaline hydrolysis (to a lesser extent in acidic medium), these cross-links are cleaved so that single-chain polypeptides are formed.

Gelatin is produced by hydrolysis of collagen, predominantly from pig skin (predominantly used for Type A), from calf and cow skin, and pretreated bones from slaughter cattle (predominantly for Type B). Depending on the production method two types are distinguished:

Type A is formed during hydrolysis with acids and has an isoelectric point at pH 7–9.

Type B is formed during alkaline hydrolysis and has an isoelectric point at pH 4.7–5.

At pH values below their isoelectric point, both types have a positive and above it a negative charge excess.

Gelatin of Type A has the best gelling capacity at pH values around 3.2., while Type B gelatin can best be used at pH values of 7–8. When solutions of both types are mixed, a colloidal turbidity can be formed at low concentrations, depending on pH. Also with ionic active agents or excipients pH-dependent incompatibilities can arise. In cold water and in glycerol, gelatin swells and subsequently dissolves upon heating. At concentrations $\geq 1.5\%$ it forms with water a thermo-reversible, transparent, elastic gel.

Due to an increased incidence of the animal disease BSE (Bovine Spongiform Encephalopathy) in the 1990s and the occurrence of a new variant of Creutzfeldt-Jacob's disease in humans, probably resulting from consumption of meat from BSE-infected cattle, the potential infection risks arising from drug ingredients of animal origin moved into focus in the pharmaceutical domain.

Like all other diseases of the TSE group (Transmissable Spongiform Encephalopathies), BSE is most likely caused and transferred by prions. Being proteins, prions are inactivated neither by conventional sterilization methods nor by virocidal procedures. Therefore, based on risk assessments, measures were introduced regarding not only the nutritional domain, but also the use of raw animal material for the pharmaceutical sector. The production of gelatins for pharmaceutical products from raw material derived from TSE-relevant animal species (especially cattle, sheep, and goats) has to proceed under observation of EU directive

2011/C 73/01 (Note for guidance on minimizing the risk of transmitting animal spongiform encephalopathy agents via human and veterinary medicinal products (EMA/410/01 rev.3)). This directive describes measures to minimize risks, including the geographic origin of the animals, the type of processed tissue, the production method, and the quality control system of the manufacturer. In accordance with this, bones are currently considered safe starting material. In addition, the harsh reaction conditions applied during the hydrolytic degradation of collagen for gelatin production, also bring along an effective depletion of prion proteins. Pharmagelatin produced under observance of currently applied instructions, are considered safe with respect to TSE-related infection risks (see also "WHO Guidelines on Tissue Infectivity Distribution in Transmissible Spongiform Encephalopathies, 2006" and "Guidance for Industry: The Sourcing and Processing of gelatin to Reduce the Potential Risk Posed by Bovine Spongiform Encephalopathy (BSE) in FDA-Regulated Products for Human Use," FDA Guidance FR Doc. 97-26501 October 7 1997).

Applications: gel former, thickener, binder for granules, base material for capsules and pessaries, coating material for micro-encapsulation.

Assessment of Gel Strength (Bloom Value)

The gel-forming strength of gelatins is measured according to the internationally common procedure of Bloom, the so-called Bloom test. It is expressed as the weight of a mass (in g) that is required for a stamp of 12.7 mm diameter to leave an impression of 4 mm depth in a 6.67% gelatin gel that has aged for about 17 hours at 10°C. To that end the stamp is lowered with a speed of 0.5 mm/s till it is immersed exactly 4 mm into the gel. The pressure, expressed as Bloom grams, that on that moment is exerted on the stamp is a measure of the gel-formation capacity. Commercial gelatin qualities have gel-forming strengths between 30 and 300 Bloom grams. Ph. Eur. and NF require that the measured value deviates no more than ±20% from the declared value.

5.3.4.6 Tragacanth (Tragacantha)

Tragacanth (Ph. Eur., NF, JP; Powdered Tragacanth, JP) is a gummy exsudation from a variety of Astralagus species, which has hardened during air drying. It is composed mainly of a mixture of heteropolysaccharides containing 20% to 40% water-soluble tragacanthin ($M_r > 10,000$) and 50% to 60% water-insoluble strongly swellable bassorin ($M_r > 100,000$). Additionally, tragacanth contains 10% to 20% of water, about 3% starch (high-quality products are starch-free) and about 4% cellulose. Tragacanthin, a polymer of D-xylose, L-fructose, D-galactose, and D-galcturonic acid (partially as methyl ester), is a weak acid by virtue of its free carboxyl groups. As a natural product, its composition and properties are subject to variations.

Tragacanth is commercially available as thin, transparent horny ribbons of a pale yellow to white color or as a white pulverized or spray-dried powder. The product is practically odor- and tasteless.

With water, at concentrations >2% pseudoplastc mucilages are formed. For the production of tragacanth gels, swelling can be accelerated by pasting it with ethanol or a plasticizer (glycerol). Subsequently, water is slowly added. The consistency of the resulting gels is quite susceptible to pH changes. Stable preparations are obtained in the pH range 4–6.5. Arabic gum and bismuth salts cause reversion of swelling and reduction of viscosity. Also, electrolytes and polyols (glycerol, sorbitol) affect viscosity at higher concentrations.

Applications: suspension stabilizer, emulsifier and thickener, gel former, tablet binding agent.

5.3.4.7 Gum Arabic (Acacia, Gummi arabicum)

Gum arabic (Acacia, Ph. Eur., NF, JP; Powdered Acacia, JP) is the dried gummy exsudate of *Acacia senegal* and a number of other Acacia species. About 80% to 90% of it consists of a mixture of various polysaccharides and up to 15% is protein. The main constituents are calcium, magnesium and potassium salts of arabonic acid, a branched acid heteropolysaccharide (structural units: D-galactose, L-rhamnose, L-arabinose, D-glucuronic acid). The dry plant material consists of rounded, whitish-yellow opaque pieces with cracked surfaces and conchoidal fractures. It is odor- and tasteless.

Gum arabic is also available in a spray-dried form and described in a separate monograph in the Ph. Eur. (Spray-dried gum arabic, Acaciae gummi dispersione desiccatum, no separate monograph in USP/NF). The substance dissolves completely but slowly, in double the amount of water, leaving behind only a small residue of undissolved plant-derived particles while no gel formation occurs. Spray-dried material dissolves without residue. The resulting slimy solution is a colorless to light yellowish, slightly acidic, thick and sticky fluid. In ethanol and ether, the substance is practically insoluble. It contains oxidases and peroxidases, which have to be inactivated prior to application as a formulation excipient. The heat exposure during spray drying generally suffices already for that purpose. Gum arabic possesses true emulsifier properties.

Applications: suspension stabilizer, emulsifier for O/W emulsions, binding agent for granulation, coating material for micro-encapsulation.

5.3.4.8   Pectin (Pectinum)

Pectins (Pectin, NF) occur as constituents of plant cell walls (water-insoluble proto-pectins), as a main component of the middle lamellae (water-insoluble calcium pectinates) as well as in the cytosol (water-soluble pectins). Chemically, they are polygalacturonides with 1,4-α-glycosidic linkages ($M_r = 30,000$ to $150,000$). About half of the carboxyl groups are esterified with methanol. Pectins have a high gel-formation capacity. They are mainly used in the food industry.

Applications: thickener, emulsifier, tablet binding agent.

5.3.4.9   Xanthan (Xanthan Gum, Xanthani gummi)

Xanthan (Ph. Eur., NF) is a branched anionic polysaccharide that is obtained through fermentation by means of the bacterium *Xanthomonas campestris*. It is available in the form of a white to yellow-white easily flowing powder that is soluble in cold as well as hot water. The molecule ($M_r \sim 2,000,000$) consists of a main chain of β-glycosidically linked glucose units, of which every second one is substituted with a tri-saccharide side chain of two mannose units and one glucuronic acid unit, carrying a terminal pyruvate residue. In solutions of low ionic strength and at elevated temperatures, xanthan molecules have a random-coil bundle structure, as the anionic side chains are mutually repelling each other. Already low concentrations of electrolytes reduce this repulsion, causing the side chains to coil around the main chain and to interact with the latter through hydrogen bonds. As a result, the polymer chain forms a stiffened, helical, rod-shaped structure, which by heating or dilution reversibly converts again into a random-coil conformation. Inter-molecular hydrogen bonds cross-link the helical rods to a gel skeleton. Based on this rigid molecular conformation, electrolyte-containing xanthan solutions have a higher viscosity and a higher yield point than equally concentrated solutions of many other polysaccharides. At the same time, xanthan solutions display a pronounced shear thinning, because mechanical disaggregation of the cross-linked rods is accompanied by a more radical structure change than the disruption of hydrogen bonds between non-organized bundles of molecules. Also the viscosity drop caused by heat sterilization is smaller in comparison to many other polysaccharides. The viscosity of the solution is stable within a wide pH range (2–12). Even in highly concentrated sugar solutions (up to 60%) xanthan can be hydrated, which makes it a suitable thickener for syrups and also suitable for the manufacture of dry syrups because of its rapid solubility.

Applications: thickener, gelation and suspension enhancer, sustained release excipient for hydrocolloid matrix tablets.

5.3.4.10   Alginates (Acidum alginicum)

Alginic acid (Ph. Eur., NF) is a polymer consisting of mannuronic and guluronic acid, with a molecular weight of about 120,000 to 200,000. It is obtained from brown algae, which contain up to 40% of mucilages, by heating with alkali and subsequent precipitation with hydrochloric acid. Alginic acid and calcium alginate are insoluble in water; the sodium, potassium, and ammonium alginates are readily soluble in water. They are incompatible with alcohols, balsams, tars, and salicylic acids. Addition of salts (phosphates, carbonates) causes a concentration-dependent reduction in viscosity. Calcium ions (e.g., calcium citrate) have a gelling effect that is based on the formation of calcium bridges between individual poly-mannuronic acid chains. In order to save alginate during the manufacturing of spreadable gels it is possible to convert soluble alginates partly into calcium alginate by addition of calcium salts.

alginic acid chain (section)

For pharmaceutical purposes mainly sodium alginate (Ph. Eur., NF) is used; aqueous solutions of it are weakly acidic. In concentrations of 3-6% ointment-like gels are formed. They are produced by pasting the material with a humectant (e.g., glycerol) and slowly adding lukewarm water. Alginate preparations are most stable in the pH range 6–7; at pH values <4.5 the free acid precipitates. Strong and long heating, especially above 70°C, should be avoided, as this causes strong viscosity losses as a result of depolymerization.

Applications: viscosity enhancer, emulsion and suspension stabilizer, binding substance for granulation, disintegration enhancer for tablets.

5.3.4.11   Guar Galactomannan (Guargalactomannanum)

Guar galactomannan (Ph. Eur.; Guar gum, NF) is a polysacchararide mixture from the mucilaginous endosperm of the seeds of the Indian guar bean (Cyamopsis tetragonolobus). It is available as a white to yellowish odorless powder. The polymer consists of a main chain of α-1,4-glycosidically linked D-mannose units, which, in turn, are substituted with α-1,6-linked galactosyl residues in a 1:1.4 to 1:2 mannose:galactose ratio. The molecular mass adds up to between 80,000 and 160,000.

Applications: In up to 10% concentrations it serves as a binding substance for granulates, as disintegration enhancer for tablets and can be deployed at higher concentrations to facilitate sustained release for hydrocolloid matrix tablets. Based on its viscosity enhancing effect it is used as emulsion stabilizer at 1% concentration and to some extent, at concentrations up to 2.5%, as a thickener for creams and lotions.

5.3.4.12   Carrageenan (Carrageenanum)

Carrageenan (Ph. Eur., NF) is a polysaccharide mixture that is obtained from certain species of red seaweeds (Rhodophyceae) by extraction with hot water or alkali solutions. The linear polymer consists of 1,3-linked β-D-galactose and 1,4-linked α-D-galactose units, either in free form or carrying sulfate groups. The α-D-galactose unit can occur as the 3,6-anhydro derivative. Carrageenan with a small proportion of 3,6-anhydrogalactose (λ-carrageenan) forms viscous solutions with water, while substances with a high proportion of anhydro units (κ- and τ-carrageenan) are capable of gel formation. The latter occurs only in presence of cations, which compensate for the negative charges of the sulfate groups. In addition, they exert a stabilizing (K^+, NH_4^+, Ca^{2+}) or destabilizing (Na^+, Li^+) effect on the helical conformation of the molecule and the gel structure. The formation and properties of carrageen gels are thus strongly dependent on the nature and the concentration of the cations that are present.

Applications: carrageen is mainly used as thickener, suspension stabilizer, pseudo-emulsifier and as a gel builder. With water it forms highly viscous solutions. κ- and τ-carrageens form thixotropic gels at concentrations of 0.3% to 1% in the presence of potassium ions.

5.3.4.13   *Shellac (Lacca)*

Shellac (Ph. Eur., NF; Purified Shellac, JP; White Shellac, JP) is a resin of animal origin, which in raw form is obtained from trees in South Asia. The female lac insect (*Taccardia lacca*) secretes for the protection of their brood, a resin-like substance on the twigs of the host tree, which is then harvested and processed into shellac by purification (separation form solid material and wax components and bleaching). As a natural product, shellac has a highly heterogeneous composition. About 75% of the substance consists of partially esterified hydroxycarboxylic acids, mainly aleuritic acid (9,10,16-trihydroxypalmitic acid) and shellolic acid (a tricyclic dihydroxy-dicarboxylic acid), which renders shellac insoluble in acids. In alkaline media, it dissolves under the formation of salts.

Applications: In the past, shellac was used as a release-delaying coating of tablets and pellets because of its resistance against gastric juice. Numerous shellac-coated products are currently still commercially available. However, the variable composition of shellac barely allows satisfactory standardization of the protective and release-sustaining function and from a biopharmaceutical perspective a pH-dependent prolongation of drug is not recommended anyhow. Shellac also provides the basic ingredient of numerous printing dyes for the lettering of tablets and capsules.

5.3.5 Semisynthetic Macromolecular Excipients

5.3.5.1 Semisynthetic Cellulose Ethers and Esters

Each glucopyranose unit of cellulose contains three hydroxyl groups. By etherification or esterification of these moieties cellulose derivatives with altered physicochemical properties can be synthesized. Generally, only a fraction of the available hydroxyl groups are substituted. The product is characterized by the so-called average degree of substitution (DS), which indicates how many OH groups of individual glucopyranose units are, on average, etherified or esterified. For example, when on average one out of the three available OH groups is etherified, DS equals 1. The chain length of the molecule is characterized by the average degree of polymerization (DP). It indicates of how many glucose units the macromolecule is composed on average. These two parameters determine the properties of the semisynthetic derivatives. The product type is indicated by a post-positioned number to the name, specifying the viscosity of a 2% (m/V) aqueous solution in mPa·s.

The basic raw material commonly used for derivation is cellulose that has been transformed into alkali cellulose by treatment with sodium hydroxide. Ether derivation is achieved with the aid of alkyl halogenides, according to the following general reaction equation.

Synthesis of cellulose ether

Cellulose or cellulose ether chain (section)

Cellulose	R:H
Methylcellulose	R:CH_3
Ethylcellulose	R:C_2H_5
Hydroxyethylcellulose	R:CH_2–CH_2OH
Hydroxypropylcellulose	R:CH_2–CH(OH)–CH_3 CH_2–CH(O–CH_2CH(OH)–CH_3)–CH_3
Hydroxypropylmethylcellulose	R:CH_2–CH(OH)–CH_3 CH_2–CH(O–CH_2CH(OH)–CH_3)–CH_3 CH_3
Carboxymethylcellulose Sodium	R:CH_2–COONa
Cellulose acetate phthalate	R:O–CO–CH_3 O–CO–C_6H_4–COOH
Hydroxypropylmethylcellulose acetate phthalate	R:CH_2–CH(OH)–CH_3 CH_2–CH(O–CH_2CH(OH)–CH_3)–CH_3 CH_3 O–CO–CH_3 O–CO–C_6H_4–COOH

Table 5-4 Etherifying Reactants

Derivative	Etherifying Reactants
methylcellulose	methyl chloride, dimethylsulfate
ethylcellulose	ethyl chloride
hydroxyethylcellulose	ethylene oxide
ethylhydroxyethylcellulose	ethyl chloride together with ethylene oxide
carboxymethylcellulose sodium	monochloroacetic acid

Specifically, the etherifying reactants listed in Table 5-4 are applied for this purpose.

The ether substitution occurs primarily at the primary hydroxyl group on the C-6 carbon, to lesser extents also at the secondary OH groups on the C-2 and C-3 carbons. During the reaction, partial cleavage of the cellulose chain occurs, yielding products with a lower degree of polymerization.

Only the partially etherified products possess the pharmaceutically important water solubility, while the more extensively etherified products are soluble in nonpolar organic solvents. All products share the ability to swell. While cellulose is swellable in water only to a limited extent, many of the etherified products display unlimited swellability—that is, they adopt the sol structure in the presence of sufficiently high amounts of water. This is surprising, as cellulose would be expected to be completely swellable with its three free OH groups per unit. This anomalous phenomenon can be explained by the consideration that the glycosidic chains of the cellulose are pushed away from each other so that the available free OH groups become better accessible for solvatation by water molecules (hydration).

Table 5-5 presents an overview of commonly used cellulose derivatives.

5.3.5.2 Methylcellulose (MC, Methylcellulosum)

Methylcelluloses (Methylcellulose, Ph. Eur., NF) are methyl ethers of cellulose with molecular masses varying from 10,000 to 220,000. Pharmaceutically applicable products are soluble in cold water. Upon heating to >55°C methylcellulose precipitates, but redissolves during subsequent cooling (thermo-reversible coagulation). Whereas water cannot penetrate into native cellulose due to its partially crystalline structure, the methyl groups effectuate a disordering of the lattice and thus enhance solubility. But only products with a degree of substitution of 1.4 to 2.0 are soluble in cold water. Both higher and lower degree of substitution diminish water solubility.

Like other nonionic cellulose ethers, methylcellulose can be considered an emulsifier. For example, 0.5% solutions display an interfacial tension *vs.* paraffin oil of 15.8 mN·m^{-1} at 35°C, as compared to 30.5 mN·m^{-1} for the water/paraffin interface. Also the surface tension of water is diminished by methylcellulose. This causes foaming when aqueous methylcellulose solutions are shaken. While methylcellulose concentrations of <1% yield aqueous solutions, concentrations of 3% to 16% lead to the formation of gels of plastic consistency, which can also be used for dermatological preparations. Methylcellulose gels are plastic and thixotropic and form, upon dilution with water, permeable transparent films on the skin. Because of the non-ionic character of these preparations they are stable in the pH range 2 to 12 and compatible with most pharmaceutical agents. Addition of high concentrations of electrolytes (>10%) causes flocculation due to reversible dehydration. Tannins and phenols act similarly.

Applications: binding agent for wet granulation (1%–5%), dry binder for direct tablet compression (10%–25%), disintegration enhancer (highly viscous types, 2%–10%), release sustaining agent in hydrocolloid matrix tablets (15%–80%), film former for film-coated tablets, additive in coating suspensions, matrix substance for solid solutions/dispersions, suspension stabilizer, gel former, viscosity enhancer.

5.3.5.3 Ethylcellulose (EC, Ethylcellulosum)

Ethylcellulose (Ph. Eur., NF) is an ethyl ether of cellulose and is insoluble in water. However, it dissolves in a number of organic solvents, including alcohols, ethers, and chlorinated hydrocarbons. With increasing degree of substitution, solubility increases.

Table 5-5 Cellulose Derivatives

Cellulose Derivative	Abbreviation	Trade Names (Examples)	Monograph	R $O{-}CH_3$	R $O{-}CH_2{-}CH_3$	R $O{-}CH_2{-}CH_2{-}OH$	R $O{-}CH_2{-}CH(OH){-}CH_3$	R $O{-}CO{-}CH_3$	R $O{-}CO{-}C_3H_7$	R $O{-}CH_2{-}CO{-}O^-\,Na^+$	R (phthalyl)	R (succinyl)
Methylcellulose	MC	Tylose® MH and MB, Methocel® MC	NF JP Ph. Eur.	27.0–31.5% 26.0–33.0% no information								
Ethylcellulose	EC	Aquacoat®, Ethocel®	NF Ph. Eur.		44.0–51.0% 44.0–51.0%							
Hydroxyethylcellulose (Hyetellose)	HEC	Ethoxose®	NF Ph. Eur.			no information no information						
Hydroxyethylmethylcellulose (Hymetellose)	MHEC, HEMC	Culminal™ MHEC	NF Ph. Eur.	no information no information		no information no information						
Hydroxypropylcellulose	HPC	Klucel®	NF JP Ph. Eur.				53.4–80.5% 53.4–77.5% no information					
Low substituted Hydroxypropylcellulose	HPC		NF, JP				5.0–16.0%					
Hydroxypropylmethylcellulose (Hypromellose)	HPMC	Pharmacoat®	Ph. Eur., NF, JP	Type 1828¹: 16.5–20.0% Type 2208: 19.0–24.0% Type 2906: 27.0–30.0% Type 2910: 28.0–30.0%			23.0–32.0% 4.0–12.0% 4.0–7.5% 7.0–12.0%					
Carboxymethylcellulose Sodium (Carmellose Sodium)	Na-CMC	Tylopur® C	NF Ph. Eur. JP							6.5–9.5% Na⁺ 6.5–10.8% Na⁺ 6.5–8.5% Na⁺		
Carboxymethylcellulose Sodium 12 NF			NF							10.4–12.0% Na⁺		
Low-substituted Carboxymethylcellulose Sodium			NF, Ph. Eur.							2.0–4.5% Na⁺		
Carboxymethylcellulose Calcium			NF, Ph. Eur.							no information		
Carboxymethylethylcellulose	CMEC		no monograph		no information					no information		
Cellulose acetate phthalate (Cellacefate)	CAP	Aquateric®	NF, Ph. Eur., JP					21.5–26%			30–36%	
Cellulose acetate butyrate (Cellaburate)	CAB		NF Ph. Eur.					1.0–41.0% 2.0–30.0%	5.0–56.0% 16.0–53.0%			
Hydroxypropylmethylcellulose phthalate (Hypromellose phthalate)	HPMCP	HP 50®, HP 55® (Shin-Etsu)	NF, Ph. Eur. JP Type 220824 JP Type 200731	no information 20.0–24.0% 18.0–22.0%			no information 6.0–10.0% 5.0–9.0%				21.0–35.0% 21–27% 27–35%	
Hydroxypropylmethylcellulose acetate succinate (Hypromellose acetate succinate)	HPMCAS	AQOAT (pronounced "Ay-coat") (Shin-Etsu)	NF, JP	12.0–28.0%			4.0–23.0%	2.0–16.0%				4.0–28.0%

¹ The type designation results from the digit sequence of the rounded average values of the concentration limits. Example: first substituent 16.5%–20.0% rounded average: 18, second substituent 23.0% to 32.0% rounded average 28, type designation 1828.

Applications: film former for water-insoluble coatings for diffusion-controlled drug release (the permeability of the film can be regulated by addition of water-soluble cellulose ethers), matrix substance for solid solutions/dispersions.

5.3.5.4 Hydroxyethylcellulose (HEC, Hyetellose, Hydroxyethylcellulosum)

Hydroxyethylcellulose (Ph. Eur.; Hydroxyethyl Cellulose, NF) is a hydroxyethyl ether of cellulose. It is produced by conversion of alkali cellulose with ethylene oxide. In that process the primary hydroxyl groups of the glucose units react preferentially. By this reaction new primary OH groups are formed, which are more reactive than the secondary OH groups of the glucose. In this way short polyethylene glycol chains are formed at the 6-positions of the glucose units. Thus, the average degree of substitution does not suffice to characterize the product, as this merely indicates the number of substituted OH groups in each glucose unit. The average molar substitution (MS) that is used for products with hydroxyl substituents expresses the total number of substituents units per glucose unit. For water-soluble products this should amount to a minimum of 1.

Hydroxyethylcellulose resembles methylcellulose in its essential properties. In contrast to most other cellulose ethers, hydroxylethylcellulose does not display heat coagulation. In concentrations of about 2.5% it forms crystal-clear, spreadable gels. For gel preparation the fine powder is pasted with a small amount of alcohol, followed by slowly adding water of 20°C under continuous stirring. Similar to methylcellulose, the swelling is enhanced by allowing it to stand at low temperatures. The preparations show stable viscosity during storage. Aqueous hydroxylethylcellulose solutions do not flocculate by addition of electrolytes, acids and alkali, but they are incompatible with tannins and Ichthyol®. Such mucilaginouos preparations are, however, miscible with ethanol, due to their high content of secondary hydroxyl groups.

Applications: thickener, suspension and emulsion stabilizer, gel former, binding substance for granulates and coatings of sugar-coated tablets and pellets.

5.3.5.5 Methylhydroxyethylcellulose (Hymetelose, Methylhydroxyethylcellulosum)

Methylhydroxyethylcellulose (Ph. Eur.; Hymetellose, NF) is a partly O-methylated and O-hydroxyethylated cellulose. It has similar properties to methylcellulose but is more readily soluble in water and the solutions are more tolerant of salts. In contrast to hydroxyethylcellulose, it displays heat coagulation. The coagulation temperature of about 60°C is higher than of methylcellulose.

Applications: tablet binder, suspension stabilizer, gel former for topical preparations

5.3.5.6 Hydroxypropylcellulose (HPC, Hydroxypropylcellulosum)

Hydroxypropylcellulose (Ph. Eur.; Hydroxypropyl Cellulose, NF) is a partially hydroxypropylated cellulose that is formed by conversion of alkali cellulose with propylene oxide. Like we saw for hydroxylethylcellulose, the etherification of already formed hydroxylpropyl groups causes the formation of side chains. For good water-solubility a substitution grade between 1 and 4 is required. Aqueous HPC solutions undergo heat coagulation at temperatures of 40-45 °C. Besides in water, the substance dissolves in alcohols, propylene glycol and chloroform. With tannins and phenols, precipitates are formed. In addition to "Hydroxypropyl Cellulose" (with 53.4% to 80.5% of hydroxypropoxy groups, calculated to the dry basis) also a "Low-Substituted Hydroxypropyl Cellulose" is monographed in the NF (containing 5.0% to 16.0% of hydroxypropoxy groups).

Applications: thickener, suspension and emulsion stabilizer, binding substance for granulates, coating substance for film tablets.

5.3.5.7 Hydroxypropylmethylcellulose (HPMC, Hypromellose, Hypromellosum)

Hydroxypropylmethylcellulose (Hypromellose, Ph. Eur., JP; Hydroxypropyl Methylcellulose, NF) is a methyl- and hydroxypropyl-substituted cellulose with properties largely similar to HPC. Four types with different amounts of methoxy- and hydroxypropoxy groups are distinguished in the NF (see Table 5-5).

Applications: thickener, viscosity enhancer for ophthalmic preparations, binding agent, film former, matrix substance for solid solutions/dispersions, alternative to gelatin as a basic substance for hard capsules (e.g., Vcaps®).

5.3.5.8   Carboxymethylcellulose Sodium (Na-CMC, Carmellose-Sodium, Carmellosum natricum)

Carboxymethylcellulose Sodium (Carmellose Sodium, Ph. Eur., JP; Carboxymethylcellulose Sodium, NF) is the sodium salt of a partially O-carboxymethylated cellulose (glycolic acid ether of cellulose). The substance as described in the Ph. Eur. contains 1.15 to 1.45 carboxymethyl groups per glucose unit (resulting in a sodium content of 10.4%–12.0%) and corresponds to the NF monograph "Carboxymethylcellulose Sodium 12." The type of substance described in the NF as "Carboxymethylcellulose Sodium," however, is characterized by a lower amount of sodium between 6.5% and 9.5%. The white powder is insoluble in the common organic solvents, but can readily be dispersed in water to form a colloidal solution.

Aqueous solutions react practically neutral and barely display surface activity. Depending on the preparation method, pharmaceutically used products contain variable proportions of NaCl, which is responsible for the slightly salty taste. In contrast to Na-CMC, the acid form of the substance, known as Carmellose (Ph. Eur., NF, JP), can be swollen and suspended in water, but forms a colloidal solution only after alkalization. Numerous types of Na-CMC are commercially available and distinguish themselves by varying degrees of polymerization and substitution ($M_r = 80,000$ to 600,000). Depending on the degree of polymerization the viscosity of aqueous Na-CMC solutions or gels varies widely; for 1% preparations it ranges from <10 to about 10,000 mPa·s. The average degree of substitution (DS) determines the water-solubility of Na-CMC. The substance described in the Ph. Eur. under "Carmellose sodium" with an DS of 1.15 to 1.45, is water-soluble, while types with DS values of 0.13 to 0.38 (2.0%-4.5% sodium), monographed in the Ph. Eur. and NF as "Low-substituted Carmellose sodium" (Carmellosum natricum substitutum humile), are insoluble in water.

Another low-substituted type is "Enzymatically-Hydrolyzed Carboxymethylcellulose Sodium" (NF) in which the glycolic acid residues were partly removed by enzymatic hydrolysis with Trichoderma reesei cellulase to a degree of substitution of 0.20 to 1.50 (sodium content 2.6%-12.2%).

Another factor that has an effect on the rheological behavior is the uniformity of the substitution. While solutions of Na-CMC types with homogeneously substituted molecules along the entire length of the chains possess pseudo-plastic flow properties, types that, in addition to substituted sections, also possess non-substituted sections, form thixotropic solutions. The non-substituted sections can form hydrogen bridges with neighboring molecules and thus build a solid but reversibly destructible gel skeleton.

The dissolution of Na-CMC in water proceeds in several stages. The initially suspended polymer particles subsequently swell under uptake of water, causing viscosity to increase rapidly. Only during further hydration, the polymer becomes molecularly dispersed which goes along with a drop in viscosity of the solution. Depending on the dissolution technique, the Na-CMC type and the electrolyte content of the solvent, the latter step often proceeds very slowly. The process may also persist in the swollen stage and lead to solutions with enhanced viscosity. This is particularly the case for Na-CMC types with a low substitution grade; as a rule, these therefore form solutions with high viscosity.

During dissolution Na-CMC tends to form clumps. It is therefore important to ensure, by taking suitable measures, that a rapid dispersion of individual particles is achieved before the onset of swelling. It is recommended to dissolve the Na-CMC before any other excipient or active ingredient is added. For the production of a gel, the powder is pasted with a wetting agent, water is added in portions under constant stirring and the mixture is allowed to stand and swell. The swelling process is only weakly temperature-dependent. In contrast to methylcellulose, Na-CMC is soluble in cold as well as hot water. Furthermore, aqueous solutions of Na-CMC are heat-stable and tolerate temperatures of 100°C for extended periods of time without coagulation.

The anionic character of Na-CMC is responsible for the relatively large number of incompatibilities as compared to non-ionic cellulose ethers. Heavy metal ions cause precipitations due to the formation of insoluble, sometimes colored salts. Similarly, cationic compounds form poorly soluble precipitates with Na-CMC. Na$^+$ ions display a viscosity-enhancing effect, in particular on the CMC types with a low degree of substitution. Lowering pH to values <3.5 causes precipitation of the CMC in its acidic form. Tannins and phenols (pyrogallol, Peru balsam) show incompatibilities with most cellulose ethers, however are relatively compatible with Na-CMC.

Applications: viscosity enhancer, suspension and emulsion stabilizer (0.25-1%), also for parenterals, gel builder (3-6%), binding substance and disintegration enhancer for tableting (1-6%), hydrocolloid-matrix builder in tablets (5-10%).

By drying a suspension of Na-CMC and microcrystalline cellulose combination products are obtained, which the Ph. Eur. describes, under the name "Microcrystalline Cellulose and Carboxymethylcellulose Sodium" (*Cellulosum microcristallinum et carmellosum natricum*), in a monograph. The proportion of Na-CMC, amounting to 5-22%, promotes the dispersibility of the cellulose particles, as it decreases the adhesion between the micro-crystallites. The aqueous dispersions have a low yield stress as well as a pronounced thixotropic behavior, which makes the substance a good stabilizer for suspensions and emulsions.

In contrast to the sodium salt, the calcium salt of CMC (**Carmellose Calcium**, Ph. Eur., NF, JP) is water-insoluble. By virtue of its swelling properties it is applied as a binding agent and disintegration enhancer of tablets at concentrations up to 15%.

5.3.5.9 Croscarmellose Sodium (Carmellosum natricum conexum)

Croscarmellose Sodium (Ph. Eur., NF, JP) is a cross-linked carmellose sodium in which oxymethyl-carboxy groups of one chain are esterified with hydroxyl groups of another. The average substitution grade is about 0.7. The substance presents a grey-whitish powder, which is soluble neither in water nor in organic solvents. Nonetheless, it is able to take up large amounts of water in a short time under strong swelling (200%).

Applications: it is used, in concentrations of 1-5%, as disintegration enhancer for tablets and granules. For that purpose it can be added to the granulate matrix as well as to the "external phase" of tableting mixtures.

5.3.5.10 Cellulose Acetate (Cellulosi acetas)

Cellulose acetate (Ph. Eur., NF) is either a partially or fully O-acetylated cellulose that is obtained by treatment of cellulose with acetic anhydrate. The qualities registered by the Ph. Eur. have a degree of substitution of 1.9 to 3.0. The white to yellowish or greyish white powder is insoluble in water, but soluble in some solvents, including certain esters and ketones.

By analogy, **cellulose acetate butyrate (Cellaburate, Cellulosi acetas butyras)** (Ph. Eur., NF) is formed by acylation of cellulose with a mixture of acetic and butyric anhydride. Compared to cellulose acetate this substance is harder, has a higher mechanical strength and a lower water absorption.

Applications: cellulose acetate is employed in the manufacture of water-insoluble tablet films, in particular for OROS (oral osmotic systems).

5.3.5.11 Cellulose Acetate Phthalate (CAP, Cellulosi acetas phthalas)

Cellulose acetate phthalate (Ph. Eur., NF, JP) is a mixed acetate/phthalate cellulose ester. The bifunctional phthalic acid forms a semi ester so that one carboxyl group remains available for salt formation. As a result, CAP is water-soluble in alkali from pH 6 and above. It is insoluble in many organic solvents, except some ketones, esters and solvent mixtures.

Application: film former for gastric juice resistant, small-intestine soluble coatings

5.3.5.12 Hydroxypropylmethylcellulose Phthalate (HPMCP, Hypromellose Phthalate, Hypromellosi phthalas)

Hydroxypropylmethylcellulose phthalate (Ph. Eur.; Hypromellose Phthalate, NF, JP) is a mixed ester of cellulose of which part of the free hydroxyl groups are esterified with phthalic acid and the rest with methyl- and hydroxylpropyl groups. Like for cellulose acetate phthalate, the free carboxyl group of the phthalic acid is available for salt formation. Two types of this substance are commonly used, which are distinguished by the molar ratio of their substituents. Grade HP-50 (phthalyl content 21-27%) is soluble in aqueous solutions with pH values above 5.0 and HP-55 (phthalyl content 27-35%) dissolves above pH 5.5. HPMCP is also soluble in methanol and methylene chloride. Tablet coatings made of HPMCP dissolve earlier in the gastro-intestinal tract than those made from CAP.

Application: film former for gastric-juice resistant, small-intestine soluble coatings.

5.3.5.13   Sodium Starch Glycolate (Carboxymethyl Starch Sodium Salt, Carboxymethylamylum natricum)

The three different types (A, B and C) of sodium starch glycolate that are described by the Ph. Eur. (types A and B also in NF and JP) are sodium salts of cross-linked, partially carboxymethylated starch (in case of Types A and B potato starch). The average degrees of substitution (DS) are in the lower range (0.1-0.5). The cross-links are accomplished either via phosphate groups (e.g., Primojel®) or directly, without cross-linker, by ester formation between carboxyl groups of one chain with hydroxyl groups of another (Vivastar®). The three types are distinguished by their substitution and degree of cross-linking. Sodium starch glycolate displays strong swelling capacity in water, which is most pronounced for type C. Upon swelling, types A and B form suspensions, while type C swells up to a highly viscous to gel-like consistency. All substances are available as a white powder and are strongly hygroscopic.

Applications: At concentrations of 2-8% types A and B serve as disintegration enhancers for tablets. Thus, they are effective in much lower concentrations than non-modified starch, which relates to their much higher swelling volume. The sodium starch glycolates are also applied as additives in granulates as well as direct tablet compression. In the former case they can be applied at the intra-granular level as well as mixed with the external phase of the tableting mixture. Type C is furthermore used as a suspension and emulsion stabilizer and is also a suitable binding agent for wet granulation.

5.3.5.14   Hydroxyalkylstarches

Hydroxyalkylstarches are hydoxyalkylethers of starches. Incorporation of hydroxyalkyl groups in the starch chains, primarily in the amorphous regions, facilitates the penetration of water into the starch granules and the gelatinization. With an increasing degree of substitution, the temperature at which initial swelling of starch granules takes place (pasting temperature) is lowered, until the product swells and disperses in cold water. As hydroxyalkylation inhibits ordered structures of the molecule chains it leads to more fluid starch pastes with improved clarity.

The following types of hydoxyalkylstarches are listed in the pharmacopeias:

- Starches, hydroxyethyl (Ph. Eur.)
- Starch, hydroxypropyl (Ph. Eur.)
- Starch, hydroxypropyl pregelatinized (Ph. Eur.)
- Hydroxypropyl corn starch (NF)
- Pregelatinized hydroxypropyl corn starch (NF)
- Hydroxypropyl pea starch (NF)
- Pregelatinized hydroxypropyl pea starch (NF)
- Hydroxypropyl potato starch (NF)
- Pregelatinized hydroxypropyl potato starch (NF)

Applications: Hydroxypropyl starch: binder, disintegrant, emulsifying agent, thickening agent and viscosity-increasing agent, aqueous film coating for immediate release, solid oral dosage forms (Lyocoat®), food additive.

Hydroxyethyl starch: intravenous plasma volume expander, bulking agent and lyoprotectant in freeze-dried products.

5.3.6   Synthetic Macromolecular Excipients

5.3.6.1   Polyacrylic Acids (Carbomers, Carbomera)

The polyacrylic acid qualities described in the monograph **Carbomers** of the Ph. Eur. and in the monograph **Carbomer homopolymer** of the NF are high molecular weight anionic polymers of acrylic acid, which are cross-linked to a low extent (0.75-2%) with allyl ethers of sugars (Ph. Eur.) or polyols (Ph. Eur., NF). The NF contains two further carbomer monographs:

Carbomer copolymer is a high molecular weight copolymer of acrylic acid and a long-chain alkyl methacrylate cross-linked with allyl ethers of polyalcohols. **Carbomer interpolymer** is a carbomer homopolymer or copolymer that contains a block copolymer of polyethylene glycol and a long-chain alkyl acid ester.

$$\left[-CH_2 - \underset{\underset{COOH}{|}}{CH} - \right]_n$$

All these substances appear as white, light, hygroscopic powders, having a slightly sour smell. Pharmaceutically applied types have a molecular mass which is estimated to range between 700,000 and $4 \cdot 10^9$ g/mol (Carbomer Homopolymer, NF, type A: 1,250,000 g/mol, type B: 3,000,000 g/mol, type C: 4,000,000 g/mol). For the preparation of gels weakly cross-linked polyacrylic acids with average molecular masses of 3 million to 4 million g/mol are suitable. In former times, benzene was commonly used in the synthesis of carbomers and residues of the solvent remained in the final product. Nowadays for pharmaceutical purposes only carbomer types produced by benzene-free synthesis and containing less than 2 ppm benzene are approved (e.g., Carbomers, Ph. Eur., Carbomer Copolymer, NF, Carbomer Homopolymer, NF, Carbomer Interpolymer, NF). However, the NF also includes older monographs of carbomer types with higher benzene limits. 1% aqueous suspensions have pH values of 2.5-3.2 and nearly the same viscosity as water. Only upon neutralization with inorganic or organic bases, gel formation occurs and highly viscous products are formed. In that process the originally convoluted polymer chains stretch out as a result of intra-molecular repulsion forces caused by the negative charges arising. For gel formation concentrations of 0.5% to 1% are required. The preparation involves gentle stirring of the fine powder in water and neutralization of the formed suspension with a precalculated amount of alkali. Neutralization can also be achieved by basic agents such as Tromethamine (Tris), Meglumin, and Dexpanthenol. Triethanolamine is not recommended for this purpose because of potential nitrosamine formation. Polyacrylic acid preparations do not change viscosity in the pH range 6–10. At pH values >10–11, a rapid drop in viscosity occurs. Also during storage viscosity changes can be expected. Polyacrylic acid preparations are sensitive to salts. Already at low concentrations cations such as Na^+, Ca^{2+} and Al^{3+} have a deteriorating effect on the gels, including the occurrence of coagulation. Polyacrylic acid is not toxic and is well tolerated by the skin. In contrast to many other gels, polyacrylate gels can penetrate into the skin.

The following types of carbomers are listed in the phamacopeias:

Monograph	Type	Viscosity of Aqueous Solution (mPa·s)	Carboxylic Acid Content (%)	Max. Benzene Content (%)	Brand Name (Examples)
Carbomers, Ph. Eur.		-	56.0–68.0	0.0002	Carbopol 971 P NF Carbopol 974 P NF Carbopol 980 NF
Carbomer Homopolymer, NF	Type A Type B Type C	4,000–11,000 (0.5%) 25,000–45,000 (0.5%) 40,000–60,000 (0.5%)	56.0–68.0	0.0002	Carbopol 971 P NF Carbopol 974 P NF Carbopol 980 NF
Carbomer Copolymer, NF	Type A Type B Type C	4,500–13,500 (1%) 10,000–29,000 (1%) 25,000–45,000 (1%)	52.0–62.0	0.0002	Permulen TR-2 NF Permulen TR-1 NF -
Carbomer Interpolymer, NF	Type A Type B Type C	45,000–65,000 (0.5%) 47,000–77,000 (1%) 8,500–16,500 (0.5%)	52.0–62.0	0.0002	Carbopol Ultrez 10 NF Carbopol EDT 2020 NF -
Carbomer 934, NF		30,500–39,400 (0.5%)	56.0–68.0	0.5	Carbopol 934 NF
Carbomer 934P, NF		29,400–39,400 (0.5%)	56.0–68.0	0.01	Carbopol 934P NF
Carbomer 940, NF		40,000–60,000 (0.5%)	56.0–68.0	0.5	Carbopol 940 NF
Carbomer 941, NF		4,000–11,600 (0.5%)	56.0-68.0	0.5	Carbopol 941 NF
Carbomer 1342, NF		9,500–26,500 (1%)	52.0-62.0	0.2	Carbopol 1342 NF

Applications: thickener, gel former, emulsion and suspension stabilizer, binding agent.

5.3.6.2　Copolymers of Methacrylic Acid and Methacrylate Esters (Eudragit® Types)

Copolymers of methacrylic acid and its esters are available as film formers for tablet coatings under the trade name Eudragit®. Table 5-6 presents an overview of the most common commercial Eudragit types. Eudragit® E contains basic groups that are responsible for its solubility in gastric juice. Eudragit® L and Eudragit® S contain acidic groups which cause the substance to dissolve only in the environment of the small intestine. Eudragit® RL and RS possess quaternary ammonium groups. These types are suitable for the manufacturing of drug formulations with sustained release of the active ingredient.

Soluble drugs are released through diffusion and the velocity of release can be controlled by varying the permeability of the film coating. The number in the type designation represents an indication of the concentration of the polymer and the nature of the solvent. Types designated 12.5 are organic solutions with a polymer content of 12.5%. The acrylic polymers are dissolved in mixtures of isopropanol and acetone. Similarly, the designation 30D indicates 30% of solid material in an aqueous dispersion. The designation 100 indicates that the substance is a virtually pure (95-98%) powder.

5.3.6.3　Aqueous Latex Dispersions

Polymeric film formers are dissolved either in organic solvents or processed as aqueous dispersions. The latter are fine, stable suspensions of microscopic spherically shaped particles (latex particles) of 0.01−1 μm diameter in water. They are obtained by emulsion polymerization. In this polymerization process the polymerization is initiated in the aqueous phase of a monomer emulsion. The polymerization takes place in the outer phase of the emulsion and starts with the formation of polymerization seeds that are stabilized by adsorbed emulsifier and gradually grow into latex particles by uptake of monomers dissolved in the aqueous phase and those which are supplied from the emulsion droplets. Aqueous polymer dispersions are colloidal systems and as such susceptible to external influences (electrolytes, pH changes, organic solvents, strong shear forces), which may lead to coagulation. Coagulated dispersions cannot be redispersed and thus are no longer useable. Usually emulsifiers and stabilizers are added to mitigate such events.

5.3.6.4　Polyvinylpyrrolidone (PVP, Polyvidone, Povidone, Povidonum)

Polyvinylpyrrolidone (Povidone, Ph. Eur., NF, JP) is obtained by polymerization of N-vinylpyrrolidone and is a strongly hygroscopic powder, readily soluble in water, alcohols, methylene chloride and chloroform.

Depending on the degree of polymerization its average molecular weight amounts to 20,000 to 700,000. It resembles polyvinyl alcohol with respect to its colloid-physical properties. The aqueous solution reacts neutral to weakly acidic and it is compatible with ethanol. Addition of significant amounts of salt (NaCl, Na_2SO_4) causes coagulation. The various povidone types are distinguished by the viscosity of their solutions, expressed as K-value ("intrinsic viscosity") according to Fickentscher (ISO 1628-1). The K-value offers the possibility to characterize the average molecular mass of polymers. In the case of PVP it can be calculated from the following formula:

$$M_r = 22.22(K + 0.075\ K^2)^{1.65}.$$

Polyvinylpyrrolidone is frequently used to enhance the dissolution rate of poorly water-soluble pharmaceutics. For this application it is used in solid as well as in fluid drug formulations, including formulations for parenteral administration. PVP is able to form solid solutions with numerous active ingredients; in such preparations the active ingredient is colloidally or, in the ideal case, molecularly dispersed in a solid matrix. Because of the high glass

Table 5-6 Eudragit® Types

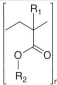

Ph. Eur./NF Monograph	Brand Name	Application	R	Solubility/Permeability
Basic butylated methacrylate copolymer (Ph. Eur.) Amino methacrylate copolymer (NF)	Eudragit® E 12,5, Eudragit® E 100, Eudragit® E PO	Rapidly disintegrating film coatings, taste masking, smell-tightness, colored or transparent, protection from abrasion and dust	$R_1 = -CH_3$ $R_2 = -CH_2-CH_2-N(CH_3)_2$, $-C_4H_9$, $-CH_3$ (2:1:1)	Soluble in gastric juice at pH up to 5, swellable and permeable above pH 5
Methacrylic acid – methyl methacrylate copolymer (1 : 1) (Ph. Eur.), Methacrylic acid and methyl methacrylate copolymer (1 : 1) (NF)	Eudragit® L 12,5, Eudragit® L 100	Gastric juice resistant coatings, tropic-proof coatings, lozenges, isolation layers	$R_1 = -CH_3$ $R_2 = -H, -CH_3$ (1:1)	Soluble in intestinal juice; from pH 6 up.
Methacrylic acid – ethyl acrylate copolymer (1 : 1) Type A (Ph. Eur.), Methacrylic acid – ethyl acrylate copolymer (NF)	Eudragit® L 100-55		$R_1 = -CH_3$ $R_2 = -H, -C_2H_5$ (1:1)	Soluble in intestinal juice from pH 5.5 up
Methacrylic acid – ethyl acrylate copolymer (1 : 1) dispersion 30 per cent (Ph. Eur)., Methacrylic acid copolymer dispersion (NF)	Eudragit® L 30 D-55, Kollicoat® MAE 30DP			
Methacrylic acid – ethyl acrylate copolymer (1 : 1) Type B (Ph. Eur.)	Kollicoat® MAE 100P		$R_1 = -H, -CH_3$ $R_2 = -H$ or Na, $-C_2H_5$ (1:1)	Soluble in intestinal juice from pH 5.5 up
Partially-neutralized methacrylic acid and ethyl acrylate copolymer (1 : 1) (NF)				
Methacrylic acid – methyl methacrylate copolymer (1 : 2) (Ph. Eur.), Methacrylic acid and methyl methacrylate copolymer (1 : 2) (NF)	Eudragit® S 12,5, Eudragit® S 100	Gastric juice resistant coatings, pH-dependent drug release, colon-targeting	$R_1 = -CH_3$ $R_2 = -H, -CH_3$ (1:2)	Soluble in intestinal juice from pH 7 up
Ammonio methacrylate copolymer (Type A) (Ph. Eur., NF)	Eudragit® RL 12,5, Eudragit® RL 100, Eudragit® RL PO, Eudragit® RL 30 D	Sustained-release formulations coatings, matrix structures	$R_1 = -H, -CH_3$ $R_2 = -C_2H_5$, $-CH_3$, $-CH_2-CH_2-N^+(CH_3)_3$ (1:2:0.2)	high permeable, pH-independent
Ammonio methacrylate copolymer (Type B) (Ph. Eur, NF)	Eudragit® RS 12,5, Eudragit® RS 100, Eudragit® RS PO, Eudragit® RS 30 D		$R_1 = -H, -CH_3$ $R_2 = -C_2H_5$, $-CH_3$, $-CH_2-CH_2-N^+(CH_3)_3$ (1:2:0.1)	low permeable, pH-independent
Polyacrylate dispersion 30 per cent (Ph. Eur.), Ethyl acrylate and methyl methycrylate copolymer dispersion (NF)	Eudragit® NE 30 D Eudragit® NM 30 D	Sustained-release formulations, coatings, matrix structures, additive to other Eudragit®-dispersions	$R_1 = -H, -CH_3$ $R_2 = -C_2H_5, -CH_3$ (1:2)	swellable, permeable, pH-independent
Variation on solid substance content of the abovementioned type	Eudragit® NE 40 D			
	Eudragit® FS 30 D	Colon-targeting	$R_1 = -H, -CH_3$ $R_2 = -H, -CH_3$ (1:10)	Soluble in intestinal juice from pH 7 up
	Plastoid B	Spray dressings, bioadhesive films	$R_1 = -CH_3$ $R_2 = -CH_3, -C_4H_9$ (1:1)	pH-independent

transition temperature of most PVP types, the T_g of such solid solutions often lies above room temperature. The resulting glass-like state offers an effective protection from recrystallization during storage.

PVP forms water-soluble molecular complexes with a host of active ingredients (e.g., iodine, ajmaline, amphotericin). Despite the good solubility of the complexes, only a small proportion of the active ingredient is in an unbound state, meaning its toxic action is diminished while its pharmaceutical activity remains constant. PVP also improves the complex formation as well as the solubilization efficiency of β-cyclodextrin inclusion compounds of numerous active ingredients. Only for a few phenolic compounds (e.g., tannin), complex formation with PVP negatively affects solubility.

Povidone contains traces of peroxides and peroxide content may further increase during storage. When it is processed with oxidation-susceptible active ingredients, it should be kept in mind that this may affect storage stability (e.g., in case of Raloxifen). In such cases one may revert to peroxide-poor special quality products such as Kollidon 30 LP).

Applications: solubilization of active ingredients, freeze-drying, stabilization of suspensions (up to 5%), thickener, adhesion enhancer for topical formulations, wet and dry binding agent for granulation and tableting, respectively (0.5%–5%), additive for tablet coatings.

Copovidone is a polymer made from N-vinylpyrrolidone and vinyl-acetate in a 6:4 ratio, with a molecular mass varying from 45,000 to 70,000. The water-soluble substance is utilized as a binding agent for granulation (2%–5%) as well as for direct tablet compression and is also used as film former in coatings.

Crosspovidone (Ph. Eur., NF, JP) is a largely physically (i.e., by entanglement) cross-linked PVP. It is completely insoluble in water. Due to its porous structure (popcorn polymer) it possesses a high hydration and swelling capacity. Specifically, it develops a high swelling pressure, which makes it one of the most effective and most frequently used tablet disintegrants.

5.3.6.5 Poly(Vinyl Acetate) (Poly(vinylis acetas))

Poly(vinyl acetate) (Ph. Eur., NF) is a water-insoluble polymer with an average molecular mass of up to 1,500,000.

Application: It serves as a film former for the manufacturing of sustained release coatings. For this purpose, a 30% dispersion (*Poly(vinyl acetate) dispersion 30 percent*) is listed in the Ph. Eur. and the NF, which is commercially available under the name Kollicoat SR 30 D. In contrast to other film formers, poly(vinyl acetate) has a very low minimal film-forming temperature of 15°C to 18°C ($T_g = 28$°C) and can therefore theoretically be processed without addition of plasticizers. Nonetheless, adding a plasticizer will enhance the flexibility of the films.

A combination of 80% poly(vinyl acetate), 19% povidone, 0.8% sodium lauryl sulfate and 0.2% silicon oxide is commercially available under the name Kollidon SR, as an excipient mixture for the manufacturing of sustained release matrix tablets by the direct tablet compression method. By virtue of its good plastic deformability, poly(vinyl acetate) at low compression forces yields a coherent, water-insoluble matrix in which the water-soluble povidone is embedded. When the latter is gradually dissolved by digestive juices, a porous structure is formed through which the likewise embedded active ingredient is slowly released.

5.3.6.6 Poly(Vinyl Alcohol) (PVA, Poly(alcohol vinylicus))

Poly(vinyl alcohol) (Ph. Eur., NF) is produced by hydrolysis of poly(vinyl acetate). In addition to nearly completely hydrolyzed types, partially hydrolyzed types are available for numerous application purposes; these may contain up to 15% (m/m) acetyl groups, corresponding to 18 mol%. The most frequently used types contain an 11% proportion of acetyl groups.

$$\left[\begin{array}{c} -CH_2-CH- \\ | \\ OH \end{array} \right]_n$$

The molecular mass amounts to 20,000–200,000, depending on the degree of polymerization. The hygroscopic powder (water content at 20°C 7%–10%) is moderately soluble in water and insoluble in nearly all organic solvents. Aqueous solutions react neutral to weakly

Table 5-7 Polyvinyl Derivatives

$-CH_2-\underset{\underset{R}{|}}{\overset{\overset{H}{|}}{C}}-$

	Abbreviations, Synonyms and Trade Names	Monograph	R −OH	R (pyrrolidone)	R (acetate)	R (phthalate)
Polyvinylpyrrolidone	PVP, Povidon, Kollidon®, Plasdone®	Ph. Eur., NF, JP		11.5–12.8% N		
Poly(vinyl acetate)	Copovidone, Copolyvidone, vinylacetate-vinylpyrrolidone copolymer, Kollidon® VA64	Ph. Eur., NF		7.0–8.0% N	35.3–42.0% Vinylacetate	
Polyvinyl acetate phthalate	PVAP, Opadry®, Enteric®, Coateric®	NF	Percentage not specified in NF		Percentage not specified in NF	55.0–62.0%

acidic. The viscosity of the solutions depends on the concentration, the molecular mass and the extent of hydrolyzed acetyl groups. Viscosity increases with increasing molecular mass and decreasing acetylation. The effect of the latter is caused by an intermolecular association of nonsubstituted chain segments. Completely hydrolyzed types have a higher viscosity than partially hydrolyzed types of comparable molecular mass. Only products with high molecular masses are suitable for hydrogel formation. At concentrations of 12% to 15%, spreadable and physiologically well-tolerated gels are formed, which are commonly used in cosmetic preparations. Alternating acetylated and non-acetylated chain segments are also responsible for the surface-active properties of partially hydrolyzed PVA types. The acetyl residues facilitate the adsorption of the esterified segments to hydrophobic interfaces (e.g., oil droplets), while the nonacetylated chain segments between these contact sites are shaped into well-hydrated loops protruding into the aqueous solution. Preparations made from poly(vinyl alcohol) are not compatible with acids, salts, tannin, and polyacrylic acids. Gelation occurs in the presence of borax or boric acid.

Applications: thickener, viscosity enhancer (e.g., for eye drops); partially hydrolyzed types: emulsifier. Table 5-7 presents an overview of the pharmaceutically applied polyvinyl derivatives.

5.3.6.7 Macrogols (Polyethylene Glycols, Polyethylene Oxides, Macrogola)

Macrogols (Macrogols, Ph. Eur.; Polyethylene glycol, NF; Macrogol 400, Macrogol 1500, Macrogol 4000, Macrogol 6000, Macrogol 20000, JP) are mixtures of polymers of the general formula $H-(O-CH_2-CH_2)_n-OH$. Types with a polymerization grade >10 have a meander shape while short-chain macrogols have a zig-zag shape, such as is characteristic for fatty acids.

polyethylene oxide chain (section)

They are produced by polymerization of ethylene oxide in the presence of acidic or alkaline catalysts ($SnCl_2$, CaO). Dependent on the selected reaction conditions, products with various polymerization grades are obtained. They are characterized by their average molecular weight, which is added as a number to the designation "Macrogol." Occasionally, in literature instead an indication of the degree of polymerization can be found.

With increasing molecular size the consistency increases. Macrogols up to a molecular mass of 600 are viscous fluids. Products with a molecular weight between 600 and 1,000 are semi-solid substances and those with molecular weights between 1,000 and 20,000 have wax-like character. Depending on their molecular size, solubility in water can vary, determined by the hydration of the ether oxygen and the terminal OH groups. They are easily soluble in acetone, dichloromethane, and ethanol and practically insoluble in ether and in fatty as well as mineral oils. Macrogols form complexes with a large variety of phenolic compounds. In this way, they liquefy, for example, by mixing with phenol, tannin, acetylsalicylic acid, or salicylic acid. Based on this complex formation Macrogol 300 is applied as an antidote in the case of phenol contamination (NRF-Antidote 19.7 according to the German New Prescription Formulatory). Also, the activity of penicillins can be diminished by macrogols.

Applications: solvent (e.g., for soft capsule fillings and injection solutions; concentrations up to 30% are possible for $M_r \geq 300$, without risk of hemolysis), ointment bases, water-soluble bases for suppositories (mostly mixtures of two macrogols of different molecular mass, e.g., M_r 1,000 + M_r 6,000 or M_r 600 + M_r 5,000; macrogols display a strong shrinkage of up to 7% upon cooling), embedding agent, for example, for melt extrusion and melt granulation, binding agent for wet granulation, matrix component for solid solutions and solid dispersions, plasticizer for film coatings (5% to 30% related to the film-forming polymer), lubricant for tableting (e.g., for lozenges and effervescent tablets).

5.3.6.8 Macrogol Poly(Vinyl Alcohol) Grafted Copolymer (Copolymerum macrogolo et alcoholi Poly(Vinylico) Constatum)

Macrogol poly(vinyl alcohol) grafted copolymer (Ph. Eur., NF) is a graft polymer consisting of a macrogol main chain on to which on average two to three poly(vinyl alcohol) side chains are grafted. The ethylene glycol: vinylalcohol ratio in the molecule amounts to 1:3, the molecular weight is around 45,000. The substance is readily soluble in water and has a glass transition temperature of 45°C.

Applications: water-soluble film coating for tablets (the substance can be processed without addition of a plasticizer), matrix substance for solid solutions and dispersions for the enhancement of dissolution rate of poorly soluble dugs (the polymer can also be processed by melt extrusion; the PEG moiety then acts as an internal plasticizer).

5.3.6.9 Polyesters of Lactic Acid and Glycolic Acid

Polylactides, polyglycolides, and their copolymers are thermoplastic biodegradable polymers. They are synthesized either by a direct condensation reaction of the monomers, lactic acid, and glycolic acid or by a ring-opening polymerization of lactide or glycolide, respectively. Their properties are determined by the molecular weight, the degree of crystallization and the monomer ratio. Products with molecular weights of 60,000 up to 150,000 are available.

While polyglycolic acid (PGA) invariably occurs in semi-crystalline form, in the case of polylactic acid (PLA) the stereochemical purity determines the crystallinity. Thus, while poly(D-lactic acid) and poly(L-lactic acid) are semi-crystalline, the racemic poly(D,L-lactic acid) appears as an amorphous substance. By virtue of the methyl groups, poly(lactic acid) is more hydrophobic than poly(glycolic acid). The delayed water uptake that comes with that is responsible for the slower hydrolytic degradation. Notwithstanding their stronger hydrophilicity, particularly the highly crystalline PGA and the PLGA copolymers with high glycolic acid content display poor hydration because water can hardly penetrate into the tightly packed ordered molecular structure. PLGA co-polymers with a glycolic acid content of less than 70% occur, on the other hand, in an amorphous form and are therefore readily hydrolysable.

A novel group of biodegradable polyesters are the PEG copolymers, in which a hydrophilic polyethylene glycol block is coupled to a hydrophobic PLA, PLG, or PLGA block or links two such blocks together. This leads to a strongly enhanced water uptake capacity of the material, which is therefore much more susceptible to biodegradation. By the same token, as a drug carrier it distinguishes itself strongly from the common PLG/PLA types with respect to encapsulation properties for hydrophobic and hydrophilic drugs, respectively.

During the hydrolytic degradation of polyesters of lactic and glycolic acid, oligomeric and monomeric degradation products with acidic character are formed, which may facilitate further acid hydrolysis of the polymer. Under certain conditions, when the degradation products are not diffusing out and no neutralization occurs, this leads to autocatalytic acceleration of the degradation. This process may under certain conditions damage acid-sensitive drugs.

Applications: Absorbable implants and suture material, microparticles, and other implantable drug carriers with prolonged release, stent coatings.

5.3.7 Lipids

5.3.7.1 Petrolatum (Vaseline, Soft Paraffin, Vaselinum)

Petrolatum is a mixture consisting of purified, mostly saturated solid and fluid hydrocarbons. The fluid phase, representing 70-90% of the mixture, consists of n- and iso-paraffins and a small amount of unsaturated hydrocarbons. Together, these amount to 0.3%–5.8% for white petrolatum (White Soft Paraffin Ph. Eur., White Petrolatum, NF, JP) and to 6.5%–12.8% for the less thoroughly purified yellow petrolatum (Yellow Soft Paraffin, Ph. Eur.; Petrolatum, NF, Yellow Petrolatum, JP). The unsaturated fraction consists of olefins (alkenes) with average molecular weights between 400 and 800. The solid phase is composed of a *crystalline component* (n-paraffin, 10%–20%) and a *microcrystalline component* (iso-paraffin and small proportions of alicyclic compounds. Only a well-balanced ratio between microcrystalline and crystalline paraffins on the one hand and fluid paraffins on the other hand ensures that the high-quality demands required of a pharmaceutically applied petrolatum (plasticity, thixotropy) are met. Particularly important in this connection are the microcrystalline paraffins. They form a fine-mesh network that effectively and tightly entraps the fluid components. A higher proportion of n-paraffins, on the other hand, results in a more coarsely structured framework. During storage the network becomes looser, ultimately falling apart and releasing the entrapped fluid components (bleeding, syneresis).

Also the ductility, that is, the desired ropiness of the petrolatum, traces back to the proportions of microcrystalline and iso-paraffin. The stiffness of the products is determined by the presence of the n-paraffins. Petrolatum types with relatively high n-paraffin content display the so-called *ice effect*. That is the formation of a solid surface during the solidification of melted petrolatum, which can only be perforated by applying pressure.

Slack wax is obtained from ointment-like residues of mineral oil refining, which, when required, can be turned into a spreadable consistency by addition of fluid paraffins. Subsequently the substance is refined: double bonds are catalytically hydrogenated and aromatic substances turned into water-soluble sulfonic acids by means of sulfuric acid and removed. Finally, by treatment with bleaching clay or activated coal, a pharmaceutically applicable product is obtained. Depending on the degree of bleaching, yellow and white petrolatum are distinguished (vaselinum flavum and vaselinum album, respectively). Both types are transparent when applied in a thin layer and nearly odorless.

Also, artificial petrolatum can be used for pharmaceutical purposes, when of pharmacopeia-conforming quality. It can be manufactured from components of petrolatum or by combined melting of microcrystalline gel formers and fluid paraffins. By incorporation of microcrystalline waxes or ceresin into a mixture of paraffin and mineral oil raffinate, satisfactory petrolatum products with a good oil-retaining capacity can be obtained. Artificial petrolatum produced by combined melting of solid and fluid paraffins is of lower quality. Due to the fact that paraffin mixtures with a high n-paraffin content are usually used, the artificial products often possess a low ropiness and tend to become grainy. Furthermore, they display a pronounced ice effect and tend to separate the oil phase.

Since it is a mixture of different hydrocarbons, petrolatum does not have a distinct melting point. The Ph. Eur. requires the verification of the drop point, which for white petrolatum must lie between 35°C and 70°C and for yellow petrolatum between 40°C and 60°C (NF, JP: melting range for yellow petrolatum and white petrolatum: 38°C–60°C). It should be indicated on the label of the storage container.

Petrolatum does not have emulsifying properties. The water uptake capacity is therefore very low (water index maximally 10–15). However, by addition of emulsifiers substantial

Table 5-8 Common Names and IUPAC
Names of Saturated Fatty Acids

General molecular formula: $C_nH_{2n+1}COOH$		
n	**Common Name**	**IUPAC Name**
5	Caproic acid	Hexanoic acid
7	Caprylic acid	Octanoic acid
9	Capric acid	Decanoic acid
11	Lauric acid	Dodecanoic acid
13	Myristic acid	Tetradecanoic acid
15	Palmitic acid	Hexadecanoic acid
17	Stearic acid	Octadecanoic acid
19	Arachidic acid	Eicosanoic acid
21	Behenic acid	Docosanoic acid

amounts of water can be incorporated. Petrolatum was prepared for the first time in 1871 by the Chesebrough Manufacturing Company in New York. In 1878, it was introduced in dermatological therapy. Nowadays, it has a prominent place in the range of bases for the manufacturing of ointments. Petrolatum is chemically and physically relatively inert and thus quite compatible with active and auxiliary ingredients, it is inexpensive and, if protected from light, practically indefinitely stable.

Application: ointment base.

5.3.7.2   Liquid Paraffins (Mineral Oils, White Oils)

Liquid paraffins are purified mixtures of fluid, saturated hydrocarbons obtained from mineral oil. They are composed almost exclusively of branched alkanes and cycloalkenes, with boiling points above 300°C. Unsaturated and aromatic hydrocarbons are removed during processing.

Monographs of the Ph. Eur., USP, and JP:

- Liquid paraffin, Ph. Eur., JP (Mineral oil, USP; Paraffinum liquidum, Paraffinum subliquidum)
- Light liquid paraffin, Ph. Eur., JP (Light mineral oil, USP; Paraffinum perliquidum)

Applications: consistency adjustment of ointment bases, skin cleaning, oily nose drops, oil phase in dermatological emulsions.

The NF includes two additional monographs: "Rectal mineral oil" and "Topical light mineral oil."

5.3.7.3   Hard Paraffin (Paraffinum solidum)

Hard paraffin (Ph. Eur; Paraffin, NF, JP) is a mixture of purified, solid and saturated hydrocarbons, predominantly n-paraffins with chain lengths C_{18}–C_{32}. The colorless to white, transparent, fatty to the touch and tasteless mass often displays a crystalline structure.

Application: consistency-increasing additive in ointments bases.

5.3.8   Fats (Triglycerides)

Fats are mixed-chain triglycerides with a consistency that depends on the ratio between saturated and unsaturated fatty acyl groups. Triglycerides predominantly containing unsaturated acyl groups are semi-solid to fluid. Important fatty acid components of natural fats are presented in Tables 5-8 and 5-9.

For the structure of fats, the steric configuration of the triglycerides and of the unsaturated acyl chains (cis- or trans-configuration) is relevant.

In semi-solid fats the major fraction of the solid, long-chain triglycerides prevail in a crystalline state. This crystalline structure pervades the entire substance in the form of a fine-mesh three-dimensional network and accommodates the fluid triglycerides by way of a capillary action. Thus, the semi-solid triglycerides may be envisaged as having a gel character. That is why they are also referred to as lipogels. During storage, the crystallites of the solid, wax-like domains may grow out to larger particles that may confer a granular structure to the product.

Table 5-9 Common Names and IUPAC Names of Unsaturated Fatty Acids

General molecular formula: $C_nH_{2n-x}COOH$			
n	**x**	**Common Name**	**IUPAC Name**
10	1	Undecylenic acid	Δ10-undecenic acid
15	1	Palmitoleic acid	Δ9-hexadecenic acid
17	1	Oleic acid	Δ9-octadecenic acid
17	3	Linoleic acid	Δ9, 12-octadecadienic acid
17	5	Linolenic acid	Δ9, 12, 15-octadecatrienic acid
19	7	Arachidonic acid	Δ5, 8, 11, 14-eicosatetraenic acid

5.3.8.1 Natural Fats

Natural fats belong to the oldest bases of ointments. Nowadays, solid fats of animal origin, such as porcine lard, are hardly applied anymore. A natural solid fat of vegetable origin that is currently still used is cocoa butter.

Fluid fats are referred to as oils and are frequently applied additives in the manufacture of pharmaceutical products. They are skin-friendly and well tolerated. Oils such as peanut oil, olive oil, sunflower oil, and rapeseed oil serve as solution and suspension media as well as to smooth the structure of lipophilic preparations. Fats containing unsaturated fatty acids tend to autoxidize under the influence of light and oxygen, causing the formation of peroxides, aldehydes, ketones, and acids followed by polymerization reactions. This process leads to oxidative drying and resinification. Depending on the extent to which this behavior occurs, drying, semi-drying, and nondrying fatty oils are distinguished. Vegetable oils are less susceptible to autoxidation because they commonly contain small amounts of antioxidants such as tocopherols.

Ph. Eur., USP/NF, and JP monographs are devoted to the following natural fats and oils, including their refined or hydrogenated derivatives. The most important of these, in the context of their application as pharmaceutical additives, are described in more detail in the following sections of this chapter. In addition to that, some other fats and oils with pharmaceutical relevance, which are not subject of a monograph, will be discussed:

- Hydrogenated cotton seed oil (Gossypii oleum hydrogenatum) (Ph. Eur., NF)
- Refined arachis oil (Arachidis oleum raffinatum) (Ph. Eur.; Peanut oil, NF, JP)
- Hydrogenated arachis oil (Arachidis oleum hydrogenatum) (Ph. Eur.)
- Refined coconut oil (Cocois oleum raffinatum) (Ph. Eur.; Coconut Oil, NF, JP)
- Hydrogenated coconut oil (NF)
- Virgin linseed oil (Lini oleum virginale) (Ph. Eur.; Flax seed oil in USP/NF chapter dietary supplements)
- Refined corn oil (Oleum raffinatum) (Ph. Eur.; Corn oil, NF, JP)
- Virgin almond oil (Amygdalae oleum virginale) (Ph. Eur.)
- Refined almond oil (Amygdalae oleum raffinatum) (Ph. Eur.; Almond oil, NF)
- Refined evening primrose oil (Oenotherae oleum raffinatum) (Ph. Eur.; Evening primrose oil in USP/NF chapter dietary supplements)
- Virgin olive oil (Olivae oleum virginale) (Ph. Eur.)
- Refined olive oil (Olivae oleum raffinatum) (Ph. Eur.; Olive oil, NF, JP)
- Palm oil (NF)
- Hydrogenated palm oil (NF)
- Palm kernel oil (NF)
- Refined rapeseed oil (Rapae oleum raffinatum) (Ph. Eur.; Rape seed oil, JP)
- Fully hydrogenated rapeseed oil (NF)
- Hydrogenated castor oil (Ricini oleum hydrogenatum) (Ph. Eur., NF)
- Virgin castor oil (Ricini oleum virginale) (Ph. Eur.)
- Refined castor oil (Ricini oleum raffinatum) (Ph. Eur.; Castor oil, NF, JP)
- Refined safflower oil (Carthami oleum raffinatum) (Ph. Eur.; Safflower oil, NF)
- Refined sesame oil (Sesami oleum raffinatum) (Ph. Eur.; Sesame oil, NF, JP)
- Hydrogenated soya-bean oil (Soiae oleum hydrogenatum) (Ph. Eur.; Hydrogenated soybean oil, NF)
- Refined soya-bean oil (Soiae oleum raffinatum) (Ph. Eur.; Soybean oil, NF, JP)
- Refined sunflower oil (Helianthi annui oleum raffinatum) (Ph. Eur.; Sunflower oil, NF)
- Hydrogenated vegetable oil (NF)
- Virgin wheat-germ oil (Tritici aestivi oleum virginale) (Ph. Eur.)
- Refined wheat-germ oil PhEur (Tritici aestivi oleum raffinatum) (Ph. Eur.)

5.3.8.2 Synthetic Fats

In addition to natural fats, hydrogenated fats (e.g., Hydrogenated vegetable oil, NF; Hydrogenated oil, JP) and synthetic fats are used as bases for ointments.

As precursors for the production of synthetic triglycerides, vegetable oils and fats are used. In order to obtain ointment-like products with spreading quality, two approaches are followed.

Saponification of Natural Triglycerides and Specific Re-Esterification with Glycerol
The saponification of triglycerides is achieved by alkaline or acidic ester hydrolysis. The fatty acids obtained are separated and subjected to fractionation (distillation). In this way, fatty acid fractions with defined chain lengths are obtained, which, after optional hydrogenation, are blended in an appropriate ratio and re-esterified with glycerol. This esterification is performed in presence of metallic catalysts (ZnO and SnO) and an excess of acids under continuous removal of the reaction water by distillation. If desired the reaction conditions can be chosen such that the final product contains a fraction of mono- and di-glycerides, which possess emulsifying properties. As a rule, at higher reaction temperatures partial esters are preferentially formed, while at lower temperatures triglyceride formation is favored.

Transesterification of Natural Triglycerides
For many purposes, transesterifications can be performed in one step, without the need for fractionation of the fatty acids (e.g., a homogeneous triglyceride should be produced from a mixture of high- and a low-melting triglycerides). In this case, a randomized inter- and intramolecular relocation of the fatty acids takes place in the reaction mixture. If one of the reaction products has a higher melting point than the initial triglycerides, the reaction can be directed toward formation of this product by applying low reaction temperatures at which the high-melting product separates by crystallization. In this way, fully saturated triglycerides can be obtained by transesterification from mixtures of partially saturated vegetable oils.

5.3.8.3   Cocoa Butter (Theobroma Oil, Cacao oleum)

Cocoa butter is the fat that is obtained by pressing cocoa beans (the shells and embryonic roots of *Theobroma cacao*) or the cocoa mass obtained after grinding the beans. Commercially, the substance is available in the form of pale yellowish, solid, brittle slabs or pieces, or as grated material. It has a weak, pleasant, cocoa-like flavor and a mild, characteristic taste. Approximately 78% of it consists of glycerol-1-palmitate-2-oleate-3-stearate, glycerol-1,3-distearate-2-oleate, and glycerol-1,3-dipalmitate-2-oleate. The remainder is composed of other triglycerides.

Based on its special triglyceride composition, cocoa butter displays a very distinct polymorphism: α, β', and β modifications are distinguished, which differ in melting temperature range:

α-modification 21°C–22°C
β'-modification 28°C–31°C
β-modification 34.5°C

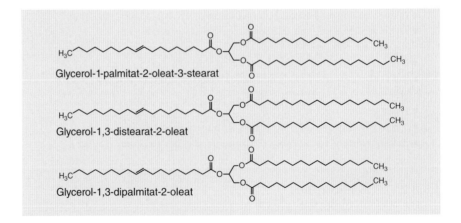

Glycerol-1-palmitat-2-oleat-3-stearat

Glycerol-1,3-distearat-2-oleat

Glycerol-1,3-dipalmitat-2-oleat

Fig. 5-10 Triglycerides of cocoa butter.

The α- and β'-modifications are unstable and are slowly converted to the more stable β-modification. During cooling of a clear melt, initially the unstable α- and β'-modification are formed. The stable β-modification is subsequently formed only slowly. It can take days before the cocoa butter completely solidifies at room temperature.

For a long time, cocoa butter was the only base for suppositories. Like all natural fats, however, it has the disadvantage, to eventually become rancid. Shelf life can be prolonged by using favorable storage conditions (dry, cool, light-protected, absence of air and storage as slabs rather than in grated form). Less oxidation-sensitive bases have nearly completely replaced cocoa butter. The Ph. Eur. no longer features cocoa butter; however, monographs are included in the NF and in some national pharmacopeias like the BP or the German Pharmacopeia.

5.3.8.4   Peanut Oil (Arachis Oil)

Peanut oil (NF, JP; Refined arachis oil, Ph. Eur.) is the refined fatty oil obtained from the peeled seeds of *Arachis hypogeae*; 80% to 87% of the fatty acids of this triglyceride mixture are unsaturated. Among these, linoleic acid predominates (20%–40%). Besides that, small proportions of long-chain saturated fatty acids are present (arachidic acid (C20), behenic acid (C22) and lignoceric acid (C24)), which are responsible for the formation of a gel-like structure when peanut oil is cooled to temperature below 10°C. Peanut oil belongs to the semi-dry oils.

Applications: carrier substance in oily solutions, oily injection solutions, soft capsules.

5.3.8.5   Sesame Oil

Sesame oil (NF, JP; Refined sesame oil, Ph. Eur.) is the fatty oil that is obtained from the seeds of *Sesamum indicum* by cold pressing or extraction. Because of its high content of linoleic and oleic acid, each amounting to 35%–60%, sesame oil belongs to the semi-dry oils. In opened containers, the substance can therefore be stored only for a limited time.

Applications: Oily solvent for drugs, carrier substance in oily injection solutions or suspensions, ground substance for ointments.

5.3.8.6   Soybean Oil

Soybean oil (NF, JP; Refined soy-bean oil, Ph. Eur.) is obtained as a fatty oil by extraction and subsequent refining (deacidification, bleaching, deodorizing) of soybeans (*Glycine soja*, *G. max*). It is a clear, pale-yellow liquid. The fatty acid spectrum of this nondrying oil includes predominantly unsaturated (linoleic, oleic, linolenic) and saturated (stearic) C_{18} acids. When the substance is to be used for the preparation of parenteral formulations, the peroxide value should not exceed 5.0 and water content should be below 0.1%.

Applications: emulsions for parenteral nutrition, lipid component for semi-solid preparations, and oil baths.

5.3.8.7   Hydrogenated Soybean Oil

Hydrogenated soybean oil (Ph. Eur.; Hydrogenated soybean oil, NF) closely resembles refined soybean oil with respect to origin and production, but it is converted into a solid substance by hydrogenation. It is a white powder that melts at about 70°C into an oily substance.

Applications: fatty component of ointments, creams and soft capsules.

5.3.8.8   Olive Oil

Olive oil (NF, JP; Refined olive oil, Ph. Eur.; Virgin olive oil, Ph. Eur.) is obtained from the stone fruits of *Olea europaea* (olives). With 80-85%, oleic acid is the main fatty acid component. By virtue of its minor content of polyunsaturated fatty acids it does not dry or resinify. Olive oil has a yellow to greenish-yellow color and it becomes turbid at temperatures between 5 and 10°C and solidifies at 0°C.

Application: carrier substance for oily solutions and suspensions.

5.3.8.9   Almond Oil

Almond oil (NF; Refined almond oil, Ph. Eur.; Virgin almond oil, Ph. Eur.) is the cold-pressed fat from the seeds of *Prunus dulcis, var. dulcis* or *var. amara*. The predominant component in the fatty acid spectrum is oleic acid with 80%. Because of its low polyunsaturated fatty acid content it belongs to the non-drying fatty oils.

Application: oily carrier for pharmaceuticals for topical, enteral or parenteral administration.

5.3.8.10   Castor Oil

Castor oil (NF; Refined castor oil, Ph. Eur.; Virgin castor oil, Ph. Eur.) is the cold-pressed oil from the seeds of *Ricinus communis*. The fatty acid fraction of this oil contains 85% to 90% ricinoleic acid (12-hydroxy-9,10-cis-octadecenic acid), in addition to oleic and linoleic acid. The toxic compounds of ricinus seeds (the lectin ricin and the pyridine alkaloid ricinin) do not end up in the oil upon cold-pressing. The high proportion of ricinoleic acid determines the viscosity of this oil and is responsible for it having the highest density of all the vegetable oils. In nonpolar solvents such as petroleum ether castor oil is poorly soluble as a result of the polar character of its main constituent. It is, on the other hand, miscible with ethanol, which makes it suitable as a lipid component in alcohol-containing externally applied preparations such as hair spirits. Castor oil hardly undergoes oxidative drying. The ricinoleic acid that is enzymatically released in the intestine during lipolysis inhibits the resorption of water in the intestinal mucosa. Thus, castor oil acts a laxative upon oral administration in doses of 15 mL and higher (adults).

By treatment with adsorbents, refined castor oil acquires a bright color. It is used for eye drops and in parenteral medications.

Applications: oily carrier substance for pharmaceutics, lipid component of alcohol-containing preparations for external use, eye drops, injection solutions and suspensions.

5.3.8.11   Hydrogenated Castor Oil

Hydrogenated castor oil (Ph. Eur., NF) is a triglyceride mixture obtained by hydrogenation of castor oil. The main constituent (85%–90%) is the triglyceride of 12-hydroxy-octadeceneic acid. The substance is available as a white powder or in flakes or pearls. Its melting point lies around 80°C to 88°C. Like castor oil, its hydrogenated derivative is insoluble in petroleum ether, but slightly soluble in ethanol.

Applications: consistency enhancer for ointments, creams and stick-shaped preparations, viscosity enhancer, mold-release agent for tableting, sustained-release agent, and embedding agent for hygroscopic substances.

5.3.8.12   Medium-Chain Triglycerides (Triglycerida mediocatenalia)

Medium-chain triglycerides (Ph. Eur., NF) are a liquid triglyceride mixture containing saturated fatty acids with a chain length C_6–C_{14}, predominantly ($\geq$95%) octanoic and decanoic acid (Miglyol® 810: 65%–80% C_8, 20%–35% C_{10}; Miglyol® 812: 50%–65% C_8, 35%–50% C_{10}). For their preparation, palm kernel or coconut oil are hydrolyzed and from the released fatty acid mixture the medium-chain saturated fatty acids are obtained by means of fractionated distillation, following which they are re-esterified with glycerol. Thus, the substance obtained is a colorless, nearly odor- and tasteless, oily liquid. It is characterized by a good stability and a pronounced capacity to dissolve lipophilic substances. Furthermore, it is miscible with ethanol.

Applications: carrier for pharmaceutical substances in suspensions, emulsions, solutions, drops, soft capsules and parenteral products, anti-sticking agent in tableting and sugarcoating, excipient for dermatological preparations and suppositories. Medium-chain triglycerides are also applied in dietetics, due to their ability to bypass the classical C_2 degradation pathway.

5.3.8.13   Hard Fat (Adeps solidus, Ph. Eur, NF)

The various hard fat qualities consist of mixtures of mono-, di-, and triglycerides of saturated C_8-C_{18} fatty acids in different, type-specific compositions ($\sim$50% lauric acid, C_{12}). They are prepared from vegetable oils of coconut and palm kernels, which contain high proportions of lauric acid. The fatty acids are hydrolytically cleaved off and, after the small amount of unsaturated acids with less than 10 C-atoms is hydrogenated, the mixture is separated into individual fractions by means of distillation. The fractions are purified and then esterified with excess glycerol in such a way that small amounts of emulsifying partial esters (nonionic emulsifiers) are formed.

Hard fat is primarily used as a base for suppositories and has, as such nearly completely replaced the earlier widely used cocoa butter because of its nearly ideal properties for that purpose. The product is a white, brittle, nearly odor- and tasteless mass, which feels fatty to the touch, is insoluble in water and has a melting point of 33°C to 36°C. The melting range is smaller than for cocoa butter. Because the formation of unstable modifications occurs only to a very limited extent, solidification occurs much faster. The viscosity values of melted hard fat are somewhat lower than for cocoa butter. In melted form, it can accommodate about equivalent amounts of warm water, which is bound so as to form a genuine emulsion. This phenomenon is accounted for by the proportion of mono- and diglycerides.

Such emulsifiers, which are included particularly in types of hard fat for pharmacy use, improve the suspension of pharmaceuticals, as well as the wetting and spreading of the melted mass in the rectum. This, in turn, promotes the absorption of active ingredients to nearly the same extent as could be achieved with cocoa butter.

Hard fat has only a minor tendency to become rancid (iodine index maximally 3, as compared to 35–39 for cocoa butter). The contractibility is high, so that pregreasing of the casting molds is not necessary to facilitate removal of the suppositories. Commercial products are, for example, Witepsol®, Massa Estarinum® and Novata®. In addition to standard types there is a large variety of different trade products available for different purposes, e.g., for easy and fast manufacturing of pharmacy-prepared suppositories. Others are tailored for incorporation of drugs that are highly lipid-soluble, which suppress the melting range, or which require bases with special emulsifying, dispersion or viscosity properties.

Application: base for suppository production, consistency modifier for ointments and creams, sustained-release agent.

A semi-solid synthetic triglyceride blend, meeting the Ph. Eur. and NF requirements for hard fat is available under the trade name Softisan 378®. It is composed of saturated fatty acids with chain lengths C_8-C_{18}, in particular caprylic, capric, lauric and stearic acid, and it is therefore not very susceptible to oxidation. Delayed hardening during storage occurs to a lesser degree than with other saturated triglycerides, such as lard or hydrogenated peanut oil.

Application: base for ointments.

5.3.9 Waxes

Chemically, waxes (*cera*) are mixtures of esters of long-chain monovalent, rarely divalent, alcohols or sterols with long-chain, mostly saturated fatty acids. Depending on the melting point, they are either fat-like products, which at room temperature have solid or semi-solid consistency or are oily liquids. They are pharmaceutically predominantly applied as consistency-increasing (for solid substances) or spreadability-enhancing (for fluid substances) additives in ointments and creams. The following waxes are listed in the pharmacopeias:

Cetyl palmitate (Cetylis palmitas, Ph. Eur., NF) (solid)
Cetostearyl isononanoate (Cetostearylis isononanoas, Ph. Eur.) (fluid)
Cocoyl caprylocaprate (Cocoylis caprylocapras, Ph. Eur.) (fluid)
Decyl oleate (Decylis oleas, Ph. Eur.) (fluid)
Ethyl oleate (Ethylis oleas, Ph. Eur., NF) (fluid)
Isopropyl myristate (Isopropylis myristas, Ph. Eur., NF) (fluid)
Isopropyl palmitate (Isopropylis palmitas, Ph. Eur., NF) (fluid)
Carnauba wax (Cera carnauba, Ph. Eur., NF, JP) (solid)
White beeswax (Cera alba, Ph., Eur.; White beeswax, JP; White wax, NF) (solid)
Yellow beeswax (Cera flava, Ph. Eur.; Yellow beeswax, JP; Yellow wax, NF) (solid)
Oleyl oleate (Oleylis oleas, Ph. Eur., NF) (liquid)

5.3.9.1   Cetyl Palmitate (Cetylis palmitas)

Cetyl palmitate (Ph. Eur., NF) is a mixture of esters of saturated fatty acids (C_{14}–C_{18}) and saturated alcohols (C_{14}–C_{18}). The main component is hexadecyl hexadecanoate, however, not all types of cetyl palmitate contain more than 50% of it. The substance occurs as white, odorless and tasteless scraps, flakes, or spherules, which are fatty to the touch. It is practically insoluble in water and cold ethanol. The melting range, determined as drop point, lies between 46°C and 49°C. Cetyl palmitate serves as a replacement of spermaceti—a similarly composed animal wax from sperm whale oil, which is obtained from the cranial cavity and the spine of the sperm whale and in earlier days was applied for pharmaceutical purposes.

Applications: consistency enhancer in creams and other semi-solid pharmaceuticals and for formulations in stick form.

5.3.9.2   Oleyl Oleate

Oleyl oleate (Ph. Eur., NF) contains, in addition to the main component octadecenyl octadecenoate some smaller amounts of esters of other fatty alcohols. It is a clear, yellowish, oily substance with a characteristic smell and taste. It becomes turbid below 10°C and solidifies below 5°C into a semi-solid mass. Oleyl oleate (*Oleylis oleas*) is practically insoluble in water, poorly soluble in 90% ethanol and readily soluble in nonpolar solvents and fatty oils. Because the substance is able to overcome the skin barrier and thus facilitates the penetration of solubilized pharmaceuticals, it is applied as a penetration enhancer.

Applications: Carrier substance for lipid-soluble pharmaceuticals, (skin) penetration enhancer.

5.3.9.3   Beeswax

Yellow beeswax (Cera flava, Ph. Eur.; Yellow beeswax, JP; Yellow wax, NF) is purified bees wax. It is obtained by melting out emptied honeycombs. By bleaching this with purified bleaching clay or hydrogen peroxide white beeswax (Cera alba, Ph. Eur.; White beeswax, JP; White wax, NF) is obtained. Beeswax contains 35% to 75% long-chain esters with 40 to 52 carbon atoms. The main component is the myristyl ester (C_{14}) of palmitic (C_{16}) and cerotic (C26) acid. The substance occurs as pieces, slabs or drops, characteristically smelling of honey and, in the case of yellow wax, a light to dark yellow color due to pollen pigments and resins. Under hand-warm conditions, it is soft and kneadable. Beeswax is insoluble in water, partially soluble in hot ethanol, and completely soluble in fatty oils.

Applications: consistency enhancing additive to ointments, creams and suppository materials, polishing wax for sugar-coated tablets.

5.3.9.4   Wool Fat

Wool fat (Adeps lanae, Ph. Eur.; Anhydrous lanolin, NF; Purified Lanolin, JP) is a complex mixture, mainly consisting of waxes. It contains up to 95% esters, 1-2% hydrocarbons and free acids and about 3% alcohols. The major fraction is composed of cholesterol fatty acid esters (cholesteryl-24-methyl hexacosanoate, cholesteryl-26-methyl octacosanoate, cholesteryl-28-methyl tricosanoate). Table 5-10 presents the most important components.

The basic substance for the production of pharmaceutically applicable wool fat is the so-called suint, a secretion product of the skin for the protection of the wool from external influences. The wash liquor that arises during the cleaning of the wool can be processed by two methods (Table 5-11). Because of the mild processing conditions, the *centrifugation process* (procedure II) yields high-quality products, characterized by a soft consistency and favorable processing times.

The crude wool fat that arises from the *acidic procedure* (procedure I) is a sordid brownish, tough, and bad-smelling mass, which was used in ancient times under the name Oesypus for application on the skin. Nowadays it is considered obsolete and is only an intermediate in the manufacturing of wool alcohols.

Purified wool fat is characterized by a high water uptake capacity. It can, for example, take up 200% to 300% water in the form of a stable W/O emulsion. This can be attributed mainly to the content of sterols, in particular cholesterol. Also, the other components of

Table 5-10   Fractions of Wool Fat

Acid fraction
  – n-Fatty acids with chain lengths C_{10} to C_{26}
  – Hydroxy acids with chain lengths C_{14} and C_{16}
  – Iso-fatty acids with chain lengths C_{10} to C_{28}
  – Anteiso-fatty acids with chain lengths C_9 to C_{29}

Alcohol fraction
1. Aliphatic alcohols
   Monohydric n-alcohols with chain lengths C_{18} to C_{30}
   1,2-Diols with chain lengths C_{16} to C_{24}
   Isoalcohols with chain lengths C_{17} to C_{27}
2. Cyclic alcohols
   Cholestane derivatives
       – Cholesterol ~15–20% (free 2.0–2.5%)
       – Cholestane-3,5,6-triol ~2%
       – Cholestanol (dihydrocholesterol)
       – Cholestane-3,5-diene-7-one ~2%

   7-Oxocholesterol ~2%
   Lanostane derivatives
       – Lanosterol ~10%
       – Dihydrolanosterol ~10%
       – Dihydroagnosterol ~4%

Further components
   Hydrocarbons ~1-2%

wool fat, such as aliphatic alcohols, possess a certain water uptake and emulsifying capacity (Table 5-11).

Wool fat can undergo autooxidative decomposition and for that reason should be stored protected from light in completely filled containers. The decomposition can be slowed down by addition of stabilizers. The Ph. Eur. has set a limit of 200 ppm on the permitted amount of butylhydroxytoluene. Because wool fat as such has a tough and sticky structure, it is therefore not suitable for direct application on the skin, and is used for the manufacture of water-absorbing ointments and hydrophobic creams. When mixed with 15% liquid paraffin and 20% water, a W/O emulsion is obtained that is monographed in the German pharmacopeia (DAB) under the name Lanolin.

Application: additive to ointment bases, fat component of cosmetic powders.

Table 5-11   Production of Wool Fat

Crude wool	
Rinsing with alkaline wash liquor	
Procedure I	**Procedure II**
Acidification with sulfuric acid, pressing out	*Centrifugation*
wool sludge (containing fatty acids and wax esters)	**crude wool fat** (containing water and fatty acids)
extraction with petroleum ether	*neutralization with alkali, extraction with aqueous ethanol*
extract	**neutral wool fat**
treatment with alcoholic KOH and water-containing alcohol	*treatment with bleaching agents*
purified extract	**wool fat**
removal of extraction liquid (distillation)	
crude wool fat (Oesypus)	
treatment with bleaching agents	
wool fat	

Table 5-12   Water Uptake Capacity of Preparations with Different Wool Fat Components (basic substance is fluid paraffin, wool fat components are added in a concentration of 5%)

Component	Water Index	Emulsion Stability after 4 Weeks
Wool alcohols	650	good
Fraction of monovalent acohols	110	poor
n-Octadecanol (C_{18})	40	good
n-Docosanol (C_{22})	60	good
Fraction of divalent alohols	65	good
Cholestane-3,5,6-triol	60	poor

5.3.10   Silicones

Silicones, chemically denoted polysiloxanes, are silicone-containing organic compounds characterized by the presence of a skeletal structure of alternatingly linked silicon and oxygen atoms. The Si atoms carry organic residues, predominantly methyl- but also phenyl groups.

Depending on the extent of cross-linking the following structures are distinguished:

- Silicone oils (linear polysiloxanes, in part also as ring structure)
- Silicone rubbers (medium-cross-linked polysiloxanes, at RT in rubber-elastic state)
- Silicone resins (highly cross-linked polysiloxanes)

The partly inorganic, partly organic nature provides the silicones with favorable properties such as:

- High chemical stability, particularly against oxidative and hydrolytic influences
- Pronounced hydrophobicity
- Heat stability
- Little temperature dependence on viscosity
- Odorlessness and tastelessness

The following types are listed in the pharmacopeias:

- **Cyclomethicone**, NF (Cyclopolydimethylsiloxane, a fully methylated cyclic siloxane with four to six repeating $-O-Si(CH_3)_2-$ units)
- **Dimeticone**, Ph. Eur., NF (Poly(dimethylsiloxane), a fully methylated linear siloxane polymer containing repeating $-O-Si(CH_3)_2-$ units and trimethylsiloxy end-blocking units $-O-Si(CH_3)_3$, degree of polymerization as specified in Ph. Eur.: 20–400)
- **Simeticone**, Ph. Eur., NF (Mixture of Poly(dimethylsiloxane) with 4% to 7% SiO_2)

$$H_3C-\underset{\underset{R}{|}}{\overset{\overset{CH_3}{|}}{Si}}-O-\left[\underset{\underset{R}{|}}{\overset{\overset{CH_3}{|}}{Si}}-O\right]_n\underset{\underset{R}{|}}{\overset{\overset{CH_3}{|}}{Si}}-CH_3$$

$$R=CH_3 \text{ oder } C_6H_5$$

Silicone oils are water-clear liquids, distinguished by their viscosity at 25°C. For example, the designation silicone oil 500 means that the kinematic viscosity of this product amounts to approximately 500 $mm^2 \cdot s^{-1}$ (500 cSt). Viscosity increases with increasing polymerization grade (Table 5-13). The low temperature dependence of the viscosity of silicone oils as compared to mineral oils is illustrated in Fig. 5-11.

The low surface tension of silicone oils (at 20°C approximately 18 to 22 $mN \cdot m^{-1}$) guarantees good ointment spreading. For skin protection ointments, dimethylsiloxanes (Dimeticon 350) are utilized, with amphiphilic creams or hydrophilic creams serving as bases.

To achieve protection from slightly aggressive skin-damaging influences, such as daily domestic work, silicone oil concentrations of 2% to 5% will suffice (caveat: rinsable!). For optimal protection from noxious substances used in working life, higher concentrations of

Table 5-13   Dependence of Viscosity of Polydimethylsiloxanes on Degree of Polymerization (*n*)

n	Viscosity ($mm^2 \cdot s^{-1}$ at 20°C)
50	60
110	140
280	680
400	1440

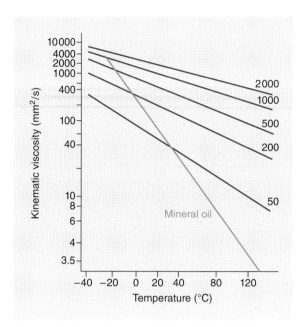

Fig. 5-11 Viscosity temperature-dependence of silicone oils.

about 25% are required. Silicone oils do not negatively affect the physiological skin functions, in particular perspiration, nor do they leave fatty traces on the skin. In addition, they display good heat conductivity and they can also be used safely on extended surface areas of skin (e.g., protection against decubitus).

Ph. Eur. 2.2.14 Melting Temperature—Capillary Method _____

The melting temperature according to the capillary method is to be understood as the temperature at which the last solid particles of a compact substance column in a melting point capillary passes over into the fluid phase.

Procedure:

■ Dry finely pulverized substance for 24 hours *in vacuo* over silicagel.
■ Fill up the melting point capillary up to 4-6 mm.
■ Heat up the heating bath to about 10°C below the expected melting temperature.
■ Set heating rate at about 1°C per minute.
■ Insert the glass capillary when the temperature is approximately 5°C below the expected melting temperature.

Ph. Eur. 2.2.60 Melting Temperature—Instrumental Method _____

The detection of the melting temperature according to the capillary method can be performed in an automatized manner. The sample capillary is placed in a metallic heating block while the tip, filled with sample, is positioned in a light beam. In method A, the transmission of the beam is measured while in method B its reflection is detected. The first deviation of the sensor signal from the starting value marks the onset of the melting process. The temperature at which the sample is completely molten and at which the signal has reached its final value, is defined as the melting temperature.

USP <741> Melting Range or Temperature _____

Two apparatus are described in the USP for determination of the melting range or temperature in analogy to Ph. Eur. 2.2.14 and 2.2.60. Apparatus I consists of a heated fluid bath in which a capillary tube containing the substance is immersed. By contrast, apparatus II transfers the heat via a block of metal into which the capillary tube is inserted.

Typically, the melting process is monoitored by means of a beam of light and a detector. Eight different procedures are described, which are applied in dependence of the nature of the substance.

Ph. Eur. 2.2.15 Melting Point—Open Capillary Method (Slip Melting Point)

This method is especially relevant for solid fats.
Procedure:

- The fat is introduced as an approximately 10-mm high column into a glass capillary (length 80 mm, inner diameter 1.0–1.2 mm) that is open at both ends and then allowed to stand for a defined time at a defined temperature.
- The capillary is then attached to a thermometer such that the sample is positioned at the mercury reservoir. Subsequently it is placed vertically, with the lower end reaching to about 1 cm from the bottom, into a glass beaker, which is filled with water to a height of 5 cm.
- The water temperature is increased at a rate of about 1°C per minute.
- The temperature at which the level of the sample in the capillary starts to rise is recorded (5 parallel measurements).

Ph. Eur. 2.2.16 Melting Point—Instantaneous Method

The instantaneous melting point is determined by repeated dropping of particles of a pulverized substance on the surface of a metal heating block, while the block is being heated (1°C/min). The temperature at which the substance melts for the first time upon contact with the metal is recorded. Subsequently, the heating is stopped and during the following cooling phase the highest temperature is recorded at which instantaneous melting is no longer observed. The instantaneous melting temperature is calculated as the average of the two recorded temperatures.

Ph. Eur. 2.2.17 Drop Point

The drop point serves to characterize fat-like substances with a broad melting interval (e.g., wool fat or macrogol stearate 400). A specially designed metal cup with a 3-mm wide outflow orifice is filled with the (solid) substance to be examined and is subsequently heated. The temperature at which the first drop of the melting substance falls through the orifice is measured. The procedure largely conforms to the standard methods of the German Association for Fat Research, the CEN (Comité Européen de Normalisation) recommendations, and the ASTM (American Society for Testing and Materials) standard methods. Besides the manual method (A), the Ph. Eur. also describes an automatized method (B) in which the falling drop is recorded photo-electrically.

DAB (German Pharmacopeia) 2.2. N3 Determination of the Congealing Point by Means of a Rotating Thermometer

Semi-solid hydrocarbon mixtures, fats and waxes do not display a precise freezing point but rather a wide or narrow temperature interval within which the congealing process evolves. A conventional method to determine a temperature, which characterizes the congealing interval, involves the rotating thermometer. This is a thermometer with a typically shaped bulb (diameter 5.5 mm, length 11.0 mm), which reaches into a stoppered test tube through a stopper hole. The thermometer, test tube and the substance to be examined are warmed up to about 10°C above the expected rigidification temperature. Then the bulb is briefly dipped in the molten substance and immediately placed back in the stoppered test tube (air bath). The thermometer together with the surrounding test tube is rotated steadily around its longitudinal axis (about 1 rotation every 2 seconds). The congealing temperature is the temperature at which the first rigidified droplet begins to follow the rotation of the thermometer.

Ph. Eur. 2.2.18 Freezing Point _____

The freezing point is the maximum temperature occurring during the solidification of a supercooled liquid. It is determined by means of a device which, in order to achieve a steady gradual cooling of the molten substance, ensures a slow heat exchange between the sample and the cooling liquid. For this purpose, the test tube filled with the sample is mounted in a second, 15 mm wider test tube, leaving an air space between the tubes. The external test tube is dipped in to a cooling liquid with a temperature of about 5°C below the expected freezing point. Before starting the measurement, the inner test tube containing the sample is heated to a temperature of about 5°C above the freezing point. After the substance has completely melted, it is placed back in the cooled outer tube. During cooling the molten substance is vigorously stirred by moving up and down a bar formed into a horizontally positioned ring at its end. The highest temperature occurring during solidification is read on a thermometer that is immersed in the test sample.

JP 2.60 Melting Point Determination _____

The JP describes three methods for the determination of the melting point. Method 1 is a capillary method similar to Ph. Eur. 2.2.14 used for substances that can be pulverized. Method 2 is an open capillary method similar to Ph. Eur. 2.2.15, which is applied to water-insoluble substances that cannot be readily pulverized. Method 3 is a drop point method applied to petrolatum.

5.4   Surfactants

Surfactants are surface-active substances. Their molecules contain at least one hydrophilic and one lipophilic group. We distinguish nonionic and ionic surfactants and the latter are, in turn, subdivided in to anionic, cationic, and amphoteric surfactants.

5.4.1   Anionic Surfactants

Anionic surfactants are salts containing an amphiphilic anion and an inorganic or organic cation. In aqueous solutions they are dissociated. The anion accounts for the emulsifying action.

5.4.1.1   Alkali Soaps

Alkali soaps are alkali salts of saturated or unsaturated fatty acids with a chain length of minimally 6-7 carbon atoms. Although in these compounds only a small COO^- group (which, nonetheless, can be strongly hydrated) is opposed by a long lipophilic hydrocarbon chain, the hydrophilic character prevails. The volume ratio of the lipophilic hydrocarbon chain to the carboxyl group is decisive for its emulsifying capacity. Alkali salts (Na^+, K^+, NH_4^+) of short-chain fatty acids (molecularly dispersable) do not display emulsifying potency. Only the longer-chain members of the homologous series (colloidally soluble), particularly C_{12}, display good emulsifying properties. Prominent representatives of the alkali soaps are the salts of palmitic and stearic acid.

Examples:

$C_{15}H_{31}COO^-Na^+$
Sodium palmitate
$C_{17}H_{35}COO^-Na^+$
Sodium stearate (Ph. Eur, NF)

The surface activity can be further enhanced by introduction of additional hydrophilicity-enhancing groups (double bonds, hydroxyl groups, sulfate groups).

Examples:

$CH_3(CH_2)_7CH = CH(CH_2)_7COO^-Na^+$
Sodium oleate

$CH_3(CH_2)_5\underset{\underset{\displaystyle OH}{|}}{CH}CH_2CH = CH(CH_2)_7COO^-Na^+$

Sodium ricinoleate

$CH_3(CH_2)_5\underset{\underset{\displaystyle OSO_3^-H^+}{|}}{CH}CH_2CH = CH(CH_2)_7COO^-Na^+$

Sodium ricinoleate sulfate

Type: O/W-Emulsifier

Application: exclusively for externally applied pharmaceutics (liniments)

Advantage: excellent emulsifiers

Disadvantages: alkaline reaction, electrolyte-sensitive, precipitation of alkaline earth metal soap by hard water.

5.4.1.2   Metal Soaps

Metal soaps are salts of multivalent metals (alkaline earth metals, heavy metals) and fatty acids. Depending on the valence of the cation, either two or three hydrocarbon residues are linked.

Examples:

$(C_{15}H_{31}COO^-)_2\ Ca^{2+}$
Calcium palmitate

$(C_{17}H_{35}COO^-)_2\ Ca^{2+}$
Calcium stearate (Ph. Eur., NF, JP)

$(C_{17}H_{35}COO^-)_3\ Al^{3+}$
Aluminum stearate (Aluminum tristearate) (Ph. Eur.)

$(C_{17}H_{35}COO^-)\ (OH^-)_2\ Al^{3+}$
Aluminum monostearate, NF, JP

Type: W/O emulsifier

Application: Exclusively for externally applied pharmaceutics (liniments)

5.4.1.3   Amine Soaps

Amine soaps are ammonium salts of fatty acids; at the nitrogen atom, up to four of the hydrogens can be substituted by organic residues.

Example:

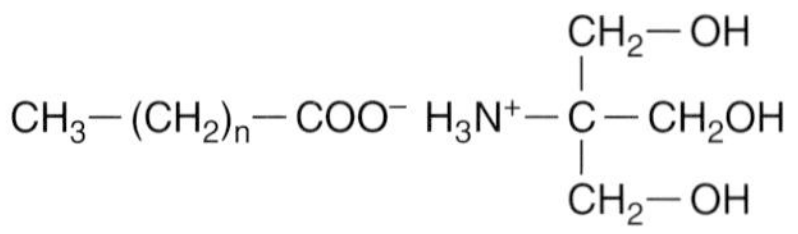

$$CH_3-(CH_2)_n-COO^-\ H_3N^+-\underset{\underset{\displaystyle CH_2-OH}{|}}{\overset{\overset{\displaystyle CH_2-OH}{|}}{C}}-CH_2OH$$

Tromethamine – fatty acid salt

Type: O/W emulsifier

Application: for externally applied pharmaceutics, maximally 2.5 wt.%.

Advantages: stronger emulsifying action compared to alkali soaps, leading to finely dispersed and very stable emulsions. Low electrolyte sensitivity.

5.4.1.4   Sulfate Esters

By conversion of higher alcohols with sulfuric acid, esters are formed, whose sodium salts (alkyl sulfates) represent important pharmaceutically applied emulsifiers. Essentially, these are the corresponding derivatives of lauryl-, cetyl-, and stearyl- alcohols. By this conversion, the hydrophilic character of these compounds is substantially increased and thus their surface activity enhanced.

Examples:

$C_{12}H_{25}$–O–SO_3^- Na^+

Sodium dodecyl sulfate (Sodium laurilsulfate, Ph. Eur.; Sodium lauryl sulfate, NF, JP), e.g., Texapon K12

$C_{16}H_{33}$–O–SO_3^- Na^+

Sodium cetyl sulfate

$C_{18}H_{37}$–O–SO_3^- Na^+

Sodium stearyl sulfate

Sodium cetostearyl sulfate (Ph. Eur., NF) such as Lanette E® (consisting of equal parts of sodiumcetyl sulfate and sodiumstearyl sulfate) Type: O/W emulsifier

Application: particularly for ointments, creams and liniments.

Advantages: Nearly neutral reaction; very insensitive to electrolytes; calcium salts are water-soluble.

5.4.1.5 Sulfonic Acids

Among the sulfonic acids, Dioctyl Sulfosuccinate Sodium Salt (Docusate sodium Ph. Eur., NF) has gained importance as a pharmaceutical excipient. It is the sodium salt of sulfosuccinic acid bis(2-ethylhexyl) ester (Sodium 1,4-bis(2-ethylhexoxy)-1,4-dioxobutane-2-sulfonate). The product occurs as a white, waxy, poorly water-soluble mass. With its HLB (Hydrophilic-Lipophilic-Balance) value of 40, it acts as an O/W emulsifier.

Application: Docusate sodium salt is mainly used for oral pharmaceutics (e.g., as a wetting agent for granulation), and in tablets and capsules as a wetting enhancer for the improvement of dissolution.

5.4.1.6 Bile Acid Salts

The alkali salts of bile acids (oxidation products of cholesterol) are physiologically very important. By virtue of their surface activity, they can emulsify water-insoluble substances like fats and in this way render those better accessible to enzymatic degradation. The bile acids do not occur in vivo in the free form, but rather, are conjugated in a peptide-like way to amino acids (e.g., glycine (glycocholic acid) or taurine (taurocholic acid)).

Example

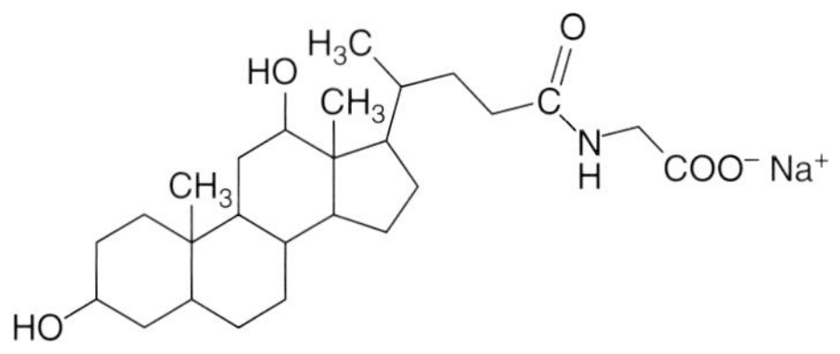

Sodium glycocholate

Type: O/W emulsifier

Application: for the preparation of mixed micelles with lecithin to solubilize poorly water-soluble substances (e.g., Konakion® MM, Cernevit®).

5.4.1.7 Saponins

Also saponins possess high surface activity. Corresponding to the nature of the aglycon moiety, they are categorized into steroid saponins and triterpene saponins. Pharmaceutically they are not favored as emulsifiers (except in liquor carbonis detergens). Not all saponins are anion active.

5.4.2   Cationic Surfactants

Cationic surfactants are salts of an amphiphilic cation and an inorganic or organic anion. In aqueous solutions they are dissociated. Unlike for soaps, it is the cation that is responsible for the emulsifying action. Most commonly, it is a quaternary ammonium compound in which the hydrogen atoms of the ammonium group are substituted by similar or different organic residues (e.g., alkyl groups, such as $-CH_3$, $-C_2H_5$ or a heterocyclic function). The Cl^- or Br^- ion acts as the anion. These compounds are also known as invert soaps (*cation soaps*) or as *quats*. Despite their high interfacial activity, they don't display much cleansing activity. However, at alkaline pH values ($\sim$pH 9), they show strong disinfecting properties, which are pharmaceutically used (preservation).

Example

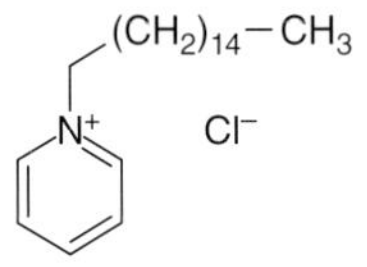

Cetylpyridinium chloride (CPC)

Type: O/W emulsifier

Application: disinfection agent, preservative

Advantage: no precipitation by Ca and Mg ions, implying full retention of activity in hard water.

Disadvantages: Invert soaps cannot be used simultaneously with anionic soaps because the cationic alkyl group interacts with the anionic residue of the soap to form an insoluble compound lacking surface activity.

5.4.3   Amphoteric Surfactants

Amphoteric (ampholytic) surfactants are compounds with both cationic and anionic groups. They are ionized in aqueous solutions and can, depending on the conditions, display either an anionic, neutral, or cationic character.

5.4.3.1   Proteins

Proteins are built up of amino acids and as such may possess COOH- and OH- functions as well as NH_2- or -NH- groups. Proteins or protein-containing material with pharmaceutical relevance are gelatin, casein, skim-milk powder, egg yolk (emulsifying properties additionally caused by lecithin) and malt extracts. In acidic solutions they serve as cationic, in alkaline solutions as anionic emulsifiers.

Type: essentially O/W emulsifiers.

Advantage: applicable in pharmaceuticals for oral administration

Disadvantages: As a result of hydrolytic processes, stability may be jeopardized. Ready flocculation at the isoelectric point. Formation of agglomereates from emulsion droplets. When this phenomenon occurs the emulsion droplets as such remain intact, but their surfactant coatings stick together.

5.4.3.2   Lecithins

Lecithins (Lecithin, NF) are mixtures of different phospholipids of which phosphatidyl-choline (often referred to as lecithin in the stricter sense) is the main component (66%–76%

in egg lecithin; 21%–33% in soy lecithin). Other constituents are phosphatidyl ethanolamine and phosphatidyl inositol.

Lecithins are predominantly obtained from egg yolk and soybeans and purified to higher phosphatidylcholine contents, to an extent that is related to the type of application. Depending on the fatty acid composition and the degree of purification and bleaching, the appearance ranges from a brown to light yellowish semi-fluid viscous mass, to a powder-like product in the case of highly purified material. Lecithins are insoluble in water and fatty oils, but in water, they form O/W emulsions upon a certain swelling period. The minor components in the phospholipid mixture contribute to the stability of the product.

Applications: lecithins are applied in ointments, soft capsule fillings, film coatings for tablets, oral suspensions, and emulsions as well as in suppositories (lowering of the melting temperature range and reduction of brittleness). Because it is a substance naturally occurring in the body (constituent of cell membranes), lecithin is well tolerated upon oral and parenteral use and it is readily metabolized. A major application is therefore its function as a stabilizer of parenteral fat emulsions. For this purpose, highly purified types of phospholipids (70% to 80% phosphatidylcholine, e.g., Lipoid E 80) are essential constituents of liposomes. For this application, oftentimes even pure phosphatidylcholines with well-defined fatty acid compositions are employed.

> Egg lecithin, derived from a natural product, is defined differently in the main pharmacopeias for parenteral use.
>
> USP/NF: Egg phospholipid is a mixture of naturally occurring phospholipids obtained from the yolk of hen's eggs that is suitable for use as an emulsifying agent in injectables.
>
> Ph.Eur: Mixture of natural phospholipids of egg yolk, and fractions thereof, for injection.
>
> JP: Purified Yolk Lecithin is a purified lecithin obtained from hen's egg yolk.

Example

R—COO—CH$_2$
R—COO—CH   O$^-$ CH$_3$
         | | |
        CH$_2$—O—P—CH$_2$—CH$_2$—N$^+$—CH$_3$
                    ‖ |
                    O   CH$_3$

R = saturated or unsaturated hydrocarbon chain

Lecithins

Type: O/W emulsifier

Advantage: emulsifier for preparations intended for internal use (e.g., emulsions for injection and infusion purposes).

5.4.4 Nonionic Surfactants

While in ionic surfactants the charge-carrying functional group represents the hydrophilic moiety of the molecule, in the nonionic emulsifiers these are hydroxyl- and ester groups, or macrogol chains, that is, mostly oxygen-containing molecular domains. Compared to the ionic surfactants, the nonionic surfactants feature some essential advantages. They are therefore of outstanding importance for pharmaceutical application. They react neutral, are hardly affected by electrolytes and largely indifferent toward chemical influences. On the other hand, the polarity of nonionic surfactants containing polyoxyethylene groups as their hydrophilic domains, is strongly temperature-dependent. With temperature rising, hydrophilicity of these surfactants decreases as a result of weakening hydrogen bonds, until ultimately they are no longer soluble as micelles, but separate out from the solution in a surfactant-rich phase. The temperature at which this separation occurs is called cloud point because of the cloud-like turbidity that can then be observed.

5.4.4.1 Higher Straight-Chain Fatty Alcohols

Although the higher fatty alcohols (lauryl-, cetyl-, and stearyl-) possess some surface activity, their surfactant effect is low. In the pharmacopeias the following alcohols of this category are monographed:

- Cetyl alcohol (Alcohol cetylicus) (Ph. Eur., NF; Cetanol, JP)
- Cetostearyl alcohol (Alcohol cetylicus et stearylicus) (Ph. Eur., NF)
  (a mixture of aliphatic alcohols consisting mainly of stearyl and cetyl alcohols)
- Stearyl alcohol (Alcohol stearylicus) (Ph. Eur., NF, JP)
- Oleyl alcohol (Alcohol oleicus) (Ph. Eur., NF)

Examples

$CH_3(CH_2)_{14}CH_2OH$
Cetyl alcohol (Ph. Eur., NF)
$CH_3(CH_2)_{16}CH_2OH$
Stearyl alcohol (Ph. Eur., NF)
  Type: W/O emulsifier
  Application: mostly used as emulsifier or stabilizer

5.4.4.2   Higher Branched-Chain Fatty Alcohols

Pharmaceutically relevant branched fatty alcohols are the fluid Guerbet alcohols

- Octyldodecanol (Ph. Eur., NF) (2-octyldodecane-1-ol, Eutanol G®)
- 2-Hexyldecane-1-ol

Applications: component of W/O creams, lipid-replenishing components in foam bath formulations, permeation enhancer, enhancement of spreading capacity.

5.4.4.3   Sterols

For a long time, cholesterol (Ph. Eur., NF, JP) (5-cholestene-3β-ol), the most widely occurring sterol in animal organisms, has been applied for pharmaceutical purposes. It is an unsaturated, monovalent hydroaromatic alcohol that is a major component of wool fat. Its high interface activity unconditionally requires the hydroxyl- as well as the C-19 methyl group to be in the cis configuration. Together with digitonin a precipitate is formed, which is a characteristic of the 3β-OH group of the emulsifying sterols.

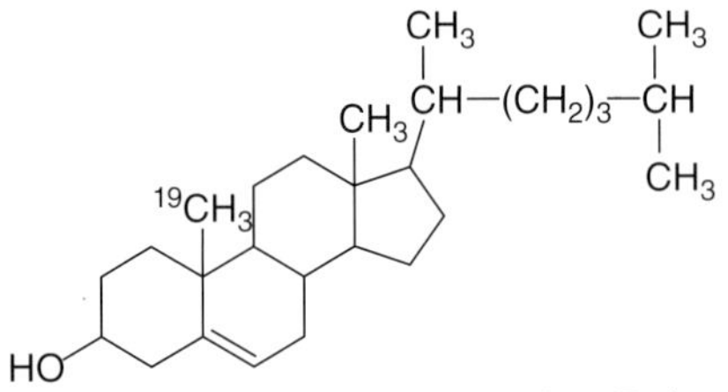

Cholesterol   (Ph. Eur)

  Type: W/O emulsifier
  Advantage: applicable for preparations intended for internal use (e.g., emulsions for injection and infusion purposes).

5.4.4.4   Lanolin Alcohols

Lanolin alcohols (Alcoholes adipis lanae) (Wool alcohols, Ph. Eur.; Lanolin alcohols, NF) are a mixture of sterols and higher aliphatic alcohols from wool fat. The substance consists of 30% cholesterol and furthermore contains cholestane- and lanostane derivatives, C_{18} to C_{20} n-alcohols and C_{16}-C_{26} i-alkane-1,2-diols. It presents itself as a bright to brown-yellow brittle mass, which becomes kneadable upon warming. Qualities of high purity are bright yellow and nearly odorless. Lanolin alcohols are insoluble in water, but readily soluble in lipophilic solvents such as dichloro-methane and ether. They are obtained by alkaline saponification of wool fat followed by extraction of the non-saponifiable residues with an organic solvent. In another procedure, the esters in wool fat are catalytically hydrogenated to alcohols. This procedure yields products with double the amount of aliphatic alcohols and half the amount of sterol alcohols as compared to the saponification method. The crude products are subsequently purified by extraction deodorizing and bleaching steps. Lanolin alcohols act as W/O emulsifiers and enhance the emulsification of lipophilic substances in aqueous environments. According to the Ph. Eur. the water uptake capacity is satisfactory when 20 mL of water can be accommodated in a mixture of 0.6 g lanoline alcohols and 9.4 g white petrolatum, such that the water does not separate out again within 24 hours. Lanoline alcohols are compatible with most pharmaceutical agents with the exception of phenolic substances.

  Applications: W/O emulsifier, particularly for water absorbing ointments and creams.

5.4.4.5 Partial Fatty Acid Esters of Multivalent Alcohols

Esterification of glycols (ethylene glycol, propylene glycol) with one or two fatty acid molecules leads to mono- or diesters of these divalent alcohols, both of them possessing emulsifying capacity. When, instead, one or two hydroxyl functions of trivalent alcohols like glycerol are esterified, stronger surface-active effects are to be expected. If, in the case of monoglycerides, only one OH group is esterified, the surface activity depends not only on the chain length of the fatty acid but also on the degree of unsaturation and, when applicable, on the stereo-isomeric form. Unsaturated monoglycerides are superior to saturated monoglycerides with respect to emulsifying capacity.

Of the following substances, monographs are available in the pharmacopeias:

- Glycerol behenate (Glyceryl behenate, NF)
- Glycerol dibehenate (Glyceroli dibehenas, Ph. Eur.; Glyceryl dibehenate, NF)
- Glycerol distearate (Glyceroli distearas, Ph. Eur.; Glyceryl distearate, NF)
- Glycerol monocaprylate (Glyceroli monocaprylas, Ph. Eur.)
- Glycerol monocaprylocaprate (Glyceroli monocaprylocapras, Ph. Eur.)
- Glycerol monolinoleate (Glyceroli monolinoleas, Ph. Eur.; Glyceryl monolinoleate, NF)
- Glycerol mono oleate (Glyceroli mono-oleas, Ph. Eur.; Glyceryl monooleate, NF)
- Glycerol monostearate (JP; Glyceryl monostearate, NF)
- Glycerol monostearate 40-55 (Glyceroli monostearas 40-55, Ph. Eur.; Mono- and di-glycerides, NF)
- Ethylene glycol monopalmitostearate (Ethylenglycoli monopalmitostearas, Ph. Eur.)
- Ethylene glycol stearates (NF)
- Diethylene glycol palmitostearate (Diethylenglycoli palmitostearas, Ph. Eur.)
- Diethylene glycol stearates (NF)
- Propylene glycol dicaprylocaprate (Propylenglycoli dicaprylocapras, Ph. Eur.; Propylene glycol dicaprylate/dicaprate, NF)
- Propylene glycol dilaurate (NF; Propylenglycoli dilauras, Ph. Eur.)
- Propylene glycol monocaprylate (NF)
- Propylene glycol monolaurate (NF; Propylenglycoli monolauras, Ph. Eur.)
- Propylene glycol monopalmitostearate (NF; Propylenglycoli monopalmitostearas, Ph. Eur.)
- Propylene glycol monostearate (Ph. Eur., NF)
- Superglycerinated fully hydrogenated rapeseed oil (NF)

The numerical specification of glycerol monostearate refers to the content of mono-acyl glycerols of 40% to 55%. The Ph. Eur. distinguishes three types of this substance with different stearic acid contents: Type I: 40% to 60%; Type II: 60% to 80% and Type III: 80% to 99%. The remaining fatty acids are represented mainly by palmitic acid.

Exceptional emulsifying potency is assigned to unsaturated monoglycerides with cis-configuration. Also in case of diglycerides the nature of the esterified fatty acids has a strong influence on the emulsifying capacity, but as a rule this is substantially lower than that of monoglycerides. Commercially available products are most often mixtures of mono- and di-esters. Also pentaerythrityl fatty acid esters, in particular pentaerythrityl-monostearate, have obtained pharmaceutical relevance.

Type: W/O emulsifier.

5.4.4.6 Partial Fatty Acid Esters of Sorbitan

Esters of higher fatty acids and higher multivalent alcohols derived from sorbitol (or from the cyclic ethers with a tetrahydropyrane or tetrahydrofurane structure formed from sorbitol by dehydration) have gained extraordinary prominence. The latter are referred to as sorbitans. From the tetrahydrofurane compound, a bicyclic anhydride can be formed called sorbide.

The corresponding lauryl-, palmityl-, stearyl- and oleyl- esters are commercially available as Span® (Arlacel®, Crill®) (Table 5-14). These surfactants are by no means pure substances, but rather mixtures. The esterification of the sorbitan-sorbide mixture is controlled in such a way that on average each sorbitan residue carries one, one and a half or three fatty acid residues.

Table 5-14 Partial Fatty Acid Esters of Sorbitan

Commercial Name	Chemical Name	HLB Value ± 1
Span® 20	Sorbitan monolaurate (Ph. Eur., NF)	8.6
Span® 40	Sorbitan monopalmitate (Ph. Eur., NF)	6.7
Span® 60	Sorbitan monostearate (Ph. Eur., NF)	4.7
Span® 65	Sorbitan tristearate (DAC/NRF)	2.1
Span® 80	Sorbitan monooleate (Ph. Eur., NF)	4.3
Span® 83 or Arlacel™ C	Sorbitan sesquioleate (Ph. Eur., NF, JP)	3.7
Span® 85	Sorbitan trioleate (Ph. Eur., NF)	1.8

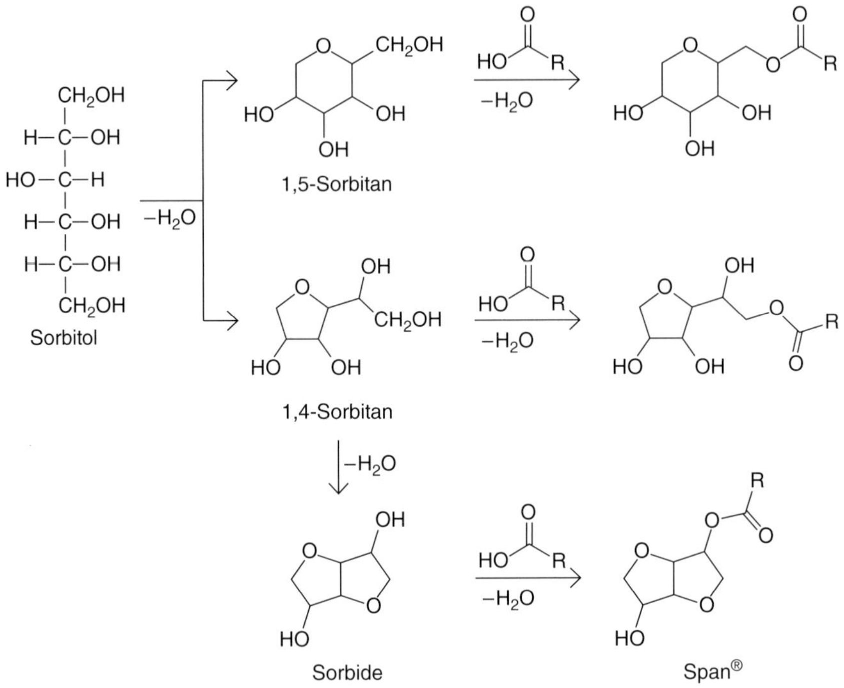

5.4.4.7   Partial Fatty Acid Esters of Polyoxyethylene Sorbitan

The pronounced lipophilic character of the Span® types makes them suitable as W/O emulsifiers. By conversion of the free hydroxyl groups of the sorbitan fatty acid esters with ethylene oxide, macrogol ethers are obtained, which are more hydrophilic emulsifiers, displaying O/W characteristics. The length of the polyoxyethylene chains determines the degree of hydrophilicity. The pharmacopeias designate these polyoxyethylene sorbitan fatty acyl esters as polysorbates; they are commercially available under the name Tween® (Table 5-15). For the most common Tween® types (20, 40, 60, and 80) used in pharmaceutical practice the sum of all ethylene oxide groups (w + x + y + z) amounts on average to 20.

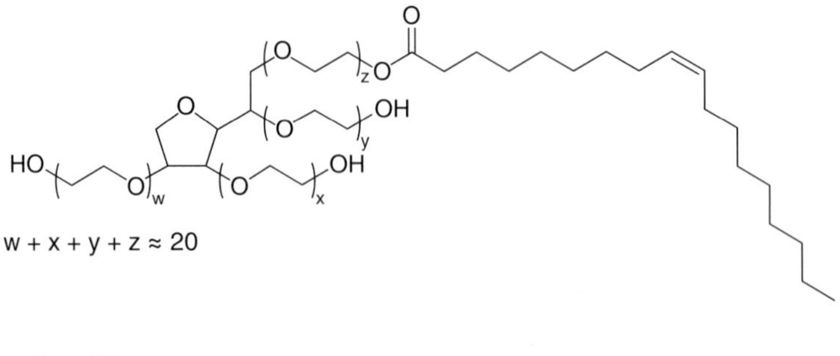

$w + x + y + z \approx 20$

Polysorbate 80
Type: O/W-emulsifier
Disadvantage: bitter taste

Table 5-15 Partial Fatty Acid Esters of Polyoxyethylene Sorbitans

Commercial Name	Chemical Name	HLB-Value ±1
Tween® 20	Polyoxyethylene (20) sorbitan monolaurate* (Ph. Eur.; Polysorbate 20, NF)	16.7
Tween® 21	Polyoxyethylene (4) sorbitan monolaurate	13.3
Tween® 40	Polyoxyethylene (20) sorbitan monopalmitate (Ph. Eur.; Polysorbate 40, NF)	15.6
Tween® 60	Polyoxyethylene (20) sorbitan monostearate (Ph. Eur.; Polysorbate 60, NF)	14.9
Tween® 61	Polyoxyethylene (4) sorbitan monostearate	9.6
Tween® 65	Polyoxyethylene (20) sorbitan tristearate	10.5
Tween® 80	Polyoxyethylene (20) sorbitan monooleate (Ph. Eur., NF; Polysorbate 80, JP)	15.0
Tween® 81	Polyoxyethylene (5) sorbitan monooleate	10.0
Tween® 85	Polyoxyethylene (20) sorbitan trioleate	11.0

*(20) = 20 mol of ethylene oxide per mol sorbitan or sorbitol anhydride.

Applications: Polysorbates are widely used surfactants in pharmaceutical practice, especially in creams, tablets (enhancer of bioavailability of the active agent), suspensions and parenteral preparations. Polysorbate 20 and 80 are often applied as stabilizers in protein solutions (biopharmaceuticals) for the purpose of preventing surface adsorption, di- and oligomerization as well as aggregate and particle formation. Because polysorbates are prone to rapid oxidation, care must be taken to exclude oxygen and light during storage and processing, in order to avoid damage to the proteins by peroxide-contaminated surfactants. For manufacture of biopharmaceuticals, highly purified polysorbate qualities are available.

5.4.4.8   Fatty Acid Esters of Polyoxyethylene Sorbitol

Besides the fatty acid esters of polyoxyethylene sorbitan, the Ph. Eur. also describes a fatty acid ester of a largely non-cyclic polyoxyethylated sorbitol in the monograph **Macrogol-40-sorbitol heptaoleate**. It is a mixture of fatty acid esters of mainly oleic acid, and sorbitol that is ethoxylated with 40 mol ethylene oxide per mol sorbitol. The molar ratio of fatty acids and sorbitol amounts to 7:1. The mixture contains in addition also macrogol fatty acid esters. It is dispersible in water and soluble in oil. The HLB value amounts to 9.5. Fatty acid esters of macrogol-sorbitol are well tolerated by the skin and are mainly employed in cosmetics.

5.4.4.9   Polyoxyethylene Glycerol Fatty Acid Esters

Polyoxyethylene glycerol fatty acid esters are mixtures of mono-, di-, and tri-esters of glycerol and di- and mono-esters of macrogols with molecular masses between 200 and 4000. They are produced either by partial alcoholysis of saturated oils (containing the triglycerides with the fatty acids that determine their name) with macrogol, or by mixing of glycerol esters with PEG esters. That is why it is mandatory that the origin of the surfactant is known, as completely different substances can result, despite identical monographs.

The following monographs for compounds of this group are listed in the pharmacopeias:

- Macrogol 6 glycerol caprylocaprate (Macrogol 6 glyceroli caprylocapras) (Ph. Eur.)
- Macrogolglycerol caprylocaprate (Macrogolglyceridorum caprylocaprates) (Ph. Eur.), Caprylocapryl polyoxylglycerides (NF)
- Macrogolglycerol cocoate (Macrogolglyceroli cocoates) (Ph. Eur.)
- Macrogolglycerol hydroxystearate (Macrogolglyceroli hydroxystearas), (Ph. Eur.), Polyoxyl 40 hydrogenated castor oil (NF) Kolliphor® RH 40, previous brand name: Cremophor® RH 40
- Macrogolglycerol laurate (Macrogolglyceridorum laurates) (Ph. Eur.), Lauroyl polyoxylglycerides (NF)
- Macrogolglycerol linoleate (Macrogolglyceridorum linoleates) (Ph. Eur.), Linoleoyl polyoxylglycerides (NF)
- Macrogol 20 glycerol monostearate (Macrogol 20 glyceroli monostearas) (Ph. Eur.)

- Macrogolglycerol oleate (Macrogolglyceridorum oleates) (Ph. Eur.), Oleyl polyoxyl-glycerides (NF)
- Macrogolglycerol ricinoleate (Macrogolglyceroli ricinoleas) (Ph. Eur.), Polyoxyl 35 castor oil (NF), Kolliphor® EL, previous brand name: Cremophor® EL
- Macrogolglycerol stearate (Macrogolglyceridorum stearates) (Ph. Eur.), Stearoyl poly-oxylglycerides (NF)

In addition, the following two substances can be found in the German Pharmaceutical Codex (DAC/NRF):
- Macrogol 20 glycerol monolaurate
- Macrogol 20 glycerol monooleate

Macrogolglycerol ricinoleate (Kolliphor EL) is also used as a solubility enhancer for injection and infusion preparations. The substance can cause leaching of the softener DEHP (di(2-ethylhexyl) phthalate)) from PVC-containing infusion bags or administration sets. Therefore, preparations containing this emulsifier should be packed in PVC-free material and equipped with PVC-free infusion sets only.

5.4.4.10   Fatty Acid Esters of Macrogols

Also esterification products of fatty acids and polyoxyethylenes of different chain lengths are used as emulsifiers. The pharmacopeias list the following compounds:
- Macrogol oleate (Macrogoli oleas) (Ph. Eur.), Polyoxyl oleate (NF)
- Macrogol stearate (Macrogoli stearas) (Ph. Eur.), Polyoxyl stearate (NF), Polyoxyl 40 stearate (JP)
- Macrogol-15-hydroxystearate (Macrogoli 15 hydroxystearas) (Ph. Eur.), Polyoxyl hydroxystearate (NF)
- Macrogol-30-dipolyhydroxystearate (Macrogoli 30 dipolyhydroxystearas) (Ph. Eur.)

The number in the name of these substances indicates the number of ethylene oxide units per molecule (nominal value). Commercial products are sold under the brand names Myrj™, Cremophor® S9 (Table 5-16) and Kolliphor® HS15.

Example

$CH_3-(CH_2)_{16}-CO-(O-CH_2-CH_2)_9-OH$
Polyoxyethylene (9) stearate (Macrogol stearate 400)
   Type: O/W emulsifier

5.4.4.11   Fatty Alcohol Ethers of Macrogols

Compounds formed by reaction of macrogols with monovalent higher alcohols have an ether structure (Table 5-17). The pharmacopeias list the following of such compounds:
- Macrogol cetylstearyl ether (Macrogoli aether cetostearylicus) (Ph. Eur.), Polyoxyl 20 cetostearyl ether (NF) (2-33 mol EO)
- Macrogol lauryl ether (Macrogoli aether laurilicus) (Ph. Eur.), Polyoxyl lauryl ether (NF) (3-23 mol EO), Polyoxyethylene lauryl alcohol ether (JP)

Table 5-16 Fatty Acid Esters of Polyoxyethylene

Commercial Name	Chemical Designation (Ph. Eur.: Macrogol stearate, NF, JP: Polyoxyl stearate)	HLB Value ±1
Myrj™ S8, Cremophor® S9	Polyoxyethylene (8) stearate	11.8
	Polyoxyethylene (9) stearate	11.6
Myrj™ S20	Polyoxyethylene (20) stearate	15.0
Myrj™ S40	Polyoxyethylene (40) stearate	16.9
Myrj™ S50	Polyoxyethylene (50) stearate	17.9
Myrj™ S100	Polyoxyethylene (100) stearate	18.8

Table 5-17 Fatty Alcohol Ethers of Polyoxyethylene

Commercial Name	Chemical Designation	n	HLB-Value ± 1
Brij® L4	Polyoxyethylene lauryl ether	4	9.7
Brij® L23	Polyoxyethylene lauryl ether	23	16.9
Brij® C2	Polyoxyethylene cetyl ether	2	5.3
Brij® C10	Polyoxyethylene cetyl ether	10	12.9
Brij® C20	Polyoxyethylene cetyl ether	20	15.7
Brij® S2	Polyoxyethylene stearyl ether	2	4.9
Brij® S10	Polyoxyethylene stearyl ether	10	12.4
Brij® S20	Polyoxyethylene stearyl ether	20	15.3
Brij® O2	Polyoxyethylene oleyl ether	2	4.9
Brij® O10	Polyoxyethylene oleyl ether	10	12.4
Brij® O20	Polyoxyethylene oleyl ether	20	15.3
Cremophor® A6	Polyoxyethylene cetostearyl ether	6	10–12
Cremophor® A25	Polyoxyethylene cetostearyl ether	20	15–17

n = number of ethylene oxide units.
Type: Depending on HLB value, O/W or W/O emulsifier.

- Lauromacrogol 400 (Lauromacrogolum 400) (Ph. Eur.) (9 mol EO)
- Macrogol oleyl ether (Macrogoli aether oleicus) (Ph. Eur.), Polyoxyl 10 oleyl ether (NF) (2-20 mol EO)
- Macrogol stearyl ether (Macrogoli aether stearylicus) (Ph. Eur.), Polyoxyl stearyl ether (NF) (2-20 mol EO)

The Ph. Eur. requires that the number of ethyleneoxide units is indicated on the container of the substance. Commercial products are Brij® and Cremophor® A.

5.4.4.12 Polyoxypropylene-polyoxyethylene Block Copolymers (Poloxamers, Ph. Eur.; Poloxamer, NF; Poloxamera)

Block polymers are macromolecules in which blocks (i.e., fragments containing several monomer units) are chemically linked to one another in a linear manner, either directly or via low-molecular weight coupling groups.

Poloxamers are block polymers that are formed by copolymerization of propylene oxide and ethylene oxide and consist of one central lipophilic polyoxypropylene chain that is linked at both ends to hydrophilic polyoxyethylene residues.

$$HO-[CH_2-CH_2-O]_a-[CH-CH_2-O]_b-[CH_2-CH_2-O]_c-H$$
$$\qquad\qquad\qquad\qquad CH_3$$

Polyoxypropylene-polyoxyethylene block copolymer
(a, c = 2 to 130; b = 15 to 67)

A large number of differerent poloxamers are commercially available under the brand names Pluronic®, Superonic®, and Lutrol®. They come as fluid (Pluronic® L), paste-like (Pluronic® P), or powder-like/flaky (Pluronic® F) substances.

Type: O/W emulsifier

Applications: viscosity enhancer for the production of transparent surfactant gels. Poloxamer 188 (Pluronic® F68), like macrogol glycerol ricinoleate, polysorbate 80 and lecithin, belong to the few emulsifiers which can also be used for parenteral application.

5.4.4.13 Fatty Acid Esters of Sucrose

Especially in the United States, sucrose-based surfactants have gained strong interest because they represent the most economically mass-produced nonionogenic surfactants. The synthesis of sugar surfactants is based on the trans-esterification of a sugar with the methyl esters of

Table 5-18 Fatty Acid Esters of Sucrose

Sucrose Fatty Acid Ester	HLB-Value
Sucrose distearate	7.0
Sucrose dioleate	7.2
Sucrose dipalmitate	7.4
Sucrose monostearate	11.2
Sucrose monopalmitate	11.7
Sucrose monooleate	11.2
Sucrose monomyristate	12.3
Sucrose monolaurate	13.0

fatty acids in the presence of potassium carbonate as a catalyst. Dependent on the reaction conditions, a mixture of mono- and di-ester is formed, which by an excess of sucrose can be converted to a large extent to the mono-ester. Predominantly the primary hydroxyl group of the glucose ring is esterified. Further esterification of sucrose occurs on the fructose ring and leads to the formation of di- and higher esters (Table 5-18). In the Ph. Eur. monographs, it can be found under sucrose monopalmitate (sacchari monopalmitas) and sucrose stearate (sacchari stearas), the NF lists sucrose palmitate and sucrose stearate and the JP contains a monograph with the title "sucrose ester of fatty acids."

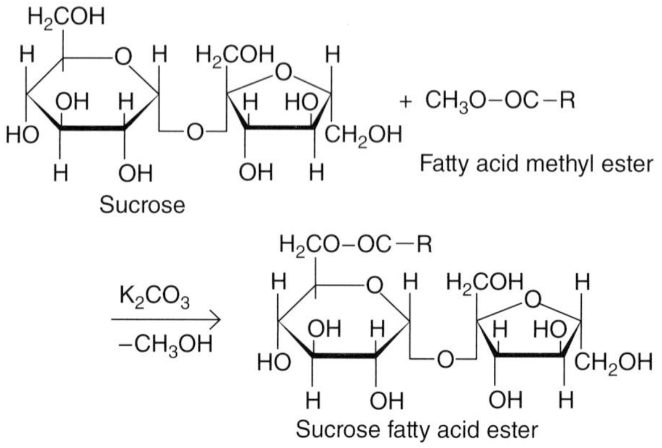

Sucrose

Fatty acid methyl ester

Sucrose fatty acid ester

Type: O/W-emulsifier

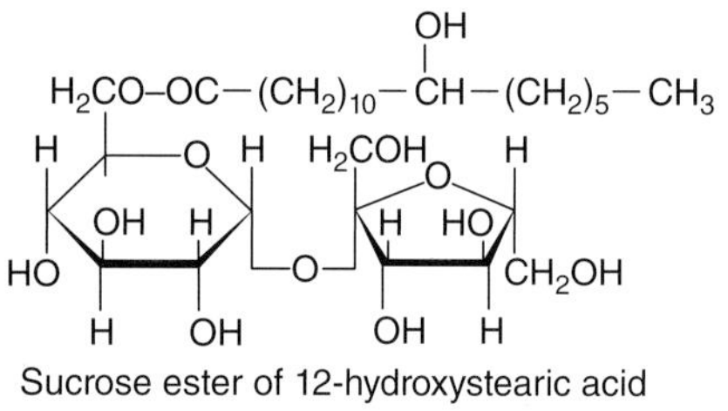

Sucrose ester of 12-hydroxystearic acid

Long-chain sugar esters are white to yellowish powders, which are insoluble in water (except the monolaurate, which is up to 30% soluble) but can be readily dispersed in water. They are partially soluble in ethanol. The introduction of hydrophilic groups like $-OH$ or $-NH_2$ in the hydrophobic moiety effectuates a substantially better water solubility. For example, the 12-hydroxystearyl ester of sucrose is readily soluble in water at 57°C to 60°C, while the corresponding stearate ester is virtually insoluble under those conditions.

5.4.4.14   Fatty Acid Esters of Polyglycerol

Polyglycerols are obtained by polycondensation of glycerol in alkaline medium. The dehydration reaction yields polymers of up to 30 glycerol units. By esterification of the OH groups with fatty acids, fluid to waxy, saturated or unsaturated, hydrophilic or hydrophobic polyglycerol esters are formed, depending on the number of esterified OH groups and the nature of the fatty acid residues. Concomitantly, their solubility varies gradually from fully oil-soluble to fully water-soluble. Polyglycerol esters are considered physiologically safe; they are metabolized completely to glycerol and fatty acids.

Pharmaceutically applied examples of this emulsifier type are **polyglyceryl dioleate (NF)**, polyglyceryl 3 diisostearate (NF), and **polyglycerol poly-12-hydroxystearate**. As W/O emulsifiers, these substances are, for instance, constituents of soft-capsule fillings, suppositories and various skin-care products. The Ph. Eur. describes **triglycerol di-isostearate** as a water-insoluble viscous fluid that, with a HLB value of 4.5, acts as a W/O emulsifier.

Application: emulsifiers for oral dosage forms and nutrition technology, skin-care bath additives and shampoos; thickener.

5.4.4.15   D-α-Tocopherol polyethylene glycol 1000 succinate

D-α-Tocopherol polyethylene glycol 1000 succinate is obtained by esterification of the free acid group of D-α-tocopheryl hydrogen succinate with macrogol 1000. It is a faintly yellowish waxy solid with a melting range of 37°C to 41°C and is soluble in water. It is rapidly absorbed in the gastrointestinal tract and is used as an absorption enhancer of poorly soluble pharmaceutics.

D-α-Tocopherol polyethylene glycol 1000 succinate
Type: O/W emulsifier (HLB-value: 13.2).

Application: emulsifier, solubilization enhancer for poorly soluble substances, absorption enhancer, vehicle for lipid-based drug delivery systems.

5.4.5   Complex Emulsifiers/Mixed Emulsifiers

5.4.5.1   Emulsifying Cetostearyl Alcohol (Type A) (Alcohol cetylicus stearylicus emulsificans A) (Ph. Eur.)

Emulsifying cetostearyl alcohol is a mixture of minimally 80% *Cetostearylalcohol* and minimally 7% sodium cetostearyl sulfate. It is a complex emulsifier as the fatty alcohols represent the factor that is responsible for its consistency, while the sodium salt of the sulfated esters acts as the actual emulsifying component. The substance comes as white granules, flakes, slabs or as a wax-like mass. In pure water it is practically insoluble, but in hot water, it forms an opalescent solution.

Type: O/W emulsifier.

Application: production of O/W creams.

5.4.5.2   Emulsifying Cetostearyl Alcohol (Type B) (Alcohol cetylicus stearylicus emulsificans B)

Emulsifying cetostearyl alcohol is a mixture of minimally 80% cetostearyl alcohol and, in contrast to Type A, minimally 7% sodium dodecyl sulfate. Optical appearance and properties correspond to those of Type A.

Type: O/W emulsifier.

Application: production of O/W creams.

5.4.5.3   Nonionic Emulsifying Alcohols

Nonionic emulsifying alcohols (*Alcoholes emulsificantes nonionici*) (monograph in the German Pharmaceutical Codex (DAC/NRF), commercial product: Rofetan® NS) are a mixture of cetostearyl alcohol, polyethylene glycol (80) cetyl/stearyl ether and glycerol monostearate 40-55 Type I. They are a white, waxy substance or can be obtained in the form of flakes.

Type: O/W emulsifier.

Application: production of O/W creams, e.g., nonionic hydrophilic cream SR DAC, nonionic aqueous liniment DAC.

5.5   Chemically Heterogeneous Groups of Substances with Special Functions

5.5.1   Dyes and Pigments

Coloring pharmaceuticals do not just serve aesthetic purposes. In addition, they help prevent mix-ups on the side of the manufacturer as well as on that of the consumer and, last but not least, the psychological effect has to be taken into consideration. For example, certain formulations of antidepressive drugs are colored yellow because of the stress-relieving effect of this color.

The application of colorants in pharmaceutics is regulated by law. In the European Union, the directive 2009/35/EC (coloring matters which may be added to medicinal products) regulates that only the substances specified in annex 1 of directive 94/36/EC (colors for use in foodstuffs) are accepted for the purpose of coloring pharmaceutics. Color additives approved in the USA for the use in drugs and medical devices are listed in parts 73 and 74 (subparts B and D) of Title 21 of the Code of Federal Regulations. Table 5-18 presents the permitted dyes.

In the European Union substances that may be used as food additives are coded as E numbers. The numbering scheme is identical to the International Numbering System for Food Additives (INS) as determined by the Codex Alimentarius committee, which was established by the Food and Agrigultural Organization of the United Nations (FAO) and the World Health Organization (WHO). Though it is widely used in many countries (outside the EU, without the "E"), this numbering scheme is still uncommon in the United States. When the first digit of the E-number of a substance is 1, the substance is a colorant. The second digit provides information on its color. Yellow substances are denoted 0, orange ones 1, red ones 2, and so on. The digit 7 represents inorganic pigments. The colorants can be of natural or synthetic origin. Naturally occurring colorants may also be obtained by chemical synthesis.

According to US regulations, all listed food and drug colorants fall into two categories: those that are subject to an FDA certification process and those that are exempt from it. Natural colorants, derived from plant or mineral sources, belong to the second category and do not need any certification. By contrast, a batch certification is required for synthetic organic dyes, lakes, or pigments (derived primarily from petroleum). Each batch of those colorants intended to be used in a food, drug, or cosmetic product has to pass analytical tests for its composition and purity in an FDA approved laboratory.

5.5.1.1   Azo Dyes

Azo dyes form the largest group of accepted dyes. Those that are approved for application in pharmaceutics are hydrophilic and strongly acidic compounds. In this way, they are distinguished from the oncogenic lipophilic, alkaline azo dyes. Because of the presence of aromatic sulfonic acid groups, the approved dyes are readily soluble in water and thus hardly absorbed in the gastrointestinal tract. Besides, modern azo dyes do not give rise to the formation of oncogenic aromatic amines. However, azo dyes, in particular Tartrazine, are suspect for causing pseudo allergies, childhood neurodermatitis, and hyperkinetic syndrome. Therefore, special declaration requirements are prescribed for its application in pharmaceutical products (EU: CPMP/463/00 "Excipients in the label and package leaflet of medicinal products for human use," USA: 21CFR201.20 "Declaration of presence of FD&C Yellow No. 5 and/or FD&C Yellow No. 6 in certain drugs for human use").

5.5.1.2   Triarylmethane Dyes

As for azo dyes, the pharmaceutically applied triarylmethane dyes contain aromatic sulfonic acid groups and thus are readily soluble in water and hardly absorbed in the gastrointestinal tract. Erythrosine is an iodine-containing example of this group of dyes. The release of the iodine from erythrosine and its potential effect on thyroid function has not yet been clarified definitively.

5.5.1.3   Natural Dyes

Natural dyes occur in numerous fruits, vegetables, and other plant parts that form part of human diets. Anthocyans can be isolated from a variety of red and blue fruits; carotenoids occur in many red and yellow fruits and vegetables. Chlorophyll is abundantly available in all green parts of plants. Carmine is a substance occurring in the lac insect that serves as a defense against ants. The dye is obtained from dried fertilized females. Nonetheless, because of its high price, it is largely replaced nowadays by the synthetic azo dye cochenille red A.

Chlorophyll has only weak coloring capacity and is light-sensitive. By replacing the central magnesium ion with a copper ion, the compound acquires higher color intensity and becomes less light-sensitive.

Caramel color is produced by heating sucrose, invert sugar, or glucose at 120°C to 160°C in the presence of reaction accelerators. Depending on the nature of the used accelerator (sodium hydroxide, sulfite, ammonia) four different products are obtained:

- Plain caramel = Caustic caramel (E 150 a)
- Caustic sulfite caramel (E 150 b)
- Ammonia caramel (E 150 c)
- Sulfite ammonia caramel (E 150 d)

In ammonia caramel, two toxic compounds (2-methylimidazole and 4-methylimidazole) have been identified. Their contents are under the control of relevant limit values. Plain caramel is obtained when sugar is heated without accelerator. The products obtained in this way are mixtures of various substances, which, among others, contain alcohols, aldehydes, and ketones and melanoidine-type compounds.

5.5.1.4   Pigments

Coloring pigments are dyes that are not soluble in any solvent. Whether a substance is designated a dye or a pigment depends on its solubility in the surrounding medium:

- In view of their insolubility in any applicable medium, inorganic coloring substances are called pigments.
- Water-soluble organic dye salts are converted in lake pigments by precipitation (see below).

Titanium dioxide is the most widely applied coloring pigment. It is toxicologically considered completely safe. Aluminum powder, silver foil and gold foil are rather of inferior importance for the application as coloring pigments.

Like titanium oxide, iron oxides, and hydroxides are largely considered toxicologically safe, Three iron-based pigments are distinguished:

- Yellow iron oxide: $FeO(OH)Fe_2O_3 \cdot H_2O$
- Red iron oxide: Fe_2O_3
- Black iron oxide: $FeO_xFe_2O_3$

Lake pigments are produced by adsorption of water-soluble dye salts on freshly precipitated aluminum hydroxide. The complexes obtained are therefore insoluble in water. For the preparation of freshly precipitated aluminum hydroxide, sodium carbonate is dissolved in water, aluminum chloride is added and precipitation is induced by lowering pH to 5.5. The water-soluble dye with free acid function is added and once again mixed with another portion of aluminum chloride. Directive 94/36/EC explicitly allows the application of the aluminum lake pigments mentioned in Table 5-19. In the USA lake pigments, with the exception of carmine (a lake made from cochineal extract), are only "provisionally listed" (21CFR82), which means they can be used on an interim basis. Initiatives are underway to establish their safety by scientific data as a prerequisite for permanent listing.

5.5.2   Preservatives

5.5.2.1   Phenols

Phenol and its derivatives (Table 5-20) belong to the oldest antimicrobial (bactericidal, fungicidal) products. Their antimicrobial effect is connected with the free phenolic group. Alkylation and chlorination, yielding cresols and chlorocresols, result in a substantially enhanced activity. All representatives of this class of compounds, except p-hydroxybenzoic acid esters, are characterized by an intense odor and taste, which puts severe limits to their applicability. They provoke a mild burning sensation on mucosal tissues.

Phenolic compounds are predominantly applied as disinfectant agents and to a small extent as additives to vaccines and sera. They are also used for the preservation of insulin preparations. The antimicrobial activity strongly depends on pH. The highest activity is associated with the nondissociated form (acid pH range); the phenolate ion is relatively inactive.

The antimicrobial action relates to a nonspecific toxicity. Phenols are typical cytotoxins, which at high concentrations cause coagulation of cellular proteins. Chlorinated derivatives

Table 5-19 Dyes and Pigments

Color	E no.	Name	Production	Origin and Chemical Classification
yellow	E 100	Curcumin	from the root of *Curcuma longa* or synthetic or by fermentation	natural yellow dye
	E 101	Riboflavin	from whey or synthetic or by fermentation	natural flavin
	E 102	Tartrazine	synthetic	artificial azo dye
	E 104	Quinoline yellow	synthetic	artificial chinophthalon dye
orange	E 110	Sunset yellow FCF, Orange yellow S	synthetic	artificial azo dye
red	E 120	Carmine, Carminic acid, Cochineal	from *Dactylopius coccus* [syn. *Coccus cacti*] or synthetic	animal anthrachinon
	E 122	Azorubine, Carmoisine	synthetic	artificial azo dye
	E 123	Amaranth	synthetic	artificial azo dye
	E 124	Ponceau 4R, Cochineal red A	synthetic	artificial azo dye
	E 127	Erythrosine	synthetic	artificial triphenylmethane dye
	E 128	Red 2G	synthetic	artificial azo dye
	E 129	Allura red AC	synthetic	artificial azo dye
blue	E 131	Patent blue V	synthetic	artificial triphenylmethane dye
	E 132	Indigo carmine, Indigotine	synthetic	artificial indigo dye
	E 133	Brilliant blue FCF	synthetic	artificial triphenylmethane dye
green	E 140	Chlorophylls and Chlorophyllins	extraction from green plant parts	natural porphyrin dye
	E 141	Copper complexes of chlorophylls and chlorophyllins	substitution of Mg^{2+} in chlorophyll or chlorophyllin by Cu^{2+}	artificial porphyrin dye
	E 142	Green S	synthetic	artificial triarylmethane dye
brown	E 150	Caramels	from sugars, particularly glucose syrups by heating with or without a catalyst, e.g., ammonium hydroxide, sulfite or ammonium metabisulfite	natural dye
	E 150a	Plain caramel		
	E 150b	Caustic sulfite caramel		
	E 150c	Ammonia caramel		
	E 150d	Sulfite ammonia caramel		
black	E 151	Brilliant black BN, Black PN	synthetic	artificial azo dye
	E 153	Vegetable carbon (Carbo medicinalis vegetabilis)	Vegetable carbon with properties of medicinal charcoal	black pigment
	E 154	Brown FK	synthetic	azo dye
	E 155	Brown HT	synthetic	azo dye
Various colors	E 160	Carotenes:		
	E 160a	β-Carotene	extraction from fruits or algae	natural dye (carotene)
	E 160b	Annatto extracts – bixin-based – norbixin-based	extraction of the seeds of the achiote tree (*Bixa orellana*). The major dye in Annatto extracts in oil is the carotinoid bixin. Norbixin is the major dye of aqueous extracts of Annatto	natural dye (apocarotinoid)
	E 160c	Paprika oleoresin (= Paprika extract)	extraction of Capsicum fruits; main colouring compounds are capsanthin and capsorubin among other carotenoids	natural dye (xanthophyll)
	E 160d	Lycopenes	by extraction from tomatoes of from the fungus Blakeslea trispora or produced synthetically	natural dye (carotene)
	E 160e	β-Apo-8′-carotenal	in spinach and citrus fruits	natural dye (apocarotinoid)
	E 160f	β-Apo-8′-carotenic acid ethyl ester	natural occurrence in some plants, mainly produced from apocarotenal	natural dye (apocarotinoid)
	E 161	Xanthophylls		
	E 161b	Lutein	extraction of the oleoresin (E161b(i)) or of the dried petals (E161b(ii)) of Tagetes erecta	natural dye (xanthophyll)
	E 161g	Canthaxanthin	natural occurrence in green algae, bacteria, and crustaceans; mainly produced synthetically	natural dye (xanthophyll)
	E 162	Beet Red, Betanin	extracted from the root of the red beet (*Beta vulgaris* var. conditiva)	natural dye (betalain)
	E 163	Anthocyanins	extraction from consumable fruits and vegetables, e.g., grape skins	natural dyes (flavonoids)
	E 170	Calcium carbonate $CaCO_3$	precipitation from calcium hydroxide with carbon dioxide	inorganic pigment
	E 171	Titanium (IV)-oxide, TiO_2 (Titanium dioxide)	from Ilmenite ($FeTiO_3$)	inorganic pigment
	E 172	Iron oxide and -hydroxide $xFe_2O_3 \cdot yFeO \cdot nH_2O$	from iron minerals	inorganic pigments
	E 173	Aluminum	from bauxite	inorganic pigment
	E 174	Silver	from silver ores	inorganic pigment
	E 175	Gold	from natural deposits	inorganic pigment
	E 180	Lithol rubine BK	synthetic	azo dye

Table 5-20 Phenols as Preservatives

Formula		Name	Pharmacopeia	Common Concentration (%)	Fields of Application
Phenol structure		Phenol	Ph. Eur., NF, JP	max. 0.25 in vaccines	According to the FDA Inactive Ingredients Guide: injections (e.g., sera and vaccines). Otherwise obsolete because of low effectiveness and high toxicity
Cresol structure		Cresol	Ph. Eur. (as reagent), NF, JP	0.2–0.4	According to the FDA Inactive Ingredients Guide: i.m., i.v., s.c., intradermal injections. Also used for disinfection,
Hydroxybenzoate ester structure	R = CH₃	Methyl-4-hydroxy-benzoate	Ph. Eur., JP (Methyl parahydroxybenzoate), NF (Methylparaben)	0.05–0.2	According to the FDA Inactive Ingredients Guide: i.m, i.v, s.c. injections; inhalation preparations; ophthalmic preparations; oral capsules, tablets, solutions and suspensions; otic, rectal, topical, vaginal preparations. Also used for Aqua conservans (DAC)
	R = C₂H₅	Ethyl-4-hydroxy-benzoate	Ph. Eur., JP (Ethyl parahydroxybenzoate), NF (Ethylparaben)	0.05–0.1	According to the FDA Inactive Ingredients Guide: oral, otic, topical preparations. Also used for Aqua conservans (DAC)
	R = C₃H₇	Propyl-4-hydroxy-benzoate	Ph. Eur., JP (Propyl parahydroxybenzoate), NF (Propylparaben)	0.03 (often in combination with methyl-4-hydroxy-benzoate)	According to the FDA Inactive Ingredients Guide: i.m., i.v., s.c. injections; inhalations; ophthalmic preparations; oral capsules, solutions, suspensions, tablets; otic, rectal, topical, vaginal preparations. Also used for Aqua conservans (DAC)
	R = C₄H₉	Butyl-4-hydroxy-benzoate	Ph. Eur., JP (Butyl parahydroxybenzoate), NF (Butylparaben)	peroralia: 0.006–0.05 dermatics: 0.02-0.4	According to the FDA Inactive Ingredients Guide: injections, oral capsules, solutions, suspensions, syrups and tablets, rectal, and topical preparations
Chlorocresol structure		Chlorocresol	Ph. Eur., NF, JP	0.1–0.2	According to the FDA Inactive Ingredients Guide: topical creams and emulsions. Also used for parenteral dosage forms and for disinfection.

Also the sodium salts of methyl-4-hydroxybenzoate, ethyl-4-hydroxy-benzoate and propyl-4-hydroxybenzoate are monographed in the Ph. Eur.

(e.g., chlorocresol, hexachlorophene) are quite suitable for the preservation of parenteral and topical dosage forms. Chlorinated phenols are extensively adsorbed by elastomers.

p-Hydroxybenzoic acid esters are presumed safe when orally administered, and they are approved as preservatives for food stuffs. Nonetheless, their application may bring along a risk of para group allergy (also known from local anesthetics with similar structure). Chronic exposure of mucosal tissue may lead to contact eczema and sensibilization. It is therefore not recommended to use these compounds to preserve ophthalmic preparations. They are also unsuitable for parenteral use. However, although there are numerous reports of delayed hypersensitivity to their topical use, the FDA believes that, at present there is no reason for concern about the use of parabenes in cosmetics and pharmaceutical preparations for topical administration to the skin. Like all phenols, they display their maximal activity in acid environment. They adsorb only to marginal extents to elastomers, but their activity might be reduced by polyoxyethylated nonionic surfactants and proteins.

5.5.2.2   Aliphatic and Aromatic Alcohols

Similar to the phenols, the activity of aliphatic and aromatic alcohols, as well as that of the more active chlorine-containing derivatives, is based on their primary toxicity. Already, the short-chain aliphatic alcohols, like ethanol (active at concentrations ≥15%) display a preservative effect. The compounds presented in Table 5-21 all are characterized by a typical odor and taste and have a certain local anesthetic effect. At the usually applied concentrations

Table 5-21 Alcohols as Preservatives

Formula	Name	Pharmacopeia	Common Concentration (%)	Fields of Application (according to the FDA Inactive Ingredients Guide)
H_3C—C(OH)(CH_3)—CCl_3	Chlorobutanol	Ph. Eur., NF, JP	0.5	i.m, i.v., s.c. injections, inhalations, nasal, otic, ophthalmic, and topical preparations
phenyl-CH_2OH	Benzyl alcohol	Ph. Eur., NF, JP	1.0–2.0	dental injections, oral capsules, solutions, tablets, topical and vaginal preparations
C_6H_5—O—CH_2—CH_2—OH	Phenoxyethanol	Ph. Eur., NF	0.5–1.0	topical preparations

they can be considered physiologically non-irritating; at higher concentrations irritation may occur, especially in case of mucosal applications. The chlorinated compounds are very well adsorbed by elastomers. Since chlorobutanol is chemically quite unstable and also volatile, it is likely to be highly sensitive to heating, and can only be used for very special preparations. Maximal activity of these compounds is obtained in the acid pH range. Above pH 6 chlorobutanol is inactive.

5.5.2.3   Organic Mercury Compounds

Organic mercury compounds (Table 5-22) are strong preservatives which, at extremely low concentrations (0.001% to 0.002%), are bacteriostatically and fungistatically active. At room temperature the onset of activity proceeds slowly (3–24 hours). The microbiostatic activity, which is strongly pH-dependent, is caused by specific reactions with thiol groups of enzymes in microorganisms. The resulting enzyme inhibition can be reversed by addition of compounds containing thiol groups. Cationic compounds of the phenyl mercury type are maximally active in the alkaline pH range. Phenyl mercury compounds display satisfactory stability. However, they need to be stored protected from light in order to prevent the splitting off of the mercury atom, which causes discoloration of solutions of these substances. Additionally, thiomersal is not very stable in neutral and alkaline conditions. Organic mercury compounds are used for the preservation of ophthalmological, rectal and cutaneous pharmaceutics.

Table 5-22 Organic Mercury Compounds as Preservatives

Formula	Chemical Designation	Pharmacopeia	Common Concentration [%]	Fields of Application
phenyl—Hg—O—C(=O)—CH_3	Phenylmercuric acetate	Ph. Eur., NF	0.002–0.005	According to the FDA Inactive Ingredients Guide: ophthalmic preparations
phenyl—Hg—O / phenyl—Hg—O : B—OH	Phenylmercuric borate	Ph. Eur.	0.002–0.005	Ophthalmic, nasal, otic preparations
phenyl—Hg—NO_3	Phenylmercuric nitrate	Ph. Eur.	0.002–0.005	According to the FDA Inactive Ingredients Guide: i.m. and ophthalmic preparation. Also used for nasal and otic preparations.
[O=C—O⁻ / phenyl—S—Hg—C_2H_5] Na^+	Thiomersal	Ph. Eur., NF	0.002	According to the FDA Inactive Ingredients Guide: i.m., i.v., s.c. injections; ophthalmic, otic, and topical preparations

Phenyl mercury compounds are incompatible with anionic drugs and excipients, in particular with halogenides, with which they form insoluble phenyl mercury halogenides. While in presence of chloride ions, high concentrations are required to form precipitates, iodide and bromide ions cause precipitates at commonly used concentrations. Similarly, tetracycline and chlortetracycline, in high concentrations also barbiturates, theophylline and sulfathiazol, turn turbid in presence of phenyl mercury compounds, culminating in the formation of precipitates after a couple of days. Thiomersal shows a lower tendency for incompatibility. Only with silver nitrate and heavy metal salts, as well as acidic compounds, precipitates are formed.

In heterogeneous drug formulations, particularly suspensions and emulsions, reduction of activity should be taken into account, caused by sorption at the interphases. Pronounced sorption occurs to rubber and artificial polymers.

5.5.2.4   Quaternary Ammonium Compounds

Quaternary ammonium compounds (invert soaps, quats) are cationic surfactants. Their antimicrobial action is based on their surface activity, which facilitates their accommodation in the plasma membrane of cells, thus causing these to become permeable to fatal extents. Also, interference with the enzyme systems of the cellular respiratory system and carbohydrate metabolism has been postulated.

Quaternary ammonium compounds have a broad activity spectrum, including bacteria, protozoas, and lower fungi. Sporocidal activity has not been confirmed. The onset of activity proceeds rather quickly, usually within a few hours. At commonly applied concentrations they act microbiostatically to microbiocidally. Their low activity toward gram-negative bacteria (in particular, *Pseudomonas aeroginosa*) can be enhanced by combination with sodium edetate. The activity of quaternary ammonium compounds is hardly dependent on pH; their activity is higher in neutral and weakly alkaline media than in strongly acidic media.

Because of their cationic nature, they experience numerous incompatibilities, which limit the number of applications:

- With anionic agents such as soaps and phenols (e.g., p-hydroxybenzoic acid esters, salicylic acid derivatives), as well as benzoic, citric, and tartaric acids and their salts, both masked and in part also visible incompatibilities occur.
- Electrolytes (e.g., nitrates, silicates, iodide, zinc-, iron- and silver salts) lead to activity-affecting complications.
- They are decomposed by oxidative agents such as iodine, potassium permanganate, and hydrogen peroxide, especially at elevated temperatures.
- Harmful concentration-dependent, interactions occur with nonionic surfactants of the Tween® and Span® type as well as with ephedrine, pilocarpine, and saponines.

In fluid multiphase pharmaceutical systems such as emulsions and suspensions, inactivation due to the distribution and accumulation of the amphiphilic preservative at the interface should always be taken into account. Also, the presence of macromolecular substances such as cellulose derivatives may cause loss of activity as a result of complex formation.

In the concentration range commonly applied for preservation purposes, quaternary ammonium compounds are physiologically well tolerated. They are particularly applied for the microbial stabilization of mucosally administered pharmaceuticals such as nose and eye drops, but also for ointments and other preparations to be applied on the skin. Like all surface-active substances, they display hemolytic activity and as such they are in general prohibited for injection purposes. Upon nasal administration, they may cause inhibition of cilia activity.

The number of commercially available surface-active substances suitable for use as preservatives is very large. Generally speaking, all the individual products have more or less similar properties and application domains. Table 5-23 presents a selection of the most important representatives of this type.

5.5.2.5   Carbonic Acids

For pharmaceutical applications, predominantly benzoic and sorbic acid are deployed; in food technology also formic, propionic and to some extent salicylic acid are used. The antimicrobial acitivity of carbonic acids is based on their primary toxicity, in particular their

Table 5-23 Quaternary Ammonium Compounds as Preservation Agents

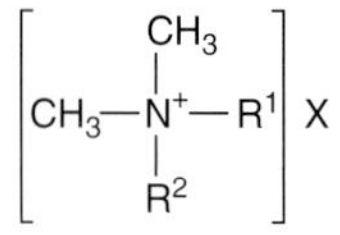

$$\left[\begin{array}{c} CH_3 \\ | \\ CH_3-N^+-R^1 \\ | \\ R^2 \end{array} \right] X$$

Formula	Name	Pharmacopeia	Common Concentration (%)	Fields of Application
R^1 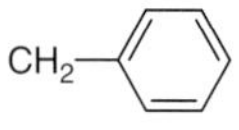 CH$_2$—⟨benzene⟩ R^2 C$_8$H$_{17}$ bls C$_{18}$H$_{37}$ X Cl$^-$	Benzalkonium chloride	Ph. Eur., NF, JP	0.002–0.02	According to the FDA Inactive Ingredients Guide: inhalations, i.m. injections, nasal, ophthalmic, otic, and topical preparations
R^1 CH$_3$ R^2 C$_{16}$H$_{33}$ X Br$^-$	Cetrimonium bromide/Cetrimide	Ph. Eur. (Cetrimide), NF (Cetrimonium bromide)	0.005–0.01	ophthalmoic, nasal, cutaneous and oral preparations
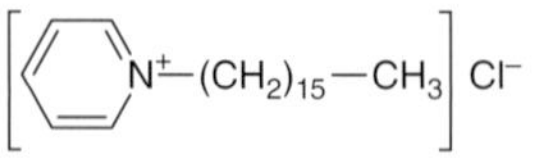 ⟨pyridinium⟩N$^\pm$—(CH$_2$)$_{15}$—CH$_3$ Cl$^-$	Cetylpyridinium chloride	Ph. Eur., NF, JP	0.001–0.01	According to the FDA Inactive Ingredients Guide: inhalation and oral preparations

interference with the basic metabolic processes of the microorganisms. Sorbic acid, for example, is assumed to inhibit the oxidation of fumarate. The activity spectrum of these substances is quite narrow and is essentially limited to lower fungi and certain bacteria; in case of sorbic acid, even only to catalase-active microorganisms. Advantages are the physiological tolerance and the lack of odor and taste. They are therefore predominantly used for the preservation of aqueous and oily peroral dosage forms, but are also used for dermatological preparations. The preservative action of carbonic acids is strongly pH-dependent. In the concentration range commonly applied for preservation purposes, the antimicrobial activity is accounted for only by the nondissociated acid. This prohibits application in neutral or alkaline environments.

Sorbic acid (Ph. Eur., NF)

CH3–CH=CH–CH=CH–COOH
Sorbic acid

Sorbic acid (hexa-2,4-dienecarbonic acid) has fungistatic and bacteriostatic action in the concentration range 0.05%–0.2% (pH < 4.5). Its activity spectrum is not very broad. It is applied for the preservation of peroral and cutaneous pharmaceutics. The FDA Inactive Ingredients Guide lists its use for ophthalmic solutions, oral capsules, solutions, syrups, tablets as well as for topical and vaginal dosage forms. Because of its oxidation sensitivity it should be stored protected from light.

Benzoic acid (Ph. Eur., NF, JP)

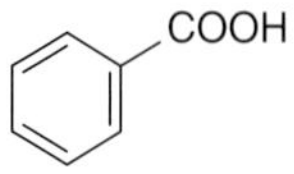

⟨benzene⟩—COOH

Benzoic acid

Benzoic acid (benzene carbonic acid), preferably applied as sodium salt, serves, similar to sorbic acid, preservation of aqueous as well as oily peroral and cutaneous pharmaceuticals. The FDA Inactive Ingredients Guide reports its use for i.m. and i.v. injections, irrigation solutions, oral solutions, suspensions, syrups, and tablets, as well as for rectal, topical, and vaginal dosage forms. It is commonly used in the concentration range 0.1% to 0.2% (pH ≤ 4.5). It should be stored protected from light.

5.5.2.6   Other Compounds

Chlorhexidine (Ph. Eur., JP)

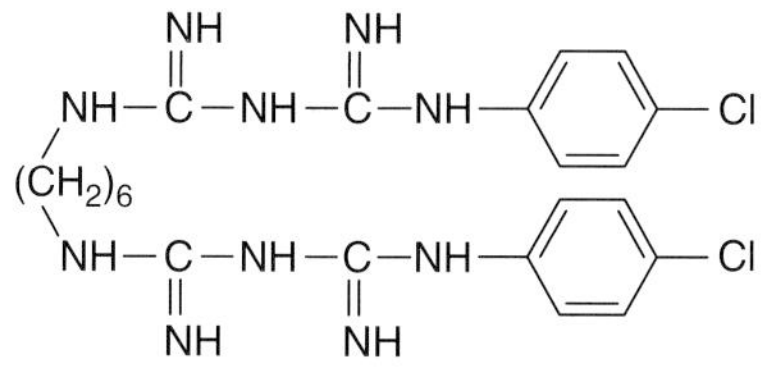

Chlorhexidine

The properties of chlorhexidine (bis-[p-chlorophenylguanidyl]-1,6-hexane dihydrochloride or diacetate, Hibitane®) resemble those of the quaternary ammonium compounds, although its surfactant character is less pronounced. It has a wide action spectrum although concerns have arisen with respect to its effectiveness toward some problematic species of the gram-negative bacteria. Chlorhexidine is predominantly used for the preservation of aqueous preparations (eye drops, cutaneous and peroral dosage forms in concentrations of 0.001 to 0.01%. It suffers from the occurrence of incompatibilities similar to those of the quaternary ammonium compounds. There are also reports of an increasing occurrence of allergies.

5.6   Antioxidants

Table 5-24 presents a list of the pharmaceutically most relevant antioxidants. They need to be physically indifferent and free from adverse effects. Depending on the specific application purpose, different requirements with respect to their organoleptic properties (appearance, smell, taste) have to be met.

5.6.1   Antioxidants for Hydrophilic Preparations

Ascorbic acid (Ph. Eur., NF, JP) and its sodium salt (Sodium ascorbate, Ph. Eur., NF) possess stabilizing properties due to their redox potential of −0.04 V (pH 7.30). They act

Table 5-24 Classification of the Antioxidants

For Lipophilic Systems	For Hydrophilic Systems

1. Natural compounds
  – tocopherols
2. Synthetic compounds
  – butylhydroxyanisole
  – butylhydroxytoluene
  – gallic acid esters
  – ascorbic acid esters
	1. Ascorbic acid
	2. Inorganic sulfur compounds
	  – sodium hydrogen sulfite
	  – sodium sulfite
	  – sodium metabisulfite (= sodium pyrosulfite)
	3. Organic sulfur compounds
	  – cysteamine
	  – thiolactic acid
	  – glutathione
	  – cysteine
	4. Others
	  – methionine
	  – tryptophane
	  – benzyl alcohol

synergistically (see below). Ascorbic acid is physiologically well tolerated and is quite suitable for the stabilization of parenteral and cutaneous dosage forms and peroral preparations at concentrations of 0.01% to 0.1%. As such, it is one of the most frequently used antioxidants. Certain oxidation products of ascorbic acid have a brownish color and thus may change the color of the preparation in the course of time. One of the end products of its oxidative degradation is oxalic acid (see for more section 25.4.1).

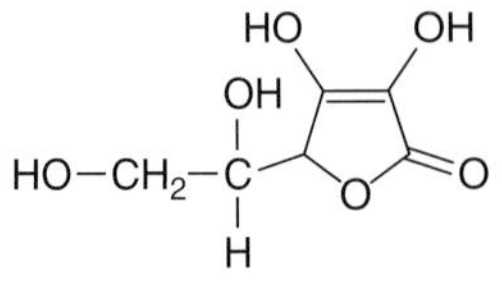

Ascorbic acid

5.6.2   Inorganic and Organic Sulfur-Containing Compounds

Because of their bad odor and taste and the potential reaction with active agents, sulfur-containing compounds, be it organic or inorganic, are now less and less frequently applied.

5.6.2.1   Inorganic Sulfur-Containing Compounds
Typical representatives of this group are sulfites and disulfites.

$NaHSO_3$, $KHSO_3$
Sodium hydrogen sulfite, Potassium hydrogen sulfite
Na_2SO_3, K_2SO_3
Sodium sulfite (Ph. Eur., NF), Potassium sulfite (Ph. Eur.)
$Na_2S_2O_5$, $K_2S_2O_5$
Sodium metabisulfite (Ph. Eur., NF), Potassium metabisulfite (Ph. Eur., NF)

These compounds decompose in acid solutions into sulfurous acid, which represents the actual active agent. They all therefore possess, the same reduction potential of +0.12 Volt. Because of their unpleasant odor and taste, they are only under certain conditions suitable for the stabilization of orally administered formulations. An additional disadvantage is the relatively high volatility of sulfurous acid. Applications that bring along elevated temperatures (sterilization) are therefore problematic. In addition, sulfites are able to react with drugs and other ingredients (sulfonation, e.g., epinephrine, see section 25.4.3.6). The common concentration range is 0.05% to 0.15%. The widely occurring sulfite intolerance, in particular in asthmatics, has meanwhile caused a further reduction in their use.

5.6.2.2   Organic Sulfur-Containing Compounds
The following compounds are applied for pharmaceutical purposes:

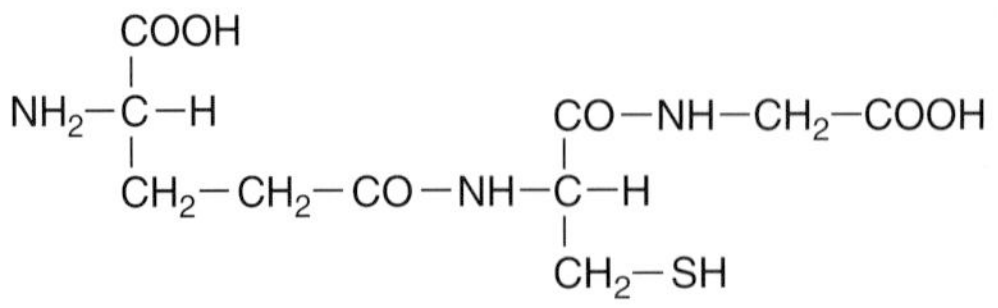

Glutathione

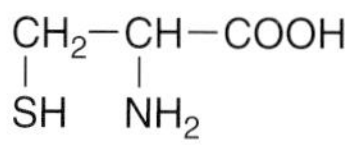

$$CH_2-CH-COOH$$
$$SH \quad NH_2$$

Cysteine

Their activity is based on the "easy" conversion (redox potential 0.14 V, pH 7, 25°C) into the corresponding di-thio compound (e.g., cysteine → cystine).

Commonly used concentrations vary from 0.05% to 0.15%. Disadvantages are, also in this case, the appalling odor and taste, which prohibit peroral and cutaneous applications.

5.6.3 Antioxidants for Lipophilic Preparations

In addition to being applied in pharmaceuticals, the compounds listed below are predominantly used as stabilizers of fats and oils in the food industry.

5.6.3.1 Natural Antioxidants

Tocopherols

Tocopherols are obtained from vegetable oils. They are mixtures of isomers (α- to δ- tocopherol) and are mostly applied as antioxidants at concentrations of 0.05% to 0.075%. At higher concentrations tocopherols can act pro-oxidatively. They are particularly suited to stabilize animal fats (pork fat), essential oils (e.g., orange oil), and vitamin A. Tocopherols are also physiologically safe.

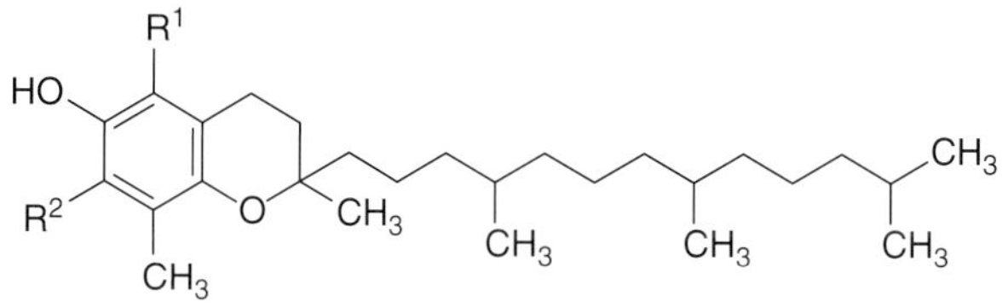

R^1, R^2 H or CH_3
Tocopherols

5.6.3.2 Synthetic and Semi-Synthetic Antioxidants

Ascorbic Acid Esters

Most widely applied are the lipid-soluble esters ascorbic acid myristate, palmitate and stearate. For the antioxidative protection of vegetable oils (e.g., sunflower, olive, cotton seed, and peanut oil) they are used at concentrations of 0.01% to 0.015%. Ascorbyl palmitate is listed in the Ph. Eur. and the NF. The FDA Inactive Ingredients Guide reports its use for oral, rectal, and topical preparations.

Gallic Acid Esters (Gallates)

Predominantly applied are the propyl, octyl, and dodecyl esters, at concentrations of 0.05% to 0.1%. All three substances are monographed in the Ph. Eur., propyl gallate also in the NF. Besides their antioxidative action, which can be significantly enhanced by addition of synergists (citric acid, lecithin), they also have weak fungistatic properties. Propyl gallate is used, according to the FDA Inactive Ingredients Guide for i.m. injections as well as for oral, and topical dosage forms.

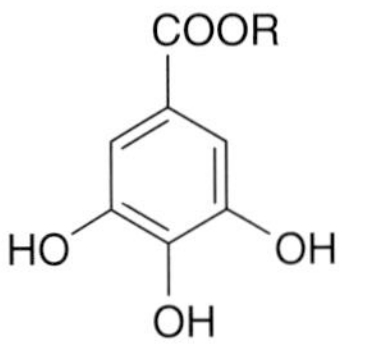

COOR

Propyl ester   R C_3H_7
Octyl ester   R C_8H_{17}
Dodecyl ester   R $C_{12}H_{25}$

Gallic acid esters (gallates)

Butylhydroxyanisol (BHA)

Butylhydroxyanisole (Ph. Eur.; Butylated hydroxyanisole, NF) is a mixture of the 2- and 3-isomers, of which the 3-isomer is the most active. Butylhydroxyanisol shows pronounced antioxidative properties at concentrations of as low as 0.005% to 0.02%. It is mostly employed for the preservation of animal fats and the stabilization of vitamin A. According to the FDA Inactive Ingredients Guide it is used for injections, oral capsules, solutions, suspensions, syrups and tablets, rectal, and topical dosage forms. At the indicated concentrations, it is physiologically safe.

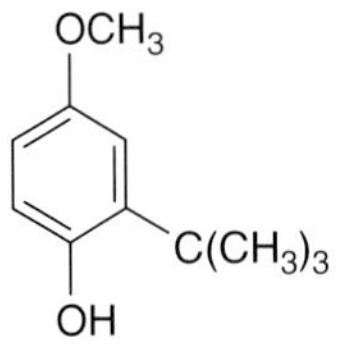

OCH_3

$C(CH_3)_3$

OH

Butylhydroxyanisol

Butylhydroxytoluene (BHT)

Butylhydroxytoluene (Ph. Eur.; Butylated hydroxytoluene, NF) resembles butylhydroxyanisol and is used at similar concentrations (0.01% to 0.02%), for similar stabilization purposes. It is believed to be particularly active as a preservative of vitamin A and carotenoids. However, it is apparently not as physiologically indifferent as was earlier assumed. The FDA Inactive Ingredients Guide reports its use for i.m. and i.v. injections, nasal sprays, oral capsules, and tablets as well as for rectal, topical, and vaginal preparations.

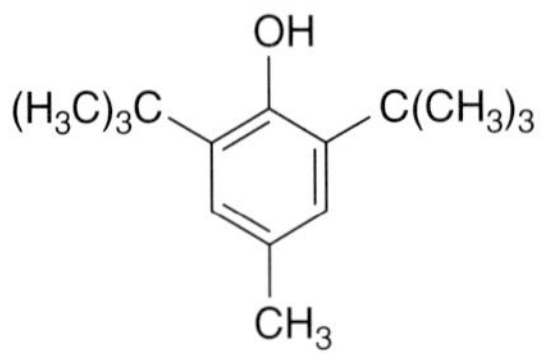

OH

$(H_3C)_3C$ $C(CH_3)_3$

CH_3

Butylhydroxytoluene

5.6.3.3   Synergists

The activity of antioxidants is supported by addition of synergists. These are compounds that are able to enhance the activity of antioxidants in a super-additive (synergistic) way. Their action is ascribed to the regeneration of consumed antioxidants, the creation of a favorable pH environment and, to some extent, their complex-forming properties (inactivation of heavy metal ions). For the selection of a suitable synergist, both the stabilizing system and the applied antioxidant have to be taken into consideration. Table 5-25 presents an overview of

Table 5-25 Pharmaceutically Applied Synergists

Compound	Common Concentration (%)	Remarks
Citric acid	0.005–0.01	especially active for vegetable oils
Citraconic acid	0.03–0.45	
Tartaric acid	0.01–0.02	
Phosphoric acid derivatives: neutral and acid monophosphates, polyphosphates	0.005–0.01 0.005–0.01	particularly active in combination with BHA and BHT
Organic phosphates	0.005–0.01	in particular dodecyl phosphate and hexose phosphate

the most important pharmaceutically applied synergists and the concentrations at which they are used.

Further Reading

Elder, D. P., Kuentz, M., and Holm, R. "Pharmaceutical Excipients—Quality, Regulatory, and Biopharmaceutical Considerations." *Eur J Pharm Sci* 87 (May 25, 2016): 88-99.

Rowe, R. C., Sheskey, P. J., and Quinn, M. E. *Handbook of Pharmaceutical Excipients*, 6th ed. London: Pharmaceutical Press, 2006.

Basic Principles of Probability and Statistics

Statistical methods are ubiquitous in pharmaceutical practice. The fabrication process of a pharmaceutical product is subject to random variations, which in the most favorable case can be minimized but never completely eliminated. Consideration of these variations is an essential element in the implementation and control of production processes and research activities. Like in many other areas, the use of statistical methods in pharmacy is influenced by the rapid development of computer-assisted data processing. Modern hardware and user-friendly software seem to turn highly complex manufacturing and assessment processes into a black box, yielding results that include a full statistical evaluation. However, meaningful application of statistical methodology requires a solid understanding of these matters. Even when a piece of equipment or software appears to relieve you from all statistics-related hands-on activities, it remains essential to understand what it is doing for you. That applies to statistical assessment as it does, say, to the use of a microwave oven (as evidenced by the need to place the warning sign "Do not use for drying pets" on the oven). In this introductory chapter we will deliberately refrain from presenting an overview of the numerous modern statistical test procedures in pharmaceutical technology. Instead, we find it more relevant to equip the reader with a conceptual understanding of probability and statistics and to emphasize that one should not only apply but also understand these methods.

6.1 Simple Calculations with Probabilities

6.1.1 Definition of Probability

Many events cannot be predicted to occur with certainty. Will it snow tomorrow in Fargo ND? How many students are able to correctly spell the word *deoxyribonucleic acid*? Will a certain medication work in a certain patient? We do not know with certainty. Nonetheless, quantitative statements are often possible. They are based on the classical probability concept, first introduced by the French mathematician Pierre-Simon Laplace (1749–1827). According to this concept, the probability $P = P(E)$ that a particular event E occurs in a test or in an experiment can be calculated by dividing the number of possibilities that event E does occur by the total number of possible test outcomes.

$$P(E) = \frac{N_E}{N_M} \qquad (6\text{-}1)$$

E a particular event

$P(E)$ probability of event E to occur

N_E number of outcomes leading to event E

N_M total number of possible outcomes

Voigt's Pharmaceutical Technology, First Edition. Alfred Fahr.

© 2018 John Wiley & Sons Ltd. Published 2018 by John Wiley & Sons Ltd.

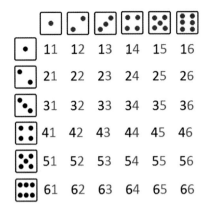

Fig. 6-1   All possible outcomes for rolling two dice.

Consider now not only a particular event but *all possible* events. For each of these events there is a certain number N_E of test outcomes, which lead to this particular event. When adding all these numbers we recover the very number $N_M = \Sigma \, N_E$ of all possible test outcomes. Accordingly, the sum of the probabilities of all possible events is $\Sigma \, P(E) = 1$.

We illustrate Laplace's idea by a simple example. The distribution of resources in the popular board game "Settlers of Catan" is derived from simultaneously throwing two dice. Each die has a number of dots on each of its six faces: 1, 2, 3, 4, 5, and 6. The probability of each individual number to end up on top after rolling the die is the same. Such a regular, non-manipulated die is called "fair." All $6 \cdot 6 = 36$ possible outcomes upon rolling two dice are listed in Fig. 6-1. Below, in section 6.3, we refer to the set of all possible outcomes as a statistical population. Each combination represents a possible outcome. Consequently, $N_M = 36$. We identify the total number of dots on top of the two dice as an event; that number varies from 2 to 12 for each outcome. Different events occur however with different frequencies. Among the $N_M = 36$ possible outcomes of one throw, there are, for example, $N_4 = 3$ possibilities $(3 + 1, 2 + 2, \text{and } 1 + 3)$ to obtain a total number of dots equal to four $(E = 4)$. According to Laplace, the corresponding probability for this event, $P(4)$, is therefore equal to $N_E/N_M = 3/36 = 0.083$, or 8.3%. The probabilities P of all other events E (i.e., the other total numbers of dots on top of the two dice) are calculated analogously:

E	2	3	4	5	6	
P	1/36	2/36	3/36	4/36	5/36	

E	12	11	10	9	8	7
P	1/36	2/36	3/36	4/36	5/36	6/36

E	total number of dots upon rolling two dice
P	corresponding probability

The sum $\Sigma \, P(E) = [2 \cdot (1 + 2 + 3 + 4 + 5) + 6] \, / 36$ of the probabilities of all possible events is precisely 1. The classical probability concept of Laplace comes with a concrete instruction on how to calculate probabilities of events. To that end, the tests (in our example the acts of rolling two dice) should be reproducible under approximately identical conditions. Many tests are, however, unique and cannot be repeated, at least not credibly frequent and under identical conditions. How likely was the fall of the Berlin Wall in 1989? How likely is it that humans will ever colonize planets outside our solar system? For such events the classical definition of probability becomes meaningless; there are, however, extensions of the probability concept.

6.1.2   Addition of Probabilities

What is the probability of obtaining a total number of either six or seven dots with one throw of two dice? Mathematically the word *or* is represented by the symbol $\cup$. The corresponding probability to obtain event E_1 or E_2 is thus expressed as $P(E_1 \cup E_2)$.

$P(E_1 \cup E_2)$: probability to obtain either event E_1 or event E_2

The individual probabilities to throw six dots or to throw seven dots are simply added up $P(6 \cup 7) = P(6) + P(7) = 5/36 + 6/36 = 11/36$ (i.e., about 30.6%). The reason why this is so simple is that the two results (six or seven dots) are mutually exclusive. The two events cannot occur simultaneously. We can also use our example of throwing two dice to discuss probabilities for events that are not mutually exclusive. To this end we consider the probability that for one throw of two dice at least one of the two displays four dots? This probability too can be expressed mathematically as $P(E_1 \cup E_2)$ if we identify the event "the first die displays four dots" as E_1 and "the second die displays four dots" as E_2. Before proceeding with the discussion it is meaningful to also introduce the probability that the

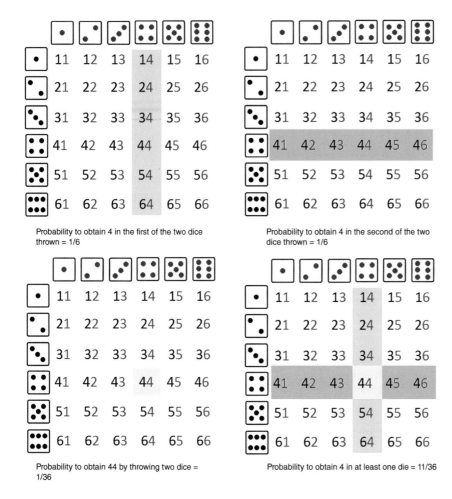

Probability to obtain 4 in the first of the two dice thrown = 1/6

Probability to obtain 4 in the second of the two dice thrown = 1/6

Probability to obtain 44 by throwing two dice = 1/36

Probability to obtain 4 in at least one die = 11/36

Fig. 6-2   Counting probabilities upon rolling two dice.

two events occur simultaneously. This simultaneous occurrence is denoted by the symbol ∩ and the corresponding probability by $P(E_1 \cap E_2)$.

$P(E_1 \cap E_2)$: probability to obtain events E_1 *and* E_2 simultaneously

In our example, the simultaneous events E_1 and E_2 correspond to the single output combination 44 of the two dice, implying $P(E_1 \cap E_2) = 1/36$. Please refer to Fig. 6-2 as you read the present and following paragraph.

In our example of mutually exclusive events discussed above, $P(E_1 \cup E_2)$ was calculated as the sum of the individual probabilities. The probability that the first die displays four dots is $P(E_1) = 1/6$. For the second die the same holds true: $P(E_2) = 1/6$. However, the probability $P(E_1 \cup E_2)$ cannot be calculated as the sum of the individual probabilities because this would imply that the simultaneously occurring event, the combination 44, would be counted twice. The double-counting immediately suggests calculating the probability by means of

$$P(E_1 \cup E_2) = P(E_1) + P(E_2) - P(E_1 \cap E_2) \tag{6-2}$$

That is, we subtract the double-counted probability from the sum of the individual probabilities. This undoes the double-counting of the combination 44. For the probability of finding four dots on at least one die equation 6-2 yields $P(E_1 \cup E_2) = 1/6 + 1/6 - 1/36 = 11/36$. The 11 possibilities to throw four dots with at least one of the two dice are highlighted in Fig. 6-2.

6.1.3   Multiplication of Probabilities

We will look once more at the probability $P(E_1 \cap E_2)$ of the simultaneous occurrence of events E_1 and E_2. In our previous example of the simultaneous occurrence of four dots on each of the two dice, we argued that $P(E_1 \cap E_2) = (1/6) \cdot (1/6) = 1/36$. The individual probabilities were simply multiplied. That is correct as long as events E_1 and E_2 are mutually independent—they are not influencing each other. This should be the case when rolling dice, unless the dice have been tampered with, for instance, by hidden magnets inside or the like. Accordingly, statistically independent outcomes imply

$$P(E_1 \cap E_2) = P(E_1) \cdot P(E_2) \tag{6-3}$$

With the multiplication rule we can for example calculate the probability that upon rolling two dice neither one will show four dots. To that end, we identify the events E_1 and E_2 as the nonoccurrence of four dots on either one of the two individual dice. Then $P(E_1) = P(E_2) = 5/6$ and thus $P(E_1 \cap E_2) = P(E_1) \cdot P(E_2) = 5/6 \cdot 5/6 = 25/36$. The probability that at least one of the two dice shows four dots is therefore $1 - 25/36 = 11/36$. Recall that we had already obtained the same result using equation 6-2. The multiplication rule in equation 6-3 analogously applies to more than two independent events: all individual probabilities are simply multiplied one by the other. For example, what is the probability that upon rolling ten dice none of them shows four dots? Since we are dealing here with independent events, the answer is simply $(5/6)^{10} = 0.162$ (i.e., 16.2%).

Example

What is the probability that by randomly selecting one out of five alternative options in each of the 20 questions of a multiple-choice exam all answers are incorrect?

Solution: By randomly choosing, the chance of selecting an incorrect answer for each individual question is $4/5$ (80%). Since the answers to the questions are mutually independent, the probability to give 20 incorrect answers equals $(4/5)^{20} = 0.0115$ (1.15%). Sadly enough, this occasionally happens in real multiple-choice exams.

Equation 6-3 applies only if the events E_1 and E_2 are statistically independent. How can we calculate $P(E_1 \cap E_2)$ if the events are not independent? To that end, let us consider another simple example. An egg carton contains six eggs (Fig. 6-3) of which two are spoiled and four are fresh.

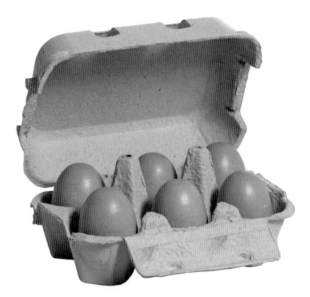

Fig. 6-3 An egg carton contains six eggs, two of which are spoiled and four are fresh. The chances of taking two fresh eggs from the box are 40%. Having to take out three fresh eggs reduces the chances to 20%.

In order to prepare a cake, we take two eggs out of the box. How likely is it that both of these are fresh, unspoiled eggs? When taking the first egg (E_1), the chances it is fresh are $4/6$. The removal of one fresh egg reduces the probability $P(E_2|E_1)$ to take another fresh egg (E_2) to $3/5$. The notation $P(E_2|E_1)$ stands for the conditional probability of the occurrence of event E_2 in case event E_1 has already occurred.

$P(E_2|E_1)$:   Probability of the occurrence of event E_2 under the condition that event E_1 has already occurred

Thus, the probability that we pick two fresh eggs from the box is $4/6 \cdot 3/5 = 2/5$ (i.e., 40%). In mathematical terms, this can be expressed by the equation

$$P(E_1 \cap E_2) = P(E_1) \cdot P(E_2|E_1) \tag{6-4}$$

This is the multiplication rule for the simultaneous occurrence of events E_1 and E_2. This rule can also be applied recursively. Upon taking three eggs from the box, the probability to have selected three fresh eggs is $(4/6) \cdot (3/5) \cdot (2/4) = 1/5$ (20%). Multiplying probabilities according to equation 6-4 is the key to the solution of numerous interesting problems.

Example

What is the probability P that among N randomly chosen individuals there are at least two whose birthday falls on the same day of the year?

Solution: The first person's birthday falls on one out of 365 days (ignoring leap years). The second person has her/his birthday on a different day with a probability of $364/365$. For the third person the probability is $363/365$ that the birthday falls on yet another day. For $N = 3$, we thus find

$$P = 1 - \frac{365}{365} \cdot \frac{364}{365} \cdot \frac{363}{365} = 1 - \prod_{i=363}^{365} \left(\frac{i}{365}\right) = 0.0082$$

This corresponds to less than 1%. Note that the symbol $\prod$ is defined analogous to the sum symbol Σ, yet it asks for a multiplication instead of an addition. For example

$$\prod_{i=1}^{4} i = 1 \cdot 2 \cdot 3 \cdot 4$$

Now it is straightforward to express the probability for larger values of N. For example, for $N = 23$ we obtain

$$P = 1 - \prod_{i=343}^{365} \left(\frac{i}{365}\right) = 0.5073$$

This already amounts to 50.7%. For $N = 50$, we find the surprisingly large value of 97%. Because of this high probability, the problem is sometimes referred to as the birthday paradox. Yet, the paradoxical appearance quickly fades once we realize that multiple birthday occurrences can fall on any day of the year instead of having to occur on a particular day.

It is also instructive to consider the following situation known as the Monty Hall problem: In a popular television game show, a candidate is given the chance to win a car. To that end, she/he has to pick one out of three doors. A car is waiting behind one of the three doors; the other two doors hide a goat. Let's assume the candidate chooses door 1; before opening it, the host Monty Hall, who knows what is behind each door, opens door 3, obviously revealing the presence of a goat, and asks the candidate if she/he wants to stick to the original choice of door 1 or prefers to switch and go for door 2. The question is: Does switching the doors make it more likely to get the car? The perhaps somewhat unexpected answer is: Yes, it becomes more likely. In fact, the chance to win the car increases from 1/3 to 2/3 if the candidate switches to door 2. This can be explained as follows: When making the original choice, the candidate's chance was 1 out of 3. The chance that the car is behind door 2 *or* door 3 was

2 out of 3. But after the host opened door 3, the candidate knows that the car is not behind that door. Thus, the 2/3 probability of the car being behind door 2 *or* door 3 has turned into the same 2/3 probability, but now applying to one door only: door 2. Therefore, the candidate should switch to door 2, now that she/he knows the car is not behind door 3. This increases the chance of winning the car from 1/3 to 2/3.

6.2   Probability Distributions

The total number of dots showing up after rolling a pair of dice is a *random variable*. Upon a single throw with two dice we do not know beforehand which one of the possible outcomes (2–12) will result. By throwing the two dice many times, we will, however, approach a well-defined distribution of outcomes. Similarly, a well-defined distribution may represent a certain feature in a batch of a pharmaceutical product. Our reasoning here is quite general: Many random variables reflect the existence of well-defined underlying probability distributions. A probability distribution refers to all possible outcomes that the random variable can adopt (the so-called *statistical population* or, simply, *population*), not only to a subset. That is, a property of the entire *population* is characterized, clearly distinct from the properties of a *random sample*, which is a subset of the population selected by chance (see section 6.3).

Random variables can be either *discrete* or *continuous*. For example, the total number of dots thrown by a pair of dice is discrete; the weights of the elephants within a species or of the tablets within a batch are continuous. Fig. 6-4 shows the probability distribution P(N) of a discrete random variable N, with values in the range 0 to 20.

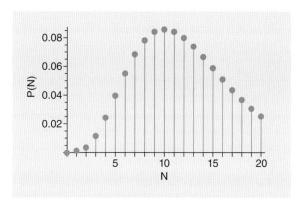

Fig. 6-4   The probability of a certain basketball player to score *N* times out of 20 attempts. Each discrete value *N* is assigned a probability *P(N)*. The probability distribution *P(N)* represents the *capability of that basketball player*. A set of actual numbers of scores out of 20 attempts represents a *sample* of that capability.

This could represent, for example, the probability of a certain basketball player to score N times after 20 attempts. Consistent with the notation P(E) in section 6.1.1, we can consider each N in P(N) as an *event*; e.g., that a basketball player scores N times. Clearly, all of the possible events can be expressed as numbers ranging from 0 to 20, which is the population on which P(N) lives.

Probability distributions are often characterized by certain specific values. Two of these are particularly important and will therefore be introduced in the following: The *mean value* (μ) is the most common (but not the only) way to extract from an entire distribution an expected event outcome (i.e. an *expectation value*). It is defined as the first moment

$$\mu = \Sigma N \cdot P(N) \tag{6-5}$$

in which the sum runs over the entire range of possible event outcomes. Variations of event outcomes are related to the width of a probability distribution. They are most commonly calculated based on

$$\sigma = \sqrt{\Sigma (N - \mu)^2 \cdot P(N)} \tag{6-6}$$

which is known as the *standard deviation* (σ). This value can also be calculated through

$$\sigma = \sqrt{\Sigma\, N^2 \cdot P(N) - \mu^2} \qquad (6\text{-}7)$$

Equation 6-7 simply follows from equation 6-6 upon multiplying out the quadratic term and taking into account that the sum of the probabilities of all possible events equals 1, that is, $\Sigma\, P(N) = 1$. Using equation 6-7 instead of 6-6 is convenient because μ and σ are directly obtained from the straightforward calculation of the two numbers $\Sigma\, N \cdot P(N)$ and $\Sigma\, N^2 \cdot P(N)$.

The probability distribution in Fig. 6-4 yields the values $\mu = 11.34$ and $\sigma = 4.20$. Because of the asymmetry of the distribution the mean value μ does not coincide with the most likely number $N = 10$. The number N with the highest probability $P(N)$ is called *modal* value. Additional characteristic values of a probability distribution that one may encounter occasionally are the *skewness v* (asymmetry) and the *kurtosis ω* (curvature). They are defined as follows

$$v = \frac{\Sigma(N - \mu)^3 \cdot P(N)}{\sigma^3} \qquad \omega = \frac{\Sigma(N - \mu)^4 \cdot P(N)}{\sigma^4} \qquad (6\text{-}8)$$

Left-skewed and *right-skewed* distributions yield $v < 0$ and $v > 0$, respectively. The data in Fig. 6-4 produce $v = 0.15$. That means the distribution is right-skewed (i.e., on the right-hand side it drops off less steep than on the left-hand side, thus producing a tail on the right-hand side). For the kurtosis of Fig. 6-4 we find $\omega = 2.25$. Distributions with kurtosis values smaller than 3 are referred to as "*platykurtic*" and those with values larger than 3 as *leptokurtic*.

6.2.1   Binomial Distribution

Many random events (the birth of a boy or a girl, the decision to go voting or stay at home, to buy a textbook for a pharmacy course or to try succeeding without it, etc.) result from binary decisions: One out of two possibilities materializes. When a sequence of individual binary events is, in addition, statistically independent, a binomial distribution emerges. Let us consider, for example, the possible outcomes "heads" or "tails" when flipping a coin. What is the probability of finding N times "heads" when flipping M coins? To answer this question, we use once more the Laplace definition of probability. For one coin there are 2, for two coins $2 \cdot 2 = 4$, and for three coins $2 \cdot 2 \cdot 2 = 8$ possible outcomes. Accordingly, for M coins we find 2^M possible outcomes. Of these, precisely

$$\binom{M}{N} = \frac{M!}{N! \cdot (M - N)!} \qquad (6\text{-}9)$$

outcomes show N times heads. The expression to the left of the equal sign in equation 6-9 is called the *binomial coefficient* (pronounce "M over N"). The binomial coefficient expresses the number of possibilities to distribute N indistinguishable objects among M indistinguishable places, where each place can host only one or no object. The right-hand side of the equation makes use of the binomial coefficient, in which

$$M! = 1 \cdot 2 \cdot 3 \cdot \ldots\ldots \cdot (M - 1) \cdot M$$

stands for the product of the integer numbers from 1 to M. For example, $4! = 1 \cdot 2 \cdot 3 \cdot 4 = 24$. The function $M!$ is called "M factorial." It increases very rapidly: The number $42!$ Is already larger than the total number of atoms making up our planet. It should be noted that $0! = 1$. It follows that the probability to find N heads upon throwing M coins is

$$P(N) = \binom{M}{N} \cdot \frac{1}{2^M}$$

To illustrate the correctness of this relation for the example of tossing three coins, implying $M = 3$, we simply write down all $2^3 = 8$ possible outcomes (heads $= 1$, tails $= 0$)

$$
\begin{array}{cccc}
000 & 001 & 010 & 011 \\
100 & 101 & 110 & 111
\end{array}
$$

The sum of occurrences of the digit 1 in each three-digit combination corresponds to the number of heads. This gives us the probabilities $P(0) = 1/8$, $P(1) = 3/8$, $P(2) = 3/8$, and $P(3) = 1/8$. The expression

$$
P(N) = \binom{M}{N} \cdot \frac{1}{2^M}
$$

leads us to the same prediction. For example

$$
P(2) = \binom{3}{2} \cdot \frac{1}{2^3} = \frac{3!}{2! \cdot 1! \cdot 8} = \frac{3}{8}
$$

When tossing one single coin, the two outcomes heads or tails are equally probable. Both possible outcomes have thus the same probability of $p = 1/2$. However, often the probability deviates from $p = 1/2$. For example, the probability to draw a spade from a deck of cards is $p = 1/4$. In the general case of an arbitrary probability p for the individual binary event, the binomial distribution is

$$
P(N) = \binom{M}{N} \cdot p^N \cdot (1 - p)^{M-N} \tag{6-10}
$$

Obviously, if in equation 6-10 we choose $p = 1/2$, we recover the result discussed above

$$
P(N) = \binom{M}{N} \cdot \left(\frac{1}{2}\right)^N \cdot \left(1 - \frac{1}{2}\right)^{M-N} = \binom{M}{N} \cdot \frac{1}{2^M}
$$

Fig. 6-5 shows two distributions for $M = 20$, one curve refers to $p = 0.5$ (squares) and the other to $p = 0.8$ (circles). The mean value and standard deviation of the binomial distribution $P(N)$ in equation 6-10 can be calculated by applying equations 6-5 and 6-6, respectively. The results are

$$
\mu = M \cdot p \quad \text{and} \quad \sigma = \sqrt{M \cdot p \cdot (1 - p)} \tag{6-11}
$$

The two binomial distributions displayed in Fig. 6-5 yield $\mu = 10$ and $\sigma = 2.24$ (for $p = 0.5$, squares) as well as $\mu = 16$ and $\sigma = 1.79$ (for $p = 0.8$, circles).

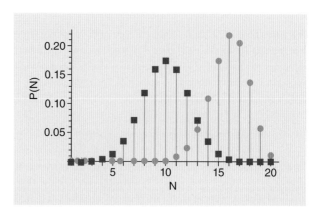

Fig. 6-5   Binomial distribution according to equation 6-10 for *M* = 20. The two data sets refer to *p* = 0.5 (squares) and p = 0.8 (circles).

Example

The average fail rate for an oral exam in pharmaceutics is 20%. One day the course instructor administers an exam for 10 students. How likely is it that no more than three students fail the exam?

Solution: We apply equation 6-10 with $p = 0.2$ and $M = 10$. The choice $N = 3$ corresponds to the probability that precisely three students fail the exam. This amounts to $P(3) = \binom{10}{3} \cdot 0.2^3 \cdot 0.8^7 = 0.20$. Similarly, we obtain $P(2) = 0.30$, $P(1) = 0.27$ and $P(0) = 0.11$. The sum is $P(3) + P(2) + P(1) + P(0) = 0.88$. Consequently, the probability that no more than three students fail is 88%. This calculation assumes the statistical independence of the individual oral exams, which in real college life is not always the case.

6.2.2 Hypergeometric Distribution

The binomial distribution rests on the assumption of statistically independent events. When flipping coins this condition is typically fulfilled. Very often, however, one event influences the next one. For example, once all the prizes available at a raffle game have been claimed, it makes no sense to buy additional tickets.

Events that are not independent have already been discussed above when introducing the concept of *conditional probability*. The reader may recall the example involving a carton containing six eggs of which two were spoiled. We had discussed the probability that upon taking, say, three eggs from the box none of them is spoiled.

Let us approach this problem in a more general sense. A population of size m (m eggs in an egg carton) contains n faulty elements (n spoiled eggs). We are asking for the probability to randomly take N faulty elements from a subpopulation of M elements. The answer to our question is the hypergeometric distribution

$$P(N) = \frac{\binom{n}{N} \cdot \binom{m-n}{M-N}}{\binom{m}{M}} \tag{6-12}$$

In the spirit of Laplace's definition (see equation 6-1), the number of favorable events (numerator) is divided by the number of possible event outcomes (denominator). The numerator multiplies the number of possibilities to pick N from n faulty elements with the number of possibilities to pick $M - N$ from $m - n$ nonfaulty elements (give that some thought!). This yields the total number of possibilities that at the end we are left with N spoiled eggs. The binomial coefficient in the denominator specifies how many possibilities there are altogether to pick M elements from a total of m elements. The denominator corresponds, therefore, to the total number of possible event outcomes.

Let us return to the egg carton example. With $m = 6$ (six eggs in the carton), $n = 2$ (two eggs are spoiled), and $M = 3$ (three eggs are picked), we obtain, according to equation 6-12,

$$P(0) = \frac{\binom{2}{0} \cdot \binom{6-2}{3-0}}{\binom{6}{3}} = 0.2$$

and similarly $P(1) = 0.6$ and $P(2) = 0.2$. As expected, $P(0) + P(1) + P(2) = 1$. Recall that we had already discussed the result for $P(0)$ (20% chance that none of the three picked eggs is spoiled) following equation 6-4.

The hypergeometric distribution also shows up in the calculation of probabilities in a lottery. Similarly to picking unspoiled eggs from an egg carton, in a lottery it is all about guessing a few selected "correct" numbers from a given range of numbers. The hypergeometric distribution is applied because each individual number is available only once. For example, in the American lottery game Powerball, 5 balls from a set of 69 numbered balls are randomly selected. To calculate the probability of predicting the numbers for 3 of the 5 balls correctly, we insert into equation 6-12 the values m = 69, n = M = 5 and N = 3. That results in a probability of 0.00179, or slightly less than 0.18%.

Which one is the more fundamental distribution, the hypergeometric or the binomial distribution? For very large values m of the underlying population and a comparatively small number M of selected elements (i.e., $m \gg M$) the ratio n/m remains practically unchanged upon removing elements. Each withdrawal then turns into a statistically independent event and the hypergeometric distribution becomes identical to the binomial distribution with p = n/m. The binomial distribution is thus a specific case of the hypergeometric distribution.

The mean value and the standard deviation of the hypergeometric distribution follow from applying equations 6-5 and 6-6 to 6-12

$$\mu = M \cdot p \text{ and } \sigma = \sqrt{M \cdot p \cdot (1-p) \cdot \left(\frac{m-M}{m-1}\right)} \tag{6-13}$$

in which we used the abbreviation p = n/m for the sake of comparing with the binomial distribution. Here too we see that the results of the binomial distribution (see equation 6-11) appear as a special case of the hypergeometric distribution for $m \gg M$.

Example

A pharmacist has to sample a batch of 10,000 ampules. We know (but she doesn't) that 1,000 of those ampules contain particles of unacceptably large size. What is the probability that the pharmacist, when randomly selecting 10 ampules, samples only correct ampules? And what is the probability that her finding exactly matches 10% of the ampules to be not acceptable?

Solution: Apparently, this problem is very much like that of the egg carton. The population m equals 10,000, containing n = 1,000 faulty elements. The probability of finding among the M = 10 randomly collected ampules no faulty elements (i.e., N = 0) is, according to the hypergeometric distribution (Equation 6-12)

$$P(0) = \frac{\binom{1,000}{0} \cdot \binom{10,000-1,000}{10-0}}{\binom{10,000}{10}} = 0.349$$

Hence, with a probability of 34.9% the pharmacist is tempted to assume the entire batch is OK. The probability of finding 1 faulty element in a sample of 10 ampules is

$$P(1) = \frac{\binom{1,000}{1} \cdot \binom{10,000-1,000}{10-1}}{\binom{10,000}{10}} = 0.388$$

With a probability of 38.8% she will correctly estimate the batch to contain 10% faulty ampules. In all other cases (i.e., with a probability of $100 - 34.9 - 38.8 = 26.3\%$) she will find more than one faulty ampule. Because with m = 10,000 and M = 10, the population m is much larger than the sample size M, we can solve the problem more efficiently using the binomial distribution (see equation 6-10), with p = n/m = 1,000/10,000 = 0.1. For example, for P(0) we calculate

$$P(0) = \binom{10}{0} \cdot 0.1^0 \cdot 0.9^{10} = 0.9^{10} = 0.349$$

As expected, we find the same result as when using equation 6-12. In fact, the results are not exactly the same. A more accurate calculation yields P(0) = 0.34850 using the hypergeometric distribution and P(0) = 0.34868 based on the binominal distribution.

6.2.3   Poisson Distribution

The two probability distributions discussed so far are fairly general and apply to a large class of problems. Yet, they are also somewhat cumbersome to deal with. Not only do they depend on multiple parameters (4 parameters for the hypergeometric and 3 parameters for the binomial distribution), they also require the calculation of potentially large factorials in the binomial coefficients. That is not particularly convenient.

If there are many possible outcomes with rare events, the situation simplifies substantially. Then, the binomial distribution adopts the limiting behavior of a Poisson distribution (Siméon Denis Poisson, who lived 1781–1840, was a student of Laplace). Applicability of the Poisson distribution requires that in the binomial distribution (equation 6-10) M is large ("many possible outcomes") and p is small ("rare events"), but in such a way that $M \cdot p$ is neither infinitely large nor vanishingly small. In practice, the Poisson distribution may be used already when $M > 10$ and $p < 0.1$. The mathematical expression for the Poisson distribution is

$$P(N) = \frac{(M \cdot p)^N}{N!} \cdot e^{-M \cdot p} \tag{6-14}$$

in which $e = 2.71828$ is Euler's number and N a binary random variable that can adopt zero or positive integer values without an upper limit. As with the binomial distribution, the events need to be statistically independent. For the mean value of a Poisson distribution we find $\mu = M \cdot p$, the standard deviation is $\sigma = \sqrt{M \cdot p} = \sqrt{\mu}$. Thus, the Poisson distribution depends, besides the random variable N, on only one additional parameter—its mean value μ. It is convenient to incorporate μ directly into the expression for the Poisson distribution

$$P(N) = \frac{\mu^N}{N!} \cdot e^{-\mu} \tag{6-15}$$

Fig. 6-6 shows a graphic representation of the Poisson distribution for $\mu = 3$, according to equation 6-15.

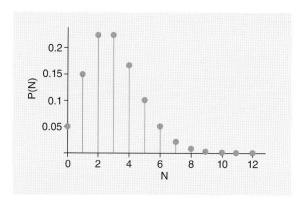

Fig. 6-6   The Poisson distribution for $\mu = M \cdot p = 3$.

The Poisson distribution has a multitude of applications. It describes, for instance, the number of typographical errors per page in a newspaper, the annual frequency of family holiday trips, or the number of leucocytes per mL of blood. Let us consider two concrete examples:

1.   Assume it is known that, on average, one out of one thousand patients will not tolerate the injection of a particular serum. What then is the probability that out of 2000 patients there are exactly three who will not tolerate the injection of that serum?

     Solution: This question can be answered based on the Poisson distribution, because $p = 0.001$ is very small and $M = 2,000$ is very large. The only relevant parameter then is the mean value $\mu = p \cdot M = 2$. The probability we wish to find is therefore according to equation 6-15

$$P(3) = \frac{2^3}{3!} \cdot e^{-2} = 0.18, \text{i.e.,} 18\%.$$

2. A rural pharmacy is visited on average by three customers between 9 a.m. and 10 a.m. every day. How likely is it that on one particular day no more than one customer will show up between 9 a.m. and 10 a.m.?

Solution: On average 3 customers within one hour, that truly makes a rare event! The probability that precisely one customer enters is according to equation 6-15

$$P(1) = 3^1 \cdot e^{-3}/(1!) = 0.15$$

In a similar manner we obtain $P(0) = 3^0 \cdot e^{-3}/(0!) = 0.05$. The sum $P(0) + P(1) = 0.20$ yields a probability of 20% that between 9 a.m. and 10 a.m. at most one customer will enter the pharmacy. The same result can also be extracted from Fig. 6-6 as the sum of the two values $P(0)$ and $P(1)$.

6.2.4   Normal Distribution

The *normal distribution* (also known as the Gaussian bell curve after the mathematician Johann Carl Friedrich Gauss (1777–1855)) is of special significance because it emerges according to the *central limit theorem* from the superposition of a large number of arbitrarily distributed random processes. Many statistical tests therefore assume a normal distribution. We illustrate the fundamental significance of the normal distribution by mentioning a few examples for its applicability: the birth weight of babies, the filling volume of milk in cardboard containers, the dollar amount of tip earned by a waiter on a busy day, the number of words per page of a novel, and the daily reading of the temperature on a thermometer over many years. The normal distribution describes the probability distribution of a continuously changing random variable. Like the Poisson distribution, it emerges as a special case of the binomial distribution. More specifically, we will find a normal distribution when the number of possible test outcomes M is very large, while the probability p of the binary individual event becomes neither too large nor too small.

As a rule of thumb for when a normal distribution is a good approximation of a binomial distribution, the following should apply

$$\sqrt{M \cdot p \cdot (1 - p)} \geq 3$$

Example

When tossing 100 coins simultaneously, we obtain a binomial distribution with $M = 100$ and $p = 0.5$ for the number of "heads" showing up. The mean value and the standard deviation are

$$\mu = 50 \text{ and } \sigma = \sqrt{M \cdot p \cdot (1 - p)} = 5, \text{respectively.}$$

Thus, instead of the binomial distribution, we may use the normal distribution. According to the rule of thumb, we can decrease the number of coins to 36 and still apply the normal distribution.

In mathematical terms, the normal distribution is given by

$$P(N) = \frac{1}{\sigma \cdot \sqrt{2 \cdot \pi}} \cdot e^{-\frac{1}{2} \cdot \left(\frac{N-\mu}{\sigma}\right)^2} \tag{6-16}$$

The range of values for the continuous random variable N is $-\infty < N < \infty$. The normal distribution $P(N)$ depends on the two parameters μ and σ. As the symbols already suggest, these are precisely the mean value and the standard deviation. Thus, the following applies: $\Sigma N \cdot P(N) = \mu$ and $\Sigma (N - \mu)^2 \cdot P(N) = \sigma^2$, where the sum Σ must be interpreted as the integral $\int_{-\infty}^{\infty} dN$. Note that also the normalization condition $\Sigma P(N) = 1$ is satisfied by Equation 6-16. That is, $\frac{1}{\sigma\sqrt{2\pi}} \int_{-\infty}^{\infty} e^{-\frac{1}{2}\left(\frac{N-\mu}{\sigma}\right)^2} dN = 1$.

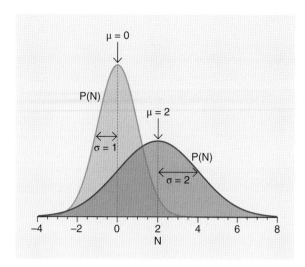

Fig. 6-7   The normal distribution for the two instances $\mu = 0$, $\sigma = 1$, and $\mu = 2$, $\sigma = 2$. The former case corresponds to the standard normal distribution.

Fig. 6-7 displays the normal distribution P(N) for the two instances $\mu = 0$ and $\sigma = 1$, as well as $\mu = 2$ and $\sigma = 2$. In the former case, for $\mu = 0$ and $\sigma = 1$, the distribution is also called *standard normal distribution*. When considering an arbitrary normal distribution as a function of the variable $x = (N - \mu)/\sigma$, we obtain the standard normal distribution. We denote it by $u(x)$; its mathematical representation is

$$u(x) = \frac{1}{\sqrt{2 \cdot \pi}} \cdot e^{-\frac{x^2}{2}} \tag{6-17}$$

Every normal distribution is symmetric. Its skewness v (defined in equation 6-8) thus vanishes. For the kurtosis ω (also defined in equation 6-8) of the normal distribution we find $\omega = 3$. That is, the expressions *platykurtic* ($\omega < 3$) and *leptokurtic* ($\omega > 3$) use the normal distribution as reference. The area under the curve P(N) is a measure for the probability. Specifically, the probability to find the random variable N within a certain range $N_{min} \leq N \leq N_{max}$ is

$$P_{tot} = \int\limits_{N_{min}}^{N_{max}} P(N)dN$$

Consider, for example, the ranges of ± 1, ± 2, or ± 3 standard deviations σ around a mean value μ. For the corresponding probabilities we find

N_{min}	N_{max}	P_{tot}
$\mu - 1 \cdot \sigma$	$\mu + 1 \cdot \sigma$	0.6827
$\mu - 2 \cdot \sigma$	$\mu + 2 \cdot \sigma$	0.9545
$\mu - 3 \cdot \sigma$	$\mu + 3 \cdot \sigma$	0.9973

Accordingly, 95.45% of all events (e.g., the results of a measurement) fall within a scatter range of two standard deviations. Often, a 95% scatter range is applied. This corresponds to 1.96 standard deviations around the mean value. That is to say, the value of a normal-distributed random variable N lies with a probability of 95% within the interval

$$\mu - 1.96 \cdot \sigma \leq N \leq \mu + 1.96 \cdot \sigma \tag{6-18}$$

This interval is also called the *95%-confidence interval*. The remaining $100\% - 95\% = 5\%$ (the *significance level*) corresponds to the probability of finding the random variable outside the confidence interval. Generally, a significance level of α corresponds to a $(1 - \alpha)\%$ confidence interval.

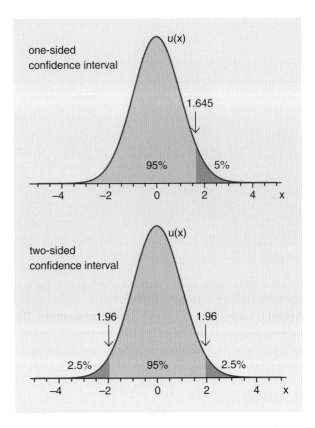

Fig. 6-8　One- and two-sided 95%-confidence intervals of the standard normal distribution $u(x)$.

In contrast to the *two-sided* confidence interval, as discussed in the foregoing, we can also define a *one-sided* confidence interval, where one of the two interval boundries remains at infinity. For example

N_{min}	N_{max}	P_{tot}
$-\infty$	$\mu + 1.645 \cdot \sigma$	0.9500

Accordingly, the value of a normal-distributed random variable N falls with a probability of 95% within the interval

$$-\infty < N \leq \mu + 1.645 \cdot \sigma$$

One-sided confidence levels are used, for example, when we wish to know the probability that a measured value will not exceed a certain limit. Fig. 6-8 illustrates the one- and two-sided 95%-confidence interval of a standard normal distribution.

Example

The distribution of the total number of dots showing up on 1000 dice in one single throw can very well be described by a normal distribution. The mean value will be $\mu = 3,500$ and the standard deviation $\sigma = 54$.

It follows that 95% of all throws deviate no more than $1.96 \cdot \sigma = 106$ from the mean value and, therefore, will be found within the range from $N_{min} = 3,394$ to $N_{max} = 3,606$. Likewise, the probability that the total number of dots in one throw is smaller than $\mu + 1.65 \cdot \sigma = 3,500 + 89 = 3,589$ is 95%. Moreover, 90% of all throws will deviate not more than $1.65 \cdot \sigma = 89$ from the mean value. That is, they will fall into the range from $N_{min} = 3,411$ to $N_{max} = 3,589$.

6.3   Sampling

A sample is defined as a subset of a statistical population such as, for example a subset of the 36 possible event outcomes displayed in Fig. 6-1. The term can be used generally when an entire population is characterized based on properties of only a limited number of representatives. Of particular usefulness are random samples because they are unbiased and thus form a convenient basis to draw quantitative conclusions about the entire population. That is, the probability for each element of the underlying population to be present in the sample is the same. The selection of a representative sample is by no means a simple and straightforward process. That is clearly illustrated by the widely discussed difficulties to design meaningful opinion polls prior to elections. In the following, we will assume that samples truly are random samples.

6.3.1   Characteristic Parameters of Samples

Samples can be characterized by certain parameters. Of particular relevance are the *mean value* and the *spread*. The mean value is a measure of location. When we say: The average (or mean) weight of an elephant is 5 tons, we are stating such a location parameter. The spread tells us something about the extent by which the weights of individual elephants deviate from the mean value. Mean and spread do not provide information about the details of distributions. We distinguish for example the heavier African elephant and the lighter Asian elephant. This would become apparent from a sufficiently large sample size taken from all elephants, but not from mean and spread alone. Often, we can describe the data set resulting from a sample by means of a list of numbers x_i with $i = 1 \ldots n$, in which n indicates the size of the sample. For example, when determining the weights of nine randomly chosen elephants (in tons, $t = 1000$ kg), we may obtain the following data set: 6.68, 4.16, 3.04, 6.87, 6.08, 5.61, 5.41, 4.96, 4.72. In this case $n = 9$, and $x_1 = 6.68t$, $x_2 = 4.16t$, etc. The most commonly used mean value is the *arithmetic mean*

$$\bar{x} = \frac{1}{n} \sum_{i=1}^{n} x_i \qquad (6\text{-}19)$$

and the most important parameter characterizing the spread is the *standard deviation*

$$s = \sqrt{\frac{\sum_{i=1}^{n} (x_i - \bar{x})^2}{n - 1}} \qquad (6\text{-}20)$$

Our example of the 9 elephants yields $\bar{x} = 5.28t$ and $s = 1.22t$. We may ask why in equation 6-20 we divide by $(n - 1)$ rather than by n, like in equation 6-19. In case the sample size was limited to one single value ($n = 1$), there would be no spread at all. From the statement that an extraterrestrial creature on another planet is 1.80 m tall, we can draw no conclusions as to how much the tallness of other extraterrestrial creatures (if there are any!) deviates from 1.80 m. We need at least two of them to obtain one piece of information about the spread of the tallness. For a sample size n we therefore obtain $(n - 1)$ "pieces of information." It is precisely these $(n - 1)$ so-called degrees of freedom of a spread measurement by which we divide in equation 6-20. An equivalent, but for practical purposes often more convenient method for the calculation of the standard deviation is

$$s = \sqrt{\frac{1}{n - 1} \left[\sum_{i=1}^{n} x_i^2 - \frac{1}{n} \left(\sum_{i=1}^{n} x_i \right)^2 \right]} \qquad (6\text{-}21)$$

As for the transition from equation 6-6 to equation 6-7, equation 6-21 follows from equation 6-20 by expanding the square in equation 6-20 and applying the definition of the mean value.

What we have introduced in equation 6-19 is the arithmetic mean. There are, however, other mean values which one can (and, as the associated examples show, often should) use as location parameters. The *harmonic mean* is produced by the reciprocal value of the average of the reciprocal data values

$$\bar{x}_H = \frac{n}{\sum\limits_{i=1}^{n} \frac{1}{x_i}}$$

Example

Of two different liquids with densities $\rho_1 = 0.80$ g/cm^3 and $\rho_2 = 1.20$ g/cm^3 aliquots of one gram (m = 1.0 g) are mixed. What is the density of the resulting mixture?

Solution: The density $\rho = m/V$ is the ratio of the mass m and the volume V. Thus, for the two liquids we may write $\rho_1 = m_1/V_1$ and $\rho_2 = m_2/V_2$, respectively, where according to our example $m_1 = m_2 = m$. The density of the resulting mixture $\rho_{av} = (m_1 + m_2)/(V_1 + V_2) = 2/(1/\rho_1 + 1/\rho_2) = 0.96$ g/cm^3 results from the harmonic mean of the individual densities.

For the *geometric mean* we take the nth root of the product of all n individual values

$$\bar{x}_G = \sqrt[n]{\prod_{i=1}^{n} x_i}$$

Example

A pharma start-up company grows in the first year by 2% and in the second year by 98%. What is the mean annual growth rate?

Solution: If S denotes the starting value of the company, then after two years the value is $S \cdot 1.02 \cdot 1.98$. Using the average growth rate $\bar{x}_G$ should yield the same result through $S \cdot \bar{x}_G \cdot \bar{x}_G$. From $S \cdot 1.02 \cdot 1.98 = S \cdot \bar{x}_G \cdot \bar{x}_G$ follows $\bar{x}_G = \sqrt{1.02 \cdot 1.98} = 1.42$. Hence, the average growth rate of 42% follows from the geometric mean of the individual growth rates.

There are a number of other characterizing parameters that are occasionally employed. When sorting data according to their numerical values and separating them into parts that contain the same number of data points, *quantiles* are obtained. For example, we may separate a data set into two size-equal parts. The value that separates two size-equal parts is called *median*. Differently expressed, the median is a value that lies in the middle of a distribution of observed values such that there is an equal probability for the other observed values to fall either above or below it.

The division into a lower, middle, and upper third, each containing the same number of data points, leads to *tertiles*. The perhaps most frequently used form are *quartiles*; that is, the division into four size-equal parts, separated from each other by the values $Q_{0.25}$, $Q_{0.50}$ and $Q_{0.75}$. The value $Q_{0.50}$ corresponds exactly to the median. Quantile distances serve as convenient scatter parameters. Specifically, the value $Q_{1.00} - Q_{0.00}$ (i.e., the difference between the largest and the smallest value) is referred to as the *range* of the data set.

An example for the application of quartiles is the box-and-whisker plot, which is often used to construct a graphic representation of a data set. In its most simple form, the median $Q_{0.50}$ is located inside a box that spans the positions $Q_{0.25}$ and $Q_{0.75}$ and is marked by two antennas (whiskers) at positions $Q_{0.00}$ and $Q_{1.00}$. Thus, the box hosts 50% of the data, whereas the whiskers contain the other 50%. Fig. 6-9 shows a box-and-whisker plot for the data on elephant weights just presented.

Box-and-whisker plots are quite well suited for a visually appealing comparison of different data sets, because the asymmetries of the distributions are easily recognized. This is illustrated by an example in Fig. 6-10. It shows a series of box-and-whisker plots representing the elevation above sea level of all cities with a population of more than 100,000 in five European countries.

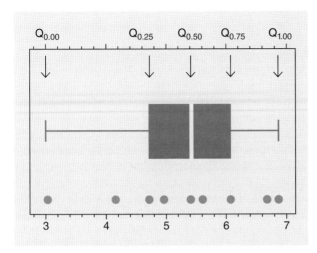

Fig. 6-9 Box-and-whisker plot of the elephant weight data set. The individual weights of the animals are specified in the lower part of the figure (filled circles). The locations of the smallest ($Q_{0.00}$) and the largest ($Q_{1.00}$) weight as well as the quartiles $Q_{0.25}$, $Q_{0.50}$, and $Q_{0.75}$ are indicated by vertical arrows on top of the diagram.

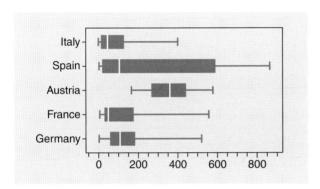

Fig. 6-10 Box-and-whisker plot of the elevations above sea level (in meters) of all cities with a population over 100,000 in five European countries. For the example of Austria, these are Vienna (166 m), Graz (360 m), Linz (267 m), Salzburg (443), and Innsbruck (578 m).

6.3.2   Distribution of Samples

Let us assume that we know the probability distribution $P(N)$ of a random variable N, where N represents an entire statistical population. What can we expect from a sample? For instance, if we repeatedly toss 100 coins simultaneously, the number of heads will vary around a mean value of all tosses. The probability distribution $P(N)$ is given by a binomial distribution with $M = 100$ and $p = 0.5$. If we could carry out an infinite number of tosses, we would find, according to equation 6-11, the exact values $\mu = M \cdot p = 50$ and $\sigma = \sqrt{M \cdot p \cdot (1 - p)} = 5$ for, respectively, the mean and the standard deviation of the entire statistical population. Although, strictly speaking, the probability distribution $P(N)$ is a binomial distribution, we can represent it as well by a normal distribution with $\mu = 50$ and $\sigma = 5$; see the example on page 252.

If we toss our set of 100 coins only 10 times and count the number of heads each time, how accurately will we reproduce the exact values $\mu = 50$ and $\sigma = 5$? The result of such a tenfold coin-tossing experiment could be for instance: 55, 56, 42, 59, 49, 46, 56, 51, 51, 51. We denote the individual values of the sample by x_i (i.e., $x_1 = 55$, $x_2 = 56$, etc.) and the size of the sample by n (i.e., $n = 10$ in our example). According to equations 6-19 and 6-20, the calculation of the mean value and the standard deviation of our data set yields $\bar{x} = 51.6$ and $s = 5.125$, respectively.

Recall that in equation 6-17 we have condensed all normal distributions $P(N)$ into a standard form $u(x)$ by switching to a new scaled variable $x = (N - \mu)/\sigma$. In a similar manner, we can calculate from s a new scaled variable, pronounced "chi square", through

$$\chi^2 = (n - 1) \cdot \frac{s^2}{\sigma^2} \tag{6-22}$$

which, as shown below in equation 6-24 and section 6.4, is of principal relevance. For our example, we obtain the numerical value $\chi^2 = (10 - 1) \cdot (5.125/5)^2 = 9.456$. We are now in the position to ask an important question: Assume we repeat the tenfold throwing of 100 coins many times and from the observed number of heads we calculate each time the mean value $\bar{x}$ and the standard deviation s (and from that the derived parameter χ^2), how will these be distributed?

One possibility to track down the distributions is by means of a computer simulation. To that end, we have generated 50,000 samples and calculated each time $\bar{x}$ and s and from those χ^2. Let us first consider the distribution of the obtained means $\bar{x}$. The relative frequency of the means $\bar{x}$ is displayed in Fig. 6-11 in the form of a *histogram* based on our 50,000 samples. The dashed curve in Fig. 6-11 shows the probability of the underlying statistical population—that is, the normal-distributed number of heads upon throwing 100 coins.

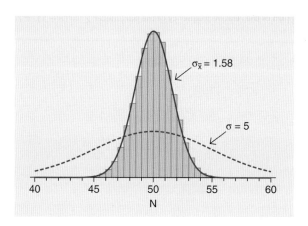

Fig. 6-11   The number of heads upon simultaneously throwing 100 coins varies around 50. The dashed curve shows the probability distribution $P(N)$, which is to a good approximation a normal distribution with mean value $\mu = 50$ and standard deviation $\sigma = 5$. If we take a sample of size $n = 10$ of 100 coin throws, the mean of the sample also adopts a normal distribution (solid line), but now with a mean value $\bar{x} = \mu = 50$ and a standard deviation $\sigma_{\bar{x}} = \sigma/\sqrt{n} = 5/3.16 = 1.58$. The histogram shows the relative frequency of the mean values for 50,000 computer-generated random samples, each of size $n = 10$.

As we already know, the mean and standard deviation are $\mu = 50$ and $\sigma = 5$, respectively. The distribution of the sample mean in the histogram is clearly distinct from that. Nonetheless, also here we are dealing with a normal distribution, with the same mean value $\bar{x} = \mu$ but with a smaller standard deviation $\sigma_{\bar{x}}$. Just how much smaller the standard deviation of the mean becomes depends on the size n of the sample in the following way

$$\sigma_{\bar{x}} = \frac{\sigma}{\sqrt{n}} \tag{6-23}$$

We can rationalize this result as follows: The standard deviation of a single throw of M coins (with $p = 1/2$) is $\sigma = \sqrt{M \cdot p \cdot (1 - p)} = \sqrt{M}/2$. The standard deviation of an n-fold throw of M coins is equal to the nth part of the standard deviation of throwing $n \cdot M$ coins: $\sigma_{\bar{x}} = (1/n) \cdot \sqrt{n \cdot M}/2$. Thus; $\sigma_{\bar{x}} = \sigma/\sqrt{n}$, exactly as stated in equation 6-23. Instead of $\sigma = 5$ we find in Fig. 6-10 therefore $\sigma_{\bar{x}} = 5/\sqrt{10} = 1.58$.

The solid curve in Fig. 6-11 shows the corresponding normal distribution with $\mu = 50$ and $\sigma_{\bar{x}} = 1.58$. Based on equation 6-18 we can now conclude that the sample mean $\bar{x}$ lies, with a probability of 95%, within the range $\mu - 1.96\,\sigma/\sqrt{n} \leq \bar{x} \leq \mu + 1.96\,\sigma/\sqrt{n}$. Thus, in order to reduce the distribution width of the sample mean to one half, the sample size has to be quadrupled.

We will now turn to the standard deviation of the sample mean distribution. We have calculated the parameter χ^2, as defined in equation 6-22, from the 50,000 samples. The relative frequency of χ^2 is displayed as a histogram in Fig. 6-12.

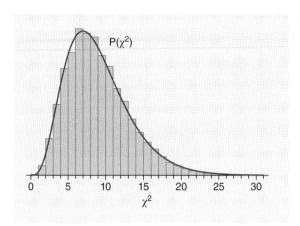

Fig. 6-12 Histogram of the relative frequency of the parameter $\chi^2 = (n-1) \cdot s^2/\sigma^2$, as defined in equation 6-22. To that end, 50,000 samples of size $n = 10$ for throwing 100 coins simultaneously were generated by a computer and the corresponding standard deviation s was calculated. The standard deviation of the underlying population is $\sigma = 5$. The solid curve marks the chi-square distribution, $P(\chi^2)$ for $n = 10$.

A visual inspection reveals that we are no longer dealing here with a normal distribution. Instead, we refer to this distribution as the χ^2 (chi-square) distribution. It describes the distribution of the sum of squared random numbers, where the random numbers by themselves are normal-distributed. Inserting the definition of s (equation 6-20) into the definition of χ^2 (equation 6-22) yields

$$\chi^2 = \sum_{i=1}^{n} \left(\frac{x_i - \bar{x}}{\sigma} \right)^2 \tag{6-24}$$

Equation 6-24 reveals that, indeed, χ^2 equals the sum of squared, normal-distributed random numbers, which are described with respect to their mean value and are scaled by the standard deviation. Because we now have eliminated two parameters, mean value and standard deviation, the χ^2 distribution depends only on one single parameter, the sample size n. Frequently, instead of the sample size n, the number of degrees of freedom $f = n - 1$ is indicated. Fig. 6-13 shows the χ^2-distribution for $f = 1$ to $f = 15$. For arbitrary n the χ^2 distribution can be described by a rather cumbersome mathematical formula. We will refrain

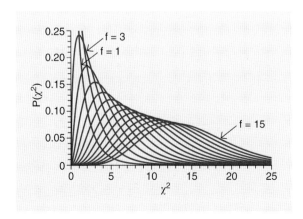

Fig. 6-13 The chi-square probability distribution $P(\chi^2)$ for different numbers of degrees of freedom from $f = 1$ to $f = 15$ as indicated. The number $n = f + 1$ specifies the size of the sample. For large values of f, the shape of the distribution approaches that of a normal distribution.

from writing that down in the general case; suffice it to specify the relation for our example with sample size n = 10 or, equivalently, f = n − 1 = 9 degrees of freedom

$$P(\chi^2) = \frac{(\chi^2)^{\frac{7}{2}} \cdot e^{-\frac{\chi^2}{2}}}{\sqrt{2 \cdot \pi} \cdot 105}$$

This function is displayed in Fig. 6-12; see the solid green line. The agreement with the "experimentally" (i.e., by means of a computer simulation) obtained frequencies in the histogram is quite satisfying. In paragraph 6.4 we will look in more detail into the case f = 1 and demonstrate how to find the corresponding distribution

$$P(\chi^2) = \frac{e^{-\frac{\chi^2}{2}}}{\sqrt{2 \cdot \pi \cdot \chi^2}}$$

Note that knowledge of the χ^2 distribution gives us access to the distribution of the standard deviations from equation 6-20, as

$$s = \sigma \cdot \sqrt{\chi^2/(n-1)}$$

Thus, we have accomplished our goal to describe the distribution of the mean values $\bar{x}$ and the standard deviations s. How can we now apply the χ^2 distribution to calculate the probability that the standard deviation of a sample lies within a certain range? For example, when we cut off, both to the left and to the right, 2.5% of the area under the χ^2 distribution, we obtain the 95% confidence interval. (Note that, as we cut off on both sides of the curve, we are dealing with a two-sided confidence interval. Obviously, we can also consider one-sided confidence intervals, depending on the nature of the problem we are investigating). Where do we find the limits of the confidence interval, when the significance level α and the number of degrees of freedom f = n − 1 are known? These values are tabulated on the Internet; see for example https://en.m.wikipedia.org/wiki/Chi-squared_distribution. Below is an excerpt of such a table, in which the numbers used in our examples are highlighted in gray:

α	2.5%	5.0%	50.0%	95.0%	97.5%
f = 1	0.001	0.004	0.45	3.84	5.02
f = 2	0.05	0.10	1.39	5.99	7.38
f = 3	0.22	0.35	2.37	7.81	9.35
f = 4	0.48	0.71	3.36	9.49	11.14
f = 9	2.70	3.33	8.34	16.92	19.02

From the table we extract for n = 10 (i.e., f = 9) the quantiles $\chi^2_{2.5\%}$ = 2.70 and $\chi^2_{97.5\%}$ = 19.02. For better visualization, we have marked the 95% confidence interval in Fig. 6-14.

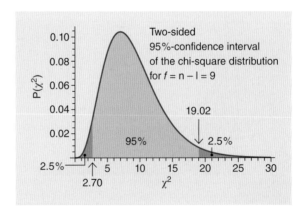

Fig. 6-14 The chi-square probability distribution $P(\chi 2)$ for $f = n − 1 = 9$. The two-sided 95%-confidence interval is marked. The quantiles $\chi^2_{2.5\%}$ = 2.70 and $\chi^2_{97.5\%}$ = 19.02 are adopted from the accompanying table.

For a known χ^2 we can calculate from equation 6-22 the confidence levels of the standard deviation $s = \sigma \cdot \sqrt{\chi^2/(n-1)}$. We obtain

$$S_{2.5\%} = \sigma \cdot \sqrt{\frac{\chi^2_{2.5\%}}{n-1}} = 5 \cdot \sqrt{\frac{2.70}{10-1}} = 2.74$$

$$S_{97.5\%} = \sigma \cdot \sqrt{\frac{\chi^2_{97.5\%}}{n-1}} = 5 \cdot \sqrt{\frac{19.02}{10-1}} = 7.27$$

The standard deviation for the number of heads in a tenfold throw of 100 coins lies with a probability of 95% within the range from 2.74 to 7.27. With a probability of 2.5%, it will be smaller than 2.74, and with a probability of 2.5%, it will be larger than 7.27.

Example

The filling weight of a marigold ointment follows a normal distribution with a mean value $\mu = 100.00$ and a standard deviation $\sigma = 2.00$ (in units of grams). This means that the filling weight of 95% of the ointments lies within a range of 100.00 ± 3.92 (see equation 6-18). The mean filling weight value of a sample of four ointments will lie, with a probability of 95%, within a range of $100.00 \pm 3.92/\sqrt{4} = 100.00 \pm 1.96$. We also wish to calculate the distribution of the standard deviations of the sample size $n = 4$. From the corresponding table we obtain the quantiles $\chi^2_{2.5\%} = 0.22$ and $\chi^2_{97.5\%} = 9.35$, which cut 2.5% off on either side of the χ^2 distribution with $f = 3$ degrees of freedom. Thus

$$S_{2.5\%} = \sigma \cdot \sqrt{\frac{\chi^2_{2.5\%}}{n-1}} = 2 \cdot \sqrt{\frac{0.22}{3}} = 0.54$$

$$S_{97.5\%} = \sigma \cdot \sqrt{\frac{\chi^2_{97.5\%}}{n-1}} = 2 \cdot \sqrt{\frac{9.35}{3}} = 3.53$$

Therefore, 95% of the standard deviations of the samples (each with $n = 4$) lie within the range $s_{2.5\%} = 0.54$ to $s_{97.5\%} = 3.53$. For a sample size of $n = 10$ we would find a range of $s_{2.5\%} = 1.10$ to $s_{97.5\%} = 2.91$. The following table shows how the scatter range of the standard deviations diminishes with increasing sample size n and approaches the value $\sigma = 2.00$ of the underlying normal distribution.

n	$s_{2.5\%}$	$s_{97.5\%}$
4	0.54	3.53
10	1.10	2.91
100	1.72	2.28
1,000	1.91	2.09
10,000	1.97	2.03

6.4 Functions of Random Variables

6.4.1 Introductory Example

The blood level value of a drug drops exponentially after a rapid initial increase following oral administration. The drop can be described as a function of time t by a first-order reaction kinetics: $dc/dt = -k \cdot c$. In this equation $c = c(t)$ represents the measured concentration in the blood at time t and k the elimination constant. If we denote the initial blood concentration of the drug (i.e., the highest concentration obtained following the rapid initial increase) as

$c(t = 0) = c_0$, we find for the exponential decrease of the drug concentration $c(t) = c_0 \cdot e^{-kt}$. The area under the $c(t)$-curve (*AUC*) is obtained by integration

$$AUC = \int_0^\infty c(t)dt = c_0 \cdot \int_0^\infty e^{-k \cdot t}dt = \frac{c_0}{k} \tag{6-25}$$

The initial concentration c_0 of the drug can be expressed as the ratio between the *dose D* (i.e., the total amount of drug in the blood at $t = 0$) and the *blood volume V*: $c_0 = D/V$. Furthermore, we define the *clearance* as $CL = k \cdot V$. This is a convenient definition because from equation 6-25 we obtain the simple relation

$$AUC = D/CL \tag{6-26}$$

The clearance CL is a drug-specific entity, which furthermore depends on a number of influences and varies from patient to patient. Because of the numerous potential factors that affect CL we may expect CL values to display a normal distribution, with a certain mean value μ and a standard deviation σ (see equation 6-16).

An interesting question now arises: given the clearance, CL, in equation 6-26 obeys a normal distribution, what then is the statistical distribution of the area under the curve, *AUC*? In order to answer this question we have carried out another computer experiment. To that end, we assumed the clearance has a mean value $\mu = 3.0$ and a standard deviation $\sigma = 0.5$, both with a unit of liter/hour $(L \cdot h^{-1})$. Using a computer we have produced 500,000 normal-distributed random numbers (with $\mu = 3.0$ and $\sigma = 0.5$); their frequencies are displayed as a histogram in Fig. 6-15. In addition, the continuous curve in Fig. 6-15 represents the normal distribution

$$P(CL) = \sqrt{\frac{2}{\pi}} \cdot e^{-2 \cdot (CL-3)^2} \tag{6-27}$$

(see equation 6-16 with $\mu = 3.0$ and $\sigma = 0.5$).

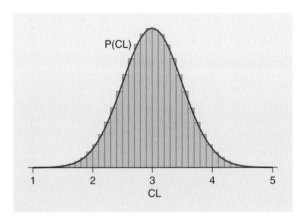

Fig. 6-15 Histogram of 500,000 normal-distributed random numbers (with $\mu = 3.0$ and $\sigma = 0.5$), representing the statistical variations of the clearance (CL). The continuous curve shows the corresponding normal distribution P(CL) according to equation 6-27.

Assuming a dose of $D = 1$ (in mg), we can determine *AUC* from equation 6-26 (in h $\cdot$ mg $\cdot$ L^{-1}). We have carried out this calculation for each of the normal-distributed clearances. The resulting relative frequencies of the 500,000 values for *AUC* are displayed again as a histogram in Fig. 6-16. For example, the value $CL = 4$ in Fig. 6-15 corresponds to an *AUC* value of $D/CL = 0.25$.

Apparently, when it comes to the distribution of *AUC* values, we are no longer dealing with a normal distribution. Hence, the inverse value of a normal-distributed random

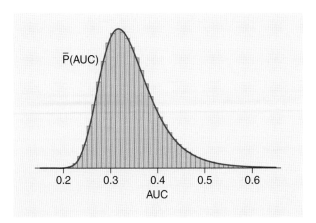

Fig. 6-16 Histogram of 500,000 normal-distributed random numbers (with $\mu = 3.0$ and $\sigma = 0.5$) representing the clearance CL, from which each time the function $AUC = D/CL$ was calculated. $D = 1$ is the administered drug dose. The continuous curve corresponds to the probability distribution $\bar{P}(AUC)$ according to equation 6-28.

variable follows no longer a normal distribution. The probability distribution we found in the histogram of Fig. 6-16 can be quantified mathematically (in paragraph 6.4.2. we will discuss how to do that) as follows

$$\bar{P}(AUC) = \sqrt{\frac{2}{\pi}} \cdot \left(\frac{1}{AUC}\right)^2 \cdot e^{-2 \cdot \left(\frac{1}{AUC} - 3\right)^2} \tag{6-28}$$

The function $\bar{P}(AUC)$ is displayed in Fig. 6-16 as a continuous curve. Obviously, we can relieve ourselves from carrying out elaborate and time-consuming computer simulations if we know how to calculate from both the probability distribution P(CL) and from the function $AUC = D/CL$ the new probability distribution $\bar{P}(AUC)$. In fact, such calculations form the most central part of statistics; they constitute the key to the understanding and application of statistical distribution functions. In the following section 6.4.2, we sketch the mathematical principle of such calculations.

Regarding our introductory example, we mention that the specific distribution function $\bar{P}(AUC)$ (see Fig. 6-16) can be converted into a new distribution function that somewhat resembles a normal distribution by considering $\bar{P}$ as function of ln AUC; that is, by presenting the distribution function on a logarithmic abscissa scale (see Fig. 6-17).

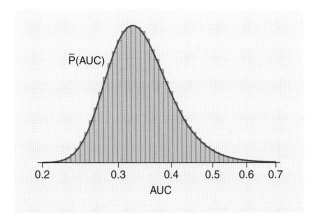

Fig. 6-17   The same histogram and the same distribution function as in Fig. 6-16, but here with a logarithmic scale on the abscissa.

6.4.2   Functions of a Random Variable

Following our introductory example of a normal-distributed clearance, CL, from the inverse of which we calculated AUC, we will now address the general problem of calculating functions of a random variable x with a probability distribution $P(x)$. We ask the following question: What is the probability distribution $\bar{P}(y)$ of a new random variable y that is calculated from the original random variable x by means of a known function $y = y(x)$? Fig. 6-18 illustrates this question.

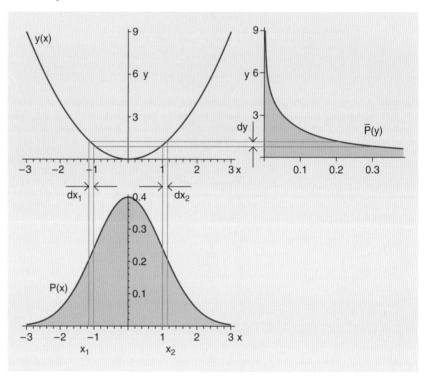

Fig. 6-18   **A random variable x has a probability distribution $P(x)$. From x we construct a new random variable y by means of the function $y(x)$. The latter satisfies the probability distribution $\bar{P}(y)$. By applying equation 6-30, we can calculate $\bar{P}(y)$ from both $P(x)$ and $y(x)$. The three diagrams $P(x)$, $y(x)$ and $\bar{P}(y)$ illustrate the conversion from $P(x)$ to $\bar{P}(y)$. Note that the right top diagram actually shows y as function of $\bar{P}(y)$. The displayed example for $P(x)$ is that of a standard normal distribution and that for $y(x)$ is the square function $y = x^2$. This leads for $\bar{P}(y)$ to the chi-square distribution $\bar{P}(y) = e^{-y/2} / \sqrt{2 \cdot \pi \cdot y}$, with one degree of freedom (also see the curve marked $f = 1$ in Fig. 6-13).**

The lower diagram shows the probability distribution $P(x)$. Above that, to the left, we see the function $y(x)$ and to the right the resulting probability distribution $\bar{P}(y)$.

To illustrate how the distribution $P(x)$ gives rise to $\bar{P}(y)$, abscissa and ordinate in the diagram for $\bar{P}(y)$ (on the top right) have been interchanged. Note that the function $y(x)$ only redistributes the probability from $P(x)$ to $\bar{P}(y)$; nothing is being lost by this operation. We point out that in Fig. 6-18 we are presenting the specific example of a standard normal distribution for $P(x)$ and a square function for $y(x)$. Obviously, we could consider any other functions $P(x)$ and $y(x)$. The probability to find the random variable in a narrow range between y and $y + dy$ is $dy \cdot \bar{P}(y)$. Which part (or parts) of the original probability $P(x)$ contributes to the probability $dy \cdot \bar{P}(y)$, depends on the function $y(x)$. Note that in the example displayed in Fig. 6-18, each value of y can be adopted by choosing two distinct x values, denoted by x_1 and x_2. Therefore we also have two contributions to the probability $dy \cdot \bar{P}(y)$, denoted $dx_1 \cdot P(x_1)$ and $dx_2 \cdot P(x_2)$. Hence,

$$dy \cdot \bar{P}(y) = dx_1 \cdot P(x_1) + dx_2 \cdot P(x_2) \tag{6-29}$$

The widths of the infinitesimal intervals dx_1 and dx_2 depend on the corresponding steepness of the function $y(x)$ and can be expressed by the two relations $dx_1 = dy \cdot |dx_1/dy|$ and

$dx_2 = dy \cdot |dx_2/dy|$. Because probabilities are always positive, we are using absolute values. Upon inserting the expressions for dx_1 and dx_2 into equation 6-29, we can eliminate dy from that equation. Finally, when regarding the two points $x_1 = x_1(y)$ and $x_2 = x_2(y)$ as functions of y, we obtain

$$\bar{P}(y) = P(x_1(y)) \cdot \left| \frac{dx_1}{dy} \right| + P(x_2(y)) \cdot \left| \frac{dx_2}{dy} \right| \tag{6-30}$$

Thus, in order to calculate $\bar{P}(y)$, we must use the inverse function $x(y)$ as well as its first derivative at the positions x_1 and x_2. It amounts to two terms that contribute to the right hand side of Equation 6-30 because in Fig. 6-18 we have considered for $y = y(x)$ a square function, which assigns the same value for two different choices of x. In general, we need to include as many terms into the calculation of $P(y)$, as there are values of x for which $y = y(x)$ is satisfied. Accordingly, we write for the general case

$$\bar{P}(y) = \sum_i P(x_i(y)) \cdot \left| \frac{dx_i}{dy} \right| \tag{6-31}$$

in which the index i runs over all possible values x_i that produce a given value y through the function $y = y(x_i)$.

Let us now return briefly to our introductory example. There we had considered a normal distributed random variable CL and, from that, defined the new random variable $AUC = D/CL$. Because this function is injective (it assigns exactly one single value of CL to any choice of AUC) we can simply calculate the probability distribution for AUC by means of $\bar{P}(AUC) = P(CL(AUC)) \cdot |dCL/dAUC|$. Because $|dCL/dAUC| = D/AUC^2$ and $D = 1$, we indeed obtain the result in equation 6-28.

The conversion of the random variable in equation 6-31 has numerous applications and leads to a series of important probability distributions. We list just a few examples:

1. The case shown in Fig. 6-18 is $y = x^2$, and $P(x)$ satisfies the standard normal distribution (see equation 6-17). For the distribution of $\bar{P}(y)$ we then obtain the chi-square distribution $\bar{P}(y) = e^{-y/2}/\sqrt{2 \cdot \pi \cdot y}$ for a single degree of freedom $f = n - 1 = 1$ (i.e., for a sample size $n = 2$). This function is displayed both in Fig. 6-18 (diagram on the right) and in Fig. 6-13 (the curve marked $f = 1$).

2. When considering the function $y = e^x$ of a normal-distributed random variable we obtain the log-normal distribution. Among the random processes it describes are the length of fingernails, the weight of sunflower seeds, the income distribution of a nation, the distribution of damage claims in insurance cases and the elevation of cities above sea level (see Fig. 6-10).

3. Another example is the function $y = x^\alpha$ of the exponential distribution $P(x) = \lambda \cdot e^{-\lambda \cdot x}$ (with $x \geq 0$), where α and λ are positive constants. For $\bar{P}(y)$ we obtain the so-called Weibull distribution, which describes, for example, the distribution of the life-time of lightbulbs (and several other technical devices) as well as the wear and failure of materials.

4. If a random variable x satisfies a normal distribution (with mean value μ and standard deviation σ) and if another random variable $y = a \cdot x + b$ is linearly dependent on x (a and b are arbitrary constants), then also y is normal-distributed, albeit with mean value $a \cdot \mu + b$ and standard deviation $\sigma \cdot |a|$. Linear functions generally lead to stretching (or compression) of probability distributions, without changing their principle character.

6.4.3   Functions of Several Random Variables

We will now take our discussion one step further and consider functions of more than one single random variable. If, for example, x_1 and x_2 are random variables with a corresponding probability distribution $P(x_1, x_2)$, we may ask which probability distribution $\bar{P}(y)$ will be satisfied by the new random variable $y = y(x_1, x_2)$. The answer can be found in analogy to our reasoning for a function of only one single random variable. We will, however, not enter into any of the mathematical details of the derivation for the general case, but instead provide the reader with a number of specific examples:

1. If two statistically independent random variables x_1 and x_2 are normal-distributed (with corresponding mean values μ_1 und μ_2 and standard deviations σ_1 and σ_2, respectively, then also the sum $y = x_1 + x_2$ is normal-distributed. The resulting mean value amounts to $\mu_1 + \mu_2$, and the standard deviation is $\sqrt{\sigma_1^2 + \sigma_2^2}$. In section 6.4.4 we will rediscover this result in the context of error propagation.

2. Assume we are dealing with n statistically independent, standard normal-distributed random variables x_i with $i = 1 \ldots n$ (i.e., $\mu_i = 0$ and $\sigma_i = 1$ for each of the normal-distributed random variables). Then, the new random variable $y = \sum_{i=1}^{n} x_i^2$ defines the chi-square distribution for $f = n - 1$ degrees of freedom. The chi-square distribution is displayed in Fig. 6-13 for $f = 1$ to $f = 15$.

3. A random variable x_1 is standard normal-distributed (see equation 6-17). Another statistically independent random variable x_2 satisfies the chi-square distribution with $f = n - 1$ degrees of freedom (see Fig. 6-13). The new random variable $y = x_1 \cdot (n - 1)/x_2$ is then distributed according to the Student's t-distribution for $f = n - 1$ degrees of freedom. The Student's t-distribution was introduced in 1908 by William Sealy Gosset, who published, as an employee of the Guinness Brewery in Dublin, under the pseudonym "Student." It is used for the analysis of the distribution of means of samples (particularly small samples) of normal-distributed data when the standard deviation of the underlying normal distribution is not known beforehand. The corresponding probability distributions for 1–5 degrees of freedom are graphically displayed in Fig. 6-19. In the limit of an infinite number of degrees of freedom the Student's t-distribution becomes exactly identical to the standard normal distribution. In practice, the two can be considered identical already for about 30 (or more) degrees of freedom.

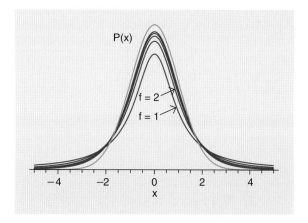

Fig. 6-19 The probability $P(x)$ according to the Student's t-distribution for 1–5 degrees of freedom (f). In the limit of an infinite number of degrees of freedom the t-distribution becomes identical to the standard normal distribution; the latter is displayed by the curve colored light-green.

6.4.4   Error Propagation

Assume we wish to determine a quantity y that depends on a measurable quantity x through a function $y = f(x)$. During the measurement of x, a random observational error occurs, implying that x, and thus also y, are random variables. To make our reasoning more specific, let us consider the surface area $y = \pi \cdot x^2/4$ of a circle, which we determine by means of measuring the diameter x. The following sequence of five measurements is recorded

i	1	2	3	4	5
x_i/m	2.0093	1.9404	1.9878	1.9837	1.9752

We may view the set of measured diameters as a sample of size $n = 5$. The sample represents a random sample, unless our measurement involves not only random but also systematic errors. From the individually measured values x_i we determine the mean value $\bar{x} = 1.979$ m and the standard deviation $s_x = 0.025$ m. When we repeatedly take samples of size $n = 5$, each time the mean value $\bar{x}$ will vary to some extent. We already know from equation 6-23 that we can calculate the statistical variation of the mean value through $s_{\bar{x}} = s_x/\sqrt{n} = 0.011$ m. We can compactly express the mean diameter together with its statistical variation as $\bar{x} \pm s_{\bar{x}} = (1.979 \pm 0.011)$ m. The uncertainty of a measured quantity is often indicated by one or two significant digits. In addition, the values of the mean and its variation should be specified with the same number of decimals.

The question now is how we determine the surface area of the circle and how the statistical uncertainty of the diameter x relates to that of the surface area y. Even without knowing anything about error propagation, we can answer this question. To that end, we simply calculate from each individual measurement x_i the corresponding area $y_i = \pi \cdot x_i^2/4$

i	1	2	3	4	5
y_i/m^2	3.1708	2.9571	3.1033	3.0906	3.0640

and subsequently calculate the mean area $\bar{y} = 3.077$ m^2 and its variation $s_{\bar{y}} = s_y/\sqrt{n} = 0.079\,\text{m}^2/\sqrt{5} = 0.035$ m^2. So, the final result of our calculation is

$$\bar{y} \pm s_{\bar{y}} = (3.077 \pm 0.035) \text{ m}^2 \tag{6-32}$$

This method comes with the disadvantage that the function $y = f(x)$ has to be applied to each individual measurement, which especially for involved functions is not convenient. In addition, we often do not even have access to all the individual function values. So the question arises whether we can deduce $\bar{y}$ and $s_{\bar{y}}$ directly from the mean value $\bar{x}$ and its variation $s_{\bar{y}}$, combined with our knowledge of the function $y = f(x)$. The answer is: yes, we can! And this is not even difficult if we assume that the individual values $y_i = f(x_i)$ are not very far from the mean value $\bar{y}$. We can then calculate the values $y_i = f(x_i)$ approximately via

$$f(x_i) = f(\bar{x}) + \left(\frac{df}{dx}\right)_{\bar{x}} \cdot (x_i - \bar{x}) \tag{6-33}$$

Equation 6-33 is known from calculus as a Taylor series expansion, carried out up to the linear order. It rests on the simple idea to approximate the behavior of $f(x)$ in the vicinity of the position $\bar{x}$ by a linear function; that is, by a tangent line that touches the function $f(x)$ at the point $\bar{x}$. This is illustrated graphically in Fig. 6-20. The slope of the tangent is given by the first derivative $(df/dx)_{\bar{x}}$ of the function $f(x)$ at position $\bar{x}$. Equation 6-33 describes the dashed straight line in Fig. 6-20.

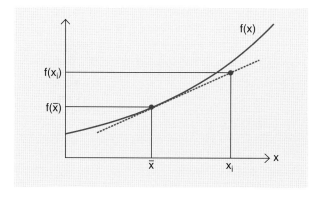

Fig. 6-20 The function $f(x)$ can be approximated close to the point $\bar{x}$ by a tangent (displayed as a dashed line). Equation 6-33 presents a mathematical expression of this tangent line.

Using equation 6-33, we are now ready to calculate the mean value

$$\bar{y} = \frac{1}{n}\sum_{i=1}^{n} y_i = \frac{1}{n}\sum_{i=1}^{n} f(x_i)$$

$$= \frac{1}{n}\sum_{i=1}^{n} \left[f(\bar{x}) + \left(\frac{df}{dx}\right)_{\bar{x}} \cdot (x_i - \bar{x})\right] = f(\bar{x})$$

In general, the simple relation $\bar{y} = f(\bar{x})$ only applies to linear functions $f(x)$. It is the Taylor series expansion that has provided for this linearization. We also still wish to calculate the statistical variation $s_{\bar{y}}$ from $s_{\bar{x}}$. To this end, we recall the calculation of the mean-value deviations

$$s_{\bar{x}} = \sqrt{\frac{1}{n \cdot (1 - n)} \cdot \sum_{i=1}^{n} (x_i - \bar{x})^2}$$

$$s_{\bar{y}} = \sqrt{\frac{1}{n \cdot (1 - n)} \cdot \sum_{i=1}^{n} (y_i - \bar{y})^2} \qquad (6\text{-}34)$$

Using the relation $\bar{y} = f(\bar{x})$ derived above, we insert equation 6-33, that is,

$$y_i - \bar{y} = \left(\frac{df}{dx}\right)_{\bar{x}} \cdot (x_i - \bar{x})$$

into equation 6-34. This gives rise to

$$s_{\bar{y}} = \sqrt{\left(\frac{df}{dx}\right)_{\bar{x}}^2 \cdot s_{\bar{x}}^2} = \left|\left(\frac{df}{dx}\right)_{\bar{x}}\right| \cdot s_{\bar{x}} \qquad (6\text{-}35)$$

The final result we obtain is thus

$$\bar{y} \pm s_{\bar{y}} = f(\bar{x}) \pm \left|\left(\frac{df}{dx}\right)_{\bar{x}}\right| \cdot s_{\bar{x}} \qquad (6\text{-}36)$$

Returning to our example in equation 6-32 and to the function $f(x) = \pi \cdot x^2/4$, we obtain $f(1.979 \text{ m}) = 3.077 \text{ m}$ and $(df/dx)_{\bar{x}} = 3.109 \text{ m}$, or $(df/dx)_{\bar{x}} \cdot s_{\bar{x}} = 0.035 \text{ m}$. Thus, we indeed reproduce the result in equation 6-32. The reason is that we can approximate the function $f(x)$ within the scattering range of the x_i very well by a linear function (even though $f(x)$ is actually a quadratic function).

Based on equation 6-35 we are now in the position to discuss how variations of a measured quantity x translate into variations of a quantity y that depends on x through a known function $y = f(x)$. For example, $f(x) = 1/x$ leads to $s_{\bar{y}} = s_{\bar{x}}/\bar{x}^2$, and thus $s_{\bar{y}}/\bar{y} = s_{\bar{x}}/\bar{x}$. Here, the relative error $s_{\bar{x}}/\bar{x}$ is transmitted. Another example is $f(x) = e^x$, leading to $s_{\bar{y}}/\bar{y} = s_{\bar{x}}$. In this case the absolute value of the statistical variation of $\bar{x}$ produces the relative statistical variation of $\bar{y}$. We encourage the reader to analyze additional examples.

Consider now the presence of two random variables x_1 and x_2 that represent independently measured quantities. We wish to calculate a new quantity $y = f(x_1, x_2)$ from these two measured quantities. How do we calculate the mean value $\bar{y}$ from the mean values $\bar{x}_1$ and $\bar{x}_2$? And how do we find the statistical variation $s_{\bar{y}}$ of the mean value $\bar{y}$ from the statistical variations $s_{\bar{x}_1}$ and $s_{\bar{x}_2}$ of the mean values $\bar{x}_1$ and $\bar{x}_2$? The answers for two independent random variables can be found by the same method as was used for one independent random variable. When the two measured values x_1 and x_2 deviate only slightly from the mean values, $\bar{x}_1$ and $\bar{x}_2$, we find $\bar{y} = f(\bar{x}_1, \bar{x}_2)$ and

> Hint: To take the partial derivative of a function $f(x_1, x_2)$ with respect to one of its two variables, say x_1, we simply calculate the usual first derivative $df(x_1)/dx_1$ of f with respect to x_1 while keeping the other variable, x_2, constant. For example, for $f(x_1, x_2) = x_1^2 + x_1 \cdot x_2$ we find the partial derivative $(\partial f/\partial x_1) = 2 \cdot x_1 + x_2$. Similarly, $(\partial f/\partial x_2) = x_1$. To calculate the partial derivative at a certain position $x_1 = \bar{x}_1$ and $x_2 = \bar{x}_2$, we simply introduce this, after calculating the derivative, into the obtained mathematical expression: $(\partial f/\partial x_1)_{\bar{x}_1, \bar{x}_2} = 2 \cdot \bar{x}_1 + \bar{x}_2$ and $(\partial f/\partial x_2)_{\bar{x}_1, \bar{x}_2} = \bar{x}_1$.

$$s_{\bar{y}} = \sqrt{\left(\frac{\partial f}{\partial x_1}\right)_{\bar{x}_1, \bar{x}_2}^2 \cdot s_{\bar{x}_1}^2 + \left(\frac{\partial f}{\partial x_2}\right)_{\bar{x}_1, \bar{x}_2}^2 \cdot s_{\bar{x}_2}^2} \qquad (6\text{-}37)$$

Equation 6-37 is known as the *Gaussian error propagation rule*. In this equation, $(\partial f/\partial x_1)_{\bar{x}_1, \bar{x}_2}$ signifies the partial derivative of the function $f(x_1, x_2)$ with respect to x_1, taken at the position $x_1 = \bar{x}_1$ and $x_2 = \bar{x}_2$ (and analogously for $(\partial f/\partial x_2)_{\bar{x}_1, \bar{x}_2}$).

In case $f(x_1, x_2)$ does not depend on two but rather on one single variable—for instance, $f(x_1, x_2) = f(x_1)$, then $(\partial f/\partial x_2) = 0$ and equation 6-37 reduces to

$$s_{\bar{y}} = \sqrt{\left(\frac{df}{dx_1}\right)_{\bar{x}_1}^2 \cdot s_{\bar{x}_1}^2} = \left|\left(\frac{df}{dx_1}\right)_{\bar{x}_1}\right| \cdot s_{\bar{x}_1}$$

This is exactly the result from equation 6-35. The latter can therefore be viewed as the Gaussian error propagation rule applied to the presence of only one single random variable. Conversely, we can generalize the Gaussian error propagation rule of equation 6-37 in a straightforward manner to an arbitrary number of independent random variables.

When two random variables x_1 and x_2 are added, $y = x_1 + x_2$, then the statistical variations "add" according to

$$s_{\bar{y}} = \sqrt{s_{\bar{x}_1}^2 + s_{\bar{x}_2}^2}$$

Assume, for example, that milk bottles are filled with (1.000 ± 0.010) Liters (L) of milk per bottle. Then two filled bottles will contain a total volume of (2.000 ± 0.014) L of milk. Similarly, 100 bottles contain (100.0 ± 0.1) L, not (100.0 ± 1.0) L.

Another interesting example is $y = x_1 \cdot x_2$. In this case, we find

$$\frac{s_{\bar{y}}}{\bar{y}} = \sqrt{\frac{s_{\bar{x}_1}^2}{\bar{x}_1^2} + \frac{s_{\bar{x}_2}^2}{\bar{x}_2^2}}$$

So, when we measure the two sides of a rectangle as $x_1 = (1.00 \pm 0.01)$ m and $x_2 = (2.00 \pm 0.10)$ m, the area of the rectangle is $A = x_1 \cdot x_2 = (2.00 \pm 0.10)$ m^2. The scatter of the surface area determination is, in this case, almost exclusively determined by the uncertainty of only one of the two measured input parameters. This kind of error mismatch is frequent; its recognition can help to carry out error estimations efficiently.

Example

(4.50 ± 0.30) g sodium chloride is dissolved in water to a final volume of 0.500 ± 0.020 L. What is the (molar) concentration of this salt solution?

Solution: We know the mean value of the sodium chloride mass, $\bar{m} = 4.50$ g and the standard deviation $s_{\bar{m}} = 0.30$ g. Furthermore, we know the mean value $\bar{V} = 0.500$ L and the standard deviation $s_{\bar{V}} = 0.020$ L of the volume of the solution. The concentration c of the solution is calculated from the mass m of the salt and the volume V of the solution via $c = m/(V \cdot M)$, in which $M = 58.4$ g/mol is the molecular mass of NaCl. For the mean value of the concentration, we find $\bar{c} = \bar{m}/(\bar{V} \cdot M) = 0.154$ mol/L. The standard deviation is calculated according to the Gaussian error propagation rule (equation 6-37)

$$s_{\bar{c}} = \sqrt{\left(\frac{dc}{dm}\right)_{\bar{m}, \bar{V}}^2 \cdot s_{\bar{m}}^2 + \left(\frac{dc}{dV}\right)_{\bar{m}, \bar{V}}^2 \cdot s_{\bar{V}}^2}$$

This leads us to

$$s_{\bar{c}} = \sqrt{\left(\frac{1}{\bar{V} \cdot M}\right)^2 s_{\bar{m}}^2 + \left(\frac{\bar{m}}{\bar{V}^2 \cdot M}\right)^2 \cdot s_{\bar{V}}^2}$$

$$= \frac{1}{\bar{V}} \cdot \sqrt{\left(\frac{s_{\bar{m}}}{M}\right)^2 + (\bar{c} \cdot s_{\bar{V}})^2} = 0.012 \frac{mol}{L}$$

Thus, the result is $c = (0.154 \pm 0.012)$ mol/L. By the way, this is an isotonic sodium chloride solution.

6.5 Statistical Tests

A large number of statistical tests have been developed, many of which are listed in textbooks or can be found on the internet. In the following section we merely aim to explain what a statistical test is and what we can do with it. To that end, we present two related tests, the Z-test and the Student's t-test.

6.5.1 Example of a *Z*-test

It is convenient to introduce the underlying idea and the procedure of performing a statistical test using a specific example: We recall our coin throw experiment in which we threw 100 identical coins simultaneously (or one coin 100 times). The obtained number of heads follows a normal distribution with mean value $\mu_0 = 50$ and standard deviation $\sigma = 5$. Now we wish to know whether it will make a difference if we cover the tails side of all coins with honey or another sticky substance. Although the coins are now no longer symmetric, it is not quite obvious whether the honey will actually shift the mean value μ away from μ_0. (A related scenario, the dropping of a buttered slice of toast, has actually been analyzed by a team of scientists). Assume we have subjected our 100 tail-coated coins to a statistical test and thrown all of them. The result was 59 times heads and 41 times tails. Now what?

In the field of statistical testing, it is customary to perform hypothesis tests. That is, we test an assumption about a statistical relationship between data sets. Typically, we postulate a null hypothesis (H_0), which asserts that the observed data result from statistical variations of the sample, but do not reflect a change in the underlying statistical distribution. The null hypothesis is juxtaposed by an alternative hypothesis (H_1), which postulates that the observed data originate from a different statistical distribution. The aim of the statistical test is to accumulate evidence that contradicts the null hypothesis with high probability. When this fails, we will have no reason to abandon our assumption that the null hypothesis is correct. It is important to emphasize that the validity of the null hypothesis can never be proven. By the way, the same reasoning applies to all physical laws. The correctness of a physical law cannot be proven. We can only assume it is correct as long as it is not shown to be incorrect.

In our coin example, the null hypothesis is that the honey has no effect on the mean value: that the number of heads in a given sample is not precisely $\mu_0 = 50$ is simply the result of statistical variations in how many heads shown up after throwing symmetric coins. We write for the null hypothesis $H_0: \mu = \mu_0$. The alternative hypothesis says in its most general form that the honey does have an effect on the mean value; we express this by writing $H_1: \mu \neq \mu_0$. This includes both possibilities: the honey either favors or suppresses the occurrence of heads. More restricted alternative hypotheses are possible. Below, we will come back to that. Now, once again, our null hypothesis and the alternative hypothesis are

$$H_0: \mu = \mu_0, \qquad H_1: \mu \neq \mu_0$$

It remains to set a significance level α. Often $\alpha = 0.05$ is chosen (that is, 5%). The significance level α corresponds to the probability that the sample provides us with a result that makes us reject the null hypothesis even if it is correct. Such an error is commonly referred to as an *error of the first kind*. Obviously, we prefer α to be as small as possible because we do not want to reject the null hypothesis in case it actually is correct. On the other hand, if we choose a value for α that is too small, there is a high probability that we will fail to reject the null hypothesis although it is incorrect. This error is called an *error of the second kind*, and the probability that it occurs is denoted β.

Error of the first kind: rejecting the null hypothesis although it is correct.
Error of the second kind: not rejecting the null hypothesis although it is incorrect.

In order to conduct a meaningful test, we need a test statistic z: a function that condenses the data into a single numerical value that we can compare with a known statistical distribution. In our coin-throwing example, the choice of the test statistic is quite simple. We have already drawn a sample (i.e., throwing 100 coins that have their tails coated with honey) and counted $\bar{x} = 59$ times heads. Recall that the single throw of 100 symmetric coins represents a sample from a normal distribution with a mean value $\mu_0 = 50$ and a standard deviation $\sigma = 5$. Consequently, $z = (\bar{x} - \mu_0)/\sigma$ would be a meaningful test statistic. In case the null hypothesis is correct, the statistical distribution of z corresponds to a standard normal distribution (see equation 6-17). We can generalize the test statistic also to the case of an n-fold throwing of 100 coins. As we know from equation 6-23, for n samples the standard deviation of the sampled mean decreases from σ to $\sigma/\sqrt{n}$. Therefore, we choose for a sample size n a test statistic

$$z = \frac{\bar{x} - \mu_0}{\sigma} \cdot \sqrt{n} \qquad (6\text{-}38)$$

In our example (59 times heads for a single sample), we find $z = (59 - 50)/5 = 1.80$. We compare this value with the standard normal distribution. As we already know from the diagram in Fig. 6-8, the two-sided confidence interval from -1.96 to $+1.96$ corresponds to a significance level of $\alpha = 0.05$. As our test statistic $z = 1.80$ lies within this range, we have no reason the reject the null hypothesis. Only for results larger than 59 or smaller than 41 observed heads would we have rejected the null hypothesis, as these occur with a probability of less than 5%. In the foregoing, we have conducted a Z-test, which is defined as a statistical test in which, under the assumption of the null hypothesis, the test statistic derives from a standard normal distribution of the underlying population. Two additional points deserve attention:

1. Had we chosen a significance level $\alpha = 0.1$ (or 10%), the two-sided confidence interval would have ranged from -1.645 to $+1.645$. In this case our test statistic $z = 1.80$ would have been outside the confidence interval and, thus, would have triggered a rejection of the null hypothesis. We see that our decision to reject the null hypothesis depends on our choice of the significance level. That rightly strikes us as quite unsatisfactory, because the question whether or not the underlying statistical distribution changes by putting honey on one face of the coins obviously does not depend on α.

2. One might argue that the honey on the tails of the coins, in case it would affect the distribution of heads *vs.* tails (i.e., in case it would alter the underlying statistical distribution), affects the distribution in such a way that on average "heads" would occur more frequently than "tails." This additional knowledge influences the statistical test, because it can now be conducted one-sidedly. In this case, we would by no means accept the occurrence of, for example, only $50 - 15 = 35$ times "heads" as an indication to reject the null hypothesis, but insist on interpreting it as a statistical variation. In contrast, observing instead $50 + 15 = 65$ times "heads" could very well mean that, depending on our choice of the significance level α, we would say good-bye to the null hypothesis. Null hypothesis and alternative hypothesis now read $H_0 : \mu = \mu_0$ and $H_1 : \mu > \mu_0$. Let us choose once more a significance level $\alpha = 0.05$. The one-sided 5% confidence interval of a standard normal distribution is displayed in the upper diagram of Fig. 6-8. It extends from $-\infty$ to 1.645. Our test statistic $z = 1.80$ now lies outside the confidence interval. Therefore, we reject the null hypothesis and accept the alternative hypothesis that the honey increases the average number of thrown heads. Our additional knowledge has sharpened our test and, in this case, changed our interpretation of the observed sample.

Let us assume that the honey indeed modifies the underlying statistical distribution as is illustrated in Fig. 6-21.

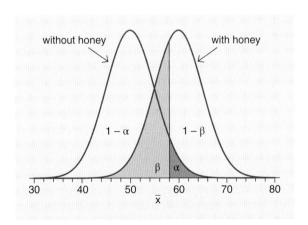

Fig. 6-21 The statistical probability distribution for the example of throwing 100 coins with and without honey covering the "tails" side. Only the distribution for the case without honey is known. It corresponds to the null hypothesis. Increasing the significance level α also increases the probability of making an error of the first kind, that is, of rejecting the possibly correct null hypothesis. Conversely, upon decreasing α, the probability increases that we do not reject a possibly incorrect null hypothesis. This error of the second kind has a probability β. A change of α in one direction implies a change of β in the opposite direction.

The distribution on the left-hand side corresponds to our null hypothesis and represents therefore a normal distribution with $\mu_0 = 50$ and $\sigma = 5$. At a significance level of $\alpha = 0.05$, the one-sided confidence interval reaches from 0 to $50.0 + 1.64 \cdot 5 = 58.2$. A sample result outside this range (i.e., larger than 58) would therefore lead to a rejection of the null hypothesis. Assume the distribution on the right-hand side corresponds to the new honey-induced probability distribution. Of course, in reality we do not know what distribution this is, and it may not even be a normal distribution. As discussed, for a sample result equal or smaller than 58, we would not reject the null hypothesis, despite the fact that it is incorrect. This error of the second kind is made with a probability β. The probability β is indicated in Fig. 6-21 (roughly 40%). As a consequence, making the correct decision, rejection of the null hypothesis, occurs with a probability of only $(1 - \beta)$. The parameter $(1 - \beta)$ is called the *statistical power* (or, briefly, *power*) of the test. A high power corresponds to a small β. However, as already mentioned above, we wish to keep both α and β small. From Fig. 6-21 it becomes clear, however, that it is not possible to realize both at the same time. A decrease of α inevitably leads to an increase of β (and *vice versa*). The smaller α, the more difficult it is to detect a potential effect (of the honey on the heads' frequency). The fundamental problem is that the two distributions in Fig. 6-21 overlap each other. A large overlap implies a generically high uncertainty when deciding between the null and the alternative hypothesis. A potential way out of this dilemma is offered by increasing the sample size n. If we conduct the coin experiment (throwing 100 coins with their tails honey-coated) not only once but multiple times ($n > 1$), the standard deviation σ of the distribution will decrease, while its mean will stay the same. Fig. 6-22 illustrates the impact of the smaller standard deviation. As in Fig. 6-21, here too we have chosen a significance level of $\alpha = 0.05$. However, the probability β of making an error of the second kind has now become much smaller because the two distributions show little overlap. Unfortunately, we do not know the actual distribution. Occasionally, however, it is possible to predict roughly how large a potential effect is, allowing us to estimate an optimal sample size.

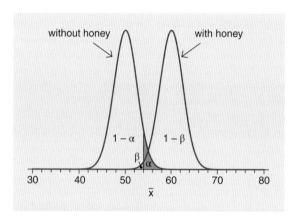

Fig. 6-22   The same scenario as in Fig. 6-21, but now for throwing the 100 coins four times each with and without honey on the tails side. The increase of the sample size from *n* = 1 to *n* = 4 reduces the width of the distributions to one half, without changing the mean values. The probabilities α and β of making an error of the first and second kind both diminish upon increasing the sample size.

6.5.2   Student's *t*-test

In our previous example of a Z-test, the standard deviation σ of the underlying normal distribution was known. In other cases, the standard deviation of a normal-distributed random variable may be known as an empirical parameter (e.g., as the result of excessive preceding sampling). Most often, however, this is not the case. In the absence of such knowledge, we apply the Student's t-test (or, briefly, t-test) instead of the Z-test. A multitude of t-tests is known. All of them are based on a normal-distributed random variable with unknown standard deviation, and all of them compare a test statistic calculated from the available sampling data with the Student's t-distribution introduced in section 6.4.3. Recall that the Student's t-distribution $y = x_1 \cdot \sqrt{(n - 1)/x_2}$ results from a combination of two random variables—one standard normal-distributed variable x_1 and a second variable x_2 that satisfies a chi-square distribution with $n - 1$ degrees of freedom. Let us assume we take a sample x_i of size n (i = $1, \ldots, n$) from a normal-distributed population (with known mean value μ and unknown standard deviation σ) and calculate from this the usual sample parameters, the mean value $\bar{x}$ (according to equation 6-19) and the standard deviation s (according to equation 6-20).

Motivated by equations 6-38 and 6-22 let us now identify the parameter $(\bar{x} - \mu_0) \cdot \sqrt{n}/\sigma$ with the random variable x_1 and the parameter $(n - 1)s^2/\sigma^2$ with the random variable x_2. Thus, we can write for the t-distribution

$$y = x_1 \cdot \frac{\sqrt{n - 1}}{\sqrt{x_2}} = \frac{\bar{x} - \mu_0}{\sigma} \cdot \sqrt{n} \cdot \frac{\sqrt{n - 1}}{\sqrt{(n - 1) \cdot s^2/\sigma^2}} = \frac{\bar{x} - \mu_0}{s} \cdot \sqrt{n}$$

From this consideration, we conclude that the parameter $z = [(\bar{x} - \mu_0)/s] \cdot \sqrt{n}$ satisfies the Student's t-distribution. The latter is therefore identified with our test statistic z. While with known standard deviation σ we compare the test function $[(\bar{x} - \mu_0) \cdot \sqrt{n}]/\sigma$ with the standard normal distribution, in the t-test the test function $[(\bar{x} - \mu_0) \cdot \sqrt{n}]/s$ is compared with the Student's t-distribution. The Student's t-distribution is plotted in Fig. 6-19 for various degrees of freedom $f = n - 1$. It is broader than the standard normal distribution, because it has to take into account the uncertainty of not knowing the standard deviation. Instead of the standard deviation σ, the standard deviation of the sample s is used in this case. For a significance level of $\alpha = 0.05$ the two-sided confidence interval of the standard normal distribution reaches from $= -1.96$ to $+1.96$. For the Student's t-distribution the confidence interval depends on the sample size n (or the number of degrees of freedom $f = n - 1$). For example, in case of $n = 4$ and a significance level $\alpha = 0.05$ the two-sided confidence interval of the t-distribution stretches from -3.182 to $+3.182$. This range is depicted graphically in Fig. 6-23. As for the normal distribution, we can, of course, also consider a one-sided confidence interval. Whether we apply a one- or a two-sided confidence interval depends on the nature of the question we are asking.

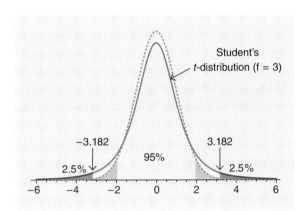

Fig. 6-23 The two-sided 95%-confidence interval of the Student's *t*-distribution with $f = 3$ degrees of freedom for a significance level $\alpha = 0.05$. 95% of the total probability falls within the interval -3.182 to 3.182 and 2.5% each lie in the regions smaller than -3.182 or larger than 3.182. For the sake of comparison, the broken line shows the standard normal distribution with its 95% confidence interval highlighted.

The limits of the confidence interval for a given significance level α can be obtained from the Internet—for instance, at https://en.m.wikipedia.org/wiki/Student%27s_t-distribution. Below is an excerpt of such a table:

α	two-sided confidence interval				
	50%	10%	5%	2%	1%
α	one-sided confidence interval				
	25%	5%	2.5%	1%	0.5%
f=1	1.000	6.314	12.706	31.821	63.657
f=2	0.816	2.920	4.303	6.965	9.925
f=3	0.765	2.353	3.182	4.541	5.841
f=4	0.741	2.132	2.776	3.747	4.604
f=5	0.727	2.015	2.571	3.365	4.032

The table shows the limits of the one- or two-sided confidence interval of different significance levels α. Different rows in the table correspond to the different degrees of freedom $f = n - 1$, where n denotes the sample size. The value that we have discussed above (for $f = 3$ and $\alpha = 0.05$) is highlighted in gray (see also Fig. 6-23).

If we take a sample of size $n = 4$ and calculate from this the mean value $\bar{x}$ and the standard deviation s, the mean value μ_0 of the underlying normal distribution satisfies with a probability of 95% the inequalities $-3.182 \leq [(\bar{x} - \mu_0)/s] \cdot \sqrt{n} \leq 3.182$. Upon isolation of μ_0, we obtain

$$\bar{x} - 3.182 \cdot \frac{s}{\sqrt{n}} \leq \mu_0 \leq \bar{x} + 3.182 \cdot \frac{s}{\sqrt{n}} \tag{6-39}$$

Now we only have to introduce concrete numbers for $\bar{x}$ and s in order to obtain an estimate of the mean value μ_0 of the underlying normal distribution. If, for example, we found upon analysis of a batch of tablets the following values for their content of an active ingredient in a sample of four tablets—64 mg, 66 mg, 89 mg, and 77 mg—we calculate $\bar{x} = 74$ mg and $s = 11.5$ mg. By introducing these values into equation 6-39 we obtain: $(74 - 18)$ mg $\leq \mu_0 \leq (74 + 18)$ mg. The average mass of the active agent for the entire batch therefore lies with 95% probability within the range $\mu_0 = (74 \pm 18)$ mg.

Now we discuss the actual t-test. As mentioned above, the term t-test refers to an array of statistical tests in which an appropriately defined test statistic is compared with the Student's t-distribution. The most simple one is the single-sample t-test (also referred to as one-sample t-test). It tests whether the calculated mean value $\bar{x}$ and standard deviation s of a sample likely originate from another underlying normal distribution than that corresponding to a pre-specified mean value μ_0. In the example presented above, we found for the content of active ingredient of four tablets the values 64, 66, 89, and 77 mg. We wish to find out whether these values are consistent with an underlying normal distribution with, say, $\mu_0 = 58$ mg, or whether they originate from another underlying normal distribution with a mean value $\mu \neq \mu_0$. In other words, does the mean value of the entire batch (of which we know only a sample of size n concur with the target value $\mu_0 = 58$ mg? Corresponding to the null hypothesis H_0 and the alternative hypothesis H_1 this is, respectively, true or not true. The mathematical formulation of the two hypotheses is $H_0: \mu = \mu_0$ and $H_1: \mu \neq \mu_0$. As we will not preclude either one of the two alternatives $\mu > \mu_0$ and $\mu < \mu$, we conduct the test two-sidedly. With a standard deviation $s = 11.5$ mg and a sample size $n = 4$ we calculate for the test statistic $z = [(\bar{x} - \mu_0)/s] \cdot \sqrt{n} = [(74 - 58)/11.5] \cdot \sqrt{4} = 2.78$ and compare this with the two-sided confidence interval $-3.182 \ldots\ldots 3.182$ of the Student's t-distribution with $n - 1 = 4 - 1 = 3$ degrees of freedom. As the test statistic 2.78 lies within the confidence interval, we do not reject the null hypothesis. This means that, at a significance level $\alpha = 0.05$, we have not been able to demonstrate that the sample (with values 64, 66, 89, and 77 mg) originates from an underlying normal distribution whose mean value μ differs from $\mu_0 = 58$ mg.

Let us assume that we know in our example of the active ingredient analysis the standard deviation σ of the underlying normal distribution and that, incidentally, it is equal to the standard deviation $s = 11.5$ of the sample of four tablets. Again, we can ask the question whether the sample originates from an underlying normal distribution with a mean different from the target value $\mu_0 = 58$ mg. As we now know the standard deviation $\sigma = 11.5$ mg, we conduct the Z-test, implying we use the test function $z = (\bar{x} - \mu_0) \cdot \sqrt{n}/\sigma = 2.78$ and compare this with the two-sided 95% confidence interval (from -1.96 to 1.96) of the standard normal distribution. In this case the test statistic lies outside the confidence interval. Therefore, we reject the null hypothesis. Hence, depending on whether we do or we do not know the standard deviation of the underlying normal distribution, while otherwise the sample values are identical, we either reject or accept the null hypothesis in our example. Quite generally, we can say that additional knowledge makes statistical tests more predictive and thus lends them more validity.

Another application of the Student's t-distribution is the two-sample t-test. As the name already suggests, in this case we compare two normal-distributed samples with respect to the question whether both have been taken from the same population. Specifically, the question is if there is a significant difference between the mean values $\bar{x}_1$ and $\bar{x}_2$ or if they only differ by chance. If, in addition, we know (or assume) the two underlying normal distributions have

Note

For sufficiently large sample size n (practically $n \geq 30$), it makes no difference whether the Z- or the t-test is used because in that situation the Student's t-distribution can barely be distinguished from the standard normal distribution. Thus, the t-test becomes most relevant when we are dealing with small sample sizes.

the same standard deviation σ (implying their mean value the only potential difference), we apply the two-sample t-test. Note that we can also statistically test the equality of the standard deviations by means of performing a F-test. If the standard deviations are different, the Welch test is used instead of the two-sample t-test. Most illustrative is the case when the two samples are mutually independent and have the same sample size n. If both conditions are fulfilled, we apply the test statistic

$$z = \frac{(\bar{x}_1 - \bar{x}_2)}{\sqrt{s_1^2 + s_2^2}} \cdot \sqrt{n} \tag{6-40}$$

in which $\bar{x}_1$ and $\bar{x}_2$ denote the two sample means. The term $\sqrt{s_1^2 + s_2^2}$ in the denominator is obtained from the two standard deviations s_1 and s_2 of the samples (see equation 6-20). It represents, so to speak, the mean standard deviation of the two samples; see also section 6.4.3. The test statistic is compared with the Student's t-distribution in the same way as for the single-sample t-test. Depending on the problem to be solved, the test can be conducted either one- or two-sidedly.

Example

We would like to find out if the amount of a pharmaceutical encapsulated in a batch of nano-capsules changes during storage. To this end, a suitable dimensionless loading parameter has been measured four times before and after storage. The individual values of this parameter before the storage were 3.4, 3.7, 4.6, and 4.7. The values after storage were 3.1, 3.2, 3.6, and 4.3. We are expected to make a statistical statement with a significance level of 5%.

Solution: Our null hypothesis is that the storage has no influence on the mean value of the loading parameter: $H_0: \mu_1 = \mu_2$, in which μ_1 and μ_2 represent the mean values of the underlying statistical distribution before and after storage. The alternative hypothesis states there is an influence of the storage: $H_1: \mu_1 \neq \mu_2$. The mean values and standard deviations before (index 1) and after (index 2) storage are $\bar{x}_1 = 4.10, \bar{x}_2 = 3.55, s_1 = 0.65, s_2 = 0.54$. From this we obtain via equation 6-40 the test statistic $z = 1.30$. We compare this value with the two-sided 95%-confidence interval of the t-distribution for $f = n - 1 = 3$ degrees of freedom. As we already know (see Fig. 6-23), this ranges from -3.182 to $+3.182$. Because the test statistic lies inside the confidence interval, we will not reject the null hypothesis. Thus, based on the two sets of four samples, we cannot substantiate the statement that storage induces a change in loading.

Note that in case the two mutually independent samples differ in size, we apply the test statistic

$$z = \frac{(\bar{x}_1 - \bar{x}_2)}{\sqrt{\dfrac{s_1^2 \cdot (n_1 - 1) + s_2^2 \cdot (n_2 - 1)}{(n_1 - 1) + (n_2 - 1)} \cdot \left(\dfrac{1}{n_1} + \dfrac{1}{n_2}\right)}} \tag{6-41}$$

Of course, for $n_1 = n_2 = n$ equation 6-41 reduces to equation 6-40. We once again emphasize that the application of the Z-test as well as the t-test is based on samples taken from underlying normal distributions. There are statistical tests that allow us to determine whether the data of a sample originate from a normal distribution. Nonetheless, distribution-independent or nonparametric tests have also been developed; these only require independence of the data, but do not presume a specific underlying probability distribution. To explore this subject, we refer the reader to specialized literature sources.

6.6   Linear Regression

Linear relations between two parameters are often encountered in natural sciences, for example the dependence of the electric current on the applied voltage in an Ohmic resistor. In fact, relations generally become linear when being observed within a sufficiently small interval. Although the world human population will not grow linearly in the next 20 years, it will do so in the next 20 days. Linear relations also appear upon presenting nonlinear relations as a function of an appropriately chosen non-linear variable. The following example illustrates this.

Example

When light of a given wavelength and intensity I_0 travels through an aqueous solution of thickness d that contains a light-absorbing substance of concentration c, the light intensity will decay according to Lambert-Beer's law, $I = I_0 \cdot 10^{-\varepsilon \cdot c \cdot d}$. Here, ε denotes the decimal *attenuation coefficient*. To determine ε experimentally, the light intensity I is measured as a function of the length of the path that the light travels through the solution (in other words, the thickness d of the layer of liquid) for a fixed concentration c (or, alternatively, as a function of the concentration c for a fixed layer thickness). If we now consider the decadic logarithm of the measured intensity, $\log I$, as a function of the product $-c \cdot d$, that is, $\log I = \log I_0 - \varepsilon \cdot c \cdot d$, we obtain a *linear relation* in which the *intercept* with the y-axis represents $\log I_0$ and the *slope* of the function the extinction coefficient ε.

Data sets based on measurements contain random errors. Data points describing linear relationships are therefore not going to be located precisely on a straight line. The question arises then how we can find the underlying linear relationship corresponding to a given set of data as, for instance, in the example presented in Fig. 6-24. We describe the relationship of these data by the linear equation

$$y(x) = a + b \cdot x \tag{6-42}$$

in which the two constants a and b correspond to the intercept with the y-axis and to the slope of the straight line, respectively. But how do we find this straight line? Specifically, which values for a and b best describe the data set? To that end, we must first specify what we mean by "best". We are facing here an optimization problem which demands from us to locate a straight line in such a way as to minimize a certain penalty function F. We encounter optimizations all the time, not only in many science areas but also in daily life (for example, when trying to take the shortest way to work in order to save time). To find the "best" straight line, we consider for a given data set (x_i, y_i) with n data points $i = 1, \ldots, n$ the sum of the squares of the distances to the data points

$$F = \sum_{i=1}^{n} [y(x_i) - y_i]^2 = \sum_{i=1}^{n} (a + b \cdot x_i - y_i)^2 \tag{6-43}$$

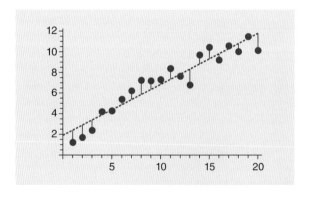

Fig. 6-24 Twenty data points describing a linear relationship. The straight line $y = a + b \cdot x$ which "best" approximates the data points minimizes the sum of the squares of the distances to the data points. The function $y = y(x)$ is represented by the dashed line. The distances between $y(x)$ and the individual data points are marked by vertical lines. For the presented data set we obtain the regression coefficients $a \pm \sigma_a = 1.90 \pm 0.45$ and $b \pm \sigma_b = 0.49 \pm 0.04$; see equations 6-42 and 6-48. The differences of the data points from the straight line can be characterized by the standard deviation $\sigma_y = 0.975$ (equation 6-46) or the coefficient of determination $R^2 = 0.905$ (equation 6-47).

Here, the function $y(x)$ is the straight line specified in equation 6-42; it contains the two unknown parameters (the so-called regression coefficients) a and b. Why do we take the squares of the distances instead of another function such as, for example, the distances as such? There is no compelling answer to this question. One could as well consider other functions, and for certain problems that is actually useful. Nonetheless, there is a strong argument in favor of the squares: It makes the solution of the problem very simple!

The penalty function in equation 6-43 depends on the two unknown regression coefficients a and b. We express this therefore as $F = F(a, b)$. The parameters a and b should now be chosen such that the penalty function $F = F(a, b)$ becomes as small as possible. Finding the minimum of a function requires the first derivative at the position of the minimum to be zero. Thus, we take the derivatives of $F = F(a, b)$ with respect to the parameters a and b and set the resulting expressions equal to zero

$$\frac{\partial F}{\partial a} = 2 \cdot \sum_{i=1}^{n} (a + b \cdot x_i - y_i) = 0$$

$$\frac{\partial F}{\partial b} = 2 \cdot \sum_{i=1}^{n} x_i \cdot (a + b \cdot x_i - y_i) = 0$$

We have obtained two linear equations for a and b, which can be solved without much effort. The solution can conveniently be written down in terms of the mean values

$$\bar{x} = \frac{1}{n} \cdot \sum_{i=1}^{n} x_i$$

$$\bar{y} = \frac{1}{n} \cdot \sum_{i=1}^{n} y_i$$

After some algebra (give it a try!), we obtain

$$b = \frac{\sum_{i=1}^{n} (x_i - \bar{x}) \cdot (y_i - \bar{y})}{\sum_{i=1}^{n} (x_i - \bar{x})^2} \tag{6-44}$$

and

$$a = \bar{y} - b \cdot \bar{x} \tag{6-45}$$

First b is calculated according to equation 6-44 and then a according to equation 6-45. Evidently, the calculation of the regression coefficients a and b from an actual data set is carried out for us by a computer. Nonetheless, it is useful to be aware of the origin of the regression coefficients. Moreover, we can apply the same method also for other regressions. For example, for a data set describing a quadratic relation, we can find the "best" parabola by using the same method. In that case, we obtain three equations for the three parameters (i.e., regression coefficients) by which a quadratic function is fully defined.

After determining the regression coefficients a and b, we also wish to know the degree our data scatter around the linear regression curve. To this end, we use the standard deviation

$$\sigma_y = \sqrt{\frac{\sum_{i=1}^{n} [f(x_i) - y_i]^2}{n - 2}} = \sqrt{\frac{\sum_{i=1}^{n} (a + b \cdot x_i - y_i)^2}{n - 2}} \tag{6-46}$$

In this equation we divide, as in the calculation of the standard deviation in equation 6-20, by the number of degrees of freedom f. The latter is in this case smaller by two than the number of data points n (i.e., $f = n - 2$) because a linear function is fully determined by two parameters (a and b). Furthermore, we notice that in the application of equation 6-46 the standard deviation along the regression curve is assumed to be constant. That may, however, not always be the case.

Another frequently used measure for the quality of the regression is the coefficient of determination

$$R^2 = \frac{\left[\sum_{i=1}^{n} (x_i - \bar{x}) \cdot (y_i - \bar{y})\right]^2}{\sum_{i=1}^{n} (x_i - \bar{x})^2 \cdot \sum_{i=1}^{n} (y_i - \bar{y})^2} \tag{6-47}$$

The R^2 value always lies between zero and one. The closer it is to one, the better the data points correlate with the regression curve. Note that the existence of a correlation (such as, for example, that we find a disproportionally large number of smokers among bingo players) by no means implies that there is a causal relationship between the two (like "smoking enhances the desire to play bingo"). We would, finally, like to mention the degree of scatter for the regression coefficients a an b

$$\sigma_a = \sigma_y \cdot \sqrt{\frac{\sum_{i=1}^{n} x_i^2}{n \cdot \sum_{i=1}^{n} (x_i - \bar{x})^2}}$$

$$\sigma_b = \sigma_y \cdot \frac{1}{\sqrt{\sum_{i=1}^{n} (x_i - \bar{x})^2}} \tag{6-48}$$

in which σ_y is given by equation 6-46. Using the degree of scatter allows us to estimate that the regression coefficients lie within the range between $a \pm \sigma_a$ and $b \pm \sigma_b$. For the data set in Fig. 6-24, we obtain $a \pm \sigma_a = 1.90 \pm 0.45$, $b \pm \sigma_b = 0.49 \pm 0.04$, $\sigma_y = 0.975$, and $R^2 = 0.905$.

Further Reading

Bolton, S. (1984). *Pharmaceutical Statistics, Series on Drugs and the Pharmaceutical Sciences*, 25, New York: Marcel Dekker Inc.

Wonnacott, T. H., and Wonnacott, R. J. (1990). *Introductory statistics*. Singapore: John Wiley & Sons.

7

Basic Principles in Biopharmaceutics

You often see something a hundred times, a thousand times before you see it really the first time.
Christian Morgenstern.

7.1   General Considerations on Biopharmaceutics

This chapter is not meant to replace the numerous comprehensive textbooks on biopharmaceutics that are already available, but is rather intended to offer the reader a technologically oriented introduction into this important aspect of the manufacturing of drugs. More than ever before, the process of drug development depends on the effects that have to be taken into consideration concerning the interaction of the drug with the target system—that is, the diseased tissue or the patient as such. The preceding decades have seen a growing awareness that for a therapeutic effect not only the drug itself and the applied dose are relevant, but the formulation of the drug is also influential. The factors responsible for these influences are to be found in the interplay of the active substance itself, the type and amounts of basic ingredients and excipients, as well as the techniques of the manufacturing process, all governed by physiochemical principles.

As a consequence, a highly complex fabric of interactions between drug formulation and the body emerges. Thus, preparations that by appearance as well as by content of active ingredient are fully identical may display very substantial differences with respect to therapeutic value. Although we know how some excipients and formulations may affect the pharmacokinetic behavior of the drug, we need much more experimental information than that, in order to answer all the questions still existing concerning drug formulation—answers that will be required to optimize drug formulation by appropriate rational modifications.

Let us consider, for example, the problems that may arise upon the administration of a tablet or capsule. To that end, we start by having a look at the organs that are involved in the dissolution and absorption of the drug. (Fig.7-1). Fractions of active ingredients may already be absorbed in the mouth to very low extents. In case of lozenges or sublingual tablets, this is desirable, as the oral mucosal tissue is here the main absorption site. Substances that are not absorbed in the stomach can be taken up by the major absorption organ, the mucosa of the small intestine.

The physiological conditions in the stomach are dynamic; presence of food, individual differences and daily variations, not to speak of pathological deviations, prevent making generally valid statements. Normally, in the stomach a strongly acid environment prevails, which favors the solubility of weakly basic agents. Nonetheless, pH values are strongly dependent on the nutrient intake. For example, protein-rich food leads to a shift toward the weakly acid range. Elderly individuals and those with gastric ailments often have sub-acidic gastric juice,

Voigt's Pharmaceutical Technology, First Edition. Alfred Fahr.
© 2018 John Wiley & Sons Ltd. Published 2018 by John Wiley & Sons Ltd.

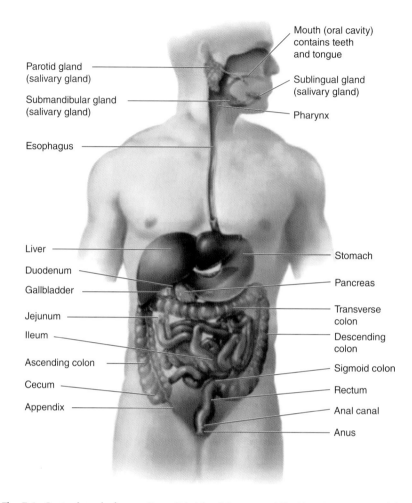

Fig. 7-1 Gastro-intestinal tract. From *Principles of Anatomy and Physiology,* Tortora & Derrickson, 12th edition, Wiley 2009.

which may substantially affect the ionization and solubility of an active agent. In such cases also the gastric juice-resistance of special drug formulations (see e.g. section 10.5.3.2) may no longer be guaranteed. On the other hand, for such pharmaceuticals it should also be taken into account that in the upper small intestine weakly acid conditions may still prevail. For the duodenum, pH values of 3.8 to 6.6 have been reported, and even in the 5-m long jejunum, weakly acidic conditions may be encountered. Furthermore, the residence time of a drug may be influenced by the degree of filling of the stomach.

To promote optimal action of the drug, it is desirable that the drug formulation (especially in case of modified release (MR) formulations, see chapter 12) travels steadily through the digestive tract. Any dysfunction of the digestive process may bring along a change in the residence time in the stomach and thus may lead to complications. Oral dosage forms usually leave the stomach after 15 minutes to 3 hours. Occasionally, residence time is extended to 8 to 10 hours. On the other hand, granulates (from e.g. multiparticulate systems) are able to pass the closed pylorus and may thus leave the stomach after 15 minutes. The half-time residence period of the contents of the small intestine amounts to 2.5 to 3 hours, on average. The passage through the colon commonly takes 4 to 20 hours. Because the residence time of preparations in the digestive tract is affected by a variety of factors, it is not possible to give an accurate average travel time. In literature, usually 10 to 12 hours is taken as a mean value.

Table 7-1 presents an overview of the physiological conditions in the gastrointestinal tract. The given values should be taken as general indications.

In the entire gastrointestinal tract mucous glands or single scattered cells are encountered which produce mucous to cover the intestinal surface. The main constituent of this secretion

Table 7-1 Physiological conditions in the digestive tract (see also Fig. 7.1)

Organ	Digestive Liquids	Amount (l/d)	pH-Value	Components	Residence Time (h)	Absorption Conditions
Mouth (Os)	Saliva	1-2	Approx. 6	Ptyalin	Short-term	
Stomach (Stomachus)	Gastric juice	2-4	1.2-1.6	Hydrochloric acid, Pepsin, Chymosin, Kathepsin, Lipase	1/4-3	Hydrophilic drugs: bad, lipophilic drugs: good
Small intestine (Duodenum, jejunum, Ileum)	Intestinal juice	Approx. 2.0	4.7-7.3	Amylase, Maltase, Lactase, Saccharase	1-10	Good
	Pancreatic juice	Approx. 7	7.5-8.8	Lipase, Erepsin, Enterokinase, Trypsin, Chymotrypsind, Amylase, Carbooxypeptidases, Nucleases		
	Bile	0.7-1.2	7.4-7.7	Bile acids, Cholesterol, Lecithin		
Colon (Colon)			4.6-8.8	Bacteria, Mucus, Stercobilin	4-20	Poor
Rectum	Mucilage		Approx. 7.3			See suppositories

consists of proteins and hexosamine-containing mucopolysaccharides. During the absorption process, active agents are initially taken up from the lumen of the stomach of the intestine by epithelial cells of the mucosa. Following passage through these cells the active agents arrive in the fluid of the *lamina propria* (layer of connective tissue below the mucosal cell lining) and from there in the blood capillaries, from which they are further transported.

The plasma membranes of the epithelial cells present a formidable barrier to hydrophilic and even more so to ionized agents, when such agents have no affinity to any of the transport systems in the epithelial membranes. Substances with molecular weights <100 (e.g., water, urea) can pass the epithelium through narrow channels between individual cells. This permeability depends on the tightness of the interaction between cells (tight junctions).

The membranes of gastric mucosa and of intestinal epithelium will allow only lipid-soluble agents to permeate. Because the majority of the known active agents are weak acids or bases, they occur to higher or lower extents in ionized form, depending on pH. In principle, only the nonionized form is permeating through the lipid barrier of cell membranes. Weak acids bases can be absorbed in the stomach because they are predominantly non-dissociated in the acid conditions of the gastric juice but the small stomach area (about $0.1-0.27$ m^2) may limit the total amount of absorbed drug. In contrast, weak bases are nearly ionized in the stomach and absorption in the stomach plays a minor role, except for very weak bases. In the intestine higher pH values prevail and thus the non-ionized form dominates. However, the drug has to be also soluble in order to reach the gut wall in solution. Arriving there, the nonionized part of the agent will disappear by permeation across the gut wall membranes and according to the equilibrium reaction, new nonionized drug will be formed from the ionized one (see section 7.6.5). As a consequence, even if the fraction of nondissociated agent is relatively small, satisfactory absorption rates in the intestine will result, the more so because of the latter's large absorption area (about $100-200$ m^2).

When we now look at the dissolution and absorption processes in some more detail, we will ultimately draw closer to a physicochemical approach of this process (Fig. 7-2).

After administration of a tablet or capsule, the active agent first needs to be released from the carrier and become available in dissolved form before it can diffuse into the blood and ultimately reach the site of action. In the simplest case, the active agent dissolves either directly in the intestinal juice (3) or only after further disintegration (2) of larger aggregates (1) after interaction with the intestinal juice. When developing a new active agent, it is commonly assumed that at least the uncharged form of the agent diffuses into the blood across the gastrointestinal barrier, which is mainly represented by the plasma membranes of the cells of the intestinal wall. Once in the blood, the ionized form is formed again due to the changed chemical equilibrium.

Let us now consider some situations that may affect the pharmacokinetics of the active agent also influenced by the formulation (Fig. 7-3). First of all, food intake may strongly affect the action of the active agent. The tablet or capsule will dissolve slower or faster depending on

The ileum contains lymphoid tissue consisting of lymphoid follicles (Peyer's patches; gut-associated lymphoid tissue (GALT)) which may provide an entry for drugs (e.g. peptides) and particles to the lymphatic system (see Weston & Yeboah 2013).

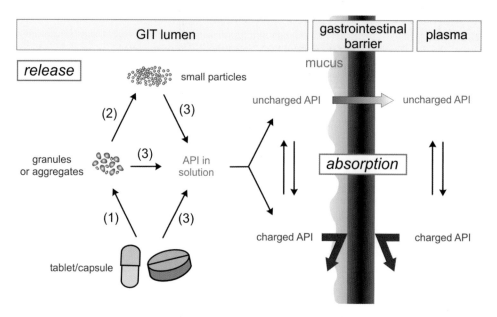

Fig. 7-2 Physical-chemical processes following after the administration of a tablet or capsule. Redrawn from Blanchard (1978), Am. J. Phar. 150, 132.

whether or not the patient has eaten shortly before (2). Particularly after a fatty meal bile salts (cholates) will be released by the gall bladder into the intestinal juice. Their surface-active properties affect not only the dissolution rate (1) but also cause the formation of micelles (3), which may accommodate lipophilic agents in their interior. The lipophilic agent is thus solubilized and transported through the lumen towards the mucus layer. After diffusing through this layer the agent reaches the epithelial cells of the intestinal wall. The agent will subsequently reach the blood compartment surrounding the intestine, either by passive diffusion (see Fig. 7-2) or by active transport (for example by the cholesterol transporter) across the cell membrane. Once in the blood, lipophilic agents will bind typically to plasma constituents such as albumin and lipoproteins to be further transported in the body. The portal vein will then carry the drug to the liver where, especially for the free form, a major fraction may unfortunately be metabolized before it reaches the systemic blood circulation (see "first-pass effect").

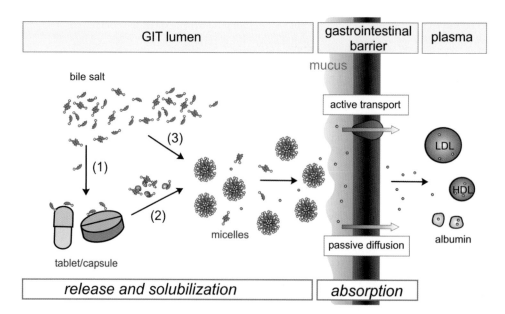

Fig. 7-3 Physiological processes following administration of a tablet or capsule.

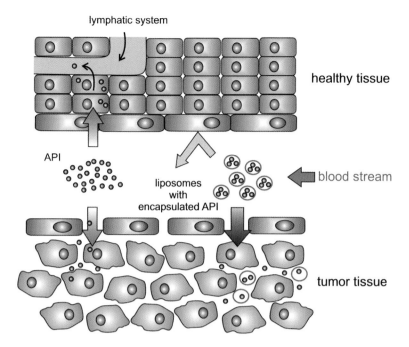

Fig. 7-4 The EPR effect.

Bioavailability and therapeutic effect can both be improved by manipulating the rate of release of the drug and its absorption by means of excipients (see also section 7.7.1). For oral formulations, the possibilities of pharmaceutical technology to create effects like targeting to the diseased site end in most cases at the intestinal wall.

This targeting can be achieved by particulate systems, which, however, do not cross the intestinal wall and therefore have to be administered by injection. This opens up entirely different possibilities, for example, targeted treatment in anti-tumor therapy (Fig. 7-4). A growing tumor (from 2 mm up) sends out angiogenetic signals that allow the body to form blood vessels to provide the tumor with nutrients and oxygen. These newly formed vessels have a peculiar property in that they possess relatively wide gaps between the rapidly growing endothelial cells that form these micro-vessels. These gaps may be up to several hundred nm in size, depending on the particular tumor type. Colloidal systems such as nanoparticles or liposomes (see chapter 20) can diffuse from the blood compartment through these gaps into the periphery of tumor. An active agent encapsulated in these particles can then be released and exert its anti-tumor action. Since such *extravasation* processes will not occur in normal (healthy) vascular endothelium, the healthy tissue will not or much less be burdened by the cytotoxic contents of the particles. Another tumor-specific condition that favors the effectiveness of particulate drug carrier systems in anti-tumor therapy is the lack of signals to form a lymph drainage system. That causes such particles to remain in the tumor for some time (Fig. 7-4). The entire process of extravasation and retention is an example of *passive targeting* and is also known as the *enhanced permeation and retention* (EPR) effect. It was described for the first time by Matsumura and Maeda in 1986. The principle was already exploited in some marketed particulate drug formulations (e.g., doxorubicin-containing liposomes, Doxil®).

From these examples, it becomes clear that therapeutic success of a drug depends to a large extent on its formulation. That is why technological approaches to influence drug action through formulation are in the focus of biopharmaceutical research. Such research efforts belong to the realm of pharmaceutical technology.

7.1.1   Biopharmaceutics

Biopharmaceutics concerns the connections between physical-chemical properties of a pharmaceutical and its formulations and the biological action it displays as a function of its formulation. The task of biopharmaceutics is sometimes also seen in a somewhat broader perspective. In addition to the release of the drug from the dosage form and its absorption, it also includes the fate of the drug in the organism (distribution, metabolism, and excretion) and the dependence thereof on anatomical, physiological and pathological factors.

7.1.2   Pharmacokinetics

The term pharmacokinetics was used for the first time in 1953 by the pediatrician F.H. Dost to describe the interactions between the organism and an administered medicine. Although Buchanan already described the correlation between drug dose, absorption and distribution in anesthesia in 1847, it was Dost who published a book on pharmacokinetics as we now understand it. Dost was motivated by the fact that until then, children were looked upon as small adults when it came to drug dosing. Due to him, the distinction of biopharmaceutics for children (and with that the difference in pharmacokinetics and dosage forms) were taken into account more and more extensively.

The main concern of pharmacokinetics is the quantitative assessments of the processes of drug absorption, metabolism and excretion. For that purpose sensitive methods are required to assess concentration changes of the drug and/or its metabolites as a function of time, particularly in blood (plasma) or urine.

7.1.3   Pharmaceutical Availability

7.1.3.1   Experimental Approaches and Evaluations

The release characteristics of a drug from its dosage form, as determined by *in-vitro* assessment, are called *pharmaceutical availability* (or in-vitro availability or content availability). This is defined as the percentage of a drug in a formulation that is released and the rate at which this occurs.

The instrumentation that is used for these purposes is often designed in such a way that, in addition to data on the dissolution of the active ingredient and its release (dissolution models), information can be obtained concerning the absorption (absorption models) by taking into account subsequent distribution processes in the body. Such instrumental designs allow the recognition of regularities, not so much to ascertain an accurate imitation of the natural process but, rather, to make the basic principles of the latter more accessible by means of applying normalized conditions.

Among the test fluids used for *in-vitro* assays are the following:

- Artificial gastrointestinal juices mimicking real intestinal juices (e.g., FESSIF or FASSIF, see Dressman et al. 1998; additions of enzymes or viscosity enhancers are possible)
- Buffer solutions (e.g., phosphate buffers)
- Simple solutions (e.g., of NaCl, NaOH, Na_2CO_3)
- Most simple: water

Drug release is substantially affected by composition and amount of the test medium, the kind and extent of stirring and the temperature, as well as the properties of the membrane, when applied.

Numerous natural as well as artificial membranes have been used as models for the barrier function of human cell membranes. With the exception of some special cases, lipid-(especially phospholipid)-containing membranes are particularly suited as general models to predict the permeation potential of drugs, because phospholipids are essential and major constituents of most biomembranes and display special polar as well as nonpolar interactions with active ingredients. Consequently, such artificial membranes show the closest similarity with natural membranes and as such are important elements of absorption models (see section 9.9.2). Besides for absorption experiments on membrane models, lipids or liposomes are often used to study the binding of drugs (IAMC; immobilized artificial membrane chromatography and LEKC; liposome electro-kinetic chromatography).

In the IAMC method, phospholipids are attached to HPLC gel particles, and the binding of drugs to these particles is assessed by measuring the retention time of the drug on a column of such particles. Most of these methods are not suited for use in routine labs because of the sensitivity of the fragile lipid "membranes." Instead, the so-called PAMPA method (parallel artificial membrane permeation assay) is often applied in such cases. This involves the use of filter materials that are soaked in a lipid-containing dodecane solution, to serve as a stable surrogate of a cell membrane (Kansy et al. 1988). The described methods often (but not always!) provide useful indications for the real permeability of the tested agent through cell membranes. When the drug engages in too strong an interaction with the lipids, the cell membranes may represent an effective retention barrier for the drug.

In theory, cell culture experiments, particularly with the CaCo-2 cell line, represent an almost ideal permeation model. However, for routine application, this complex method is not suitable. Besides, it is questionable whether this cell line, which was developed from colon epithelial cells, presents a good model for studies on absorption processes in the small intestine. By the same token, this model is not suited for testing of drugs based on surfactants, as these cells lack the mucus layer that in the intestine serves to protect the cell membranes from dissolution by the detergents. On the other hand, the model is well suited for the detection and characterization of active transport systems for active agents or pro-drugs.

The predictive value of in-vitro results has often been overestimated. Although in some cases quite satisfactory accordance with in-vivo results have been reported, generalization is by no means warranted. Nonetheless, such methods can provide important indications.

In-vitro tests allow comparative studies of test samples with different release characteristics and thus will permit a classification of such samples. The aim is obviously to develop in-vitro methods yielding results that correlate to in-vivo observations. The in-vitro vs. in-vivo correlation has been extensively investigated and discussed in literature. In recent years, the tendency has been toward an increasingly critical appraisal of such a correlation, if not judged unrealistic. We can understand that it is virtually impossible to simulate the complex processes in the human body, even when using highly sophisticated experimental arrangements. We purposely refrain from making explicit qualifications on correlation methods in this context. More detailed information on this controversial theme can be found in specialized books on biopharmaceutics (see the list of recommended literature at the end of this book).

The significance of in-vitro experiments in this context is not affected by the statements made in the foregoing. This is illustrated by the following:

- For the development of new and the optimization of existing medicines, release tests are indispensable. Before elaborate assessments of bioavailability and subsequent extensive clinical testing can even be considered, it is mandatory to first confirm, by appropriate pharmaco-technical measures, that a desirable, sufficiently high pharmaceutical availability has been attained or that proper adjustment to desired requirements has been reached MR formulations.
- Drug release tests ascertain the uniformity within a batch (batch homogeneity) and from batch to batch (batch conformity), and thus the consistency of the drug release during the production cycle or in case of discontinuous production. In addition, bioavailability assessments confirm that a drug formulation with certain release characteristics results in optimal (pharmacological) action, in-vitro tests of quality control, will serve to confirm conformity of activity.
- Release tests can be involved in solving durability problems. When for a certain formulation increasingly lower release rates are found during prolonged storage, failing stability is probably at hand. This may concern the active ingredient itself but also be caused by age-dependent changes in basic ingredients or interactions between drug and excipients or packing material.

For drug formulations with concurring pharmaceutical availability, the term *pharmaceutical equivalence* has been coined. This is defined as the equality of two preparations yielding identical release rates of the same active ingredient from the same dosage form and that have been developed in accordance with the best available technology.

7.1.4 Presentation of Results

When we cumulatively plot the amount of drug released at certain time intervals in a coordinate system (released amount m of drug in percent (m[%]) against time (t) and connect

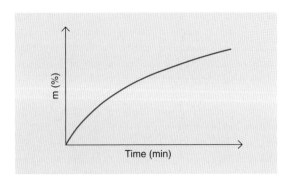

Fig. 7-5 Dissolution or release profile.

the measured points, we obtain a curve which is known as the dissolution or release profile (Fig. 7-5).

Although such graphic representations are quite informative, they are not well suited for quantitative comparison. For that reason, it is customary to characterize the release process by a few parameters including rate and magnitude of the release (*curve parameters*). We distinguish in this connection quantity or percent parameters (fraction of active agent released after a certain time interval) and time parameters (time required to release a certain fraction of active agent, maximal release rate, time at which maximal release rate is attained), and designate those as *empirical, model-independent parameters*. It speaks for itself that for a precise description of the progression of the curve several parameters are required. When it concerns merely a test to confirm that a preparation meets the quality demands of certain regulations or the testing conditions of a pharmacopeia, often a single content assay suffices to determine whether in a certain time interval a defined percentage of the formulation has gone into solution. The U.S pharmacopeia subjects tablet and capsule preparations to a dissolution test. Individual monographs provide instructions on whether to use the blade-stirrer or the rotating-cup method, as well as on preparation-specific requirements concerning the percentage of released drug within a defined time interval. In most cases at least 75% release within 45 minutes is required in water as a test fluid (Fig. 7-6).

A further option to characterize the dissolution process is the mean dissolution time t_{diss}. It represents a statistical parameter and concerns the arithmetic mean of the residence time of the drug molecule in the dosage form (Fig. 7-7). It can be calculated from equation 7-1:

$$t_{diss} = \frac{ABC}{Y} \tag{7-1}$$

ABC = area between the curves
Y　 = total amount of released drug

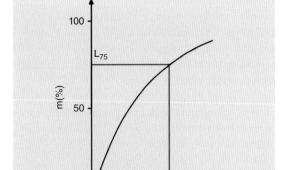

Fig. 7-6 Dissolution curve with solubility parameters.

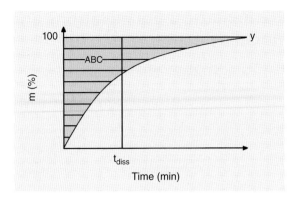

Fig. 7-7 Mean dissolution time.

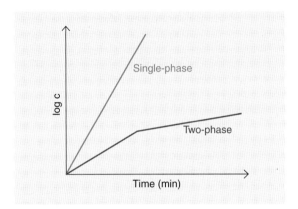

Fig. 7-8 Linearization of dissolution and release curves.

Quite frequently it may be useful to linearize the curve. Such a transformation can be readily obtained by plotting the amount of released agent logarithmically against time (Fig. 7-8). When this results in a straight line with a break point, we are dealing with a bi-phasic course of the release (Fig. 7-8). In such a case we can derive from the slopes of the straight lines that the drug is released faster in the first phase than in the second phase of the process (e.g., by a starting dose).

One of the common options for linearization is the *Sigma-Minus plot*. For this plot, the (time-dependent) released amount of drug (m) is subtracted from the total amount of drug (sigma, sum) m_0. The amount of non-dissolved drug thus obtained ($m_0 - m$) is then plotted semi-logarithmically against time.

What results is a declining straight line whose slope represents the dissolution constant (Fig. 7-9).

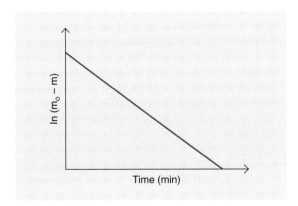

Fig. 7-9 The Sigma-Minus plot.

7.2   Mathematical Formulations and Model Systems

7.2.1   Biokinetic Models—Pharmacokinetics

In spite of the complexity of the processes involved in tablet dissolution, the release of a drug from a tablet, the distribution in the intestinal lumen, the diffusion through the intestinal wall, the distribution in blood and the subsequent elimination (Figs. 7-2 and 7-3), the models required to describe the changes in drug concentration in the different compartments are relatively simple. It is assumed, for example, that the intestinal lumen and the blood compartment represent well-stirred volumes in which reactions and interactions between drug and body obey first-order kinetics. Under normal conditions it is further assumed that for instance drug absorption and elimination are directly proportional to the prevailing drug concentration (in intestinal lumen or blood). This linear relationship between concentration and reaction velocity is known as *linear pharmacokinetics*. Mathematically formulated:

$$\frac{dc}{dt} = -k \cdot c \tag{7-2}$$

C = drug concentration
k = reaction constant

By simply separating the variables, knowing that integration of dc/c yields the natural logarithm, and applying the corresponding simplifications (equation 7-3), we see that the linear pharmacokinetics lead to exponential functions:

$$\frac{dc}{dt} = -k \cdot c(t) \Rightarrow \frac{dc}{c} = -k \cdot dt$$

$$\int_{c_0}^{c(t)} \frac{1}{c} dc = -k \cdot \int_0^t dt \Rightarrow \ln(c(t)) - \ln c_0 = -k \cdot t \tag{7-3}$$

$$\ln \frac{c(t)}{c_0} = -k \cdot t \Rightarrow c(t) = c_0 \cdot e^{-k \cdot t}$$

It is remarkable that this model, based on relatively simple assumptions, can describe most pharmacokinetics in pharmaceutical science.

This correlation applies in any case to the elimination processes and likewise to the dissolution and absorption processes of most oral dosage forms (tablets, capsules). On the other hand, for the release mechanism from sustained release or other special dosage forms (e.g., film tablets, OROS), as well as for infusions, a zero-order reaction (constant release) is observed. Active agents that are released in this way will subsequently be removed by reactions of the first order. The complex mathematical derivations fully describing these processes may be found in the corresponding textbooks. In the following, we will limit ourselves to the solution of the equations of first-order kinetics for dissolution, absorption, and elimination.

Incidentally, evolution biologists like to "explain" the first-order elimination reactions in a teleological way by pointing out that the body eliminates drugs according to the same principle as it does for toxins and thus has "learned" to bring high concentrations of such substances back to lower, less toxic levels as quickly as possible (see equation 7-2: high concentrations correspond to high dc/dt values), giving the body time to subsequently eliminate the lower, possibly less toxic concentrations. Furthermore, we would have to have large amounts of enzymes to ascertain zero-order reactions and we would thus have been a slow-moving protein-rich target for prehistoric predators.

The following section will further clarify the events in the organism and the descriptive mathematical formulation of a sustained release drug formulation by means of a simple biokinetic model as described here:

$$D \xrightarrow{k_r^0} G \xrightarrow{k_g} B \xrightarrow{k_e} E \tag{7-4}$$

D = sustained-release formulation

G = gastro-intestinal tract (absorption site)

B = distribution fluid (blood)

E = excretion organs

k_{r0} = rate constant for the release of active agent

k_a = rate constant of the absorption

k_e = rate constant of the elimination

The MR form delivers the drug to the gastrointestinal tract G for absorption, from where it reaches the transport medium B by means of diffusion, cell penetration, and permeation and ultimately becomes subject to elimination E. In order to sustain a constant drug concentration in blood and organs for a prolonged period of time, the drug should continuously enter the blood and organs in constant amounts; thus, a zero-order release from the MR form is required. Nonetheless, in many cases, including the one considered below, release kinetics of the first-order will be observed.

7.2.2   Application of a Single Oral Dose

Presuming a certain dose D_0 of a drug in G, which travels consecutively from G to B and E, the following equation applies, assuming first-order kinetics:

$$c_p = \frac{D_0 \cdot F}{V} \cdot \frac{K_a}{k_a - k_e} \cdot \left(e^{-k_e \cdot t} - e^{-k_a \cdot t} \right) \tag{7-5}$$

c_p = plasma concentration

D_0 = applied dose

F = absorbed fraction

V = distribution volume

This is the Dost basic equation of pharmacokinetics, also known as Bateman function, after H. Bateman, who first described this in 1910 for a mother-daughter-granddaughter isotope decay scheme. Dependent on distribution volume and the other factors, we obtain the plasma concentration c_p of the drug as a function of time. The absorbed fraction F (varying from 0 to 1) can be determined by independent experiments. The distribution volume often is a computational parameter. Only for large hydrophilic molecules, which leave the blood circulation not by way of diffusion but rather by an elimination process, the distribution volume equals the blood volume.

Fig 7-10 shows a curve corresponding to equation 7-5, based on the values $k_a = 2.0$ h^{-1} and $k_e = 0.2$ h^{-1}. After rapidly reaching a maximum, the drug concentration decreases from

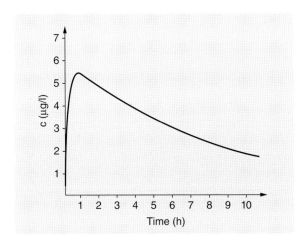

Fig. 7-10 Blood level after oral application of a single dose.

there on and exponentially approaches zero. The slopes of the ascending and descending limb of the curve depend on k_a and k_e. Also, the maximal concentration and the time to attain this value are functions of these two parameters.

7.2.3   Application of a MR Dosage Form

The MR formulation can deliver a drug according to a zero-order process—that is, with a constant rate, in the gastrointestinal tract; absorption and elimination then proceed as a first-order process.

$$b_t = \frac{k_{r^0}}{k_e} \left(1 - e^{-k_e t}\right) \frac{k_a \cdot D_0 - k_{r^0}}{k_e - k_a} \left(e^{-k_a t} - e^{-k_e t}\right) \tag{7-6}$$

In equation 7-6 b_t is the amount of drug in blood at time t, which initially rises rapidly from 0 at time t = 0 and then more slowly, to theoretically reach a constant limit value at time t = ∞.

The attainable constant maximal concentration c_{max} can be calculated from equation 7-7:

$$c_{max} = \frac{k_{r^0}}{k_e} \quad \text{for } t \to \infty \tag{7-7}$$

From this and k_a and k_e, which are given by the drug properties, k_{r^0} can be used to fix the maximal drug level. As a result, the limit value turns into the desired optimal level c_{opt} as follows:

$$c_{opt} = \frac{k_{r^0}}{k_e} \quad \text{for } t \to \infty \tag{7-8}$$

While the desired release constant k_{r^0} becomes the product of k_e and the desired optimal blood level (equation 7-9).

$$k_{r^0} = k_e \cdot c_{opt} \tag{7-9}$$

Furthermore, the release constant results as the product of k_e and the single dose D_0 that provides the desired blood level, so that the following relation can be derived (equation 7-10) using the known relation between k and $t_{1/2}$ (half-life) for an exponential decay function:

$$k_{r0} = \frac{0{,}693 \cdot D_0}{t_{1/2}} \tag{7-10}$$

The amount of drug that has to be incorporated in the MR formulation as the maintenance dose, D_m, complies with the time span during which the optimal drug concentration needs to be sustained in the organism:

$$D_m = k_{r0} \cdot h \tag{7-11}$$

h = time during which the desired drug level should be sustained

Fig. 7-11 shows a curve image corresponding to equation 7-6, in which the k_a and k_e values match with those of Fig. 7-10. In order to calculate k_{r^0}, we assume that the maximal concentration that is obtained by the single dose D_0 also represents the optimal concentration. As is apparent from Fig. 7-11, the optimal drug concentration, represented by the straight horizontal line, has not yet been attained after 10 hours. As a consequence, it can hardly be expected that optimal blood levels will be reached and sustained within a reasonable time frame. After all, the intestinal tract will be eliminating the drug during this time. It is worthwhile noting in this connection, that bioadhesive drug formulations that can stick to the intestinal wall are in a developmental stage.

Bioadhesion occurs either to the epithelial cell lining or to the mucus. Polymers with hydrogen bonding groups (like carbomers, starch, HPC, HPMC) or charges (like chitosan) can bind to the mucus layer in the intestine. This seems to apply not only to tablets, but also to multiparticulates (Tao et al. 2009) and osmotic pump systems (Alam et al. 2015).

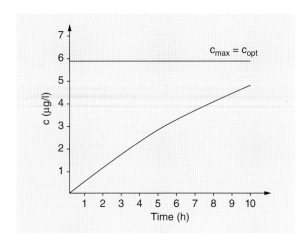

Fig. 7-11 Blood level after application of a MR dosage form.

7.2.4 Application of an Ideal Peroral Modified Release Dosage Form

From the foregoing, it follows that an ideal oral MR dosage form should consist of two parts:
1. The initiating part contains an instantaneously available initial dose D_i that, like a single dose, results in rapid attainment of the desired dug concentration.
2. The depot (reservoir) part contains the maintenance dose D_m, which, by means of the steady release of its active principle, sustains the desired concentration for the desired length of time.

The total drug content of the MR formulation D_{tot} is composed of $D_i + D_m$.

$$D_{tot} = D_0 - (k_{r^0} \cdot t_{max}) + k_{r^0} \cdot h$$

7.2.5 Calculation of Initial, Maintenance, and Total Dose

The total quantity of drug to be incorporated in a MR formulation can be calculated as follows:

$$D_{tot} = D_0 + \frac{0,693}{t_{1/2}} D_0 \cdot h \tag{7-12}$$

D_{tot} = total amount of drug to be incorporated
D_0 = amount of drug required to attain the desired blood level when given as a single dose

This formula has been criticized as being incorrect, since the initial dose D_i of a sustained-release preparation cannot be considered equal to the single dose D_0, which is required to attain the optimal blood level, because the release of the drug from the initiating part and that from the depot part start simultaneously, resulting in a higher blood level than desired.

By differentiation of equation 7-12 and determining the zero value, we obtain the time t_{max}, which elapses until the maximal amount of drug after a single dose has been released.

$$t_{max} = \frac{2,303}{k_a - k_e} \lg \frac{k_a}{k_e} \tag{7-13}$$

After input of the time t_{max} and the desired optimal concentration c_{opt} in equation 7-9, D_i can be calculated. A suitable correction of the immediately available dose between $t = 0$ and t_{max} is recommended. This correction equals $k_{(r^0)} t_{max}$ so that we find for D_i:

$$D_i = D_0 - (k_{r^0} \cdot t_{max}) \tag{7-14}$$

Because $D_{tot} = D_i + D_m$ and

$$D_m = k_{r^0} \cdot h$$

the total amount of drug D_{tot} can be calculated according to equations 7.15 and 7.16:

$$D_{tot} = D_0 - (k_{r^0} \cdot t_{max}) + k_{r^0} \cdot h \tag{7-15}$$

$$D_{tot} = D_0 + k_{r^0} \cdot (h - t_{max}) \tag{7-16}$$

Keep in mind, however, that only insignificant proportions of the depot part will have been released before the initial dose has been absorbed, and that the problem of the immediate and the delayed release of the MR dose depends on practical conditions (e.g., of coated tablets the depot part becomes available only after release of the initiating dose has taken place).

In the case of delayed release of the MR dose, we obtain:

$$D_i = D_0$$
$$D_m = k_{r^0} (h - t_{max}). \tag{7-17}$$

In industrial development and production of pharmaceutics, the application of these models can be difficult, as in vitro/in vivo correlations are not reliable (in the case of parenteral depot formulations, were the same equation hold, sometimes even an in vivo experiment has to be done to qualify an industrial batch).

7.3   Bioavailability

7.3.1   Definition

The central concern of biopharmaceutics is the influence of pharmaceutical technology on bioavailability. This is defined as follows: The bioavailability (BA) of a pharmaceutical is the rate and the quantity at which the active agent is absorbed from the formulation or presents itself at the site of action.

Thus, bioavailability indicates what fraction of the active agent (%) is absorbed from the formulation by the organism and represents the pharmaceutical activity of the drug as determined by the formulation.

Bioavailability characterizes the amount of drug that arrives in the blood circulation after administration. The term is also used in case of substances that are not absorbed—for example, in case of the transfer of a drug from a dermally applied formulation into the skin tissue.

7.3.2   Detection of Drug Concentrations in Body Fluids

Bioavailability studies analyze the absorbed drug, taking into account that it is often present in only very low concentrations, which can often bring along serious difficulties. It would be desirable that the therapeutic effect of the drug on the organism could be measured and/or when the drug concentration at the site of action (e.g., a receptor) could be determined. In general, this is not possible; instead, the bioavailability of the absorbed drug is predominantly determined in blood plasma (blood without red and white cells and platelets, but including fibrinogen) or in serum (fibrinogen-free plasma). Although bioavailability is not assessed by determining the pharmaco-dynamic effect but rather by assaying the amount or concentration of the drug, it is assumed that the blood concentration thus obtained reflects the concentration at the site of action and thus represents a criterion for the therapeutic effect.

It should be kept in mind, however, that we will not always find an unambiguous correlation between blood or plasma concentration and clinical activity of a drug. The pharmacodynamic activity may persist long after the drug has reached undetectable levels in blood (e.g., for beta blockers). The onset of corticosteroid action occurs only after the blood concentration has reached its maximum. We must also take into account that results obtained with healthy volunteers cannot always be extrapolated to the situation in patients.

The previous discussion illustrates that bioavailability can only be assessed by *in vivo* experiments. Such experiments can be conducted in animals as well as in humans. For the development of new pharmaceutics, animal experiments are indispensable, particularly to determine optimal compositions of drug formulations and to establish process parameters. However, results thus obtained can only be extrapolated to a limited extent to the conditions prevailing in humans. Therefore, bioavailability is commonly understood as to result from experiments in humans, unless explicitly indicated otherwise.

As a common procedure, the absorption of a test preparation (e.g., a suppository) is determined by comparison with a standard preparation. When the standard preparation is an i.v. injection fluid, whose availability may be set at 100%, we speak of *absolute bioavailability*.

On the other hand, often two different drug formulations containing the same active ingredient at according doses and identical routes of administration are compared, one of them representing the standard preparation. A novel suspension preparation can, for example, be compared with a therapeutically proven tablet preparation. Such a comparison between two arbitrary drug formulations (except i.v. injection fluids) will give us the *relative bioavailability*.

Active ingredients undergoing a first-pass effect (metabolized at the first liver passage) will show poor availability, even in case of complete absorption, because only small quantities of unchanged active ingredient will appear in the general blood circulation.

Generally, bioavailability is determined by means of blood level curves. For that purpose, we compare the areas under the blood or plasma concentration *vs.* time curves (AUC, area under the curve). The area under the curve equals the dose fraction that arrives in the systemic circulation divided by the distribution volume and the elimination rate constant (metabolism and excretion). Because we apply identical doses for test and standard preparation, distribution volume and elimination rate constant remain the same, and thus bioavailability (BA, in %) results from the following equation:

$$BA\,(\%) = \frac{AUC_{(x)}}{AUC_{(s)}} \cdot 100 \qquad\qquad (7\text{-}18)$$

$AUC_{(x)}$: area under the plasma concentration-time-curve after administration
     of the test formulation,

$AUC_{(s)}$: area under the plasma concentration-time-curve after administration
     of the standard formulation.

The area under the curve can be assessed planimetrically, gravimetrically (*by cutting out the plotted area on paper and weighing it; an ancient but effective and instructive method*) or by calculation. The evaluation requires that we are dealing with closed curves, implying that the blood level values should be determined down to complete elimination of the drug from the blood compartment. For an accurate assessment of a blood level curve at least 15 assay points are required.

The area under the blood level curve alone does not provide sufficient information; equally important are height of the maximum of the curve and the time required to reach this maximum (slope of the curve). This is illustrated by Figs. 7-12 to 7-14. The AUC's I-III in Fig. 7-12 are identical, yet only curves I and II exceed the minimal effective concentration (MEC) and therefore lie within the therapeutically effective range, albeit with different therapeutic intensities (T.I.), while curve III remains entirely below this range.

In Fig. 7-13, the AUCs I to III are not identical. All three curves attain the same maximum, implying identical therapeutic intensities, yet considerable differences are manifest in duration (T.D.) of the therapeutic effect of the drug.

Often drug concentrations have to be determined in whole blood. Especially if the drug binds strongly and variably to red blood cells, as in the case of cyclosporine. 70% of the cyclosporine in blood is bound to a protein called cyclophilin located inside red blood cells (Foxwell et al. 1988)

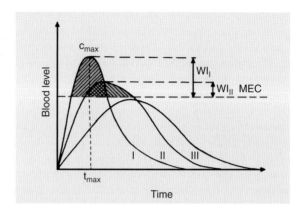

Fig. 7-12   Blood level curves (differences in therapeutic intensity).

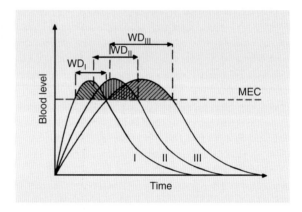

Fig. 7-13   Blood level curves (differences in duration of effect).

In Fig. 7-14, again the AUCs of all three curves are approximately identical while in addition therapeutically effective concentrations are attained. In this case we see, however, significant differences in the time of onset of the effect (T.O.).

To characterize bioavailability, the following parameters are used:

- Area under the blood level curve (AUC)
- Maximum height of the blood level C_{max} (Fig. 7-12)
- Time required to reach the curve maximum t_{max} (Fig. 7-12)

Bioavailability tests are done in the following cases:

- All drug formulations with systemic action
- For novel active ingredients

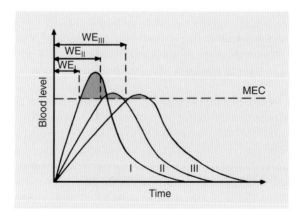

Fig. 7-14   Blood level curves (differences in onset of effect).

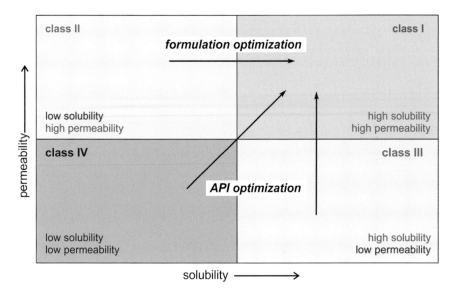

Fig. 7-15 Biopharmaceutical Classification System (BCS).

- New formulations of existing drugs
- Drugs with poor solubility (<0.3%) or low dissolution rate
- Occurrence of drug-excipient or drug-drug interactions that may alter solubility
- Drugs with steep dose-activity curves and/or a narrow therapeutic range
- Drugs with high first-pass effect
- Formulations with modified drug release (all MR and gastric juice resistant formulations or therapeutic systems)

As a rule, bioavailability studies are imperative for pharmaceutics intended for specific application areas such as coronary therapeutics, cytostatics, anti-diabetics, immune-suppressives, and virostatics.

After small alterations in the formulation, there is no absolute need to conduct renewed testing of the bioavailability. In individual cases the necessity to do that will have to be considered critically. Such tests are not required for example when a new formulation is made, based on an existing preparation whose activity is secured by a bioavailability test, with the same drug and identical excipient composition, but higher dose, while both preparations show identical in vitro release pattern (i.e., same kinetics, but of course different amount).

In other situations, such as listed here, bioavailability assays are not required:

- Exclusive i.v. application
- Aqueous solutions without excipients for oral, subcutaneous or intramuscular application
- Peroral, rectal, or vaginal applications, if the active ingredient is not absorbed or in case of topical application without a strong systemic effect
- Nonretarded solid or semi-solid peroral formulations when no bioavailability problems are foreseen (i.e., when the applied drug is not known as a problem substance)

Drugs that by empirical observation are known to cause difficulties in ascertaining satisfactory bioavailability and whose presence in a formulation necessitates a bioavailability test are considered problem substances. This concerns primarily drugs with poor solubility, dissolution rate, and permeability. But also substances with a steep dose-activity curve or with a narrow therapeutic window fall in this category. Their number has increased substantially in the last few years; about 40% of the drugs currently on the market are poorly soluble. A few examples are presented in Table 7-2. Particularly solubility and permeability are critical parameters for the bioavailability. According to the FDA, the solubility of an active agent may be considered high when the highest dose solubilizes in less than 250 mL in a pH range between 1 and 7.5—that is, in all environments the drug may encounter in

Table 7-2 Examples of Problematic Drugs

Aminophyllin	Nitrofurantoin
Ampicillin	Prednisolon, methylprednisolon
Chinidin	Reserpin
Chloramphenicol	Spironolacton
Digoxin	Tetracyclin, oxy-, chlortetracyclin
Indomethacin	Theophyllin
Meprobamat	Tolbutamid

the gastrointestinal tract. The FDA considers a drug highly permeable when the absorbed fraction is higher than 90% of the applied dose.

Occasionally, urine excretion curves are used to determine bioavailability. In those cases, urine collection has to be continued until the drug has been completely excreted from the body.

When determining bioavailability, it is essential to take into account that numerous physiological and pathological factors may exert a substantial influence; these include age, gender, body weight, nutritional state, food intake, pregnancy, genetic factors, intestinal and renal function, disease, environmental influences and more. To eliminate such factors to allow drawing justified conclusions, blood and urine data of at least 6, more commonly 12, individuals should be collected. The test subjects (aged 18–40 years) should be healthy, have a body weight deviating not more than 10% from ideal weight and not have taken any medicine for at least one week preceding the test. The time interval between administration of reference and test preparation should likewise amount to about one week. An interval of approximately five to six half-lives is considered the minimal space between two consecutive administrations in order to exclude interference by the preceding administration. Individual variations are eliminated by applying the crossover technique—that is, that each individual receives consecutively the standard as well as the test preparation.

When investigations on bioavailability in healthy persons are ethically not acceptable, such as in the case of cytostatics or opiates, the study will be conducted on patients who are therapeutically treated with these medicines.

7.3.3   Assessment of Pharmacological or Therapeutic Effects

Assessment of bioavailability by determination of the drug concentration in blood or urine represents currently the most important method to evaluate bioavailability. Only occasionally other pharmacological or therapeutic parameters are called on to evaluate bioavailability. This will become particularly important when assessment of drug concentrations in body fluids is not possible. However, even when suitable assay methods to determine therapeutic and pharmacological effects are available, they will in most cases suffer from a large error width. Statistical significance of results thus obtained can only be achieved by using large numbers of test subjects. The application of such pharmacological methods on patients commonly fails due to a lack of sufficient numbers of patients with uniform pathological symptoms/diagnosis. Up to now, the evaluation of bioavailability is based, for example, on the following pharmacological or diagnostic parameters: blood pressure, blood glucose level, pupil diameter, internal eyeball pressure, and body temperature, as well as ECG or EEG data.

7.4   Bioequivalence

Generic drugs are drug preparations that are made available by pharmaceutical firms other than the original manufacturer, but containing identical active ingredients in the same dosage and dosage form and for largely the same applications as the original preparation. Such preparations may be considered as *pharmaceutically equivalent*. The question is whether they are also *therapeutically equivalent*. We speak of therapeutic equivalence when two preparations containing the same active ingredient show identical therapeutic activity and/or toxicity when administered in identical doses to identical test subjects.

As the parameter, therapeutic equivalence is not easily accessible to objective measurement—often, the term *bioequivalence* is used instead. This is defined as the equivalence of two preparations containing the same active ingredient displaying the same bioavailability when administered to identical test subjects at identical dosages.

The large number of internationally distributed generics explains the high interest attributed in recent years to bioequivalence research. Worldwide, a multitude of pharmaceutical companies process several hundred active ingredients into pharmaceutical formulations and are bringing them to the market under different brand names.

The decision of whether such products are bioequivalent is taken on the basis of assays on relative bioavailability. According to EU guidelines, two formulations may be considered bioequivalent when, under identical experimental conditions (including identical administration route for test and reference preparation), rate and extent of absorption (bioavailability) differ only within acceptable limits. The test procedure requires experimental planning and statistical evaluation according to specified regulations. The statistical processing that should lead to the decision to accept or reject bioequivalence constitutes the bottleneck in the procedure. Up until now no method exists that is statistically sufficiently secured to fully exclude incorrect interpretations.

Despite this limitation, the 75%/125% rule recommended by the FDA is considered favorable for a provisional approximation of bioequivalence. According to this rule, a test preparation should yield a relative bioavailability between 75% and 125% relative to the reference product in minimally 75% of the tested subjects. For example, the reference preparation is administered to 12 subjects and the AUC value of the drug is determined in each subject. Each individual value thus obtained is set at 100%. After the appropriate time interval, each person then receives the test preparation, and the AUC values are determined again and are related for each subject to that of the reference preparation. In at least nine (75%) of the subjects, this value should lie between 75% and 125%.

> FDA defines bioequivalence as follows: the absence of a significant difference in the rate and extent to which the active ingredient or active moiety in pharmaceutical equivalents or pharmaceutical alternatives becomes available at the site of drug action when administered at the same molar dose under similar conditions in an appropriately designed study.

Example

In 8 (out of 12) individuals, a relative bioavailability for the test preparation is found between 124.6% and 76.3%, (in accordance with the 75%/125% rule), the values for the other four are 70.8%, 68.8%, 73.2%, and 144.7%. This means that four values (33.3%) lie outside the set limits. For this reason the test preparation will not receive recognition as being bioequivalent to the reference preparation.

An alternative procedure to arrive at a bioequivalence decision is based on two interlocked t-tests (see section 6.5.2); this method requires that the averaged parameters lie within a precisely defined confidence interval. Besides the AUC values, in specified cases also c_{max} and t_{max} may be called upon for an evaluation of bioequivalence.

7.5 Absorption of Active Ingredients

7.5.1 Absorption Mechanisms

For the development of optimally active drug formulations a clear perception of the absorption process is mandatory. The absorption process consists of a series of individual events, which do not occur separated in time, but rather overlap each other. It should not be considered as a static but rather as a dynamic process.

Absorption is understood as the uptake of a substance from the body surface or from locally confined sites of the body interior into the lymph or blood compartment. In this chain of events diffusion, as a voluntary movement of a dissolved substance driven by a concentration gradient in a solid or fluid solvent phase, is the major process. A compelling condition for absorption is the release of the active ingredient, i.e. its release out of the formulation or disintegration products thereof, and the diffusion of the dissolved drug to the site of absorption. This is followed by the following events:

- *Penetration*: the intrusion of a substance *into* membranes, lipid films, or organs
- *Permeation*: the movement of a substance *across* a membrane—whose normal function is to rather prevent such movement—into absorption organs

After uptake of the drug in the vascular system (circulation) the subsequent step is the *distribution* in the transport medium (blood), allowing the drug to distribute along the concentration gradient between blood and tissues further into the entire organism. The combined absorption and distribution processes in the organism is called *invasion*.

Finally, the drug will exert its typical activity, commonly involving interaction with a receptor, which requires a certain minimal local concentration. The duration of the effect depends on how long the active concentration, the so-called *therapeutic blood level*, is sustained.

The processes discussed above are already overlapped by subsequent phases, such as *biotransformation* (metabolism) and *inactivation*, taking into account different variants of the latter. For example, the drug might migrate into other organs and tissues. Furthermore, inactivation of the drug may be brought about by depot formation, binding to serum components, sorption, or storage events. Finally, inactivation may take place by (chemical) biotransformation catalyzed by complex enzyme systems. The overall process culminates ultimately in the *excretion* of the drug or its metabolites from the body. This is mediated either by the urinary or the intestinal tract. Volatile substances are eliminated through the lungs. The concentration decrease by biotransformation and elimination is achieved according to the rules of reaction kinetics, like the absorption processes.

Opposite to earlier viewpoints, it is not only the drug dose by itself that is responsible for the therapeutic effect. Additional factors, starting with the **L**iberation of the drug from the formulation, via the **A**bsorption, onto the **D**istribution, **M**etabolism, and **E**xcretion (the **LADME** scheme), have a decisive role in the ultimate therapeutic effect, which is commonly based on a drug-receptor interaction phenomenon in the biophase.

The release of the drug from the formulation represents a particularly important parameter in the entire absorption process. The release capacity determines the rate of release thus time to reach maximum blood levels. The release phase for drug formulations is equally important, except in case of intravenous administration, when the active ingredient is directly introduced in the blood compartment. The extent of release is determined above all by the solubility and the dissolution rate of the drug. When the drug is present in solution, no problems are to be expected with respect to the absorption process. For readily water-soluble drugs, the release from the formulation will predictably proceed at a high rate. However, many drugs are poorly water-soluble. It may be safely assumed that for all active agents with a solubility of < 0.3%, the dissolution rate is slower than the absorption rate. This will cause the release process to be the rate-limiting and controlling factor for the entire absorption process.

The importance of the release phase lies above all in the various possibilities to manipulate the release rate by means of pharma-/technological measures during the formulation process of the drug. This can be effectuated for example by choosing a particular physical of chemical form (particles of different sizes, crystalline *vs.* amorphous, salt or base etc.) as well as by the proper selection of the excipients and the manufacturing technology. For poorly soluble agents ("problem drugs," Table 7-2) it is often important to achieve higher release rates in order to improve the bioavailability. Additionally, by taking such measures we can achieve maximally fast release of an initial dose, while securing a prolonged and largely constant blood level due to the subsequently released maintenance dose. The ideal worth striving for is a formulation with absorption properties that can be manipulated with respect to onset, intensity and duration of activity.

The action of a drug requires the drug to enter cells in the body. These cells are by no means washed around by blood, but are rather bathing in an aqueous tissue fluid containing proteins like albumine, which can also transport some lipophilic drugs. As a consequence, water-solubility presents an essential requirement for the effective permeation and activity. On the other hand, drugs (need to) penetrate into cells via cell layers that have a fundamentally lipid nature, therefore lipid-soluble characteristics are also required. As a rule, drug absorption involves simple distribution processes between aqueous solutions and biomembranes possessing predominantly lipophilic properties (Fig. 7-16). These processes are dictated by physicochemical rules such as the dependence on lipid-solubility and pH for alkaline and acidic compounds. Predictably, the distribution (the result of flowing media, e.g., blood), proceeds rapidly. By contrast, diffusion or permeation through membranes and boundary layers represent slow processes, due to the natural resistance these structures offer against penetration. As in the latter case, the drug has to travel to the site of action via multiple successively positioned volumes separated by semi-permeable membranes. The concentration gradients gradually level off from volume to volume and are protracted in time.

The transport of molecules across membranes occurs basically either by *diffusion* or by *convection*.

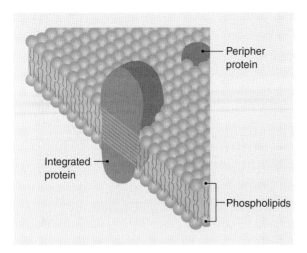

Fig. 7-16   Schematic structure of biological membranes.

The diffusion process is explained as follows (Fig. 7-17a): The transport of the dissolved molecule (solute) occurs without noticeable displacement of the solvent. The driving force is the difference in concentration of the drug between the outside (c_o) and the inside (c_i) of the membrane (passive diffusion). When the transport proceeds across a membrane without pores, the transport flow q is proportional to the distribution coefficient f of the molecule in question between the membrane material and the solvent. Furthermore, the transport flow is proportional to the membrane surface A and inversely proportional to the thickness d of the membrane. The diffusion constant D characterizes the specific diffusion of the molecule in the membrane material. In this situation, only those molecules are able to diffuse that are soluble in the basic material of the membrane. Only lipid-soluble, nonionized molecules are capable of diffusing across lipid membranes, while ionized molecules essentially cannot penetrate such membranes.

Diffusion-driven transport is described by the following mathematical equation (modified after Fick's law):

$$q = D\frac{A}{d}f(c_a - c_i) \tag{7-19}$$

In case of advection, the transport of the dissolved molecules occurs together with displacement of the solvent (Fig. 7-17b). Amount and direction of the transport are determined by the hydrostatic pressure gradient between the outside (P_o) and the inside (P_i) of the membrane. When the transport takes place by laminar flow through circular pores, as we assume for the cause of simplicity, then q is proportional to the number of pores n and the fourth

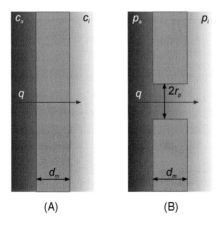

$$(A) \qquad\qquad (B)$$

**Fig. 7-17   Diffusion and convection as basic mechanisms of drug transport through membranes:
(A) diffusion; (B) advection (convection).**

power of the radius r of the pores and inversely proportional to the length of the pore, which corresponds to the thickness d of the membrane. The viscosity constant η characterizes the specific resistance of the solution against convective shift. Convective transport is described by the following equation (modified Hagen-Poiseuille law):

$$q = \frac{1}{\eta} \cdot \frac{n \cdot \pi \cdot r^4}{8 \cdot d} (P_a - P_i) \qquad\qquad (7\text{-}20)$$

All lipid-containing membranes in the body possess pores, which vary in size and number for different membranes. Basically, only small hydrophilic molecules are able to penetrate. Furthermore, it has to be taken into account that the pores may have charges at the inside, which can influence the movement of cations and anions.

For membranes that display transport characteristics that cannot be explained by the laws of diffusion or convection, permeation results from special mechanisms—for example, by facilitated carrier-mediated transport. The carrier hypothesis assumes the presence in the membrane of cell-specific carrier molecules that stereo-specifically bind the substance to be transported. The complex thus formed is translocated to the inside face of the membrane where the molecule to be transported is released. The carrier then diffuses back to the outside of the membrane so that the process can be repeated. Generally speaking, this transport mechanism has not yet been of great significance for the absorption of drugs. However, currently drugs are under development, which are supposed to be translocated across membranes via this very transport system.

With respect to membrane permeation, four functional membrane types can be distinguished (Fig. 7-18):

- *Type* 1: The membrane consists of material that is impermeable to dissolved molecules; it has water-filled pores through which diffusion as well as convection may occur.
- *Type* 2: The membrane consists of a closed layer without pores. In this case, only diffusion can occur, but this will be restricted to molecules that are soluble in the membrane material.
- *Type* 3: The membrane material is like that of type 2, but now it has pores. Molecules can then cross the membrane through the membrane material and through the pores.
- *Type* 4: Membranes with carrier transport systems.

Additional absorption mechanisms are known and proven to be operational for several drugs. In a quantitative sense, however, these absorption mechanisms are of lower significance. *Active transport* is defined as the energy-consuming permeation of substances through membranes against a concentration gradient. This type of absorption has been demonstrated for instance for amino acids and some sugars. *Pinocytosis* is the process by which liquid droplets

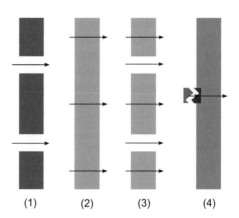

   (1)   (2)   (3)   (4)

Fig. 7-18   Membrane types.

are taken up by means of an invagination of the cell membrane in the same way solid particles are taken up in a process called *phagocytosis*. When ultra-small particles are crossing a cell layer through small gaps in between the cells (particularly epithelial cells), we speak of *persorption*. Finally, molecules may be absorbed by the dissociation of compounds by *ion-pair diffusion*.

7.5.2 Distribution Balance, Biological Half Life

In order to determine for each individual active agent the proper type of administration and the corresponding drug formulation, absorption in humans must be determined, using different administration methods, by means of assaying blood concentrations at certain time intervals. Whenever possible, the active agent is administered without addition of excipients—that is, merely dissolved in water or suspended or processed into a lipid base or in gelatin capsules. Absorption and distribution of the administered pharmaceutical in the volumes of blood, tissue fluid, organs, and the flow rate therein leads to a concentration at the active site that determines the speed and the realization of the pharmacological action. With the help of sensitive analytical methods, it is possible to determine the concentration in blood plasma and tissues after certain time intervals. From such data, the amount of absorbed, metabolized, and eliminated substances can be obtained, allowing us to make up a quantitative distribution balance concerning the fate of the pharmaceutical in the organism. Fig. 7-19 presents the course of the blood levels and the tissue concentration of a drug following intestinal absorption. It shows the distribution in the body as well as the inactivation and elimination. In this case, maximal blood concentration is reached rapidly after the administration of the drug, and then diminishes exponentially. Maximal concentration in tissues is attained later than in blood. Inactivation and excretion cause a steady decrease of the drug concentration in blood and tissues. The terminal part of the descending limb of the blood level curve in Fig. 7-19 usually follows the kinetics of a first order reaction (see section 25.2.2), which, after taking the logarithm, can be rearranged to:

$$k_e = \frac{2.303}{t} \lg \frac{c_0}{c} \tag{7-21}$$

k_e = elimination constant (h^{-1}),
c = drug concentration at time t,
c_0 = drug concentration at time t $= 0$

For a graphic evaluation, equation 7-22 is rearranged algebraically to

$$\lg c = -\frac{k_e}{2.303} t + \lg c_0 \tag{7-22}$$

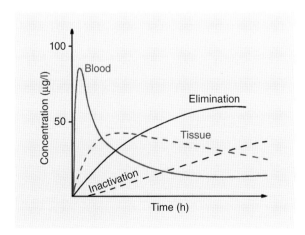

Fig. 7-19 Distribution balance of a pharmaceutical.

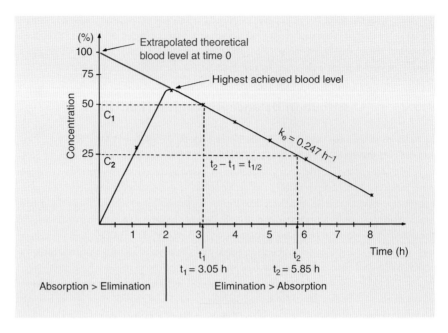

Fig. 7-20 Blood level curve (semi-logarithmic presentation).

The evaluation follows now after plotting the experimentally determined blood level values in a coordinate system (ordinate: c (μg/mL) or (%) logarithmically; abscissa t (h) linearly). The result is a straight line (see Fig. 7-20) from whose slope ($-k_e/2.303$) the elimination constant is obtained. The intercept with the ordinate yields the drug concentration at t = 0. The half-life $t_{1/2}$ can be calculated as

$$t_{1/2} = \frac{0.693}{k_e} \qquad\qquad (7\text{-}23)$$

The half-life can also be obtained directly from the graphic presentation ($t_2 - t_1 = t_{1/2}$).

In the given example t_1 ($c_1 = 50\%$) = 3.05 h and t_2 ($c_2 = 25\%$) = 5.85 h; from this follows $t_{1/2} = 2.80$ h.

By introducing the value for $t_{1/2}$ in the converted equation the excretion rate constant can be calculated:

$$k_e = \frac{0.693}{2.8\,\text{h}} = 0.247\,\text{h}^{-1} \qquad\qquad (7\text{-}24)$$

The exact number of drug *disappearing* per h is not 24.7%, but $(1 - e^{-k}) * 100\% = 21.9\%$ per h as calculated for a one-compartment model (see next section). For the usually small k_e the difference becomes negligible.

This implies (after some calculations) that each hour approx. 22% of the amount of drug that is present at the start of that hour disappears from the blood. The majority of the investigated active agents display comparable behavior, that is, elimination follows, as a rule, first order kinetics. In identical time intervals identical proportions of the drug still present in the blood are excreted. Accordingly, the biological half-life (elimination half-life) is understood as the time in which half of the amount of drug is present in biologically active form, while the other half has already been inactivated (metabolized and excreted). The biological half-life is a statistical parameter. It differs between individuals and can also vary within one and the same subject. Basically, when interpreting this pharmacokinetic parameter, a number of factors have to be taken into account; these include dose level, urine pH, age of subject, simultaneous administration of another pharmaceutical, protein binding, and nature of the disease. The straight line in Fig. 7-20 intersects the abscissa in a certain point. The smaller the angle at which this occurs (i.e., the shallower the course of the line), the longer the action of the drug lasts. When $t_{1/2}$ is long, a small maintenance dose will suffice to sustain the achieved therapeutic concentration. When, by contrast, $t_{1/2}$ is short, higher doses will be required to achieve this. The biological half-lives of various drugs are very different (Table 7-3).

7.5.3   Pharmacokinetic Compartment Models

Table 7-3 Biological Half-Lives of Drugs in Humans

Drug	$t_{1/2}$
Tubocurarin	13 min
Penicillin	28 min
Hexamethonium	1.5 h
p-Aminosalicylic acid	1.9 h
Glutethimide	10 h
Phenazone	11 h
Thiopental	16 h
Sulfamerazine	26 h
Pentobarbital	42 h
Barbital	4 to 8 d
Vitamin D	40 d

In order to obtain pharmacokinetic information concerning the course of absorption, distribution, metabolism, and excretion of pharmaceutics from measured blood and urine values, *compartment models* are used, which allow us to illustrate and describe the processes in the human organism. Compartments are delimited fictitious distribution spaces in which we assume the agent to be homogeneously distributed (blood, tissues etc.). We distinguish one-, two-, and multi-compartment models.

The one-compartment model requires that the drug be distributed quickly and homogeneously in the body fluids and tissues. An arbitrary volume of blood contains an amount of drug that is proportional to the amount present at any time in any other body fluid. Thus, shortly after administration, the drug is present only in blood or evenly distributed between the blood compartment and the body tissues and other body fluids, so that at any time the amount excreted in the urine is proportional to the amount absorbed by the body. In such cases the body can be envisaged as a single reaction chamber or as one compartment.

The following correlation emerges:

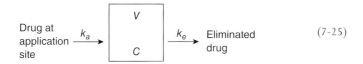

$$(7\text{-}25)$$

V = volume of the compartment

C = drug concentration in the compartment

k_e = elimination rate constant

k_a = absorption rate

Because the elimination of active agents or their metabolites from the human body proceeds in most cases with first-order kinetics, a drug-time diagram will show an exponentially declining curve (Fig. 7-19). When, instead of the concentration itself, the value of its logarithm is plotted in the diagram, we obtain a straight line (Fig. 7-20) with a slope that represents k_e. For absorption as well as elimination processes, a multitude of blood concentration versus time correlations can be described by the so-called Bateman function, which originally was developed for the decay of radioactive isotopes. Often, however, other apparent k values are observed, for instance when one follows the time-dependent blood levels of a drug following a single-dose intravenous administration. In such cases, the blood level curve initially drops steeply for a short time, to evolve subsequently into a more shallow straight line with a slope that, again, is a measure for the elimination rate. This phenomenon is caused by the rapid distribution of the drug in quickly accessible spaces of tissue fluid, from which the drug then gradually returns in the central compartment. These conditions can best be described by a *two-compartment model*.

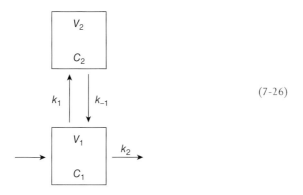

$$(7\text{-}26)$$

V_1 = volume of the central compartment (blood)
C_1 = drug concentration in the central compartment
V_2 = volume of the peripheral compartments (tissue fluid)
C_2 = drug concentration in the peripheral compartment
k_1 = rate constant for the drug entering the peripheral compartment
k_{-1} = rate constant for the return of the drug into the central compartment
k_2 = elimination rate constant

In case of multiple fluid spaces with unequal diffusion rates into and out of these spaces we have to take into account a corresponding number of compartments when modeling this situation. As a rule, such complex models (multiple compartment models) can only be effectively described on the basis of measured blood levels following intravenous administration. The compartment with the lowest drug efflux rate is termed the deep compartment and determines its terminal half-life.

7.5.4   The Clearance Concept

Besides the calculation of drug kinetics by means of the compartment models discussed in the preceding paragraphs, the concept of clearance has gained acceptance, particularly in the field of clinical pharmacokinetics. This concept was first used in renal physiology (Homer Smith, 1895–1962, New York University) and later introduced in general pharmacokinetics. It has the advantage that also in case the drop in drug concentration does not precisely follow first-order kinetics (e.g., in patients), the elimination factors can be assessed quantitatively.

In addition to the kidney as the most important excretion organ, the liver, lungs, and some other organs are also involved in the metabolism of drugs. The integral drug removal process is known as body clearance or as total plasma clearance.

Instead of determining the elimination rate, like in the compartment analysis, the clearance concept calculates the volume of plasma that is freed (cleared) from drug per unit of time. Fig. 7-21 further clarifies this concept. When the drug-containing blood flows through an eliminating organ, it is freed of a fraction of the drug. This could be interpreted as a reduction in drug concentration, but may also be seen as a certain plasma volume fraction that is completely freed of the drug.

When the plasma flow rate (mL/min) through the organ is known, we can simply calculate the amount of drug eliminated by the organ per unit of time.

The basic equation (7.27) shows that the drug elimination per unit of time depends on the plasma concentration and the elimination capacity (expressed as clearance). The unit of clearance in this formula we thus obtain is mL/min or l/h, in other words the complete removal of drug from a certain fractional volume of plasma, as already discussed.

$$\frac{dm}{dt} = -Clearance \cdot c_p \qquad\qquad (7\text{-}27)$$

dM/dt = drug elimination per unit of time
c_p = plasma concentration (amount of drug/volume)
clearance = volume of plasma completely cleared of drug per unit of time

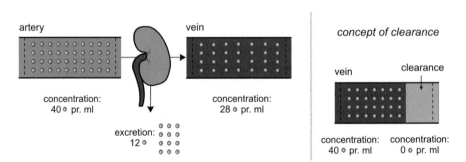

Fig. 7-21 The clearance concept.

Like for the compartment analysis (equation 7-2), we also notice here the basic principle that the absolute amount of eliminated drug depends on the plasma concentration. When we compare the clearance model with the one-compartment model, we see (equation 7-28), after adjustment of coefficients, that the total clearance Cl in the clearance concept represents the product of elimination constant k and distribution volume V or better even: $k = Cl/V$. Thus, the elimination constant k depends on the distribution volume of the drug in the body and the elimination capacity of the body.

$$
c = \frac{M}{V}
$$
$$
\frac{dM}{dt} = -k \cdot c_p \cdot V \equiv \frac{dM}{dt} = -Clearance \cdot c_p
$$
$$
Clearance \cdot c_p = k \cdot c_p \cdot V
$$
$$
Clearance = k \cdot V
$$

(7-28)

The advantage of the clearance concept is that the clearance can be calculated relatively easily when the amount of drug that arrives in the blood after administration is precisely known. In case of intravenous injection this is given by definition, for oral administration the total absorbed amount must be known. We "only" have to know the AUC of the total blood concentration versus time curve and the absorbed drug dose to calculate the total clearance (see equation 7-29).

$$
-\frac{dM}{dt} = c_p \cdot Cl_{tot} \Rightarrow -dM = Cl_{tot} \cdot c_p \cdot dt
$$
$$
integrated: -M = D = Cl_{tot} \cdot AUC
$$

(7-29)

Cl_{tot} = total or body clearance
$-M$ = total eliminated amount of drug, which equals D (*eliminated = removed from the system, therefore the "-" sign*)
D = injected or absorbed dose
AUC = area under the plasma concentration-time curve

As pointed out before, the advantage of the clearance concept is that clearance always applies when the given dose appears entirely in the central compartment (e.g., upon intravascular administration). It is, however, independent on the shape of the plasma concentration-time curve, meaning it is irrelevant, whether the drug is given as a bolus injection or slowly infused and whether or not the elimination follows an exponential function, as long as linear pharmacokinetics prevail (i.e., no saturation processes are involved).

7.5.5   Diffusion Coefficient

As the release of active agent is essentially based on diffusion processes, Fick's first diffusion law constitutes the basic foundation of the various diffusion conditions. The diffusion rate, or the amount of material passing a given cross section in a very short time, is proportional to the area of the cross section and the concentration gradient:

$$
dQ = -D \cdot A \left(\frac{dc}{dx} \right)_t dt
$$

(7-30)

dQ = amount of drug
A = cross-sectional area
D = diffusion coefficient
$\left(\frac{dc}{dx} \right)_t$ = concentration gradient at time t

The minus sign indicates that the diffusion proceeds in the direction of the concentration gradient. The diffusion coefficient indicates the amount of material that diffuses across the cross-sectional unit in a unit of time at a concentration gradient 1. Its dimension is $cm^2 \cdot s^{-1}$.

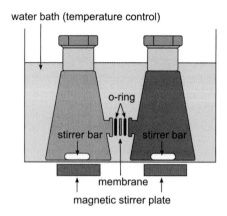

Fig. 7-22 **Equipment to measure diffusion coefficients (after *Goldberg and Higuchi* 1968).**

The diffusion coefficient of a substance depends on the temperature, the viscosity of the medium, and the molecular size of the diffusing substance, as given in equation 7-31:

$$D = \frac{R \cdot T}{6 \cdot \pi \cdot \eta \cdot r \cdot N_A}$$

(7-31)

R = gas constant
T = absolute temperature
η = viscosity of the solvent
r = radius of the solute molecule
N_A = Avogadro constant

In general, the diffusion coefficient of electrolytes in aqueous solution decreases with increasing dilution. Diffusion is decelerated by other dissolved substances. However, when both dissolved substances are electrolytes, diffusion may be accelerated.

Because direct assessment of diffusion coefficients (implying just overlaying two layers of liquid) is not a simple affair, this is mostly accomplished by using a system consisting of two chambers separated by a membrane, such as the double-flask system depicted in Fig. 7-22 (silver membrane with pore width 1.2 μm, thickness 50 μm).

Diffusion coefficients can be determined with such equipment within two hours. As a metallic membrane is used, reproducibility and stability is better than in systems using membranes of biological origin. Flask 1 is filled with water, flask 2 with drug solution. The system is calibrated (cell constant) with a substance having a known diffusion coefficient.

To calculate the diffusion coefficient, the following equation is applied:

$$D = \frac{G}{L\,(c_2 - c_1)}$$

(7-32)

L = cell constant
D = diffusion coefficient
G = transport rate from flask 2 to flask 1
c_1, c_2 = concentrations

Strictly speaking, we are dealing here with dialysis coefficients. Because the size of the pores in the membrane permits unrestricted diffusion, in this case, the term *diffusion coefficient* is justified. Experimental setups of this kind are likewise suitable for the assessment of diffusion of drugs in aqueous systems containing mucilage, surfactants as well as lipidic systems.

7.6   Factors Affecting Release and Absorption

7.6.1   Dosage Form and Type of Application

The drug dosage form and, connected with that, the route of administration we choose, depend primarily on the medical indication and on the absorption, toxicity, and stability of the active ingredient. Often, a prompt but long-lasting and possibly constant activity is desired. In this connection, the *prolonged intravenous infusion* must be considered the ideal dosage form, which can only be applied as an in-patient mode. After the initial dose, the drug is infused by continuous drip infusion at a rate that parallels the rate of elimination. In this way, the blood and tissue levels of the drug may be set at a constant value. *Intravenous injection* leads to a rapid distribution of the drug in the entire organism, resulting in prompt onset of activity and a high intensity of drug action as long as the drug is given as a solution (no release phase, optimal availability of the active ingredient). The duration of activity depends, in essence, on the specific elimination rate of the drug, but usually, it does not last long. *Subcutaneous or intramuscular injection* leads to a gradual onset of activity because the drug first has to emerge from the depot at the injection site before it can be absorbed. The intensity of action is not very distinct, but, on the other hand, prolonged blood levels are accomplished. This particularly applies to intramuscularly administered drug formulations.

For *rectal drug formulations* absorption depends on the vehicle (aqueous micro-enema, suppositories with water-soluble or fusible basic substances), as well as on the solubility of the active ingredient. Rapid absorption can be expected when a readily water-soluble active agent is suspended in a suitable lipophilic ground substance.

Also for *percutaneous drug formulations*, the action of the drug varies and depends on its structure and on the vehicle. Drugs in solution, in lotions, in powders, and in some ground substances of ointments only act on the upper skin layers, while other ointment types facilitate diffusion of the drug through the skin.

For peroral drug formulations, we may, in general, expect shallower blood and tissue levels curves than for parenteral formulations. There is no general rule with respect to the absorption conditions. The latter are influenced by the nature of the drug, the type of formulation (tablets, solutions, suspensions, etc.), and the physiological conditions in the gastrointestinal tract. From the point of view of pharmaceutical technology, in this case absorption can be varied in many different ways.

With inhalation formulations, a rapid onset of action and high action intensity are obtained, but are mostly accompanied by a short time span of action.

7.6.2   Physical–Chemical Properties of the Drug

7.6.2.1   Solubility and Dissolution Rate

The release and absorption behavior of a drug is particularly determined by its solubility and dissolution velocity. For readily water-soluble drugs, rapid dissolution ensures rapid absorption. In case of lower solubility, the time factor becomes particularly relevant. Thus it may be that during the travel of the drug through the absorption zone of the gastro-intestinal tract the time available is not sufficient to achieve complete dissolution and absorption. For poorly soluble drugs, the release and absorption conditions are simply unfavorable. In section 3.10.4, the principles that may lead to improvement of dissolution properties of a drug are discussed.

Particle size is significant because, by diminishing this parameter, resulting in an increase of surface area, an increase in dissolution rate can be achieved and thereby absorption enhancement. It is also essential to take particle size distribution into consideration. Homogeneity in particle size yields a higher dissolution rate than when the particles significantly differ in size, even when the specific surface area in both cases is the same. Because the onset of drug action and its intensity as well as duration are all strongly dependent on the degree of dispersion, particle size reduction is mandatory for poorly soluble agents in order to achieve better

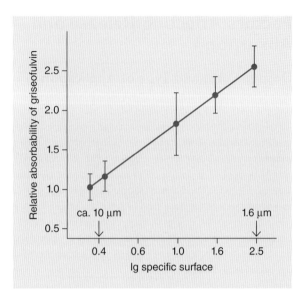

Fig. 7-23   Dependence of griseofulvin absorption on specific surface area. The relative absorbability of griseofulvin is correlated to the area under the blood level curve (with standard errors). Given in μm are the corresponding particle sizes for the given logarithmic specific surface.

absorption. Beyond that, minimal particle size is decisive for patient tolerance (eyedrops, ointments) and for accurate dosing (tablets, suppositories). Finally, it plays an important role with respect to homogeneity and stability of drug formulations (powders, suspensions).

In the following, we will demonstrate the effect of particle size on absorption by means of a few examples. A conspicuous case is the particle size dependence of the absorption of griseofulvin. This antimycotic is practically insoluble in water. It was demonstrated that 125 mg micronized griseofulvin has the same antimycotic activity as 250 mg of coarse powder and that there is a linear correlation between the logarithm of the specific surface area and the absorption of griseofulvin (Fig. 7-23). This finding has led manufacturers of the drug to use micronized griseofulvin in their formulations, resulting in a reduction of the dose, leading in turn to a substantial reduction in treatment costs. Similar differences were observed for other poorly soluble drugs when formulated in either micronized or microcrystalline form (e.g., antidiabetic sulfonylureas). Not only was reduced particle size leading to higher blood level values, but maximal concentrations were attained faster. Moreover, absorption proceeded more uniformly in time. We must take into account, however, that the rapidly attained high plasma levels resulting from micronization also decline again rapidly. Although medium-fine or coarsely powdered drugs may require more time to be absorbed and thus result in lower plasma levels, they are retained over longer periods of time.

The toxicity of a drug depends on particle size: Micronized drug formulations may display a lower lethal dose than a coarsely disperse formulation. Especially for drugs with a narrow tolerance range, it is essential to pay special attention to particle size.

Treatment failure with pharmaceutics is sometimes due to insufficient reduction of the particle size of the active agent. This is not to say that activity enhancement will always be achieved by reduction of particle size, but by doing so we may at least count on a faster onset of activity if this is desired. From a certain grain size up, coarsely disperse agents will no longer display significant improvement of absorption behavior. It may also occur that an organism takes up an active agent independent of particle size; this is, for instance, the case for tetracyclin.

On the other hand, extensive particle size reduction is not always indicated. This is, for instance, the case when slow absorption is required (depot drugs). Furthermore, for drugs that dissolve in gastric juice but are absorbed only in the intestine, substantial particle reduction is not mandatory. A very small size of particles may also be unfavorable in terms of upscaling formulations and storage, as very small particles due to their large curvature and their large specific surface will interact and react with other particles or other matter in close vicinity probably causing, for example, size increase. Combination of particles with different sizes can be used, if a rapid onset combined with a prolonged activity is desired.

7.6.2.2   Crystallinity, Amorphous State, and Solubility

Crystal form and crystal size are factors of general importance in drug manufacturing. They significantly affect the physical properties of a powder, which in turn may have an effect on the technological processes as well as on the quality of the ultimate preparation (see section 3.2.1).

By choosing the appropriate conditions, specified crystal structures can be obtained during crystallization. Many active ingredients are commercially available in different crystal forms. As these often have different dissolution velocities, depending on the ratio between volume and surface area, they may also affect drug absorption. The more uniform the crystal form, the more reproducible the activity will be. As a rule, crystal forms with blunt, rounded-off edges are preferred, as they approximate spherical shape. Unfortunately, manufacturers rarely succeed in manipulating the crystallization, precipitation, and grinding process to the extent that such forms are obtained. Often, it is possible to achieve prolongation of activity with a combination of larger and smaller crystals by mixing different crystal forms of a substance.

As a rule, amorphous forms of a substance dissolve more rapidly and are better absorbed than the corresponding crystalline forms. However, amorphous materials often have a tendency to transform into the lower-energy crystalline state, so that special stabilization measures are necessary to keep the amorphous state.

The differences in activity between crystalline and amorphous substances can be quite distinct. Zinc-insulin occurs in a crystalline and an amorphous form, depending on the manufacturing conditions. While the amorphous form is rapidly absorbed as a result of the high dissolution rate, the crystalline form displays delayed activity onset but its activity is sustained for extended periods. Preparations containing 70% crystalline and 30% amorphous zinc-insulin ensure a rapid onset of activity and an intermediate duration of action.

7.6.3   Polymorphism

Likewise, the occurrence of different crystalline modifications (polymorphism) of active agents (see section 3.2.1.1) may substantially affect biopharmaceutical behavior, particularly of poorly soluble agents. A striking example is methyl prednisolone that exists in two enantiotropic forms that distinguish themselves in melting point (difference more than 25 K) and solubility. Strong influences of polymorphism are manifest for chloramphenicol-palmitate suspensions. Chloramphenicol-palmitate forms multiple polymorphous variants of which only one is cleaved by intestinal esterases at a sufficient rate to make adequate amounts of the active chloramphenicol available for absorption. The gradual conversion of the originally present metastable modification into the stable form causes complete inactivation of chloramphenicol-palmitate preparations. The addition of macromolecular excipients can prevent this conversion. In addition to differences in dissolution rate, also differences in reactivity can explain the disparity in bioavailability. Possibly, the active modification of chloramphenicol-palmitate has a favorable stereochemical configuration that makes it more susceptible to the enzymatic ester cleavage required for an adequate absorption rate.

7.6.4   Pseudopolymorphism

Pseudopolymorphism is the phenomenon wherein a compound is obtained in crystalline forms that differ in the nature or stoichiometry of included solvent molecules. Many active ingredients (e.g., steroids, antibiotics, barbiturates, sulfonamides, and phenylbutazone) display pseudopolymorphism and, as a result, marked differences in dissolution and absorption rates (see also section 3.2.1.2). In general, water-free drugs show higher dissolution rates than the corresponding hydrates. Examples are prednisolone, quinine, caffeine, theophylline, and barbiturates. Based on serum level values in humans, it was demonstrated that the water-free compound provides a more favorable availability than the tri-hydrate. It should be taken into account that during the processing of water-free ingredients hydrate formation may occur during storage or upon application. In case of poorly soluble drugs this may lead to a further limitation of the absorption perspectives. Solvate-containing crystals often display the opposite situation in that they have higher dissolution rates than the solvate-free counterparts. This has been demonstrated for hydrocortisone esters (ethanol), succinyl-sulfathiazol (n-pentanol) and a few other drugs. Such differences in absorption may also be caused by the nature of the crystallization medium.

7.6.5   Degree of Ionization and pK_a Value

The majority of drugs have an acidic or alkaline character. Depending on pH, these compounds can occur in ionized or nonionized form. The permeability of a drug through the lipid barrier of membranes depends on the fraction of the drug that is not ionized—that is, the degree of ionization α. The latter can be calculated from the acidity constant K_a or the pK_a value, whereby pK_a, analogous to pH, stands for the negative logarithm of the acidity constant K_a:

For acids:

$$\alpha_s = \frac{K_a}{K_a + [H^+]} = \frac{1}{1 + 10^{pK_a - pH}} \tag{7-33}$$

For bases:

$$\alpha_B = \frac{[H^+]}{[H^+] + K_a} = \frac{1}{1 + 10^{pH - pK_a}} \tag{7-34}$$

In the graphic presentation (Fig. 7-24) we obtain sigmoid curves, which clarify the pH-dependence of the ionization conditions. For weak acids the degree of ionization increases with increasing pH value, whereas it diminishes in case of weak bases. When pK_a equals pH, 50% of the substance is present in its ionized form. In the pH range around the pK_a value (i.e., the steepest part of the curve) a small change in proton concentration causes a severe shift in α.

From the above, it follows that the pH value of the absorption environment has a decisive influence on the absorption of drugs, as the nondissociated form is subject to other uptake conditions than the dissociated form. But the two forms may also differ in biological activity. Furthermore, the proton concentration has effects on solubility and distribution coefficients of the drug as well as on the membrane potential and interface activity. Water-solubility increases with the concentration of the ionized form, whereas lipid solubility usually increases with the concentration of the nonionized form (Fig. 7-25). This implies that a weak acid with low pK_a value is better absorbed in the stomach, as ionization is strongly suppressed at the low pH prevailing there and therefore exists predominantly in its nondissociated form. In the alkaline environment of the intestine, on the other hand, weak bases

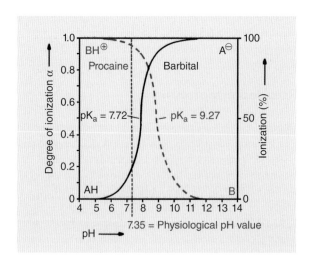

Fig. 7-24 Correlation between pH value and degree of ionization of procaine (base) and barbital (acid).

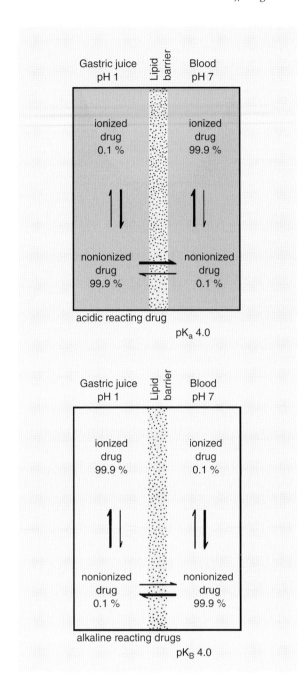

Fig. 7-25 Dependence of drug absorption on the degree of ionization.

are better absorbed. In summary, assuming that the lipid-water distribution coefficient of the nondissociated form is relatively large, we can make up rules of thumb as presented in Table 7-4. However, these rules should by no means be considered generally applicable.

Besides for solubility and absorption, the ionization degree is relevant for the stability and compatibility of active ingredients and excipients, as well as for the activity of preservation agents and antioxidants (see chapters 25 and 26).

7.6.6   Distribution Coefficient

The absorption rate of organic drugs strongly depends on the extent of the lipophilic character of the compound. The more lipophilic the compound, the better it will penetrate the lipophilic membranes of the organism. Thus, the lipid-water distribution coefficient

Table 7-4 Absorbability of Acid and Basic Drugs

Character of the Drug	Absorption in the Stomach	Absorption in the Intestine
very strongly acidic	poor	poor
strongly acidic, pK_a values 0–3	good	little
weakly acidic, pK_a value > 3	good	less good
basic, pK_a value < 8	little	good
strongly basic, pK_a value > 8	poor	poor

is essential for penetration and absorption processes. It provides information on the distribution equilibrium of a compound in two immiscible fluids. According to Nernst's distribution rule, the following correlation applies, at constant pressure and temperature:

$$\frac{c_1}{c_2} = k \tag{7-35}$$

c_1 = concentration in phase 1 (lipophilic phase)
c_2 = concentration in phase 2 (hydrophilic phase)
k = distribution coefficient (constant)

According to this equation, the ratio of the concentrations (more precisely: of the activities) of a compound in the two phases is independent of the absolute concentrations in the two phases. This independence does not apply, however, when the distributed compound in one phase occurs in another form than in the other (e.g., as a dimer). The distribution coefficient serves as a characteristic parameter of a drug and permits predictions about its absorption behavior. It has been demonstrated that absorption improves with increasing distribution coefficient (Table 7-5). Drugs with a very low distribution coefficient are not at all absorbed in the stomach. This confirms that the stomach wall has the character of a lipid membrane through which drugs permeate in a passive way, in accordance with their lipid solubility. Similar conditions prevail in the rectum and in most part of the intestine. Also, the outer skin layers likewise function as lipid membranes, but having a different construction of the layers.

The distribution coefficient is also an interesting parameter for the distribution behavior of active ingredients and excipients in multiphase systems (creams, emulsions), and as such often represents an important predictor of the biological activity of a substance.

The distribution behavior of ionizable drugs depends on the proton concentration (pH) because the nondissociated compound possesses higher lipid solubility than the dissociated

Table 7-5 Drug Absorption in Rat Intestine Compared with the Distribution Coefficient *k* for Heptane/Water and Chloroform/Water Mixtures

Drug	Absorption %	*K* Heptane	*K* Chloroform
Thiopental	67	3.30	> 100
Benzoic acid	54	0.19	2.9
p-Hydroxypropiophenone	61	0.12	5.1
Salicylic acid	60	0.12	2.9
Acetyl-salicylic acid	21	0.03	2.0
Theophylline	30	0.02	0.3
Barbital	25	< 0.002	0.7
Theobromine	22	< 0.002	0.4
Sulfanilamide	24	< 0.002	0.03
p-Hydroxybenzoic acid	23	< 0.002	0.01
Barbituric acid	5	< 0.002	0.008
Sulfaguanidine	< 2	< 0.002	< 0.002
Mannitol	< 2	< 0.002	< 0.002

form. Distinct from the *true distribution coefficient*, which relates to the nonionogenic form of the molecule, in daily practice mostly the *apparent distribution coefficient* is determined. This represents the concentration ratio of the drug in the two phases, independent of which form of the drug prevails in each phase.

7.7 Assay Method

In the lipophilic phase, mostly organic solvents are used, including octanol, hexane, benzene, toluene, ethers, fatty oils, and others (see e.g. Malkia et al. 2004). The hydrophilic phase consists of water or a buffer solution of a certain pH. For the assay, identical volumes of the two phases, one of which containing the active ingredient, are shaken at constant temperature (commonly 20° or 37°C) until the drug has equilibrated between the two phases (in most cases several hours) and then the drug concentration in the aqueous phase is determined. In some cases, liposomes are used as a model distribution system. The lipid-water distribution coefficient k can now be calculated:

$$k = \frac{V_2 \left(c_2^0 - c_2^t \right)}{V_1 \cdot c_2^t} \qquad (7\text{-}36)$$

V_1 = volume of the lipophilic phase
V_2 = volume of the aqueous phase
c_2^0 = drug concentration in the aqueous phase before start of the experiment (in case the drug was added to the aqueous phase)
c_2^t = drug concentration in the aqueous phase after shaking, when the two phases have separated again (in case the drug was added to the aqueous phase)

Depending on the applied solvent and the composition of the aqueous phase the distribution coefficient may have different values.

This classical experimental design is more and more often supplemented by measuring the binding of the drug to liposomal membranes, predominantly consisting of phospholipids. In contrast to octanol, phospholipids contain phosphate and other charged groups, with which the drug can interact in an entirely different way than with octanol. Besides, lipid membranes do not contain a lipophilic bulk phase as in the solvent/water systems, but rather, a thin (ca. 4 nm) lipid phase composed of the fatty acid tails of the phospholipid. Consequently, the lipid membranes represent large areas of lipophilic/hydrophilic interfaces, to which dipole-like or amphiphilic drug molecules may associate in a totally different way than at a bulk octanol phase for instance.

This is illustrated by Fig. 7-26. The binding of a drug to lipid membranes (LEKC method, see section 7.1.3.1) correlates very well with its absorption in humans, but not with the

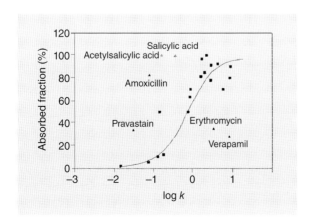

Fig. 7-26 Relation between drug-lipid membrane interaction and drug absorption in man (after Liu et al. 2011).

classical partition coefficient (data not shown here). The sigmoidal shape of the curve is caused by the logarithmic scale on the abscissa. Some values deviate, however, strongly from the correlation as illustrated by the triangles in Fig. 7-26. The open triangles refer to substances with low (<200) molecular mass that can diffuse in between cells (paracellularly); the filled triangles represent drugs that can be transported actively by an energy-requiring process—some of them obviously back into the intestinal lumen by p-glycoprotein transporters.

7.7.1   Excipients

Each substance used in the manufacturing of a drug formulation can affect in some way or another the onset, intensity and duration of drug action. It is not possible to make general statements in this connection, because of the vast number of possible combinations of a drug and the other substances required for its formulation. In 1968, the field was shocked by a spectacular affair drawing exceptional attention to the interaction between drug and excipient. In an Australian clinic, numerous patients who were treated with phenytoin capsules suddenly presented toxic symptoms. It was eventually found that this phenomenon was caused by replacing the commonly used filling substance calcium sulfate by lactose. Although the latter was considered to be as inert as calcium sulfate, it appeared that it enhanced the bioavailability of the drug to such an extent that toxic symptoms occurred.

There are various possibilities to enhance drug absorption by the use of excipients. For example, faster disintegration of peroral medicines will in general promote the absorption. An optimal disintegration rate can be obtained for instance by addition of agents that promote disintegration or hydrophilization, or alternatively, by diminishing the proportion of binding agent or the pressure during compression (see section 9.2.3; 9.5). For other drug formulations, buffer substances or sorbitol are often deployed as absorption enhancers. In case of formulations to be applied externally, 1,2-propylene glycol or hyaluronidase, among others, are applied.

Furthermore, we are pointing to the existence of typical absorption-delaying agents. Also, here we are dealing with a large variety of possibilities. In aqueous environment macromolecular substances, in particular, material capable of swelling, may lead to more or less distinct reduction of absorption due to viscosity enhancement. Similar effects are obtained with oils, whose viscosity can be further enhanced by additional substances such as aluminum monostearate.

Complex formation as a result of interactions between drug and excipient may affect the absorption process in very different ways. Among factors involved here we have: changes in molecular size, drug solubility, distribution coefficient, viscosity and drug mobilization (micellar localization, type of inclusion compound) and effects of the excipient on membrane permeability.

Surface-active compounds (detergents, surfactants) play an ever-increasing part in the manufacturing of medicines because of their potential to enhance the absorption of drugs when applied in suitable concentrations. One well-known surfactant that improves drug absorption is saponin. Narrowly defined statements on whether addition of a detergent will cause faster or perhaps also more intensive absorption, cannot be given as yet.

Absorption enhancement may also have different causes. Improved wetting of the particle surface may lead to better dissolution, which in turn may cause better absorption. For example, improvement of the solubility of the drug by solubilization may be responsible for the stimulatory effect. Furthermore, detergents facilitate the absorption of fats and fat-like substances due to better wetting and emulsification. On the one hand, it is assumed that detergents enhance the permeability of tissue membranes. On the other hand, it has been shown that, depending on type and amount, detergents are capable of delaying absorption. It is also conceivable that inclusion of the drug in large micellar structures, preventing membrane penetration or causing protracted drug release, plays a role to this effect. In contact with water, detergents may, in special compositions with active ingredients, spontaneously form micro-emulsions. From the latter, drugs such as cyclosporine are absorbed more effectively than from emulsions.

Several detergents have a specific activity by themselves. Others are, at least at higher concentration, physiologically not harmless. Consequently, when developing detergent-containing formulations, toxicity tests are mandatory.

Not only macromolecular and surface-active substances and excipient, but also inorganic excipients may engage in interactions with the active ingredient. Adsorbents such as bolus alba (white clay or kaolin, etc.) lead to delayed drug release and absorption due to adsorption of active ingredient. Generally, this is considered to be an undesirable effect; nonetheless, such excipients are deployed when aiming at a depot effect.

The mutually interactive effect that is observed when two drugs are combined in one formulation, and that may lead to either enhancement or reduction of activity, may also occur when excipients in one formulation interact with each other.

In several cases, the drug complex will not be able to penetrate membranes because of its size or because its physicochemical properties are decisively different from those of the free drug. In such cases, the drug can become active only after cleavage of the complex in the organism, either enzymatically or by pH change. The interaction between drug and excipients substance may, however, be so strong that cleavage occurs only very slowly—or even not at all. That will bring along a strongly delayed drug action, which, in case of MR preparations, may even be desirable, or may cause a lack of drug action altogether.

By contrast, it has also been observed that the complex traverses the stomach wall more readily than the drug as such. But increased drug action will only be observed when the drug is quickly and quantitatively released from the complex further on in the organism.

7.7.2 Manufacturing Technology

All stages in the manufacturing process may affect bioavailability. It is not uncommon that even the order of the various steps in the process is significant. Drug formulations produced in the laboratory setting or in a pilot study do not always display biopharmaceutical parameters identical to those of the mass-produced product. The type and brand of involved equipment and machines are liable to alter bioavailability. Tablet form and diameter, granulate form and size, type of granulation technique—these all play a role. But also, the type of tableting machine (single punch or rotary press, speed of tablet production, pressure force, etc., are of decisive importance for the quality parameters of the final product (physical firmness, susceptibility to disintegration, dissolution rate).

For emulsions, the dispersion grade depends on whether they are prepared manually or by mixing or homogenization equipment, high-performance colloid mills or ultrasound.

For many drug formulations the dispersion grade and the release and absorption process resulting from it constitute a central manufacturing problem. There is a risk of change in particle size and distribution during manufacturing of a drug, with loss of activity as a result. This has to be taken into account for example during tablet production when moist granulation is applied (see section 8.4.2), or when during pressing relatively high temperatures occur (high-speed press), which may induce sintering phenomena. In suspensions, high stirring velocities or temperature elevation may alter particle size.

When manufacturing suppositories by means of a pressing procedure, the dispersion grade should be kept strictly constant. By contrast, in the more common pouring procedure, during which the active ingredient is dissolved in the fatty mass by heating, crystallization occurs upon cooling, accompanied by a substantial increase in particle size.

An analogous situation occurs during manufacturing of ointments. Here, the release rates strongly depend on the manufacturing procedure, both for suspension and solution ointments. Substantial differences are observed between ointments where the active ingredient is processed into the molten basic substance and those where the incorporation is achieved by manual or machine-operated stirring. The release rate increases considerably with increasing mechanical stress causing perturbation of the gel framework. Consistent validation (see section 1.2) is an effective quality control instrument to largely exclude discrepancies in activity of drug formulations as a result of manufacturing technology.

The specific biopharmaceutical aspects of individual drug formulations are summarized in separate chapters: tablets (section 9.9); peroral MR formulations (section 12.7.3); rectal preparations (section 13.9); semi-solid preparations (section 15.6); solutions (section 17.4); injection and infusion preparations (section 21.9); ophthalmics (section 22.6).

Further Reading

Alam, N., Beg, S., Rizwan, M., Ahmad, A., Ahmad, F. J., Ali, A., et al. "Mucoadhesive elementary osmotic pump tablets of trimetazidine for controlled drug delivery and reduced variability in oral bioavailability." *Drug Dev Ind Pharm* 41 (4) (2015): 692–702.

Bateman, H. "The solution of a system of differential equations occurring in the theory of radioactive transformations." *Proc. Cambridge. Philos. Soc.* 15 (pt V) (1910): 423–427.

Dost, F. H. *Grundlagen der Pharmakokinetik.* Stuttgart: Thieme, 1968.

Dressman, J. B., Amidon, G. L., Reppas, C., Shah, V. P. "Dissolution Testing as a Prognostic Tool for Oral Drug Absorption: Immediate Release Dosage Forms." *Pharmaceutical Research* 15 (1) (1998): 11–22.

Foxwell, B. M. J., Frazer, G., Winters, M., Hiestand, P., Wenger, R., Ryffel, B. "Identification of cyclophilin as the erythrocyte ciclosporin-binding protein." *Biochim. Biophys. Acta* 938 (1988): 447–455.

Goldberg, A. H., Higuchi, W. I. "Improved Method for Diffusion Coefficient Determinations Employing the Silver Membrane Filter." *Journal of*

pharmaceutical sciences 57 (9) (1968): 1583–1585.

Kansy, M., Senner, F., and Gubernator, K. "Physicochemical high throughput screening: parallel artificial membrane permeation assay in the description of passive absorption processes." *J Med Chem* 41 (7) (1998): 1007–1010.

Liu, X., Testa, B., and Fahr, A. "Lipophilicity and Its Relationship with Passive Drug Permeation." *Pharmaceutical Research* 28 (Oct. 30, 2011): 962–977.

Malkia, A., Murtomaki, L., Urtti, A., Kontturi, K. "Drug permeation in biomembranes: in vitro and in silico prediction and influence of physicochemical properties." *Eur. J. Pharm. Sci.* 23 (1) (2004): 13–47.

Shargel, L., Yu, A. *Applied Biopharmaceutics & Pharmacokinetics, 7th ed.* New York: McGraw Hill Professional, 2015.

Tao, Y., Lu, Y., Sun, Y., Gu, B., Lu, W., Pan, J. "Development of mucoadhesive microspheres of acyclovir with enhanced bioavailability." *Int. J. Pharm.* 378 (1) (2009): 30–36.

Weston, G. S., Yeboah, K. G. "Site-Specific Drug Delivery to the Gastrointestinal Tract." *Journal of Molecular Pharmaceutics & Organic Process Research* 1 (2) (2013): 3 pages.

Solid Dosage Forms

PART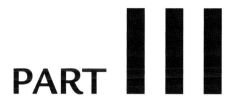

Powders and Granules

8

8.1 General Considerations and Definitions

Powders are air-dried materials consisting of solid particles. They can be considered solid-in-gas dispersions, in which the particles of the internal, dispersed phase are in mutual contact. In most cases, the contact between individual powder particles is not direct but via air or solvate layers adsorbed to the particle surface. The coherence of the internal phase is at least in part abrogated when the powder is induced to flow. The individual particle is defined as the smallest unit within a powder, while individual particles may differ in shape, size and mass. The shape of the particle depends on the manufacturing and size-reduction procedures. The particles may be crystalline, amorphous, or form aggregates that cannot be disaggregated by sieving or mixing methods. Such aggregates may be formed by processes such as sintering or crystal growth. They are distinguished from agglomerates, which also contain multiple particles sticking together but in this case under the influence of secondary or mechanical binding forces (adhesion, electrostatic forces, friction). In contrast to aggregates, agglomerates can be readily disrupted—for instance by sieving, wetting, shaking, or gentle friction. By granulation of a powder, a material with coarser grains (granules) is obtained. Each granule represents a dry aggregate of solid individual particles that is sufficiently firm to allow further handling. The surface of granules is mostly rough and irregular, while the granules are to a greater or lesser extent porous. Pellets are ideally spherical, slightly porous with a smooth surface and narrow size distribution.

In general, granules have some advantages over powders:

- Better compressibility because of higher porosity
- Better flow characteristics because of larger size
- Lower compaction tendency and thus higher dosing accuracy
- Less dust formation during further processing
- Optimal and uniform distribution of active ingredient within the granules
- Preservation of mixing degree due to approximately equal density and size of the granules
- Avoidance of incompatibilities because of the possibility to perform separate granulation of incompatible components followed by mixing of the two preparations
- Feasibility to adjust and control drug release properties by coating the granules

However, granules and granulations also present some disadvantages:

- The production of granules (granulation) is more time-consuming and cost-intensive.
- The active ingredients are embedded in the granules, necessitating measures to ensure efficient drug release, except when slow drug release is anticipated.

Voigt's Pharmaceutical Technology, First Edition. Alfred Fahr.
© 2018 John Wiley & Sons Ltd. Published 2018 by John Wiley & Sons Ltd.

Both powders and granules have only minor importance as dosage forms, but they play a major role as starting and bulk materials for the manufacturing of other dosage forms such as tablets, suspensions, and capsules.

8.2   Powders and Granules as Dosage Form

8.2.1   Powders for Cutaneous Application

The solid particles in powders commonly have a particle size of less than 100 µm in order to prevent irritation. Furthermore, powders should possess good adhesive and spreading properties as well as the capacity to adsorb fluids (water as well as oils). Moreover, chemical inertness and high chemical stability are required. Finally, they should tolerate sterilization processes. Different vehicles, often in combination, can be used to formulate pharmaceutical powders with suitable properties. Powder vehicles can be classified in organic and inorganic vehicles. Due to their longer shelf lives, inorganic vehicles are usually preferred.

8.2.1.1   Inorganic Powder Vehicles
Talc (Talcum) (section 5.2.5.2)
Talc is a natural magnesium hydroxide polysilicate that feels greasy to the touch. It is chemically inert and practically insoluble in water and acids. It is commonly used as the major ingredient in cutaneous powders due to its excellent adhesiveness on the skin and fair flow properties. Admixture of talcum can improve the flow characteristics of other powders and has fairly good lubrication properties due to its layered lattice structure (Fig. 8-1). The weak Van der Waals forces between the layers facilitate shifting of the layers with respect to each other. Water absorption is low, but oil absorption capacity is considerable. The absorption of hydrophilic fluids can be enhanced significantly by addition of other substances such as colloidal silica. Occasional cases of granuloma formation (*talcum granuloma*) have been reported after application of talcum for wound treatment or after use of talcum in rubber gloves for surgery or gynecology. Therefore, the general use of talcum is no longer recommended. If used, talcum should not contain any asbestos fibers. Talcum is often substantially contaminated with microorganisms. This is why dry heat sterilization is required before its use in pharmaceutical formulations.

Zinc Oxide (section 5.2.4.2)
Zinc oxide is a noncrystalline powder with good absorption capacities of both water and oil. It has satisfactory flow properties, but practically no adhesiveness. It acts as a mild disinfectant

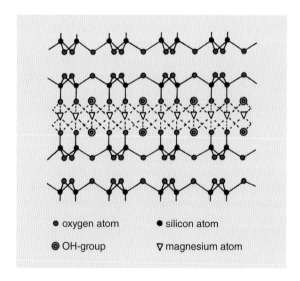

● oxygen atom   ● silicon atom

◉ OH-group   ▽ magnesium atom

Fig. 8-1 Crystal structure of talcum.

and astringent and is able to neutralize malodorous organic acids due to its weakly alkaline character.

White Clay (Bolus Alba) (section 5.2.5.4)
White clay is a natural water-containing aluminum silicate, which is characterized by its insolubility in water, acids, and alkali; chemical inertness; and appreciable adhesive properties. It has high absorption capacity for water and a moderate oil-absorption capacity.

Titanium Dioxide (sections 5.2.4.1 and 5.5.1.4)
This possesses an excellent opacity. Flow capacity and adhesive properties are satisfactory. It is chemically inert and aqueous dispersions react neutral.

Magnesium Oxide (section 5.2.4.3)
Magnesium oxide has appreciable water absorption capacity, but flow properties are poor.

Magnesium Carbonate
This has quite substantial adhesive properties and a good water-absorption capacity. However, flow properties are poor.

Natural Silica (Diatomite)
Natural silica has a high capacity to absorb both water and oil, but flow characteristics and adhesive properties are poor.

Colloidal Silica (section 5.2.5.1)
Colloidal silica is commercially available as, for example, Aerosil®, Cab-O-Sil®, and hydrophobized Aerosil®. Colloidal silica has good adhesion properties and can absorb considerable quantities of water as well as oil without becoming sticky. It is mainly used as an additive (0.5% to 3%) to other powders to improve their flow properties.

8.2.1.2   Organic Powder Vehicles

Stearates (section 5.3.2.2)
Most commonly applied are aluminum-, magnesium, and zinc stearates. All three are greasy and have a slight cooling effect on the skin. Noteworthy is their excellent adhesiveness. They serve as additives (3% to 5%) to other vehicles in order to improve the adhesiveness of powders. Stearates have practically no absorptive capacity.

Starch (section 5.3.4.1)
Common starch preparations are obtained from potatoes, wheat and rice. They are characterized by excellent adhesiveness, good flow properties and good absorption capacity for water and oils. Starch provides a good substrate for microbial growth under moist conditions. By etherification and cross-linking of natural starch, products that do not swell or gelatinize upon heating are obtained. These starch derivatives can therefore be sterilized. Since starch derivatives can be absorbed by the body, they have found application in some medical products (e.g., Biosorb®). *Amylum non mucilaginosum* (ANM powder) is obtained by enzymatic degradation and has similar properties (e.g., it is readily adsorbed by the body).

Lactose and Glucose (section 5.3.3)
These absorbable sugars are applied as vehicles for the manufacturing of wound powders (absorbable powders).

8.2.1.3   Special Powders

Cooling Powders
These powders produce a cooling sensation on the skin. This effect is predominantly produced by some types of starch and is attributed to their water content. Also stearates have a slight cooling effect.

Fatty Powders

Fatty powders are applied on dry skin or may be required when dermatological interventions such as treatment with fat-dissolving formulations result in defatting of the skin. Fatty powders contain 2% to 10% lipidic material (fatty oil, lanolin, etc.), which is mixed with the powder vehicle either after dissolution in an adequate solvent or by heating and grinding together with the vehicle. Many cosmetic powders as well as several wound powders and powders for children contain lipophilic additives.

Astringent Powders

Corresponding active ingredients such as tannin and other tanning agents as well as bismuth salts are mixed with the powder vehicle. Talcum, starch and white clay (bolus alba) are predominantly used as powder vehicles for this purpose.

Anti-Itching and Analgesic Powders

The powder vehicle can be mixed with 1% to 2% menthol to produce a cooling sensation on the skin and alleviate itching. In case of strong itching or pain, local anesthetics are used.

Disinfecting Powders

Frequently used active ingredients for disinfecting powders are thymol, salicylic acid, bismuth compounds, and various other disinfecting agents.

Antibiotic Powders

These are especially used for the treatment of infected wounds and in surgery. As antibiotics in powders occasionally remain active only for limited time periods, shelf life is an issue to be taken into account for these products.

8.2.2   Powders and Granules for Oral Use

Generally, simple powders (*pulveres simplices*) consist only of one component and mixed powders (*pulveres mixti*) consist of multiple active ingredients and/or excipients. As a rule, powders and granules are dissolved or suspended in water before use or, alternatively, swallowed with water. To ensure rapid dissolution of the powder or granules, effervescent components such as bicarbonate together with an organic acid may be added (effervescent powder or granules). Powders and granules can be packed in single- or multiple-dose packages. By intensive grinding of active ingredients with inert excipients, for example in a porcelain mortar or with special mills such as mortar mills (section 2.1.4.2), fine and homogeneous triturations can be obtained depending on the processing time. Triturations with lactose as vehicle present a homeopathic dosage form. Triturations of sucrose with oils are known as *oily sugars*. They are, for example, used for taste masking and as mild adjuvants in stomach powders. As essential oils tend to evaporate upon prolonged storage, these products always need to be freshly prepared. It has become more and more common to convert powder mixtures into granules in order to achieve higher dosing accuracy. Addition of taste masking agents or coating provide conditions facilitating oral administration. Coating of granules may also be applied to affect the release of the active ingredient. Granulates with "instant" properties dissolve rapidly and are especially intended for instant preparation of ready-to-take solutions that are prepared with water by the patient self. Granules may be coated to obtain gastro-resistant properties (enteric coating) or to obtain depot formulations with delayed drug release (section 10.5.3).

8.2.3   Powder Formulations in Other Dosage Forms

Powders and granules are also applied for the preparation of liquid formulations—for example, when the components only have a limited stability in solution (e.g., powders for the preparation of injections and infusions, powders for eyedrops or eye washes, powders, and granules for the preparation of solutions or suspensions for oral or cutaneous application). Finally, powders are used for several topical administration routes such as ear and nasal powders as well as powders for inhalation; section 23.4).

8.3   Production of Powders and Active Substances in Powder Form

The production of powders can be achieved in a number of different ways. In most cases, this is done by mechanical downsizing. This involves fine or ultra-fine milling of material previously subjected to coarse grinding. Various types of machines may be used for this purpose. Depending on the amount of material, its solid-state properties and the required degree of fineness, particularly ball, hammer, pin, pounding, and jet mills are used (section 2.1.4).

For the manufacturing of micropowders (micronized powders with particle size <10 μm), air jet mills have proven their usefulness. It should be kept in mind that size reduction is accompanied by a substantial increase in surface area. The specific surface area of cyproterone acetate, for example, increases from 1 000 to 26 000 cm^2/g upon micronization (Table 3-14). The heat produced during the milling process should be kept minimal. Moreover, possible contamination of the final product with metal traces by abrasion is another point of concern. Besides the dry milling procedure discussed above, wet milling also plays an important role in pharmaceutical technology (section 2.1.3.1).

Powdered products and substances can also be obtained by means of spray-drying. With this method, particle size may be controlled in many ways by adjustment of the processing parameters such as nozzle size, inlet and outlet temperature, and pump rate. Another technique to obtain powders is freeze-drying (lyophilization), which is particularly useful for processing of thermo-labile agents (section 2.4.3.11).

Some drug formulations can be produced by crystallization. By appropriately controlling the crystallization process, particles with desired form and size may be obtained. A number of powdered agents (salicylic acid, benzoic acid, and others) can be obtained as very small particles by sublimation. Finally, it is possible to obtain finely dispersed powders by precipitation from a solution by changing the solvent properties.

Simple powders (unmixed powders, *pulveres simplices*) consist of only one substance of adequate fineness; this implies that milling of the starting material may be required, depending on the route of administration. During the production of mixed powders (*pulveres mixti*), consisting of more than one component, problems may arise. Mixing is achieved with the devices discussed in section 2.2.3. For the mixing of small quantities, a mortar and pestle may suffice, or the powder can be mixed with a special mixing box (also named Wolsiffer box). This is a manually rotated light-metal can containing, as a rule, three steel or glass balls. It is necessary to ascertain that all components are uniformly distributed within the powder.

Mixing efficiency is a function of time and further depends on the properties of the individual components, the applied technique, and the efficiency of the mixing device (section 2.2). After exposure of a small powder sample on a smooth surface, no agglomerates or other irregularities should be observable by the naked eye. When the individual components of the powder have different grain sizes or densities, this requirement is not always easily fulfilled.

Problems may also arise during mixing when one or more components of the powder are hygroscopic (tendency to adsorb water) or have a tendency to agglomerate. Dry extracts, for example, are highly hygroscopic and tend to become cloggy. To avoid that, intensive mixing with lactose or colloidal silica is recommended. Also, essential oils are added to powders as lactose triturations. In principle, powder mixtures should only be prepared from well-dried substances. To prevent powder mixtures containing inorganic salts from getting moist, the salts should not contain crystal water. Hygroscopic, strongly smelling, or volatile substances must be packaged in airtight containers. In order to obtain high dosage accuracy, powders should allow appropriate weighing accuracy—that is, the total mass of one powder dose should not be lower than 0.2–0.5 g. When required, lactose can be added as a filler to obtain minimum weight.

The *powder dispenser*, which is used to divide a powder into separate doses, is rather inaccurate and should only be used when the active ingredient has a wide dose range, if at all. As dosing is based on volume, which depends on powder characteristics such as flow behavior and packing density, rather than on mass, unacceptable mass deviations cannot be excluded. A similar challenge applies to other powder-dispensing equipment and powder-packaging

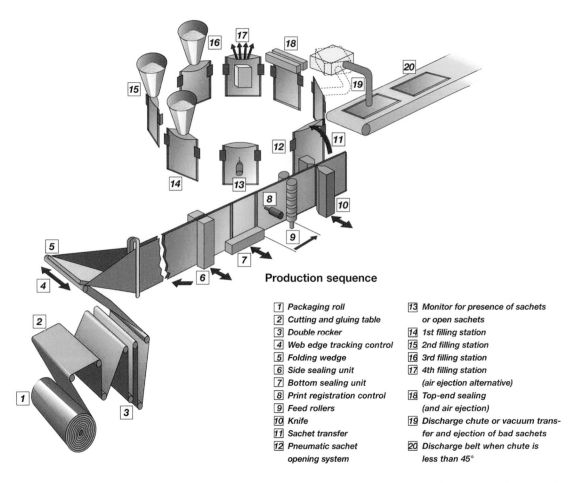

Production sequence

1. Packaging roll
2. Cutting and gluing table
3. Double rocker
4. Web edge tracking control
5. Folding wedge
6. Side sealing unit
7. Bottom sealing unit
8. Print registration control
9. Feed rollers
10. Knife
11. Sachet transfer
12. Pneumatic sachet opening system
13. Monitor for presence of sachets or open sachets
14. 1st filling station
15. 2nd filling station
16. 3rd filling station
17. 4th filling station (air ejection alternative)
18. Top-end sealing (and air ejection)
19. Discharge chute or vacuum transfer and ejection of bad sachets
20. Discharge belt when chute is less than 45°

Fig. 8-2 Powder packaging machine. Reproduced with permission from Harro Höfliger Verpackungsmaschinen GmbH © 2016.

machines (Fig. 8-2). When using such equipment, dosing accuracy may be obtained by normalizing the powder properties, by addition of glidants to improve flow properties, or by granulation.

8.4 Granulation

8.4.1 General Considerations

Granulation refers to a process whereby primary powder particles agglomerate into larger, multiparticulate aggregates (granules) of different sizes. Granules as dosage form are usually mechanically more robust and have a somewhat larger granule size than granules that are to be processed into tablets.

One distinguishes bottom-up and top-down granulation processes, while the latter can be further divided into wet and dry granulation (Table 8-1). By wet top-down granulation, aggregation is obtained by wetting a dry powder with a granulation liquid. The wet mass is then further sized down into granules of suitable size. In contrast, in bottom-up granulation techniques, the granules are built up separately by subsequent agglomeration of single powder particles, such as when a powder is wetted with the granulation liquid in a fluid bed. Bottom-up granulation can be achieved by either a continuous or a discontinuous process.

Table 8-1 Granulation Processes

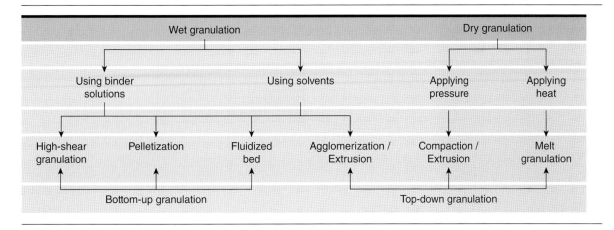

8.4.2 Top-Down Wet Granulation (Reverse Wet Granulation)

8.4.2.1 Binding Mechanisms

In reverse wet granulation, the dry powder material is wetted with a granulation liquid in such a way that the powder becomes sticky, mainly due to capillary forces of the liquid layer of granulation fluid between the individual powder particles. After sizing down by forcing the wet mass through, for example, a sieve, the granulation liquid is removed by drying. Depending on the nature of the granulation liquid and the type of solid bridges formed, two types of granules are distinguished.

Granules Bonded by Recrystallized Material ("Crusty" Granules)

As granulation liquid water or ethanol-water mixtures are usually employed but also isopropanol is used for this purpose. The latter has the advantage that it is completely removed upon drying and thus is absent in the final granules. A prerequisite to obtain crusty granules is that the powder material (or part of it) dissolves in the granulation liquid. This results in the formation of a concentrated solution on the particle surface and formation of solid bridges due to recrystallization upon drying. Thus, a solid crust is formed upon the removal of the granulation liquid by air drying at 30° to 40°C or by means of drying by infrared light, microwaves or hot air, depending on the nature of the granulation fluid. Of decisive importance is the solubility of the powder in the applied granulation liquid. Lactose, for example, can be granulated directly with water, because it is only slightly (but sufficiently) soluble in water. On the other hand, for the granulation of sugars that are more readily soluble in water (e.g., sucrose), ethanol-water mixtures are more suitable. Organic solvents must be recovered upon drying according to the air pollution legislation. Due to their crystalline nature, the solid bridges in crusty granules are usually stiff and not very elastic.

Solubility of sugars in water at 25°C	
Glucose	90.9 g/100 mL
Lactose	18.9 g/100 mL
Sucrose	210 g/100 mL

Granules Bonded by Polymers ("Gluey" Granules)

For the production of gluey granules, a binder (usually a polymer with adhesive properties) is employed. Typical binders for wet granulation include starches, polyvinylpyrrolidone (povidone, PVP), gelatin and cellulose ethers. Starches (corn, wheat, potato, pregelatinized starches) are used as 10% to 25 % aqueous mucilages, PVP (Kollidon®) as 1% to 5% solution (both in water and ethanol) and gelatin as 2% to 20% aqueous solution. The most important cellulose ethers (section 5.3.5) used as binders in wet granulation are hydroxypropylcellulose (HPC), methylcellulose (MC), hydroxypropylmethylcellulose (HPMC) and carboxymethylcellulose sodium (Carmellose Sodium) as 1% to 6% aqueous solutions. Ethylcellulose (EC) can only be used in ethanolic solutions, because it is insoluble in water. During drying of downsized wet granules, solidified bridges of the binder are formed between the aggregated primary particles. These solid polymeric bridges usually have a higher elasticity than the solid crystalline bridges formed in crusty granules.

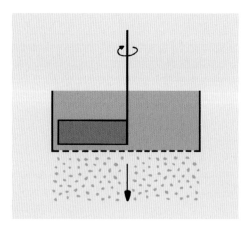

Fig. 8-3 Device for producing pressed granules.

8.4.2.2   Production Procedures

After aggregation of the powder by wetting with the granulation liquid, the resulting wet mass is disaggregated in such a way that granules with a suitable size are obtained. Granule formation can be achieved by different methods and, depending on the specific process, granules with different shapes are obtained. However, all methods have in common that the wet material is forced, either manually or automatically, through a sieve or a perforated disk with adequate mesh size.

Granulation by Applying Pressure

For the production of pressed granules, the wet material is forced through a sieve or a perforated disk. For manual granulation, plastic or stainless steel scrapers may also be applied. For automatic granulation in a sieve-type granulation machine, a stirring device forces the wet material through a sieve or perforated plate, resulting in the formation of worm-shaped particles with defined cross section (Fig. 8-3). It may be necessary to cut the formed granules to the desired length by applying a knife or a scraper directly underneath the sieve or perforated plate (Fig. 8-4). For small-scale production, the Erweka wet granulator (Fig. 8-5) may be applied. The pore size can be adjusted to the amount of moisture in the material. The more moisture, the larger the mesh size of the sieve needs to be. Pressed granules are usually characterized by the presence of elongated, rod-shaped structures (Fig. 8-7).

Granulation by Shaking

Granules can also be obtained by passing the wet granulation material through a sieve or a perforated plate by shaking. Even when using sieves with identical mesh size, granules produced by shaking have a smaller diameter than those produced by pressing the mass through the sieve. Granules obtained by shaking methods are characterized by a more or less

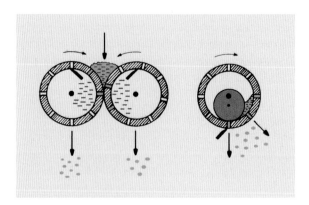

Fig. 8-4 Types of machines for producing pressed granules.

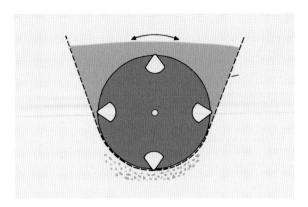

Fig. 8-5 Wet granulator.

spherical or ellipsoid shape (Fig. 8-7), resulting in better flow properties and thus improved dosing accuracy. Nonetheless, large-scale production with this method is barely feasible.

Perforated-Disk Granulates

The granulation material is forced through a perforated disk—for example, through two perforated cylinders rotating in opposite directions (Fig. 8-6). The granules produced are thus similar in shape to the rod-like pressed granules, but they commonly display a smoother surface (Fig. 8-7).

8.4.2.3 Drying of Wet Granules

The granules are spread out in thin layers and dried at a temperature usually not exceeding 40°C, either by warm air, infrared radiation, microwaves, or by using an air stream. Alternatively, granules can be dried in a drying oven with or without applying a vacuum or in fluidized-bed dryers. In the latter, the granules are kept in a fluidized bed in a warm air stream while being dried (section 2.4.3).

Based on differences in drying behavior, *hydrophilic* and *areophilic* substances are distinguished. *Hydrophilic substances*, including active pharmaceutical ingredients (API) as well as excipients such as sodium chloride, ascorbic acid, codeine phosphate, starch and others,

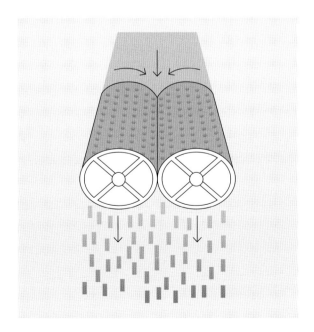

Fig. 8-6 Perforated-disk granulator.

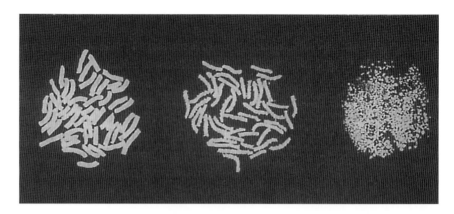

Fig. 8-7 Granule shape depending on granulation method: perforated-disk granules (left), pressed granules (middle), and granules obtained by shaking (right).

are water-soluble and may have the capacity to swell. They can bind water, either by absorption or adsorption, depending on relative humidity. Moreover, they can have distinct hygroscopic properties. Even upon adequate drying, a certain amount of residual moisture is usually retained in the granules. This is desirable for tableting, as completely dried granules may lose their binding capacity. *Aerophilic substances* such as talcum and sulfonamides are, on the other hand, poorly soluble in water. Their pronounced lipophilic properties almost completely prevent water adsorption. Such granules lose nearly all their water during the drying process, which is undesirable because granules containing too little water will cause problems during tableting, such as the occurrence of "capping" of the tablets (section 9.6.4). However, complete drying of granules containing aerophilic substances can be prevented by the addition of humectants such as glycerol, which strongly binds water and prevents too high loss of moisture during the drying process.

The drying rate depends, generally, on the porosity of the granules.

8.4.3   Dry Granulation

Dry granulation (compacting with subsequent size reduction of the compressed material) is widely applied in pharmaceutical industry, particularly for granulation prior to tableting. Dry granulation has several advantages over moist granulation:

- □ The process is less time- and cost-consuming.
- □ There is a lower moisture burden for hydrolysis-sensitive substances.
- □ There is no need for solvent recovery.
- □ no need for drying.

As the recovery of organic solvents (e.g., ethanol, isopropanol) is cost-intensive, direct compaction or dry granulation often is the first-choice approach during development of new products. However, when processing thermolabile compounds, the risk of locally high temperatures during the compaction process must be taken into account.

A commonly used dry granulator is the roller compactor. The mixed powder is fed from a hopper by a rotating screw to two oppositely rotating rollers where the powder is forced through the narrow gap between them (Fig. 8-8). Subsequently, the compressed material is downsized to the desired granule size. This can be achieved, for example, by conventional milling equipment or by using a fine granulator (Fig. 8-8).

8.4.4   Melt Granulation

In this procedure, the active ingredients are processed in a melt process together with a suitable thermoplastic polymer or a solid lipid (e.g. waxes) in such a way that the active agents

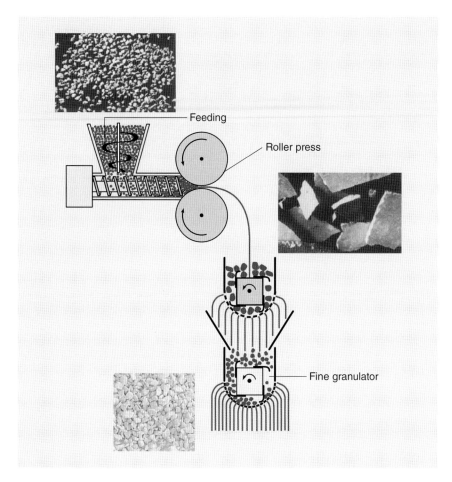

Fig. 8-8 Dry granulation by compaction.

are embedded in the polymer or lipid. After introduction of the mixture of polymer and drug into the funnel, it is transported by single or twin screws through the barrel to the spray nozzle. Barrel and screw can be heated and are usually designed in such a way that the highest temperature occurs near the spray nozzle. In this way the thermoplast thoroughly melts at the end of the barrel and when passing the nozzle. Immediately upon solidification, a strand is formed that is cut into pieces of appropriate size by a rotating knife behind the nozzle. Size reduction may also be carried out separately by using conventional milling equipment. Thermoplastic granules predominantly serve the manufacturing of depot formulations and taste masking, but melt granulation (hot-melt extrusion) is also increasingly employed for immediate release granules to improve dissolution and thus bioavailability of poorly soluble drugs.

Melt extrusion has been in use for over 100 years in the plastics industry. Suitable polymers can be extruded, e.g., in a twin-screw extruder (Fig. 8-9), together with an incorporated, molecularly dispersed drug. To produce granules, the spaghetti-like extrudate can be cut by the machine into small pieces (Fig. 8-9). The peroral formulations developed from this material enhance the bioavailability of the corresponding drugs (Wilson et al. 2012). Melt extrusion can also be used to produce melt films for poorly soluble drugs. Melt films have a thickness of 20 to 500 μm with surface areas varying from 2 to 10 cm^2. They are placed on or underneath the tongue, where they are rapidly dissolved by the saliva.

8.4.5   Bottom-Up Wet Granulation

In bottom-up granulation processes, bigger aggregates are gradually built up resulting in more or less spherical granules with a relatively smooth surface. The size of the final granules

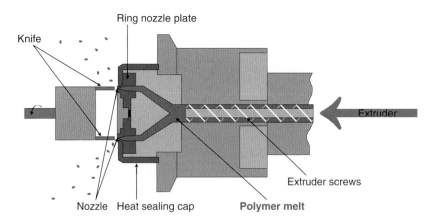

Fig. 8-9   Micro Pelletizer (hot melt extrusion principle). Reproduced with permission from Evonik Nutrition & Care GmbH, Darmstadt, Germany.

depends on the fineness of the starting material, the droplet size and the amount of granulation fluid. There are generally two different ways in which granules can be built up by bottom-up granulation: (1) particle growth and (2) particle agglomeration.

Particle growth may follow when the starting material (often preformed starting pellets) is wetted with the granulation fluid containing suspended powder particles. In this way, the initially present particles continuously grow in mass and size upon evaporation of the granulation fluid, while the number of particles does not change.

In the *particle agglomeration* method, powder particles are wetted directly with the granulation fluid, resulting in agglomeration of the wet particles. This also results in an increase in mass and size, however—in this case, by agglomeration of individual powder particles.

Bottom-op granules can be produced by various techniques including spray drying or spray solidification.

8.4.5.1   Granulation in the Granulation Drum

The granulation drum is the classic device for bottom-up granulation. The dry powder material is introduced into one side of the drum and is subsequently transported in an axial direction through the inclined rotating drum, while the material gradually moves along the inner surface of the drum. At the same time, the granulation fluid is sprayed from the top of the drum onto the powder (Fig. 8-10). The formed granules are spherical in shape, but may vary in size, which requires separation and classification. Particles that have attained a certain size are transported out of the drum, depending on the inclination angle of the drum and its rotation speed. Size classification can also be achieved by positioning a sieve at the outlet of the drum. Finally, the obtained granules are dried, when required, under reduced pressure.

8.4.5.2   Kettle Granulation

A rotating coating kettle (inclination angle 60°) equipped with collision plates is filled with the powder material, which is initially mixed in dry form. Upon spraying the granulation fluid onto the powder, spherical granules are formed. Subsequently, the granules are dried by hot air or by heat conduction and ready-to-use granules are obtained when a tableting powder is added in the final step. With this procedure, a substantial reduction in processing time can be attained.

8.4.5.3   Fluidized-Bed Granulation

Currently, procedures in which the processes of mixing, wetting, and drying are combined in one single cycle are now common practice. In the fluidized-bed technique, the powder particles are kept floating by an upward-directed air flow while being wetted with the granulation fluid (solution or suspension) and thus become coated with the granulation fluid (section 10.6.4). The granulation liquid (solvent) evaporates in the warm air stream. Fluidized-bed

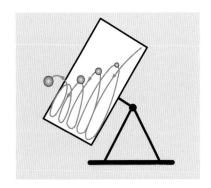

Fig. 8-10   Granulation drum.

processes are often discontinuous, but equipment for continuous processing is also available. In an alternative method, wet but still flowing granulation material is introduced into the fluidized-bed granulator, where particles up to a defined size are kept floating by an upward air stream. Particle agglomeration occurs by mutual contact between the wetted particles, and granules are subsequently obtained by drying in the warm air stream. When the granules have reached a certain critical size and mass, they can no longer be kept floating in the fluid bed and fall down, ultimately resulting in spherical granules (pellets, section 8.4.6). Both bottom spray (*Wurster* principle) and tangential spray devices (section 10.6.4) are used for this purpose. The process can be optimized by controlling temperature and humidity of the inlet and outlet air as well as the air flow rate, temperature being the most crucial parameter for the wetting process. In a subsequent step, the pellets can be coated in the fluidized-bed device to modulate the drug release properties.

The flow characteristics of these granules are often so good that they can be used for tableting without any further treatment.

8.4.5.4 Spray Granulation

By spray-drying, a solution or suspension is converted into a dry powder by applying a stream of hot air (section 2.4.3). The liquid is sprayed through a nozzle or by a rotating nebulizing disk into a hot air stream (Fig. 8-11). Drying occurs very rapidly but nonetheless gently in spite of the supply of hot air, since heat is dissipated by evaporation of the solvent during drying. Thus, solutions or suspensions of fillers, binders, disintegrants, and lubricants can be converted into spherical granules that can be tableted upon, for example, addition of the active pharmaceutical ingredient.

Spray solidification can be conducted in the same device, but, instead of hot air, cold air is blown into the device to solidify the sprayed molten material. This procedure can be used for embedding of powdered active ingredients in, for example, fats and waxes. Granulates thus obtained represent the depot dose in formulations with delayed or prolonged action.

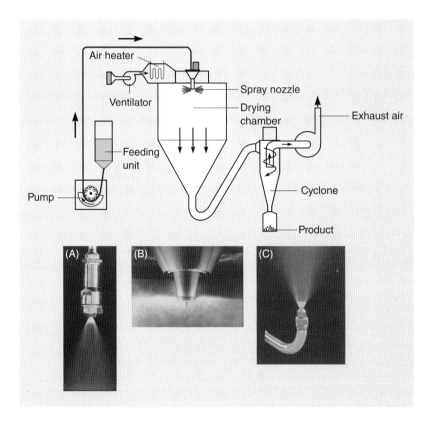

Fig. 8-11 Spray-drying plant. Schematic view and nozzle types: (A) direct-flow principle; (B) centrifugal atomizer; and (C) fountain principle with double-stream nozzle.

8.4.5.5   Single Pot Granulation

Bottom-up granulation with high-speed mixers is based on the principle that the granulation material (e.g., a powder) is kept in constant movement in optimal relation to the addition of the granulation fluid. A large variety of high-speed granulators working according to this principle are commercially available. Examples are the rotating double-coned and the V-blenders and the so-called batch shear mixer (section 2.2.3), all equipped with choppers to avoid clumping and deposition of material on the wall of the machine. As the name implies, both blending of the starting material and granulation are carried out in the same machine. Drying of the granules often proceeds separately, but the number of devices carrying out mixing, granulation, and drying in one operational step is increasing. Vacuum rotatory drum dryers provide a very gentle drying of granules.

The DIOSNA high-shear granulator is equipped with a sensor, which measures flow resistance of the flowing wet material and thus provides information about granule properties (grain size, density). In this way, granule formation can be monitored, and the end point of the granulation process can be directly determined. The recorded values also present a basis for the operation parameters in the production of following batches. The chopper of the device operates at high speeds, varying from 1,500 to 3,000 rpm. Due to the special shape of the slowly rotating stirrer blade, freely flowing granules are obtained.

The TOPO vacuum granulator consists basically of a cylindrical drum that can be heated and tilted and is suitable for batches of 500 to 600 kg. A spiral stirrer, which reaches the entire internal surface of the drum, can operate in both directions at a continuously adjustable rotation speed. The powder is sucked into the drum by reduced pressure, which also provides for optimal distribution of the granulation fluid and drying of the granules. A sieve at the outlet of the device is used to break up agglomerates. The hermetically closed system prevents environmental hazards caused by dust (including toxic substances such as hormones) or solvents (separated by a condenser). Energy consumption is low as the produced heat is nearly completely recycled in the drying process.

8.4.6   Pellets

Pellets are defined as spherical granules with a smooth surface and a size between about 0.1 and 2 mm. Due to their spherical shape and narrow size distribution, pellets have very good flow properties.

Homogeneous pellets consist either of one single substance or of a homogeneous mixture of active ingredient and excipients. *Heterogeneous pellets* generally contain a starter particle (usually without active ingredient) that is surrounded by one or several drug-containing or drug-free layers (Fig. 8-12).

Pellets (particularly heterogeneous pellets) can be manufactured by bottom-up granulation in the granulation drum, fluidized-bed devices or in special pelleting devices (section 8.4.6). As starter particles for the production of heterogeneous pellets, mostly rounded spherules of different size consisting of sucrose-starch mixtures are commonly used. However, also sieve-sized coarse particles consisting of active or excipients can be applied as starter particles. The resulting pellets are subsequently compressed into tablets or filled into capsules. Pellets may be coated in the fluidized-bed devices in order to modify drug release properties (chapter 10). It is also possible to fill pellets with different drug-release properties into capsules—for example, to achieve a sustained drug release followed by an initial "burst" dose.

Production of homogeneous pellets is often achieved by spheronization of granules obtained by a conventional wet granulation procedure such as extrusion (section 8.4.2). Important parameters for spheronization are optimal moisture content of the powder material and plasticity of the excipients. The quality of the pellets (size distribution) after spheronization depends furthermore on the properties of the extrudate. By roller granulation, for example, granules of high porosity are obtained. This may result in irregular fracturing of the granules during spheronization, which, in turn, may lead to a broader size distribution.

A Spheronizer® consists of a fast rotating bottom plate with a rippled surface. In the Spheronizer, the pellets travel in spiral movements and are thus rounded (spheronized) on the rotating bottom plate and the static wall until they reach the desired size (Fig. 8-13).

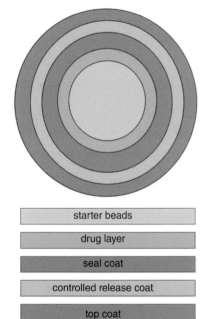

starter beads
drug layer
seal coat
controlled release coat
top coat

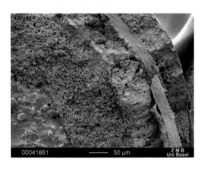

Fig. 8-12 Heterogonous pellet (schematic drawing and realization). The top coat could be, for example, a taste-masking coat or an enteric coat. Reproduced with permission from Glatt GmbH Binzen © 2016.

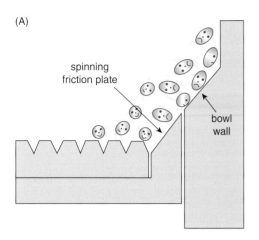

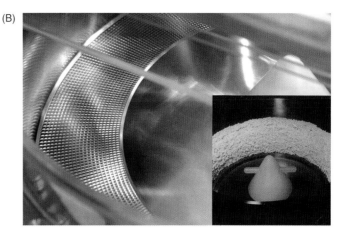

Fig. 8-13 **Spheronizer®: (A) Schematic drawing of the Spheronizer operation (after an idea of Dr. Stahl, GEA); (B) photography of a spheronizer; inset: spheronizer in action.** Reproduced with permission from GEA Group AG © 2016.

Prolonged rotation times may lead to disintegration of the pellets into powder and should therefore be avoided.

8.4.7 Binding Mechanisms in Granules

The mechanical strength of aggregates such as granulates can be obtained by various binding mechanisms (Table 8-2).

Solid Bridges

Sinter bridges and solid bridges obtained by chemical reactions or partial melting are of limited importance in pharmaceutical granules. Formation of *sinter bridges* involves molecular diffusion from particle to particle. Diffusion is strongly dependent on temperature and pressure and increasing temperature and higher pressure favor the strength of the binding. Binding through *chemical reaction*, determined by the degree of moisture, is in general not desirable. *Partial melting* may occur in substances with low melting temperature as a result of a temperature increase due to the applied pressure. Due to friction, fluid bridges of molten material are formed at the contact points, which rapidly solidify upon cooling.

During wet granulation, the binding is essentially achieved by a *hardening binder* (gluey granules), by a *recrystallizing binder* (crust granules) and/or by *deposition of suspended particles* at the contact areas between the particles. The strength of the formed solid bridges depends on several factors, including crystallization/solidification velocity and the solid-state structure of the solid bridge. From a biopharmaceutical point of view, crystal growth during the agglomeration process is not desirable but cannot always be avoided when using granulation fluids. Although rapid drying (high temperature) results in finer crystal structures lending the granules high mechanical strength, this often impedes disintegration of the granules.

Adhesion and Cohesion Forces in Non-Freely Moving Binder Films

Highly viscous binding agents act through adhesion forces at the solid–liquid interface as well as by cohesion forces within the binder. However, in the manufacturing of pharmaceutical granules they play only a minor role. Binders such as starch, on the other hand, improve the binding and at the same time the disintegration of the granules, due to their disintegrative effect. Thin *adsorption layers* can be formed by uptake of moisture from the air. They are not freely moving, but are able to lower the distance between the contact points of the particles and thus improve binding. In layers thinner than 3 nm, the molecular forces are fully transferred from particle to particle, whereby deformations at contact points may occur and strong binding is achieved.

Interfacial and Capillary Pressure at Freely Moving Fluid Surfaces

This binding mechanism plays a dominant role during agglomeration of solid particles. Upon addition of small amounts of granulation fluid, fluid bridges are formed, initially point-wise.

Table 8-2 Binding Mechanisms in Granules

1. Solid bridges
   1. sinter bridges
   2. chemical reaction
   3. partly melting
   4. hardening binder
   5. a) crystallization of dissolved substances
   5. b) deposition of suspended particles
2. Adhesion and cohesion forces in not freely moving binding agents
   1. highly viscous binder
   2. adsorption layers (below 3–5 nm thickness)
3. Interfacial and capillary pressure at freely moving fluid surfaces
   1. fluid bridges
   2. capillary forces at the surface of liquid containing aggregates
4. Attractive forces between solid particles
   1. Van der Waals forces, free chemical valences
   2. electrostatic forces
5. Interlocking bindings

By adding more granulation fluid, the spaces between the particles are completely filled with fluid. Concave menisci are then formed at the wall of the pores, and the powder particles stick together due to capillary forces.

Attractive Forces between Solid Particles
Van der Waals forces, as typical short-range forces, only act at close proximity of the particles, but then may become quite strong. Free chemical valences may occur at freshly formed solid surfaces (e.g., during particle fragmentation). These are, however, quickly saturated by chemical reactions. This type of binding is of subordinate significance for powder agglomeration.

Interlocking Binding
This binding mechanism is not typical for powdered materials, but it occurs between fibrous or strongly irregular shaped particles as a result of pressure and shear forces. These cause the particles to intertwine, to be engulfed or entangled with each other. The firmness of such binding depends on the type of material.

8.5   Flow Properties of Bulk Materials

8.5.1   Significance and Parameters

Flow properties of powders and granules are of crucial importance, not only for the way in which these materials flow out of storage containers but also for dosing accuracy during manufacturing of volume-dosed drug formulations (e.g., capsules, tablets), as well as for their mixing behavior and for their processing properties in general. Regarding the movement of bulk materials, one can distinguish primary (determined by gravity) and secondary (movement of particles relative to each other) movements. Inter-particulate interactions such as Van der Waals forces (enforced by moisture), capillary forces (wet products), and electrostatic forces (especially in case of small, dry particles) result in impairment of the flow properties of bulk materials. These interparticulate forces are dependent on:

- Particle shape
- Particle size
- Surface properties
- Particle size distribution
- Porosity
- Degree of moisture
- Interparticulate friction

Weight load generally promotes the flow. Since the weight load increases more with increasing size than the adhesion forces ($F_G \sim r^3$, but $F_A \sim r$), weight load predominates for larger particles. That explains why bulk materials with particle sizes above about 250 μm usually have good flow properties, whereas flow properties become poorer for particles smaller than about 100 μm where adhesion forces become more prominent. Nonetheless, each powder has a critical particle size limit at which adhesion forces outweigh weight load, resulting in poor flow properties. This is due to the fact that, in addition to size, the particle shape (strongly anisometric particles result in poor flow), surface properties, and particle density strongly influence the flow properties. A small proportion of fine material may have a beneficial effect on the flow behavior of the bulk material.

8.5.2   Measures to Improve Flow Properties

The following parameters provide starting points to improve the flow properties:

- Addition of glidants or flow-regulating agents (smoothening of surface irregularities, distance keepers, adsorption of moisture)
- Increase of particle size (e.g., by granulation)
- Alteration of particle shape (ideally spherical)
- Reducing moisture content (drying, addition of colloidal silica)

As glidants and flow-regulating substances, colloidal silica and talcum are often used. To elucidate the effect of glidants and to select the best suited one, flowability of the powder with and without the glidant is compared (section 8.6.2). When determining the mass m of the material flowing out of the funnel within a defined period of time, the flow factor f can be calculated by equation 8-1:

$$f = \frac{m_{(material+glidant)}}{m_{(material)}} \tag{8-1}$$

A factor f > 1 indicates an improvement of the flow properties of the material.

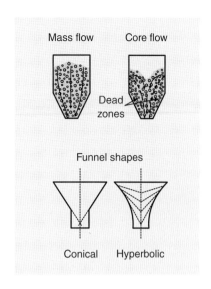

Fig. 8-14 Mass and core flow during outflow of bulk material from storage containers (top) and dependency of bridge-formation on the funnel geometry (bottom).

8.5.3   Mass and Core Flow

Depending on the flow properties of the material, either mass or core flow is observed during the outflow of the material from a funnel (Fig. 8-14). Materials with good flow properties give rise to mass flow, implying that all particles are moving at the same time and thus the funnel empties uniformly, while only minor friction forces occur. However, materials with poor flow properties often cause core flow, which is characterized by inhomogeneous flow, preferentially proceeding along shear planes. As a result, increased friction occurs along the wall and a meniscus is formed in the center of the funnel. Only the material in the center (core) of the funnel is moving, and dead zones may form near the funnel walls. Basically, core flow is an undesirable phenomenon, which can be diminished or even prevented by the following measures:

- Improvement of the flow properties of the material
- Steeply inclining funnel wall
- Asymmetric or hyperbolic funnel shape
- Smooth funnel wall

Another problem that may occur during flow of a material out from a funnel is the so-called bridge formation by compaction of parts of the material. This phenomenon can even lead to complete flow interruption. Although this is typical for poorly flowing materials, occasionally it is also observed with freely flowing materials, especially when a funnel with a narrow orifice is used. Bridge formation can be diminished by applying a wider orifice, a hyperbolically shaped funnel (Fig. 8-14), or by incorporation of chicanes and other mechanical aids.

8.6   Test Methods for Powders and Granules

Powders and granules can be characterized by their specific properties (see chapter 3). In powder technology, evaluation proceeds on the basis of dimensional properties (particle size and particle size distribution, section 3.3), surface and density properties (surface, density, porosity, section 3.5) as well as by their flow properties. With regard to biopharmaceutical parameters, solubility and dissolution rate (sections 3.9 and 3.10), solid-state properties such as crystallinity and polymorphism (section 3.2.1) are of crucial importance. For single-dose powders or granules, uniformity of mass or content must be assessed.

8.6.1   Bulk and Tapped Density

The volume and the assembly of the powder bed are determined by particle size and shape. Needle- and rod-shaped particles mostly produce a loose packing, as they only contact each other by their edges and protrusions with air-filled spaces between them are prevalent. Also

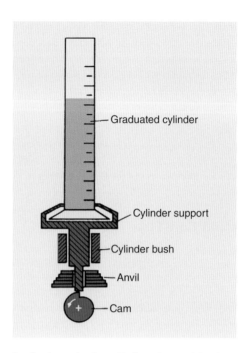

Fig. 8-15 Apparatus for the determination of bulk and tapped density.

the presence of equal electrical charges leads to such arrangements due to mutual repulsion between the particles. In contrast, spherical and disk-shaped particles results in a denser packing.

Powders and granules can be characterized by their bulk and tapped densities (or the corresponding volumes). To determine these parameters, 100 g of powder or granules is carefully filled into a graduated cylinder and the surface of the material is smoothened without causing any compaction. The volume thus obtained (including the interparticulate void volume) is the bulk volume (or specific bulk volume [mL/g]) and the bulk density (or specific bulk density [g/mL]) can be calculated. The tapped density (or volume) is determined by defined vertical movements of the cylinder (e.g., in a settling device) (Fig. 8-15). The tapped volume of a material is defined as the volume that is occupied by a mass unit (e.g., 100 g) in maximally packed arrangement without affecting the shape of the particles. In the settling device, the graduated cylinder with the material is held in a cylinder support mounted on an anvil. The mechanical tapping is achieved by up-and-down movements of the cylinder resulting from the rotating cam underneath the anvil.

The number of lifts is registered by a counter device. The volume of the packed sample is read on the scale of the calibrated cylinder. Comparison of bulk and tapped densities (or volumes) provides information about compaction tendency of the material, which also gives an indication of the flow properties (section 8.6.2). The smaller the compaction tendency, the better are the flow properties (Table 8-3). The Hausner factor (HF) and the compressibility

Table 8-3 Flow Properties as Quantified by the Hausner Factor and Compressibility Index (Ph. Eur. 2.9.36)

Compressibility Index (%)	Flow Behavior	Hausner Factor
1–10	excellent	1.00–1.11
11–15	good	1.12–1.18
16–20	fair	1.19–1.25
21–25	moderate	1.26–1.34
26–31	poor	1.35–1.45
32–37	very poor	1.46–1.59
> 38	unsatisfactory	>1.60

index (also called Carr index, CI) can be calculated from bulk and tapped densities according to equations 8-2 and 8-3:

$$HF = \frac{\rho_{tapped}}{\rho_{bulk}} \tag{8-2}$$

$$CI = 100\ \% \cdot \frac{\rho_{tapped} - \rho_{bulk}}{\rho_{tapped}} \tag{8-3}$$

Examples

The volume of 100 g of a powder is 80 mL. The specific bulk volume is 0.80 mL/g and the reciprocal value (1.25 g/mL) is the specific bulk density. After compaction in a settling device, the powder volume was reduced to 43 mL. The tapped density is 100 g/43 mL = 2.325 g/mL, while the specific tapped volume is 0.43 mL/g.

Ph. Eur. 2.9.34 Bulk and Tapped Density of Powders

USP ⟨616⟩ Bulk Density and Tapped Density of Powders
JP 3.01 Determination of Bulk and Tapped Densities

Bulk Density

The bulk density is determined either by measuring the volume of a powder sample of known mass (method 1) or by weighing a sample of known volume (methods 2 and 3). In all cases, the powder samples are passed through a sieve (mesh size 1.0 mm) before the measurement in order to break up agglomerates.

Method 1: Approximately 100 g powder, weighed to 0.1% accuracy, are gently introduced into a graduated cylinder (commonly 250 mL, readable to 2 mL), taking care not to cause any compression and the volume is read to the nearest graduated unit.

Method 2: An excess of powder is allowed to flow through an apparatus, consisting of a top funnel fitted with a 1.0 mm sieve and a baffle box, mounted below the funnel, into a sample receiving cup of known volume (16.39 or 25.00 mL) until it overflows. Excess powder is scraped away from the top of the cup and the mass of the powder is determined. The bulk density is calculated as the average of three determinations of three different powder samples.

Method 3: The powder is allowed to flow freely into a cylindrical 100-mL stainless steel vessel of predetermined weight. After scraping the excess powder from the top of the vessel, the cylinder is weighed again and the density is calculated as the average of three independent determinations.

The pharmacopeias recommends giving preference to methods 1 and 3.

Tapped Density

Methods 1 and 2: Approximately 100 g powder, weighed to 0.1% accuracy, is introduced into a 250 mL graduated cylinder (readable to 2 mL) and the unsettled apparent powder volume V_0 is read. Subsequently, 10, 500, and 1,250 taps are carried out on the same powder sample (Method 1: 250 ± 15 taps/min from a height of 3 ± 0.2 mm or 300 ± 15 taps/min from a height of 14 ± 2 mm; Method 2: fixed drop of 3 ± 0.2 mm at a rate of 250 taps/min) and the corresponding volumes (V_{10}, V_{500}, and V_{1250}) are read. When V_{500} and V_{1250} differ by more than 2 mL, tapping is repeated in increments of, for example, 1,250 taps until the difference between successive measurements is less than or equal 2 mL. The tap volumeter described in the Ph. Eur. meets the ISO 787 Part 11 and ASTM requirements. The tapped density is calculated as the ratio of the powder weight and the tapped volume. If method 1 is used, the drop height is indicated with the results.

Method 3: On top of the vessel used in Method 3 of the bulk density test, a metal tube of identical inner diameter is mounted and the powder is allowed to flow in. By means of a suitable tapped density tester, 200 taps are carried out, the metal tube is removed, and excess powder is scraped from the top of the vessel. The vessel is weighed and tapping is repeated in increments of 200 taps until the difference between successive measurements is less than or equal to 2%. The tapped density is calculated as the average of three independent determinations.

8.6.2   Flowability

A variety of methods is available to evaluate of flow properties of bulk materials, with variable experimental setups:

- □ Angle of repose
- □ Compressibility index or Hausner factor (section 8.6.1)
- □ Flowability
- □ Shear cells

8.6.2.1   Angle of Repose

The angle of repose is observed when a flowing powder or granules flows out from a funnel on a flat surface to form a cone (Fig. 8-16). The angle of repose is the angle between the base and the slope of the cone. The flatter the cone (i.e., the smaller the inclination angle), the better are the flow properties of the powder or granules. The angle of repose α can be calculated from equation 8-4 in which h is the height of the powder cone and r the radius of the base of the cone:

$$\tan \alpha = \frac{h}{r} \tag{8-4}$$

h = height of powder conus
r = radius of base area of the cone

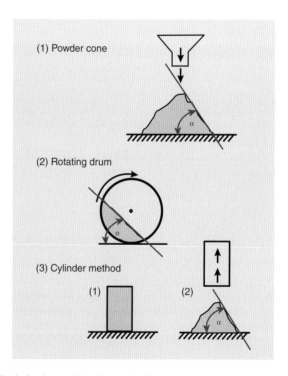

Fig. 8-16   **Methods for determining the angle of repose.**

Different experimental setups are used to determine the angle of repose (Fig. 8-16), while the experimental setup has a considerable influence on the final measured result.

To determine the angle of friction by the tilting table, the powder bed is tilted until the powder starts to flow (Fig. 8-17). In contrast to the other methods, where the angle of repose is determined from the moving material, here the powder is at rest and the onset of flow is determined. Therefore, the angle of friction determined by the tilting table method is mainly determined by interparticulate friction. Compression of powder upon filling it into the cylindrical container may have a considerable effect on the result.

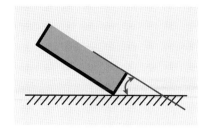

Fig. 8-17 Method for determining the angle of friction.

8.6.2.2   Flowability

Another method to evaluate flow properties of powders and granules refers to their flowability. Two test methods can be distinguished:

1. Measuring the time required for a defined amount of material to flow out from a funnel
2. Measuring the amount of material that flows out from the funnel within a defined time interval

---

Ph. Eur. 2.9.16 Flowability _____

In accordance with the Ph. Eur., powder fluidity may be measured as the time required for 100 g powder to flow out of a funnel. Without restricting the size and shape of the funnel to certain specifications, two typical apparatuses with, without a stem, and with different angles and orifice diameters are shown in the Ph. Eur. One of these apparatuses is a glass funnel with a stem (diameter 12 mm); the other is a steel funnel with three exchangeable stemless nozzles (10, 15, 25 mm).

8.6.2.3   Shear Cells

With the help of shear cells, the flow properties of powders can be investigated precisely and reproducibly. In all types of shear cells, the powder sample is initially compressed in a controlled way and then flow is induced under defined conditions. The shear cell according to Jenike (Fig. 8-18) consists of two concentric flat cylindrical rings positioned one on top of the other. The rings have identical diameters, while the upper (shear) ring can be shifted horizontally. The material is filled into the assembled double ring, and the cell is covered by a cover plate. By applying a defined force on the cover plate, the material is compressed in a defined manner. Subsequently, the force needed to shear the powder by moving the upper ring is determined. Shear stress is then determined at different degrees of compaction. A disadvantage of the method is the limitation of the shear distance. Furthermore, the equipment needs to be readjusted after each measurement and requires frequent refilling.

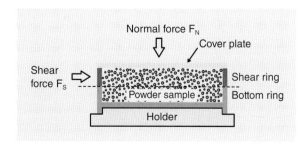

Fig. 8-18 Jenike shear cell.

Ph. Eur. 2.9.36 Powder Flow _____

USP ⟨1174⟩ Powder Flow

JP G2 Solid-State Properties, Powder Flow

In a harmonized chapter the Ph. Eur., the USP, and the JP describe four methods to determine powder flow.

Angle of Repose

Two test methods are mentioned in the pharmacopeias: the drained angle of repose and the dynamic angle of response.

The drained angle of repose is determined by allowing an excess quantity of material positioned above a fixed diameter base to "drain" from the container. The angle (relative to the horizontal base) assumed by the cone-like pile of powder is a characteristic related to interparticular friction, or resistance to movement between particles. As the angle of repose is influenced by the nature of the base surface, it is recommended to form the cone on a layer of powder. Such a powder layer can be retained on the surface by using a base with a protruding outer edge. In the procedure recommended by the pharmacopeias, the powder is allowed to flow from a funnel onto a fixed base with a retaining lip. The funnel is moved upward during the procedure, keeping it all the time approximately 2 to 4 cm above the top of the increasing powder pile, in order to minimize the impact of falling powder on the tip of the cone. From the height of the cone the angle of repose α is calculated, using the following equation: $\tan \alpha = \text{height} / (0.5 \cdot \text{base diameter})$.

The dynamic angle of repose is determined by filling a powder sample into a cylinder, which is equipped with a clear, flat cover on one end, and rotating the cylinder in a horizontal position at a specified speed. The dynamic angle of repose is the angle (relative to the horizontal) formed by the flowing powder.

Compressibility Index and Hausner Ratio

These two parameters may be calculated from the bulk volume (V_0) and the tapping volume (V_f) or alternatively from bulk density (ρ_0) and tapping density (ρ_f), see equations 8.2 and 8.3 (page 337).

Flow through an Orifice

For free-flowing powders the determination of the flow rate through an orifice is a particularly informative method. The flow rate can be measured as the time required for a certain mass to flow through a defined orifice, as the powder mass flowing through an orifice during a certain period of time or as a continuous record of the flowing mass per unit of time. Instead of the mass flow rate, the volume flow rate may be determined, however, measurement of the mass flow rate is the easier of the methods. Maximal information is obtained by continuous recording of a mass-time profile, since this will detect any irregularities such as pulsating flow patterns or changes in flow rate as the container empties. In order to make flow properties largely independent of powder-wall friction but primarily a function of powder-over-powder movement, a cylinder-shaped geometry is recommended. The orifice should be circular and its diameter at least six times larger than the size of the particles and maximally half that of the container vessel.

Shear Cell Methods

Powder rheological methods provide the most detailed data on powder flow. Ph. Eur., USP and JP refer to three different shear-cell types but gives no recommendations or detailed operation instructions. In all cases the powder bed is consolidated in the shear cell, using a well-defined procedure, and the force necessary to shear the powder bed by horizontal movement is measured. One type of shear cell is the cylindrical shear cell (Jenike shear tester), in which two stacked rings enclosing the consolidated powder bed are displaced with respect to one another by applying a horizontal shear force. Annular shear cells (e.g., the Schulze ring shear tester) operate by means of a ring-shaped chamber in which the powder is subjected to a normal force, applied through an annular lid, and a shear force, exerted by rotating the shear cell relative to the lid. The torque necessary for shearing is measured. Plate-type shear cells consist of a thin sandwich of powder between a lower stationary rough surface and an upper rough surface that is movable. For evaluation, shear stress / displacement diagrams may be recorded at various normal forces. Characteristic parameters of bulk materials, like the yield locus (yield limit of a consolidated bulk solid) and the unconfined yield strength (stress required to deform or break a material when it is not confined by a container) can be derived from normal stress vs. shear stress diagrams.

8.6.3 Friability of Granules

Granulates must have satisfactory mechanical stability in order to withstand further handling and processing. In the friability test, the granules are submitted to defined mechanical stress and the loss of material (abrasion and/or fragmentation) is determined.

8.6.4 Special Tests of Powders

8.6.4.1 Adhesive Strength

The simplest device to determine adhesive strength of a powder consists of a wooden board covered with a metal, glass, or glossy paper sheet, mounted in a tilted manner and equipped with a manually operated tapping mechanism. The powder is uniformly spread on the surface and after a tenfold operation of the tapping mechanism, the powder that is still adhering on the surface is quantitatively collected and weighed.

Such conventional methods, however, are often quite error-prone. Moreover, the materials of the support plate are rather poor models for human skin. Much more relevant information is obtained when the powder is tested on human skin.

8.6.4.2 Absorption Capacity for Fluids

To characterize the absorption capacity of powders for liquids (e.g., uptake of aqueous wound secretions or lipophilic drugs in a fluid state), the Enslin-Neff device can be used (Fig. 8-19). It consists of a ceramic frit (diameter 2 cm) connected via 20 cm long flexible tubing to a graduated burette (graduation of 0.02 ml). The frit is adjusted in such a way that its bottom is at the same height as the horizontally positioned pipette. For the determination of the absorption capacity of a substance, the tubing and pipette are filled with an appropriate amount of test fluid (e.g., water or oil) and 1 g of powder is uniformly distributed on filter

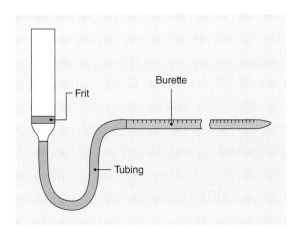

Fig. 8-19 Enslin-Neff device.

paper on the frit, thus bringing it into contact with the fluid. The test is terminated when the meniscus of the fluid in the pipette remains constant. The absorption capacity of a powder (Enslin number, W for water and O for oil) is defined as that amount of liquid [g or mL], which is maximally taken up by 1 g of the substance in a maximum of 15 minutes.

Ph. Eur. 2.9.41 Friability of granules and spheroids

Friability of granules and spheroids is defined as a reduction in the mass or in the formation of fragments, for example, by abrasion, breakage or deformation, occurring when the granules or spheroids are subjected to mechanical strain, like tumbling, vibration, fluidization, and so on. The Ph. Eur. describes two methods to quantify this process:

Method A (fluidized bed apparatus): The apparatus consists of a conically tapered glass cylinder (diameter 5 cm) which at the top is covered by a sieve lid. The conical end is connected to a U-shaped glass tube. After loading with an exactly weighed sample of about 8.0 g of granules or spheroids, which beforehand have been freed from fine material by sieving, the cylinder is flushed from bottom to top with pressurized air to cause swirling of the particles. After 15 minutes, the material is collected from the cylinder and weighed again to determine loss of mass. In order to remove all dust by the airflow, it is recommended to spray the inside of the apparatus with an antistatic agent every three determinations to prevent electrostatic charging. The mean value is calculated from the results of three measurements.

Method B (oscillating apparatus): The apparatus consists of a cylindrical glass container with a volume of 107 mL. It is mounted on a 15.2-cm long arm, which is oscillating at an angle of 37°. The frequency can be adjusted to a value in the range 0 to 400 oscillations per minute. The material to be examined is freed from fine particles below a certain size by means of sieving. About 10.00 g of the granules or spheroids are exactly weighed and transferred to the container. The container is shaken for 40 seconds at the highest frequency for hard granules or spheroids or for 120 seconds at lower frequency (e.g., 140 oscillations/min) for soft particles. The sample is sieved, using the same sieve as before shaking, and weighed again. The mean value of three measurements is calculated.

Both methods may require correction for potential water uptake by heating the material at 105°C before each weighing procedure.

Ph. Eur. 2.9.43 Apparent Dissolution

The Ph. Eur. describes a special flow-through cell to determine the dissolution rate of pure solid substances. This cell may also be used for the determination of the apparent dissolution rate of active substances in preparations presented as powders or granules. The cell consists of three parts that fit into each other. The lower part supports a system of grids and filters on which the powder is placed. The middle part contains an insert that sieves the sample when the dissolution medium flows through the cell. A second grid and filter assembly is placed on the top of the middle part before fitting the upper part through which the dissolution medium flows out of the cell. The flow-through cell is connected to an apparatus as described under 2.9.3 Method 4, which forces, by means of a pump, a dissolution medium at a temperature of 37° ± 0.5°C upward though the cell. Samples of the dissolution medium are collected at the outlet of the cell. The samples are filtered immediately and the amount of dissolved substance is analyzed in the filtrate.

Ph. Eur. 2.9.35 Powder Fineness

USP ⟨811⟩ Powder Fineness
JP G2 Solid-State Properties, Powder Fineness

Where the cumulative particle size distribution has been determined by analytical sieving or by application of other methods, particle size may be characterized by the 90%-, 50%-, and 10%-quantiles (x_{90}, x_{50}, x_{10}, often also designated as d_{90}, d_{50}, d_{10}).

x_{90}: 90% of all particles are smaller than this size.

x_{50}: 50% of all particles are smaller than this size.

x_{10}: 10% of all particles are smaller than this size.

$Q_r(x)$ is the symbol for a cumulative distribution, in which r specifies the type of distribution:

r	Distribution Type
0	number
1	length
2	surface
3	volume

Therefore, by definition:

$Q_r(x) = 0.90$ when $x = x_{90}$

$Q_r(x) = 0.50$ when $x = x_{50}$

$Q_r(x) = 0.10$ when $x = x_{10}$

An alternative but less informative method of classifying powder fineness is by use of the following descriptive terms:

Descriptive Term	x_{50} (μm)
coarse	>355
intermediate	180–355
fine	125–180
very fine	≤125

Ph. Eur. 2.9.27 Uniformity of Mass of Delivered Doses from Multidose Containers

Oral dosage forms that are supplied in multidose containers provided at manufacture with a measuring device must be deliverable with a sufficient degree of uniformity of the measured doses. Not more than two individual masses out of 20 doses, taken at random from one or more containers with the measuring device, are allowed to deviate from the average mass by more than 10% and none by more than 20%.

Further Reading

Masuda, H., Higashitani, K., Yoshida, H. eds. Powder Technology Handbook, 3rd ed. Boca Raton: CRC Press, 2006.

Shanmugam, S. "Granulation techniques and technologies: recent progresses." *Bioimpacts* 5 (1) (2015): 55–63.

Wilson, M., et al. "Hot-melt extrusion technology and pharmaceutical application." *Therapeutic Delivery* 3 (6) (2012): 787–797.

Tablets

9

Great things are done by a series of small things brought together.

Vincent van Gogh

9.1 General Considerations

Among the different dosage forms, tablets (*compressi*) and other oral solid dosage forms are undoubtedly the most commonly used. Traditional formulations for oral administration such as pills, spherules, boluses, and lozenges can be considered as the precursor of modern tablet formulations. The rapid development of tablet formulations started as early as 1843 with the invention of the first tablet machine by William Brockedon in Great Britain, followed by the patent application of tablet machines in the United States by J. A. McFerran (1874), J. P. Remington (1875), and J. Dunton (1876). Remarkably, around 1,900 machines for tablet coating (chapter 10) have been developed.

Nowadays, one can expect that at least 40% of all pharmaceutically active ingredients are processed into tablets. A major advantage of tablets over other dosage forms is that they can be mass-produced at relatively low cost. Tablets can be accurately dosed and are easy to pack, transport, and store. Due to their dry, solid state, tablet formulations usually provide a long shelf life of the active ingredient. Finally, tablets are easy to administer and are usually the dosage form preferred by patients.

The word tablet (tabuletta, tabletta) derives from the Latin word *tabuletta*, meaning a fragment, small strip, platelet, or small table (tabula = table). Some pharmacopeias, among them the Ph. Eur., designate tablets as *compressi*, thus referring to the most common manufacturing process of tablets.

Tablets are single-dose, solid formulations. They are normally formed from dry powders or granules, usually containing suitable excipients, and produced by application of high pressure (compaction, compression). The shape of tablets may be cylindrical, cubic, oblong, or discoidal, but can also be oval or spheroid. Cylindrical forms in particular, but convexly curved and oblong tablet forms as well, have gained largest acceptance. In general, tablet diameters vary between 5 and 17 mm and masses between 0.1 and 1 g.

The shape of the tablet largely affects the ease of transport and storage stability. Biplanar cylindrical tablets, for example, may easily be damaged at their edges. Tablets with a faceted edge are much more resistant to such damage. Biconvex tablets contact each other in a tablet chute only at their thickest and mechanically most insensitive side and are thus less vulnerable to mechanical damage than biplanar tablets (Fig. 9-1). Tablet disintegration may also be affected to some extent by their shape. Table 9-1 presents an overview of the different tablet types described in the Ph. Eur., together with their main characteristics and applications.

Voigt's Pharmaceutical Technology, First Edition. Alfred Fahr.
© 2018 John Wiley & Sons Ltd. Published 2018 by John Wiley & Sons Ltd.

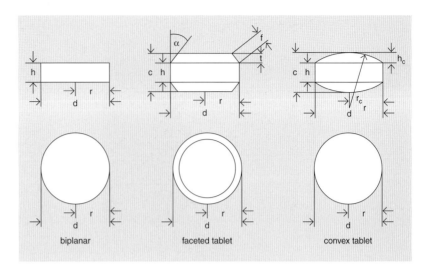

Fig. 9-1 Important tablet shapes and designations. h band height, c thickness, d diameter, r radius, f facet edge, t facet depth, α facet angle, h_c height of the curvature, r_c radius of curvature.

Table 9-1 Overview of Tablet Types in the Ph. Eur. (for comparison with USP and JP see Table A-1, page 758).

Uncoated tablets	Single- or multi-layer tablets, no specific effect of drug release due to applied excipient.	Rapid disintegration within 15 min. Disintegration requirements do not apply to chewing tablets.
Coated tablets	Tablets with various coatings, e.g., sugar or thin polymer film (film tablets).	Disintegration requirements dependent on type of coating (film tablets within 30 min; tablets with other coatings within 60 min). Requirements do not apply to coated chewing tablets. Except for film tablets, a test of uniformity of drug content is always required, independent on the amount of active ingredient.
Effervescent tablets	Uncoated tablets that in contact with water release CO_2. Contain acids and carbonates/bicarbonates. Administration after dissolving/dispersing in water.	Disintegrate within 5 min under gas formation. Effervescent tablets are sensitive to moisture.
Soluble and dispersible tablets	Uncoated or film-coated tablets. Ingestion after dissolving/dispersing in water.	Rapid disintegration within 3 min; produce a clear or opalescent solution or a homogeneous dispersion.
Orodispersible tablets (Melting tablets)	Uncoated tablets, rapidly disintegrating in the mouth before swallowing. Production by compression or melt extrusion.	Disintegrate within 3 min. The designation "melting tablet" is confusing, as the tablets do not really melt but just dissolve or disintegrate rapidly upon contact with water.
Modified-release tablets	Film-coated tablets or uncoated tablets containing special excipients or prepared by special procedures, or both, determining the rate, site and time of release of the active ingredient; prolonged, delayed or pulsatile-release tablets.	Tablets can have release-modifying coatings or a matrix controlling drug release (matrix tablets). Tablets with release-modifying coatings must not be divided. The modified drug release should be confirmed by means of an appropriate test.
Gastro-resistant tablets	Tablets with delayed drug release are resistant to gastric juice, as they release only in the small intestine; film-coated or matrix tablets.	No disintegration in 0.1 m HCl within 2 h; rapid disintegration in phosphate buffer ph 6.8, within 60 min; film-coated gastro-resistant tablets must not be divided.
Tablets for use in the mouth	Usually uncoated tablets; Lozenges: solid single-dose preparations for sucking in order to achieve a local or systemic effect; sublingual or buccal tablets: solid, single-dose preparations for application under the tongue (sublingual) or in the buccal cavity to achieve a systemic effect.	Must conform to the monograph "oromucosal preparations"; slow release of active ingredient in the oral cavity; for sublingual or buccal tablets the release of active ingredient must be confirmed by proper testing.
Oral lyophilisates	Solid preparations for application in the oral cavity or to be dispersed/dissolved in water before administration; preparation by lyophilization.	Disintegrate within 3 min.

9.2 Excipients in Tablet Manufacturing

9.2.1 General Considerations

The range of excipients used in tablet formulation and production is large. A strict classification in groups is not always possible because many excipients have more than one function. Tablet excipients should be inert, odorless, tasteless, and, whenever possible, colorless (exceptions are, of course, for example, sweeteners or colorants). Whether or not excipients have to be added and in which concentration must be evaluated in each individual case.

9.2.2 Diluents (Fillers)

When only very small quantities of the active pharmaceutical ingredient are required (e.g., alkaloids, hormones, vitamins, etc.), the addition of a diluent (or filler) is necessary to provide a certain powder volume that can be processed into a tablet. Diluents ensure that the tablet is within the required mass range (0.1–1 g).

Diluents should be chemically and physiologically inert. Lactose, cellulose, and starches (corn, potato, and wheat starch) are predominantly used as diluents in tablet formulations in Europe. Spray-dried lactose possesses better compaction properties than crystalline lactose. The former, as well as microcrystalline cellulose (e.g., Avicel®), can also be used for direct tableting (section 9.3). Other diluents, particularly used in lozenges and vaginal tablets, are glucose, mannitol, and sorbitol. Calcium dihydrogen phosphate is commonly used in North America.

9.2.3 Binders

This group of excipients provides tablets with mechanical strength. They also result in stable aggregation of the powder particles in granules (section 8.4.7). The hardness of a tablet is affected by the applied pressure as well as by the properties of the binder. Keep in mind that tablet hardness and disintegration are opposing properties, and therefore the amount of binder should be kept to a minimum (if fast disintegration is required). The diluents discussed in section 9.2.2 can to some extent also function as a binder. The binder is added during granulation (section 8.4) or to the tableting powder for direct compression (section 9.3). Typical binders for wet granulation are polyvinyl pyrrolidone (Povidon, Kollidon®), starch mucilages and cellulose ethers such as sodium carboxymethylcellulose (Nymcel®), hydroxyethyl cellulose (Cellosize®), and methylcellulose (Methocel®).

Microcrystalline cellulose (Avicel®, Emcocel®, Vivacel®) is a typical dry binder. Also, polyethylene glycols (macrogols) with molar masses between 4,000 and 6,000 have good binding properties, but are incompatible with many active pharmaceutical ingredients.

9.2.4 Flow-Regulating Agents (Glidants)

Flow-regulating agents improve the flow characteristics of powder mixtures by reducing the inter-particulate friction and thus enhance the flow of the tableting powder mixture from the feed shoe into the filling cavity (die) of the tablet machine. In this way, glidants (section 5.2.5) improve dosing accuracy. A widely used glidant is colloidal silicon dioxide (Aerosil®), usually used in a concentration of 0.05% to 0.5%.

The effect of glidants can be explained by mainly three mechanisms:
- Adhesion of the glidant onto the surface of the powder particles creates new surfaces, resulting in weaker friction and adhesion forces in the powder mixture.
- Reduction of moisture in the powder mixture.
- For small, round particles (such as in Aerosil®), a "ball-bearing effect" resulting in reduction of friction forces between the powder particles has been suggested.

However, problems concerning powder flow of tableting masses cannot always be solved by addition of a glidant. When the powder or granules gets stuck in the funnel or feed shoe due to excessive moisture in the powder or granule mass, the material must be dried further. Air-conditioning during processing of powders or granules may effectively reduce the air humidity and facilitate maintenance of powder flow properties.

9.2.5   Lubricants

Lubricants are used to prevent sticking of the tablet mass on the die and punches of the tablet machine:

- They facilitate expulsion of the tablet from the cavity (die) by reducing friction between the inner wall of the die and the tablet.
- They reduce friction between the punches and die of the tablet machine, thus preventing jamming.

Processing of hygroscopic substances may cause problems due to their tendency to stick on punches and the die. Compounds with a melting range below 75°C tend to stick strongly and are not suitable for compaction without additional measures. First choice of suitable excipients is addition of magnesium stearate, calcium behenate, or glycerol monostearate (Precirol®). Among the second-choice excipients are stearic acid and hydrogenated plant fats such as hydrogenated castor oil and cotton seed oil (Sterotex®). All these lubricants share a distinct hydrophobicity. This implies that these substances will reduce wettability of the tablets and may thus impair tablet disintegration. Therefore, these lubricants are used in the lowest possible concentration and added just before compaction to the powder or granule tablet mass.

For tablets that are dissolved prior to use (effervescent tablets, tablets for solution), water-soluble lubricants such as PEG 4000, sodium dodecyl sulfate, and magnesium dodecyl sulfate are used. Their effect on tablet disintegration is much lower than that of hydrophobic lubricants, because the wettability is not compromised and may even be improved.

The frequently used talcum is a rather poor lubricant. It can only improve lubrication to a certain extent when suboptimal magnesium stearate concentrations are used.

9.2.6   Disintegrants

Disintegrants are added to tablet formulations to ensure efficient and rapid disintegration of the tablet in the gastrointestinal fluids, as a prerequisite of dissolution of the active pharmaceutical ingredient. A number of factors affect the disintegration process. The nature and the amount of the active pharmaceutical ingredient, added excipients such as binders (especially binders used in wet granulation), and hydrophobic lubricants may all have a negative effect on the disintegration process. Improvement of disintegration can often be achieved by minimizing the amount of these excipients or replacement by other excipients. The size and shape of granules should also be taken into consideration. Another important parameter is the applied pressure during compaction. A slight reduction in compaction pressure may have a distinct beneficial effect on tablet disintegration. Finally, the size and shape of the tablet, as well as its age, may also influence the ease of disintegration.

Disintegrants can enhance tablet disintegration by the following mechanisms:

1. Enhancing water absorption into the table by enhancing capillary activity, resulting in swelling and disintegration of the tablet.
2. Production of a gas (usually carbon dioxide) when the tablet comes into contact with water (effervescent tablets).
3. Improvement of tablet wettability (hydrophilizing excipients).

Most disintegration enhancers belong to group 1. These compounds generally swell in the presence of water. Important for disintegration is the swelling pressure, which counteracts and may even overcome the binding forces within the tablet. The porosity of the tablet also plays an important role, as it will promote water uptake into the tablet. Tablet porosity can be increased by reducing the compaction pressure, although disintegrants may further improve capillarity of the tablets. In this regard, not only is high porosity important, but it is also adequate wettability. Disintegrants have a higher potency when their ability to swell is limited, exhibiting a high swelling pressure and creation of a highly wettable pore system within the tablet

The complexity of the disintegration process becomes apparent in the case of starches, the oldest and most often used disintegration enhancers. Often pregelatinized starches (Lycatab®) are employed. Corn starches are most widely used in a concentration of about 5% to 10% and result in tablets with satisfactory disintegration behavior. Starches swell to a considerable extent in water undergoing a substantial increase in volume. Starch grains undergo substantial plastic deformation during compaction, which may alter their swelling properties. Starches also belong to the hydrophilizing agents, that is, they enhance both porosity and wettability of the tablet and facilitate water uptake into the tablet (*wicking action*), thus accelerating tablet disintegration.

In addition to starches, alginic acid and its salts and derivatives are commonly used disintegration enhancers. The water-insoluble alginic acid can take up a multiple of its own mass of water. Thus, it swells and enhances the disintegration process. Its swelling capacity is retained even after multiple wetting and drying cycles. Due to its acidity, alginic acid is not suitable for all tablet formulations and its calcium or sodium salts are often used instead.

Disintegrants with high potency (e.g., only comparatively small amounts (1%–4%) are needed to ensure efficient tablet disintegration) are called *super-disintegrants*. Examples of this group of disintegrants are sodium carboxymethylcellulose (Carmellose, Nymcel®), cross-linked polyvinyl pyrrolidones (Crospovidon, Polyplasdone® XL, Kollidon® CL), cross-linked sodium carboxymethylcellulose (Croscarmellose, Ac-Di-Sol®, Solutab®), and cross-linked sodium carboxymethylstarch (Primojel®, Explotab®). These super-disintegrants possess considerable swelling capacity as well as high capillary activity. Moreover, there is no slime formation, as is typical for starches. Furthermore, super-disintegrants may also function as binders, providing tablets with both a high mechanical strength and adequate disintegration properties.

An example of group 2 disintegrants is sodium bicarbonate. Tablets containing this substance disintegrate rapidly in water in the presence of an acid (such as in the stomach) due to carbon dioxide formation. To ensure rapid disintegration in water or in the stomach of people with sub-acidic gastric juice, acidic excipients such as citric or tartaric acid are added. Understandably, tablets whose disintegration depends on moisture-induced gas formation are very sensitive to moisture and require suitable storage conditions (e.g., integration of a desiccant in the tablet tube).

Excipients mentioned in group 3 are not disintegrants in the strict sense, as they do not have a direct effect on tablet disintegration. However, they serve to optimize the effectiveness of the actual disintegration agent by increasing tablet wettability. Tablets containing hydrophobic substances often possess insufficient disintegration. Due to poor wettability, the effect of added disintegration enhancers is delayed or even completely compromised. Addition of surface-active agents, which will hydrophilize the tablets and facilitate water permeation into the tablet matrix and thus aid the effect of added disintegrants, is recommended in such cases. The anionic detergent sodium lauryl sulfate and nonionic detergents such as polysorbates (section 5.4.4.7) are used for this purpose. Although such surface-active substances are known to have some physiological activity, serious pharmacological objections have not been raised so far.

Pronounced disintegration can also be achieved by colloidal silica. It promotes, like microcrystalline cellulose, water penetration into the tablet.

No single disintegrant can generally be recommended and the most suitable type and quantity of a disintegrant must be determined empirically for each tablet formulation.

9.2.7   Humectants

In some cases, addition of moisture-binding excipients (humectants) to tablet formulations may be necessary. Humectants prevent dehydration of the tablet powder or granule mixture (which potentially may result in "capping" of tablets during the compaction process) and the tablet itself (traces of moisture accelerate disintegration). Addition of glycerol or sorbitol to tablet formulations has proven to be effective in this context. Starch is also considered to be useful for this purpose as it can adsorb moisture and functions as a "water regulator" in the tablet.

9.2.8   Adsorption Agents

When fluid or viscous active ingredients (essential oils, lipophilic vitamins, fluid extracts) are to be compressed into tablets, they must first be adsorbed on a suitable solid compound. Lactose, starch and derivatives, bentonite, and colloidal silica (Aerosil®) can be used for this purpose. Most frequently the active pharmaceutical ingredient is dissolved in a suitable organic solvent, such as ethanol, followed by spraying the solution onto a suitable carrier.

9.2.9   Dissolution Inhibitors

Dissolution inhibitors are only required for tablets for which too rapid disintegration is undesirable (lozenges, buccal tablets, implantation tablets, etc.).

In addition to sucrose, Arabic gum, tragacanth, dextrins, hydrophobic substances such as hydrogenated fats, stearin, and paraffin, are used for this purpose. Polyethylene glycols may also retard disintegration when applied at suitable concentrations.

9.3   Direct Compression

9.3.1   General Introduction

In direct tableting (direct compression), a powder mixture is compressed as such—that is, without previous granulation. As direct compression is not very labor-intensive, it provides an economical advantage over production and compaction of granules and is gaining increasing interest in the pharmaceutical industry. A disadvantage is that excipients, which are suitable for direct compression, are often expensive. Direct compression becomes especially advantageous when moisture- and heat-sensitive active ingredients, whose stability may be compromised during granulation, are processed.

Only few active pharmaceutical ingredients can be directly compressed without any pretreatment or without addition of suitable excipients. Depending on the physical properties of the active pharmaceutical ingredient and its crystal structure, the pressure required to achieve a product with appropriate mechanical stability will vary. The crystal structure influences the compaction process where a cubic crystal structure offers a clear advantage. Furthermore, coarse crystalline substances allow easier compaction than fine powders. With the latter, inclusion of air can further counteract the formation of tablets with sufficient mechanical stability. Ammonium chloride and iodide, potassium chloride and chlorate, sodium chloride and citrate and zinc sulfate are examples of substances that can be effectively compressed without any additives.

The (generally) rather weak binding forces between powder particles, possibly resulting in tablets with unsatisfactory mechanical stability, as well as in poor flow properties of bulk powders, present a serious challenge in direct compaction. Nonetheless, modification of the powder particle properties (shape, size, and size distribution), addition of suitable excipients (dry binders, glidants, lubricants), as well as alteration of the compaction parameters (application of higher pressure, equipment of hopper shoes with stirring devices to facilitate die filling) may aid in direct compression. A particle size of approximately 0.5 mm is generally considered as optimal. A spherical particle shape is an advantage in powders intended for direct compaction due to their good flow properties (roll friction < slip friction). Suitable particle properties, for excipients for direct compression, such as shape, are usually obtained by spray drying. Molten substances can be transferred to powders with adequate flow properties by spray freezing.

A general prerequisite for direct compression is a low moisture content of all excipients used. Satisfactory miscibility of active pharmaceutical ingredients and the excipients is another important prerequisite for direct compression. Since powder mixtures tend to segregate (e.g., due to differences in particle size and density), powder homogeneity needs to be tested in each step of the direct compression procedure.

9.3.2   Dry Binders

Excipients (dry binders) for direct tableting should improve flow properties, facilitate compaction by their plastic deformation properties, and lead to a product with sufficient mechanical strength. Microcrystalline cellulose (MCC, Avicel®, Vivapur®) and special cellulose powders (Elcema®, Rehocel®) are mainly used as dry binders. MCC is widely considered as an excellent binder in tablets and is particularly well suited for direct compression due to its excellent deformation properties and usually yields tablets with high mechanical strength. Compared to other products, it can be compressed at relatively low pressure. MCC is also suitable as a carrier substance for fluid, semi-solid and hygroscopic substances and as a diluent. Its relatively high bulk density prevents mass deviations. Moreover, its hydrophilic properties result in short disintegration times. Due to hydrogen bonding, flow properties are only moderate but can be considerably improved by addition of Aerosil®. Silica-modified microcrystalline cellulose (SMCC, ProSolv®) is produced by processing a mixture of 98% MCC and 2% Aerosil and results in a powder with improved flow and compaction properties. Due to their rather poor flow properties, native starches are less well suited for direct compression. However, modified and pretreated starches, such as pregelatinized starch (Lycatab PGS®) and hydrolyzed starches such as dextran (Emdex®) and maltodextrin (Maldex®) are suitable for direct compression. Other excipients suitable for direct compression include spray-dried lactose (SpheroLac®, Tablettose®, SuperTab®) and tribasic calcium phosphate (TRI-TAB®). Also, copovidon, a co-polymer of polyvinyl pyrrolidone and vinyl acetate (Kollidon VA64®), can be used in low concentrations (2%–5%) as a dry binder. In recent years, a gradual increase in the use of processed mixtures of two or more excipients for direct tableting has developed. Such products have better flow and compaction properties than the physical mixtures of the individual components. Most commercially available processed mixtures of different excipients contain a large proportion of a rather brittle excipient, such as lactose, and a smaller quantity of an excipient with high plastic deformability, such as MCC. Examples of such ready-to-use mixtures are Microcelac® 100 (75% lactose and 25% microcrystalline cellulose), StarLac® (85% lactose and 15% corn starch) as well as Ludipress LCE® (96.5% lactose and 3.5% Povidon). Ludipress® is a processed mixture of three components (lactose, povidone K30, and Crospovidone).

9.4   Granulation

In most cases it remains necessary to process the active pharmaceutical ingredient and the required excipients via granulation (section 8.4) prior to compaction. Granulation results in a product with coarser grains having better flow and compaction properties than powders. Due to the better flow capacity, a more continuous and uniform filling of the die in the tablet machine is achieved, resulting in low variability in tablet mass and thus high dose accuracy. A granule is defined as a conglutinated asymmetric aggregate of powder particles (whole crystals, crystal fragments, drug particles) and often does not have a uniform shape. It is rather described as a more or less spherical, rod-shaped or cylindrical powder aggregate. The surface is usually irregular, jagged or roughened and the granule is often more or less porous.

During granulation, the total surface area of all powder particles is reduced resulting in a decrease in adhesive forces. Porosity of the granules facilitates plastic deformation upon compaction and a tablet with sufficient mechanical strength is formed (section 8.4.7).

The requirements for granules that are suitable for compaction can be summarized as follows. The granules should:

- Be as uniform as possible in shape and size.
- Contain no more than 10% powder.
- Have good flow properties.
- Possess satisfactory mechanical strength.
- Be not too dry (3%–5% residual moisture is considered as optimal).
- Easily disintegrate in water.

The production and testing of granules is discussed in sections 8.4 and 8.6, respectively.

9.5   Compaction

9.5.1   Compaction Procedure

The compaction procedure is generally the same in all tablet machines. They all have two movable punches. While the lower punch continuously moves within the die, the upper punch enters the die only during the compaction step. The following four steps can be distinguished:

- The die matrix takes up the powder to be compressed. The amount of powder is determined by the position of the lower punch.
- The upper punch moves into the die and compresses the powder into a tablet.

Thickness, mechanical strength, and surface properties of the tablet depend on the compaction pressure. The depth of penetration of the upper (single-punch tablet machines) or both punches (rotary tablet machines) and thus the compaction pressure can be regulated.

- The position of the lower punch within the die determines the filling volume of the die. In rotary tablet machines, the lower punch is also involved in the compression step. When compression is complete, the lower punch moves upward and ejects the tablet from the die. As soon as the lower punch is back in its lower position, the die is ready to be filled again.
- The filling funnel—the lower section of which is called the feed shoe—contains the tableting mixture. The bottom of the feed shoe is partially open so that the tableting mixture can flow into the die space during its forward movement (single-punch machine), where at the same time the ejected tablet of the previous compression step is removed, for instance, onto a transport belt.

9.5.2   Tablet Machines

Two types of fully automatic tablet machines are distinguished: single-punch and rotary presses.

9.5.2.1   Single-Punch Tablet Machines

The upper punch is moved by a cam wheel in this type of tablet machine (Fig. 9-2). The rotary movement of the drive shaft is converted into a translational movement, that is, the up and down movement of the upper punch. By adjusting the point of the deepest position of the upper punch by adjustment of the eccentric screw, the pressure can be regulated. Adjustment of the volume in the die space is achieved by adjusting the position of the lower punch. One typical characteristic of single-punch machines is that the die is fixed while the hopper shoe is moving. It slides back and forth on the die and ensures constant refilling of the die. However, movements of the hopper shoe may result in partial segregation when nonuniform granules or powder mixtures are processed. Segregation in granule or powder mixtures will result in erroneous dosing.

Some definitions of shoes:

The **hopper** describes in compaction science the funnel, which is the intermediate container for the material (powder, granules) to be pressed. The **feed shoe**, also often called **fill shoe**, is connected via the **fill tube** to the hopper. The feed (fill) shoe is designed for the filling of the die. In tabletting manufacturing, hopper, fill tube and fill shoe are often one unit and called **hopper shoe**.

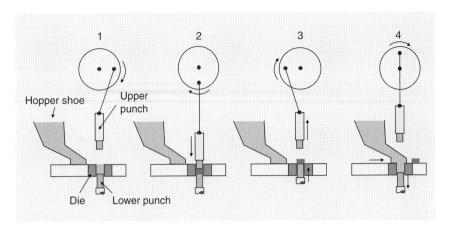

Fig. 9-2 Schematic presentation of the compression process in a single punch tablet machine.

The following steps can be distinguished in a single-punch tablet machine (Fig. 9-2):

Phase 1: The upper and lower punch and the fill shoe (or hopper shoe) are in the starting position and the die space is filled with the tableting material.

Phase 2: The upper punch moves down into the die and compresses the powder or granules into a tablet.

Phase 3: The upper punch moves upward and returns to its starting position. At the same time, the lower punch moves upward and ejects the tablet from the die.

Phase 4: The lower punch falls back into its starting position and the feed shoe slides forward, moving the finished tablet on the transport belt and filling the die with material for the next compression step.

In single-punch presses only the upper punch is actively involved in the compression process; the pressure is built up abruptly. A typical characteristic of tablets produced by this type of tablet machine is that the two sides of the tablet differ in hardness (~10%–30%, depending on pressure). Single-punch tablet machines usually produce approximately 2,000 tablets per hour, but high-capacity machines are capable of producing up to 4,000 tablets per hour.

9.5.2.2   Rotary Presses

In this type of tablet press, the hopper shoe is fixed while the die table moves. The circular horizontal plate (die table) carries a number of dies; typically 3 to 5 in small machines, but up to 115 in high-capacity machines. Each die has its own pair of upper and lower punches and both the die and the punches rotate together.

The punches are moved by tacks passing over cams and rolls so that the punches in each phase of the compression cycle are in a different vertical position (Fig. 9-3). Upon rotating the horizontal die table, the dies are filled with the tableting mixture when the die is positioned in the filling position. The hopper shoe may be equipped with a rotating device (the force-feeding device) to improve reproducibility of die filling. Upon subsequent rotation of the die table, the tableting mixture is compressed by up (lower punch) and down (upper punch) movement of the pair of punches. Movement over pressure rollers provides the required pressure.

During the compression cycle, the two punches usually contribute equally to the compaction pressure. As a result, tablets with similar hardness on both sides are obtained. Fig. 9-3 illustrates schematically the function of a rotary press. In the ejection phase, the tablets are pushed upward by the lower punch and pushed away, when the die moves into the filling position.

In double rotary presses with two compression stations, only half a rotation of the die table is used for one working cycle (filling, compression, ejection). During the other half rotation, another, second cycle proceeds in the same order. Rotary presses with up to four working cycles upon one rotation of the die table are available.

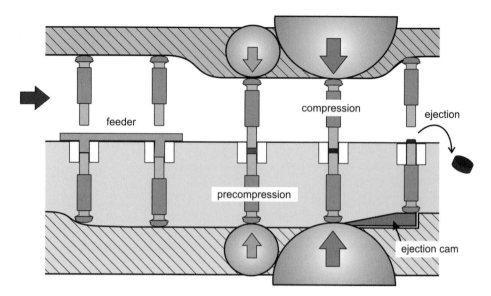

Fig. 9-3 Working principle of an advanced rotary press.

Depending on the number of dies, the capacity of rotary presses varies. Capacity can furthermore be substantially enhanced when, instead of single-punch equipment (one pair of punches and die), multiple punches and dies are working in parallel. Capacities between 20,000 and 60,000 tablets per hour are not unusual for such machines. High-speed presses work according to the same principle but may produce over 100,000 tablets per hour. Ultra-high-capacity machines can produce up to 1,600,000 tablets per hour.

The maximal pressure applied varies from machine to machine, but is generally between 500 and 1,000 MPa (in practice, expressed as force: 5 kN to 100 kN; even up to 160 kN).

9.5.2.3   Advanced and Special Devices

Multiple technical improvements in tableting machines facilitate the compression process, providing uniform flow of the filling material into the die and thus ensuring constant die filling. A stirring blade mounted directly above the hopper shoe pushes the filling material homogeneously into the die. It also regulates the flow process and prevents powder segregation. Unsatisfactory flow behavior can also be significantly improved by placing a magnet into the hopper shoe, resulting in vibration. Even simple eccentrically working stirring devices, such as a shaft rotating in the hopper shoe, loosen up the powder or granules and break down large aggregates. The mixing device may be equipped with several spikes to improve its efficiency. Such force-feeding devices are positioned directly above the opening of the hopper shoe and ensure a uniform filling of the die (Fig. 9-4).

A special problem is air inclusion within the tablet mixture during compression. When such air inclusions do not have a chance to escape, irregularities in the tablet such as capping and low mechanical strength are likely to occur. Many tablet machines therefore are equipped with a configuration to stepwise or progressively increase pressure. This implies that compression proceeds in single individual phases, so that included air may escape. Another advantage of stepwise compression is the production of harder tablets. For many formulations, several compression steps with lower pressure deliver an altogether harder tablet, as obtained in many modern tablet machines with two or even three pressure roller systems for the same compression cycle.

Modern tablet machines are provided with force-monitoring systems. Microprocessor-controlled monitoring devices facilitate automation of the manufacturing process and at the same time provide information for in-process controls. In such monitoring systems, the compression pressure is displayed with percentage deviation and tablet masses are controlled within predetermined limits. Tablets with masses outside the preset mass interval are automatically discarded. The entire machine, including punches and dies, is monitored and stopped when measured values are out of the preset limits. A batch protocol, documenting all process variables, is obtained for all tablet batches.

(A)

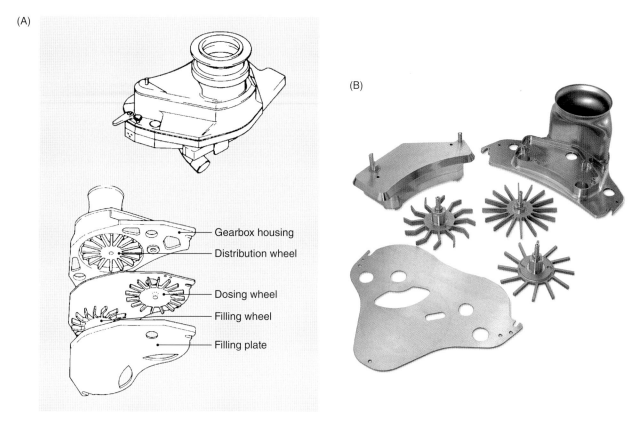

(B)

Fig. 9-4 Force feeder: (A) Overview; (B) Single parts in an exploded view. Reproduced with permission from LMT Group © 2016.

According to GMP guidelines, the following measures must be taken to protect product, personnel, and environment:

- Isolation of the tablet press to avoid dust contamination
- Clean-air system to keep the production location free of dust
- Air conditioning
- Noise reduction measures

9.5.2.4 Instrumentation of Tablet Machines

All tablet presses used today in industry employ a complete instrumentation, which was formerly only the case for presses used in method development. Forces occurring during the compression process are measured as a function of time (pressure-time profiles) and as a function of the distance covered by the punches (force-displacement profiles). As the compression pressures vary within different tablet machines, pressure-time profiles are usually only used to document the maximal pressure occurring during compression. In force-displacement profiles, the movements of the upper and lower punch in the die are monitored. A force-displacement relationship can be recorded digitally and further processed. The instrumentation of tablet presses comprises a strain gauge, a piezoelectric force transducer, or an inductive displacement sensor. The force sensor can be positioned on moving (punch holder, die) or stationary (pressure roller, ejection cam, material, or tablet scraper) parts, whereas the sensor is most commonly placed on the punch holder, as this position provides highest sensitivity.

Strain gauges are polymeric foils with a meandering metallic conductance track. Such strips are glued with a special glue onto a relevant part of the machine (such as the punch holder in tablet machines) in the direction of the force. Because an applied force will evoke a directly proportional compression or expansion of the particular part of the machine, the strips will be deformed accordingly to the forces applied. Changes in length and cross section of the conductance track produce a change in electric resistance that, through a corresponding circuit, can be converted into an electric signal. Unless a special type of strain gauge (providing

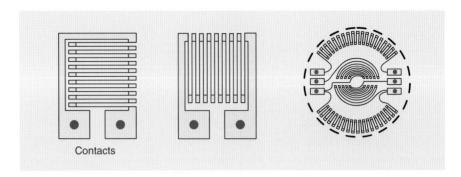

Contacts

Fig. 9-5   Strain gauge.

correction for changes in temperature) is used, the influence of temperature changes can be abolished by positioning a second strip perpendicular to the longitudinal direction of the part of the machine. There is a large variability in arrangement of conductive parts in commercially available strain gauges. Some commonly used types of strain gauges are shown in Fig. 9-5.

Piezoelectric force transducer. Upon the action of a force on a piezoelectric crystal, a shift of positively and negatively charged crystal lattice units occurs. These cause the occurrence of electric charges on the surface of the crystal. The arising electric potential can be detected, amplified, and recorded. Piezoelectric crystals mostly consist of pure quartz. For the purpose of force measurement, they must be incorporated in the relevant machine parts.

Inductive Displacement Sensor. When a metal pen is moved into a coil, the inductivity of the coil changes, depending on the penetration depth of the pen. This phenomenon can be used for the registration of movements of the punches, where the change in impedance (alternating-current resistance) of the coil is measured.

9.5.3   Physical Processes during Compression

During compression, the tableting material (powder or granules) can undergo three deformation stages:

1. Elastic deformation
2. Plastic deformation
3. Fracture and fragmentation

When the punch exerts a pressure on the tableting material, initially an elastic deformation occurs. This is characterized by the fact that the powder or granules resume their original shape upon removal of the force.

Upon increasing the pressure, the elastic limit of the material is exceeded, which results in plastic deformation and the particles remain irreversibly deformed upon removal of the applied pressure. The plastic behavior of a crystalline substance is mainly determined by defects in the crystal structure, called *dislocations*. These are irregularities in the distance between the lattice elements, which expand linearly or spirally along the crystal over a certain distance. During deformation, these irregularities move through the crystal.

When the force (and thus the pressure) is further increased, fragmentation of the compressed material may result. Fragmentation occurs when the energy of the crystal defects is higher than the binding energy between the lattice elements.

The aim of compaction is to exert a high enough pressure to plastically deform the material, but low enough to prevent fragmentation, or, in the case of brittle substances, to prevent brittle fractures occurring after exceeding the elastic deformation range. Fragmentation generally occurs more readily with brittle substances than with ductile materials.

Normally, mixtures of substances are used in tablet formulations. As the different materials may possess different deformation properties, tableting mixtures usually have a complex deformation behavior, and elastic and plastic deformations, as well as (partial) fragmentation, may occur simultaneously.

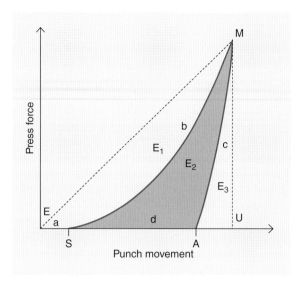

Fig. 9-6 Press force as a function of upper punch movement at a single-punch tablet machine (see explanation in text).

9.5.4   Stages and Energy of the Compression Process

During compaction, the following phases can be distinguished (Fig. 9-6):

- After forceless precompression (phase a), by moving the upper punch from the insertion point (E) into the die until an increase of the force is observed (S), the granules or powder particles are pushed together by the punch without deformation.
- In the next phase (b), pressure increases strongly and deformation of the granules or powder particles occurs. Pressure becomes maximal (M) when the upper punch has reached its lowest position (U). Initially, elastic deformation occurs followed by plastic deformation when the elastic limit of the material is exceeded. In the case of so-called visco-elastic behavior, the deformation depends on the deformation velocity, as well as on exposure time of the force.
- Finally, the elastic deformation of the compressed material and the machine (elastic recovery of the punches and other challenged components of the machine) is relieved upon withdrawal of the punch (c), until the punch loses contact with the tablet (A).
- Phases (d) and (a) designate the forceless movement of the punch to the insertion point (E). The usual further expansion of the tablet after the punch has moved up, is not registered in the force-displacement profile.

One particle can pass through these processes several times. Ultimately, the particle surfaces are pushed together so closely that interparticulate attraction forces are established. Alternative hyperbolic curve shapes can occur, for example, by:

- Changes in the crystal structure of the compressed material
- Sintering
- Change in particle size distribution
- Change in compression velocity
- Change in tablet dimensions (filling depth or diameter of the die)

From the observations described above, it becomes clear that not only the maximal pressure but also the pressure history and the time course determines the quality of the compression. Particularly critical are residual tensions of elastically deformed compounds, which, for example, can lead to capping of the tablets. By connecting points (E), (M), and (U) in the force-displacement profile by straight lines, a rectangular triangle (EMU) is obtained. The area of the triangle is proportional to the total amount of energy that has been used during compression, under the theoretical assumption of a linear pressure increase. This energy is designated E_{max} and contains the energy contributions of the areas E_1, E_2 and E_3. Area E_2 corresponds to the energy required for plastic deformation of the tablet mixture and for the friction at the die wall. Area E_3 is a measure of the elastic behavior of the compressed material and the challenged parts of the machine. It represents the energy of elastic recovery that is returned by the compressed tablet to the upper punch.

For the evaluation of the compression characteristics of substances, the individual plane areas are considered in relation to each other. The aim is to obtain a maximal value for the ratio $(E_2 + E_3)/E_1$, which represents a quality parameter for compressibility. A curve corresponding to the line EM has merely theoretical relevance, but it should be close to the measured curve (b). Area E_1 should be as small as possible in favor of the largest possible area E_2, which represents the deformation energy residing in the tablet (e.g., plastic deformation). Similarly, a small area E_3, corresponding to a small distance between U and A, is desirable.

Based on the force-displacement profiles, practically useful conclusions can be drawn. For example, substances with poor compression properties are often characterized by displaying a strong elastic rebound (slope of section (c) in Fig. 9-6). Often, they are also characterized by a long precompression stage. The dose-dependence of the maximal forces can be used in production control to monitor dosing accuracy, especially in rotary presses. Today's rotary tablet machines are equipped with a digital control system.

The energy consumed during compaction of a substance can be determined by the force-displacement profile. On average, energies between 4.2 and 21 J/g are observed. By far, the largest proportion of the mechanical energy is released as heat. Corresponding to the specific heat of the substances and the high heat dissipation of the tablet machines, temperature increase in the final tablet as compared to the starting material can vary between 5 K and 20 K. An important factor that may affect the compression process is the friction at the die wall. As a result of this friction, counterforces occur at the die walls. These forces increase with increasing compression of the tablet mixture. As these counterforces must also be overcome by the punches, additional energy is necessary for compression in comparison with friction-less compression. Moreover, high friction may also result in a distinctly higher tablet temperature. Even more important is that the friction at the die wall may compromise a homogeneous density distribution within the tablet. As this may lead to reduced mechanical strength of the tablet and even to capping, minimal die wall friction is generally sought for. This can be achieved by special tools within the tablet machine (e.g., punches with minimal band height for coated tablets, etc.) on one hand and the use of suitable lubricants on the other.

The compression forces affect the physical properties of the tablet in multiple ways, while greater force invariably results in higher mechanical strength. As this may reduce disintegration ability, one usually aims for a compromise between mechanical strength and adequate disintegration. On the other hand, cases have been reported where application of higher compression forces resulted in changes of the crystal structure of the active pharmaceutical ingredient, as a result of which an improvement of the dissolution rate and absorption of the drug was obtained.

9.6   Complications during Compaction

9.6.1   General Introduction

Multiple complications can occur during compaction, which may disturb the process and lead to tablet defects. The causes of such problems may lie in the material to be compressed, but may also be found in the tablet machine. A number of particularly serious and commonly occurring complications during compaction are listed in this section.

9.6.2   Squeaking

A squeaky noise emerging from the machine is caused by air inclusions or friction noise, arising by sticking of the tablet mass to the die wall or lower punch. High humidity, insufficient lubrication, or improperly adjusted or worn equipment may be responsible for these problems.

9.6.3   Sticking to the Punches

This phenomenon can prevent continuity of production and leads to production of tablets with rough surfaces. Among the causes of this problem are too much moisture in the tablet mass, formation of eutectics, insufficient lubrication, damaged punches or engravings (especially when very small or with narrow bends or loops), or too low pressure.

9.6.4   Capping

Shedding or scaling of one or more layers from the tablet surface during ejection from the die or during storage, as well as cracking of the surface of the tablet, is called *capping*. It always occurs when the elastic stress during the compression process is insufficiently released due to brittle fracture or plastic flow. Capping of tablets is triggered by the following conditions:
  – Too low or too high moisture content of the tablet material
  – Insufficient binder effect
  – Unsuitable crystal forms
  – Strongly aerophilic substances
  – Too high porosity
  – Too high powder fraction
  – Too strong interparticulate binding between granules
  – Unsuitable granule shape

Machine-dependent parameters that may result in capping include:
  – Too high pressure
  – Poorly adjusted or worn equipment
  – Too high compression speed
  – Air inclusions

9.6.5   Insufficient Mechanical Strength

Insufficient mechanical strength includes poor abrasion resistance, poor bending strength and insufficient pressure resistance. Causes of insufficient mechanical strength include:
  – Unsuitable granule shape
  – Unsuitable granule size
  – Too high porosity
  – Insufficient binder effect
  – Too low or too high moisture content
  – Insufficient or unsuitable lubrication

Among machine-dependent parameters, insufficient pressure and unfavorable choice of tablet shape are important.

9.6.6   Unsatisfactory Disintegration

Tablet disintegration is unsatisfactory when it does not fulfill the requirements of tablet disintegration prescribed in the Ph. Eur. for the given tablet type. Factors that might result in poor disintegration include:
  – Insufficient disintegrant effect
  – Excessive binder effect
  – Too much lubricant
  – Unsuitable particle size and shape
  – Insufficient wettability
  – Too low porosity
  – Too high pressure (machine-dependent)

9.6.7   Dose Variability

Dosage variabilities exceeding the limits set by the Ph. Eur. may have the following causes:
- Unsuitable granule size and shape
- Too high powder proportion
- Unfavorable Hausner ratio (for definition of Hausner factor see chapter 8)
- Insufficient glidant
- Too high moisture content

Machine-dependent factors include the following:
- Too high compression speed
- Loose lower punch
- Too strong vibration or agitation of the material in the hopper shoe

Finally, attention should be paid to errors or flaws like double filling of the matrix or unsuitable engravings.

9.6.8   Failing Maintenance

Many machine-derived complications during compaction can be avoided by regular thorough maintenance of the tableting machine and tools. Lubrication should be carried out exactly according to the manufacturer's instructions. Thorough cleaning of all parts of the machine and punches after each compaction cycle is mandatory. The punches must be demounted from the machine and all adhered materials must be carefully removed. Metal parts must not be used for cleaning of the punches, as they can easily cause scratching of the highly sensitive pressing surfaces. Once damage has been inflicted, this will not only be transferred to the surface of each individual tablet, but may also cause tableting complications such as sticking of the tablet material to the punch. For the cleaning of punches, hot water with soap is recommended. After thorough drying, all parts need to be treated with acid-free, odorless grease (petrolatum or liquid paraffin are well suited for that purpose). Storage of the punches is best done in waxed paper or by hanging them up to prevent mechanical damage. The risk of rusting of punches and machine parts is often underestimated. Not only can moisture in the air lead to rapid rust formation, but also, and even much more likely, processed active pharmaceutical ingredients can cause rust. Rust deposits on parts that were insufficiently greased can occur within a few hours. Punches need to be polished frequently and, in the case of rotary presses, must be checked for equal length.

9.7   Special Tablet Types and Chewing Gums Containing Active Ingredients

9.7.1   Chewable Tablets

Chewable tablets do not contain disintegrants and therefore disintegrate slowly. They are intended to be chewed before swallowing. For patients experiencing difficulties swallowing, chewable tablets may be advantageous. They have a pleasant taste and contain, in addition to a relatively high proportion of binder, sugars, sugar substitutes, and aromatic substances.

9.7.2   Sublingual and Buccal Tablets

Sublingual and buccal tablets are placed in the oral cavity, under the tongue or on the gum in the cheek pocket, whereby they slowly release their active pharmaceutical ingredient. The latter is mainly absorbed via the oral mucosa, thus circumventing the gastrointestinal tract and first pass metabolism. For this reason, these tablet types are particularly suited for drugs that are inactivated in the gastrointestinal tract.

As a rule, the active pharmaceutical ingredient is released slowly so that the drug is absorbed by the mucosal tissue at a rate proportional to its release rate. However, sublingual tablets may also be employed to achieve a rapid onset of drug effect. Sublingual nitroglycerine tablets, which are administered in acute angina pectoris, are an example. Buccal tablets may contain excipients that facilitate the adhesion of the tablet to the mucosa (mucoadhesion). Sublingual and buccal tablets are generally small and without sharp edges.

9.7.3 Rapidly Disintegrating Tablets

Tablets that rapidly disintegrate or even completely dissolve in the oral cavity are becoming increasingly popular. Manufacturing procedures as well as the terminology used are not always consistent. The term *melting tablet*, often used for rapidly dissolving or disintegrating orally administered tablets, is misleading, since neither during their production nor after administration a melting process is involved. Melting tablets are produced by compaction using substances with high plastic deformability (sorbitol, maltose, trehalose and others) and highly water-soluble compounds (mannitol, glucose). During the production, a relatively low compression pressure is applied. To ensure rapid disintegration, effective disintegrants may be employed at higher concentrations than in regular tablets, such as sodium carboxymethyl starches (Explotab®) and Crosspovidon (Kollidon CL®) in concentrations of 10% to 20% w/w.

In contrast to melting tablets, oral lyophilizates, as their name suggests, are not produced by compression but by freeze-drying (lyophilization) of an aqueous solution or suspension, containing the active pharmaceutical ingredient and suitable excipients. Hydrophilic polymers such as gelatins, dextrans, or alginates are predominantly used as matrix formers. Mannitol and glycerol are added as skeleton builders and humectants. As a result of the freeze-drying process a porous matrix is formed, which rapidly dissolves or disintegrates upon contact with water.

As the lyophilizates have very low mechanical strength and are highly water-sensitive, they are packaged in special peel-off blisters. Drug-containing oral films, produced by solvent evaporation or melt extrusion, are similarly packaged in this way. Like oral lyophilizates, such films display poor mechanical stability and are strongly water-sensitive.

9.7.4 Vaginal Tablets

Vaginal tablets mostly contain active pharmaceutical ingredients for a local effect on the vaginal mucosa and are generally aimed for slow dissolution.

Only readily water-soluble excipients such as glucose, lactose, and sorbitol are used as excipients in vaginal tablets. The pH should be ~5 in order not to do disturb the vaginal micro-flora. The use of talcum should be avoided because of the risk of granuloma formation.

9.7.5 Medicated Chewing Gums

Although not a tablet formulation, chewing gums will be briefly discussed in this section. Medicated chewing gums are solid single-dose preparations consisting of an insoluble chewing mass and are intended to be chewed and not swallowed. They may be applied for local treatment or for systemic drug delivery. Natural or synthetic elastomers, active pharmaceutical ingredient(s), and suitable excipients such as fillers, plasticizers, sweeteners, taste masking compounds, and stabilizers are usually added to the tasteless chewing mass. They can be produced by a softening or melting procedure as well as by compression of a directly compressible powder containing chewing gum excipient mixtures (e.g., Pharmagum®).

Medicated chewing gums may furthermore be provided with a coating. Proper release of the active pharmaceutical ingredient is tested in special apparatus, imitating the chewing movement (Ph. Eur. 2.9.25).

9.8   Physical Testing of Tablets

The following tests also apply to coated tablets (chapter 10) and modified release tablets (chapter 12).

9.8.1   General Considerations

Tablet tests serve two purposes: first, quality testing, that is, to ensure that the tablet properties comply with pharmacopeia requirements and second, development and optimization of tablet formulations, including validation of relevant parameters of the compression process. As with all drug formulations, one can distinguish between tests on the active pharmaceutical ingredient (based on chemical, physicochemical or microbiological methods) and physico-technological tests of the dosage form.

The Ph. Eur. provides the following tests for tablets (see appendix for tests required by USP and JP):

- Uniformity of dosage units (Ph. Eur. 2.9.40)
- Uniformity of content (Ph. Eur. 2.9.6)
- Uniformity of mass (Ph. Eur. 2.9.5)
- Friability (Ph. Eur. 2.9.7, only for uncoated tablets)
- Resistance to crushing (Ph. Eur. 2.9.8)
- Dissolution test for solid dosage forms (Ph. Eur. 2.9.3)
- Disintegration (Ph. Eur. 2.9.1)

Tablets that are meant to be divided into several parts usually have a break mark, and therefore the efficiency of the break mark needs to be tested during product development to ensure that the patient receives the correct dose upon dividing the tablet.

9.8.2   Uniformity of Mass and Content

Because of international harmonization of the pharmacopeias, different methods to test uniformity of mass and content can be found in the Ph. Eur. The harmonized method "Uniformity of Dosage Units" (Ph. Eur. 2.9.40), which includes testing of both mass and content, is likely to replace the two older test methods in the near future (Ph. Eur. 2.9.5 and 2.9.6).

Depending on the type of tablet and the drug content, either only content uniformity (assay of the drug content in individual tablets) or mass uniformity is examined. Determination of mass variation is experimentally easier and less expensive, but is only acceptable when variation in mass is a proper measure of variation in drug content (noncoated tablets or film-coated tablets with a drug content ≥ 25 mg or $\geq 25\%$).

9.8.3   Mechanical Strength

9.8.3.1   General Considerations

The term *mechanical strength* refers to tablet properties of a diverse physical nature. Specifically, this concerns resistance towards pressure, pulling, beating, bending, breaking, rolling, dragging, and dropping. Characterization of mechanical strength is mandatory in order to ensure that tablets can withstand further processing, including coating, transport, and handling.

(A)

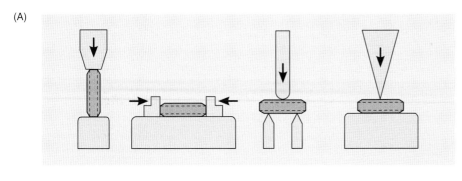

(B)

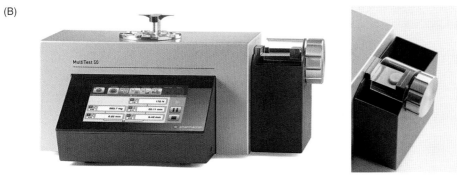

Fig. 9-7   Assessment of fracture resistance: (A) Principles of assessment: (B) Realization of one principle in a commercial device (Reproduced with permission from SOTAX Group © 2017).

Very different methods can be applied, some simple in nature, while others require the use of special equipment, yet all basically involving routine procedures. The Ph. Eur. describes methods to evaluate fracture strength (resistance to crushing, Ph. Eur. 2.9.8) and friability (Ph. Eur. 2.9.7).

9.8.3.2   Bending and Pressure Resistance

Bending resistance is defined as the resistance of a tablet against a force on one of its surfaces, without mechanical support on the opposite side. Pressure resistance is the resistance of a tablet against a diametrically acting force, causing the tablet to be crushed. A variety of devices is available to assess pressure resistance; they are commonly known as *hardness testers*. The term *hardness* used in this context is not entirely correct. Hardness is defined as the force of resistance of the surface of a solid against penetration by a pointed or conical test specimen. By definition, hardness tests are therefore tests of surface solidity. They are barely relevant for the evaluation of tablet quality.

Fig. 9-7 schematically presents various measuring principles for the assessment of pressure and bending resistance.

Ph. Eur. 2.9.5 Uniformity of Mass of Single-Dose Preparations _____

As a result of pharmacopeial harmonization, the Ph. Eur. includes two different approaches to test uniformity of dosage units. Although the harmonized text 2.9.40 (Uniformity of dosage units) was introduced for future replacement of the Ph. Eur. methods 2.9.5 (Uniformity of mass of single-dose preparations) and 2.9.6 (Uniformity of content of single-dose preparations), the Quality Working Party of the European Medicines Agency states that, from a pharmaceutical quality point of view, both approaches are considered equivalent.

For testing uniformity of mass according to Ph. Eur. 2.9.5, 20 randomly sampled dosage units are weighed and their average mass is calculated. Maximally 2 of the 20 units are allowed to have a mass deviating from the average by a higher percentage than indicated in the following table and none is allowed to deviate by more than twice that percentage.

Pharmaceutical Form	Average Mass (mg)	Percentage Deviation
Tablets (uncoated and film-coated)	≤80	10
	>80, <250	7.5
	≥250	5
Capsules, granules (uncoated, single-dose) and powders (single-dose)	<300	10
	≥300	7.5
Powders for parenteral administration* (single-dose)	>40	10
Suppositories and pessaries	all masses	5
Powders for eye drops and powders for eye lotions	<300	10
	≥300	7.5

*When the average mass is less than 40 mg, the preparation is not submitted to the test for uniformity of mass but rather to the test for uniformity of content of single-dose preparations (Ph. Eur. 2.9.6).

Ph. Eur. 2.9.40 Uniformity of Dosage Units

USP ⟨905⟩ Uniformity of Dosage Units
JP 6.02 Uniformity of Dosage Units

The Ph. Eur. monographs 2.9.5 (Uniformity of mass of single-dose preparations) and 2.9.6 (Uniformity of content of single-dose preparations) describe with nonparametric or partially parametric sample tests, in which no assumptions are made concerning the statistic distribution of the quality parameter to be tested. Monograph 2.9.40, on the other hand, describes a parametric test, which is based on a concrete distribution type (in this case the normal distribution). The applied mathematical method is a parametric tolerance interval test, which evaluates from the standard deviation of a random sample (n = 10 or n = 30) whether at least 91% of the dosage units of the whole batch do not deviate more than ±15% from the target value with a confidence level of 0.84.

Based on the mean and the standard deviation of a sample of 10 or 30 units, as well as on the target value, an absolute (positive) acceptance value is calculated that should not exceed a predetermined upper limit. The rationale of this procedure is the consideration that all individual units of a batch with a mean value deviating from the target value may nonetheless lie within the tolerance limits if the deviation of the mean is compensated by a sufficiently small standard deviation.

Thus, while the tests described in Ph. Eur. 2.9.5 and Ph. Eur. 2.9.6 take into account only the deviation of the units from the sample mean value, the test on "Uniformity of Dosage Units" (Ph. Eur. 2.9.40, USP 905, JP 6.02) considers, in addition, the deviation of the sample mean from the target value.

Depending on the formulation, either the content or the mass of the dosage unit is tested. For the dosage forms listed below a homogeneous distribution of drug substance and excipients is presumed and therefore only a mass uniformity test is carried out:

- Solutions in unit-dose containers and soft capsules.
- Solids with only one component in single-dose containers
- Solids with one or more components in single-dose containers, produced by freeze drying of a real solution
- Hard capsules, uncoated tablets and film-coated tablets containing minimally 25 mg active agent which in addition represents minimally 25% of the tablet mass or the capsule content, respectively.

For all other dosage forms a content uniformity test is required. However, based on process validation data exceptions may be permitted. Exempted from the test are suspensions, emulsions or gels in single-dose containers intended for cutaneous administration as well as multivitamin and trace-element preparations.

Ph. Eur. 2.9.47 Demonstration of Uniformity of Dosage Units Using Large Sample Sizes

Whereas in earlier times content assays were always destructive and could only be performed on small sample sizes, nondestructive procedures like NIR spectroscopy are increasingly applied and allow characterization of a batch by a large number of individual values. Modern concepts of continuous monitoring and control of manufacturing procedures, such as the Process Analytical Technology (PAT) concept are based on a high measurement frequency (on line, in line, or at line). The acceptance criteria for content uniformity as defined in Ph. Eur. 2.9.40 do not allow individual values outside the acceptance limit L2 (25% deviation from the mean value). However, even in normally distributed batches of high quality a small number of units may be expected to strongly deviate from the mean. With increasing sample sizes, the probability increases that such outliers are detected. According to 2.9.40, this would result in the rejection of the entire batch. Chapter 2.9.47 was included in the Ph. Eur. to cope with these special requirements of large sample sizes. The test can be performed parametrically or nonparametrically.

Ph. Eur. 2.9.8 Resistance to Crushing of Tablets

USP ⟨1217⟩ Tablet Breaking Force

This test determines the force required to break a tablet by application of a compressive load. In the measuring device the tablet is placed between two parallel polished platens, one of which is movable and exerts a continuously increasing force on the tablet. As soon as the tablet breaks, the force is relieved and the instrument indicates the highest force value measured before the fracture. The rate at which the compressive load is applied may significantly affect the results, because time-dependent processes may be involved in tablet failure. Currently available instruments provide a constant loading rate of ≤20 N/s or a constant platen movement of ≤3.5 mm/s. To ensure comparability of results, testing must be performed under identical conditions of loading rate or platen movement rate and the applied test settings must be specified along with the determined breaking force. As in many cases the tablets only break rather than being completely crushed, the USP prefers the term "breaking force" over "resistance to crushing," which is the designation in the Ph. Eur. When positioning the tablet in the device attention should be paid to the orientation of shape, score and embossment with respect to the direction of the force. In general, tablets are tested either across the diameter or parallel to the longest axis. In order to achieve sufficient statistical precision the USP requires testing of minimally 6 tablet samples. By contrast, the Ph. Eur. test is performed on 10 tablets and the results are expressed as the mean, minimum, and maximum force values.

A compact is always weakest in tension and strongest in compression. For this reason, the tensile strength is a more fundamental measure of the mechanical strength, as it takes into account the geometry of the tablet. USP chapter ⟨1217⟩ describes several equations to calculate the tensile strength of cylindrical flat-faced and convex-faced tablets from the breaking force as well as from the bending force in a three-point flexure test.

Ph. Eur. 2.9.6 Uniformity of Content of Single-Dose Preparations

Drug content is determined in 10 randomly sampled units. Multivitamin and trace element preparations are exempted from testing. In case of tablets, powders for injection, ophthalmic inserts and suspensions for injection the following decision tree applies:

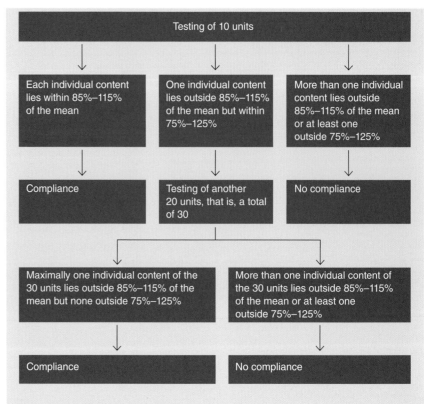

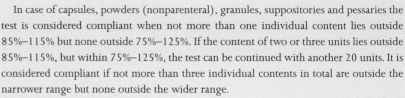

In case of capsules, powders (nonparenteral), granules, suppositories and pessaries the test is considered compliant when not more than one individual content lies outside 85%–115% but none outside 75%–125%. If the content of two or three units lies outside 85%–115%, but within 75%–125%, the test can be continued with another 20 units. It is considered compliant if not more than three individual contents in total are outside the narrower range but none outside the wider range.

For transdermal patches the mean content of 10 units should lie within 90%–110% of the label claim and no individual content outside the 75%–125% range.

9.8.3.3   Friability

Abrasion or friability is the total loss of tablet mass by powder formation during mechanical strain. It is tested in a rotating drum (Fig. 9-8), in which a weighed amount of tablets (after removal of all powder) is tumbled under defined conditions (time, rotation speed, presence of blades in the drum, etc.). After this treatment, the total mass of dust-free tablets is determined again and the percentage of tablet mass lost is calculated. Friability is only tested for uncoated tablets.

Ph. Eur. 2.9.7 Friability of Uncoated Tablets _____

USP ⟨1216⟩ Tablet Friability

JP G6 Tablet Friability Test

The friability (abrasion resistance) of tablets is measured as attrition caused by rolling and dropping. 10 tablets of an individual mass of >650 mg, or a number of as closely as possible approaching a total mass of 6.5 g in case of an individual mass of ≤650 mg are placed in a rotating drum of about 29 cm diameter. At each rotation, they are lifted by the blades in the drum until they drop at the highest point. After 100 rotations at 25 rpm, the tablets are freed from dust and weighed again. Friability is expressed as percent loss of mass. A maximum mean weight loss from the three samples of not more than 1.0% is considered acceptable for most products. However, if obviously cracked, cleaved, or broken, tablets are present in the tablet sample after tumbling, the sample fails the test.

Fig. 9-8   Device to determine friability according to Ph. Eur. (A) and (B) friability device. Reproduced with permission from SOTAX Group © 2017.

9.8.4   Disintegration

Rapid and complete disintegration of the dosage form is a prerequisite for drug dissolution and absorption and thus an important parameter for bioavailability of a drug from a tablet formulation. The disintegration test contributes to standardization of tablet formulations and in this way ensures uniformity of tablet preparations. The tablet is considered as disintegrated when it is dissolved or has disaggregated into numerous particles in a standard medium at defined conditions. The time needed to achieve complete disintegration of the tablet is measured.

Disintegration generally occurs in two, not necessarily distinctly distinguishable steps, from disintegration of the tablet into granules followed by disintegration of the granules into powder particles. Water or an artificial simulated gastric fluid of defined temperature (usually 37°C) serves as a disintegration medium. Disintegration times vary between different tablet types (Table 9-1).

For special tablets, such as gastro-resistant tablets, artificial gastric fluids are applied, which are comparable to physiological conditions in terms of pH and to some extent also in terms of surface tension and viscosity (mucous substances). The test conditions should generally mimic the physiological environment as closely as possible.

Ph. Eur. conforming devices for disintegration testing are fully automatically working instruments. They mainly consist of a basket-rack assembly provided with six, or for larger tablets three, glass tubes each of which can contain one test unit (Fig. 9-9). The tubes are open at the top while a screen sieve (2 mm mesh width) closes off the bottom end.

The basket is immersed in a beaker containing the test fluid. A temperature of 37°C is maintained by a water bath. Upon starting the apparatus, the test basket performs defined up-and-down movements. By the end of disintegration time, all parts of the tablet should have fallen through the sieve mesh. When required, disks are providing enough pressure to prevent floating of the tablets can be used.

(A)

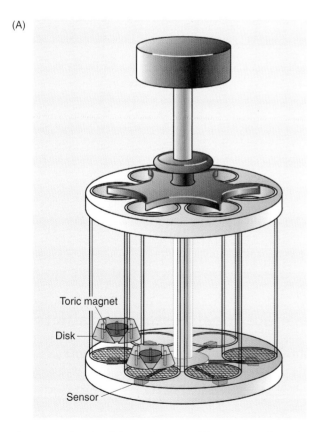

(B)

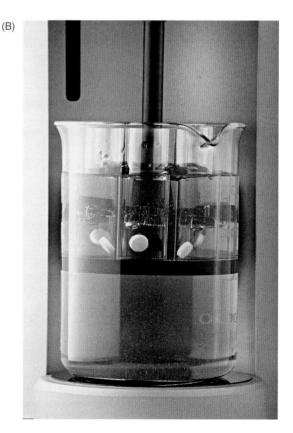

Fig. 9-9 Basket for disintegration test with evaluation electronics: (A) disk with toric magnets and Hall sensors; (B) device in operation. Reproduced with permission from SOTAX Group © 2017.

Automatic determination of disintegration time is also possible. Several methods are used to determine the endpoint. One method works through electrical contacts where rigid tiny metal rings are used to make the contact of the disks with the sieve segments. The disks approach the sieve bottom of the basket during the disintegration process. When the disk (with the mounted metal ring) touches the bottom, a contact closes, a current is induced that is recorded by the apparatus as (complete) disintegration. For sugarcoated and film-coated tablets that do not completely dissolve/disintegrate, a calibration procedure is performed where the endpoint of disintegration corresponds to the residual thickness of the tablet. Another method yields the Ph. Eur.-compliant disintegration time with the help of a toric magnet and a Hall sensor (see Fig. 9-9).

Disintegration tests cannot, however, in all cases provide sufficient information about the actual biopharmaceutical performance of the tablet formulation. Additional in-vitro procedures such as the determination of drug release (dissolution) are required for tablets with modified drug release, where the actual release of the active pharmaceutical ingredient into buffer or simulated gastric fluids is determined.

Ph. Eur. 2.9.1 Disintegration of Tablets and Capsules _____

USP ⟨701⟩ Disintegration

JP 6.09 Disintegration Test

The apparatus used to test the disintegration time of tablets and capsules consists of a basket-rack assembly, which is immersed into a 1,000-mL beaker containing a specified medium, a thermostatic arrangement for heating the fluid to the test temperature of $37 \pm 2°C$, and a device for raising and lowering the basket in the immersion fluid at a constant frequency rate between 29 and 32 cycles per minute through a distance of 55 ± 2 mm. The basket-rack assembly is an arrangement of six open-ended transparent tubes, having an inside diameter of 20.7 to 23 mm, held by two plates in a vertical position. The lower openings of the tubes are covered with a woven stainless steel wire cloth with apertures of 2.0 ± 0.2 mm. Ph. Eur. describes additionally a second basket-rack assembly, supporting only three but wider tubes (internal diameter 33 ± 0.5 mm) which is designed for testing larger dosage forms (Test B—Large Tablets and large capsules). If so specified (in monographs) or allowed (by registration authorities), the units to be tested are covered by transparent disks of defined dimensions, shape and density, which assist disintegration by exerting an additional mechanical stress. While Ph. Eur. specifies the applicable test conditions in the chapter "dosage forms," USP and JP include various instructions for immediate-release, enteric coated and some other preparations directly in the method chapters USP<701> and JP 6.09. Six units are tested (in case of Ph. Eur. Test B concurrently with two devices or consecutively three at a time). The test is considered successful when all units completely disintegrate. If ≤2 units do not fulfill the requirement, the test can be repeated with 12 additional units, all of which have to disintegrate within the required time (however, no repetition is allowed in case of Ph. Eur. Test B). JP 6.09 additionally includes an instruction for testing granules and dry syrups, using six "auxiliary tubes" of specified dimensions, which are covered at both ends with a wire gauze having 0.42-mm openings.

9.9   Biopharmaceutical Testing of Tablets

9.9.1   Release and Dissolution of Active Ingredients

9.9.1.1   General Considerations

Since the dissolution rate of the active pharmaceutical ingredient often represents the rate-limiting factor of the absorption process, a release (dissolution) test offers important information concerning the biopharmaceutical quality of drug formulations. Although the methods developed for oral drug formulations generally appear simple, it often takes several decades before they became standardized and validated test methods of the pharmacopeias.

Concerning the dissolution rate of pure compounds, a distinction is made between the intrinsic dissolution rate (Ph. Eur. 2.2.29) and the apparent dissolution rate (Ph. Eur. 2.9.43). In determination of the intrinsic dissolution rate, effects of parameters such as particle size are eliminated by the experimental setup.

Both above-mentioned methods must be distinguished from the test method to determine release of the active pharmaceutical ingredient from a dosage form. The number of proposed methods to study drug release from dosage forms is considerable. The most important models and those derived from them are introduced below, and the parameters influencing the dissolution kinetics will be explained.

In accordance with the experimental setup, two general groups of tests concerning dissolution, release, and absorption are distinguished, depending on the conditions:

1. Non-sink conditions are applicable when the concentration of the drug in the medium increases, corresponding to its dissolution or release, up to a maximal value. As a general rule, a predetermined percentage of drug(s) must be dissolved within a predetermined period of time (e.g., 60% in 30 minutes). This condition applies when during the dissolution process the active pharmaceutical ingredient, or the formulation, is in direct contact with the entire amount of solvent while the dissolution medium is neither exchanged nor replaced (closed system).

2. Sink conditions, on the other hand, apply when the concentration of the drug in the dissolution medium is kept at a low level, despite its continuous dissolution. This situation bears a similarity to the absorption process, where the drug is continuously eliminated from the gastrointestinal tract by absorption into the enterocytes and finally into blood circulation.

Sink conditions are obtained when the concentration of the dissolved drug does not exceed 10% of the saturation concentration. In model experiments, this condition is attainable by withdrawing sample volumes from the test solution for analysis and replacing them by equal volumes of fresh test solution, or by flushing the drug dosage form continuously with fresh dissolution medium (flow cell). Models operating according to the second principle (sink conditions) are called open systems.

9.9.1.2   Closed Systems

In all variations of this assay method, the tablet or capsule is positioned in a temperature-controlled vessel containing the dissolution medium, which is kept in motion by means of stirring, shaking, rotation or vibration. The amount of dissolution medium should be sufficiently large to ensure that drug concentration remains below the saturation concentration, even after complete drug dissolution. For testing of poorly soluble substances, the volume of the dissolution medium may need to be rather large.

Beaker Method

This particularly simple method (Fig. 9-10) is applied for the assessment of drug release and dissolution from tablets. The tablet is carefully placed in the middle of a beaker containing a certain volume of dissolution medium (usually 250 mL buffer) and mixed with a stirrer. Aliquots of the release medium are collected at predetermined time points and the drug content in the sample fractions is determined. At each sampling, the withdrawn sample volume is replaced with dissolution medium. The results depend on the stirring rate, the position of the tablet, and the immersion depth of the stirrer. A rotation speed of 50 rpm is considered to mimic the conditions in the gastrointestinal tract and a rotation speed of 40–60 rpm is therefore recommended for the beaker method.

Rotating Basket Method

The formulation is placed in a wire basket with defined dimensions and mesh size, rotating in the dissolution medium at a defined speed (Fig. 9-11). The method is described in several pharmacopeias (USP, Ph. Eur.).

This method has some serious challenges. The wire mesh can cause abrasion of the tablets, gelling excipients may clog the mesh compromising equilibration, and the dosage form may stick at the position of lowest agitation.

> **Intrinsic dissolution rate:** the dissolution of the (pure) active ingredient.
>
> **Apparent dissolution:** the actual dissolution of the active ingredient embedded in the formulation.

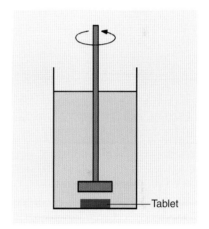

Fig. 9-10 Beaker method.

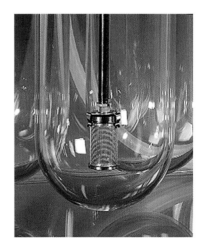

Fig. 9-11 Rotating basket method (without tablet and dissolution medium). Reproduced with permission from SOTAX Group © 2017.

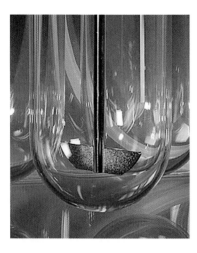

Fig. 9-12 The paddle method (without tablet and dissolution medium).
Reproduced with permission from SOTAX Group © 2017.

Paddle Method

This is the commonly preferred test method and is included in all modern pharmacopeias (e.g., Ph. Eur. 2.9.3). A number of variants of the method are known, which all share the use of a round-bottom flask with a dual blade stirrer of special shape (Fig. 9-12) and temperature-control by placing the round-bottom flask in a water bath.

Due to the round-bottom shape of the flask, the dosage form is positioned centrally under the stirring blade during the procedure. Solvent movement thus proceeds uniformly, which ensures reproducible test results.

As a rule, a flask of 1 L volume is used, while the volume of the dissolution medium is max. 900 mL. Occasionally, flasks with either smaller or larger volumes are used.

For serial testing, equipment with multiple test vessels and stirring blades can be utilized simultaneously. The rotation speed varies from 25 to 200 rpm, with an accuracy of ± 1 rpm. Modern dissolution equipment provides the option of automatic sampling in accordance with the requirements of the pharmacopeias (e.g., Erweka dissolution tester DT). Tablet reservoirs drop the tablets simultaneously in the dissolution medium, thus saving time and improving accuracy by eliminating the need to calculate delay time between individual test vessels. With a 20-chamber reservoir, a corresponding number of tablets can be tested simultaneously and be fully automated with six test specimens.

9.9.1.3   Open Systems

In open systems, aliquots of a fixed volume of solvent are continuously withdrawn and replaced by the release medium. This procedure is applied in a flow cell (sink conditions, Ph. Eur. 2.9.43).

Flow-Through Method

The test formulation is placed between two glass or ceramic frits and is continuously flushed from the bottom with the dissolution medium (water, artificial gastric, or intestinal juice) (Fig. 9-13). The amount of dissolved substance is determined in the efflux fluid, usually by a spectrophotometric assay in a flow cuvette. The method is characterized by its good reproducibility, precision, and possibility to mimic in vivo conditions (sink conditions, see section 9.9.1.1). To simulate the conditions in the gastrointestinal tract, the flow rate is adjusted to about 40 to 80 mL/min.

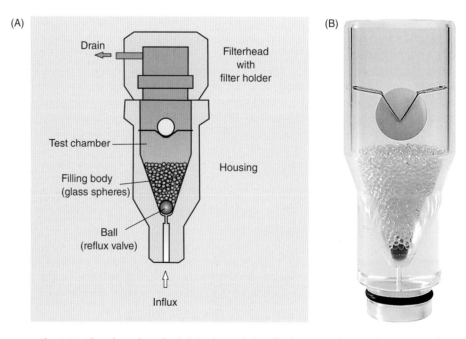

Fig. 9-13 Flow through method: (A) scheme; (B) realization. Reproduced with permission from SOTAX Group © 2017.

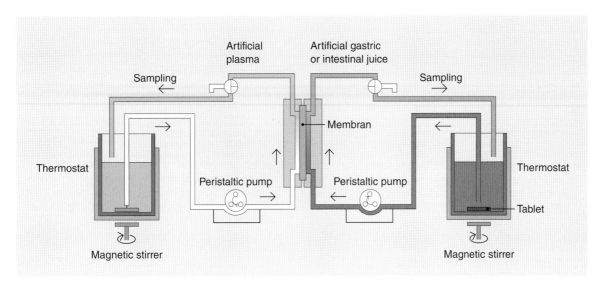

Fig. 9-14 Absorption model (according to Stricker (1973)).

9.9.2 Absorption Models

While dissolution tests are primarily used for the characterization of dissolution and release behavior, absorption models simulate the distribution of drug between the gastrointestinal fluid and the lipid-containing cell membranes. Not only dissolution rate, but also absorption rate is highly dependent on partitioning of the drug into the lipid membrane. This underscores the importance of this step for the absorption process. Literature describes many different experimental setups, but only the most representative and widely used test methods will be discussed here. In absorption models, both artificial and natural membranes are used to mimic in vivo conditions in humans. Although animal membranes correspond more closely to in vivo conditions (as a matter of fact, the porcine diaphragm, even after appropriate storage, produces quite reproducible results), artificial membranes are preferred because of their reproducibility and ease of handling. Occasionally, biological membranes are simulated by coating artificial membranes with lipids (e.g., PAMPA assay). The membrane is mounted in a diffusion cell in such a way that the membrane separates two chambers (dual chamber model). One chamber contains the drug solution (donor fluid, when appropriate also the drug formulation) and the other one the dissolution medium, where the drug accumulates after permeating the membrane (acceptor fluid). The media in both chambers are kept at constant temperature and are permanently stirred in order to keep them constant and prevent build-up of a diffusion layer on the membrane. The absorption model according to Stricker allows studies to be performed under conditions closely resembling the conditions in the gastrointestinal tract. It consists basically of a diffusion chamber (Fig. 9-14) with two compartments separated by a special lipid membrane. One compartment contains artificial gastric fluid or artificial intestinal fluid containing the dissolved drug (donor), and the other is filled with artificial plasma (acceptor). The diffusion rate of the drug into the plasma, which should be directly proportional to the in vivo absorption rate constant, can be calculated.

9.9.3 Distribution Models

In some models, the membrane is simulated by an organic solvent that is immiscible with water (distribution models). Only lipophilic or nonionic drugs will partition with a sufficiently high rate from the donor phase into the lipid phase, and from this into the (aqueous) acceptor phase. As an example, the Schulman cell is schematically presented in Fig. 9-15. The Schulman cell represents the simplest experimental set up of a distribution model.

The aqueous phases A (donor phase) and C (acceptor phase) are separated by an impermeable wall. Both phases are overlaid with the lipid phase B. All three phases are stirred at

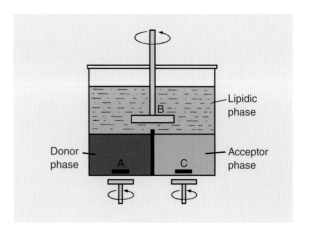

Fig. 9-15 Schulman cell.

a constant speed (phases A and C with a magnetic bar and phase B with a blade stirrer) and held at a defined temperature. Partitioning of the drug from A to B and from B to C can be monitored by assaying the drug concentrations in each phase through time-dependent sampling.

Many such models are available, some containing biological tissue, such as the "everted-sac" model. A piece of rat intestine, which is turned inside out (everted), that is, with the epithelium on the outside, is tied off at one end and filled with buffer before tying off the other end. The "sausage" thus formed is placed in a drug solution in a beaker and stirred for a few hours. The buffer in the everted sac is then collected and assayed for drug content, corresponding to the fraction of drug absorbed.

Ph. Eur. 2.9.3 Dissolution Test for Solid Dosage Forms _____

Ph. Eur. 5.17.1 Recommendations for Drug Release Tests
USP ⟨711⟩ Dissolution
USP ⟨724⟩ Drug Release
USP ⟨1092⟩ The Dissolution Procedure: Development and Validation
USP ⟨1094⟩ Capsules—Dissolution Testing and Related Quality Attributes
USP ⟨2040⟩ Disintegration and Dissolution of Dietary Supplements
JP 6.10 Dissolution Test
The Ph. Eur. and USP describe four, JP only three devices for testing dissolution or drug release from solid oral dosage forms, of which apparatus 1 and apparatus 2 are used most frequently. In addition, the USP includes another apparatus (apparatus 7) dedicated for testing of drug release from extended-release tablets.

Apparatus 1, Basket apparatus: The assembly consists of a 1-liter (USP: also 2- and 4-liter) cylindrical glass vessel with a hemispherical bottom, which is temperature-controlled (37 ± 0.5°C) by a water bath or a heating device. The vessel may be covered to retard evaporation of the test fluid. A shaft with a cylindrical wire mesh basket (inner dimensions: h = 27.0 mm. ø = 20.2 mm) mounted at the end is immersed in the fluid. The motor-driven shaft is rotated at a controllable velocity (50–100, maximally 150, rpm) with ±4% accuracy. The dosage unit is placed in the dry basket and care is taken to exclude air bubbles at the surface when the basket is immersed.

Apparatus 2, Paddle apparatus: In this assembly, a paddle formed from a blade and a shaft is used as the stirring element. The formulation to be tested is placed in the vessel before stirring is started. By virtue of the shape of the vessel's bottom, the formulation is always centered underneath the stirrer, which ends at 25 mm above the bottom. Formulations that tend to float are kept in position by a sinker, such as a glass or wire spiral that loosely clasps the dosage form.

Apparatus 3, Reciprocating cylinder (Not included in JP)**:** The apparatus consists of a set of cylindrical, flat-bottomed glass vessels (~300 mL), which are partially immersed in a water bath (37 ± 0.5°C) and filled with dissolution medium. The dosage forms to be tested are placed in glass cylinders, which are covered with screens at their tops and bottoms. The dosage forms are moved up and down in the test fluid by a motor and drive assembly at a specified dip rate through a distance of 10 cm. Apparatus 3 has been found especially useful for chewable tablets, soft gelatin capsules, delayed-release dosage forms, and products of a nondisintegrating type, such as coated beads.

Apparatus 4, Flow-through-cell: The assembly consists of a reservoir, a pump, a water bath for the dissolution medium and a set of flow-through cells, for which two dimensionally different construction types are described. The vertically mounted tubular cells, made of transparent material, are flushed from bottom to top with temperature-controlled (37 ± 0.5°C) dissolution medium. The cells narrow conically towards the lower ends; the upper part contains a filter system to retain undissolved particles. The diameter of the middle part is approximately 23 mm in one type and about 12 mm in the other. The bottom cone is usually filled with small glass beads and the test formulation is placed on top of the beads. Alternatively, the specimen can be placed on a wire carrier mounted inside the cylindrical middle part of the cell. Either fresh dissolution medium is continuously flushed through the cells or the release medium is circulated in a closed loop circuit (4–16 mL/min). Apparatus 4 may offer advantages for dosage forms that contain active ingredients with limited solubility but also for multiple dosage form types such as soft gelatin capsules, beaded products, suppositories, or depot dosage forms, as well as suspension-type extended-release dosage forms.

USP Apparatus 7, Reciprocating holder (Not included in Ph. Eur. and JP): Apparatus 7, described in USP ⟨724⟩ ("Drug release") for testing of osmotic pump tablets, consists of a set of preferably transparent solution containers, a set of sample holders, and a motor and drive assembly to move the system up and down and to automatically index the system horizontally to a different row of vessels, if desired. The solution cylinders are partially immersed in a water bath to maintain a temperature of 37° ± 0.5°C inside the containers. Oral extended-release tablet holders are designed either as acrylic rods with the tablets glued to their tips or as stainless steel tubes with stainless steel springs at their tips to accommodate the tablets. The sample holders are moved up and down at a frequency of about 30 cycles per minute with an amplitude of about 2 cm. At each sampling time point (at least three), the solution containers are removed, and before analysis, a sufficient volume of solvent is added to correct for evaporation losses.

For each apparatus 1 to 4, the pharmacopeias describe test procedures for immediate-release, prolonged-release (termed "extended-release" in the USP), and delayed-release dosage forms. In case of apparatus 1 to 3, samples are taken from the test medium at predetermined time intervals. Each time the withdrawn volumes are replaced with fresh medium or the loss of volume is corrected for by calculation.

Delayed-release formulations require a change in pH after 2 hours (JP: 2 hours for tablets and capsules, 1 hour for granules). In case of the basket or paddle apparatus, this can be achieved by addition of sodium phosphate and subsequent pH adjustment (method A, not accepted by JP) or by complete exchange of the dissolution medium (method B).

Interpretation of the test results:

For immediate-release dosage forms, the duration of the dissolution procedure is typically 30–60 minutes; in most cases, a single time point specification is adequate for pharmacopeial purposes.

The requirements are met if the amount of drug released exceeds the value specified in the individual monograph by at least 5% (as a rule, ≥80% released in 45 min). For method development, however, a sufficient number of time points should be selected to adequately characterize the ascending and plateau phases of the dissolution curve (however, no profile comparison is considered necessary for dosage forms of BCS Class 1 drugs if they release ≥85% of the drug substance within 15 minutes).

For prolonged-release dosage forms, the release profile is specified by upper and lower acceptance limits at multiple test time points and the requirements are met if no individual value lies outside each of specified ranges and no individual value is less than the specified amount at the final test time. Typically, at least three time points are required to define the curve profile: the first one usually when 20% to 30% of the drug has been released, which should reveal the occurrence of an unintended rapid release of a major fraction of the drug (dose dumping). The second point should be set around the time when 50% of the drug has been released and at the third point, the drug release should be above 80%.

Delayed-release dosage forms usually require specifications for at least two time points. In the case of enteric-coated dosage forms, the functionality of the coating is proven by challenge in an acid medium, followed by a demonstration of dissolution in a higher-pH medium. No single unit should release more than 10% of the drug during the acidic test phase and must have released at least 80% at a predetermined time in the buffered phase.

The test is first performed with 6 units and is passed if all individual values meet the requirements. If the results do not conform, the test is repeated with another 6 units and under certain circumstances once more with 12 units. In these extended test stages, all 12 or 24 units must comply with the specifications.

In addition to the general information on methods, equipment and acceptance criteria given in Ph. Eur. 2.9.3 and USP ⟨711⟩, a variety of detailed instructions and recommendations on test design, equipment selection, and qualification and validation of the procedure is provided in Ph. Eur. 5.17.1 (Recommendations for drug release tests) and USP chapter ⟨1092⟩ (The dissolution procedure: development and validation). Amongst others, the following aspects require special attention:

Filters: Undissolved drug particles have to be removed immediately from the withdrawn solution, as otherwise they will continue to dissolve and will bias the results. This is achieved by filtration, commonly using pore sizes from 0.20 to 70 μm. The filter material must be compatible with the drug and potential drug adsorption to the filter material must be evaluated during development of the test.

Dissolution medium: Typical media for dissolution may include diluted hydrochloric acid, buffers (phosphate or acetate) in the physiological pH range of 1.2 to 7.5, simulated gastric or intestinal fluid (with or without enzymes), and water. Proteolytic enzymes such as pepsin (at low pH) or pancreatin (at pH 6.8) may be favorable for testing gelatin capsules if the capsule shell does not dissolve in ordinary aqueous media because of cross-linking. Routinely, the dissolution medium is buffered. Water is only recommended when it is proven that pH variations do not have an influence on the dissolution characteristics. The stability of the drug substance in the dissolution medium at 37°C should be investigated during method development. In order to ensure that the material already in solution does not exert a significant modifying effect on the rate of dissolution, the goal is to maintain sink conditions during the whole dissolution procedure, defined as maintaining a volume of medium that is at least 3 to 10 times the saturation volume. For the testing of poorly water-soluble substances, addition of a surfactant (e.g., sodium dodecyl sulfate (SDS) or polysorbate) may be necessary to enhance solubility of the drug. Air bubbles, which may arise from dissolved atmospheric gases, may affect the dissolution process by acting as a barrier between the solution and the surface, by causing particles to cling to the vessel walls or by increasing the buoyancy of the dosage form. To avoid this, the medium is usually deaerated prior to the test, which can be achieved for instance by heating, filtering, or vacuum methods. Usually, commercially available media preparation stations are used, which degas, preheat, and dispense the medium.

9.10   Concluding Remarks

Each single stage in the manufacturing of tablets may have a decisive influence on the disintegration and the release and absorption of the active ingredient. The major impact of excipients, the size and shape of the granules or powder particles and the compaction procedure (especially pressure) may all have a enhancing or inhibitory effect on drug release and thus on absorption and therefore must all be taken into consideration.

A prerequisite for favorable release and absorption behavior is the complete disintegration of the tablet, with the exception of drugs released via diffusion across a rate-limiting membrane or matrix (modified release formulations, chapter 10). The first step in the disintegration process is the breakdown of the tablet into granules, which further disintegrate into powder-like components. The disintegration process proceeds, therefore, in the opposite order of the aggregation process during tablet manufacture, where granules are first prepared from a powder and then the granules are subsequently compressed into a tablet.

Although to a small extent the active pharmaceutical ingredient can be released directly from the intact tablet, release rates from granules are considerably higher due to their larger surface area. Further disintegration into powder particles is, however, required to achieve fast and complete dissolution of the drug, given that the API is readily water-soluble. Even when slowly swelling polymers were used as wet-binders for granulation, or when lipophilic excipients such as magnesium and calcium stearate or talcum were added as lubricants, impeding diffusion and wetting, this should not result in a significant delay in drug release and absorption. In general, tablets and granules should disintegrate rapidly so that absorption of the drug (at least of readily water-soluble drugs) can occur without delay.

When a drug dissolves only slowly from the disintegration products of a tablet, either because of its low dissolution rate (poor water solubility) or because it is too tightly associated with formulation components, this will result in incomplete absorption in the gastrointestinal tract, and insufficient blood concentration levels (e.g., poor bioavailability) will be the result.

For some drug formulations, it is recommended to add a buffer substance so that a favorable pH value is attained, facilitating rapid dissolution of the drug. When micronized drugs are processed into tablets, improper formulation may result in loss of the advantage of the small particle size (dissolution rate increases distinctly with decreasing particle size) during the granulation and compression processes. An example is a micronized powder of griseofulvin, which yields considerably higher blood levels when applied as a suspension compared to a tablet formulation.

Insufficient drug absorption from a tablet or insufficient drug solubility can also be due to complex formation between drug and excipients. The formation of adsorptive bonds between the active pharmaceutical ingredient and excipients, particularly occurring with, for example, talcum, colloidal kaolin, calcium carbonate, magnesium tri-silicate, magnesium hydroxide, magnesium oxide, zinc stearate, stearic acid, and aluminum hydroxide, is a well-recognized phenomenon. Thus far, it has not been possible, however, to define potential specific physical processes involved in each individual case. For example, tetracycline forms complexes with Al^{3+} ions, but also with Ca^{2+}, which in the case of administration of this drug together with milk (high Ca^{2+} content!) may cause a serious reduction in activity.

The conclusions already drawn also apply to formulations discussed in chapter 10 (coated formulations). These also consist of a tablet as a core, whose rapid disintegration is a prerequisite for appropriate absorption. In this case however, the surrounding coating must first be dissolved (e.g., by salt formation with ions in the stomach or intestinal contents), cracked (by swelling of the core after diffusion of fluid through the coating layer), or become permeable to the drug. While nonretarding film coatings barely cause any delay in release of active pharmaceutical ingredients, sugarcoatings, because of their considerable thickness, require some time to dissolve. In both cases, it must be made sure that adequate disintegration of the tablets occurs during the absorptive gut transit time (e.g., by adding suitable disintegrants).

Further Reading

Gad, S. C. "Pharmaceutical manufacturing handbook: production and processes." John Wiley & Sons, Hoboken, New Jersey, 2008.

Kuentz, M., Holm, R., and Elder, D. P. "Methodology of oral formulation selection in the pharmaceutical industry." *Eur J Pharm Sci* 25 (87) (May 2016): 136–163.

Stricker, H. "Die Arzneistoffresorption im Gastrointestinaltrakt-In vitro-Untersuchung lipophiler Substanzen." *Pharm Ind* 35 (1) (1973): 13–17.

Coated Oral Dosage Forms

10

10.1 General Introduction

Coating of drug formulations, particularly of pills, has been performed for a long time, being first practiced by Mal von Rhazes (850–923) by means of plant seed mucilage from *Plantago Psyllium*. Recipe collections from the early twentieth century list the following coating materials: chocolate, collodium, silver leaf, gelatin, keratin, and sugar. Coated oral dosage forms (tablets, sugarcoated tablets, pills etc.) were termed *compressi obducti, tabulettae obductae*, and earlier, more broadly as dragées. They were swallowed, sucked (Lozenges) or chewed (chewing dragées). Coated dosage forms consist of a core (tablet, granules) covered by a complete and uniform layer (coating). In the past, sugarcoated formulations were predominantly used, however procedures were gradually developed allowing the application of sugar-free materials. In such formulations, the coating consists of only a thin film (film coating). Of special interest are coatings that are stable in the gastric fluid (gastro-resistant tablets), thus allowing the dosage form to disintegrate only after arrival in the intestine and not in the stomach. Minor diffusion of the active ingredient across the film in the digestive tract may occur, even if undesired.

Classical (sugar) coating is performed in a rotating bowl or pan (*kettle*). The coating solution or suspension is added to the core material (tablets or granules) either manually or by spraying. Nowadays, more modern methods are applied, such as fluidized-bed coating (section 10.6.4) or spray coating in a pan coater (section 10.6.1).

10.2 Reasons for Coating Dosage Forms

Although the production of coated tablets is more time-consuming and therefore more costly, it is becoming increasingly important. Coating can provide the following advantages:

- Masking of unpleasant taste or smell (the original reason for coating)
- Protecting the active ingredient from external influences (oxygen, moisture)
- Improving mechanical stability (e.g., higher resistance against mechanical strain, friability)
- Protecting the active ingredient against inactivation by gastric fluid (gastro-resistant tablets)
- Protecting patients against ingredients that may harm the oral or gastric mucosa (gastro-resistant tablets)
- Improving the ease of swallowing the dosage form due to smooth, nonsticking surfaces and the lack of sharp edges

Voigt's Pharmaceutical Technology, First Edition. Alfred Fahr.

- Psychological and aesthetic effects (color, shine, and shape), thereby improving patient compliance
- Ability to distinguish and identify preparations by the use of different colors (decreased risk of mixing up)
- Ability to control drug release (modified release (MR) dosage forms)
- Masking of process-related irregular color of the tablets (e.g., when granules of different colors are compressed into tablets)

10.3   Starting Material

The starting material (the core) can be tablets, granules, pellets, or even capsules. Only cores with sufficient physical stability that are able to withstand the mechanical stress in the coating pan (roll and shear forces) or the fluidized-bed (bumping) are suitable. On the other hand, satisfactory disintegration in the gastrointestinal tract should also be ensured. With sugar coating in particular, the cores gain substantially in mass by the coating procedure and the size of the final product requires special attention in order to avoid problems with administration. The mass of the core should not be larger than 0.5 g. It is essential for the cores to roll easily in the pan and not stick together, like a roll of coins—for this reason, they should not have flat surfaces. Instead, biconvex round or biconvex oval tablet shapes with low band height are most suitable. Convex tablets roll easily in the pan and tend to have low friability.

Furthermore, the cores must be free of adhesive powder material and should not swell, in order to avoid premature disintegration. Also, the core material should not be too soft. Highly porous cores should be avoided since a porous surface favors undesired entrance of the coating fluid and may result in premature disintegration.

10.4   Sugarcoating

10.4.1   General Introduction

Originally, the term coating exclusively referred to the application of a sugar coating. The importance of sugar coating in drug manufacturing, however, has greatly diminished in recent decades due to high production costs and cumbersome process automation, in favor of the development of film coating technology. The production of one batch of sugarcoated tablets (dragées) may take up to a week to complete. The sugar coating may be applied either at room temperature or at elevated temperatures (up to 60°C).

10.4.2   The Coating Pan

Sugarcoating is usually performed in a coating pan. Small pans with diameters between 30 and 50 cm are used for development and small-scale production. For larger batches, pans with diameters of 100 to 120 cm are available. In one batch a maximum of 600 kg dragées can be produced. Coating pans are made of stainless steel or copper. In general, coating pans rotate clock-wise for the convenience of the (mostly right-handed) *coating master* who, in this way, can more easily manually interfere with the process. They are mounted on an inclined axis with adjustable inclination in the smaller types. The rotation speed can also be regulated. Additionally, the pan should be provided with a cover to close it and should preferably be provided with a heat source. In small-scale equipment heating is often performed by means of a blower or infrared lamp, but at the industrial scale a hot air supply (hot air blowers, 60°C) with a higher capacity is used. Appropriate exhaust provisions permanently remove dust. The internal surface of the pan is first coated with a layer of sugar in order to make the wall less smooth and to enhance rolling efficiency of the cores. Ribs on the pan surface (baffles) improve the circulation of the cores and thus coating efficiency. The pan is filled to a maximum of two thirds.

Table 10-1 Typical Stages of the Coating Process

Layer	Function	Composition
Sealing (optional)	□ Protection of light-, moisture- and/or oxidation-sensitive substances against external influences that may compromise stability □ Preventing bitter-tasting substances or water-soluble dyes penetrating the coating layer, thus avoiding the production of unevenly colored or bitter-tasting products.	□ Ethanolic *cellulose acetate phthalate* and *shellack solutions* containing plasticizers (e.g., castor oil, mono-olein, propylene glycol) □ Etheric-alcoholic tolu balsam, acetonic silica resin solutions □ Spray-dried mixed polymers of vinyl derivatives (vinyl pyrrolidone/vinyl acetate 60:40, Luviskol VA 64®, in organic solvent)
Subcoating	□ Enhancing mechanical strength □ Protection of the core against moisture □ Prevention of diffusion of bitter-tasting substances into the coating □ Protection of the core from dyes present in the coating solution/dispersion □ Rounding off the core material	□ *Subcoating syrup:* sugar syrup (50%–65%) with Arabic gum, colloidal silica, sodium carboxymethylcellulose, calcium carbonate, gelatin □ *Subcoating powder:* mixtures of talcum, powdered sugar, calcium carbonate, colloidal silica
Coating	□ Actual coating process	□ *Sucrose syrup* with colloidal silicon dioxide, sodium carboxymethyl-cellulose, starch and others □ *Coating suspension* □ *Coating powder:* like subcoating powder
Coloring	□ Physiologically compatible and in accord with legal regulations	□ *Inorganic dyes:* titanium dioxide, calcium carbonate, iron oxide □ *Organic micronized pigment suspensions* □ *carotenoids* □ *Dispersing agents* coating syrups, polyvinyl pyrrolidone (Kollidon 25®), cellulose derivatives
Smoothing		□ *Smoothing syrup:* like coating syrup, with glucose if desired (10%–15%) □ *Smoothing paste:* binding dye (solution of binder and pigment) and coating powder
Polishing		□ *Polishing wax* (polishing fat mixture): carnauba wax or mixtures of beewax, cacao butter, ceresin, and paraffin □ *Polishing solution:* carnauba wax, beewax, etc., in organic solvents □ *Polishing emulsion:* fat emulsion with talcum □ *Polishing talcum:* talcum-containing polishing fat mixture

10.4.3 The Coating Procedure

The classic procedure consists of six stages (Table 10-1):

1. *Sealing.* The aqueous coating solution or suspension may interact in an unfavorable way with the core material. Therefore, the core is often initially sealed with a thin water-insoluble polymeric film. Shellac has traditionally been used as film-forming polymer, but nowadays, synthetic polymers are more often used for this purpose.

Example

Composition of a moisture-sealing layer:

cellulose acetate phthalate	4.5 g
glycerol triacetate	1.0 g
isopropanol	94.5 g

2. *Subcoating (3–8 layers).* The subcoating layer is intended to protect the core mechanically and from permeating moisture. The subcoating syrup contains, besides sugar, binders (e.g., polyvinyl pyrrolidone, cellulose derivatives, and gelatin), anti-sticking agents (e.g., talc) and diluents (e.g., calcium carbonate). The subcoating syrup is added to the cores in small quantities, alternating with a subcoating powder.

   To begin, the cores are heated in the pan and subcoating syrup is added until the cores become sticky. Subcoating powder is then added until the cores begin to move freely again. The procedure is repeated until the required subcoating layers are obtained. During the whole procedure the cores and the added coating layers are dried with hot air.

Example I

Composition of a subcoating syrup (1000 g):

I	gelatin	20.0 g
	purified water	55.0 g
II	Gum arabic (Acacia)	50.0 g
	purified water	80.0 g
III	sucrose	550.0 g
	Tween® 80	10.0 g
	purified water ad	1000.0 g

Example II

Composition of a subcoating powder (1000 g):

Gum arabic (Acacia)	40.0 g
sucrose	200.0 g
talcum	250.0 g
calcium carbonate	350.0 g
colloidal silica	160.0 g

3. *Coating (up to 40 layers).* The coating layer makes up the majority of the coating. Through the coating procedure, the core gains weight and becomes more rounded. The coating syrup has a low viscosity and contains less binder than the subcoating syrup.

   Coating syrup is added step-wise, alternating with addition of coating power under drying until the mass of the coating reaches about 30% to 50% of the mass of the core and all sharp edges (*band*) have disappeared.

Example

Composition of a coating syrup (100 g):

sodium carboxymethylcellulose	0.8–1.8 g
purified water	41.2–31.0 g
sucrose	55.0–58.0 g
colloidal silicon dioxide	1.0–3.0 g
titanium dioxide	0.0–0.2 g
rice starch	2.0–6.0 g

4. *Coloring.* Coloring is generally performed together with the last coating layer. About 1% to 3% of dye is added to the coating syrup in the last coating step.

Example

Composition of a dye suspension (1000 g):

I	dye powder	380.0 g
II	potassium sorbate	2.0 g
	purified water	q. s.
III	Polyvidon (e.g. Kollidon® 25)	3.0 g
	sodium carboxymethylcellulose	9.0 g
IV	Tween® 80	1.0 g
	glucose solution Ph. Eur.	10.0 g
	sodium hydrogen phosphate	14.0 g
	sugar syrup	395.0 g

Dye powder is a mixture of dyes or pigments (section 5.5.1.4), most commonly combined with titanium oxide and powdered sugar.

5. *Smoothing (3–5 layers).* The principle of smoothing involves the slow evaporation of water following the addition of smoothing syrup, surface erosion, and the filling of small cavities in the surface. Moreover, crystallization of sugar on the surface results in surface glazing. This step is carried out without supplied heat. After addition of the smoothing syrup, the dragées are rolled further in the rotating pan under closed cover for about 10 to 30 minutes.

Example

Composition of a smoothing syrup:

dye suspension	1 part
sugar syrup	1 part

6. *Polishing.* Polishing is usually done in a special polishing pan—that is, a pan lined with sail linen or similar on the inside. The polishing solution or emulsion is then added. Alternatively, a polishing wax (e.g., cetylpalmitate granules) can be added directly to the polishing drum. No heat is applied in this step, and the dragées must retain a certain moisture content.

Example

Composition of a polishing emulsion (100 g):

cetyl palmitate	16.0 g
Gum arabic solution 40%	38.0 g
sugar syrup	20.0 g
liquid glucose (Ph. Eur.)	7.0 g
purified water ad	100.0 g

10.4.4   Physical Processes during Sugarcoating

Since the middle of the last century, researchers have made an increasing effort to elucidate the physical aspects of the sugarcoating process. Detailed knowledge of the coating process is of high scientific and practical interest, as it presents a prerequisite for the automatic control of the coating process in industry.

10.4.4.1   Determination of the Optimal Amount of Syrup

Finding the optimal amount of syrup per batch is of particular importance. Generally, the amount of coating syrup should be chosen in such a way that the core material is uniformly wetted. Too much syrup may lead to irreversible cohesion of the individual cores, resulting in formation of twin or multiple dragées (twinning). Upon correct dosing of syrup, the kinetic energy of the rotating core material is just sufficient to prevent them from sticking together. Irreversible sticking of the core material is induced by evaporation of the solvent (water) causing crystallization of the sugar. The thickness of a sugar layer in each step after addition of sugar syrup is about 10 to 14 µm. Pigment particles suspended in the sugar syrup should therefore not exceed this size, in order to ensure a sufficiently smooth and shiny surface of the final product.

10.4.4.2   Motion and Localization of the Added Syrup

The motion of the core material in the coating pan is influenced by several parameters, such as shape of the pan, amount and moisture of the core material, rotation speed, and the inclination angle of the coating pan. By using slow-motion recordings, movements on the surface of the rotating core material can be examined and different zones of movement can be distinguished (Fig. 10-1).

Zone I

In the so-called *whirling zone*, the movement of the core material is characterized by a more-or-less circular rotation around its own axis, without inversion of the upper and lower sides.

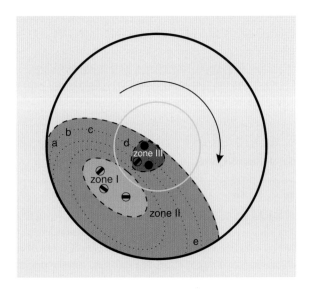

Fig. 10-1 Rolling processes in the coating pan (pan coater).

The circulating cores pass this zone in a curling line and remain in zone 1, as compared to the other zones, for a relatively long time at the surface of the rotating core material.

Zone II

This zone surrounds zone I and has about double the surface area of zone 1. This zone is the most important one for the coating process. It includes the following movements:

- *Motion patterns.* A single core remains for extended periods in an ordered, nearly elliptic path within the rotating core material. These elliptic pathways are partly visible at the surface of the rotating mass and partly hidden in its depths. In this process, the cores tumble steadily with continuous inversion of the upper and the lower sides. Moreover, a velocity gradient has been detected within the moving core material. The core material moving along the narrower elliptic pathways close to the rotation center of zone I completes one rotation within the same time as the material moving on the broader elliptic pathways closer to the walls of the coating pan.
- *Energetic considerations.* Centrifugal forces press the moving core material onto the wall of the rotating coating pan. From there it is moved upward (zone IIa) until it disengages from the pan wall due to gravitational forces (zone IIb). At its highest position in the pan, it has its maximal potential energy (zone IIc) and subsequently, it starts to fall down (zone IId). Due to gravity, the core material is accelerated until it collides either with other cores or with the wall of the pan, thus losing most of its kinetic energy (zone IIe). Finally, it is moved upward again on the wall of the pan and the whole cycle starts again.

Zone III

This small but important zone is found at the surface of the coating mass facing the coating master (Fig. 10-1). The core material has a high kinetic energy in this zone and is in a disordered falling motion. In this position, the risk of aggregation of cores is minimal. Zone III is therefore the most suitable position to add the coating syrup. After leaving the surface-located zone III, the wetted core material immerses into the depths of the coating mass (zone IIe).

10.4.5   Sugarcoating Defects

The following important rules will help to avoid problems during the production of sugar-coated tablets (dragées):

- Careful drying of the core material by hot air or infrared radiation before addition of the next coating layer is essential. Any twin products should be removed from the pan, not just separated, as this would further enhance twin formation.

□ The syrup should be added in a thin stream. It is important not to add too much coating syrup in the single coating steps (just enough to wet all core material) and to add the syrup slowly to ensure uniform wetting of the core material.

□ While coating is carried out with the pan in a tilted position, polishing is preferably performed with a smaller tilt angle of the pan axis.

Generally, it is difficult to achieve a uniform color distribution on the dragées. The most common difficulties are:

□ *Cloud formation* in the case of water-soluble dyes. The surface of the dragée should be perfectly smooth before application of the next layer, to avoid this defect.

□ Water-soluble dyes may penetrate the coating layer and reach the core, where undesirable interactions may occur.

□ As a result of the rotatory and circular movement, of the core material in the coating pan, centrifugal forces may act on suspended dye particles in the pigment syrup, which may force them to move to the edges of the dragée. This leads to the *moon formation*, a well-known dragée defect characterized by accumulation of pigments on the edges and opaque shimmering in the middle of the dragée. Rapid drying and increased viscosity of the coating medium (containing the dye suspension) counteracts the tendency of moon formation.

□ Cracks and fissures indicate permeation of moisture into the core, inducing swelling of the disintegrants.

10.4.6 Rapid Sugarcoating

Efforts to shorten the time-consuming classic sugarcoating process resulted in the development of *rapid sugarcoating* procedures. Despite saving time due to the reduction of coating thickness (thin-layered dragée, coating mass of only 10% to 30% of core mass), this could not replace classical sugarcoating completely.

In order to achieve a rapid coating process, more concentrated coating suspensions containing sucrose, wheat starch, sodium carboxy methyl cellulose, dyes, and water are used. As a result, the use of a coating powder is no longer required. In this way, a batch of dragées can be manufactured within 4 to 5 hours.

Further significant reduction of production time could be achieved by the use of rapidly drying coating syrups and replacing water-soluble dyes by (water-insoluble) pigments. The pigments are suspended in the coating syrup in the last coating steps. In addition to the numerous advantages of pigments (better and more uniform staining), the use of pigments also permits polishing without a preceding smoothing step. Pigment suspensions contain, for example, polyvinyl pyrrolidones (Kollidon® 25), sodium carboxy methyl cellulose, talcum, colloidal silica (Aerosil®), powdered sugar, water and starch syrup from partially hydrolyzed corn starch, or glucose syrup. Addition of bentonite can stabilize the suspension.

10.5 Film Coating of Tablets

10.5.1 General Introduction

Time- and material-consuming sugarcoating, which is also connected with an increase in volume and mass of the dragée, potentially leading to high packing and transport costs, has created an incentive to develop alternative tablet coating procedures. Film-coated tablets are characterized by the presence of a thin film of suitable material coating the core material. The coating does not change the original shape of the core, including complete preservation of engravings. Nonetheless, the coating layer should be able to mask a poor taste, enhance stability of the active pharmaceutical ingredient against environmental factors and provide mechanical strength. In addition, film-coated tablets should be of similar (or better) quality with respect to appearance and drug release properties when compared to dragées and noncoated tablets, respectively. From an industrial point of view, film-coated tablets offer the advantage of an essentially shortened production time as well as providing multiple options to modify tablet properties.

Film coatings, whose primary function is not to modify drug release, predominantly serve to improve patient compliance. Bitter taste of active ingredients can be effectively masked, and swallowing is facilitated by the smooth surface of coated tablets. In addition, psychological effects, caused, for example, by an attractive color, should not be underestimated.

Gastro-resistant film coatings serve, on the one hand, to protect active pharmaceutical ingredients against degradation under gastro-intestinal conditions and, on the other hand, to protect the gastric mucosa against irritation caused by the drugs. By dissolution of the film coating in the weakly acidic or neutral environment in the small intestine, enhanced bioavailability is often achieved.

By providing prolonged drug release, sustained availability of the active pharmaceutical ingredient (retarded effect) is obtained through film coating. The film coating swells, for example, in the intestinal fluid, and the drug is released by diffusion through the coating film.

10.5.2   Coating Thickness

The coating thickness, which is required to ensure gastro-resistance on the one hand and appropriate dissolution of the film in the small intestine on the other, depends on the coating material. Plasticizers and other excipients (pigments, dyes, colloidal silicon dioxide, starch, cellulose derivatives, high molecular weight macrogols, polyvinyl pyrrolidone) may alter the permeability characteristics of the film. Permeability characteristics depend on the hydrophilic versus hydrophobic balance of all film components. In any case, not only disintegration of the coated tablet but also release of the active pharmaceutical ingredient must be assessed by appropriate dissolution tests.

The calculation of the amount of coating material is based on the surface area of the core material (e.g., the tablet). For a cylindrical tablet, the surface area (A) is calculated according to equation 10-1:

$$A = 2(r \cdot h + r^2) \cdot \pi \tag{10-1}$$

Volume (V) and surface area (A) of the preferentially used convex tablets (Fig. 9-1) are calculated according 10-2 and 10-3, respectively.

$$V = (r^2 h + r^2 h_c + h_c^3/3) \cdot \pi \tag{10-2}$$

$$A = 2(r \cdot h + r^2 + h_c^2) \cdot \pi \tag{10-3}$$

From the calculated surface area of a single tablet, the number of tablets in the batch and the thickness of the coating layer, the required amount of coating material can be calculated according to equation 10-4:

$$m_{film} = N \cdot A_{tablet} \cdot D \tag{10-4}$$

m_{film}	total amount of coating for the entire batch (mg)
$N = m_{total}/m_{single}$	number of tablets
m_{total}	mass of all tablets in a batch (g)
m_{single}	mass of one tablet (g)
D	coating density per tablet (mg/cm^2)
A_{tablet}	surface area of one tablet (cm^2)

Declarations about the thickness of tablet films vary. Thicknesses of coating films between 20 and 200 µm have been reported, but they may also be distinctly thicker. As a rule, however, film coatings are much thinner than sugar coatings.

Table 10-2   Functional and Structural Classification of Film-Forming Agents

Rapidly disintegrating coatings	Basic amino groups to conceal taste and odor; swell up in saliva and are soluble in the stomach	Free carboxyl groups for gastro-resistant coatings	Insoluble but Swellable Coatings → Diffusion across permeable membrane with retardated diffusion as a result
Cellulose ethers			
MC		CMEC	EC
HPMC			
HEC			
HPC			
Na-CMC			
Cellulose esters			
		CAP	
		HPMCP	
Poly-methacrylates			
	Eudragit E	Eudragit L 100	Eudragit RS
		Eudragit S 100	Eudragit N 30 D
		Eudragit L100–55	Eudragit L
			Eudragit S
Polyvinyl derivatives			
PVP		PVAP	
PVAc			
Poly-hydroxycarboxylic acids			
		Shellac	

10.5.3   Coating Materials

Coating materials can be distinguished according to their chemical or functional properties. Classification by chemical character is provided in chapter 5 and an overview of commonly used film-coating polymers is presented in Table 10-2, together with their functional properties.

10.5.3.1   Soluble Film-Coating Materials

Cellulose Derivatives

Cellulose derivatives such as methylcellulose (MC), hydroxyethylcellulose (HEC), hydroxypropylcellulose (HPC), hydroxypropylmethylcellulose (HPMC), and sodium carboxymethylcellulose (NaCMC, carmellose) are well soluble in water and used in concentrations ranging from 5% to 10%.

Methacrylates

Methacrylates with basic amino groups (Eudragit® E) swell in saliva in the mouth, but only dissolve in the acidic pH range of the gastric fluid.

Povidon (polyvinylpyrrolidone, PVP)

Povidon is a highly hydrophilic and very hygroscopic polymer. At 70% relative humidity, Povidon becomes fluid. It is, therefore, not suited as a film-coating material alone, but is often used as an additive to adjust the permeability of insoluble film coatings.

Copovidon (Polyvidon acetate, PVAc)

Copovidon is a co-polymer Povidone and vinyl acetate in a ratio of 6:4 for Kollidon® VA64. Copovidon is less hygroscopic than Povidon and forms elastic films.

10.5.3.2   Gastro-Resistant Coating Materials

Gastro-resistant tablets are provided with a coating that is resistant to the acid environment of the stomach. At the same time, they disintegrate and dissolve relatively rapidly in the weakly acidic, neutral, or alkaline environment of the small intestine. These properties ensure that the active pharmaceutical ingredient is only released in the small intestine. With such formulations, the drug is transported safely through the stomach due to the coating, which is insoluble in the gastric fluid.

Gastro-resistant coating is applied in this conditions:

- The drug is likely to be inactivated or destroyed when exposed to the gastric environment (antibiotics, organ-derived preparations, enzymes).
- The drug may irritate or damage the gastric mucosa or cause nausea and/or vomiting (non-steroidal anti-inflammatory drugs such as acetylsalicylic acid and diclofenac, iron-, bismuth- and phosphorus-containing compounds, sulfonamides).
- High drug concentrations need to be attained in the intestine, such as in case of localized treatment (anthelminthic agents, antiseptics).
- The drug hampers the digestive process (tannins, astringent ions, formation of insoluble compounds with pepsins and peptones).
- Delayed drug release is anticipated (chapter 12).
- Optimal absorption has to be achieved by complete drug release in the intestine.

Earlier ideas about the conditions in the gastrointestinal tract were not very precise and grossly simplified representations were often used. It was assumed, for example, that in the stomach strongly acidic conditions occur, followed by an immediate switch to alkaline pH values in the duodenum. Many failures of gastro-resistant formulations could be attributed in those times to such incorrect assumptions. Although pH values in the stomach are commonly in the acidic range and in the basic range in the intestine, an abrupt transition from acidic to alkaline should not be expected; rather, slightly acidic conditions must be considered in the upper parts of the small intestine (section 7.1).

Gastro-resistant formulations should be administered at least 30 minutes prior to food intake in order to ensure unhindered passage through the stomach. According to the Ph. Eur., gastro-resistant dosage forms should withstand conditions in the stomach for at least 2 hours and disintegrate within 1 hour in an alkaline environment, which mimics the small intestine.

A common structural characteristic of gastro-resistant coating materials, which dissolve only at weak acidic or alkaline pH, is the presence of an acid function in the side chain, which is readily soluble in water only in the deprotonated form.

Pseudo latex dispersion

Pseudolatices are prepared by organic polymer solution emulsification in water followed by removal of organic solvent in vacuum.

Cellulose Acetate Phthalate (CAP)
CAP is a mixed ester of cellulose with phthalic acid and acetic acid. In an alkaline environment, salt formation of the free carboxyl group of phthalic acid occurs. CAP is only soluble in organic solvents.

Aquateric® is an aqueous pseudo latex dispersion, which can be processed without addition of organic solvents. Addition of 5% to 30% glycerol tri-acetate (plasticizer) is required due to the high glass transition temperature of the polymer (section 10.5.3.4). Also, phthalate and citrate esters can be used as plasticizers.

Hydroxypropylmethylcellulose Phthalate (HPMCP)
There are two types commercially available: HP 50® and HP 55®. The number indicates the pH value at which the film dissolves (5.0 and 5.5, respectively). HPMCP can be used as aqueous dispersions under thermal gelation. As the glass transition temperature is below 20°C, the addition of a softener is not required.

Carboxymethylethylcellulose (CMEC)
CMEC is a cellulose ether and therefore not highly susceptible to hydrolysis. The commercial powder product Duodcell® is dispersed in water for further processing. Up to 30% glycerol monocaprylate is added as a plasticizer.

Polyvinyl-Acetate-Phthalate (PVAP)
The pure substance is only soluble in organic solvents. The commercially available coating formulation (Opadry®) contains a softener and can be used without addition of other additives.

Shellac

Older drug formulations especially still contain shellac as a gastro-resistant or release-retarding coating. This substance is often used as a sealing layer in the production of sugarcoated formulations. Shellac dissolves in the alkaline environment of the small intestine by salt formation of the polyhydroxycarboxylic acids. The addition of a softener is recommended because shellac forms rather brittle films.

Methacrylic Acid Esters

The methacrylic acid esters Eudragit® L and S allow precise control of pH-dependent drug release. Eudragit® L100-55 dissolves at pH 5.5, Eudragit® L above pH 6.0, and Eudragit® S only above 7.0. For the production of a latex dispersion in aqueous media, the aqueous dispersion or the powder is partially neutralized with NaOH. As the film tends to be brittle, triethyl citrate is added as a softener.

10.5.3.3 Insoluble Film-Forming Agents

Insoluble film-coating materials swell in the digestive tract, resulting in a higher permeability of the film and drug release from the dosage form by diffusion through the film material. For insoluble, permeable coatings predominantly ethyl cellulose and methacrylate are employed.

Ethylcellulose (EC)

EC is the only water-insoluble cellulose derivative that has found application as a film-coating substance. The solubility of EC depends on the degree of substitution. The insoluble EC derivatives with a degree of substitution of 2.3 to 2.6 are applied in pharmaceutical products. In combination with other film-coating substances, EC is used for the production of coatings with defined permeability. Addition of 20% di-butyl phthalate as a softener is mandatory. When desirable, PEG (Macrogol) may be added to modify the diffusion of the active ingredient.

Aquacoat® ECT is a 30% aqueous latex dispersion of EC, additionally containing cetylalcohol, sodium dodecyl-sulfate and di-methyl polysiloxan as additives. Addition of 25% to 30% softener is necessary in order to lower the film-forming temperature.

Surelease® contains colloidally dispersed EC (30%) in an aqueous aluminum hydroxide solution. It contains dibutyl sebacate, or fractionated coconut oil, as a softener. The dispersion is stabilized by oleic acid. Colloidal silicon dioxide acts as an anti-sticking agent.

Methacrylic Acid Esters

Eudragit® RS (poorly permeable) and RL (readily permeable) are methyl-methacrylate/ethyl-acrylate-2:1 copolymers with trimethylammonioethyl methacrylate chloride (TAMCl) groups in the side chains. The monomer (TAMCl) is very hydrophilic and by mixing both Eudragit types, permeability of the film can be adjusted independent of pH. In aqueous environments, the polymers swell and the drug diffuses through the hydrophilic domains in the coating. In most cases, addition of a softener is required. Eudragit® N 30 D is a neutral dispersion and is used for both matrix and film tablets with delayed drug release. Addition of a softener is not required. Eudragit® L and S can also be compressed directly into eroding matrix tablets while exploiting its pH-dependent dissolution behavior.

10.5.3.4 Plasticizers

Plasticizers (or softeners) are low-molecular weight fluids with a high boiling point. They enhance flexibility of otherwise stiff polymer films and reduce their brittleness. The plasticizers sit in between the polymer chains of the film-coating agents. As a result, the polymer chains can no longer strongly interact with each other and the flexibility of the chains increases. Some characteristic parameters of the polymers are altered upon addition of a plasticizer. The most important parameter of the film-coating polymers is the glass transition temperature Tg. Below Tg, the polymer is in an amorphous glassy state. At temperatures above Tg, the viscosity of the substance decreases significantly, and therefore film formation is performed at temperatures above Tg. By adding a softener, the glass transition temperature can be lowered to room temperature.

> **Film-forming temperature or minimum film forming temperature (MFT or MFFT)**
>
> This is the lowest temperature at which a polymer (or emulsion) can self-coalescence to form a continuous polymer film (e.g., at the particle surface).

Commonly used plasticizers include:

- Citrate esters (Citroflex®)
  - tributyl citrate (TBC)
  - triethyl citrate (TEC)
  - acetyl triethyl citrate (ATEC)
  - acetyl tri-n-butyl citrate (ATBC)
- Phthalate esters
  - dimethyl phthalate (DMP)
  - diethyl phthalate (DEP)
  - dibutyl phthalate (DBP)
- Other esters of organic polyalcohols
  - dibutyl sebacate (DBS)
  - glycerol triacetate (GTA) = Triacetin
  - castor oil
  - glycerides of acetylated fatty acids
- Polyalcohol
  - glycerol
  - propylene glycol
- Polyoxyethylene derivatives
  - polyethylene glycol (PEG, Macrogol)
  - polyoxyethylene-polyoxypropylene block copolymer (Poloxamers)

Polyethylene Glycol (PEG, Macrogol)
Increasing proportions of PEG enhances the permeability of film coatings. This allows control of drug release by means of varying the PEG content in the film coating.

Polyoxyethylene-Polyoxypropylene Block Copolymer (Poloxamers)
By varying the proportions of hydrophilic ethylene oxide and hydrophobic propylene oxide groups, as well as the chain lengths of the polymer blocks, the solubility of the products and thus the drug release properties can be varied.

10.5.4   Dyes and Pigments

Coloring of film-coated tablets does not merely serve aesthetic considerations. In addition to avoidance of involuntary mixing-up of medication at the level of both the manufacturer and the patient, the psychological effect of colored tablets is highly relevant. Formulations of anti-depressive drugs are, for example, colored yellow because of the known relaxing effect of this color. Dyes and pigments are listed and discussed in section 5.5.1.

10.6   Coating Techniques

10.6.1   Pan Coating

The application of a film coating can be performed in the same coating pans as used for sugar-coating (section 10.4). Instead of using a coating syrup, the coating material, either as a solution in organic solvents or as an aqueous latex suspension, is sprayed on the core material by a spray nozzle (dual jet devices).

For coating of small batches, air pressure spray pistols (two-chamber nozzles) are used, which operate at pressures between 0.15 and 0.3 MPa (1.5 to 3 bar). Careful adjustment of the jet settings and the airflow is an important requirement to prevent losses of coating material up to 20%, due to spray drying.

For larger scales, single-jet nozzles are often used. They operate at higher pressures between 5 and 15 MPa (50–150 bar), which are produced by pressurized air. However, air does not

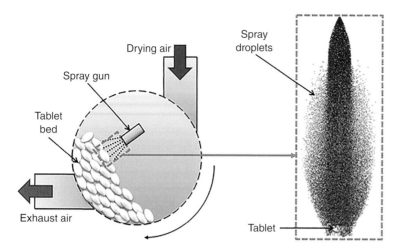

Fig. 10-2 Spray-on process. Reprinted from Suzzi et al. 2010, with permission of Elsevier (see Further reading for detailed reference).

enter the spray jet (airless systems), thus avoiding nebulization. The jet diameter (which depends on the size of the suspended particles when suspensions are used) and the spray pressure determine spray velocity. The spray jet is directed onto the falling core material in the upper part of the coating pan (zone III, Fig. 10-1), while the supply of hot air is located closely behind the spray zone. Evaporating solvents are aspirated by an exhaust supply located in the upper edge of the pan. The airflow through the exhaust device should be larger than the supply of hot air, in order to avoid escape of solvent vapor from the pan (Fig. 10-2). One tablet in the bed gets sprayed in for a fraction of a second and starts to dry immediately afterwards to avoid sticking to other tablets. To ensure proper movement of the core material (film tablets have a tendency of sliding), the pan is provided with a profile of baffles (section 10.4.2) or a movable baffle.

Film coating has become increasingly automatized, and fully automatized spray installations are usually used in the pharmaceutical industry.

Automatized spray installations accomplish the following:

- Spraying a defined amount of coating suspension or solution at predetermined time intervals.
- Control and adjustment of proper movement of the core material.
- Regulation of the subsequent air supply and drying.

Often, several coating pans are arranged in line and controlled and monitored from one control panel. To control the individual process phases, the following basic principles apply:

1. Computer-assisted regulation, based on experience obtained from time-dependent observations during manual film coating.
2. Control system to determine the dryness of the film coating by measurement of humidity in the pan or in the exhaust device. Direct moisture measurement is performed, for example, with devices measuring electrical conductivity and the lithium chloride hygrometer.
3. Control system based on temperature measurement with thermo-elements. This involves measuring the drop in temperature related to normal temperature, due to drying and evaporation. A decline in temperature is detectable as long as solvents evaporate from the freshly applied film coating layer. After complete drying of the film layer, the temperature will increase to the initial value (normal temperature) and the next addition of coating suspension or solution is initiated.

Also, combinations of these techniques can be used to control the automatized film coating process—for example, a combination of direct moisture measurement (principle 2) and the indirect moisture measurement by temperature measurement (principle 3).

10.6.2   Immersion Pipe and Immersion Sword Procedures

The so-called immersion pipe procedure (Fig. 10-3) avoids the formation of atomized spray and ensures an effective utilization of the drying air. The coating time can thus be shortened. A pipe is immersed in the rotating core material in the coating pan. The pipe is curved at its lower end and contains perforations in the direction opposite to the rotation direction. A stream of hot air enters the perforations at the lower end of the pipe and creates an "air bubble" (the core material is blown away due to the air stream) within the core material. In this air bubble, the coating suspension or solution is continuously added from a nozzle at the end of the pipe. Core material covering the edge of the air bubble is hit by the spray jet and instantaneously dried by the hot air stream within the spray zone. The drying air subsequently passes the mass of core material, resulting in further drying of core material before it leaves via the pan opening. Due to the permanent change of core material at the border of the air bubble, all core material is gradually and uniformly film coated.

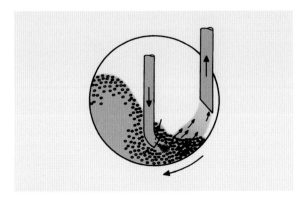

Fig. 10-3 Immersion pipe procedure.

The *immersion sword technique* (Fig. 10-4) provides some advantages for both sugar and film coating, and film coating process times can be reduced to a few hours. The sword presents a double-chamber system that is introduced into the core material, facilitating an intensive air exchange between air supply and exhaust through its perforated outer wall. During film coating, the nozzles are positioned to the left and the right of the immersion sword, approximately 20 cm above the moving core material. During sugarcoating, a thin-walled stainless-steel tube with perforations at the lower side is used to apply the coating syrup, however, a spray device may also be applicable.

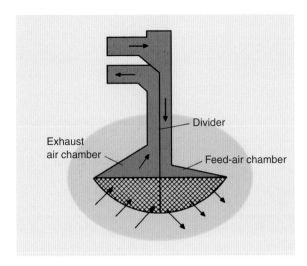

Fig. 10-4 Immersion sword procedure.

10.6.3   Drum Coating (Accela-cota®) Procedure

Reduction of the drying time by about 50% can be achieved by using perforated coating drums (Fig. 10-5), also called side-vented coating pans. In these devices, air is forced through the perforated wall of a rotating cylindrical drum, which is also equipped with a spray installation. Mixing blades may help to keep the core material in optimal movement. An exhaust device ensures appropriate dust removal. The use of perforated drums is nowadays the standard procedure for the film coating of tablets of larger sizes, and there are several drum coaters available—for example, the Premier Coater (Bosch Packaging) or Hi-Coater (Freund-Vector Corp).

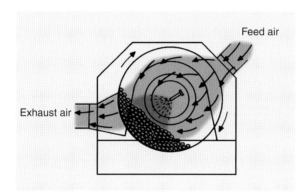

Fig. 10-5   Accela-cota® device.

10.6.4   Fluidized Bed Coating

Air suspension processes (fluidized bed techniques) have a special position among the various process techniques. They can be implemented in modularly constructed systems by exchange of individual elements so that only a basic device, to produce the airflow, is required. Fluidized bed devices (Fig. 10-6) are available in different sizes, starting with a batch size of 1.5 liters up to more than 3,000 liters.

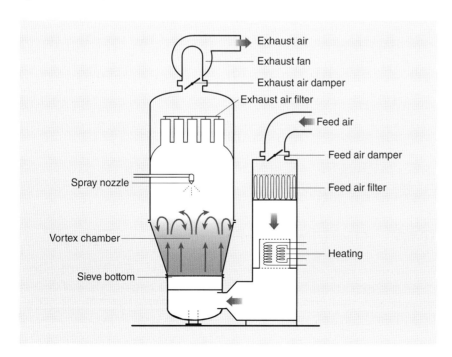

Fig. 10-6   Fluidized bed coater (Glatt GmbH, D-Binzen).

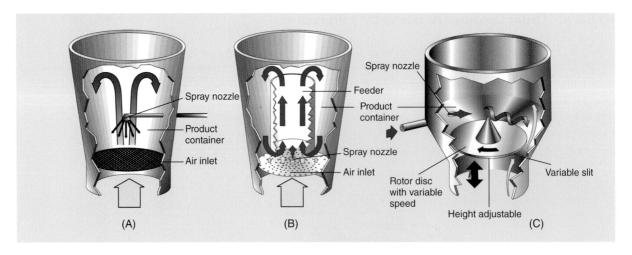

Fig. 10-7 Setups for the fluidized bed coater:
A: Top-spray-setup; B: Bottom-spray-setup (Wurster setup); C: Rotor-setup.

In small devices, the airflow rate is about 750 m³/h, whilst high capacity fluidized bed machines may require airflow rates of up to 14,000 m³/h. Air is warmed in a heating device and then introduced into the vortex chamber, where it keeps the core material in constant motion, while the motion of the core material is controlled by additional devices.

A particularly important fluidized bed method for granulation and film forming is the Wurster technique—a "bottom-spray" procedure (Fig. 10-7B). The air is supplied through the perforated bottom of the "working cylinder" in which a vertical tube is mounted. A two-chamber nozzle is positioned just underneath the tube. The granulation fluid or the film coating dispersion is sprayed into the tube, where the core material is moving upwards. The material is simultaneously dried by the flow of hot air. After leaving the vertical tube, the core material falls down outside the vertical tube to the bottom where it is coated and then transported upwards through the tube again. This circulating process is facilitated by a special construction of the bottom plate. The perforation density of the bottom plate is higher in the middle than at the edges so that the airflow is stronger in the middle. This causes flow of the core material from the edges to the center where it is accelerated and lifted upwards into the vertical tube.

A *top-spray* setup is shown in Fig. 10-7A. The core material is lifted upward by the airflow but sprayed from the top.

In the *tangential-spray* procedure (Fig. 10-7C), according to K. H. Bauer, a disk with a sharp cone in its center is rotating. Air flows into the vortex chamber through an adjustable slit in which the position of the disk determines the width. The core material is kept in a circular movement. Coating dispersion is added through a nozzle, which is positioned laterally in the instrument. The cores must have sufficient mechanical strength as they are subjected to considerable mechanical stress during the coating process.

The fluidized bed procedures are less suitable for sugarcoating. They are, however, widely used for film coating and especially for coating of smaller entities such as powders and granules.

10.6.5   Mechanism of Coating Process

In all procedures described, a polymer dispersion is sprayed to core material (Fig. 10-8A). During the coating process, water is evaporating resulting in a tighter packing of the latex particles (Fig. 10-8B). If the temperature of the process chamber is higher than the minimal film temperature, particles start to deform (Fig. 10-8C). The emulsifier film of the latex particles collapses and fragments (Fig. 10-8D). At the end of the process a homogenous film is formed (Fig. 10-8E), as visualized in Fig. 10-9.

Coating principle in the Wurster Setup. For clarity only a single spray-droplet impact on a particle is shown.

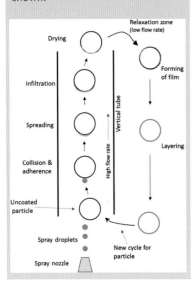

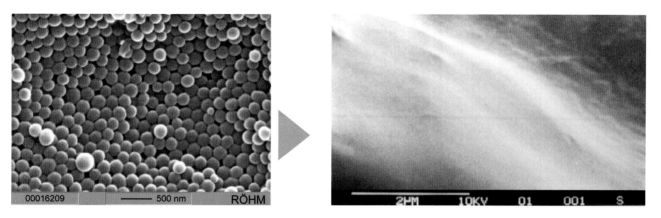

Fig. 10-9 Melting of single polymer particles to a homogenous film. Reproduced with permission from Evonik Nutrition & Care GmbH, Darmstadt, Germany © 2016.

10.7 Testing

10.7.1 Core Material

The Ph. Eur. does not require any special tests of the core material, however, as the quality of the final product depends on the quality of the starting material, the core material should meet the following quality demands:

- The mechanical strength (friability and resistance to crushing) of the core material must be higher than that of non-cooled tablets because of the mechanical strain they have to withstand during the coating process.
- Despite their high mechanical strength, the cores should possess adequate disintegration properties.
- Porosity is also an important quality criterion; low porosity favors mechanical strength and prevents penetration of the coating fluid into the core, however low porosity usually has an unfavorable effect on disintegration. In the event of extremely low porosity, added disintegrants may be ineffective.

10.7.2 Coated Tablets

The tests for coated tablets can be found in the Monograph "Tablets" and is summarized in section 9.9.

Further Reading

Bauer, K. H., Lehmann, K., Osterwald, H. P., Rothgang, G. *Coated Pharmaceutical Dosage Forms*. Boca Raton, CRC Press, 1998.

Felton, L. A. "Mechanisms of Polymeric Film Formation." *International Journal of Pharmaceutics* 457 (2) (2013): 423–427.

Suzzi, D., Radl, S., Khinast, J. G. "Local Analysis of the Tablet Coating Process: Impact of Operation Conditions on Film Quality." *Chem Eng Sci* 65 (21) (2010): 5699–5715.

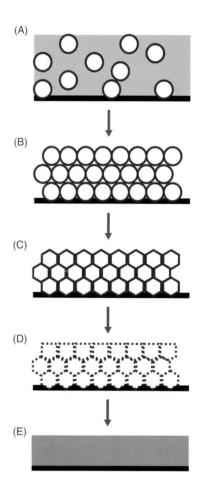

(A)

(B)

(C)

(D)

(E)

Fig. 10-8 Coating mechanism. Explanations in text. Reproduced with permission from Evonik Nutrition & Care GmbH, Darmstadt, Germany © 2016.

Capsules

11.1 General Introduction

Capsules are amongst the oldest pharmaceutical dosage forms and were commonly used already in ancient Egypt. Capsules are hollow, usually flexible, bodies of variable size designed to contain, in most cases a single-dose, solid active ingredient (powder, granules, pellets, tablets) or occasionally a viscous fluid, paste, or melting preparation. In addition, some dosed medications in which the active substance is tightly enclosed by gelatin or another similar suitable polymer, such as hydroxypropylmethylcellulose (HPMC) or pullulan, are also considered capsules (Fig. 11-1). The pharmacopeia distinguishes hard and soft capsules and cachets. In addition, gastro-resistant capsules and modified-release capsules are distinguished. Usually, for the production of hard and soft capsules gelatin is used as a starting material.

Gelatin capsules (*capsulae gelatinosae*) have a series of advantages compared to tablets and sugarcoated tablets (dragees). They are odor- and tasteless, and are easy to ingest because the surface of the gelatin capsules becomes slippery upon contact with saliva, thus facilitating swallowing. Thanks to their capability to dissolve quickly in water and biorelevant media, the active ingredients are readily released in the stomach. Numerous drugs, for example oxidation, light or heat sensitive compounds, or drugs with poor physicochemical properties that cannot readily be processed into other solid oral formulations, can be encapsulated into two-piece capsules without additional processing steps. Encapsulation comes into consideration when the active ingredient has a disagreeable taste (e.g., chloramphenicol) or odor. When stored between 15° and 25°C and 35 to 65 RH, capsule shells display high stability and remain unchanged for at least 5 years. Furthermore, modern manufacturing techniques provide high production speeds, easily serving commercial blockbuster volumes, offering high flexibility. They are considered an attractive option in the development of novel drug formulations. In contrast to granulation or compression into tablets, the gentle and relatively simple encapsulation procedure does not bring along the risk of altering the properties of the starting materials (crystallinity, occurrence of polymorphous modifications, stability) or the formulation (porosity, disintegration) and consequently, changes of drug release.

Gelatin is a well-known and well-tolerated polymer described in the pharmacopeias (see section 5.3.4 and 13.3.3). At higher concentrations warm gelatin solutions form a liquid system (sol), which upon cooling reversibly returns to a gel. Two-piece hard gelatin capsules consist of gelatin, water, SDS (sodium lauryl sulfate) and <0.5% lubricants. Colorants may also be added. They are manufactured through a dipping process and are delivered as empty capsules to be filled in filling machines.

Soft gelatin capsules are composed of gelatin, water, and a plasticizer (glycerol, sorbitol, propylene glycol) as well as colorants. Soft capsules are manufactured by fusing together two gelatin ribbons with a high water content along with the filling. The filled capsule thus formed is subsequently dried. A typical finished soft gelatin capsule shell is composed of 52% gelatin, 39% glycerol, and 9% water.

Voigt's Pharmaceutical Technology, First Edition. Alfred Fahr.

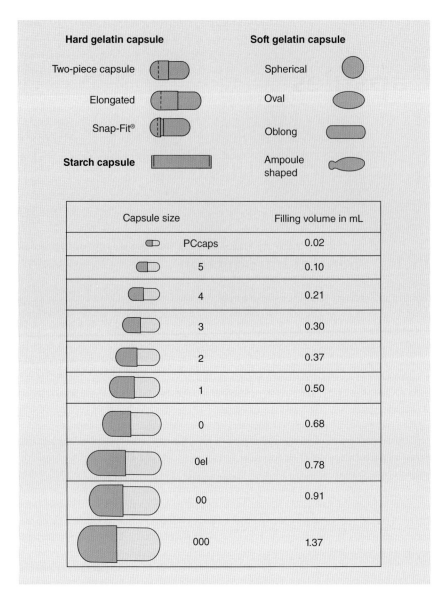

Fig. 11-1 Capsule types, shapes and sizes.

Soft gelatin capsules differ from hard capsules in that the former most often have a thicker shell and contain a plasticizer. The proportion of plasticizer determines elasticity, softness, and equilibrium water content of the shell. The residual moisture of hard capsules varies between 13% and 16%, while that of soft capsules is normally below 9%. Traditionally, soft gelatin capsules are used for liquid and semi-solid formulations, while hard gelatin capsules are used for solid fills. However, over the past few years, sealing and banding technologies have been developed which also allow filling of liquid and semisolid formulations into hard capsules.

Cachets (starch capsules, *capsulae amylaceae*) nowadays play a minor role in pharmacy because of their sensitivity to moisture and mechanical impact as well as their high production cost. Cachets consist of a pair of prefabricated flat cylindrical sections with a diameter of 15 to 25 mm and a height of about 10 mm. The parts either slide box-like into one another (slip over or dry closing type) or are closed per flange by moisturizing and applying slight pressure (flange type). They are made of unleavened bread, usually from rice flour, and are used for the incorporation of dry, powdery drugs.

Before administration, they are immersed in water for 30 seconds and allowed to swell into a soft mass before they are swallowed with water. Cachets can be filled either manually or machine-mediated at an industrial scale.

In addition to gelatin other polymers have been developed for hard and soft capsules. VegaGels™ (Swiss Caps) are vegetarian soft capsules made from potato or tapioca starch, which do not present consumer concerns about animal derived materials. Meanwhile, alternative shell materials have been developed for hard capsules. They include HPMC (Vcaps™, VcapsPlus™, (Capsugel), QualiV™ (Qualicaps)). In contrast to hard gelatin capsules, HPMC based hard capsules differ in composition and release profile. HPMC capsules manufactured by the traditional process contain a gelling system (carrageenan (QualiV™) or gellan gum (Vcaps™) that leads to a pH and ionic strength dependent in vitro dissolution behavior. HPMC capsules manufactured by a thermogellation process do not contain any additional additives and provide for fast and consistent dissolution profiles across all pH and ionic strength media in vitro. In addition to this, HPMC capsules with delayed release characteristics have been developed for both the nutritional (DRcaps™) and the pharmaceutical (Vcaps™ Enteric) market. Due to their lower and adjustable moisture content, and their constant mechanical properties even at very low moisture content (e.g., 2%) as compared to hard gelatin capsules, they are particularly suitable for encapsulation of moisture-sensitive or hygroscopic substances as well as for dry powder inhalers. Hard capsules made from the polysaccharide pullulan (Plantcaps™) offer in addition a strong barrier function toward oxygen and thus better protect their content from oxidation than gelatin or HPMC.

Cross-linking, as sometimes observed with gelatin capsules, is negligible with the newest generation of HPMC or pullulan capsules. Such cross-linking of gelatin may occur under extreme storage conditions (high temperature and humidity, strong light influence), or when in contact with reactive compounds (e.g., aldehydes). This may lead to delayed release of the active ingredient because of a thin water-insoluble layer that is formed at the interface between the capsule shell and the content of the capsule.

11.2 Hard Gelatin Capsules

11.2.1 Manufacturing of Empty Capsules

Oblong hard capsules (hard gelatin capsules, two-piece capsules, *capsulae operculatae*) are hollow bodies. They consist of two prefabricated, cylindrical sections, the body and the cap, each of which has one rounded, hemispherical closed end and one open end. The capsule is closed by slipping one section over the other.

Modern hard capsule types have an indented locking-ring on the body that snaps into a closely matching ring in the cap (Snap-Fit®); they have punctate notches (dimples) underneath the closing ring of the upper part of the capsule as a pre-closing mechanism to keep capsule cap and body together during transport and processing on high-speed filling machines. Alternatively, comparable closing mechanisms can be applied (Fig. 11-1). *Air vents*, channels in the body of the capsule, allow the rapid escape of air during capsule closing, at high speed on filling machines (Fig. 11-2).

Hard gelatin capsules, which are suited to be filled with liquid or semi-solid contents (e.g., Licaps®), do not have such air vents in order to ensure the tight closure by mechanical means.

For human applications, standardized hard gelatin capsules mostly have sizes between 000 (large) and 5 (small), with defined dimensions and filling volumes (Fig. 11-1). Furthermore, by elongating the capsules' lower sections while keeping the diameter constant, additional elongated shapes are obtained (extension "el"), which extend the variety of capsules with different fill volumes.

In addition to the standard capsule shape and dimensions, capsules have been developed with a shorter body part and a cap overlapping the cylindrical outer part of the capsules after closing. The different sizes of these capsules are AAA, AA, and A-E (e.g., DBcaps™). These capsules provide a strong tamper resistance and are particularly useful for encapsulation of tablets or capsules in double blind (DB) clinical studies, simplifying the clinical trial design by avoiding the complexity of double dummy techniques. Due to the increasing demand for flexible and easy-to-swallow formulations for pediatric and geriatric applications a capsule that can be easily opened manually, has recently been introduced (Coni-Snap™ Sprinkle

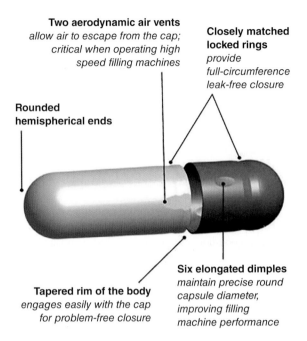

Two aerodynamic air vents
*allow air to escape from the cap;
critical when operating high
speed filling machines*

**Closely matched
locked rings**
*provide
full-circumference
leak-free closure*

**Rounded
hemispherical ends**

Tapered rim of the body
*engages easily with the cap
for problem-free closure*

Six elongated dimples
*maintain precise round
capsule diameter,
improving filling
machine performance*

Fig. 11-2 Aerodynamically designed capsules for fast machine-filling procedures (e.g., Coni-Snap®). Reproduced with permission from Capsugel® © 2016.

capsule). Moreover, with the increasing use of capsule-based dry powder inhalation systems and the advances in dry powder inhalation therapy (section 23.4), capsules based on gelatin and HPMC are customized to optimize the formulation stability. Fine-particle fraction release from the capsule, piercing or opening performance can be optimized by adjusting moisture content and surface properties of the capsules. This is normally done in collaboration with the capsule manufacturers and suppliers.

Empty capsules are produced at an industrial scale. The gelatin shell can be colored, mostly by iron oxide, or made opaque by pigments such as titanium oxide to protect light-sensitive drugs from exposure to light. Capsules for double-blind studies are colored (e.g., by Swedish Orange) such that shimmering through of contents is excluded.

11.2.1.1   The Dipping Method

The manufacturing of empty capsules nowadays proceeds exclusively according to the dipping technique. Fully automatic machines, provided with tens of thousands of stainless steel pins shaped like a capsule, serve as molds, producing in parallel the body and cap of the capsules. The pins are arranged in rows on rods and have to be produced with the highest accuracy to ensure high quality of the capsule sections. Multiple rows of immersion pins are simultaneously dipped in a temperature- and viscosity-controlled gelatin bath and pulled out at a defined velocity. By $2^1/_2$ rotations around the longitudinal axis the liquid gelatin distributes during the cooling, uniformly along the pins before it fully solidifies after a few seconds. A steady flow of temperature-controlled air provides for a residual moisture content of about 17%. The two capsule parts are then stripped away from the dipping pins, cut precisely to the required length by rotating cutting blades, joined to the pre-close position and transported to the packaging area whereby they reach their targeted moisture content of 13% to 16%. The thickness of the capsule shell is predominantly determined by the viscosity of the gelatin solution. The production capacity of such machines depends on the capsule size as well as on the type of capsule and can reach up to 100,000 capsules an hour.

Despite the constant quality improvements during the past years, some defects might still be present after the manufacturing. These defects are detected by online control systems during manufacturing or by automatic or manual visual inspection immediately following the production. They are classified in three categories according to type and relevance. Critical defects affect the subsequent filling process, for example; capsules with holes, cracks, indentations, residual cutting fragments in the capsule or defective length of the capsule body.

Major defects may become manifest during the filling process and might affect performance of the product. Examples of such flaws are: large spots, blisters or folds in the capsule shell, telescoping, or insufficient thickness of the shell. Minor defects do not affect the activity of the formulation but just their aesthetic appearance, for example; irregular color or a rough surface. The more critical defects mostly lead to dimensional changes of the capsule (e.g., ovalization). This makes it possible to separate out defective capsules by means of a sieving procedure through a vibrating metal plate with precision-made perforations, which only allows capsules of the correct dimensions to pass.

11.2.2 Capsule Content

Hard capsules are particularly suited for the incorporation of solid substances (powders, granules and pellets, mini-tablets, capsules, or combinations thereof). To ensure uniform dosing, powders need to possess good flow properties and sufficient plastic deformation to form a plug upon gentle densification on the filling machines. In general, the Carr's Index determines flow properties for encapsulation, and should be around 30 for dosator machine filling and 37 for dosing disc-filling machines (see the following different principles).

With these (and several more, see, e.g., Heda et al. 2002) stipulations a dose accuracy of $<\pm 5\%$ can be attained. In as far as no particular filling material is prescribed, it is recommended to use a mixture of 99.5 parts mannitol with 0.5 parts Aerosil® (DAC Attachment G). However, the majority of marketed hard capsule formulations are based on mixtures of a diluent (e.g., MCC, lactose monohydrate), a strong disintegrant (e.g., crosscarmellose, sodium starch glycolate), and a lubricant (e.g., Mg-stearate). Nonetheless, hard capsules can also be filled with liquid material when the gap between body and cap is adequately sealed. Aqueous solutions cannot be used to fill hard capsules as they will dissolve the gelatin. Also, low aliphatic alcohols cannot be encapsulated; ethanol for instance permeates the capsule shell and interacts with the gelatin. W/O emulsions might be acceptable, but this should be confirmed by compatibility tests. Substances that are incompatible with gelatin (ethanol, iron salts, tannins, and other protein denaturing agents) are obviously not suited for encapsulation.

For the encapsulation of low viscosity liquids in hard capsules, an effective sealing will be required to prevent leakage due to capillary forces. This can be achieved by sealing of the two-piece capsules by a capsule fusion process applying a hydroalcoholic sealing fluid (Liquid Encapsulation Microspray Sealing (LEMS)) or by applying a gelatin band around the cap-body overlapping zone (banding process). The problem may also be prevented by addition of a thixotropic agent (Thixotrop procedure) to the fill formulation. This will cause the formation of a thixotropic gel following the filling process, while during the filling a low viscosity will prevail because of stirring. This low viscosity will allow dosing with a dosing pump and thus accurate filling. Alternatively, an excipient such as higher molecular weight poly(ethylene glycol) (PEG) is added that is melted during the dosing and filling process up to a maximum temperature of 70°C, and upon cooling rapidly solidifies within the capsule (Thermocap process).

Capsules also play a role in asthma therapy (e.g., Novartis Breezehaler®). The encapsulation of the drug as engineered particles (e.g., spray drying) or carrier-based systems (pure drug often amounting to only μg, with amounts of excipients like lactose of 5 to 20 mg) in capsules protects it from agglomeration caused by the adhesive properties of the drug particles (<5 μm). Due to the low dose and the required deaggregation during the inhalation, this requires a gentle filling procedure that does not expose the formulation to mechanical stress or compaction. Therefore, special capsule filling techniques are applied for inhalation products (e.g., drum fillers, see Fig. 11-6).

11.2.3 Filling and Closing

Filling and closing of two-piece capsules is performed by manual, semi-automatic or fully automatic capsule filling machines. For use in the public pharmacy, where it may be an advantage over the prescription-based preparation of powders, pills or tablets, manual and

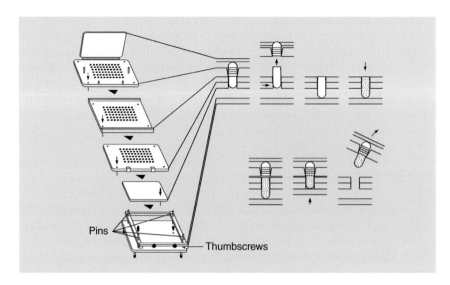

Fig. 11-3 Construction and principle of a manual capsule-filling machine.

semi-automatic equipment is used while in the industrial setting semi-automatic machines as well as high speed filling machines are deployed, efficiently covering the entire cycle from early development all the way to marketing.

The dimensions vary from such devices involving manual dosing of powdered drugs or granules, *via* devices based on body filling by gravimetry (e.g., Feton) or semi-automatic devices with a dosing auger or screw (auger or screw *dosing system*) up to the fully automated high-performance filling machines using a dosator or a dosing disc principle. These fully automated machines run in an intermittent or continuous mode whereby the operation includes empty capsule feeding, rectification, opening, filling, closing and ejection. Depending on the type of machine and the capsule size, maximal production rate ranges from 2,000 up to 400,000 filled capsules per hour.

The simple capsule-filling machine for manual filling (Fig. 11-3) consists of a frame with four pins to support perforated plates. These plates are provided with notches into which the individual preclosed capsules are inserted.

With the aid of screws, the position of the lower capsule sections can be fixed allowing the corresponding caps to be removed by lifting the upper perforated plate. The screws are then loosened causing the capsule bodies to slide downward to the bottom plate. After the filling of the body parts the upper plate holding the caps is replaced over the filled body parts and the capsules are firmly closed by pressing the two plates together.

At the industrial scale, capsule-filling technology operates fully automatic and performs the following major operations: capsule rectification, capsule opening, capsule filling, and capsule ejection. Analytical process technologies are increasingly applied to identify empty capsules as well as accurate filling. Powder filling technology traditionally uses one of two known procedures, the dosator or the dosing disc procedure.

The dosator principle (Fig. 11-4) is based on a tube dipping into a powder bed of a defined height and a piston compressing the powder at a pressure of 20–30 N to form a powder plug. The tube swings over the capsule body and ejects the powder plug into the capsule body by light pressure. For obvious reasons the powder should have a higher degree of compactability.

In contrast to this, the dosing disc procedure densifies the powder by five gentle taps through a dosing disc to build up a plug that is then ejected directly into the capsule body (Fig. 11-5). In both capsule-filling procedures, the formation of powder plugs serves to secure a clean and complete transfer of the powder into the capsule. This is generally performed at a force on the powder plug of about 1–2 N. In case of the dosing disc procedure, a lower level of added lubricant in the powder as compared to the dosator principle is sufficient.

The dose is determined by the size of dosing disc. Alternatively, hard capsules can be filled by the auger principle whereby a screw rotates moving the powder forward into the capsules and controls the dose by the number of rotations. For the filling of low dose inhalation

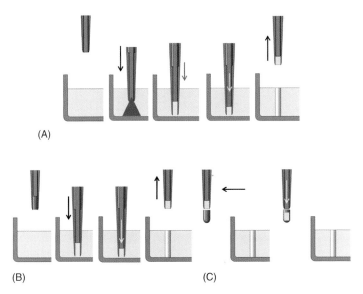

(A)

(B)   (C)

Fig. 11-4 Dosator principle. Case A. The tube with fully inserted piston is lowered into the powder bed where it exerts a pressure on the powder underneath it. The shaded cone indicates the pressure profile. Then the tube is lowered further into the powder bed until it reaches the bottom, while the piston is retained at its position. Thus, the lower part of the tube is now filled with powder. Then the piston is lowered to some extent to compact the powder in the tube. The tube containing the compressed powder is then retracted and swings over to above the capsule body where the compacted powder plug is pushed out.

Case B. The tube, with the piston fixed in a partly retracted position, is lowered into the powder bed until it reaches the bottom. Thus, the open space in the tube is filled with powder, and subsequently, the piston is lowered to slightly compress the powder in the tube. The tube containing the compressed powder is withdrawn from the powder bed and, like in case A, swings over to above the capsule body (C), where it is emptied by applying slight pressure. Reproduced with permission from Harro Höfliger Verpackungsmaschinen GmbH © 2016.

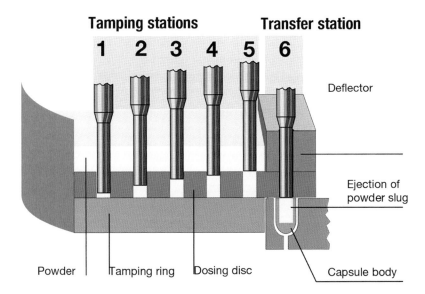

Tamping stations   **Transfer station**

1   2   3   4   5   6

Deflector

Ejection of powder slug

Powder   Tamping ring   Dosing disc   Capsule body

Fig. 11-5 Tamping pin station with compaction procedure (Harro Höfliger GmbH, Germany). Tamping station consists of 6 plunges (5 tamping pins). There are many tamping stations in this device, all functioning on the same rotating dosing disc.

The dosing disc (in green) is moving one step to the right. During this moving, all tamping pins are out of the dosing disc for about 2 cm (in the powder bed). Then each of the five tamping pins is tamping powder into its respective bore of the dosing disc. then again all tamping pins retract, the dosing disc moves one step further. Moving and tamping happens with a frequency of 140 /min. The tamping pins exert a force of about 150 N in the partly filled bores. Reproduced with permission from Harro Höfliger Verpackungsmaschinen GmbH © 2016.

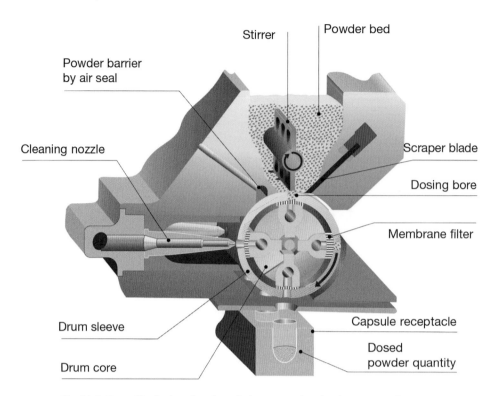

Stirrer

Powder bed

Powder barrier
by air seal

Cleaning nozzle

Scraper blade

Dosing bore

Membrane filter

Drum sleeve

Capsule receptacle

Dosed
powder quantity

Drum core

Fig. 11-6 Drum filler for low dose formulations. Reproduced with permission from Harro Höfliger Verpackungsmaschinen GmbH © 2016.

products, vacuum drum filling principles are used (see Fig. 11-6) This filling principle is based on a drum containing dosing cavities that are filled by vacuum from a powder reservoir, before rotating to the capsule bodies, ejecting the powder.

A faster way of filling capsules can be done with pellets, which are free flowing without dusting and do not have to be compressed. One of the filling machine principles for pellet filling is shown in Fig. 11-7.

Liquid or semi-solid preparations are filled by dosing pumps. A piston transports the filling material from the storage container into a dosing chamber. The filling needle is lowered while the storage container is closed and simultaneously the entrance to the filling needle is opened allowing it to deliver the filling material directly into the capsule body (Fig. 11-8).

All filling procedures can be combined as to allow for example a complicated single drug or multiple drug release profile. A selection of possible combinations is depicted in Fig. 11-9.

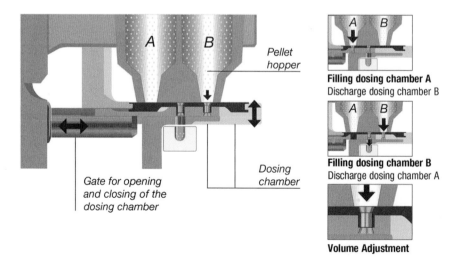

Pellet hopper

*Gate for opening
and closing of the
dosing chamber*

*Dosing
chamber*

Filling dosing chamber A
Discharge dosing chamber B

Filling dosing chamber B
Discharge dosing chamber A

Volume Adjustment

Fig. 11-7 Pellet-filling station. Reproduced with permission from Harro Höfliger Verpackungs-maschinen GmbH © 2016.

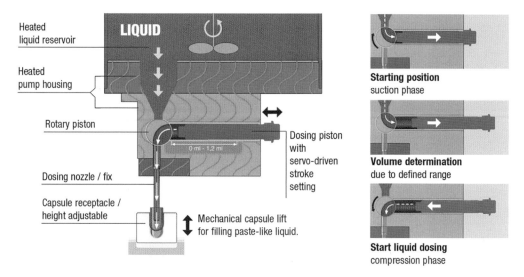

Fig. 11-8 Liquid filling of capsules. Reproduced with permission from Harro Höfliger Verpackungsmaschinen GmbH © 2016.

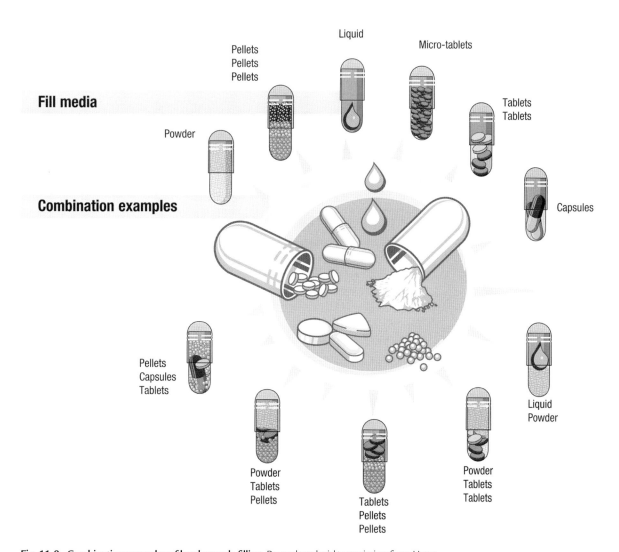

Fig. 11-9 Combination examples of hard capsule filling. Reproduced with permission from Harro Höfliger Verpackungsmaschinen GmbH © 2016.

11.3   Soft Gelatin Capsules

11.3.1   Application Forms and Filling Material

In contrast to the premanufactured two-piece hard capsule technology, soft gelatin capsules are manufactured in one step together with the filling and contain plasticizers (e.g., sorbitol, glycerol) in the shell formula. Soft gelatin capsules can be manufactured in variable sizes and shapes. Spherical, oval, and oblong capsules are the most preferred shapes. Soft gelatin capsules are specified according to their size indicated as maximal filling capacity in "minim" units (1 minim = 0.06 mL).

Soft gelatin capsules can be filled with liquid or semi solid formulations and have been shown to be also suitable for rectal administration (section 13.8). For this purpose they accomplish a significantly higher bioavailability than equally dosed suppositories with lipophilic excipients. Soft gelatin capsules for vaginal applications are favored for the same reason.

Soft gelatin capsules are also used for buccal absorption as a chewable dosage form. In this case, the shell is threefold thicker than regular capsules and contains the active ingredient. Nitroglycerin chewing capsules produce rapid absorption of the drug through the oral mucosa. Finally, single-dose drugs can be applied after opening (puncturing or cutting) tube-shaped ointment capsules by squeezing out the content (percutaneous application of nitroglycerin heart ointment). Ampoule-shaped twist-off capsules have a neck of several millimeters in length, which can be removed by twisting, which opens the capsule.

Generally, liquids or semi-solids can be encapsulated in soft capsules. Fatty oils, fluid hydrocarbons, medium-chain triglycerides (Miglyol® 812), and essential oils are particularly suited for this purpose. There are currently few drugs that cannot be encapsulated after dissolution, suspension or emulsification (W/O emulsion) in an oily liquid carrier. Vitamin A containing oils such as cod-liver oil, solutions of vitamin A, D, E, or K in inert oils and solutions of hormones can be encapsulated directly. Solids are usually dissolved or dispersed in a suitable vehicle, mostly a fatty oil, or processed together with a thickener to give a paste-like consistency, thus preventing the solid particles from sedimenting. Readily flowing mixtures are nonetheless homogenized just before filling them into the capsules. In some cases, it is preferable to use a hydrophilic solvent or carrier; poly(ethylene glycol) has proven its usefulness for that purpose. Depending on the nature of the content and the surfaces in contact with it, partial migration of constituents from the capsule content into the shell and *vice versa* may occur. Due to the different shell composition and manufacturing process, soft gelatin capsules can be filled with a broader range of liquid and semisolid formulations compared to two-piece hard capsules, for example hydrophilic compositions and compositions with solvents like ethanol. However, it should be noted that during the drying process ethanol and hydrophilic phase might evaporate, thus changing the quantitative composition of the formulation.

Usually, soft gelatin capsules are produced at an industrial scale by contract manufacturers under climate-controlled conditions (20% to 30% relative humidity, 22°C). Small scale manufacturing in public pharmacies is rarely done.

11.3.2   Production

11.3.2.1   The Globex Method

The Globex method is a fully automated procedure (Fig. 11-10) that has been used predominantly for the encapsulation of oils. It exploits the interfacial tension between two immiscible fluids, which in case of similar densities leads to a spherical shape. A pump pushes the lipophilic filling material at regular distances dropwise out of a nozzle. At the same time, a warm gelatin solution flows from a tube surrounding the nozzle into a cooling liquid (commonly fluid paraffin of 4°C) thus forming a seamless capsule around the filling material while the gelatin is solidifying. In this way spherical seamless capsules are formed, free of entrapped air, which finally undergo a washing and drying process. By exchanging or adjustment of the shell material (liquid, e.g. gelatine sol)

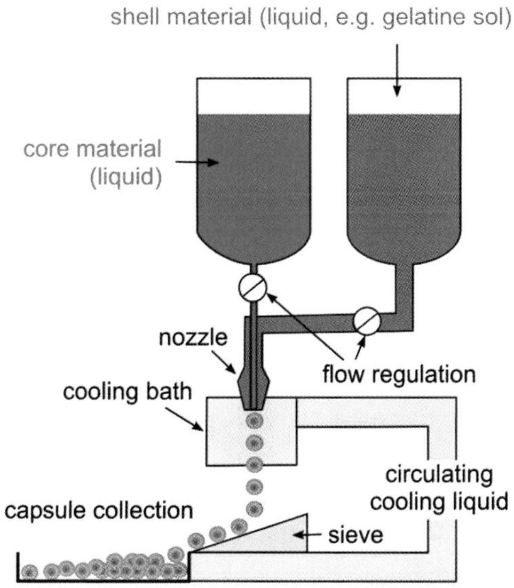

core material
(liquid)

nozzle

flow regulation

cooling bath

circulating
cooling liquid

capsule collection

sieve

Fig. 11-10 Globex method.

nozzle head, the capsule size may be varied within a wide range. The production capacity amounts to approximately 5,000 capsules per hour with a mass deviation of ±3%.

11.3.2.2 The Plate Process

Two mechanical plate procedures developed in the United States have led to a considerably increased performance in the manufacturing of soft capsules. After forming a gelatin band from a gelatin solution, the gelatin ribbon is passed over a heated metal plate provided with the relevant mold shapes, the gelatin attaches to the molds (Colton procedure) or the gelatin ribbon is sucked against the mold by means of a vacuum through a porous mold plate (Upjohn procedure) to form a mold. The filling material is injected into the mold by means of a filling nozzle before a second gelatin band is fused by a subsequent compression cycle with the other gelatin ribbon to form and eject the capsule.

More up to date is the Accogel process which, like the plate process, includes a measuring roll that holds the fill formulation in its cavities under the vacuum and rotates directly above the elasticized sheet of the gelatin ribbon. The ribbon is drawn into the cavities of the die roll by vacuum. The filling pump dispenses the required volume of the fill material into the cavity on the die roll (Fig. 11-11). The die roll then converges with the rotating seal roll covered with another gelatin ribbon. The convergence of two rotating rolls seals the gelatin ribbons to form the capsule shape and size and cuts the capsules from the fused ribbons.

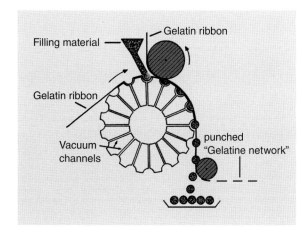

Filling material

Gelatin ribbon

Gelatin ribbon

Vacuum
channels

punched
"Gelatine network"

Fig. 11-11 Accogel process.

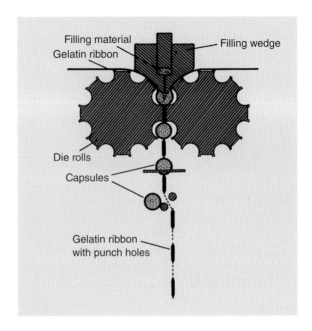

Fig. 11-12 Scherer procedure.

After releasing the vacuum, the capsule with two identical moieties is shaped and released. It is emphasized that this procedure not only allows dosing of liquid or paste-like substances, but also powdered material after precondensation by an auxiliary device. Depending on the capsule size, a production of 25,000 to 60,000 capsules per hour may be attained. Capsules produced according to this procedure show welding seams.

11.3.2.3   Scherer or Rotary Die Procedure

A decisive step forward was the invention in 1933 by Scherer in Detroit, who developed a machine for manufacturing soft capsules, which is capable of performing in one operation, both capsule formation and filling. Fully automatic high-performance machines nowadays produce up to 100,000 capsules per hour with a dose accuracy of $\pm 1\%$. The capsules have a central longitudinal welding seam and are filled without air inclusion. The manufacturing of a variety of shapes (spherical, oval, oblong, drop- and ampoule-shaped) is possible. The effective content may vary from 0.08 to 7 mL.

These machines operate according to the following principle (Fig. 11-12): An infinite ribbon of gelatin (40% gelatin, 30% glycerol, 30% water) runs between two mold rollers rotating in opposite directions (rotary dies). The rollers punch the capsule shape out from the gelatin ribbon. At the same time, a dose of the filling material is deposited between the two punched-out sheets by means of a filling wedge and a pump. The edges of the sheets are welded together by heat. The capsule thus formed is expelled, precooled, and after washing or cleaning with organic solvent, dried at 20°C in conditioned air of about 30% relative humidity until the required shell moisture or capsule hardness is achieved, which can take up to several weeks. The capsules can be made in one or two colors. To process dry powders, these have to be processed first into a suspension or paste with an inert carrier for encapsulation.

11.4   Modification of Capsules

For reasons of unmistakable identification and enhancement of compliance, prior to filling capsules may be colored and printed either radially or axially with one or more approved pharmaceutical colorants, which might further provide important information to the user.

After filling hard gelatin capsules with fine, adhesive or electrically charged powder or when overfilling the capsules, powder residues might be visible on the outside of the capsules. In such rare cases, the capsules can be dedusted and polished between counter-rotating ribbons or polishing pipes consisting of slanted cylinders provided with rotating brushes. Simultaneously, a permanent stream of air may support the dedusting procedure.

In case the hard capsules are filled with liquid or require tamper evidence (security closure), additional sealing may be achieved by applying a visible gelatin band around the seam at the cap-body interface (*banding*), closing the space between cap and body.

Alternatively, fluid sealing by microspray may be accomplished by spraying an aqueous alcohol solution onto the cap-body interface. Capillary action draws the fluid up between cap and body. Air, heated to 40° to 60°C, is gently blown across the capsule to complete melting and fusion of the body and cap (Liquid Encapsulation Microspray Sealing LEMS™ procedure), within one minute. This procedure is used in particular for filling with liquid content.

Hard and soft gelatin capsules can also be manufactured in a gastro-resistant variety. Coating of the capsules with a gastro-resistant film (section 10.5.3) is technologically challenging because the connective part between the capsule moieties is difficult to coat. Moreover, the resistant film must be sufficiently elastic in order not to break. Usually gastro-resistant capsules are normal gelatin or HPMC capsules containing gastro-resistant particles or pellets with sizes between 0.5 and 2 mm, taking advantage of the more consistent emptying of enteric multiparticulates from the stomach compared to the larger single units (tablets). Furthermore, capsules with modified drug release may be produced of which the content (by e.g. coating of the multiparticulates) or the shell or both contain appropriate excipients. Alternatively, they are prepared by a special process designed to modify the rate, the place, or the time at which the active substance(s) are released.

For reasons of identification and enhancement of compliance, capsules may be stained either radially or axially with one or more approved pharmaceutical colorants.

> **Tamper-evident** describes a device or process that makes unauthorized access to the protected object easily detected. Seals, markings, or other techniques may be tamper indicating.

> There are also gastro-retentive systems on the market, which are using capsules as containers for folded formulations e.g. polymeric systems (Bellinger et al. 2016).

11.5 Tests

Capsules must meet the following test requirements of the Ph. Eur.:
- uniformity of dosage units
- uniformity of content
- uniformity of mass
- when applicable, dissolution
- disintegration

The disintegration of hard and soft capsules is tested in water, under certain conditions in hydrochloric acid or artificial gastric juice. Capsules should fully disintegrate within 30 minutes. Capsules with a gastro-resistant shell should remain intact for at least two hours in 0.1 M hydrochloric acid. In phosphate buffer pH 6.8 the capsules should then disintegrate within 60 minutes. Modified-release capsules should demonstrate appropriate release of the active ingredient. The disintegration test may be skipped when the dissolution test is performed. It should be noticed that the disintegration test described in the pharmacopeia has an operator-dependent endpoint. This often leads to concerns about batch-to-batch variability. Using the recently introduced disintegration test for systems with an automated endpoint detection (e.g., Sotax DT3), the disintegration time of gelatin capsules has been determined to be consistently between 2 and 3 minutes.

Further Reading

Bellinger, A. M., Jafari, M., Grant, T. M., Zhang, S., Slater, H. C., Wenger, E. A., et al. (2016). "Oral, Ultra–Long-Lasting Drug Delivery: Application toward Malaria Elimination Goals." *Science Translational Medicine* 8(365): 365ra157-365ra157.

Heda, P. K., Muteba, K., Augsburger, L. L. (2002). "Comparison of the Formulation Requirements of Dosator and Dosing Disc Automatic Capsule Filling Machines." *AAPS PharmSci* 4(3), 45–60.

Mandal, U. K., Chatterjee, B., Senjoti, F. G. (2016). "Gastro-Retentive Drug Delivery Systems and Their in Vivo Success: A Recent Update." *Asian Journal of Pharmaceutical Sciences* 11(5): 575–584.

Podczeck, Fridrun, and Jones, Brian. (2014). *Pharmaceutical Capsules*. 2nd ed. London: Pharmaceutical Press.

Stegemann, S. (2011). "Capsules as a Delivery System for Modified Release Products." In C. Wilson and P. Crowley, ed. *Controlled Release in Oral Drug Delivery*. New York: Springer, pp. 277–298.

Stegemann, S. (2002). "Hard Gelatin Capsules Today—and Tomorrow."

Capsugel Library, Germany, downloadable: http://www.capsugel.com/media/library/hard-gelatin-capsules-today-and-tomorrow.pdf

Tang, E. S. K., Chan, L. W., Heng, P. W. S. (2005). "Coating of multiparticulates for sustained release." *Am. J. Drug. Deliv.* 3(1): 17–28.

Peroral Modified Release (MR) Formulations

12

12.1　General Considerations

The duration of the effect of a drug varies, but as a rule it lies between minutes and a few hours. After oral administration of one dose of a medicine, the onset of its effect occurs more or less rapidly and, after reaching its maximal blood concentration, it gradually declines (Fig. 12-1, curve A). Blood levels of the drug should not exceed the optimal therapeutic concentration range in order to exclude toxic effects (Fig. 12-1, curve B). In order to achieve a sustained effect, the drug thus will have to be administered repeatedly to compensate for the decreasing drug concentration due to biotransformation and excretion by the organism (Fig. 12-1, curves C and D). This may present a significant burden not only for the patient but also for both the nursing and medical staff, especially in long-term treatment of chronic diseases.

In these cases, oral drug formulations providing a prolonged effect of the drug present an attractive alternative (Fig. 12-1, curve E), and about 8% of solid dosage forms on today's market show this effect. Maintenance of rather constant blood and tissue levels of the drug is desirable for several clinical situations (e.g., infections, chronic cardiovascular diseases, allergies, chronic pain and hormone substitution). Drug formulations providing prolonged drug release not only ensure a consistent activity, circumventing high plasma peak levels but also often reduce side effects. In addition, therapy costs may be reduced, as the total amount of administered drug may be lower compared to administration of instant-release formulations. A further advantage is that the patient needs to take the medication only once or twice a day, thus avoiding administration of the medication, for example, during the night. It has also been demonstrated that once-a-day administration is more easily implemented by patients, particularly in the case of chronic drug use. These advantages significantly improve patient compliance.

Unfortunately, not all active pharmaceutical ingredients can be processed into a formulation with a prolonged effect. Furthermore, it should be taken into account that physiological conditions may vary distinctly between individual patients, so that a defined drug activity (e.g., constant blood levels over a defined period of time) cannot always be ensured. MR formulations may present a risk of undesired effects, since they cannot easily be eliminated to shorten drug effects. In addition, MR formulations often cannot be divided and therefore the active pharmaceutical ingredient can only be dosed in full units (e.g., one or two tablets). By chewing a MR tablet, sudden release of the total amount of administered drug (dose dumping) may result in toxic effects.

Production of MR formulations of a drug with a long biological half-life (>10 h) is pointless, since the drug by itself already has a prolonged activity. For drugs requiring a high single-dose (e.g., ≥ 200 mg, for example sulfanilamide at a single dose of 1–2 g), MR formulations would require drug quantities that are no longer compatible with peroral administration. In

Voigt's Pharmaceutical Technology, First Edition. Alfred Fahr.
© 2018 John Wiley & Sons Ltd. Published 2018 by John Wiley & Sons Ltd.

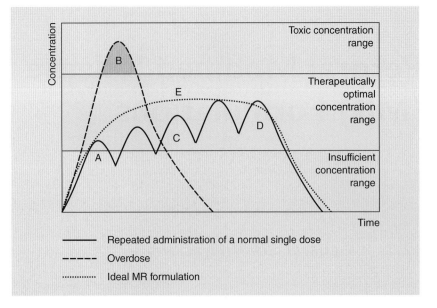

Fig. 12-1   Schematic diagram of drug concentration vs. time in the body after peroral application of single dose, overdosing and an ideal retard principle.

addition, in cases where the drug (e.g., lactoflavin) is absorbed exclusively in the upper part of the gastro-intestinal tract, MR formulations are worthless.

The plasma curve of a MR formation shown in Fig. 12-1 (curve E), represents a hypothetical ideal case. The continuous release of the drug and its degradation and elimination are balanced in this case, to sustain a therapeutically optimal blood concentration for a prolonged period of time. In the case of drug formulations with prolonged drug release, only an approximation of these ideal conditions can usually be attained. Besides Curve E (Fig. 12-1), also curve F (Fig. 12-2) represents an example of a satisfactory prolongation of drug activity, since the active drug concentration remains within the therapeutically optimal range for a prolonged time, however the onset of the effect is somewhat delayed. For this reason, an initial dose is often administered, which is frequently a "built-in" feature of retard formulations (see below). The plasma levels after repeated dosage are shown in curves G, H, and J

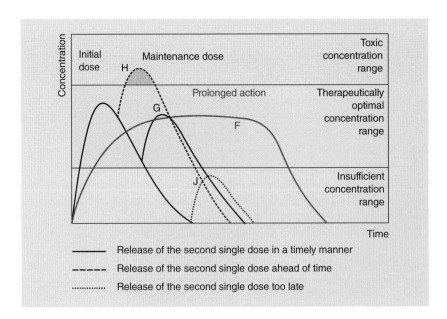

Fig. 12-2   Schematic diagram of drug concentration vs. time in the body after peroral application of retarded and phased drug release and two formulations with improper release of the second dose.

in Fig. 12-2. In the development of formulations with prolonged (or also pulsatile) drug activity, it is important to achieve drug release without large fluctuations, where blood levels of the drug should neither exceed nor fall short of the therapeutically optimal concentration range. In the case of the example curve H in Fig. 12-2, the second dose (e.g., the maintenance dose) became available too early resulting in blood levels in the toxic range, since the second dose is building on the already high blood concentration from the initial dosage. By contrast, blood levels as shown in curve J (Fig. 12-2) will result when the second dose is released too slowly or administered too late. In this case, the blood level of the drug remains below the therapeutically optimal concentration and no effect is obtained.

The development of MR formulations requires intensive collaboration of scientists in pharmaceutical technology, analytical and physical chemistry, pharmacology, and clinical therapy. Prior to performing the galenic work of dosage formulation, acquisition of extensive pharmacokinetic and clinical knowledge of the drug is necessary. Only this knowledge, together with correct interpretation of the collected data, will provide the pharmaceutical formulation scientist with the fundamental basis for successful development of MR formulations.

Based on all the above-mentioned issues, the requirements of an ideal MR formulation can be summarized by the following points:

- The formulation should result in therapeutically optimal blood levels as shortly as possible following administration.
- From then on, constant blood levels should be ensured.
- Uniform biological activity should be maintained for the entire time frame required.
- By avoiding peaks in plasma levels, that is, drug concentrations in the toxic range, intensity and prevalence of unwanted side effects should be reduced.

Peroral drug formulations with prolonged effect have been known for decades. Patents dating back to 1930 describe, for example, that lipid-coated drug particles, which become poorly soluble in the gastrointestinal fluids due to their lipidic coating material, still release the drug during passage through the gastrointestinal tract. In 1952, when D-amphetamine in the form of fat- or wax-coated pellets (Spansules) became commercially available, a new era, resulting in the development of numerous types of such drug formulations, began.

The number of formulations with prolonged drug release has increased substantially in the last decades. At the same time, however, criticism with respect to the evaluation of such preparations has also increased. All efforts have thus far been aimed at attaining continuous drug release for a maximally prolonged period of time. Little attention, however, has been paid to chronopharmacological aspects reflecting the periodically fluctuating susceptibility of physiological and pathophysiological body functions. In particular, the circadian rhythm (24-hour biorhythm) has to be taken into account. It is well known for several disorders that pain or discomfort occurs in particular in the morning hours and attenuates through the course of the day. Also, the frequency of exacerbations, such as in asthma, is often especially greater in the morning or during the night. Blood pressure values may vary greatly during the day, also in the case of hypertensive disorders. While in the morning often a higher blood pressure is observed, this usually drops to normal values during the night, making medication superfluous. These few examples illustrate that constant drug concentration in the blood for the entire day may not necessarily always be required and may even be harmful under certain circumstances. Apart from unnecessary burdening of the organism by a drug, chronic application may lead to reduction of activity due to development of drug tolerance. For these reasons, modern trends in drug development take into account biorhythms and potential drug tolerance and aim for strategies to adjust drug release patterns to the varying therapeutic requirements occurring during the day.

12.2 Options to Achieve Prolonged Drug Activity

Prolongation of drug activity may be achieved according to different principles, varying from chemical to pharmaceutical-technological measures or by exploitation of physiological or pharmacological possibilities (Table 12-1).

Table 12-1   Technical Opportunities for the Extended Action of a Drug

Chemical modification of API
- □ Salt formation
- □ Ester formation
- □ Adduct formation
- □ Coordination compounds
- □ Enlargement of molecule
- □ Introduction of functional groups

Modifications of the formulation
- □ Choice of sparingly soluble drug modifications
- □ Size and shape of particles
- □ Type and amount of excipients
- □ High fraction of binders
- □ Hydrophobic lubricants in the case of tablets
- □ Interactions with excipients
- □ Production technology (e.g., large hardness of tablets)
- □ Choice of coating or embedding
- □ Matrix formation
- □ Complexing with ion exchanger

Administration and pharmacokinetics
- □ Site of application
- □ Type of application
- □ Reaction inhibitor
- □ Vessel constrictor
- □ Excretion blocker

Chemical modification of a drug molecule may make it less soluble so that it will be absorbed more slowly or that the active moiety is slowly released from the modified drug (prodrug approach). Such modifications may be achieved by the formation of salts, esters, or ethers, use of addition compounds, or by complexation or coupling to another molecule. Examples are protamine-insulin, zinc-insulin, procaine-penicillin, and esters of the steroid hormones. Drug modification may also result in a reduction of biotransformation and elimination. Modifications of the drug molecule as such are often not a useful option as this is commonly accompanied by a change in pharmacological properties.

From a physiological or pharmacological point of view, the choice of the site of administration provides different possibilities to obtain MR effects (section 7.1). Implants, for example, provide drug activities extending for several months or even years (e.g., hormone implants). By the use of vasoconstrictors (e.g., adrenalin in solutions of local anesthetics), elimination of the active pharmaceutical ingredient may be retarded, while renal excretion may be suppressed by renal function blockers such as probenecid or p-amino hippuric acid. Application of the latter substance is, however, therapeutically not relevant.

Pharmaceutical technology and formulation offers several possibilities to prolong drug action. In essence, all these methods are based on retardation (or control) of drug release, for example, by reducing dissolution and/or diffusion rate. The various aspects of controlled and prolonged drug release from oral dosage forms will be discussed in the following paragraphs.

12.3   Definitions

The terminology used for formulations with delayed drug release is not internationally uniform. As a result, several terms are used in parallel. The terminologies used here are essentially those proposed by the European Pharmacopeia or of the international approval authorities (European Medicines Agency, EMA; Food and Drug Administration, FDA).

The Ph. Eur. defines *modified-release dosage forms* as: "... preparations where the rate and/or place of release of the active substance(s) are different from that of a conventional-release dosage form administered by the same route. This deliberate modification is achieved by a special formulation design and/or manufacturing method. Modified-release dosage forms include prolonged-release, delayed-release and pulsatile-release dosage forms." Formulations with nonmodified (immediate) drug release—*conventional-release dosage forms*—are defined in the Ph. Eur. as a "… preparation showing a release of the active substance(s), which is not deliberately modified by a special formulation design and/or manufacturing method. In the case of a solid dosage form, the dissolution profile of the active substance depends essentially on its intrinsic properties. Equivalent term: immediate-release dosage form."

In order to achieve a constant blood level *prolonged- (or extended-) release dosage forms* are applied (e.g., curve F in Fig. 12-2). These are defined in the Ph. Eur. as a "… modified-release dosage form showing a slower release of the active substance(s) than that of a conventional-release dosage from administered by the same route." The term *sustained-release dosage form* is also commonly used.

The prolonged effect of such formulations is based on the gradual release and absorption of a drug from a depot. For parenteral dosage forms this applies to drug-containing implants, intramuscular administration of oily suspensions or administration of an ester derivative of the drug from which the active drug is gradually released following hydrolysis. Peroral dosage forms often contain an initial dose and a depot dose (section 12.1). In such cases, the active drug is rapidly made available to the body via the initial dose resulting in a sufficiently, but not too high, plasma drug level to perform the desired pharmacological effect. Subsequently, the formulation should continuously release the drug at such a rate that a measurable prolongation of drug activity is obtained when compared to administration of a normal single dose.

Step-wise drug release may be achieved by *pulsatile-release dosage forms*, which are defined as a "… modified-release dosage form showing a sequential release of the active substance(s)" (Ph. Eur.). Examples of blood level curves resulting from such dosage forms are schematically presented in curve G in Fig. 12-2. This type of release pattern may also result in prolonged release, particularly when a series of consecutive single doses is given.

Another type of modified-release dosage form is represented by *delayed-release dosage forms*, which are described as a "… modified-release dosage form showing a release of the active substance(s) which is delayed. … Delayed-release dosage forms include gastro-resistant preparations …" (Ph. Eur.). Formulations with delayed release mostly represent gastro-resistant formulations, which usually are not MR formulations.

All these dosage forms with modified drug release have in common that the formulation controls the release of the drug by virtue of its composition in combination with the manufacturing process, and these are often referred to as controlled-release formulations. In a narrower sense, this term often refers to formulations with prolonged drug release. Depending on the applied control mechanism of drug release, one may distinguish diffusion-, matrix-, swelling-, membrane-, or chemically controlled drug release.

Fig. 12-3 provides an overview about the rather complex definitions in the different pharmacopeias (after K.G. Wagner, Bonn):

Modified release dosage forms (MRDF)				
prolonged (PHEur.)/ extended (USP,JP) release DF		Delayed release DF e.g. entericcoated		Pulsatile release DF
PHEur.: strong focus on release from DF	USP/JP: strong focus on prolonged availability in body + decrease of dosage frequence and side effects (only JP)	Ph.Eur.: no restriction to entericcoating	USP/JP: restricted to enteric coating	Only mentioned in Ph.Eur., not in USP/JP, as the physiological aim of this DF is identical with extended release

Fig. 12-3 Definitions of modified dosage forms in the different pharmacopeias (DF = dosage form).

In the context of modified-release dosage forms, often even further distinctions are made. Single-unit dosage forms are so-called monolithic formulations such as matrix tablets or dragées, that pass through the gastrointestinal tract without disintegration, but may become gradually smaller due to surface erosion (erosion tablets), or release the drug after arrival in the intestinal tract (gastro-resistant tablets).

Multiple-unit dosage forms (microparticulates) on the other hand, are products that disintegrate in the stomach into smaller subunits. This may concern tablets consisting of differently pretreated granules, or of microcapsules produced by coacervation or by fluidized-bed technology. Likewise, gelatin capsules containing coated pellets also belong in this category.

While in the case of single units the residence time in the stomach may show appreciable variation (from 0.5 to 4 hours in the fasted state to even more than 10 hours after food intake), the small (mostly <1-mm) subunits released from a multiple-unit dosage form continuously pass the pylorus, even in the closed state, and distribute within the entire gastrointestinal tract. Ideally, this leads to a fairly uniform passage through the gastrointestinal tract, as indicated by clinical studies reporting quite reproducible blood levels. Because such formulations perform independently of gastric emptying, excellent control of drug release is obtained. However, these dosage forms are also clearly affected by food intake. Nonetheless, increasing numbers of modified-release dosage forms based on multiple units are appearing on the market.

12.4   Manufacturing Procedures

12.4.1   Coating of the Active Pharmaceutical Ingredient

The method involves the coating of drug particles with adequate size, such as a large single crystal or crystal aggregate, usually with lipids or synthetic or semi-synthetic film formers (section 10.5.3).

Technically this is achieved, for example, by means of fluidized-bed coating (section 10.6.4) or by coacervation. The procedure can be applied in manufacturing of tablets, capsules and granules (Fig. 12-4A).

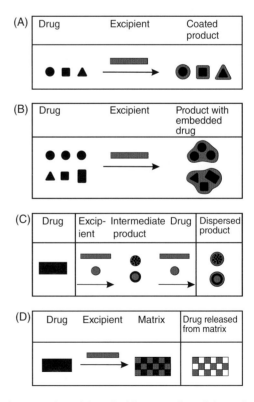

Fig. 12-4 (A) Coating procedure; (B) Embedding procedure; (C) Coating of dosage forms; (D) Matrix technologies.

12.4.2 Embedding Procedure

By this method, the active substance(s) is homogeneously dispersed in the pharmaceutical excipient(s) intended to slow down the release (Fig. 12-4B). Fats, waxes and hardened oils are preferentially used as carrier materials, as well as hydrophilic polymers such as dextran, cellulose derivatives, polyvinyl-pyrrolidone and gelatin. Embedding active ingredients in hydrophilic excipients is most often performed with spray-drying while spray-solidification is preferentially applied in case of embedding the active ingredient in lipophilic substances. The mechanism of action of embedded formulations is based on slowing down the dissolution phase and/or on the increased viscosity occurring during dissolution.

Heat-deformable synthetic polymers (thermoplasts) offer the possibility to transfer a drug-excipient mixture by melt extrusion directly into a tablet-like product (section 27.2.2).

An alternative embedding procedure is the *pearl polymerization*. In this procedure the active pharmaceutical ingredient is added to a mixture of droplets of suitable monomers. During the polymerization process the drug becomes incorporated in the polymer matrix. Depending on the functional groups of the polymer, and thus its solubility properties in the gastrointestinal fluids, products with different release properties may be obtained. Alkaline groups in the polymer matrix promote dissolution or swelling in the acidic environment in the stomach (initial dose), while acidic groups facilitate dissolution or swelling in the weakly acidic to neutral environment of the duodenum (maintenance dosage). Additional control of drug release can be obtained by combining pellets with different drug release properties in a single-dosage formulation (capsule or tablet).

12.4.3 Coating of Dosage Forms

Whilst in the aforementioned procedures drug particles (or granules, *i.e.* intermediates in the production of medicines) were coated or embedded in a matrix, the dosage form itself (usually tablets or capsules) may be coated with, for example, cellulose derivatives in order to control drug release by the formed polymeric film (film coated tablets, Fig. 12-4C). The coating process is predominantly performed by drum-coating (pan coating, section 10.6.1) or fluidized-bed coating (section 10.6.4). For the production of gastro-resistant dosage forms especially, a coating methodology is usually used.

12.4.4 Matrix Technologies

A further possibility to achieve retarded drug release involves the manufacturing of matrix tablets, which ensure continuous release. Water-soluble drugs are, either alone or in combination with suitable (usually polymeric) excipients, compressed into tablets, either directly or following granulation (Fig. 12-4D). For the granulation process, commonly used granulation binders are applied together with granulation fluids in which the matrix-forming excipient but not the active ingredient is soluble. Among the variety of water- and acid-soluble polymers used for this purpose, polyvinyl chloride, polyvinyl acetate, polyethylene and polymers and co-polymers of acrylates, and methacrylates have proven particularly useful. During compression, the matrix-forming polymer is sintered (pressure and thermo sintering) into a continuous matrix, thus incorporating a substantial fraction of the active drug in suspended form.

Table 12-2 presents an overview of the equipment and processing methods for the manufacturing of MR formulations discussed in the foregoing paragraphs. From a technological

Table 12-2 Devices and Processing Methods for the Production of MR Formulations by Different Techniques

Technological Procedure	Devices or Processing Techniques
Film-coating	fluidized-bed coating, coacervation
Embedding	Spray drying, Modified granulation
Embedding	Drum coater (pan coater), Fluidized-bed coating, Microencapsulation
Matrix technology	Tablet press

point of view, embedding and matrix technologies show similarities in production technology and are, therefore, often discussed together.

12.5   Special Products

12.5.1   Press-Coated Tablets

The production of press-coated tablets (or dry-coated tablets) can be considered as "dry coating" as the core material is coated—in contrast to the conventional coating processes—without application of moisture and heat. In contrast, the coating layer is obtained by compaction of granules onto the core material. This also allows processing of moisture-sensitive active agents. In addition, incompatible drugs may be separated in this way in the core and the coating layer. Furthermore, it is possible to separate the core and coating layer by an intermediate layer. Particularly important are press-coated MR tablets. By processing a part of the active substance in a readily disintegrating coating layer and the remainder in the slowly disintegrating core material (e.g., by embedding in a high-melting fat or insoluble polymeric matrix), the therapeutic activity may be significantly prolonged. Gastro-resistance can also be attained in this way, by using film-coated gastro-resistant core material or granules (dry-coating layer). Where the active substance is also incorporated in the dry coating layer, a better dosing accuracy may be obtained than by processing the drug with a conventional coating process applying moisture and heat. Finally, press-coated tablets usually disintegrate more slowly than film-coated tablets. The main advantages of press-coated tablets over film-coated tablets are the relatively low space requirements of high-capacity equipment, shorter production time and the smaller amounts of pharmaceutical excipients that are needed.

On the other hand, sufficiently strong binding between core and coating layer as well as accurate centering of the core within the coating may present a challenge. The production capacity is also inferior to that of modern film-coating processes.

For dry coating, essentially two manufacturing processes are commonly used. The cores may be processed by a conventional tablet machine followed by dry coating in a special press-coating machine, or core and coat are processed together in two rotary tablet machines that are coupled together, where one unit compresses the cores while dry coating is performed in the other.

Fig. 12-5 demonstrates the general operation procedure of dry coating:
1. Filling sufficient amounts of coating material (e.g., pellets) into the die
2. Positioning of the core
3. Upper punch drops down (without applying compression force) and embeds the core in coating material
4. Filling up the die with coating material
5. Pre-compression and final compression
6. Expulsion of the dry-coated tablet

By omitting step 4, tablets with half coating only, so-called bull's-eye tablets are obtained. This dosage form has no relevance in today's market.

12.5.2   Layered Tablets

In multilayer or sandwich tablets, two or three layers of different granules are combined in one tablet. Thus, incompatible active ingredients may be processed separately in different

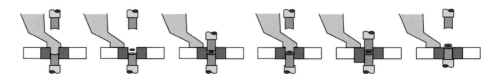

Fig. 12-5 Principle of dry coating.

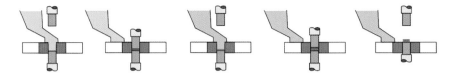

Fig. 12-6   Operation principle of a multilayer tablet press.

granules, and then directly compressed into a product. If required, separation of the different layers may be achieved by using a layer of "neutral" granules. Multilayer tablets are particularly suited to attain a prolonged effect. This is achieved by special treatment of part of the active ingredient, for instance by coating the granules with lipids or a suitable film-forming polymer. In order to obtain strict separation between the layers inside the tablet, the granules should be homogeneous in size (0.15–1 mm), and always smaller than half a layer thickness. The use of minimal amounts of lubricant and the same binder in all layers will ensure that all layers remain intact when applying mechanical strain during packing and transport.

The manufacturing of multilayer tablets requires special tablet machines, which nonetheless resemble in principle common rotary tablet machines. The granules required for the individual layers are filled into the die by separate hopper shoes. To ensure adequate separation between the layers, each individual layer is first precompressed before the granules of the next layer are filled on top of it. Only after the material for all layers has been filled into the die (and precompressed), the final compression of the entire tablet is carried out (Fig. 12-6). For double-layer tablets, the following production steps can be distinguished:

1. Filling the granules for the first tablet layer into the die
2. Precompression of the first layer
3. Filling the granules for the second tablet layer into the die
4. Precompression of the second layer and final compression
5. Expulsion of the double-layer tablet

12.5.3   Mixed-Granule Tablets

By compression of a mixture of granules with different pretreatment (e.g., coating), mixed-granule tablets are obtained. They may consist, for example, of immediate-release granules (initial dosage), together with granules providing prolonged drug release (maintenance dosage).

12.5.4   Duplex Tablets

Duplex tablets are film-coated tablets produced by film-coating procedures. The depot dose (e.g., in the tablet core) is coated with an additional layer containing the initial dosage. By analogy, a sugarcoated analogue may be produced by consecutive sugarcoating of appropriate cores (retarded or nonretarded). They are called laminated or multiple-layer dragées.

12.6   Principles of Controlled Release

An active pharmaceutical ingredient is usually rapidly absorbed from a solution (molecularly dispersed state). However, when the drug is in the solid state and released only slowly, the release step becomes the rate-limiting factor for drug absorption if drug release is slower then drug absorption. There are essentially two principles by which under these conditions retardation of drug activity may be achieved:

- slow dissolution of the active ingredient
- creation of diffusion barriers

12.6.1   Principal Release Mechanisms

After release of the initial dose, the release of the depot dose from pore-containing matrix tablets depends on two factors:

1. The amount of drug-dissolving fluid penetrating into the matrix per unit of time
2. The diffusion of dissolved drug out of the matrix

The penetration of digestive fluids into the pores of the matrix can be described by an equation representing a modification of Noyes and Whitney's equation of dissolution.

$$v = K(c_m - c)\frac{m}{M \cdot l} \tag{12-1}$$

v = amount of fluid diffusing per time into the matrix

m = mass of dissolvable drug in the cavities of the matrix

M = mass of the pure matrix

l = average length of capillaries

c_m = maximal possible drug concentration at front of the fluid intruding into the capillaries

c = drug concentration in the capillaries

K = constant

The diffusion of the dissolved drug towards the surface of the matrix tablet (e.g., diffusion out of the matrix) obeys Fick's diffusion law (section 3.10.2). According to this law, the magnitude of the diffusion depends on the diffusion coefficient of the system, the diffusion surface area, and the concentration gradient. When a drug is present in a spherical body (dosage form), drug release into the surrounding fluid is accomplished in several steps (Fig. 12-7).

- The drug dissolves in A (physical reaction) or dissociates from, for example, an ion exchanger (physical or chemical reaction). The rate is determined by the dissolution rate, cleavage rate, or exchange processes.
- The drug travels from A to B by diffusion at a rate, which is determined by the diffusion rate in the matrix.
- The drug moves from B to C by diffusion at a rate, which is determined by the diffusion rate in the solvent film.

In general, the diffusion rates from A to B and from B to C are different. The release rate is determined by the slowest of the three steps. Based on these considerations, the release process is categorized in:

- Release controlled by a reaction (occurring in A). In this case, the release rate is independent on tablet size.

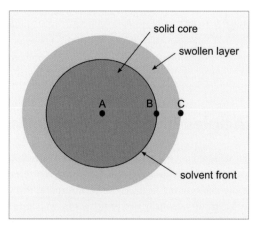

Fig. 12-7 Drug release by diffusion showing different drug locations: (A) solid core; (B) solid core surface; (C) outer surface of the swollen layer.

- Release controlled by diffusion through the matrix (diffusion from A to B). The release rate decreases inversely proportional to the square of the tablet's diameter.
- Release controlled by film diffusion (film diffusion, diffusion from B to C). The release rate decreases inversely proportional to the tablet's diameter.

Since with diffusion through the matrix the release rate decreases much more strongly with increasing size of the matrix than in the case of diffusion through a thin film. The release from larger tablets is predominantly controlled by diffusion through the matrix, whereas the release from smaller tablets is rather controlled by the diffusion through the film.

12.6.2   Slow Dissolution of the Drug

12.6.2.1   Exploitation of Poorly Soluble Drug Forms
For immediate-release formulations, special efforts are often required to ascertain rapid dissolution of the drug (minimal particle size, readily soluble salts etc., section 7.1). For MR formulations, however, such measures are only applicable with respect to the initial dosage. For the maintenance dosage, the opposite effect, that is, slow dissolution (e.g., by the use of macro-crystals, more stable crystal modifications and poorly soluble salts) is required.

12.6.2.2   Binding to an Ion Exchange Resin
Slow drug release can be achieved by binding of the drug to an ion exchange material (section 5.2.2.3). Such drug-loaded ion exchange resins are known as resinates. The resin-bound drug is exchanged for protons in the stomach and by Na^+ and K^+ ions in the intestinal tract. Particularly with alkaloids (e.g., codeine) and other alkaline drugs, retarded drug release is achieved. It has been shown, that the use of a mixture of the free base and salt or, alternatively, the use of only partly alkaline ion exchange resins can be advantageous with respect to adjustment of the initial and maintenance dose. Despite the fact that the (fairly) consistent ion concentration in the gastrointestinal tract should ensure a rapid first-order release and, in addition, that ion exchange resin granules are readily compressible into tablets, there are only few such preparations on the market. In the case of long-term therapeutic treatment (e.g., chronic diseases), alterations in electrolyte homeostasis cannot be excluded. Furthermore, only ionizable drugs are suitable for processing in ion-exchange resins, and the drug content per tablet may be low due to limited binding capacity.

12.6.3   Creation of Diffusion Barriers

12.6.3.1   Membranes as a Coating Material
When the drug (as such) or the formulation (granules, pellets, tablets) is coated with a polymer membrane which protects the active ingredient from the environment of the digestive tract, but allows the drug to permeate the membrane, prolonged and potentially retarded release will result. Generally, membranes with and without pores are distinguished (Fig. 12-8).

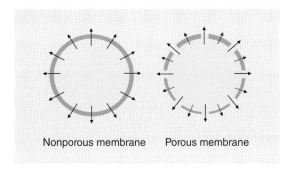

Nonporous membrane   Porous membrane

Fig. 12-8   Drug diffusion through pore-free or porous membranes.

Membranes without Pore-Formers

For water-insoluble pore-free membranes (e.g., from ethyl cellulose or methyl methacrylate) it must be ensured that the active ingredient is soluble in the film-forming material(s) and the molecular weight of the API should not be larger than 500. At the interface between the drug and membrane, the drug will first dissolve in and subsequently diffuse across the membrane to be released into the intestinal fluids. This method of membrane diffusion to control drug release requires that the distribution coefficient of the drug is in favor of the membrane. Options to control drug release are provided by adequate selection of the membrane-forming polymer (diffusion coefficient) and membrane thickness. However, only rather low release rates are usually obtained with these kind of membranes.

Membranes with Pores

Nowadays mostly porous membranes are applied because they are permeable to both water and the dissolved active ingredient. For the production of porous membranes, water-insoluble film-forming polymers (e.g., ethylcellulose) are processed together with water-soluble film-forming polymers (e.g., polyethylene glycol, water-soluble cellulose derivatives). In contact with intestinal juice, the water-soluble polymer dissolves, thus generating pores in the membrane. The extent of porosity can be accurately adjusted to the requirements by informed choice of the nature and the proportion of the hydrophilic components. A further option to control drug release is membrane thickness. The flow of liquid entering the tablet core through the pores results in dissolution of the drug and creates a concentrated solution inside the formulation. The drug is released by diffusion, ideally at a constant rate (zero order). Depending on its solubility, part of the active ingredient may also diffuse across the water-insoluble membrane, albeit at an essentially lower rate.

Disintegrating Membranes

For formulations (predominantly pellets and granules) with a water-permeable coating, water permeates across the membrane into the formulation. This results in a high internal pressure, which causes rupture of the coating membrane. The time required for the formulation to disintegrate depends on the permeability of the membrane to water but more so on membrane thickness. By mixing coated products such as granules with different coating thicknesses, in an adequate ratio, a constant drug release over an extended period is achieved, because of the time-dependent disintegration of the differently coated granules. Such mixtures of granules are usually filled into gelatin capsules.

pH-dependent Dissolution of the Membrane

Likewise, gelatin capsules may be filled with micro-formulations (e.g., pellets) that are partly untreated and partly coated with a gastro-resistant film. While the former will release the drug already in the stomach, the latter will release it only in the small intestine. For film-forming polymers with different pH-dependent solubility values, the drug will be released gradually as a function of pH along the intestinal tract. Through varying membrane thickness and proper choice of the film-forming polymers, time-controlled drug release may be achieved.

Today, membrane systems are only used for micro-formulations (e.g., pellets), as the danger of dose-dumping for monolithic tablets is too high. If the membrane is damaged, the whole dose may be then released in a short period causing side effects or intoxication.

12.6.3.2   Embedding in Matrices

Nonporous Matrices

When active ingredients are embedded in polymers (ethyl cellulose, amino-methacrylate, PVAc/PVP), nondegradable fats or carnauba wax, solubility of the drug in the matrix is a prerequisite for drug release. However, a uniform release pattern is usually not obtained in these cases. While molecules located in the matrix close to the tablet surface will be released quickly, molecules located in the inner core require a relatively long time to diffuse to the tablet surface and thus be released (Fig. 12-9).

This diffusion-controlled release can be described mathematically by the square root rule (see equation 12-2 or section 15.6.4.4).

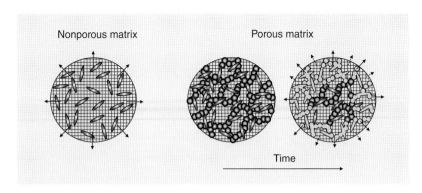

Fig. 12-9   Drug diffusion through pore-free or porous matrix systems.

Porous Matrices

For the production of porous matrices, relatively large proportions of active substance or mixtures of drug with a hydrophilic excipient (e.g., PEG) are compressed together with a matrix-forming excipient, in such a way that during compression a coherent network of drug or drug/excipient particles is formed. After administration of such a tablet, intestinal fluids rapidly dissolve the surface-located drug (initial dosage). Due to the slower dissolution of the drug (when applicable including also the hydrophilic pore-forming excipient) in the inner part of the matrix, pores are gradually formed within the matrix network. Through these pores the drug residing in the interior of the matrix is slowly released further (depot dosage). The drug-depleted framework is not digested and will be excreted as such. In contrast to other tablet types, the release rate from matrix tablets is only marginally influenced by peristaltic movement, amount of fluid, viscosity, surface tension, electrolyte concentration and is in most cases not even influenced by pH values (Fig. 12-9). The extent of release depends on the mass ratio between water-soluble components (drug or drug/excipient mixture) and the matrix-forming excipient, but also on the drug concentration as well as on the number and structure of the pores in the matrix (straight *vs.* angular). The release is also diffusion-controlled and follows the square-root rule, but the pores inside the matrix will increase the diffusion rate, depending on number, length, branches, and form of the pores.

Hydrogel Matrix

When formulations containing high proportions (20%–25%) of undigestible swelling excipients such as HPMC, HPC, or PVA are compressed (when applicable together with other suitable excipients) into tablets, hydro-colloid matrix tablets are formed. Upon contact with water or digestive fluids, initially rapid drug release occurs. At the same time, however, hydration and gel formation will occur at the interface between fluid and tablet core, resulting in the formation of a gel barrier. This hampers the contact between the drug enclosed in the tablet core and the surrounding fluids. Over the course of time, however, the tablet will become completely saturated leading to an increase in volume and an overall swelling of the matrix (Fig. 12-10). The rate of drug release depends on both the penetration of fluid into the matrix and the diffusion rate of the drug across the gel layer formed. The developing gel layer is pore-free and is the main diffusion barrier for the drug molecule dissolved in the hydrogel matrix. The thickness of the gel layer is a function of time, as the more fluid penetrates the more gel is formed. While initially the drug release proceeds rapidly, it slows down due to the increasing diffusion path length. During passage through the gut, drug release is therefore attained by diffusion as well as by the gradual mechanical erosion of the outer gel layers. This is depicted in Fig. 12-11 as Diffusion + Erosion. The release profile of this mixed effect is called *anomalous transport* and has, according to the Ritger and Peppas equation (equation 12-2), an n-value between 0.5 and 1 (Fig. 12-11).

Manufacturing of such hydrogel-forming matrix tablets—with virtually pH- and enzyme-independent drug release within a period of 6 to 8 hours—is relatively simple. A certain degree of control over the drug release can be achieved by variation of the degree of polymerization of the hydrogel-forming polymer.

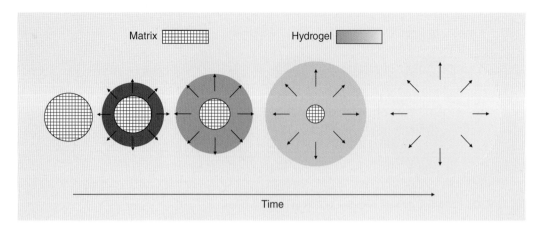

Fig. 12-10   Drug diffusion from a hydrogel matrix.

Among the most commonly used gel-forming polymers are cellulose derivatives (methyl-, hydroxymethyl-, hydroxypropyl-, sodium carboxy-methyl cellulose), copolymers of methacrylic acid (methyl-methacrylate, 2-hydroxy-methyl methacrylate), galacto-mannan, and alginates.

When an active pharmaceutical ingredient is compressed into tablets together with alginic acid in the presence of Ca^{2+} ions and water, a sponge-like, water-insoluble but swellable calcium alginate matrix is formed, because of salt formation between the carboxyl groups of alginic acid and cations. Slow release of the incorporated drug proceeds by drug dissolution and diffusion.

An interesting, but nonetheless very rarely applied variation of swelling-mediated drug release, which is not dependent on Fick's diffusion law is shown in Figs. 12-11 and 12-12 (erosion). A glass-like polymer contains an embedded active ingredient. After administration, intestinal juice slowly penetrates into the surface of the tablet. The surface becomes gel-like and erosion starts, liberating the polymer and the active ingredient is released. This erosion proceeds with a constant rate and uniform drug release can be achieved with $n = 1$ (Fig. 12-11).

Ritger & Peppas developed a simple formulae (equation 12-2), which describes the release of drugs from matrix formulations not necessarily being a sphere. It covers all release mechanism discussed here and can also be applied to parenteral depot formulations.

$$\frac{M_t}{M_\infty} = k \cdot t^n \tag{12-2}$$

$\frac{M_t}{M_\infty}$ is the fractional drug release, t is the release time, and n is the diffusional exponent.

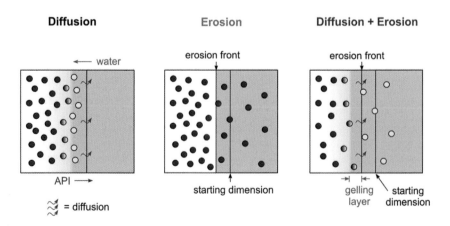

Fig. 12-11   Schematic drawing of drug release mechanisms from different matrix systems (redrawn after Wagner, 2016).

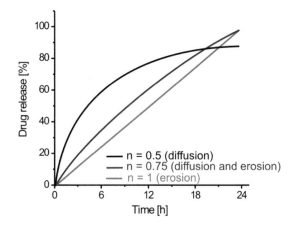

Fig. 12-12 Simulated drug release profiles for the different matrix systems (Fig. 12-11) (redrawn after Wagner 2016).

If the experimentally obtained release data are plotted over time (see Fig. 12-12 for simulated curves), the release mechanism can be estimated from the calculated value of n.

For example:

- Diffusion type (e.g., an inert (not degradable) porous matrix formulation) will yield the typical Higuchi-type of release (Fickian diffusion; square-root-law; see also section 15.6.4.4) with an n = 0.5.
- Surface erosion is typical for surface-erodible formulations and will yield a drug release–time relation with an n-value of 1, signifying a zero-order release (for about 70%–90% of the time). This zero-order release is also known as "case II" transport.
- Diffusion + Erosion (e.g., hydrogel) will yield a drug release–time relation with an n-value of about 0.75, varying between > 0.5 and 1.0 (also known as anomalous transport). If the diffusion of the water front into the matrix is considerably smaller than the erosion process, values of n close to 1 will be obtained.

Biodegradable Systems

With biodegradable drug formulations erosion occurs, that is, the diffusion barrier diminishes, based on the gradual disintegration of the matrix material and in some cases even complete dissolution of the matrix itself. A well-known tablet formulation of this type is the lozenge, which does not disintegrate but instead gradually and slowly dissolves while being sucked. Likewise, fat pellets in which the active ingredient is incorporated in a digestible fat, belong in this category and the drug is released as a result of the lipolytic activity in the gastrointestinal tract. Nonetheless, considerable differences in hydrolysis rates by intestinal lipases may occur due to the diverse (fatty acid) composition of natural fats. Therefore, exclusively synthetic triglycerides with a relatively high melting point are applied as carrier substances for this purpose. When well-defined synthetic triglycerides with a known enzymatic hydrolysis rate (short-chain glycerides are hydrolyzed much more rapidly than long-chain glycerides) are used, the enzymatically controlled drug release can be predicted within certain accuracy limits and yield zero-order release kinetics (Figs. 12-11, 12-12).

Most currently available drug formulations contain polymeric excipients and display an erosion process that may proceed according to one of the following three principles:

1. Hydrophilic polymers become insoluble due to hydrolytically unstable cross-linking.
2. Water-insoluble polymers are converted into water-soluble polymers by hydrolysis or protonation of relevant functional groups in the polymer chain.
3. Water-insoluble polymers are broken down into smaller water-soluble fragments by hydrolytic cleavage.

During the production of biodegradable systems that can be broken down uniformly under physiological conditions (pH, enzymes), the active substance and the polymer are dissolved together in an organic solvent. After removal of the solvent, the mixture is further processed (e.g., into tablets).

For peroral use, poly-anhydrides, poly-ortho-esters and synthetic tri- di- and mono-glyerides are the first choice as surface-eroding polymers allowing zero-order release kinetics. The number of oral MR formulations based on biodegradable polymers is still small, but rising. With monolithic formulations (tablets) in particular, uniform passage through the gastrointestinal tract may not always be ensured. However, biodegradable systems become more and more important for parenteral dosage forms (injectables, implants, section 21.6) using also other biocompatible polymers like polylactic acid or polyethylene carbonate.

12.6.4   Peroral Therapeutic Systems

By applying peroral therapeutic systems such as Oros®, zero-order drug release kinetics may be achieved, at least for a certain period. Oros® is an osmosis-driven system and visually resembles a conventional film tablet. In its simplest variant (Fig. 12-13), water penetrates at a constant rate through a semi-permeable membrane (usually consisting of cellulose acetate) into the tablet, reaches the solid drug inside the tablet and dissolves it up to saturation. The dissolved drug produces an osmotic pressure that remains constant as long as nondissolved osmotically active material is present in the tablet core. Other osmotically active excipients such as sodium chloride or mannitol can be added, if the drug itself does not lead to a sufficiently high osmotic pressure. The water flux into the tablet results in an overpressure inside the tablet, which dissipates via an exit opening in the tablet surface. This opening (ca. 100–250 μm) is usually burnt in the membrane with a laser beam.

As long as the osmotic pressure in the tablet remains constant, a uniform outflow of the tablet and thus drug release is achieved. When the concentration of the drug/excipient ultimately drops below the saturation level, the release rate gradually diminishes. The release rate is independent of the acidity and motility of the gastrointestinal tract. Because the membrane only allows passage of water molecules, the other components of the digestive fluid do not enter the tablet. The Oros® system remains unchanged in shape during passage through the digestive tract and is finally excreted. The solubility of the active substance plays a decisive role in the functional potential of the system. In case of too low solubility, the osmotic pressure produced will not be high enough to attain sufficient drug release. When solubility is too high, the saturated solution is diluted too rapidly, leading to a concomitant drop in release rate. A solubility range between 20% and 40% ensures a sufficiently high osmotic pressure, with a correspondingly sufficient release rate.

The limitation of single-compartment systems to drugs with appropriate solubility properties has led to the development of the push–pull system (Fig. 12-14). With such systems a continuous release pattern may also be achieved for poorly soluble drugs. The core of these tablets consists of two layers, one containing the active substance and the other a gelling agent together with an osmotically active excipient. Both layers are osmotically active and covered by a semipermeable membrane. The exit hole is located at the side of the drug-containing layer. In the drug compartment, the osmosis-driven water flow results in the formation of a drug solution or suspension. This solution is then released from the tablet through the exit opening, due to the pressure arising from the slowly expanding swelling agent in the second layer. Most such systems currently available on the market are constructed according to this principle. Examples are Cardular PP®, Jurnista®, and Concerta® containing doxazosin, hydromorphon, and methylphenidat as the active substance, respectively. The applied technology is quite flexible and allows, for example, the inclusion of an additional drug-containing layer in the core of the tablet, with a different drug concentration. By applying a coating containing an initial dose, further modification of the drug release pattern may be obtained.

12.6.5   Additional Retard Formulations

The extent of drug absorption from the gastrointestinal tract is generally limited by the residence time of the formulation in the stomach and the upper regions of the small intestine. The latter is considered the major absorption site and represents the absorption window for most drugs. As a result of a prolonged residence time in the stomach, together with a slow

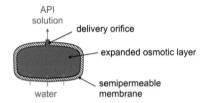

Fig. 12-13 Schematic representation of a single-compartment Oros® system.

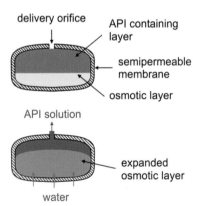

Fig. 12-14 Schematic representation of a push-pull Oros® (upper drawing) and in function (bottom drawing).

drug release, small quantities of drug will pass the absorption window, while full exploitation of the latter facilitates optimal drug absorption. Two strategies have been explored to prolong the residence time in the stomach.

The first approach aims at attaining the same blood level profile with a single dose per day using a *floating controlled release dosage form* (floating capsules), compared to three times per day with a conventional dosage form. The formulation contains hydrocolloids that swell in the gastric juice and, due to the inclusion of air, results in a lower density than that of gastric fluid, resulting in flotation of the dosage form on the gastric fluid. The Madopar®-MR floating capsule contains, among others, hydrated plant oil and the gel-forming polymer methyl-hydroxy-propyl cellulose. The *housekeeper effect* of the empty stomach (squeezing out the last remaining food from the stomach) and the assurance of reproducibility of absorption are critical parameters for the functional potential of this concept, as large variations in gastric residence time may occur (section 12.3). Moreover, the position of the patient (i.e., upright *vs.* lying position) may also have an impact.

The other strategy focuses on *adhesive drug formulations*, which adhere to the stomach wall via interaction with the gastric mucosa resulting in prolonged residence time in the stomach. However, final conclusions about safety—occurrence of local irritations cannot be excluded—and efficiency, cannot be drawn as yet.

More favorable possibilities for the design of prolonged-release dosage forms would emerge if drug absorption would occur in the colon. Up to now, however, absorption from the colon has only been demonstrated for a few drugs such as theophyllin, glibenclamid, and metoprolol.

12.7 Testing

The testing of peroral dosage forms with modified drug release is more complicated than that of immediate release formulations and also requires more time to accomplish. In principle, the methods used for conventional dosage forms (section 9.8) may also be applied in this case, except that they need to be performed at 37°C. Drug release is usually tested in media with defined pH and, when applicable, a pH change mimicking the pH change occurring in the gastro-intestinal tract. Exceptionally, artificial digestive fluids are used, including the addition of enzymes. The paddle or rotating basket method is the preferred technique to perform this test (section 9.9).

12.7.1 Methods to Simulate pH Changes

The half-change method is the oldest method to test peroral MR formulations with pH-dependent release, as well as gastro-resistant dosage forms. During the testing, at each pre-determined time point, half of the test fluid is removed and replaced by solution with another pH to mimic the situation in the gastrointestinal tract, where the pH continuously changes from strongly acid to mildly alkaline (Table 12-3). A pH change may also be accomplished by adding a solid buffer substance, for example a mixture of Tris (tris(hydroxymethyl aminomethane) and sodium acetate. When the test is performed in a flow cell, the different

> Another way to colon delivery is exploiting the bacterial metabolic potential in the colon. About 100 billion CFU/mL of bacteria in the colon have a higher metabolic power than the liver in sum. Specific polysaccharides ("resistant starch") survive pancreatic digestion but are degraded by colon bacteria. Coating of tablets with these starches (and additionally Eudragit S as a dissolvable coating for pH > 7) leads to release of the encapsulated drug after digesting of the film coat by the colon bacteria.

Table 12-3 Half-Change Method According to Ph. Eur. 7.0 (section 5.17.1)

Test Duration (h)	Ratio Test Solution pH 1.2/ Buffer Solution pH 7.5 (%)	pH Value
0-1	100/0	1.2
1-2	50/50	2.5
2–3.5	25/75	4.5
3.5–5.5	12.5/87.5	7.0
5.5->7	6.25/93.75	7.5

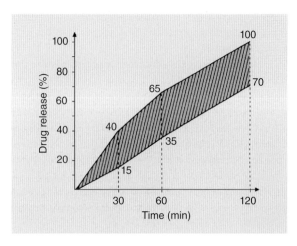

Fig. 12-15 Requirements of the USP XXIII concerning the in vitro drug release from formulations with modified release properties (example phenytoin retard capsules). The released amount of drug should be within the hatched region.

pH regions in the GIT can be simulated by pH changes of the test fluid, mostly done by a pH gradient.

12.7.2   Acceptance Criteria for the Release from Solid Peroral MR Preparations

In order to ascertain adequate availability, the pharmacopeias and approval authorities require of immediate-release tablets that a minimal amount of drug is released after a certain time (e.g., at least 75% after maximally 45 min). For prolonged-release dosage forms, the acceptance criteria for drug release are determined at different time points (at least three time points) in order to be able to assess the time profile of drug release. Meaningful time points are, for example, those at which 20% to 30%, about 50% and more than 80% of the drug is released, respectively. As a rule, not only the minimal amount but also the maximal amount of released drug at each point is defined. Thus, the amounts of released drug are fixed between a lower and an upper limit (Fig. 12-15).

12.7.3   Testing of Bioavailability and Bioequivalence

In bioavailability tests, MR formulations are characterized by the *AUC*, c_{max} value and *plateau times*. The plateau time indicates the time during which the plasma concentration of the drug lies above a certain predetermined value, for example the minimal effective concentration, MEC. The plateau time is most commonly approximated without any further mathematical effort directly from the plasma curve as the *half value duration, HVD*, representing the time at which the plasma concentration is $\geq$ 50% of the maximal plasma concentration c_{max}. Fig. 12-16 illustrates the characterization of a MR formulation in comparison with an immediate-release dosage form by the indicated plateau times. The c_{max} values of the conventional and the MR form allow conclusions to be drawn about the therapeutically required plasma levels and possible side effects.

Among the additional target values, which are suggested for MR formulations in literature, all requiring considerable mathematical efforts, we will only consider the *mean residence time* (MRT), which represents the average residence time of a drug molecule in the organism. The MRT is calculated by means of the statistical moment analysis from the plasma concentration curve according to:

$$MRT = AUMC/AUC$$

AUC is the area under the plasma concentration versus time curve:

$$AUC = \int_0^\infty C_p \, dt,$$

AUMC is the area under the plasma concentration · time versus time curve:

$$AUMC = \int_0^\infty t \cdot C_p \, dt$$

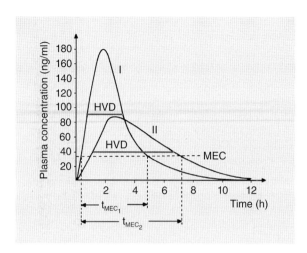

Fig. 12-16 **Comparison of plasma level profiles of formulations with rapid (I) and retarded (II) release, as characterized by half value duration (HVD).**

where AUMC (area under the moment curve) is the area under the first moment curve of the plasma concentration curve.

Conclusions about bioequivalence of MR formulations are based on the typical pharmacokinetic parameters AUC and c_{max}, as well as on comparable plateau times (or, alternatively, comparable MRT values).

Further Reading

Ibekwe, V. C., Khela, M. K., Evans, D. F., and Basit, A. W. "A new concept in colonic drug targeting: a combined pH-responsive and bacterially-triggered drug delivery technology." *Aliment Pharmacol Ther* 28 (7) (2008): 911–916.

Purves, R. D. "Optimum numerical integration methods for estimation of area-under-the-curve (AUC) and area-under-the-moment-curve (AUMC)." *Journal of Pharmacokinetics and Pharmacodynamics* 20 (3) (1992): 211–226.

Ritger, P. L., and Peppas, N. A. "A simple equation for description of solute release I. Fickian and non-Fickian release from non-swellable devices in the form of slabs, spheres, cylinders or discs." *Journal of Controlled Release* 5 (1) (1987): 23–36.

Wagner, K. G. "Perorale Retardarzneiformen." *Pharmakon* 4 (2) (2016): 107–16.

Uhrich, K. E., Cannizzaro, S. M., Langer, R. S., and Shakesheff, K. M. "Polymeric Systems for Controlled Drug Release." *Chem Rev* 99 (11) (1999): 3181–3198.

13

Rectal Preparations

13.1 General Considerations

Among the preparations intended for rectal application (*rectalia*), suppositories are by far the most widely applied. These are solid, single-dose preparations, mostly of torpedo-like shape, intended for insertion in the rectum. They melt at body temperature or dissolve in an aqueous environment. Suppositories for use by adults generally have a mass of about 2 g; those intended for children about 1 g. In addition, there are some other solid, liquid and semi-solid preparations for rectal application (see section 13.8).

Rectal drug formulations were already used in ancient Egypt and Mesopotamia and were applied both for local as well as for systemic treatment. In those days, the formulations were either based on tallow or simply were plugs of wool soaked in fat containing the active ingredient. The use of soap suppositories as laxatives was introduced by Galenus (Galen of Pergamon). The ancient Greeks already applied wax as suppository base. In the Middle Ages lard, tallow, wax, and soap were used for this purpose. Around 1750, the French pharmacist Baumé recommended cocoa butter, a substance discovered 100 years earlier, for the preparation of suppositories. Glycerol-based suppositories were invented in 1888.

Rectal therapy offers several advantages over other application routes, such as peroral administration. This seems obvious for local therapeutic treatment of rectal disorders; additional advantages include the circumvention of the first-pass effect, the prevention of stomach burden and bad taste sensation, the possibility to use it for patients with swallowing problems (children, elderly) or in case of nausea and vomiting. Of particular relevance is the use of suppositories in pediatrics. Especially in case of very young children, medication can be administered much more easily this way than orally. Potential disadvantages include possibly incomplete drug availability in case of premature emptying of the device and the higher production costs in comparison with simple tablets. In addition, it appears that the acceptance of this dosage form varies considerably by region and culture. In Southern European and Latin American countries, for example, suppositories are prescribed much more frequently than in Northern Europe and Anglo-Saxon countries. Primarily, esthetic considerations (the "shocking way of application") have thus far prohibited widespread use in these countries.

In addition to the treatment of hemorrhoids and as a laxative, both aiming at a local effect, systemically active suppositories carrying antipyretic, anti-rheumatic, analgesic drugs or sedatives are the dominating formulations of this type. Liquid preparations for rectal administration are employed for the treatment of inflammatory disease of the rectum and the lower sections of the colon, as well as to serve as a contrast agent for imaging purposes.

Voigt's Pharmaceutical Technology, First Edition. Alfred Fahr.
© 2018 John Wiley & Sons Ltd. Published 2018 by John Wiley & Sons Ltd.

13.2   Requirements of Suppositories and Their Components

Suppository bases as well as the suppositories produced from those have to meet a series of requirements. First of all, they should be physiologically inert and lack irritating effects on the rectum. The latter may be provoked by oversized dimensions of the device, irritating constituents (free fatty acids, rancidness), inappropriate hardness, but also by insufficient comminution of the active substance grains. The bases need to be chemically stable and should not display incompatibilities with the active ingredient. When relevant for the processing of the respective active ingredient, the bases should possess a certain capacity to absorb lipophilic or hydrophilic fluids.

Because suppositories are mostly manufactured by means of a casting procedure, thermal properties of the components play an important role. The interval between the slip point and the final melting temperature of the ground substance should be narrow. This is important for shape retention and also for storage stability, especially at higher temperatures. Appropriate viscosity of the melt will reduce sedimentation of suspended drug grains in the preparation vessel and thus contributes to dosing precision. The interval between melting and solidification point should be minimal in order to ensure that the melt will quickly solidify in the mold after casting. This prevents sedimentation of suspended drug particles in the mold and avoids a lengthy solidification process. A significant contraction during solidification will facilitate the removal of the suppository from the mold. The formation of unstable modifications during the solidification process that may cause unfavorable melting points should be prevented.

In the solidified suppositories, there should be no significant alterations of chemical and physical properties (e.g., as a result of polymorphic transitions, post-production hardening, softening, chemical degradation), ensuring proper storage stability. After administration, the suppository should melt or dissolve within a few minutes at body temperature, thus releasing its active component. Ideally, the suppository base should also promote uniform spreading of the melted mass on the rectal mucosa and the absorption of the active ingredient.

13.3   Suppository Bases

Suppository bases can be categorized in fats and fatty substances yielding a formulation that melts at body temperature, and water-soluble substances that release the incorporated drug by dissolution. Nowadays, suppositories for rectal administration are predominantly based on hard fat. For pessaries (chapter 14), hard fat as wells as macrogols are used. Gelatinous mixtures—for example, based on glycerol-gelatin mixtures—have lost their role almost completely and are only sometimes employed for the extemporaneous preparation of pessaries.

13.3.1   Oleaginous Bases

13.3.1.1   Cocoa Butter (Theobroma Oil)

For a long time, cocoa butter (section 5.3.8.3) served as standard suppository base and it is still referred to in many pharmacopeias. Cocoa butter is chemically inert and physiologically well tolerated. It is stable in shape at room temperature and has a favorable melting range just below body temperature (31°–34°C). Cocoa butter suppositories have an appealing appearance and melt quickly (~5 minutes) at body temperature. As a disadvantage, cocoa butter may become rancid and it displays an extremely complex polymorphic behavior, which may severely hamper handling during the casting process. Furthermore, it lacks emulsifying properties. For all these reasons it has been replaced almost completely by synthetic bases, in particular, hard fat (see 13.3.1.2).

When processing cocoa butter, care needs to be taken that no metastable modifications are formed upon solidification, as those will cause an unfavorable melting behavior. In order to ensure that solidification occurs in the stable β-modification, which has the optimal melting point of 34°C, the cocoa butter should be carefully melted. The processing temperature should not exceed 34°C in order to preserve a certain amount of nonmelted fat components (see 13.4.1). Alternatively, only 90% of the required cocoa butter is melted to clarity, and the remaining 10% is added in grated form, which then is mixed with the melted mass right before the casting procedure. Cocoa butter has a relatively low contractibility. Upon solidification, it tends to stick at the mold; therefore, this needs to be lubricated, for instance, with fluid paraffin before casting. To minimize sedimentation of suspended drug particles in the melted cocoa butter, continuous stirring during the casting process is mandatory. Certain additives, such as oils, cause a strong melting point depression. In such cases, the inclusion of consistency-enhancing excipients (wax, cetyl alcohol) is recommended. At the site of administration, the rectum, there are no enzymes to cleave fat molecules; the cocoa butter is thus not absorbed. It rather forms a fatty film on the rectal mucosa.

13.3.1.2 Hard Fat

By cleavage of natural fats, fractionation of the resulting fatty acids, hydrogenation and selective esterification to a mixture of mono-, di-, and triglycerides, products are obtained that largely meet the ideal requirements of suppository bases. In the Ph. Eur., they are designated hard fat and are described in detail in section 5.3.8.13. There are a large number of hard fat types commercially available, which can be distinguished with respect to melting range, content of partial glycerides with emulsifying and wetting properties (in partial glycerides the glycerol moieties are not fully esterified with fatty acids), and potentially further additives like emulsifiers. This makes it possible to find a suitable hydrogenated fat type for practically each possible formulation requirement. Unlike cocoa butter, hard fats can also be processed from the clear melt. Due to the contractility of the fat mass, lubrication of the molds is usually not required. Like cocoa butter, hard fat is well compatible with most active ingredients.

13.3.2 Water-Soluble High-Melting Substances (Macrogols)

In certain cases, such as application in tropical areas, the use of high-melting suppository bases may be required. Because such formulations will not melt upon administration, the incorporated drug has to be released by means of dissolution of the base. This requirement is fulfilled by substances based on high-molecular weight macrogols (poly(ethyleneglycol), section 5.4.4.9). The water solubility of these polymers is based on the formation of hydrogen bonds between the ether oxygen and water molecules. The dissolution of macrogol-based suppositories in the rectum is, however, not optimal due to the limited amounts of water available at that site: 1 to 2 mL of fluid spread out along the 16 to 20 cm long rectum. Although the dissolution of such suppositories may be enhanced by secretion of corresponding amounts of fluid into the intestinal lumen as a result of osmotic forces, this requires a relatively long time. In addition, the resulting flow of fluid proceeds opposite the direction of absorption and, furthermore, the osmotic effect may irritate the rectal mucosa.

Some commercial bases consist of highly polymeric macrogols, with an average molecular mass of 6,000 and melting points between 54° and 60°C, and dissolve only slowly. A macrogol with low melting range (47°–49°C) and better solubility contains equal parts of macrogols 1,000 and 2,000 with a water supplement of 10% to 15%. Mixtures of shorter- and longer-chain macrogols are often applied. The quite-stable macrogols (Carbowax, Polywax®) are good solvents for a variety of drugs, which may cause a retardation of drug absorption. Further disadvantages are the hardness and the post-production hardening that may occur, the risk of peroxide formation, and the potential presence of reducing substances. The latter may lead to incompatibilities with a variety of active agents (e.g., silver salts, tannins, aminophenazone, quinine, acetyl salicylic acid, ammonium bituminosulfonate, Peru balsam, penicillin, and some sulfonamides). Although the post-production hardening may be suppressed by the addition of softening agents (glycerol, wool fat), the dissolution time in water of 37°C remains long. Despite the limitations with respect to the application of macrogols, some studies report the attainment of considerable absorption rates also with bases of that type. Supplementation with an emulsifier or lactose may improve absorption from macrogol bases.

13.3.3   Water-Soluble Gelatinous Materials

The elastic glycerol-gelatin gels, which become fluid at body temperature, are the main representative of this group.

Gelatin (section 5.3.4.5) swells in water and dissolves therein upon heating. At concentrations starting at about 1.5% transparent, elastic gels are formed at room temperature, which may serve as a basis for the manufacturing of officinal gels such as, for instance, zinc gelatin. Gelatin gels show a reversible thermal gel-sol-gel conversion, i.e. during heating the gel fluidizes into a sol, while upon lowering the temperature gel formation sets in again.

Glycerol provides the gel with suppleness and promotes the cross-linking of the gelatin gel framework. Increasing proportions of glycerol enhance the consistency of the gel. Nonetheless, the glycerol content of suppository bases to be used for rectal administration should be kept as low as possible, since glycerol at larger concentrations acts as a laxative. Rectal administration of elastic glycerol-gelatin suppositories may bring along some difficulties. That is one of the main reasons why other substances have a much wider application range and glycerol-gelatin is preferably used for vaginal preparations. A commonly applied formulation consists of 1 part gelatin, 2 parts water, and 5 parts 85% glycerol.

An advantage of such bases is their rapid disintegration following administration. This is based on the gel-sol transition of the base in combination with its miscibility with the aqueous medium at the site of administration and the osmotic properties of glycerol. A disadvantage is that the suppositories (or the glycerol-gelatin gel) constitute a good substrate for microorganisms, especially at low glycerol content. Preparations based on glycerol-gelatin gels should be freshly prepared and may in certain cases be preserved with for instance 0.15% p-hydroxy-benzoic acid esters. Preparations should be stored in a cool environment and in a tightly closed container. This will help prevent microbial spoilage and gradual drying out of the material. Metal and polymer foil or polymer containers are suitable as packaging materials for glycerol-gelatin suppositories or pessaries. In the presence of incompatible components hardening or destruction of the gel network may occur. Incompatible substances include salicylic acid, tannins and tannin-containing preparations, soluble aluminum and ammonium salts, chloral hydrate as well as some stronger acids and bases. Such incompatibilities are not always immediately recognizable. Shape and elasticity of the gel may remain largely intact, but in spite of that such preparations lose their capacity to dissolve in an aqueous milieu. Glycerol-based laxative suppositories may also be produced by gelation of a glycerol-water mixture by means of alkali soaps (glycerol-soap suppositories). For example, after dissolving stearic acid and sodium carbonate in diluted heated glycerol dimensionally stable gels are formed upon cooling.

13.4   Formulation and Manufacturing

Manufacturing techniques may be distinguished in molding and compression procedures. In particular in the industrial practice nowadays, manufacturing procedures are used that simultaneously lead to optimal packaging (chapter 27).

13.4.1   The Molding Procedure

Suppositories are produced almost exclusively by the molding (casting) technique, both in manual procedures and at industrial scale.

When the base has melted and has been combined with the active ingredient, it is poured out in the molds. To ensure rapid solidification and thus to prevent sedimentation of suspended drug particles, the temperature used in the melting process should become not too high. That is achieved by very careful warming (e.g., water bath of <40°C). If required (e.g.,

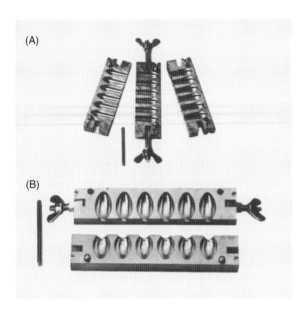

Fig. 13-1 Molds for (A) suppositories and (B) pessaries (Wepa Apothekenbedarf, Germany).

in the case of cocoa butter suppositories), the mass is not melted to complete clarity—that is, both melted and nonmelted particles of the base are present, which lends the mixture a creamy appearance and high viscosity. During the casting, the material should possess maximal viscosity and a temperature only slightly above the congealing point. Continuous and intensive stirring of the material is essential. The casting of small batches of suppositories is performed in a single cast. That is, the individual molds are filled consecutively. At the industrial or semi-industrial scale, on the other hand, simultaneous filling of multiple or all individual molds is achieved by means of suitable funnel-shaped devices.

The molds can consist of different materials. While in former days brass molds were dominating, currently for small-scale production, light metal molds are commercially available. Fig. 13-1 presents mold shapes for suppositories and pessaries. They have a capacity of ca. 2 g (adults) or ca. 1 g (children), and 3 g (vaginal preparations), respectively, and consist of longitudinally partitioned semi- molds that can be held together by screws, clamps, or straps.

While for officinal formulations molds with 6, 12, and 24 holes are common, in industrial production, molds with 500 or even more casting channels were used in earlier days. Because the release of the solidified suppositories from longitudinally divided molds may occasionally cause problems nowadays preference is sometimes given to cross-divided molds. These consist of a top and a bottom part and contain the suppositories, after opening of the mold, partly in the upper and partly in the lower half. From such molds, the products can be removed much more easily. Water should not be used to clean the molds. Using detergents is even more discouraged. They bring along the risk of surface oxidation of the molds, which may take on a gray color. To remove residues of the suppository material from the molds, a mixture of alkali soap and ethanol may be used. It is absolutely prohibited to use metal objects for cleaning. Any scratch resulting from such treatment will affect the smoothness of the suppository surface and may in addition hamper the release of the suppository from the mold. Suppositories cast in metal molds must be individually packed, such as in aluminum foil, for dispensing.

For the sake of efficiency, extemporaneously prepared suppositories are often cast in prefabricated disposable polymer molds that simultaneously act as packaging material. Immediately following the casting process, the suppositories should be cooled; if not, they will solidify too slowly. The disposable molds have a well-standardized volume, do not need to be cleaned, allow processing under strictly hygienic conditions, and at the same time lend the final product good protection. A disadvantage is that visual inspection of the product is usually impossible. In industrial production, casting proceeds exclusively in preformed package foils, which are mostly produced directly by the suppository-filling machine. The melted, medicated suppository base is poured in the molds by means of a dosing pump.

> Extemporaneous compounding is the preparation of a therapeutic product for an individual patient in response to an identified need.

13.4.2   Compression Procedure

The compression procedure can be applied both manually and at the industrial level. The starting material consists of a mixture of grated suppository base with finely powdered active agent. This starting material is filled into a suppository press and squeezed through a narrow opening into the mold by means of a piston, which is brought in motion by a shaft. A special device then expels the resulting suppository. All common commercially available suppository bases are more or less suitable for the production of compressed suppositories. When required, plasticizers (fluid paraffin, wool fat) may be added to minimize brittleness. Several suppository presses possess connections for water cooling to dissipate the heat produced by the compression. Larger machines are able to produce several suppositories in parallel. The suppository molds of such machines can be exchanged for pessary molds. It is also possible to prepare compressed suppositories in tablet press-like devices that can be cooled and are equipped with special sets of punches. The compression technique may be interesting for the processing of thermo-labile drugs. In principle, however, the compression method comes with more difficulties than the casting technique, particularly with respect to the required homogeneity of the suppositories and the achievement of appropriate fracture strength. The compression method is less suitable for fluid active agents.

13.4.3   Directions for the Processing of Particular Active Agents

When suppositories need to be produced with lipophilic fluids such as oils (castor oil, cod liver oil), essential oils, ammonium bituminosulfonate (ichthyol) and so on, it should be taken into account that such substances will lower the melting range of the base, which may lead to technological problems. In such case, it is recommended to use special suppository bases with a higher melting range. Alternatively, small but appropriate amounts of a consistency enhancer such as wax may be added to the standard base. Also, viscosity enhancers such as colloidal silica may be considered for this purpose. The latter may also be used to adsorb fluids, including hydrophilic fluids (such as fluid extracts), prior to processing them in the melted base. Small quantities of hydrophilic fluids may be readily processed in oleaginous bases spiked with an emulsifier, leading to the formation of solid(ified) W/O emulsions.

The melting process may be complicated and viscosity may be strongly increased when high proportions of powdered drugs are suspended in the fatty material. This can be counteracted by addition of small amounts of lecithin or by applying special low-melting bases.

For the processing of aggregating active ingredients such as aminophylline, phenyl butazone, papaverin hydrochloride, as well as hygroscopic substances (e.g., dry extracts), trituration with colloidal silica has shown its value.

13.5   The Suppository as a Disperse System

Depending on the distribution of the active ingredient in the base, suppositories may be classified either as a suspension or as a solution suppository. Emulsion suppositories, which are formed upon processing of immiscible fluids (e.g., fluid extracts), are rarely used and often show unsatisfactory microbiological and chemical stability.

13.5.1   Suspension Suppositories

In general, the solubility of the active ingredient in suppository bases tends to be poor. Therefore, the former is usually present in a suspended form (solidified suspension). In order to attain a uniform distribution of the active ingredient among all suppositories and thus high dose accuracy, during the casting process sedimentation of the drug particles in the melted base must be avoided. For that purpose, intensive stirring is required and the viscosity of the melted mass should be kept as high as possible. That can be achieved by keeping the temperature just above the congealing point during the casting procedure. It is furthermore important that, once in the mold, the melt solidifies rapidly, in order to prevent a nonuniform distribution of the drug particles within individual suppositories. This would cause an enrichment of the drug particles in the tip of the suppository, which, in turn, may have a substantial influence on the mechanical stability of the suppository. Keep in mind that even vigorous stirring, although diminishing sedimentation, will not prevent this process completely, as it will terminate only after the melt is completely solidified.

According to Stokes' law, the sedimentation velocity

$$v = \frac{2}{9} \frac{r^2 (\rho_1 - \rho_2) g}{\eta} \qquad (13\text{-}1)$$

| r = particle radius | ρ_1 density of the suspended phase
| ρ_2 = density of the continuous phase | η viscosity of the continuous phase
| g = gravitational acceleration.

However, Stokes' law does not apply in this case because we are dealing here with swarm sedimentation. Therefore, under these conditions, the valid proportionality equation merely reads:

$$v \propto \frac{\bar{r} \cdot (\rho_1 - \rho_2)}{\eta} \qquad (13\text{-}2)$$

| $\bar{r}$ = average radius

Accordingly, a prerequisite for satisfactory dose accuracy is a very small size of the drug particles. This is also required to exclude irritation of the rectal mucosa by coarse crystals and to facilitate the dissolution of the drug after administration. A further influential factor is the difference between the density of the suspension medium (melted base) and that of the suspended phase, that is, the active ingredient. Since the density of inorganic active agents (e.g., Bismuth salts) is substantially higher than that of organic substances, sedimentation effects will have to be specifically taken into account when processing such substances. To improve dose accuracy by affecting viscosity when using the casting procedure, viscosity-enhancing additives (e.g., glycerol mono-stearate, aluminum stearate, bentonite, colloidal silica) are recommended. These are able to considerably increase viscosity (Table 13-1), but on the other hand, they may seriously interfere with drug release due to binding of the drug to several of such additives. Finally, when applying such excipients, it should be taken into consideration that the pharmacopeia requirements concerning softening time and disintegration of suppositories need to be met.

13.5.2   Solution Suppositories

In some cases, active ingredients can be dissolved in the suppository base. However, for most drugs, solubility in an oleaginous base is low. Exceptions are: camphor 8%; procaine 1%;

Table 13-1 Viscosity Increase of Witepsol H 15® by Excipients

Suppository Base / Excipient	Apparent Viscosity (mPa · s) at 40°C
Pure suppository base with	31
2% glycerol stearate	38
5% glycerol stearate	55
2% aluminum stearate	55
5% aluminum stearate	100
2% bentonite	200
5% bentonite	400
2% colloidal silica	330
5% colloidal silica	648

chloral hydrate 5%. Marked solubility may also be observed for balsams and oils. Generally, however, solubility is so low that it becomes of minor importance. Although during the melting process solubility markedly increases, a substantial fraction of the drug molecules recrystallizes during solidification of the base. The melting and congealing points of fatty bases are depressed when relatively large quantities of active ingredient are dissolved. This may lead to production problems, while such products may also lack sufficient firmness. In these cases either the use of special bases (increased melting range) or addition of 1% to 3% colloidal silica may be recommendable. As a rule, with solution suppositories, lower drug absorption is observed than with the suspension counterpart, as the drugs tend to be retained in the base.

13.6   Dosing Methods

13.6.1   Application of Displacement Values

In this procedure the necessary amount of suppository base is determined by calculation. To that end firstly the holding capacity of the suppository mold (calibration value) is determined by filling all individual mold forms with pure base. After solidification and removal of the excess the suppositories are taken from the mold and weighed and the average mass is calculated as the calibration value. Since the various drugs to be processed into suppositories vary in density, they displace different amounts of base. This behavior is expressed by the displacement value f, which indicates how many grams of a certain base are displaced by 1 gram of active ingredient.

Factor f may be formally calculated from:

$$f = \text{density of the base / density of the active ingredient} \qquad (13\text{-}3)$$

The displacement values can be determined experimentally for the casting procedure and are listed in tables for established active agents as well as excipients. A selection is presented in Table 13-2. The values depend to a certain extent on the physical form and some other parameters of the active ingredient (water content, voluminous or compact form, solubility

Table 13-2 Displacement Values (Selection) According to a German Formularium (Suppository Base: Hard Fat; Clear Melt)

Active Ingredient	Displacement Value
Benzocaine	0.83
Bisacodyl	0.76
Bismuth gallate, alkaline	0.37
Butoxycaine hydrochloride	0.82
Codeine monohydrate	0.74
Diazepam	0.70
Diclofenac sodium	0.64
Hydrocortisone acetate	0.73
Ibuprofen	0.90
Indomethacin	0.68
Metamizole sodium monohydrate	0.70
Metronidazole	0.67
Morphine hydrochloride tri-hydrate	0.80
Nystatin	0.77
Oxazepam	0.63
Papaverine hydrochloride	0.72
Paracetamol	0.72
Prednisolone acetate	0.75
Procaine hydrochlorid	0.80
Propyphenazone	0.84
Quinine hydrochloride di-hydrate	0.76
Sulfanilamide	0.62
Theophylline	0.66
Zink oxide	0.16

in the base), but also on the nature of the base and the selected preparation procedure. That is why, for accurate dosing, it is recommended to experimentally determine the displacement value for each individual set of processing conditions. The calculation of the required amount of suppository base follows from the following formula:

$$M_n = n(\bar{E} - fA) \tag{13-4}$$

| M_n = mass of base required for n suppositories (g)
| n = number of suppositories to be produced
| E = calibration value
| f = displacement value
| A = amount of active ingredient (g) per suppository

For suppositories with multiple active ingredients Equation 13-5 applies:

$$M_n = n\left(\bar{E} - \sum f_i A_i\right) \tag{13-5}$$

| $\Sigma f_i A_i$ = sum of all products of f and A for the drugs under consideration.

To compensate for production-related losses (e.g., residues in or on casting dishes, pestle) an excess of up to 30% (active agent and base) is recommended for the production of a relatively small number of suppositories. For larger numbers the loss compensation is lower.

13.6.2 Volumetric Dosing Methods

With these methods, the amount of starting material needed for a specific formulation is determined volumetrically. This can be done in analogy to the determination of the calibration value of the casting mold and involves the assessment of the volume taken by the suppository melt, for example by means of a graded casting beaker (Fig. 13-2). Specialized beakers may be provided with a double wall serving as a water bath and a thermometer to control melting and casting temperature.

The casting material is prepared by levigation of the comminuted active ingredient with melted suppository base and later filling it up to the mark.

Also the method of double casting is based on the volumetric dosing principle. With this method the active ingredient is first mixed with only part of the required base and this mass is poured into the molds, only partly filling them. The mold is then filled up completely with pure melted suppository base. Thus, the required quantity of base is determined empirically, but no homogeneous drug distribution has been attained between drug and vehicle.

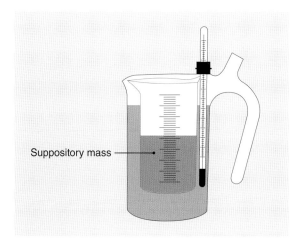

Suppository mass

Fig. 13-2 Casting beaker.

To achieve this, the solidified suppositories are removed from the molds, melted and the melt is casted once more in the molds. This method is suited for officinal production of suppositories. An obvious disadvantage is the higher expenditure of time and labor. Furthermore, the method brings along double exposure to elevated temperatures limiting application for temperature-sensitive ingredients.

13.7   Manufacturing and Packaging Procedures

13.7.1   Manual Casting

Besides the traditional casting of the medicated suppository mass into metal molds by means of pouring bowls, beakers, or bottles, the application of disposable plastic (e.g., PE or PVC) casting molds is gradually gaining acceptance. This procedure makes the removal of the suppositories from the molds and separate packaging superfluous. Prior to filling, the flexible plastic strips containing a series of molds are fitted in a metal frame and suspended in a cooling bath to ensure rapid solidification of the suppository mass. Following solidification and removal of the excess mass, the molds are closed off with a special foil.

13.7.2   Casting Pans for Suppositories

For larger amounts of starting material casting pans with a capacity of 1.5 to 3 L can be used. However, pans with a substantially larger net capacity are available. The casting pan consists of a double-walled vessel, a heating device with thermostat, and a stirrer to counteract sedimentation. The stirrer is constructed in such a way that no air bubbles are introduced in the casting mass, thus preventing the undesired formation of a porous product. Modern equipment allows fully homogeneous mixing of the preweighed added components by a built-in homogenizing device. At a later stage, the rotating speed of the stirrer is reduced to exploit merely the stirring function of the device. In the industrial setting, the individual molds are filled by a thin jet of melt while they pass underneath the casting pan and are then guided on a conveyor belt into a cooling tunnel.

13.7.3   Automatic Filling and Sealing

Separately preformed strips of foil serve as casting molds and primary packaging material. They are filled and sealed by the procedure described below. The capacity of such automatic machines varies from 5,000 to 20,000 suppositories per hour. However, the GMP-compatible storage of the shock-sensitive hollow-mold strips is quite intricate.

13.7.4   Forming, Filling, and Sealing Machines

In these high-capacity production lines with outputs of up to 25.000 suppositories per hour the functional packaging is produced in the first step of the integrated production process from foil by deformation (mostly by deep-drawing) and sealing of the mirror-imaged hemiforms (Fig. 13-3). The compounding, filling and sealing process is characterized by the following individual steps:

1. Melting the suppository base in a heated vessel.
2. Production of the casting mix in a heated container involving a stirring device (or colloid mill) to ensure a homogeneous distribution of the active ingredient.
3. Pumping the highly viscous mass into the casting pan of the filling station.
4. Filling the molds by dosing pumps via hollow needles, each cycle filling 6–15 molds simultaneously, depending on the machine type.

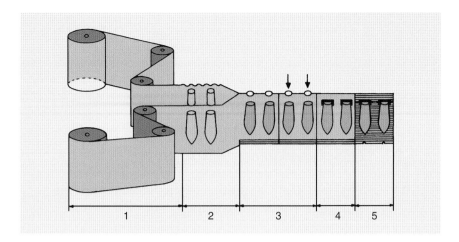

Fig. 13-3   Automatic formation, filling, and sealing of disposable suppository molds.

5. Sealing the filling holes.
6. Application of a batch stamp, bringing on stiffening ribs when required to enhance mechanical firmness, and providing grooves to facilitate withdrawal and perforations to detach the product.
7. Cooling the product by passage through a cooling tunnel.
8. Transport of the portioned strips to the cartoning machine.

Control and safety devices to monitor the functioning of the foil transport and the dosing pumps, to regulate temperature in the casting containers, in the product transport guiding systems and in the cooling tunnel ensure high reliability of the entire production facility.

13.8   Further Rectal Drug Formulations

Rectal tampons are medicated tampons intended to remain for a certain time in the lower section of the rectum. The core of such tampons may consist, for example, of cellulose, impregnated with an active agent. There are suppository-like products of this type, containing a padding mull, which fixes the product at the outer end of the rectum to achieve maximal targeting of a locally active drug. Such products are applied, for example, in the treatment of anal eczema and hemorrhoids.

Rectal capsules are usually torpedo-shaped soft gelatin capsules (section 11.3.2), often coated with a polymer film to facilitate insertion. They should be administered after lubrication with water. The water-soluble capsules cause no irritation effect on the rectal mucosa and ensure rapid drug release as far as no coating-mediated modified release mechanism is involved.

They are packed in moisture-tight glass medicine flasks or sealed polymer or aluminum foil.

Rectal solutions and suspensions are formulations that have to be instilled and are used for instance in the treatment of chronic inflammatory bowel disease or as a laxative. As a rule, these formulations constitute single-dose preparations that can be applied under hygienic conditions by means of an enema flask or bag or as a micro-enema. The latter consists for example of a polymer cannula that is inserted in the rectum up to an integrated ring-shaped bulge. Behind the bulge a small plastic balloon is mounted that contains a few ml of the drug solution. By pressing the balloon the dissolved drug is injected into the rectum. The pharmacopeia also describes rectal emulsions, but these are rarely used. The liquid preparations for rectal application can also be reconstituted immediately prior to use from solid formulations (tablets, powders).

Anti-inflammatory drugs are also applied as *rectal foams*. These belong to the group of the medicated foams. They are commonly prepared immediately before administration from a liquid preparation by means of a propellant gas and then inserted like an enema. Surface active excipients are used to induce foam formation and to enhance stability of the foam; they also contribute to a proper distribution on the intestinal mucosa.

Semi-solid rectal preparations are usually intended for the treatment of anorectal disorders such as hemorrhoids. Options are ointments, creams, and gels; for this application range, most often lipophilic preparations are employed. Depending on the very administration site, a suitable application device may be required.

13.9   Biopharmaceutical Aspects

13.9.1   Physiological Conditions in the Rectum and Their Influence on Bioavailability

The rectum has an average length of 15 to 20 cm and contains about 1 to 3 mL mucus with a pH of 7.4 at low buffer capacity. In the immediate vicinity of the rectal mucosa a pH value of 5.4 is assumed to prevail. The surface area of the human rectum represents only about 0.01% of the entire gastrointestinal tract. The upper part of the rectum, about three quarters of the total length, is called *pars ampullaris* or *ampulla recti*, the lower part is known as *pars canalis analis*. The very opening is formed by the inner and outer sphincter muscle. As a rule, in individuals not suffering from an intestinal disorder the rectum is normally empty. It is filled only shortly before defecation, which triggers the urge to defecate. The elaborate vascularization makes the rectal mucosa a suitable absorption site. The blood is drained from the rectum by three venous strands with two draining directions. While the veins in the lower one third (inferior and middle rectal vein) bring the blood to the systemic circulation (*inferior vena cava*), thus bypassing the primary liver passage, the superior rectal vein drains directly on the mesenteric vein (portal vein, *vena portae*), and thus to the liver (Fig. 13-4).

In as far as absorption occurs in the lower segments of the rectum, primary liver passage and by that also first-pass metabolism of the drug is circumvented. This is important for the bioavailability of active agents that undergo major metabolism during first liver passage. It

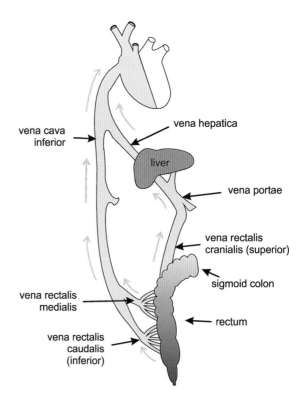

Fig. 13-4 Venous systems of the rectum.

should be emphasized, however, that the three venous systems are interconnected by anastomoses, implying that we cannot count on complete bypassing the liver of a drug absorbed by the lower section of the rectum.

Decisively important for rectal absorption is the spreading or dissolution behavior of the suppositories, as this determines the contact areas with the rectal mucosa. Suppositories are required to melt at body temperature (36.5°C), preferably even slightly (1°−2°C) below that.

When all substance-related requirements are met, appropriate absorption from the rectum should be obtained. It is subject to the rules of passive diffusion and, analogous to gastrointestinal absorption, it depends on distribution coefficients and thus on the degree of ionization. Aside from some exceptions, following rectal administration of a drug maximal blood levels are reached later than after peroral ingestion. The extent of absorption will not always coincide with that of peroral administration, but often is up to 50% lower. This does not apply however for the often used suppositories containing nonsteroidal anti-inflammatory drugs such as indomethacin, diclofenac-sodium, ibuprofen, naproxen and piroxicam, which show relative bioavailability values of 75% to 100% of those after peroral administration as solution, capsule, or tablet.

13.9.2   Directives to Influence Bioavailability

The rate and extent at which active ingredients become available from suppositories is essentially determined by the distribution of the drug in the preparations while this, in turn, will depend on the solubility in the suppository base. In principle, we may assume that in order to attain satisfactory bioavailability, the drug should be suspended in the finest possible form. Since for the production of suppositories mostly fatty bases are used, the active substance should be processed in the form of poorly lipid-soluble salts (e.g., alkaloid salts). As a result of the unfavorable distribution coefficient suppository mass / rectal mucus solution suppositories mostly show unsatisfactory bioavailability.

The influence of the suppository base and further excipients on the availability of active agents is extremely complex and does not permit to draw generally valid conclusions. Surfactants and surfactant-containing bases tend to improve wettability of the suspended drug particles as well as the spreading of the melted or largely softened suppository and in this way favor the drug's bioavailability.

It should be noted that the addition of surfactant should be optimized in correlation with the nature of the preparation, because most surfactants at higher concentrations may lead to limitations of the bioavailability. Emulsifiers may, however, also contribute to improved drug permeability by virtue of an interaction with the rectal mucosa.

13.9.3   Assessment of in Vitro Drug Release

A number of experimental approaches are known to assess the liberation of active ingredients from suppositories. They include both open and closed systems. The tests are commonly performed in aqueous buffer solutions of pH 7.4 and at 37°C, similar to the dissolution tests for solid peroral formulations (section 9.9.1). It should be kept in mind that particularly in the testing of fatty suppositories strict temperature requirements apply since release from such products is strongly dependent on the melting behavior and viscosity.

Among the multiple experimental approaches there is one that has developed into a method meeting all requirements, such as for example sink conditions, and not requiring the use of a diffusion-affecting membrane between the test product and the release medium (Fig. 13-5, Fig. 13-6). This method is also described in the Ph. Eur. The inherent disadvantage of the membrane-less test methods that the released excipient enters the release medium is largely overcome by a number of mechanical measures. For the release assay all experimental parameters need to be strictly observed; for example, the pharmacopeia prescribes for buffered media a pH value that should not deviate more than 0.05 pH units from the desired value. In order to prevent the occurrence of uncontrolled whirling in chamber A of the flow-through cell, the flow rate of the release medium should be accurately controlled (Fig. 13-6).

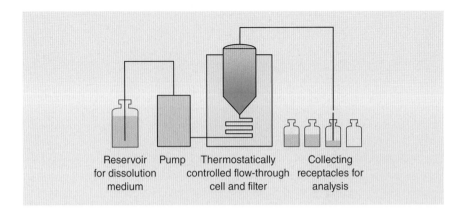

Fig. 13-5   Layout of the flow-through apparatus according to the Ph. Eur.

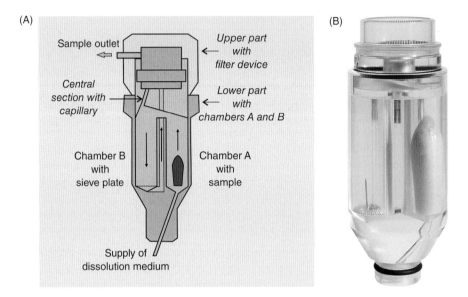

Fig. 13-6   Flow-through cell for lipophilic solid dosage forms according to Ph. Eur. (A) Schematic drawing; (B) real device. Reproduced with permission from SOTAX Group © 2017.

Ph. Eur. 2.9.42 Dissolution Test for Lipophilic Solid Dosage Forms _____

This method makes use of a flow-through cell specifically designed for the testing of lipophilic solid dosage forms such as suppositories and soft capsules. In the lower part of the cell two adjacent chambers are located. Chamber A serves to accommodate the sample. It is perfused from the bottom up with dissolution medium. The medium leaves chamber A at its upper end and passes chamber B in downward direction. A cavity on top of the two chambers collects the lipophilic excipients floating at the surface of dissolution medium. A thin capillary tube connecting the cavity with the filter holder serves to lead air bubbles out of this cavity. At the bottom of chamber B the dissolution medium flows through a small-size bore exit, which leads upwards to a filter assembly. The test medium may be flowing in an open or a closed circulation system and is maintained by a water bath at $37° \pm 0.5°C$.

Ph. Eur. 2.9.2 Disintegration of Suppositories and Pessaries _____

The disintegration test determines whether the suppositories or pessaries soften or disintegrate within the prescribed time when placed in a liquid medium. The apparatus consists of a transparent sleeve to the interior of which two perforated metal disks are attached about 30 mm apart (Fig. 13-7). The test is carried out using three such apparatuses each containing a single sample. Each apparatus is placed in a vessel with 4 L (using three devices in total) water maintained at 36°–37°C or the three apparatuses are placed together in a vessel with 12 L water. The vessels are equipped with a device that will hold the apparatuses vertically not less than 90 mm below the surface of the water and allow them to be inverted without emerging from the water. Each of three suppositories or pessaries is placed on the lower disc of a device and the latter is fixed in the sleeve. The three apparatuses are immersed into the water and inverted every 10 minutes. It is required that suppositories with a fatty base disintegrate within 30 minutes, those based on water-soluble excipients within 60 minutes, and rectal capsules within 30 minutes. Automated suppository disintegration testers—for example, Erweka ST 35 or Pharmatest PTS3E—enable an unattended and pharmacopeia-compliant performance of the test with the inversion of the test objects proceeding automatically at predetermined intervals. Particularly, suppositories with a high hydroxyl value retain their shape during softening, which hampers proper judgment of the disintegration and softening time. It is recommended, therefore, to probe the test object for the absence of a solid core by means of a glass rod.

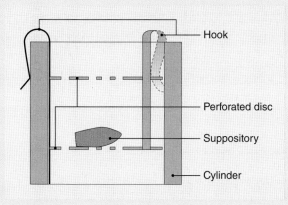

Fig. 13-7 Device for the pharmacopeia-compliant assessment of the disintegration time of suppositories and pessaries.

13.10 Testing

13.10.1 Uniformity of Dosage Units

Single-dose preparations for rectal administration must comply with the Ph. Eur. test requirements for uniformity of dosage units (Ph. Eur. 2.9.40). As a rule, this refers to content uniformity. Only in exceptional—well-substantiated—cases is it permitted to refer to older pharmacopeia tests for uniformity of mass (Ph. Eur. 2.9.5) or content (Ph. Eur. 2.9.6). In this connection, it should be taken into consideration that suppositories meeting the requirement of permissible mass deviation may exhibit substantial content deviations. To assess the distribution of drug within the suppository, the product is cut into segments perpendicularly to its main axis and the drug concentration in the single sections is determined.

> **Ph. Eur. 2.9.22 Softening Time Determination of Lipophilic Suppositories** _____
>
> The Ph. Eur. describes two devices to determine softening time of lipophilic suppositories—that is, the time period until a suppository maintained in water softens to the extent that it no longer offers resistance when a defined weight is applied. Device A is essentially a glass tube with water kept at 35.6°C. After the product has been introduced with the tip downward, a metal rod of 30 g provided with a small metal needle protruding from its broadened end, is placed on the suppository and then the time required for

the rod to touch the bottom of the glass tube is measured. Device B is identical to the test device according to Krówczynski (see Fig. 13-8).

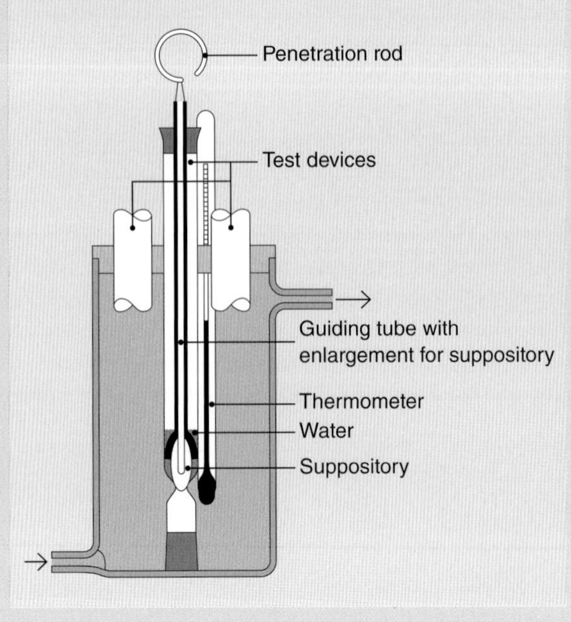

Fig. 13-8   Device for the assessment of the softening time of lipophilic suppositories according to Ph. Eur. 7.0.

13.10.2   Disintegration and Softening Time

To determine disintegration time (melting time or dissolution time for water-soluble preparations) of suppositories numerous methods are available, which produce different results, depending on methodical and instrument-related conditions. The test is commonly conducted in water of 36° to 37°C. The methods described in the following section have proven their suitability.

13.10.2.1   Pharmacopeia-Compliant Assessment of the Disintegration Time of Suppositories and Pessaries

In this method, which is also applicable to rectal and vaginal capsules, the equipment presented in Fig. 13-7 is used. Disintegration is assessed visually. For the testing of softening time of lipophilic suppositories under well-defined conditions, two experimental arrangements are described in the pharmacopeia. Both assess softening by means of a test rod that sinks through the suppository during the softening process. One of them essentially represents a simple vertically positioned glass tube filled with water in which the product is tested under temperature-controlled conditions. The other is a somewhat more complex device (Fig. 13-8), similar to the instrument designed by Krówczynski, in which the product is positioned in a more defined manner and surrounded by less water.

The tube filled with 5 mL water is placed in a jacket that is flushed by water of 36.5°C from a thermostat. After introducing the suppository to be tested in the tube the former is immediately weighted down with a glass test rod. The melted suppository material will flow upward along the rod. The melt-through time is taken as the time elapsing from the introduction of suppository and test rod till the rod contacts the constriction of the tube. The device may accommodate multiple test tubes.

13.10.2.2   Test Design According to Setnikar and Fantelli

This so-called dynamic model strives at an approximation of the physiological conditions in the rectum (Fig. 13-9). The suppository sits in a deformable cellophane tubing and is

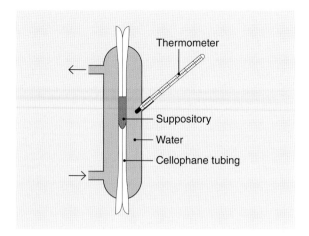

Fig. 13-9 **Suppository test equipment according to Setnikar and Fantelli.**

exposed to a hydrodynamic pressure simulating the abdominal pressure. The endpoint is reached when the test formulation is fully fluidized.

13.10.3 Resistance to Pressure and Crushing

13.10.3.1 Testing Device for the Resistance of Suppositories to Crushing

The assessment of crushing resistance of lipophilic suppositories requires accurate temperature control because the physical state of the base is strongly temperature dependent due to its very broad melting range. This has also been taken into consideration in connection with the test equipment described in previous editions of the Ph. Eur. (Fig. 13-10). It has a double-walled heating chamber mounted on the upper part of a stand that is flushed by thermostated water. The chamber contains a device with exchangeable polymer inserts for the accommodation of the suppository to be tested. This device serves at the same time as a guide for a pendant in whose upper part a likewise exchangeable polymer insert is mounted with a shape corresponding to that of the suppository. The pendant is elongated downwards and has a basic mass of 600 g. After setting the desired test temperature, a (prewarmed) suppository is inserted in the retaining mechanism with its tip pointing upward, the pendant is carefully put in position, and the test chamber is closed by a glass window.

At 1-minute intervals, disk-shaped weights of 200 g each, provided with a slit, are placed on the pendant until ultimately the suppository collapses under the collective burden of the disks. As a measure of the fracture resistance, the sum of the weights that press on the suppository at the moment of collapse is taken (including the basic weight of the pendant). A practical minimally required resistance lies between 1.2 kg and 1.4 kg.

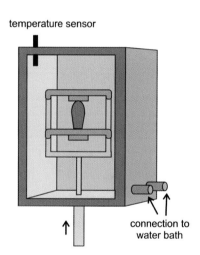

Fig. 13-10 **Suppository fracture resistance tester.**

Further Reading

Hermann, T. "Recent research on bioavailability of drugs from suppositories" *International journal of pharmaceutics* 123(1) (1995): 1–11.

Jannin, V., Lemagnen, G., Gueroult, P., Larrouture, D., Tuleu, C., "Rectal route in the 21st Century to treat children" *Adv Drug Deliv Rev* 73 (2014): 34–49.

Setnikar, I., and Fantelli, S. "Liquefaction Time of Rectal Suppositories." *Journal of Pharmaceutical Sciences* 51 (June 1962): 566–571.

Vaginal Dosage Forms and Dosage Forms to be Introduced in Body Cavities

14

14.1 Vaginal Dosage Forms

14.1.1 General Considerations

The wall of the vagina, which measures a length of 8 to 12 cm in adult women, consists of a multilayered nonkeratinized squamous epithelium, which is continuously renewed. A steadily secreted transudate, which ensures the elasticity of the cell layers and exerts a protective function, constitutes, together with the cervical secretion and shed cells, the vaginal fluid that covers the epithelium with a fluid film.

In healthy women, this film has an acidic pH due to the presence of a number of organic acids, predominantly lactic acid. The acidic environment has a protective function for the specific natural vaginal flora that is built up of a variety of microorganisms—in particular, lactic acid bacteria. Deviations from the physiological pH value (3.5–4.5) may create conditions under which pathogenic microorganisms may also colonize the mucosa.

Vaginal preparations are introduced into the vagina primarily for local therapy with anti-inflammatory, antimycotic, or other antiseptic ingredients, but also, for instance, for local hormone substitution or contraception.

14.1.2 Preparations for Local Administration

Pessaries mostly have an oval shape and a mass of 2 to 6 g. At body temperature they should soften or liquefy. Although, analogous to the rectal situation, active ingredients could be absorbed readily through the highly vascularized mucosa, this option is rarely exploited. Uniform and extended wetting of the moist vaginal mucosa is best achieved by hydrophilic bases. Once-traditional glycerol-gelatin bases are rarely used now. In marketed pharmaceuticals predominantly macrogols and, in particular, hard fat are applied as bases. The hydrophilicity and spreading properties of hard fats on the vaginal mucosa can be improved by addition of surface-active substances (such as Macrogol-25-cetylstearylether in Witepsol S 55® and Witepsol S 58®).

Pessaries are commonly produced according to the principles of the suppository technology (i.e., by melting of the excipients and casting in appropriately shaped molds). A typical cast shape for pessaries is depicted in Fig. 13-1B. Testing of dose uniformity, disintegration time and, for lipophilic pessaries, fracture resistance as well as the release of active substance are analogous to that of rectal suppositories (sections 13.9.3 and 13.10).

Vaginal tablets (section 9.7.4) are compressed products and represent an important vaginal dosage form. Their production and testing proceed as for tablets (described in Chapter 9). A special instruction exists for the testing of disintegration time, based on the equipment used for rectal suppositories. This procedure involves testing of disintegration in contact with only

Voigt's Pharmaceutical Technology, First Edition. Alfred Fahr.
© 2018 John Wiley & Sons Ltd. Published 2018 by John Wiley & Sons Ltd.

small amounts of aqueous medium (Ph. Eur. 2.9.2). Vaginal tablets are preferentially made with lactose, often in combination with cellulose as filling substance, and should not possess sharp edges. They may be provided with a water-soluble film coating.

Vaginal capsules are usually soft gelatin capsules with a shape adjusted to vaginal administration.

Medicated vaginal tampons consist of cotton, cellulose, or gauze impregnated with the active substance. They play no significant role in the pharmaceutical practice.

In contrast, *semi-solid vaginal preparations* such as ointments, creams, or gels, which mostly contain hydrophilic bases, are very often applied (e.g., O/W creams, hydrogels, see Chapter 15). The containers should be provided with a suitable applicator.

Vaginal foams are predominantly applied as a contraceptive; they are packed in a pressurized container provided with a dosing valve and a device for intravaginal application. The active ingredient is either dissolved or dispersed in an O/W emulsion. Foam formation proceeds as described in section 23.2.8.4.

Vaginal preparations may also be inserted in fluid form (solutions, emulsions, suspensions), likewise with the aid of an application device. They are either used for irrigation or to achieve a local action.

14.1.3   Intravaginal and Intrauterine Therapeutic Systems

14.1.3.1   Intravaginal Therapeutic Systems

Vaginal inserts represent advanced vaginal drug formulations with prolonged time-controlled release of their active ingredient. They include flexible polymer rings that, over time intervals of several weeks or even months, continuously release embedded hormones. They are deployed as contraceptive devices (NuvaRing®, Circlet®) or for local hormonal treatment (ESTRING®). Therapeutic Systems (TS) are characterized in that they release an incorporated active ingredient over a prolonged predetermined period of time (hours to years) at a defined rate. The active substance is contained in a reservoir and is, in most cases, released by membrane or matrix-controlled diffusion.

An example of an intravaginal TS for contraceptive purposes is the NuvaRing® (Fig. 14-1). It is a transparent flexible ring, to be applied intravaginally, containing the two active ingredients ethinyl estradiol (estrogen) and etonogestrel (gestagen) incorporated in the polymer ethyl vinyl acetate (EVA). The core of the ring, containing a large excess of both hormones, serves as a reservoir. It is enveloped by a membrane also consisting of EVA, which is responsible for release control. The two hormones diffuse along their concentration gradient across this membrane and are thus released in a time span of three weeks at a constant rate, but each at their own rate.

14.1.3.2   Intrauterine Therapeutic Systems

The history of intrauterine contraceptives dates back to early twentieth century, when German physicians inserted a nickel-bronze wire coiled around a piece of catgut in the uterus. Copper-containing intrauterine pessaries are still applied for contraceptive purposes. The first hormone-containing intrauterine contraceptive system (Progestasert®) was developed by Alza and was able to continuously release progesterone into the lumen of the uterus for

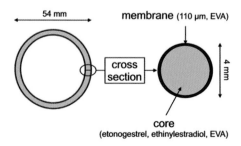

Fig. 14-1 Construction of the intravaginal therapeutic system NuvaRing®.

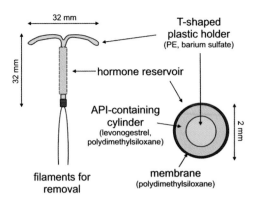

Fig. 14-2 Construction of the intrauterine therapeutic system Mirena®.

approximately one year. The intrauterine therapeutic system Mirena®, which is currently on the market, is based on the continuous release of a gestagen. The system consists of a T-shaped polymer support made of polyethylene, in which barium sulfate is incorporated for the purpose of radiographic detection (Fig. 14-2). To the stem of the support a hormone reservoir is attached that contains a mixture of poly(dimethyl siloxane) and levonorgestrel. The release of the hormone proceeds by diffusion controlled by a poly(dimethyl-siloxane) membrane. Hormone release extends over a time span of maximally 5 years, with an average release rate of 14 μg per day, varying from approximately 20 μg/day initially to minimally 10 μg/day by the end of the application period.

14.2   Medicated Sticks (*styli*)

These are solid formulations for local application, for instance, in the urethra, the vagina, the nasal cavity, and the auditory canal, as well as in wound channels or for cauterization. They have a cylindrical, rod-like, or conical shape. For insertion into the urethra or in wounds, the devices must be sterile.

Sticks may consist of pure active ingredient or of an active substance dissolved or dispersed in a suitable base. Depending on the composition, they may have a solid, soft, or flexible character; at body temperature they melt, dissolve, or swell. As a solid hydrophilic base, macrogols may be used. Suppository bases (e.g., hard fat) mainly serve as a lipophilic, melting base; when required, their consistency may be adjusted by addition of fatty oils plasticizers or wax (hardener). Elastic sticks are made with glycerol-gelatin as a base (2 parts gelatin, 1 part water, 4 parts glycerol). Soluble drug rods may also be produced on a carbohydrate base (12 parts tragacanth, 18 parts starch, 60 parts sucrose, and 10 parts gum arabic are mixed with a mixture of 2 parts glycerol and 1 part water to form a malleable mass that can be rolled out). Finally, substances like tragacanth and laminaria can be used for the production of swellable medicated sticks.

Usually, the manufacturing follows the principles of the suppository technology. The medicated base is cast in molds or aspirated in molds or tubes. In the same way, cosmetic preparations such as lipsticks are produced. Also compression into molds is a technique that is applied in this connection; in recent years, medicated sticks made of powdery substances, such as based on carbohydrates, are made like tablets in corresponding machines. Finally, sticks may be obtained by mechanical processing—for example, by lathe-shaping of crystals (alum sticks, silver nitrate, copper sulfate).

Further Reading _____

Dobaria, N., Mashru, R., Vadia, N. "Vaginal drug delivery systems: a review of current status." *East and Central African Journal of Pharmaceutical Sciences* 10(1) (2007): 3–13.

Semi-Solid Dosage Forms

PART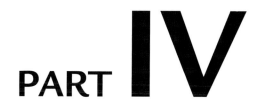

Semi-Solid Preparations for Cutaneous Application

15

15.1 General Considerations

In ancient times, semi-solid preparations for cutaneous application, popularly known as ointments, played an important role in human society. Their main usage was in skin care, and in some cultures, their application was part of welcoming ceremonies. *Salving* (the use of ointments) was commonly used in early civilizations. The Romans especially appreciated public baths and comforted themselves with aromatic oils and ointments.

In the Ebers papyrus (about 1600 BC), ointments were for the first time referred to as healing substances. Hippocrates and Galen held the use of ointments in high esteem. Animal fats (bovine and goat), oils, and bone marrow were passed down as components of ointment preparations. In the first century AD, a renowned medical school in Laodicea (in present-day Turkey) was known for eye and ear ointments. In the Middle Ages, beeswax, plant gums, and honey were employed.

The use of "magic salve" (called *witch salve* in medieval Germany) in the Middle Ages is an indication of early knowledge of the systemic effects of various alkaloids such as scopolamine, hyoscyamine, and atropine following topical application. The use of monkey, dog, and snake fat, as well as human or animal feces, urine, and glandular secretions has significantly contributed to the inglorious reputation of the baroque "mock pharmacies." The introduction of soft paraffin in the dermatological practice by Cheseborough in 1878 and purified wool fat in 1885 by Liebig signified a major leap in the innovation of the ointment therapy in those days.

An advanced scientific treatment of the theme "ointment" was set off in the late 1950s. It was only from then on that the intensive physicochemical characterization of ointments as well as the inclusion of dermatological aspects was leading to a comprehensive understanding of the various interactions between the vehicle, the active ingredient and the skin.

According to Ph. Eur., semi-solid preparations for cutaneous application are intended for application on the healthy, diseased or damaged skin. Semi-solid preparations intended to be applied to particular surfaces or mucous membranes (e.g., eyes, nose, and rectum) may be found in other general monographs on dosage forms. Pharmaceutical substances may be dissolved (e.g., solution ointments) or suspended (e.g., suspension ointments) in semi-solid basis. The inclusion of water or aqueous solutions of active substances in emulsifier-containing basis results in the formation of creams. Semi-solid systems with a high proportion of solids finely dispersed in either a semi-solid hydrophilic or lipophilic base are termed *pastes*.

Semi-solid preparations for cutaneous application are mainly employed for local therapeutic treatment.

Voigt's Pharmaceutical Technology, First Edition. Alfred Fahr.

In Italy, a 9 year old treated with daily topical application of 15% salicylic acid patches for plantar wart showed a significantly worsened health and mildly impaired mental performance. Patient's condition improved progressively upon cessation of the topical treatment and worsened again upon resuming patch for treatment of a relapsing wart. (Loraschi et al. 2008).

Screening or protecting ointments are meant to protect the healthy skin from harmful environmental influences. Antiseptic ointments serve to treat minor injuries or skin attritions. For most cutaneous applied active substances penetration into the affected upper skin layers is required for a therapeutic effect to be achieved. Transport into the deeper skin layers and adjacent tissues or even into the systemic circulation (transdermal activity) is rarely aimed for. For example, in case of topical antirheumatic drug therapy, a regional effect in tissues adjacent to the site of application is desired. When estradiol gels are applied to the skin, we want the active ingredient to travel across the skin and to be absorbed into the systemic circulation. When applied on large skin surfaces, certain active substances may even cause undesired systemic effects, culminating in toxicity. Such toxic events have been reported, for instance, in small children after cutaneous application of salicylic acid.

For the treatment of skin disorders, in many countries the prescription of extemporaneously prepared pharmaceutical preparations is still common practice (customized medication). This practice may serve to fill the therapeutic gap when, for example, a drug formulation in the desired vehicle is insufficiently stable for a longer period of time, a preservative-free formulation is required, individual dosing is necessary, or a licensed pharmaceutical preparation is not yet or no longer available.

The nomenclature and classification of semisolid dermal dosage forms are not uniform. Physicians and pharmacists often maintain different practices in this context, which may frequently lead to confusion. Often, the term *ointment* is used for all semi-solid preparations without differentiating with respect to the exact semi-solid preparations as listed in Ph. Eur.

The dermatological classification is mostly based on the *phase triangle* of the dermatological principles distinguishing between greasy ointments, ointments, creams, and gels with regard to semi-solid preparations (Fig. 15-1). The regular system used in the pharmaceutical world and the corresponding common parlance is predominantly oriented towards the Ph. Eur.

The latter maintains under the term "semi-solid preparations for cutaneous application (*praeparationes molles ad usum dermicum*)" a classification based on pharmaceutical points of view and uses as criteria polarity (hydrophilic *vs.* lipophilic) as well as physicochemical aspects (single- or multiphasic). This implies that, according to the pharmacopeia, semi-solid preparations may be single- or bi- or multiple-phasic, while each of these systems, again, may be lipophilic or hydrophilic. Extra definitions are given for pastes (semi-solid preparations with large proportions of finely dispersed solids), poultices, and medicated plasters or cutaneous patches containing an active agent. The latter are discussed in chapter 16. This chapter discusses the broader term *semi-solid preparations*, the semi-solid dermal preparations (ointments, creams, gels, pastes, compress pastes) as well as semi-solid preparations for noncutaneous application.

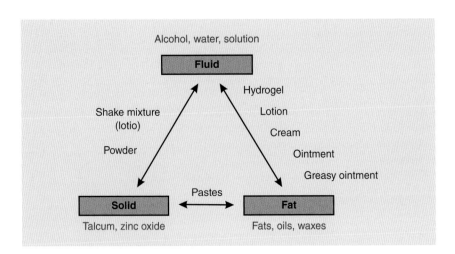

Fig. 15-1 **Phase triangle of basis for dermatics.**

15.2 Requirements of Dermal Preparations with Semi-Solid Properties

Semi-solid preparations for cutaneous application consist of a basis (vehicle) and one or more pharmaceutical actives. The vehicle may be a simple system consisting of a few components, for example soft paraffin. However, most are complex mixtures of multiple excipients, which, from a physicochemical perspective, form a multiphase system. The applied excipients include hydrophilic and lipophilic base components as well as additives such as preservatives, antioxidants, stabilizers, emulsifiers, thickening agents, and penetration enhancers.

As opposed to most other application forms, for dermal preparations a potential effect of the base, without the addition of an active agent, is explicitly taken into account. Besides a purely physical action such as cooling or simply covering the skin surface, the base, depending on its composition, may interact with the skin. This may, in particular, affect the barrier properties of the skin, in either a positive or a negative sense. This *vehicle effect* becomes decisively important in case of local therapy. For dermal therapy, one and the same active ingredient may be formulated in different vehicles because, besides the galenic properties of the active ingredient (e.g., solubility, distribution behavior), additional factors should be taken into consideration to achieve optimal activity. Among those factors is the intended site of action (e.g., upper skin layers or deeper tissue areas), but also a number of dermatological aspects. The latter include the condition of the application site (injured, diseased, or healthy skin), the stage of the disorder (acute or chronic process), skin condition (seborrhoeic or sebostatic skin), and the physiological peculiarities of the application site (mucosal tissue, hairy skin).

For semi-solid preparations, only excipients of appropriate quality are allowed. Mostly, there are individual monographs for the substances in a pharmacopeia. Otherwise, the excipients need to comply with the general monograph "Substances for pharmaceutical Use." The materials to be processed need to be stable and should not exhibit any incompatibility with other excipients and with the used active ingredient(s).

Semi-solid preparations should exhibit suitable rheological properties—in particular, fair spreading behavior—and adequate release of the active ingredient. Of essential importance is, furthermore, that these formulations are well tolerated by the skin, implying that the applied excipients should have only a very low irritation or sensitization potential. Also, a certain water uptake potential of the formulation is required and, unless therapeutically desirable, there should be no or only little effect on physiological skin functions (heat accumulation, impediment of trans-epidermal water loss).

To optimize compliance, the cosmetic properties such as skin absorption, spreading potential, and skin feel play an important role. The final preparation should have a homogeneous appearance. Particular care should be taken of a sufficiently homogeneous distribution of the active ingredient in case the latter is not fully soluble in the basis but rather, is present as a liquid (emulsion) or a solid (suspension) dispersion.

Particle size should be adjusted to the intended application; it should, for example, not cause mechanical irritation upon application on the skin (section 15.4.2).

Preparations for cutaneous application should have low microbial load. According to the Ph. Eur., a total aerobic microbial count (TAMC) of 10^2 and a combined total yeast/mold count (TYMC) of 10^1 per gram or per mL are acceptable. Furthermore, *Pseudomonas aeruginosa* and *Staphylococcus aureus* have to be absent. Preparations intended for use on severely injured skin must be sterile. In order to attain satisfactory microbiological quality, necessary precautions should be taken during the preparation. Appropriate measures should be taken to ensure maintenance of proper microbiological quality during storage and application, such as preservation and employment of suitable primary packaging.

15.3 Classification and Structure of Semi-Solid Preparations

Characteristic of semi-solid preparations is their spreading potential. This specific rheological property is based on the colloidal structure of the basis. From a physicochemical perspective,

Important general chapters in the Ph. Eur. for dermal semisolid preparations:

Sterility test (2.6.1)

Measurement of rheological properties by rotating viscometer (2.2.10)

Deliverable mass or volume (2.9.28)

Measurement of consistency by penetrometry (2.9.9)

Methods for preparation of sterile products (5.1.1)

Efficacy of microbial preservation (5.1.3)

Microbiological quality of pharmaceutical preparation (5.1.4).

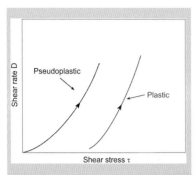

Typical flow behavior of semi-solid formulations.

semi-solid preparations can be described as gels consisting of at least two components. A solid component, which builds a three-dimensional framework (matrix), and a fluid component, immobilized as a similarly coherent medium in the matrix. IUPAC defines gels as "colloidal network or polymer network that is expanded throughout its whole volume by a fluid and that has a finite, usually rather small, yield point." For this reason, gels are not free flowing but require a certain force (shear stress) to bring the system from rest to flow.

Depending on the strength of the acting force, gels may behave in different ways: At low shear forces, they behave predominantly as a solid body (elastic), at forces higher than the yield point, rather like a fluid (viscous); they are known as visco-elastic systems. In line with their rheological properties, gels may be described as plastic bodies with Casson characteristics, that is, they display a certain yield point and, upon exceeding that limit, also a shear-thinning, because by increasing shear structural degradation ensues (section 3.12.1.3). Upon releasing the force, the system comes to a rest, and after a certain recovery time, the original consistence will be regained: We speak of a thixotropic system in such cases.

The structural properties of these gels, which form the basis of their plastic flow behavior, may be quite diverse for the different forms of semi-solid preparations. Up to now, relatively little has been known about the exact fine structure of many semi-solid preparations. This is, in part, based on the structural complexity of the base. Even the processed single components often consist of multiple chemical entities (e.g., soft paraffin). The colloidal fine structure of semi-solid preparations depends on the qualitative and quantitative composition as well as on the processing conditions. Model representations of the colloidal structure of a small number of bases have been developed, based on experimental data. The models described here are meant to help the reader to understand certain properties of semi-solid preparations: properties that are for example of major importance for the production procedures as well as for their behavior after application.

The classification of semi-solid preparations may be performed from different perspectives (e.g., based on their function or their composition). The systematic introduction in the Ph. Eur. under "Semi-Solid Preparations for Cutaneous Application" is based on structure and composition as well as on the hydrophilic and lipophilic character of the different preparations. Examples of how officinal bases may be ordered in the individual groups may be found in the box Pharmacopeial (Ph. Eur, DAB) and compendial (NRF) formulation examples.

Nonetheless, common nomenclature of semi-solid preparations among dermatologists as well as the currently still prevailing designations for formulations of licensed pharmaceutical preparations are clearly deviating from this. Table 15-1 presents the corresponding opposing designations.

A transparent nomenclature is relevant, for example, when a licensed semi-solid drug preparation shall be used in the extemporaneous preparation of a medicinal product, to properly assess the character of a licensed semi-solid drug preparation and to avoid incompatibilities (section 26.1). If no relevant information of the manufacturer is available, the type of base has to be determined from the composition or, when necessary, by performing some simple testing.

Table 15-1   Common Designations of Semi-Solid Preparations for Cutaneous Application

Commonly Used Terms for Semi-Solid Preparations for Cutaneous Application

Ph. Eur. compliant	Used by dermatologists/for licensed pharmaceutical preparations	EDQM standard term for the pharmaceutical dose form
Hydrogel	Hydrogel	Gel
Hydrophilic ointment	(Fat-free) ointments	Ointment
Hydrophilic cream	Cream/greasy cream	Cream
Lipophilic cream	Greasy cream/ointment	Cream
Water-emulsifying ointment	Ointment/greasy ointment	Ointment
Hydrophobic ointment	Greasy ointment	Ointment
Lipophilic gel (Oleogel)	Greasy ointment	Gel
Paste	Paste	Paste for cutaneous application

15.3.1   Ointments

As a rule, ointments in accordance with the Ph. Eur. are essentially water-free semi-solid preparations. They consist of a single-phase base. Solid or liquid substances (mostly active agents) may be dispersed in it. Based on their behavior toward water, they are classified in hydrophobic, hydrophilic and water-emulsifying ointments. To display spreading properties ointments must have a gel structure, that is, besides fluid components it must also contain solid (either amorphous or crystalline) components, allowing the formation of a multi-phase system of uniform polarity (hydrophilic or hydrophobic).

15.3.1.1   Hydrophobic Ointments

Hydrophobic ointments consist of nonpolar components and can thus absorb only small amounts of water. Typical basis used for their formulation are soft paraffin (although not mentioned in Ph. Eur.); hard, liquid, and light liquid paraffins; vegetable oils; animal fats; synthetic glycerides; waxes; and liquid polyalkylsiloxanes.

A further differentiation is made based on chemical structure of the base. In this way, for example, nonpolar hydrocarbon gels are distinguished from more polar lipogels. To establish specific properties (spreading, solving potential, drug penetration etc.) for the production of licensed pharmaceutical preparations, constituents of hydrocarbon gels and lipogels in addition to other lipids are mixed together.

> Practical example of a hydrophobic ointment of complex composition 1 g contains: methyl-prednisolone aceponate 1 mg. Additional components: white soft paraffin, liquid paraffin, microcrystalline hydrocarbons (40–60 C atoms), hydrogenated castor oil.

Licensed pharmaceutical preparations that belong to the hydrophobic ointments are mostly designated greasy ointments. The EDQM standard term for this pharmaceutical dose form is ointment.

Hydrocarbon Gels

These are commonly used as base of hydrophobic ointments (as well as many other semi-solid preparations). Hydrocarbon gels include the natural products yellow and white soft paraffin as well as the synthetic hydrophobic base gel DAC.

In all three hydrocarbon gels, the fluid gel phase is formed by paraffin oil, which, in turn, is composed of n- and iso-paraffins as well as nonaromatic, cyclic hydrocarbons (naphthenes).

The gel matrix (10%–30%) of yellow and white soft paraffin consists of mainly branched long-chain hydrocarbons. They form three-dimensional linked crystallites with liquid paraffin (70%–90%) incorporated in the amorphous edge regions (glass-like cover layers) and free interspaces (Fig. 15-2).

It is assumed that the long-chain paraffins, under formation of folding planes, arrange themselves side-by-side in a parallel fashion. By subsequent stacking of these structural elements, even stronger bundles are formed, and these are clearly visible in the polarized light microscope.

The higher the degree of interaction within the framework, the more intense the fluid fraction will be immobilized by lyosorption (absorption of liquid into a solid, e.g., the suspended particles). Like the ductility of a high-quality soft paraffin, this is promoted by long hydrocarbon chains and a high degree of branching. Insufficiently branched hydrocarbons form large crystals during storage. As a result, the gel framework will condense and fluid components will separate out. This syneresis of the hydrocarbon gel is also known as the bleeding of soft paraffin.

The oil retention capacity may be improved by addition of a microcrystalline wax (ozokerite, earth wax, ceresin). This is a natural mixture of high molecular weight normal or branched or cyclo-aliphatic hydrocarbons, that is, constituents of the gel matrix of soft paraffin. Microcrystalline wax belongs to the so-called mineral waxes, but is, from a chemical perspective, not a wax at all.

DAC (German Pharmaceutical Codex)

This is the supplementary book to the DAB (German Pharmacopeia), which is published collectively with the NRF (cf. other box). It has a practical orientation, in which for example the excipients are listed. We are referring here to this, as it has a long tradition and is well documented. Other countries do also have this supplementation, but because of space considerations we cannot refer to all of them here.

White soft paraffin is synonymous with Vaselinum album, white petrolatum and soft paraffin wax.

Yellow soft paraffin is synonymous with Vaselinum flavum and yellow petrolatum.

Both, white and yellow soft paraffins are obtained as fractions during refining of crude petroleum oil.

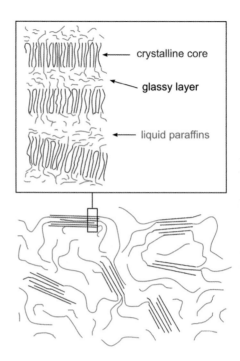

Fig. 15-2 **Model of the colloidal assembly of soft paraffin.**

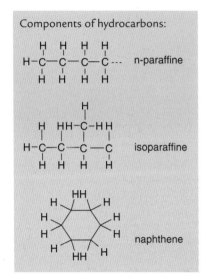

The consistency of soft paraffin diminishes with increasing temperature because the crystalline regions will melt ultimately, leading to total liquefaction. After solidification of molten soft paraffin, crystalline regions will be gradually formed again, detectable by polarization microscopy. Macroscopically, the increasing crystallinity of the system becomes apparent as a gradual increase in turbidity.

The consistency of hydrocarbon basis can be adjusted by addition of liquid or hard paraffin. For many soft paraffin-based ointments, the DAB (German Pharmacopeia) permits the addition of a certain percentage of liquid paraffin.

White soft paraffin is distinguished from yellow soft paraffin by more extensive refinement, during which unsaturated hydrocarbons are removed. Irrespective of any refinement, both types of soft paraffin are practically free from aromatic hydrocarbons, as prescribed by the relevant pharmacopeias.

For the hydrophobic base gel (DAC; the German Drug Codex), liquid paraffin is gelified in a special process with 5% high-pressure polyethylene (low-density polyethylene (LDPE), Mr ~21.000). To that end, the components are melted together at 130°C and are subsequently rapidly cooled (10 K/s). As the desired structure is obtained only by this special operation procedure, this product is manufactured only at the industrial level. The product is not as ductile and has a softer texture as soft paraffin. Furthermore, due to the usage of long-chain unbranched n-paraffins as matrix builders, its capacity to retain oil is smaller than that of soft paraffin. Nonetheless, an advantage is that its consistency barely alters in the temperature range between −15° and +60°C because of the higher melting temperature of the gel matrix. Indeed, the Ph. Eur. describes the hydrophobic basic gel as an example of a lipophilic gel (oleogel).

In hydrocarbon gels, both the matrix formers and the fluid constituents may be assigned to the same chemical class, implying that in this case we are dealing with an isogel. The restoration of its matrix structure after shearing takes a certain amount of time; therefore, it is a thixotropic system.

Soft paraffin is a nearly inert base. Only in highly sensitive patients occasional skin irritations are observed. Soft paraffin is quite suitable as a coating ointment, as a vehicle system for pharmaceuticals with peripheral activity, and as a basis for emulsifier-containing systems with water-emulsifying capacity (see section 15.3.1.2, "Water-Emulsifying Ointments"). A soft paraffin film applied on the skin is barely permeable to water vapor, resulting in enhanced local blood flow and hydration and swelling of the *Stratum corneum*. This occlusion effect promotes penetration of active agents through the horny layer. Occlusion can increase penetration of, for example, corticosteroids 100-fold, but a factor of 2 to 6 is more common for most low molecular weight drugs. For complete occlusion, however, a really thick layer (several 100 μm) needs to be applied.

Hydrocarbons are relative poor solvents for most pharmaceutically active agents, explaining why in most cases such agents prevail in suspended form in the base.

Lipogels

Lipogels are isogels made up of solid and liquid triglycerides (triacylglyceride). They are of natural origin, such as porcine lard or, in case of mixed-chain triglycerides, semi-synthetic (e.g., Softisan® 378). Nowadays, however, only in exceptional cases are animal fats still used for this purpose. This is, on the one hand, related to standardization problems and on the other to their sensitivity to oxidation, which, in spite of addition of antioxidants, cannot be entirely overcome.

The properties of lipogels are determined by the chain length of the fatty acid moieties as well as by the number of double bonds. In natural lipogels, the matrix consists of triglycerides with approximately one third unsaturated fatty acids. The liquid components of the lipogel consist of triglycerides with about two thirds unsaturated fatty acids. Semi-synthetic lipogels contain almost exclusively oxidation-resistant saturated fatty acids. In order to obtain a semi-solid mixture of liquid and solid trigylcerides, a fatty acid cut with a spectrum ranging from C8 to C18 is used.

The colloidal structure of lipogels results from the crystallization of long-chain unsaturated fatty acids. However, in view of the low uniformity of the components, no large crystals can be formed. Instead, crystallites are formed containing numerous crystal defects contributing to an extremely fine three-dimensional matrix network. Therein, the liquid triglyceride component is immobilized by lyo-sorption, capillary condensation and by mechanical means.

Because lipogels are more polar than hydrocarbon gels, they have lower occlusive potential.

15.3.1.2 Water-Emulsifying Ointments

Typically, for ointments, the water-emulsifying ointments are water-free but are able to absorb large quantities of water. The bases of water-emulsifying ointments are those of hydrophobic ointments, very often with a high proportion of hydrocarbons. In order to attain the desired water uptake, the base is supplemented by emulsifiers of the water-in-oil type such as wool alcohols, sorbitan esters and mono-glycerides or alternatively of the oil-in-water type such as sulfated fatty alcohols, polysorbates, fatty acid esters, or ethers of macrogols. Water-emulsifying ointments are also called absorption bases; depending on the applied emulsifier type, hydrophilic and lipophilic water-emulsifying basis are distinguished.

In order to achieve a homogeneous distribution, the incorporation of the emulsifiers, which often possess a high melting point, is performed at elevated temperature, followed by cold stirring. This applies in particular when the emulsifier mix contains a matrix-forming component such as cetostearyl alcohol or glycerol monostearate, which recrystallizes upon cooling. The mixture of cetyl- and stearyl-alcohol, which often forms a component of lipophilic as well as hydrophilic absorption bases, is even at relatively low concentrations (5%–10%) capable of building up three-dimensional networks of fatty alcohol crystallisates, incorporating the other components of the basis for ointments. These crystallisates may consist exclusively of the matrix-forming components, but often they form in addition, together with the further emulsifiers, mixed lamellar crystallisates, which also contribute to the structure formation (Fig. 15-3). Besides, this may result in the formation of polar regions around the hydrophilic head groups in which water can be incorporated.

For lipophilic absorption bases, however, good water absorption capacity is associated with the emulsifier molecules dissolved in the liquid components of the basis. Accordingly, in the emulsifying eye ointment, DAC cholesterol dissolved in the liquid hydrocarbon allows the incorporation of a 1.5-fold mass of water at a cholesterol content of merely 1% under moderate heating conditions.

The wool alcohols, which often are used as W/O emulsifiers in semi-solid preparations, consist of aliphatic alcohols in addition to up to 70% cholesterol-like sterols. As a quality requirement of a wool alcohol ointment the German pharmacopeia (DAB) prescribes that the basis should be capable of absorbing twice its weight in water.

Lipogels can be classified either as hydrophobic ointments (usually found in pharmacopeias) but a classification to lipophilic gels (oleogels) is also possible, as seen in Ph. Eur. 2.9.5 Uniformity of Mass of Single-Dose Preparations.

Softisan® 378 is a blend of triglycerides containing saturated, unbranched fatty acids with C8 to C18 chain lengths and meets the pharmacopeial requirement of Hard Fat in Ph. Eur. It has a soft consistency and is used often as an emollient in creams.

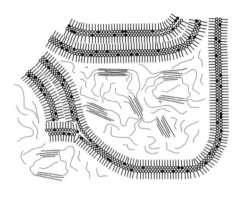

∂ paraffins   ↑ fatty alcohol   ↑ fatty alcohol sulphate

Fig. 15-3 Model structure of the hydrophilic ointment DAB.

Based on their emulsifier content water-emulsifying ointments are less occlusive than hydrophobic ointments. Lipophilic water-emulsifying ointments are not at all washed off by cold or lukewarm water, whereas hydrophilic water-emulsifying ointments are barely washed off by cold or lukewarm water. A disadvantage of the use of wool fat products is the relatively high sensitizing potential, which, however, diminishes with increasing purity or derivation. The sensitizing effect seems to be caused by additives such as alkane-β-diols and alkane-α,ω-diols, or possibly pesticide residues.

Like the hydrophobic ointments, water-emulsifying ointments are mostly called fatty ointments in the context of licensed pharmaceutical preparations. The EDQM standard term for this pharmaceutical dose form is ointment.

15.3.1.3 Hydrophilic Ointments

Hydrophilic ointments are preparations based on water-miscible basis. Usually, such bases consist of mixtures of liquid and solid macrogols (polyethylene glycols). As opposed to all other ointments, they may, according to the Ph. Eur. monograph, contain appropriate amounts of water. During the preparation, liquid and solid macrogols (e.g., macrogol 300 and 1,500) are melted at 60°C and subsequently cold stirred. During the cooling process, the higher molecular weight macrogols crystallize again. The ratio between solid and liquid components is chosen such that a homogeneous mass of soft paraffin-like consistency is formed.

Thus, the matrix structure of the macrogol ointments is based on the proportion of crystalline material. It is assumed that the chains of macrogol 1,500 arrange themselves in parallel stretches and thus form crystalline lamellae in between whose hydrophilic planes liquid macrogols can be accommodated. Alternatively, in case of longer-chain macrogols (MW > 3,000), the lamellae may be formed of folded macrogol chains with the liquid macrogols accommodated between the individual lamellae. The crystallites constructed of lamellae organize themselves starting from a seed in larger units, called spherulites, which are in contact with each other and thus build up a coherent gel matrix structure in the ointment. In this network, the remaining fraction of liquid macrogols is immobilized. Thus, macrogol ointments are isogels with a structural make-up similar to that of hydrocarbon gels or lipogels. Macrogol ointments can take up only limited amounts of water before they liquefy due to their complete miscibility with water. If it is required to incorporate larger amounts of water (>10%) a matrix-building component such as cetostearyl alcohol should be included.

Macrogol bases do not cause skin irritation, have suitable adhesive and spreading potential and do not lead to occlusion. By virtue of their hydrophilic character they easily wash off with water and can be applied on hairy skin. Because of their osmotic activity, they exert a dehydrating effect on the skin. The high absorption potential may be exploited in antimicrobial creams by absorbing the wound exudates. That is why macrogol-based bases are also applied in the realm of antiseptic (e.g., Povidone-iodide ointment) and antimycotic preparations. The osmotic activity may be adjusted by incorporating water. Macrogol ointments

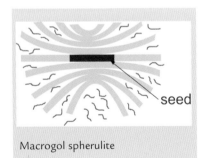

Macrogol spherulite

seed

are hygroscopic and liquefy during storage in moist environment. For that reason, but also because of the risk of autoxidation, macrogol ointments need to be tightly sealed and stored while protected from light. When processing and packaging macrogols, it should be taken into account that these substances are able to dissolve certain synthetic polymers (e.g., PVC) and lacquers. Therefore, the processing of such ointments with a polymer-lined ointment mill and the packaging in ointment jars or tubes require prior testing of compatibility.

Macrogols also represent excellent solvents for numerous active agents (e.g., salicylic acids, nitrofural). This allows the formulation of solution ointments in a therapeutically relevant concentration range, which do not bring along the risk of recrystallization or crystal growth during storage. However, a good solubility of a drug affects the partitioning of the drug into the skin negatively and thus unfavorably influences its penetration into the skin (section 15.6).

In the context of licensed pharmaceutical preparations, hydrophilic ointments are commonly designated simply as ointments or they are described as fat-free (basis for) ointments. The EDQM standard term for this pharmaceutical dose form is ointment.

Ph. Eur./DAB/DAC: Formulation Examples for Official Semi-Solid Ground Substances and Preparations

Ointments
Hydrophobic ointments
Yellow soft paraffin Ph. Eur.
White soft paraffin Ph. Eur.
Pork lard DAB

Simple eye ointment DAC
liquid paraffin	40 parts
white soft paraffin	60 parts

Water-emulsifying ointments
Lipophilic absorption bases
Wool alcohol ointment DAB
cetostearyl alcohol	0.5 parts
wool alcohols	6 parts
white soft paraffin	93.5 parts

Wool alcohol ointment SR
sorbitan- and glycerol mono-oleate	3.0 parts
wool alcohols	2.5 parts
white soft paraffin	94.5 parts

Emulsifying eye ointment DAC
cholesterol	1 part
liquid paraffin	42.5 parts
white soft paraffin	ad 100 parts

Zinc ointment DAB
zinc oxide	10 parts
wool alcohols ointment	90 parts

Hydrophilic absorption bases
Hydrophilic ointment DAB
emulsifying cetostearyl alcohol (Type A)	30 parts
liquid paraffin	35 parts
white soft paraffin	35 parts

Hydrophilic ointments
Macrogol ointment DAC
macrogol 300	50 parts
macrogol 1.500	50 parts

Creams
Lipophilic creams
Hydrous wool fat Ph. Eur.
wool fat	75 parts
purified water	25 parts

wool alcohol cream DAB
wool alcohol ointment	50 parts
purified water	50 parts

After the drug, the base constitutes the second most important component in semisolid formulations. However, other ingredients may additionally be present in a semisolid formulation depending on the nature of the drug, the therapeutic application and the characteristics of the base. Such ingredients include:

1. Preservatives
2. Antioxidants
3. Penetration enhancers
4. Humectants
5. Buffers

When selecting preservatives and antioxidants care should be taken to avoid any incompatibilities with components of the formulation base (e.g. added surfactants) as these substances often bind preservatives and antioxidants thereby diminishing their protective effects. For example, the preservative methyl paraben loses its activity in presence of 5% Tween-80.

Typical preservatives employed in semi-solid formulations include;
- methyl paraben
- ethyl paraben
- propyl paraben
- butyl paraben
- benzyl alcohol
- Phenoxyethanol
- Benzoic acid
- Sorbic acid/potassium sorbate

Some typical antioxidants employed in the semi-solid formulations are: butylated hydroxyanisole (BHA), butylated hydroxytoluene (BHT), propyl gallate

Humectants are often employed in hydrophilic creams to prevent loss of water as hydrophilic creams can lose most water within minutes after application. Typically used humectants include polyols such as glycerol, propylene glycol, sorbitol 70%, and low MW PEGs. Selection of a proper humectant is critical as it affects the consistency and texture of the cream.

Non-ionic hydrophillic cream DAB, Basic cream DAC and Anionic hydrophilic creams SR DAC are some examples of cream bases employing polyol humectants.

Buffers are important to maintain the appropriate pH especially for formulations containing high fractions of water such as gels and hydrophilic creams. Typically used buffers include citrate, and phosphate buffers. Buffer selection is important especially because ionic components of the formulations can adversely affect the buffering capacity.

In many modern formulations chemical penetration enhancers are often employed for a faster and deeper drug penetration into the skin. For a detailed overview of this topic refer to section 15.6.3.3 of this chapter.

Wool alcohol cream SR	
wool alcohol ointment SR	50 parts
purified water	50 parts

Lanolin DAB	
liquid paraffin	15 parts
purified water	20 parts
wool fat	65 parts

Hydrophobic base cream DAC	
glycerol tri-di-isostearate	3.0 parts
isopropyl palmitate	2.4 parts
hydrophobic base gel	24.6 parts
potassium sorbate	0.14 parts
anhydrous citric acid	0.07 parts
magnesium sulfate	0.5 parts
glycerol 85%	5.0 parts
purified water	6429 parts

Cold cream DAB	
yellow beeswax	7 parts
cetyl palmitate	8 parts
arachidis oil	60 parts
purified water	25 parts

Soft cream DAC	
purified water	10 parts
liquid paraffin	7.5 parts
wool fat	32.5 parts
yellow soft paraffin	50 parts

Hydrophilic creams

Anionic hydrophilic cream DAB	
hydrophilic ointment	30 parts
purified water	70 parts

Nonionic hydrophilic cream DAB	
polysorbate 60	5 parts
cetostearyl alcohol	10 parts
glycerol (85%)	10 parts
white soft paraffin	25 parts
purified water	50 parts

Base cream DAC	
glycerol monostearate 60	4 parts
cetyl alcohol	6 parts
medium-chain triglycerides	7.5 parts
white soft paraffin	25.5 parts
macrogol-20-glycerol monostearate	7 parts
propylene glycol	10 parts
purified water	40 parts

Nonionic hydrophilic cream SR DAC	
nonionic emulsifying wax	21 parts
2-ethyl-hexyl lauromyristate	10 parts
glycerol 85%	5 parts
potassium sorbate	0.14 parts
anhydrous citric acid	0.07 parts
purified water	63.79 parts

Anionic hydrophilic cream SR DAC	
Emulsifying cetostearyl alcohol (Typ A)	21 parts
2-ethyl-hexyl lauromyristate	10 parts
glycerol 85%	5 parts
potassium sorbate	014 parts
anhydrous citric acid	0.07 parts
purified water	6379 parts

Gels

Lipophilic gels

Hydrophobic base gel DAC	
high-pressure polyethylene	5 parts
liquid paraffin	95 parts

Hydrophilic gels

Aqueos carbomer gel DAB

carbomer (50.000 mPa · s)	0.5 parts
sodium hydroxide solution (50 g/l)	3 parts
purified water	96.5 parts

2-Propanol-containing carbomer gel DAB

carbomer (50.000 mPa · s)	0.5 parts
sodium hydroxide solution (50 g/l)	1 part
2-propanol	25 parts
purified water	73.5 parts

Carmellose-sodium gel DAB

carmellose-sodium 600	5 parts
glycerol 85%	10 parts
purified water	85 parts

Hydroxyethyl cellulose gel DAB

hydroxyethyl cellulose 10.000	2.5 parts
glycerol 85%	10 parts
purified water	87.5 parts

Unna's paste DAB

zinc oxide	10 parts
glycerol 85%	40 parts
gelatin	15 parts
purified water	35 parts

Pastes

Soft zinc paste DAB

zinc oxide	30 parts
liquid paraffin	40 parts
white soft paraffin	20 parts
white bees wax	10 parts

Zinc paste DAB

zinc oxide	25 parts
wheat starch	25 parts
white soft-paraffin	50 parts

Pharmacopeial recommendations for preservation are not taken into account.

15.3.2 Creams

The Ph. Eur. defines creams as multiphase preparations consisting of a lipophilic and an aqueous phase. Formally, they are formed by incorporating water in water-emulsifying ointments. Normally, creams are systems containing one or more emulsifiers. The final product is an emulsion-like system in which the water prevails either as dispersed phase (lipophilic creams) or as continuous phase (hydrophilic creams). Creams distinguish themselves from "normal" fluid emulsions (Ch. 18) by their semi-solid character, which, as in the case of ointments, is based on the presence of a colloidal matrix structures. Accordingly, creams may, in general, be considered as emulsions with a thickened, that is, congealed external phase. The semi-solid state enhances the physical stability of these dispersed preparations. This is due to the reduction of the rate of either or all creaming or sedimentation, aggregation, and coalescence as a result of the immobilization of the dispersed phase.

15.3.2.1 Lipophilic Creams

In lipophilic creams, the external phase is nonpolar—it consists typically of a hydrophobic ointment or a lipophilic gel. The dispersed phase is aqueous. For the improvement of the physical stability they commonly contain emulsifiers of the water-in-oil type such as wool alcohols, sorbitane esters and monoglycerides. Accordingly, water in oil (W/O) creams are lipophilic emulsions in which the external hydrophobic phase is a gel (hydrocarbon gel, oleogel or lipogel). This provides the formulation its good spreading properties.

A typical representative is the wool alcohol cream DAB, consisting of wool alcohol and cetostearyl alcohol, white soft paraffin and purified water.

We had chosen Ph. Eur., DAB, and NRF as reference. Of course in all pharmacopeias you will find formulation examples. Here is a selected list:

Hydrophobic Ointments

Paraffin Ointment	BP
Sulfur Ointment	USP/NF
White Ointment	USP/NF
Yellow Ointment	USP/NF
Zinc and Castor Oil Ointment	BP
Zinc Oxide Ointment	USP/NF

Water-emulsifying Ointments

Cetomacrogol Emulsifying Ointment	BP
Cetrimide Emulsifying Ointment	BP
Emulsifying Ointment	BP
Hydropilic Petrolatum	USP/NF
Salicylic Acid Ointment	BP
Simple Ointment	BP
Wool Alcohols Ointment	BP
Zinc Ointment	BP

Hydrophilic Creams

Aqueous Cream	BP
Buffered Cream	BP
Cetrimide Cream	BP
Hydrophilic Ointment	USP/NF
Rose Water Ointment	USP/NF

Lipophilic Creams

Hydrous Ointment	BP
Zinc Cream	BP

Pastes

Compound Zinc Paste	BP
Zinc and Sylicylic Acid Paste (Lassar's Paste)	USP/NF

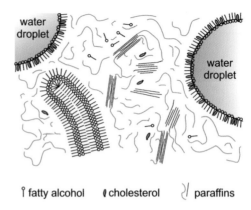

? fatty alcohol   ⸮ cholesterol   ⸮⸮ paraffins

Fig. 15-4 Model structure of the wool alcohol cream DAB.

A schematic representation of the colloidal structure is presented in Fig. 15-4. It shows a structure in which the water droplets, dispersed in the hydrocarbon gel (soft paraffin), are surrounded by a mixed film of emulsifiers consisting of fatty alcohols and sterols. These reduce the interfacial tension with the lipophilic phase and thus diminish the interfacial energy, simultaneously providing protection from coalescence.

The water-emulsifying capacity is strongly enhanced by the use of mixed emulsifiers. In addition, the semi-solid gel character of the external phase immobilizes the water droplets and thus stabilizes the dispersed system. The emulsifier molecules bound at the interface are in equilibrium with those dissolved in the liquid components of the external phase. The insoluble excess of emulsifier molecules crystallizes and the formed crystallites contribute to the structure of the basis, like in water-free systems. Due to the low emulsifier concentration, the structure of the lipophilic phase is nonetheless dominated by the matrix structure of the soft paraffin.

The preparation of the final product from the individual components is accomplished at elevated temperature in order to have the higher-melting components in the liquid state. However, when starting from the water-emulsifying ointment (e.g., wool alcohol ointment), the incorporation of the required amount of water may also be performed in the cold.

In case of manufacturing at higher temperature, it will be required to keep stirring the preparation during cooling and concomitantly occurring recrystallization process in order to obtain the desired matrix structure.

Among the lipophilic creams, the cold cream DAB takes a special position. In contrast to the "normal" lipophilic creams, it contains no emulsifiers. The disperse water phase is in this cream largely mechanically bound. This is supported by the very weakly emulsifying properties of the yellow wax. As a result the preparation is physically stable only to a limited extent and barely suitable for the incorporation of additional active ingredients. The product displays, however, the basic character of a lipophilic cream that, by virtue of its high proportion of waxes, conveys a very pleasant skin feel. A special characteristic of the cold cream is the easy water loss following application, which is responsible for the desired cooling effect on the skin.

The use of lipophilic creams brings along a limited hygiene risk. In case a contamination occurs, spread of the microorganisms in the basis is impeded since the germs can hardly survive in the continuous lipid phase. Moreover, the gelified external phase of the cream forms a mechanical barrier that barely permits proliferation from one droplet of the disperse water phase to another. In case of low water content and high dispersion grade the addition of a preservative may often be relinquished. For preparations with higher water content, preservation is regularly recommended or may even be stipulated in the concurrent extemporaneous preparations, such as for the hydrophobic base cream DAC.

Lipophilic creams show incompatibilities with hydrophilic active ingredients with an amphiphilic structure (e.g., polidocanol) (section 26.3).

Lipophilic creams have a greasing effect and are preferentially applied for dry skin types (sebostasic skin). These are partially occlusive and promote the hydration of the *Stratum corneum.* Nonetheless, because of the incorporated water the occlusion effect is not as pronounced as for hydrophobic or water-emulsifying ointments. These preparations cannot be washed off with water and leave a greasy film on the skin. In the context of licensed pharmaceutical preparations, products of this type are usually designated ointments, but in part also known as greasy creams. The EDQM standard term for this pharmaceutical dosage form is cream.

15.3.2.2 Hydrophilic Creams

In hydrophilic creams, the external phase is the aqueous phase, the lipophilic phase mostly representing the dispersed phase. The preparations contain emulsifiers of the O/W type, such as the sodium or trolamine soaps, sulfatized fatty alcohols, polysorbates, or esters of polyethoxy fatty acids and polyethoxy fatty alcohols referred to in the Ph. Eur. From a structural point of view, O/W creams may, in general, be considered mixed systems consisting of a hydrogel and an emulsion. The hydrogel may be made up of a synthetic polymer, traditionally however it represents a swollen, lamellar liquid-crystalline matrix formed by surfactant molecules.

To that end, hydrophilic creams contain a mixture of minimally two emulsifiers, *complex emulsifiers*, combining hydrophilic and lipophilic amphiphilic molecules. The hydrophilic component determines the emulsion type and stabilizes the disperse oil phase. The lipophilic component, often cetostearyl alcohol, crystallizes at room temperature, either alone or together with the hydrophilic component, and forms a matrix that lends the cream its semi-solid properties and provides stability.

Typical structural features may be found in the Anionic Hydrophilic Cream DAB.

Fig. 15-5 shows a model representation of the colloidal structure of this hydrophilic cream (ingredients: emulsifying cetostearyl alcohol, liquid paraffin, white soft paraffin, water). Part of the cetostearyl alcohol forms a mixed crystallisate with the fatty alcohol sulfates (a). The lamellae thus formed have a highly hydrophilic surface due to the enclosed sulfate groups so that between them water can be accommodated (b). The layered structure thus formed is designated hydrophilic gel phase (a + b). The remaining fraction of fatty alcohol crystallizes as a hemihydrate, likewise in a lamellar arrangement, the so-called lipophilic gel phase (c). The two gel phases together form a coherent matrix structure in which the aqueous fraction therein is immobilized as the bulk water phase (d). The water molecules in the bulk phase are freely movable, whereas the intralamellar water is firmly fixed. Bulk water and bound water are in dynamic equilibrium. They are coherent, which results in electric conductivity. The dispersed lipophilic phase (e) consisting of liquid paraffin and soft paraffin is enclosed in the cream structure via the hydrophobic chains of the fatty alcohols.

The anionic surfactants (fatty alcohol sulfates) in the hydrophilic cream may lead to incompatibilities. The hydrophilic gel phase is, for instance, highly sensitive to added salts

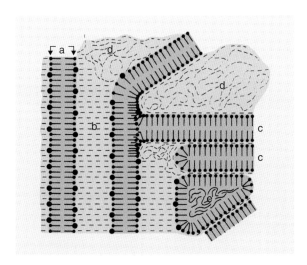

Fig. 15-5 Model structure of the Anionic Hydrophilic Cream DAB (see text for notations).

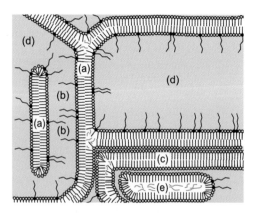

Fig. 15-6 **Model structure of the Nonionic Hydrophilic Cream DAB. (a) mixed crystals of non-ionic surfactants and cetylstearyl alcohol, (b) immobilized water, (c) lipophilic gel phase, (d) bulk water, (e) lipophilic dispersed phase.**

(expulsion of interlamellar water). Besides, incompatibilities with cationic active ingredients (e.g., antihistaminic drugs, local anesthetics, and acridine derivatives) may arise. Furthermore, skin irritations have been reported. That is why, particularly in case of licensed pharmaceutical preparations, often hydrophilic nonionic surfactants are deployed instead of anionic surfactants (e.g., polysorbate 60 in the Nonionic Hydrophilic Cream DAB or macrogol-fatty alcohol ethers in the Nonionic Hydrophilic Cream SR monographed in the DAC). For such systems, a structural buildup is assumed quite similar to that of Anionic Hydrophilic Cream (Fig. 15-6).

Stearate creams, which are particularly used in cosmetics, can be produced solely based on stearic acid or other long-chain saturated fatty acids without addition of another lipophilic component. Parts of the acidic groups are converted to the corresponding soap form by addition of a base such as sodium hydroxide or tromethamine (Tris). Following processing at elevated temperature and subsequent cold stirred, a structure is formed that is analogous to the model proposed for hydrophilic ointments, with fatty acids instead of fatty alcohols and without the lipophilic paraffin phase. Stearate crystals dispersed in the water phase are responsible for the mother-of-pearl shine of these preparations. The Ph. Helv. monographs an *Unguentum stearinicum* as an officinal formulation of this type. In the context of cosmetics, stearate creams are called vanishing creams.

Hydrophilic creams with a lamellar matrix structure are manufactured by means of a so-called hot/hot process. Lipid and water phase are first heated separately, then mixed at 70°C and subsequently cooled while being stirred because only in this way the desired colloidal structure is maintained. Even when using the corresponding water-emulsifying ointment as a starting material, cold-produced creams are less stable, clearly distinguish themselves with respect to the ratio of free bulk water and intralamellarly bound water.

The semi-solid character of traditional hydrophilic creams is due to a lamellar mixed crystallisate of the hydrophilic emulsifiers and the matrix builders. Contemporary dermal formulations are often based on macromolecular hydrogel formers such as carbomer (section 15.3.3.5) in order to obtain the desired rheological properties. The advantage is that less emulsifier and co-emulsifier is required, which are also lipids in a more common sense. This leads to formulations, which in the world of cosmetics are known as "light" creams. To distinguish them from the traditional creams they are as a brand sometimes called emulgel or emgel. However, they comply with the Ph. Eur. definition of hydrophilic creams. The risk of microbial contamination is higher with hydrophilic creams than that of lipophilic creams because in the former water forms the external phase. In order to ensure microbiological quality they are commonly preserved, mostly (in extemporaneous preparations) with sorbic acid, potassium sorbate, a mixture of p-hydroxybenzoic acid esters, or benzoic acid. Often, a humectant such as glycerol, propylene glycol, or sorbitol is added in hydrophilic creams in order to prevent rapid evaporation of the water following application on the skin.

Although hydrophilic creams are preferably used for application on seborrheic skin, they are also used in other applications. They are well tolerated and therefore are the most widely employed as a base in licensed pharmaceutical preparations. They are readily washed off by water and therefore are also applicable on hair-covered skin areas. Hydrophilic creams are practically nonocclusive, but may enhance the water-binding capacity of the skin when suitable lipids and moisturizers are incorporated.

Following application of hydrophilic creams on the skin, the water of the external phase evaporates within a few minutes. This rapidly leads to a metamorphosis of the vehicle so that shortly after application, the base bears little resemblance to the original material: The originally water-rich formulation turns into a lipid-rich, but nonetheless still hydrophilic, formulation. Because of the evaporation of the water phase, the concentration of the active ingredients dissolved in it will increase. This results in an increase in thermodynamic activity, thus creating favorable conditions for penetration of the active substance. It should be kept in mind, however, that the active substance should remain in solution and not crystallize. In order to prevent this, nonvolatile solvents such as propylene glycol may be added.

In the realm of licensed pharmaceutical preparations, hydrophilic creams are simply called creams. Sometimes, "based on O/W emulsion" is added for clarity. The EDQM standard term for this pharmaceutical dose form is cream.

15.3.2.3   Amphiphilic Creams

Amphiphilic creams have at least a bicoherent structure, that is, both the lipophilic and the aqueous phase are continuous. In most cases, they also have a similarly coherent matrix structure of a lamellar crystallisate consisting, for example, of glycerol monostearate and fatty alcohols, together resulting in a tricoherent structure. This matrix can swell to limited extents, but is already at very low water content fully hydrated and lends mechanical stability and good spreading properties to the amphiphilic cream.

A typical representative is the Base Cream DAC, which contains the matrix forming glycerol monostearate and cetyl alcohol as well as the O/W emulsifier macrogol-20-glycerolmonostearate. The structural model in Fig. 15-7 distinguishes (a) a partially swollen gel matrix (emulsifier phase), (b) a fully swollen gel matrix (aqueous phase), and (c) a coherent lipid phase; all phases are coherently entangled with one another.

According to this model, no distinction can be made between an inner and an outer phase, so that this type of formulation does not comply with the IUPAC definition of emulsions. Because of their coherent oil and water phases, amphiphilic creams can be diluted with either one component at low energy expense. That is why they comply neither with the definition of lipophilic creams nor with that of hydrophilic creams. They take an intermediate position and cannot easily be accommodated in the systematics of the Ph. Eur., but at the same time, they are not considered an independent subgroup. Based on their composition (they contain typical O/W emulsifiers) and their dermatological properties they could be counted among the hydrophilic creams. Common tests to determine the phase distribution, for instance, the wash-off or dye test, as well as the assessment of the electric conductivity,

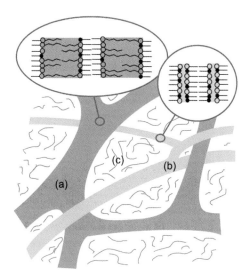

Fig. 15-7 Model structure of an amphiphilic cream (see text for notations).

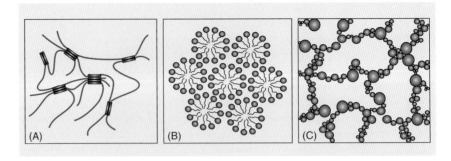

Fig. 15-8 Colloidal basic structure of gels. (A) polymer networks, (B) ordered gel mesophases, (C) particulate gel matrix

generally do not produce unambiguous results because of the bi- or tricoherent characteristics. Like hydrophilic creams, licensed pharmaceutical preparations of this type are commonly simply called creams. The EDQM standard term for this pharmaceutical dose form is cream.

15.3.3   Gels

In the Ph. Eur., gels are defined in a very broad and general sense: Gels consist of liquids gelled by means of suitable gelling agents. As a rule, gelling agents are substances such as macromolecules, associates of surfactants, or solids in the colloidal size range that immobilize the liquid. As a consequence, these preparations have—in accordance with the IUPAC definition for gels—a finite, usually rather small, yield point. To this end, the molecules or particles of the gelling agents show substantial interactions. Out of this, there exist three basic structures characterizing the colloidal makeup of gels (Fig. 15-8):

1. Gels with polymer networks: They have a predominantly nonordered structure in addition to partly ordered domains, which, by physical aggregation of polymer chains, act as the network junction points. This structure is characteristic of hydrogels containing organic macromolecules such as hydroxylethylcellulose.
2. Gels with ordered gel mesophases: The structural elements of this type are association colloids consisting of surfactant molecules. Typical representatives are the poloxamer gels.
3. Gels with a particulate gel matrix: Colloidal solid particles, mostly of inorganic nature, aggregated via weak interaction forces, serve as gelling agents. This structure is typical of gels from colloidal silica or phyllosilicates.

15.3.3.1   Lipophilic Gels

According to the definition of the Ph. Eur., lipophilic gels (oleogels) are preparations whose bases usually consist of liquid paraffin with polyethylene or fatty oils gelled with colloidal silica or aluminum or zinc soaps. Consequently, they cannot be distinguished unambiguously from hydrophobic ointments. Depending on their composition, they can be subcategorized in isogels and heterogels.

The former can even be further subdivided in hydrocarbon gels and lipogels, which should, however, rather be considered to belong to the hydrophobic ointments (section 15.3.1). Explicitly referring to hydrocarbon gels consisting of paraffin and polyethylene (hydrophobic base gel DAC) as belonging to the lipophilic gels seems to be little systematic. However, soft paraffin is mentioned neither as a lipophilic gel, nor as a hydrophobic ointment base in Ph. Eur.

Oleogels in the narrower sense are heterogels with a liquid lipophilic phase based on hydrocarbons, glycerides, polysiloxans (silicon oils), or liquid waxes. Typical gelling agents are:

– Zinc stearate, aluminum stearate
– Colloidal silica
– Organo-modified Hectorite
– Ethylcellulose

What all these substances have in common is that in the liquid phase, the gelling agents have only (very) limited solubility. By interparticulate interactions, a three-dimensional network is built in which the liquid phase is immobilized. Because the solubility of the gelling agents varies only slightly in the practically relevant temperature range, the consistency of the oleogels is only slightly temperature dependent.

Although zinc- and aluminum-stearate are soluble in lipids at temperatures above 100°C, they recrystallize upon cooling and form a three-dimensional particulate network. Colloidal silica forms hydrogen bonds in nearly all nonpolar fluids between the superficial silanol groups of the spherocolloid particles and thus aggregates into a gel matrix. Only 5% to 10% of this material suffices to form this matrix. The gel formation is strongly enhanced by short-chain additives such as Macrogol 400, because these facilitate the formation of hydrogen bonds leading to the inter-particular cross-linking of the colloid particles. Similarly positive, but less easily controlled, is the influence of small amounts of water (up to about 5%). The three-dimensional particulate network is strongly shear-sensitive, and therefore, the resulting oleogels are extremely thixotropic. For dermal applications, these gels are not well suited, as their cosmetic properties are unfavorable due to the dulling sensation on the skin. More often, the thickening effect of colloidal silica is exploited in the production of suppositories or in the lipophilic filling material for soft capsules in order to prevent sedimentation of active agents during the production process.

Organo-modified Hectorites (e.g., Bentone®) are produced by adsorption of di-stearyl, dimethyl-ammonium ions to 2:1 phyllosilicate of the Hectorite type (Bentonite). This results in the formation of *platelets* (laminar colloids) that are moistened by lipids and furthermore have the ability to aggregate and to form a three-dimensional matrix (card house structure) in fluids with low or intermediate polarity (Fig. 15-9). To accomplish this, often a small quantity of an activator such as ethanol is required. Gels with Bentone® have certain advantageous application properties, but display a brownish opaque appearance due to their intrinsic color and the particle size of the gelling agent.

Ethylcellulose is a cellulose ether soluble in polar lipids (e.g., castor oil). In less polar oils, such as octyldodecanol the substance is only partially soluble. Less well solvated fractions of the polymer chains will then build a gel matrix through polymer-polymer interactions. Thus, ethylcellulose can be counted among the cross-linked weak-interaction polymer networks with predominantly nonordered structure and partially ordered domains. When solubility in the lipid phase becomes too low, like for example in medium-chain triglycerides, the polymer precipitates and does not build a gel.

15.3.3.2 Hydrophilic Gels

Hydrophilic gels (hydrogels) for cutaneous application are bicoherent systems, consisting of a solid component building a coherent three-dimensional matrix (texture, network) and a liquid that stays as a coherent medium in the matrix.

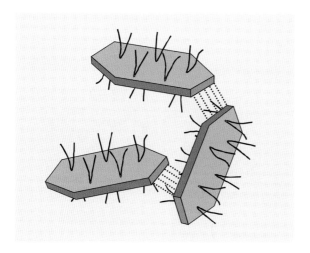

Fig. 15-9 Matrix formation with organo-modified Hectorite (Bentone®).

Hydrogels are always heterogels in which matrix and liquid component are chemically different. In order to be spreadable (semi-solid), the gelling agents interact only by physical bonds (noncovalent).

The liquid phase, which may make up 80% to nearly 100% of the preparation, is aqueous or hydro-alcoholic and may contain up to 10% of a humectant such as glycerol, sorbitol, or propylene glycol, less frequently are also pentylene glycol or hexylene glycol.

As gelling agents, rarely inorganic substances like Mg-Al silicates (Bentonite) are used. In most cases organic macromolecules that swell are used and thus form the matrix. Examples of this group as per the Ph. Eur. include starch, cellulose derivatives, and carbomer. At sufficiently high concentrations, the macromolecules form a three-dimensional coherent network and thus determine the rheological properties of the system.

In addition, surfactant gels may be considered to belong to the hydrogels, in which surfactant associates (ordered gel mesophases) build the matrix in these cases. The Ph. Eur. refers to poloxamers as suitable excipients.

The most important pharmaceutical hydrogelling agents are carbomers and cellulose ethers. Corresponding preparations are also presented in DAB (see Ph. Eur./DAB/DAC: example formulations). Particularly in licensed pharmaceutical preparations, carbomers are frequently employed.

15.3.3.3   Hydrogels with Inorganic Gelling Agents

The inorganic gelling agent for aqueous-based gels belong either to the group of swellable phyllosilicates of the montmorillonite type (Bentonite, Laponite, Veegum®) or to the colloidal silicas.

Colloidal silica consists of nanometer-sized spherical primary particles with superficial silanol groups, which are able to form cross-linked gel networks by means of hydrogen bonds (Fig. 15-10 right). In water, such strongly thixotropic gels are formed at substantially higher concentrations (about 15% to 20%) than in nonpolar fluids. This is due to the competitive interactions of water with the silanol groups that build up a gel network via hydrogen bonds. This reduces the gel stability.

Crystal clear hydrogels may be formed from amorphous silica when, by addition of polyols (glycerol, sorbitol), the refractive index of the aqueous phase is adjusted to the same value as that of SiO_2. Such formulations do not play a significant role in dermal formulations but have become more and more popular in toothpastes.

The gel-forming capacity of colloidal silica is tremendously enhanced by adsorption of surfactants (cationic or nonionic macrogol derivatives) at the surface of the silica particles. At half-maximal adsorption at the silica surface, particles are formed that will aggregate via hydrophobic interactions (Fig. 15-11), so that even at relatively low concentrations ($\sim$5%) hydrogels are formed.

Montmorillonites consist of plate-shaped particles of colloidal dimensions (90% < 1 μm) belonging to the 2:1 phyllosilicates. In montmorillonites monovalent cations are embedded in the spaces between the plates. These cations are hydrated upon the contact to water, causing the clay to swell. The individual montmorillonite plates carry negative charges on their surface, but excess positive charges on the fracture planes. This allows gel formation due to ionic aggregation and leads to a card-house-like three-dimensional network structure

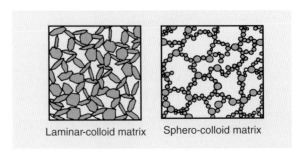

Laminar-colloid matrix   Sphero-colloid matrix

Fig. 15-10 Gel structures with inorganic hydrogel builders. Left: card-house structure with swellable phyllosilicates, Right: aggregated sphero-colloids of colloidal silica.

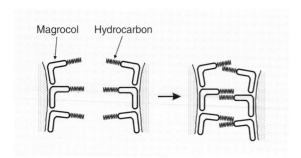

Fig. 15-11 Aggregation of SiO₂ after half-maximal surface coverage with a nonionic surfactant.

(Fig. 15-10 left). Montmorillonite gels are highly electrolyte-sensitive because the gel formation is based on ionic interactions. Bentonite gels are, typically, distinctly thixotropic, that is, they display a pronounced shear-induced isothermal gel-sol-transition (Fig. 15-12). Mechanical influences (shock, shear) destroy the structured situation causing the system to liquefy. When left to stand, the particles approach each other again by Brownian motion and thus rebuild the gel matrix causing the system to solidify again. When so desired, the thixotropic properties may be further promoted by addition of sodium carbonate. During storage of bentonite gels no changes in viscosity occur; temperature changes may have a minor effect on viscosity. They are stable within the pH range 4.5 to 10.5. As montmorillonnites act as cation exchanger, the incorporation of cationic pharmaceutical actives may give rise to quality issues (section 26.2).

To prepare bentonite gels, it is possible to add consecutively small amounts of the substance to water or disperse it after adding all at once with a high-speed stirrer. Gel formation requires a swelling time of several hours; hot water (80° to 90°C) may shorten this.

Montmorillonite gels may offer an attractive formulation option when a covering effect of clay pigments on the skin is desired (e.g., in hydrogels for acne treatment). In particular, on the American market, preparations based on bentonite play a role in the manufacturing of shake lotions. A typical example is calamine lotion consisting of calamine 8 g, zinc oxide 8 g, glycerin 2 mL, bentonite magma 25 mL, and calcium hydroxide topical solution, in a sufficient quantity to make 100 mL.

15.3.3.4 Hydrogels with Organic Gelling Agents

Organic macromolecular hydrogel formers originate from different chemical classes and may be of natural, semi-synthetic or fully synthetic origin.

Hydrogels are formed by swelling of organic molecules in water or hydro-alcoholic mixtures. In general, hydrogels for dermal preparations are not cross-linked and may swell unlimited. Water uptake proceeds under:

- Volume expansion
- Pressure development (up to 100 MPa)
- Positive heat effect (exotherm; $\Delta G < 0$)

At low water uptake, bodies with an elastic character are formed. With increasing water content, systems are formed with plastic flow behavior. At high water content, a gel-to-sol transition is characterized by pseudo-plastic flow.

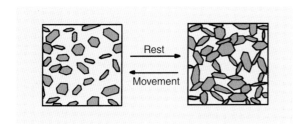

Fig. 15-12 Gel–sol transition of Bentonite preparations (Thixotropy).

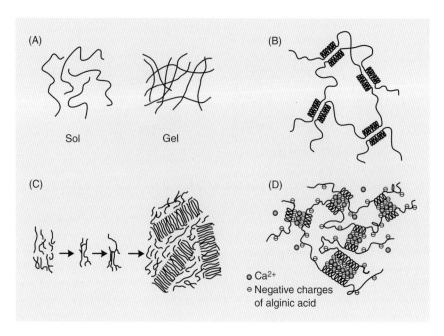

Fig. 15-13 Possible gel structures with organic hydrogel builders: (A) interlocking/ entanglement for linear macromolecules; (B) Formation of helical areas; (C) formation of crystal-like structures; (D) ionotropic gel forming.

Gel formation from organic macromolecular gelling agents may be based on different structuring mechanisms (Fig. 15-13).

Gels of Interlocking/Entangled Linear Macromolecules
These hydrogels arise at sufficiently high concentrations of an infinitely swellable linear macromolecule without the occurrence of specific interactions. The flow-inhibiting action in these gels is based on an interpenetration of the macromolecules with a subsequent mechanical interlocking or entanglement process as a result. With increasing polymer concentration, a conversion from a pseudo-plastic sol without yield point to a plastic gel displaying a certain yield point is observed. This gel-building mechanism is particularly efficient for very large and elongated macromolecules such as polyacrylic acids. When the carboxyl groups in this polymer (molecular mass >1,000,000) are neutralized with alkali in an electrolyte-poor medium, the repulsive effect of the resulting negative charges will cause the polymer to stretch extensively and results in gel formation. Typical representatives of this group of gelling agents are PVP, PVA, and carbomers.

Formation of Crystal-Like Structures
In this gel type, the interactions between the polymer chains arise from alignment of polymer segments in the form of highly ordered crystal-like structures. This gelation mechanism is typical of cellulose ethers and maltodextrins.

Formation of Helical Domains
Another possibility to link polymer chains is the formation of a double helix by two polymer strands. This interaction is very strong and only yields gels with good spreading properties provided the number of helical domains is not too large. In case of pronounced helix formation, for example with gelatin, hydrogels are formed that show the *rheodestruction phenomenon*. Upon applying a shear stress, the matrix is irreversibly destroyed and, even after a long resting phase, it is not rebuilt.

Regeneration requires newly reformed helices, which can typically be achieved by subsequent cooling of a heated mixture; the gels show a thermo-reversible sol–gel transition. Helical structures are to be encountered in hydrogels with gelatin, starch, or galactomannans.

Ionotropic Gel Formation

In ionotropic gels cross-linking of ionic macromolecules is established by means of multivalent ions. This effect can be nonspecific or, as in case of alginate, lead to a very special structure, the egg-box structure. In this structure, divalent cations, preferably Ca^{2+}, are accommodated in the zig-zag structure of the gulluronic acid moieties of the alginic acid. By virtue of this strong interaction mechanism, ionotropic gels often display only limited spreadability.

In terms of behavior following their application, hydrogels of organic macromolecules can be distinguished in film-forming and non–film-forming preparations. Film-forming gelling agents include, in particular, the cellulose ethers.

By contrast, hydrogels obtained from anionic carbomers do not leave a film on after rubbing it into the skin. This is based on the electrolyte-sensitivity of carbomer gels causing their gel matrix to collapse upon application on the skin under the influence of the salts present there; the hydrogel appears to melt and does not build a film.

15.3.3.5   Carbomer Gels

Carbomers are high-molecular-weight polyacrylic acids slightly cross-linked with polyalkene ethers of sugars or polyalcohols. For pharmaceutical purposes, only types with a residual benzene level below 2 ppm are permitted (e.g., Carbopol® 980 or 974 P). For gel building as little as 0.5% to 1% (m/m) of carbomer is sufficient.

For gel formation, carbomer is dispersed in water, and the resulting suspension is neutralized with an inorganic or organic base. Only after neutralization gel formation proceeds (Fig. 15-14). The white, loose, hygroscopic Carbopol powder consists of primary particles of weakly cross-linked polyacrylic acid, which agglomerate into units of a size within the µm range. In dry conditions, the polymer chains are strongly coiled. Upon dispersion in water, the substance takes up some water and swells, causing the chains to uncoil to some extent. The resulting dispersion has a pH of about 3 and initially remains fluid. By neutralization with an appropriate amount of base, the polymer is deprotonated. The anionic charges cause the polymer chains to repel each other and occupy maximal distance from each other. This leads to complete uncoiling and stretching of the chains, which is accompanied by strong swelling of the particles (up to 1,000-fold their original volume) and gel formation.

In addition to alkali hydroxides, organic bases such as trometamol (Tris) are employed for neutralization. Likewise, when present, basic pharmaceutical actives can be used as

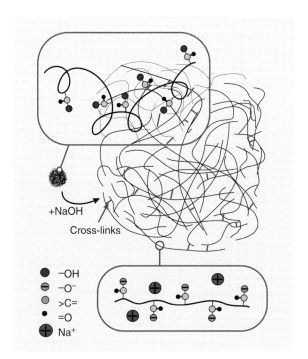

Fig. 15-14   Formation of carbomer gels.

neutralizing agent. The application of triethanolamine (Trolamine, 2,2′,2″-Nitrilotriethanol, TEA) as a base should be avoided in externally applied pharmaceutics because of the risk of nitrosamine formation, or should be limited to maximally 2.5%. The amount of potentially carcinogenic N-nitrosamines in licensed pharmaceutical preparations should not exceed 10 ppb.

Polyacrylate gels are only little thixotropic and are quite attractive because of their crystal-clear appearance. In addition, they are well tolerated on the skin and do not leave a film on the skin upon drying. The viscosity of carbomer gels is stable in a pH range from 6 to 10. At above pH 10, viscosity decreases. At pH values below 5, viscosity is rapidly lost. Therefore, if sorbic acid is used as a preservative, which is effective only at weakly acid conditions, careful pH adjustment is mandatory. Furthermore, carbomer gels are highly sensitive to the addition of salt. Even low concentrations of salt, such as sodium chloride, or even more pronounced multivalent cations, such as Ca^{2+} and Al^{3+} have a significant negative effect on the consistency of carbomer gels and could cause coagulation. For stabilization purposes, often edetate-Na is added as a chelating substance to sequester the multivalent cations. The incompatibility with salts leads to apparent melting of the gels following application on the skin, as well as to a certain stickiness. Carbomer gels are also incompatible with several cationic active substances or polymers (see section 26.2). Polyacrylate gels are subject to reaction with oxygen, which causes a permanent reduction or loss of viscosity. Sunlight and UV light catalyze this process. Therefore, the gels should be stored protected from light.

15.3.3.6   Cellulose Ethers

The cellulose ethers—which are able to swell unlimited in water—are also often used as gelling agents for aqueous-based gels. These substances (see also 5.3.5.1) are obtained by partial substitution of the three reactive hydroxyl groups in the anhydroglucose units of cellulose. The degree of substitution (DS) is given by the average number of ether bonds per anhydroglucose unit. The average molar substitution grade (MS) represents the molar ratio of substituents per anhydroglucose units. Instead of MS or DS, often the percentage of substituents in the cellulose ether molecule is given.

The most important substances for the production of hydrogels are the nonionic cellulose ethers hydroxyethylcellulose, hydroxypropylcellulose, and hypromellose (hydroxylpropyl-methylcellulose), as well as the anionic carmellose-sodium (sodium carboxymethylcellulose). In principle, the nonionic methylcellulose is suitable as well, but this is nonetheless rarely deployed as a gelling agent.

In concentrations of >2% and dependent on the chain length of the molecule, the nonionic cellulose ethers form gels with good spreading properties. Hydroxyethylcellulose forms clear gels that are compatible with low electrolyte concentrations, including multivalent cations. Hydroxypropylmethylcellulose stands out as a gel builder in that it also stabilizes hydro-alcoholic gels. Methylcellulose and hypromellose are only soluble in the cold. Above 50°C (turbidity point), these gelling agents are insoluble. Both cellulose ethers are surface active, which makes particularly hypromellose highly suitable for the preparation of hydro-dispersion gels (section 15.8.2). All nonionic cellulose ethers display, to a larger or lesser extent, incompatibilities with electrolytes at higher concentrations, tannins, and phenol derivatives.

Carmellose-sodium (sodium carboxymethylcellulose, see also 5.3.5.8) takes an exceptional position because of its approximately equal solubility in cold and hot water. Gels with good spreading properties are obtained in concentrations of 3% to 8%. Maximal viscosity is attained in the pH range between 6 and 9 and at low salt concentrations. In contrast to the nonionic cellulose ethers, carmellose-sodium is compatible with phenols, but incompatible with cationic actives.

As with most water-soluble gelling agents, cellulose ethers have a tendency to lump when first wetted with water. To prevent this, cellulose ethers can be prewetted with a water-miscible organic liquid (e.g., the moisturizer) or dry-blended with other dry materials before adding to water. This ascertains an effective separation of the cellulose ether dry powder particles prior to their contact with water and subsequently allows gel formation by addition of water without lumping. The temperature-dependent solubility of some cellulose ethers can also be exploited in the gel production process. For example, hypromellose may be quite uniformly dispersed in hot water, in which it is insoluble. The swelling process can then be induced by storing at lower temperature.

15.3.3.7   Natural Gelling Agents

Natural gelling agents are hardly deployed for the production of semi-solid preparations, but are to some extent applied in another context as excipients. For example, gelatin gels are only rarely applied for cutaneous application, e.g., as zinc glue DAB (*Unna's paste*). But in other pharmaceutical domains they play an important role—for example, in the manufacturing of gelatin capsules or of glycerol-gelatin mixtures for rectal or vaginal application.

Gelatin gels used in pharmaceuticals are highly elastic and display at room temperature a rheo-destructive behavior because the special network structure (helix formation) cannot be reconstructed by simple diffusion of the constituting molecules. Due to this, gelatin gels cannot be designated to be semi-solid. After rheo-destruction, the gel structure can only be restored by heating above the gel-sol-transition temperature and subsequently cooling.

In cosmetic preparations, xanthan and guar gum are deployed, mostly for the purpose of gel formation in the external phase of O/W emulsions.

Guar gum is the ground mucous endosperm of the guar bean and consists of nearly 80% guaran, a galactomannan with 64% mannose, and 36% galactose. Guar allows the production of highly viscous hydrocolloid solutions displaying maximal viscosity in neutral solution.

Xanthan gum is a high-molecular-weight heteropolysaccharide, produced by the fermentation of glucose, sucrose, or lactose by the microorganism *Xanthamonas campestris*. It consists essentially of β-1,4-linked glucose units with side chains of mannose and glucuronic acid. Xanthan gum is readily soluble in water and forms plastic gels with low temperature dependence. Gel building from xanthan is promoted synergetically by addition of galactomannans.

15.3.3.8   Surfactant Gels

Surfactant gels belong to the lyotropic liquid crystals (surfactant mesophases). They are formed by aggregation (self-assembly) of hydrated or solvated surfactant molecules. Dependent on concentration and structure of the surfactant different aggregates may arise (see box "Liquid-crystalline phases").

Cubic and hexagonal liquid crystals display distinct visco-elastic behavior, that is, they exhibit both the rheologic properties of a solid and of a liquid. Typical for gels, they have a distinct yield point. Upon applying a mechanical stress to cubic gel phases they react exceptionally elastic. Cubic gel phases often show the ringing phenomena when they are excited to mechanical vibrations due to energy dissipation in the acoustic frequency range. Due to their one-dimensional ordering lamellar liquid crystals have mostly better flow properties than cubic or hexagonal phases, but also show some visco-elastic behavior, although less distinct.

Thermo-sensitive surfactant gels may be obtained with poloxamers (PEG-PPG block-copolymers). In the cold, these gels are liquid and they gel at temperatures above room temperature, while at further temperature increase to above body temperature they fluidize again. To accomplish these properties, such preparations must contain up to 30% poloxamer and about 20% propylene glycol in the water phase. The solid–gel transition temperature can be adjusted in a relatively wide range by varying the amount and ratio of poloxamer and propylene glycol.

A particular application form of the surfactant gels is *thermogels*. These consist of a special combination of excipients such as poloxamer 407, medium-chain triglycerides, dimethyl-isosorbide, 2-propanol and water (e.g., in Dolgit® mikrogel, Dolobene® Ibu gel, Dolormin® Mobil gel). Due to its thermo-reversible gelling behavior, this formulation is liquid at 4°C and semi-solid at temperatures above 12°C. That is why this formulation may be easily applied to the affected body site and remains in place due to the rapid warming by the body heat. The addition of dimethyl-sorbide and 2-propanol improves the penetration for many active ingredients into the skin.

Surfactant gels can exist only at a defined ratio of water and surfactant. However, the water content of these formulations changes following application on the skin. Within a few minutes, the excess water evaporates, causing the gels to undergo pronounced changes in accordance with their phase behavior. Thus, when we apply a cubic phase on the skin, this may

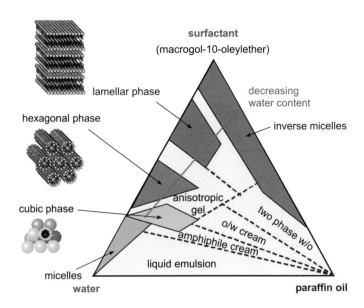

Fig. 15-15   Possible changes of the vehicle structure after application.

subsequently change into a hexagonal and further into a lamellar phase. At very low water content, an inverted micellar system may even be formed. Furthermore, multiphasic transition states may form in between (Fig. 15-15). Water release and phase changes are dynamic processes. This implies that the occurrence of individual "phenotypes" ultimately is not thermodynamically but rather, kinetically controlled, and may be strongly inhibited at high viscosity.

Most organic molecules utilized for the production of well-spreading gels (e.g., cellulose derivatives) swell unlimited—that is, in presence of sufficient solvent the gel converts to a sol. The amount of water added for the swelling process determines the rheological properties of the preparations thus formed. With small quantities of added water, the resulting material consists of swollen bodies with elastic properties. Upon further addition of water, systems with plastic deformability arise, which by virtue of their good spreadability may be applied cutaneously.

When ultimately, at very high water content, the solution state is reached, the macromolecules are spatially arranged separate from each other. Carbomer gels take an exceptional position. The gel particles can accommodate only a limited amount of water as a result of the chemical cross-linking. Additional water will merely find its place between the particles, thus creating a suspension of gel particles.

Hydrogels display structural viscosity and are mostly thixotropic; in case of Bentonite gels, these properties are quite distinct. During storage especially highly concentrated gels are subject to aging, leading to liquid loss but leaving the exterior of the gel bodies intact. This process is called *syneresis* and is attributed to the contraction of the matrix under increasing formation of more ordered or crystalline structures.

A typical hydrogel contains, in addition to the gelling agents and water, humectants and preservatives. The function of the humectant (e.g., glycerol, propylene glycol, or sorbitol in concentrations of 10% to 20%) is not only to protect the gel from drying out following application but also to lend the preparation suppleness and spreading properties (plasticizer function). When using film-forming gelling agents (cellulose ethers), humectants are mandatory to maintain extensibility. Due to their high water content, hydrogels are microbially vulnerable and must therefore be preserved, usually with sorbic acid/potassium sorbate or a parabene mixture and occasionally with alcohols. Preparations containing more than 15% ethanol, 2-propanol, or propylene glycol do not require additional preservatives because of the antimicrobial action of the alcohols. Similar to hydrophilic creams, nonpreserved hydrogels need to be prepared freshly, to be packed in a tube or dose dispenser and not to be used after one week. Tube filling not only protects from microbial contamination but also from drying out.

As nongreasy preparations, hydrophilic gels are suitable for application on the seborrheic skin and are often used as vehicle for acne therapeutics as well as for application on hairy skin. In addition, agents for the treatment of itching skin conditions (e.g., anti-histamines, corticosteroids, anti-mycotics, and anti-parasite drugs) are often formulated in a hydrogel. The cooling effect of such bases further enhances the therapeutic effect. Polyacrylate gels are used as the base for topical treatment with nonsteroidal anti-inflammatory drugs or for transdermal hormone therapy, such as with estradiol.

15.3.4   Pastes

Pastes are semi-solid preparations for cutaneous applications and contain large proportions of finely dispersed powders. The Ph. Eur. does not specify at what proportion of suspended substances to differentiate between pastes and suspension ointments. As an example from a local compendium: In the DAC/NRF (German Pharmacopeia), preparations with 20% solids are still considered ointments while the zinc pastes described have a powder content of 30% to 50%. Depending on the amount of solids, a distinction is made between soft ($\sim$30% solids) and hard ($\sim$50% solids) pastes. Liquid pastes are preparations with 50% solids in oil, but they are not counted among the semi-solid dermal formulations.

The rheological character of a paste is largely determined by its solid content, which has a distinct solidifying effect on the pure base. Particularly in highly concentrated pastes (>50% solids), the dispersed powder particles are so densely packed that interparticulate interactions occur. A large fraction of the base is in direct contact with the surface of the dispersed particles and engages in interactions with them. The particles are only separated from one another by a thin film of base through which capillary forces can be exerted on the powder particles.

The structure and the behavior of a paste depend not only on the concentration of the dispersed solid phase but also largely on the particle size. Finely dispersed particles represent a substantially larger surface area, which not only facilitates interactions but also the adsorption of continuous phase. By virtue of the interactions between the dispersed particles, highly concentrated pastes display shear-thickening flow behavior; they are dilatant bodies. Particularly during vigorous stirring, this results in a shear-induced thickening of the preparation, ultimately leading to a solid-like behavior. In systems with lower concentrations of solids or at lesser shear force, the rheologic behavior of the base becomes dominant—that is, predominantly plastic flow behavior is observed (section 3.12.1.5).

The Ph. Eur. does not explicitly distinguish between hydrophilic and hydrophobic pastes, but both formulation types are possible.

15.3.4.1   Hydrophobic Pastes

Hydrophobic pastes contain mostly zinc oxide and/or other inorganic pigments as a solid. But also starch, finely dispersed in a hydrophobic ointment (hydrocarbon gel or lipogel), or a water-emulsifying ointment is used for this purpose, an important function of hydrophobic pastes is their covering action. Only at very high solid content do they absorb liquid and act dehydrating. Soft pastes with a low content of solids instead display the properties of the basis; they have a protecting and greasing function.

15.3.4.2   Hydrophilic Pastes

In hydrophilic pastes, the solids are finely dispersed in a hydrogel—that is, they are thickened shake lotions. In practice, they are less common than hydrophobic pastes. In contrast to the traditional hydrophobic pastes, they have the advantage that, by virtue of their composition, they effectively act dehydrating, like a powder for cutaneous application.

15.3.4.3   Adhesive Pastes

Adhesive pastes (e.g., hypromellose adhesive paste 4% NRF) are special lipophilic preparations for application on mucosal tissue. They contain a high proportion of suspended hydrocolloids, such as cellulose ethers, to establish sustained contact with the moist mucosal surface. As soon as the particles of the gelling agent at the surface of the paste encounter the mucosa, they absorb moisture and swell up, which immediately leads to strong adhesion of the paste to the mucosa. The hydrophobic basis prevents rapid erosion of the preparation.

For the preparation of the paste, the finely disperse powder is suspended in the external phase. The latter may be warmed or melted. This facilitates the incorporation of the powder in case of semi-solid vehicles in which the powder is not soluble. To ensure a uniform distribution of the solid particles and, particularly to disaggregate powder clusters or agglomerates, often additional homogenization by means of kneading device or an ointment mill may be required (section 15.4.2; Fig. 15-17).

15.3.5   Poultices

The Ph. Eur. defines poultices as preparations consisting of a dispersion of liquid or solid active ingredient in a hydrophilic heat-storing basis. Only a few licensed pharmaceutical preparations fall in this category (e.g., Enelbin® paste, Kytta plasma® poultice). They are distinguished from other pastes mainly in that they may be applied not only cold but also warm. The poultice is applied as a thick layer (>1 mm) on a suitable dressing, placed on the affected body part and covered with a cloth.

Liquid-Crystalline Phases

Liquid-crystalline phases, also known as mesophases, represent an intermediate state between the crystalline-solid and the liquid state of matter. The molecules in the liquid-crystalline phase are, at least in one dimension, oriented in a regular manner (e.g., preferential orientation or regularly arranged layers) and as such experience strongly limited mobility. Nonetheless, the individual molecules in mesophases are freely motile in one or both other dimensions. Macroscopically, the character of such systems varies from viscous-fluid to relatively solid-plastic. Liquid-crystalline phases are formed from a substance suited to form liquid-crystals, a so-called mesogen, either by temperature changes (thermotropic mesophases) or by addition of a solvent (lyotropic mesophase). Upon reaching the melting point of the crystalline phase, thermotropic mesogenes initially form a slightly turbid fluid, the thermotropic liquid-crystalline phase. Upon further heating, at a defined temperature this phase converts to an isotropic melt. These phase transitions are reversible upon cooling. Important types of thermotropic mesophases are the nematic and the smectic phase. The nematic phase consists of rod-shaped organic molecules that have no positional order, but self-align to have long-range directional order with their long axes almost parallel. In the smectic phase, the paralleled molecules are, in addition, ordered in layers in which the molecular axis may be oriented perpendicular or tilted with respect to the layers. Liquid-crystalline structures were discovered more than 10 years ago in cholesterol esters, which form such thermotropic mesophases. In addition, several active substances such as fenoprofen-Na display thermotropic mesomorphism. From a practical point of view, however, this bears no relevance to the field of drug formulation.

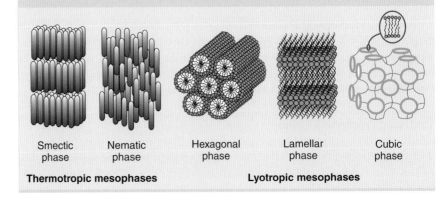

| Smectic phase | Nematic phase | Hexagonal phase | Lamellar phase | Cubic phase |

Thermotropic mesophases   **Lyotropic mesophases**

The occurrence of lyotropic mesophases, on the other hand, may be observed more often in several pharmaceutical preparations or during their manufacturing. They are formed by amphiphilic molecules that, upon contact with water, are hydrated at their head groups. This leads to swelling processes and, in conjunction with hydrophobic interactions, to a self-assembly of the amphiphilic molecules and the formation of liquid-crystalline phases.

During the dissolution of a (water-soluble) surfactant in water at very low concentrations, a molecularly dispersed solution results. Upon increasing the concentration, micelles are formed (section 3.9.9.6). When further increasing the amount of surfactant, a liquid-crystalline *hexagonal structure* may emerge (middle phase). This consists of cylindrically arranged densely packed surfactant molecules. The polar groups of the surfactant molecules form the surface of the parallel ordered cylinders, while the nonpolar chains stick out into the internal space of the cylinders in an entirely nonordered manner. Upon further increase of the surfactant concentration, a conversion into a *lamellar phase* (neat phase) is possible. This is characterized by a palisade-like arrangement of the surfactant molecules. The hydrated polar head groups of opposing molecules are pointing toward one another in one plane. In the space in between these planes, the nonpolar hydrocarbon moieties orient themselves without any order. An additional mesophase is the inverse hexagonal phase that may be formed from lipophilic surfactants (e.g., *unsaturated monoglycerides*) dissolved in oil and in the presence of a little water. In this phase the polar head groups of the surfactants shape the cylinder core, surrounded by the nonpolar outward oriented hydrocarbon chains. Cubic phases either are bicontinuous systems with a continuous bilayer structure or arise by dense packing of regular or inverse micelles. The type of lyotropic mesophase formed by a surfactant depends on its chemical structure. From this structure and in conjunction with the hydration of the hydrophilic head groups as well as the uptake of lipophilic fluids in the region of the hydrocarbon chains, a structure is finally formed, which itself determines strongly the aggregation behavior. Ternary mixtures of water, surfactant, and oil produce lyotropic mesophases in different, sometimes broad ranges of mixing ratios. A helpful tool to outline the composition regions where different phases exist is a ternary plot (see box). The formation of mesophases is strongly temperature-dependent because, especially for macrogol derivatives, their hydration and polarity varies strongly with temperature. For example, under certain circumstances a temperature change may trigger the transformation into another mesophase but it might lead as well to a crystalline or a liquid phase. Several substances—for instance, phospholipids—may form lyotropic as well as thermotropic mesophases. With the exception of cubic phases, liquid-crystalline phases are optically anisotropic. They display strong birefringence and are detectable by means of polarized light microscopy and can be distinguished microscopically on the basis of various "textures." These optical properties, which resemble those of crystals, have led to the designation "liquid crystals."

Liquid crystalline structures are involved in the matrix formation of many hydrophilic creams. For a few topical preparations, the gel character of a lyotropic liquid-crystalline phase is used as a base (section 15.3.3). The dispersion of lamellar liquid-crystalline phospholipid/water mixtures in an aqueous phase leads to the formation of liposomes. Liposomes are of particular interest as a drug carrier system in dermal preparations, but more particularly for parenteral application (section 20.3). Sometimes liquid-crystalline structures are just formed upon contact with physiological fluids. Such a phase transition may be exploited for special purposes, for instance in the case of Elyzol® dental gel, a preparation for the treatment of paradontitis. This gel, which represents a suspension of glycerol mono-oleate, sesame oil, and water, is introduced directly in the gingival pocket. At body temperature, it fluidizes initially and subsequently transforms into an inverse hexagonal phase upon water uptake. This adheres strongly to the site of action and slowly releases the active ingredient.

Three-Component Diagram (Ternary Plot)

Mixtures composed of three components (e.g., water, oil, surfactant) may be conveniently represented in a triangular diagram. The three corner points of the diagram represent the three pure components; binary mixtures are recorded as points on the sides of the triangle and ternary mixtures by points within the triangle. In this way, properties of these ternary systems such as different phase domains or miscibility gaps can be plotted as a function of composition. In the example diagram (right panel), the formulation point (a) represents a mixture of 20% component A, 30% B, and 50% C. Point (a) can be found as the intercept of the three corresponding concentration lines (the lines of equal concentration of a certain component are for each concentration the respective parallels in the diagram running to the triangle side opposite the "corner" of this component). In order to find all possible ternary mixtures with a fixed ratio of two of the components (e.g., 40 % A and 60 % C), a straight line is drawn from the formulation point of the binary mixture of these components to the "corner" of the third component (line (b)). Also, domains with particular concentration limits may thus be presented. For example, the green surface (c) represents all possible mixtures that contain more than 30% of component A and more than 20% component B, but maximally 40% of component C. Each individual triangular diagram is always only applicable for defined external conditions such as temperature and pressure. The involvement of an additional factor would require a three-dimensional representation. This also applies when a forth component should be considered. As a makeshift for the representation of mixtures of four components, in simple cases a *pseudo-ternary diagram* may be constructed in which one corner point represents not one pure component but rather, a defined ratio of two of the four components.

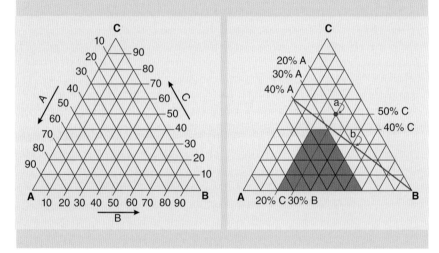

15.4   Production Technology

15.4.1   General Considerations

To ensure the quality of semi-solid preparations, a respectively designed manufacturing process, at the industrial scale as well as for extemporaneously prepared or stock formulations, is a prerequisite. Semi-solid preparations for cutaneous application are germ-poor preparations. In the manufacture, packaging, storage, and distribution of semi-solid preparations for cutaneous application, suitable measures have to be taken to ensure their microbiological quality. This calls for the processing of germ-poor raw materials and a high hygienic standard during the production process. For the industrial production corresponding standards of the Good Manufacturing Process (GMP) rules apply, including the requirements regarding personnel, raw materials, working places, instruments, method of production and documentation. Compounding in a pharmacy or any other site authorized by an appropriate jurisdiction is subject to other regulations laid down, for example, in the following:

- European Pharmacopeia (Ph. Eur.): Pharmaceutical Preparations
- United States Pharmacopeial Convention (USP): Pharmacetutical Compounding—Nonsterile Preparations
- The Pharmaceutical Inspection Cooperation Scheme (PIC/S): Guide to Good Practices for the Preparation of Medicinal Products in Healthcare Establishments

The individual steps in compounding and the industrial production of semi-solid preparations are by and large similar in principle; the major differences concern the scale size and the deployed equipment. The production procedure has to be adjusted to the type and composition of the chosen base. Furthermore, the degree of dispersion (molecular; colloidal; microscopic) of the active ingredient in the carrier substance essentially determines the production technology. Depending on their solubility characteristics, active pharmaceutical ingredients are either fully dissolved in the base or suspended (in a saturated solution); correspondingly, solution and suspension ointments and creams are distinguished. Preparations containing multiple active pharmaceutical ingredients of different solubilities may represent a solution preparation for one ingredient and simultaneously a suspension preparation for one or more of the others. Pharmaceuticals with moderate solubility in the base may yield a solution preparation at low concentrations but a suspension preparation at higher concentrations.

15.4.2   Semi-Solid Preparations with Suspended Active Ingredients

Active pharmaceutical ingredients are often not fully soluble in ointment and cream bases. In these cases, the particle size of the suspended actives is of decisive importance. Coarse particles (>180 μm) are perceived as solid particles upon application and have a sandpaper-like effect on the skin. However, prior sieving of the particles (as a rule, through sieve 180) can be done to remove these particles.

In order to achieve a homogeneous distribution, in low-dose preparations micronized particles of the active ingredient should be employed. (section 2.1.1). In addition, small drug particles promote the dissolution of the suspended particles following application and have a positive effect on bioavailability. When necessary, for compounding the particles may be further reduced in size by grinding, using a rough porcelain pestle and mortar. For the production of micronized drug powders, suitable mills are required (section 2.1.4). Extremely fine primary particles are obtained when using precipitated pharmaceutics (e.g., zinc oxide or alkaline bismuth nitrate), so that further size reduction is generally not necessary in such cases. Because ultra-finely dispersed powders (particle size <20 μm) show a strong tendency to agglomerate, prior sieving is recommended in order to fragment coarse agglomerates. The production procedure should be designed such that effective disagglomeration is guaranteed.

A highly uniform dispersion of the active ingredient may be achieved by producing a stepwise trituration of a concentrate. The finely powdered active ingredient should then be triturated with the same to twice the amount of base (or a liquid component of the base). In this way, it is possible in most cases to attain a homogeneous dispersion because, as a result of the plastic behavior of the basis and the high concentration of solid, a more intense shearing is achieved than in preparations with a lower active substance content. The drug concentrate is subsequently brought to the desired final concentration by geometric dilution with the remaining basis (step-wise processing of the drug-containing and drug-free base, each time at a 1:1 ratio). With the common compounding method using pestle and mortar dish (Fig. 15-16) (in some cases, also stirring and rolling devices), in most cases size reduction of drug particles should not be expected. Although the occurring shear forces may cause disagglomeration, they will be insufficient to reduce effectively the size of the solid particles. Moreover, the hardness of the used equipment will be in most cases insufficient to act as a grinding device.

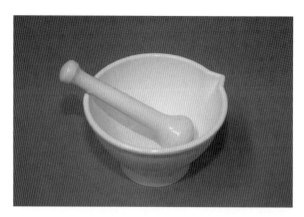

Fig. 15-16 Mortar and pestle used for compounding of semi-solid preparations. Reproduced with permission from Elsevier.

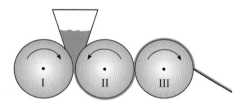

Fig. 15-17 Three-roll mill.

In highly concentrated preparations (e.g., stock triturates, pastes), by processing in a roll mill particle size reduction may be achieved. The three-roll mill (ointment mill) (Fig. 15-17) is widely used to achieve this. This consists of three motor-driven contra-rotating rollers (I, II, and III) made of hard porcelain, ceramic, stoneware, or polymer material. The efficiency of this device may be enhanced by applying different rotation speeds of the rollers (I < II < III). This causes friction and shearing forces to arise in the narrow gap between the rollers. The preparation is introduced in the device between rollers I and II and moves as a film through the gaps between the rollers along their surface and is ultimately scraped off from roller III. The width of the roller gaps can be adjusted and is usually kept slightly smaller between rollers II and III than between I and II. Gap width as small as 5 μm can be realized. The trituration effect obtained with ointment mills is accounted for by the pressure, friction, and shear forces occurring in the roller gaps, and depends on the concentration of solids in the preparation. With less concentrated preparations, the size reduction effect is less pronounced, but powder agglomerates are readily removed (disagglomerated). The employment of a three-roll mill in compounding and in small industrial scale preparations aims at breaking up powder agglomerates, disagglomeration and homogenization in suspension preparations. To obtain satisfactory homogeneity the suspension often has to be passed repeatedly through the three-roll mill. Polymer-coated rollers may be susceptible to material abrasion when the friction forces on the rollers become too strong and the drug particles are harder than the polymer material on the rollers.

Following the production of suspension preparations, potential crystal growth due to dissolution/re-precipitation processes should be taken into account when the suspended active ingredient is markedly soluble in the base (Table 15-2). This is promoted by temperature variations during storage because upon a temperature increase, drug molecules will dissolve and recrystallize again upon cooling. Particle size increase may also be induced during the production when intense shearing (e.g., in stirring devices) may cause substantial heat production. By the same token, the suspension of particles in a relative good solvent (e.g., a polar lipid), followed by subsequent dilution in a poor solvent (e.g., a hydrocarbon), may result in uncontrolled crystal growth from the then-super-saturated solution (section 25.3.1). Particle-size increase may also be the result of *Ostwald ripening*, which brings along gradual growth of larger particles at the expense of smaller ones.

Table 15-2 Solubility (%) of Some Pharmaceutics in Basis for Ointments at 20°C

Pharmaceutic	Soft Paraffin	Hydrogenated Peanut Oil
Menthol	20	18
Camphor	15	20
Thymol	6	30
Hydrocortisone	0.2	–
Benzocain	0.1	–
Salicylic acid	0.06	2

Ostwald ripening may be moderated by a narrow size distribution. In order to ensure the quality of suspension preparations produced at small industrial scale, particle size should be assessed regularly during storage.

15.4.3   Semi-Solid Preparations with Dissolved Active Agents

Among the hydrophobic and water-emulsifying ointments, preparations with fully dissolved active ingredients are rare. The reason for that is the generally insufficient solubility of active ingredients in the corresponding base (Table 15-2). An exception is formed by the essential oils and their pure constituents. By contrast, the hydrophilic ointments, that is, the macrogol ointments, are mostly solution ointments as the macrogols usually are good solvents for many active substances. The incorporation of the active ingredient in solution ointments is performed either in the cold, or the active ingredient is dissolved at the lowest possible temperature in the melted base, which then subsequently is cold stirred. The use of substantial amounts of dissolved active substance may cause a pronounced decrease in the melting point and thus result in softening of the preparation (e.g., the incorporation of camphor in soft paraffin). When, as a result, the semi-solid character of the preparation is lost, this effect may be corrected for by the addition of suitable consistency-enhancing excipients (e.g., hard paraffin or long-chain macrogols in case of hydrophilic ointments). The maximal amount of active ingredient to be processed in a solution preparation is determined by the solubility at the storage temperature rather than by a potentially increased processing temperature. In any case, super-saturation should be avoided in order to prevent the occurrence of recrystallization during storage. To be on the safe side, when the dissolution behavior of an active ingredient in the base is not precisely known, the preparation should be prepared as a suspension ointment in order to prevent later recrystallization. In hydrophilic gels, the solubility of the drug in the aqueous phase at its specific pH value decides whether a solution preparation is possible. In hydrophilic and lipophilic creams, active ingredients can be dissolved in the lipid phase as well as in the aqueous phase. That is why solution preparations are more often found in creams rather than ointments.

Mixing

The NRF describes in section I.6.9 "Preparation and Packaging Techniques" both manual and mechanical mixing devices for the compounding of dermal preparations. For the manual preparation following recommendations apply:

▢ Rough porcelain mortar and pestle	for powders
▢ mortar and pestle	for semi-solid preparations, emulsions and suspensions
▢ Beaker with glass rod	for solutions

Advanced (automized) devices are for example:

▢ Magnetic stirrer	for fluid preparations
▢ Stirring and rolling systems	for semi-solid dermal preparations

The latter include devices such as the Unguator®, the TopiTec® and the Tubag®-System. For all of these, compouding is performed directly in the primary package (for the Unguator® and TopiTec® in a special jar, for the Tubag® system in a flexible bag (to be placed in a tube)).

The suitability for a specific formulation needs to be checked in each individual case.

The following general preparation instructions are given:

For the manufacturing of suspension ointments and creams, micronized substances should be employed from which, at low dosages, a concentrated premix is prepared with about 10% of the base. Alternatively, suitable compounding concentrates may be applied. When using a rolling system, prior to the rolling procedure a "pre-trituration" may be performed by manual kneading with a small amount

More details about the Unguator can be found at https://www.unguator.com/ Information about the Topitec in English is difficult to get. But an available illustrated English manual gives sufficient information about the system. http://www.topitec.de/site/topitec/Mischsysteme/Downloads/TOPITEC%20Touch/TTT_BAL_05-2013_8Sprachen_low.pdf. For the Tubag system a patent might be informative: http://www.freepatentsonline.net/DE102004021731A1.html

of base in a transiently separated compartment of the bag. For that purpose, it is recommended to ultimately weigh the solid substances. When the preparation is performed with a stirring system, the weighed solid material is added to half of the basis and overlaid with the remainder of the base (sandwich method).

When *pre-trituration* is required, stirring is interrupted and continued after adding the remaining amount of base. When using the rolling system, it is necessary to interrupt the rolling process several times in order to squeeze the filling in the bag longitudinally and thus ensure adequate mixing perpendicular to the normal shear direction.

15.4.4   Preparation at the Pharmacy Scale

For compounding, such as in the pharmacy setting, manual processing with mortar and pestle is still a standard procedure (Fig. 15-12). When required, prior to the incorporation into the base, the active ingredients can be ground up in a rough porcelain mortar and subsequently classified by sieving. Heating is performed in a water bath or, alternatively, by means of a microwave oven. Homogenization, particularly of highly concentrated suspension preparations (e.g., stock triturates or pastes) is performed with a three-roll mill (ointment mill).

Alternative to the conventional preparation, several stirring or rolling systems have established their usefulness for the production of semi-solid preparations at this scale. These devices have in common that they are suitable for the production of semi-solid dermatics, predominantly creams and ointments, directly in the final or stock container. Mostly, pre-fabricated bulk material is used for the base rather than preparing it from the individual components.

In the Unguator® stirring system, mixing is performed with an electrically driven mixing blade. The stirring container is a specially designed jar. The special shape ensures optimal mixing. Thorough mixing in the vertical direction is achieved by up-and-down movements of the jar, which may be performed either manually or automatically. Stirring times vary, depending on the consistency of the product and the amount of material, between 5 and 10 minutes. As a rule, the individual components of the formulation are weighed out in the jar. The amount of air in the jar is minimized by shifting the bottom. Subsequently, the actual mixing process ensues. At the end of the process, product residues sticking to the stirrer are flung off by a rotational movement. After removal of the stirrer, the jar is closed with a screw cap. The amount of product is limited by the volume of the available jar (15 to 1,000 mL) and the capacity of the stirring device. As an alternative to the usual blade stirrer, a disposable blade stirrer may also be used. This remains in the jar after completion of the process, thus avoiding cleaning expenses.

In the Topitec® stirring system, the mixing process proceeds by means of a mixing disk electrically driven by a tool shaft. A jar serves as a mixing container. Thorough vertical mixing is achieved by automatic up-and-down movements of the jar by means of a carriage. Depending on the nature of the product and the amount of material, the stirring times may vary from 1 to 8 minutes at a recommended rotation speed of 500 to 2,500 rpm.

Typically, all components of the formulation are weighed out into the jar. Air is expelled by lifting the bottom of the jar. Then, the actual mixing process by means of the mixing disk follows. After the stirring shaft is removed, the jar is closed by a push-up bottom with an inserted moving screw base (metering bottom). Depending on the volume of the jar, the batch size, or the prescribed dose, the amount of processed material may vary from 20 to 500 g. As a rule, the mixing disk remains in the jar with its metering bottom after preparation, allowing for minimal cleaning time and costs.

In the TUBAG roller system (tube & bag), the mixing process is performed in a bag made from high-pressure polyethylene (low density). After completion of the preparation procedure, the bag serves as the primary packaging material. The components of the formulation are weighed out into the bag. Solid substances are added following fluid or semi-solid components. Air is expelled from the bag and the open end is simply closed by a knot. Solid components are then predispersed manually with the fluid or semi-solid components within the bag. The actual mixing process is performed in a rolling device that vigorously massages the polyethylene bag, thus ensuring a thorough mixing process. The essential longitudinal mixing is achieved while the preparation in the bag is lengthwise being spread. The mixing process usually takes only a few minutes. After termination of the mixing process, the bag is place in a standard aluminum tube, one end is pulled out from the tube orifice, and the bag is sliced off at this site. The tube is closed with a screw cap and at the other end closed by folding. When during the preparation heating is required, this can be done either in a water bath or, quite efficiently, in a microwave oven. When using the latter method, it must be taken into account that the various components may absorb different amounts of microwave energy. In order to prevent overheating, the microwave oven should be used at the lowest possible energy level. Adjustment of the amount of supplied heat to the batch size may be accomplished by variation of exposure time. The amount of energy supplied (time and intensity of stirring) depends on the nature of the formulation and the size of the batch. Relevant information is given by the manufacturer's manual.

A big advantage of compounding with stirring or rolling systems is the time-saving aspect, since there is no need to clean the device after use, and the fully automatic stirring process. Besides, improved hygiene, minimal exposure of the compounder to the constituents of the preparation and the minimal loss of material due to the closed character of the system, and the possibility to standardize the procedure based on the instrumental parameters, offer additional advantages.

A potential disadvantage is that visual in-process controls and inspection of the final product in the dispensing jar is hardly feasible. Whenever possible, for the preparation of suspension ointments or creams the solid components should be added as micronized substances because the stirring or rolling systems will not accomplish a significant size-reduction. A further advantage will be obtained when using prefabricated stock triturations and compounding concentrates. To ensure uniform distribution of the active in the base, an adequate processing technique (e.g., the sandwich method) and, when applicable, usage of pretrituration of the active agent with ~10% of the base are important. When using high-speed stirring devices, the development of substantial friction heat has to be taken into account, which may lead to uncontrolled temperature increase in the preparation (up to >40°C).

This may affect the quality of the preparation when an active ingredient (e.g., metronizadol) increasingly dissolves in the base at elevated temperatures and recrystallizes again upon cooling. Some cutaneously applied semi-solid formulations, such as, for example, hydrophilic cholorhexidine digluconate cream NRF, are highly shear-sensitive. This may lead to a distinctly lower consistency for formulations prepared by stirring or rolling techniques (producing strong shear forces) than for manually produced preparations. In each individual case, the possibility to use the alternative procedure should therefore be evaluated carefully.

15.4.5   Production at the Industrial Scale

The production of larger quantities of semi-solid preparations (up to 2,000 kg) commonly takes place in process units allowing temperature control, mixing, and homogenization as well as evacuation (Fig. 15-18). The mixers are equipped with large-size agitators, often in combination with wall-contacting scrapers, which ensure thorough mixing and good heat transport to and from a thermostated double jacket. Especially for the production of preparations containing a dispersed phase (e.g., creams or suspension ointments), the device is equipped with an additional homogenizer of the rotor-stator type (e.g., colloid mills, section 2.1.4.7), partially complemented by a dissolver disk. The latter (Fig. 15-18) possesses upward and downward bent blades, producing adequate shear forces. As far as possible, the production proceeds in a closed system to minimize the risk of (microbial) contamination. To that end, the lipid and, when applicable, water phase are prepared in separate phase vessels.

Also, these containers are double jacketed so that the individual phases of the semi-solid preparation can be heated or melted right there and mixed by means of a separate stirring device. The prepared (pre-)phases are transferred via pipelines into the processing unit. During the transfer, they may in addition be (sterile-) filtered. In the processing unit, the prephases are mixed, homogenized, and cold-stirred. In most currently available processing units, the homogenizer is centrally positioned at the bottom of the product vessel. The

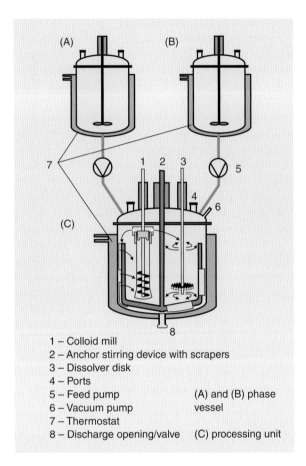

1 – Colloid mill
2 – Anchor stirring device with scrapers
3 – Dissolver disk
4 – Ports
5 – Feed pump   (A) and (B) phase
6 – Vacuum pump   vessel
7 – Thermostat
8 – Discharge opening/valve   (C) processing unit

Fig. 15-18 Equipment for batch-wise production of semi-solid preparations.

homogenized product can either be returned in the upper part of the container or withdrawn from the container via a valve (Fig. 15-19). To this end, the homogenizer simultaneously acts as a pump.

In the production of creams, the emulsification of lipid and water phases is accomplished with the homogenizer at a temperature slightly above the solidification temperature of the lipid phase. The cold-stirring step is, as for the manual preparation procedure, essential for the formation of the desired matrix structures and, with that, for the consistency and physical stability of the product. The stirring and cooling rates must be accurately coordinated in

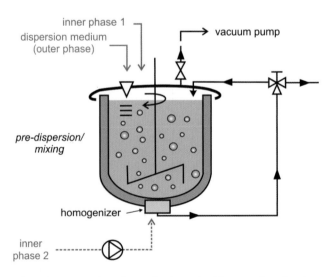

Fig. 15-19 Schematic construction of a production unit with external product loop.

order to ascertain not only the production of the required amount of mechanical stress but also an adequate temperature distribution, avoiding the formation of solidified lipid crusts on the wall of the double jacket. After the product has cooled down to ~30°C, often it is homogenized once more in order to retain the final matrix structure.

When the energy input is too intensive, shear-sensitive products may give rise to (partially) irreversible matrix destruction and thus loss of consistency. To shorten the long cooling process and thus to save energy, cold emulsification may be considered under certain circumstances for the production of creams (cryo-mix or cold-hot processing). This involves the incorporation of one phase (usually the water phase) in the cold. In the simplest way, the active ingredient can be integrated in the preparations in the form of a solution. In that case, it should be ascertained that also in the final product, the active agent remains completely dissolved.

For the production of preparations of the suspension type, the active ingredients are introduced and dispersed in the product as a powder or, preferentially, as a prefabricated suspension concentrate at as low a temperature as possible. For that purpose, processing units often offer the possibility to draw in the solid in the evacuated device in close vicinity to the homogenizer (Fig. 15-19). In addition, whenever possible, gelling agents are introduced as a homogeneous suspension in a fluid in which they hardly swell, in order to avoid formation of lumps. Additional treatment of the cooled preparation out of the production vessel (e.g., in a three-roll mill) should be avoided, as it will lead to an interruption of the closed process system.

All dispersion and stirring processes in the equipment are preferentially performed in a vacuum in order to avoid entrapment of air bubbles. These may potentially have an (unfavorable) effect on the consistency and the density but, more importantly, may also put at risk the chemical and microbiological stability of the preparation. In gels, air bubbles additionally negatively affect the optical appearance. If possible, the final product is filled into its primary packaging material in a closed system, if unavoidable after a brief storage period. In case of highly viscous preparations, manual removal from the production container may nonetheless be unavoidable.

In addition to the discontinuous procedure described above, which offers a batch-wise production procedure, semi-solid preparations may be prepared in a continuous process (Fig. 15-20). In that case, the different phases are continuously pumped from the pre-phase containers via corresponding filters into a homogenizer and, after dispersion, cooled down under stirring in a continuously operating cooler/scraper, so that a continuous flow of the final product can be withdrawn from the production line. Such production units are particularly useful for products that are produced in very large quantities. They play practically no role in pharmaceutical plants. The reasons for that are mainly:

- □ Continuous processing units offer no advantages because of costly and time consuming adjustment and cleaning procedures which might be necessary due to frequent batch change overs in case of a broad product portfolio or small batch sizes.
- □ Addition and homogeneous distribution of temperature-sensitive and/or low-dose active ingredients is often problematic.
- □ Traceability cannot be based on a specific batch but on a time period of production.

Independent of the production method, all individual steps in the production of dermal products must be performed under germ-poor conditions. Besides working in a closed system it is mandatory that all equipment used can be easily cleaned (preferably by clean-in-place (CIP): a method of cleaning the equipment without disassembly) and sanitized (preferably by steam-in-place (SIP): a method used to heat the assembled equipment to be sanitized/sterilized). If working on the open product is unavoidable, the risk of contamination can be reduced for example by the use of laminar-air-flow spaces. When the final drug product needs to be sterile, such as in case of semi-solid systems for application on seriously injured skin or in the eyes, the entire production procedure needs to occur under aseptic conditions (Class A environment), as terminal sterilization is rarely possible for semi-solid preparations. This calls for a suitable clean room to accommodate the production unit, and it should be possible to steam-sterilize the entire processing equipment (interior surfaces of pipes, vessels, process equipment, filters, and associated fittings). Furthermore, sterile or at least

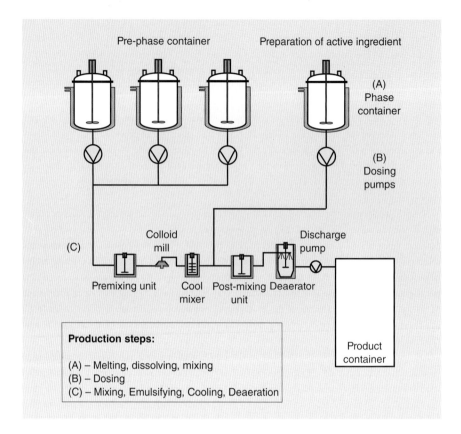

Fig. 15-20 Continuously operating unit for the production of semi-solid preparations.

germ-poor ingredients have to be used. Germ-reducing measures during the production include for example thermal sterilization of sufficiently thermo-stable pre-phases in their respective containers, and when possible subsequent filtration through a bacteria-retentive membrane. Under certain conditions, sterilization of the starting ingredients can be performed directly in the processing unit.

Consecutively, the starting material must be homogenized and cold-stirred again. Also the active ingredients has to be added as sterile material, for example, as a heat-sterilized powder or, after aseptic production, as a solution which has been passed through a bacteria-retentive filter or as an aqueous suspension which has been autoclaved. Ultimately, aseptic filling into the sterile primary sterile packaging is necessary, preferably in a closed system.

In the production of semi-solid preparations the possibilities for in-process controls are mainly limited to surveillance of the equipment and the process parameters as well as control of the environment.

Parameters to be controlled are for example the temperature of the constituting phases and of the total batch during the production, stirring and homogenization times, and speeds, as well as the order and time point of addition of individual components. Assessment of the consistency may achieved indirectly via the recording the energy consumption of the stirrer motor. Particle size of the dispersed phases can be monitored by means of suitable in-line measuring probes.

15.5   Packaging, Stability, Storage

The primary packaging material for semi-solid preparations are tubes and, for compounded formulations, (dispensing) jars. Because of high contamination risk, conventional jars should only be used when dosing from tubes or dispensing jars is practically not possible due to high consistency of the product, like, for example, in case of pastes. Whenever possible, semi-solid preparations should be filled in tubes in order to ensure effective protection from contamination and evaporation as well as from oxidation in air and effects of light. For many application fields (e.g., ophthalmic preparations), pharmacopeias recommend to use tubes as multidose containers fitted with a suitable applicator. When selecting the primary packaging material, the chemical compatibility of the preparation with the container material or components thereof should be taken into account. For example, containers of synthetic polymers are not suited for storage of macrogol ointments because macrogols may dissolve certain polymers. When carbomer gels are filled into aluminum tubes with damaged internal protection lacquer, the gel can dissolve aluminum ions from the tube, which may then cause an incompatibility leading to a loss in viscosity. When choosing appropriate tubes for ophthalmic ointments, special attention should be paid to the absence of metal splinters. For obvious reasons, ophthalmic preparations should only be filled in sterile tubes.

The shelf life of a final product depends on its chemical, physical as well as microbiological stability. All three aspects are influenced by the composition, the preparation method, and the type of packaging of the product. For licensed pharmaceutical products, which should have a shelf life of several years, storage stability is optimized while taking these factors into consideration. The shelf life of a licensed semi-solid preparation is determined based on data obtained by stability testing according to the respective guidelines. Because compounded preparations are generally intended for immediate use, relative short expiration dates are acceptable. In accordance with laws and regulations on drug safety, information on the limited shelf life, including a concrete expiration date ("to be used by *month-day-year*") should be labeled. If the formulation requires, additional information should be provided on maximal stability after first opening of the packaging.

Likewise, the expiration dating of compounded stock and base preparations that are kept in store in the pharmacy (e.g., basis for dermal preparations) should receive due attention. Guidelines on shelf life and expiration dating of compounded and stock preparations may be found in the NRF (Table 15-3). Stock and base formulations as well as formulation concentrates should always be kept in stock in amounts corresponding to the estimated consumption. Sticking strictly to the expiration date is mandatory because too long storage might substantially impair the quality. This may concern both the base (rancidity, unacceptable posthardening, unfavorable changes of the dispersion grade of emulsions) as well as the active ingredient (chemical and microbiological conversions, altered particle size). Microbiologically susceptible preparations without preservative need to be freshly prepared according to need.

Semi-solid preparations must be stored in a cool place and as much as possible under exclusion of air (containers filled to the brim). Oxidation-sensitive basis and preparations containing light-sensitive active agents such as triclosan or bismuth salts should be protected from exposure to light.

Table 15-3   Guidelines for Expiration Dating of Standardized or Chemically and Physically Stable Semi-Solid Preparations for Repeated Application in Multi-Dose Containers According to NRF

Hydrophobic Ointments, Water-Emulsifying Ointments, Lipophilic Gels, Pastes	
tube, dispensing jar	3 years
jar	6 month; exception e.g., very high consistency
Lipophilic creams	
with preservative; tube	1 year
with preservative; dispenser	6 months
with preservative; jar	4 weeks; exception e.g., incompatibility with tube
without preservative; tube, dispenser	4 weeks
Hydrophilic ointments	
tube, dispensing jar	3 years
Hydrophilic creams, hydrogels	
with preservative; tube	1 year
with preservative; dispensing jar	6 months
with preservation; jar	4 weeks; exception e.g., incompatibility with tube
without preservative; tube, dispenser	1 week; strongly dependent on pH, components and temperature 2 weeks in fridge

15.6   Biopharmaceutical Aspects

15.6.1   The Skin and Its Influence on Uptake of Pharmaceuticals

The human skin has a thickness of 1 to 4 mm and a total surface area of 1.6 to 2.0 m^2. In the skin three histologically defined layers can be distinguished: the hypodermis (sub-cutis), the dermis (corium) and the epidermis. Epidermis and dermis together build the cutis. All layers are streaked by skin adnexa such as the sweat and sebaceous glands (Fig. 15-21). The sub-cutis consists of loose connective tissue and fat cells (adipocytes, lipocytes) and has, besides its protective function, the task to store energy in the form of fat. The dermis, predominantly consisting of collagen and elastin with embedded fibroblasts, lends elasticity and mechanical stability to the skin. In this part of the skin tissue an extensive network of blood vessels and nerve fibers is laid out that provides the skin with nutrients; besides, touch sensitivity (tactility) as well as pain, heat, and cold perception are located there. The water content of this part amounts to about 70%. The epidermis (Fig. 15-22) mainly consists of keratinocytes (~95%). In addition, small numbers of other cell types can be found there, such as melanocytes (~2%) and touch-sensitive (tactile) Merkel cells (~1%). The basal cell layer

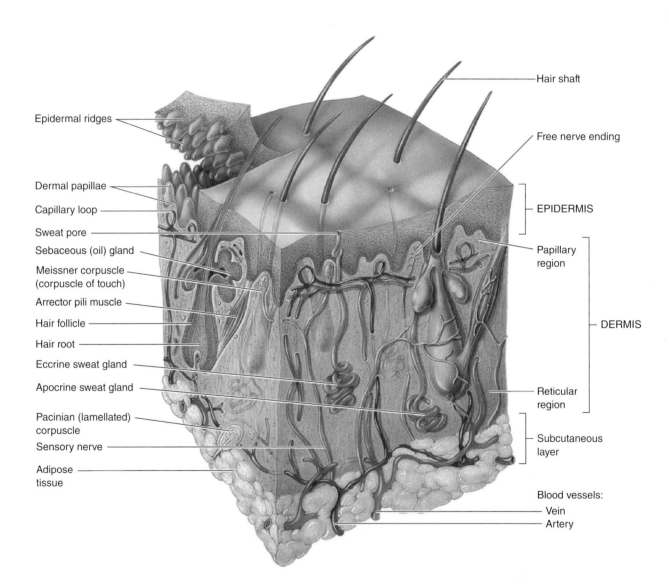

Fig. 15-21 Sectional view of the skin. From *Principles of Anatomy and Physiology*, Tortora & Derrickson, 12th edition, Wiley 2009.

(A)

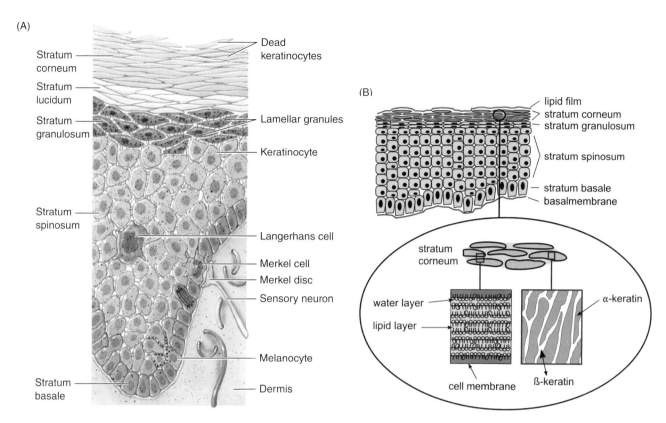

Fig. 15-22 Sectional view of the epidermis (A) and detailed view of the Stratum corneum (B).
From *Principles of Anatomy and Physiology*, Tortora & Derrickson, 12th edition, Wiley 2009.

(*Stratum basale*) harbors undifferentiated keratinocytes (basal cells), displaying mitotic activity. Their continuous division, proliferation and differentiation form the epidermal tissue. The newly formed keratinocytes travel in 20 to 30 days from the *Stratum basale* to the surface of the skin and on their way they change in shape and function. Upon arrival in the *Stratum corneum*, the keratinocytes no longer have a nucleus, but meanwhile they have accumulated a large proportion of keratin (~80%). The keratin is predominantly formed during the passage of the keratinocytes through the *Stratum granulosum* (Fig. 15-22).

The fully differentiated keratinocytes in the *Stratum corneum* are called corneocytes and are 0.5 μm thick and 20 to 40 μm wide; they have a low water content (~15% to 20%) but a high water absorption capacity by virtue of their high content of moisture-retaining substances (natural moisturizing factor, NMF). The *Stratum corneum* (horny layer) consists of about 15 to 20 layers of corneocytes, embedded in a lipid mixture. A generally accepted schematic description of the structure of the *Stratum corneum* is the brick-and-mortar model. It compares the corneocytes with bricks that, like in a wall, are arranged in a regular overlapping order and surrounded by a "mortar" layer consisting of intercellular lipids and can be seen as an oversimplification of Fig. 15-23 (lower right). The corneocytes are essential for the chemical and mechanical stability of the skin. The intercellular lipid matrix, making up ~10% of the dry mass of the *Stratum corneum*, predominantly maintains the barrier function of the *Stratum corneum* against transepidermal water loss and external noxes. The lipids of the *Stratum corneum* originate from the keratinosomes (Odland bodies, lamellar bodies) that are formed in the cells of the *Stratum spinosum* (prickle layer) and the *Stratum granulosum* (granular layer) and secreted at the upper limit of the *Stratum granulosum* in the intercellular spaces. There, the stacked lipid double-layers fuse and form up to 12 intercellular lipid double-layers between the cells. The intercellular lipids of the *Stratum corneum* have a characteristic composition.

They consist predominantly of a mixture of ceramides (35%), cholesterol (20%) and free fatty acids (25%), which together form a semi-crystalline gel phase embedded with liquid-crystalline domains.

Advantages and disadvantages of cutaneous drug delivery

Advantages:

1. Avoids first pass effect.
2. Excellent delivery route for local treatment.
3. Usually a good patient compliance is reported for these formulations compared with injectables and even orally administered formulations.
4. In case of adverse reaction to the formulation, applied drug can be easily removed by wiping off the skin.
5. Avoids any adverse effects in GIT or drug degradation in GIT.
6. Suitable to be used in patients suffering from nausea or diarrhoea.

Although not really an advantage from a patient's perspective, skin drug delivery offers some freedom or flexibility to the pharmacist as a higher number of raw materials are generally available compared to oral and parenteral drug delivery. For example ingredients like PEG-20 cetyl ether, isopropyl myristate or butyl stearate have been only approved in topical applications and not oral or parenteral formulations.

Disadvantages:

1. Only useful for a relatively small number of drugs which possess appropriate physicochemical properties for skin penetration.
2. Slow drug delivery into the systemic circulation.
3. Skin barrier properties can change based on age, location, sex and disease conditions which can have an unfavourable effect on the drug delivery potential.
4. Not useful for drugs which have potential to cause skin irritation/inflammation.

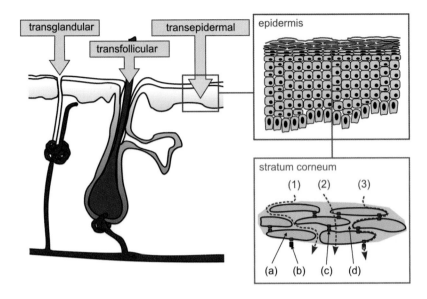

Fig. 15-23   Penetration routes of drugs in the skin: (1) intercellular path; (2) transcellular path; (3) corneodesmosomal path; (a) corneocyte; (b) desmosome; (c) corneodesmosome; (d) extracellular lipid matrix

The *Stratum corneum*, the outermost protective layer, is perforated by the efferent ducts of the sweat and sebaceous glands and by the hair follicles; together these structures make up as little as 0.1% to 1% of the skin surface, depending on the body region. The horny layer is covered by an emulsion of water and lipids (fats) known as the hydro-lipid film consisting of fatty acids, triglycerides, waxes, squalene, and the aqueous part, known as the protective acid mantle. This film reduces the wettability of the horny layer, keeps it supple and also has antimicrobial activity.

Four separate steps can be distinguished in the transport of active ingredients across the skin:

1. Liberation: release of the active ingredient from the basis on the skin surface
2. Penetration: entrance into the *Stratum corneum*
3. Permeation: dissemination in the corium and partially in the subcutis
4. Absorption: uptake in lymph and blood vessels

The extent and rate of uptake of the active substance are determined by the properties of the skin, the vehicle, the drug itself and their interaction. For example, the vehicle may interact with the skin and thus affect the skin permeability. In addition, the spreading of the substances along the skin surface has to be taken into account.

The penetration process reflects the diffusion of the substance into the skin. The following penetration routes are conceivable (Fig. 15-23):

- Intercellular
- Transcellular
- Corneo-desmosomal
- Follicular
- Glandular

Accordingly, a molecule may diffuse in two principally different ways into the human skin: along the skin appendages or transepidermally (Fig. 15-23). The former represents transport through the sweat glands (transglandular) or the hair follicles and the sebaceous glands associated with those (transfollicular).

Both alternatives circumvent direct transport across the *Stratum corneum* and are accordingly called *shunt routes*. Transport via the appendages is primarily of interest with respect to the penetration of ions and large polar molecules as those are hardly capable of diffusing transepidermally. Besides, it appears from recent research that this route also plays a special role in the application of colloidal carrier systems. Transdermal transport is defined as transport across the intact horny layer either intercellularly, intracellularly, or corneo-desmosomal. Of these, the intercellular route is the most and the transcellular route the least important.

As may be expected, large molecules penetrate more slowly than smaller ones. Strongly hydrophilic substances (mainly salts) but also extremely lipophilic compounds penetrate the skin less easily than substances of intermediate polarity.

Ideally, the drug should be lipophilic (octanol-water distribution coefficient between 10 and 1,000) but to a certain extent should also be soluble in water. Furthermore, penetration of a molecule strongly depends on the vehicle. It may be enhanced by a variety of factors, including heat, occlusion, and solvents.

Passage of the epidermal barrier proceeds very slowly; penetration into the deeper, viable layers of the skin, possibly accompanied by metabolic conversions, and the uptake into the capillary system proceeds substantially faster, though. For example, the diffusion coefficient of most pharmaceutics in the water-rich dermis is about three orders of magnitude larger than in the horny layer. Exceptions are some lipophilic substances such as corticosteroids and iodine, which accumulate in the lower cell layers of the *Stratum corneum* and build a reservoir there.

Active pharmaceutical ingredients that permeate across the horny layer may exert systemic effects. Except in case of transdermal drug administration this is not desirable because it may lead to undesired side effects or even toxic effects. Especially in case of application on large areas of severely damaged skin (associated with a loss of the skin barrier function), the possibility that such effects occur should be taken into account. Enhanced permeation of an active ingredient may also occur by heating (e.g., warm bath) or occlusion.

The extent and rate of uptake of active substances into and through the skin is determined by the properties of the vehicle, the drug itself and their mutual interaction as well as their interaction with the skin. They depend on the morphological and physiological conditions of the application site as well as on the character and the composition of the formulation. Since we are dealing with a multifactorial event, it is virtually impossible to make general statements concerning the influences of each of the factors in Table 15-4. Because drug transport

Table 15-4   Factors Influencing the Uptake in the Skin of a Pharmaceutical from a Formulation

1. Properties of the Skin

    ▫ skin condition
    ▫ skin type
    ▫ localization (pH value)
    ▫ (pre)treatment of the skin

2. Properties and Influences of the Active Pharmaceutical Ingredient

    ▫ concentration
    ▫ solubility in the base
    ▫ melting point
    ▫ molecular size
    ▫ diffusion capacity
    ▫ dissolution rate
    ▫ dissociation ability
    ▫ distribution between the phases of the basis
    ▫ distribution between ointment and skin (distribution coefficient)
    ▫ solubility in skin fat
    ▫ binding to skin proteins
    ▫ particle size and size distribution

3. Properties and Influences of the Formulation

    ▫ vehicle properties (hydrophilic, lipophilic, emulsion type)
    ▫ structuring of the matrix-forming phase (depending on production technique)
    ▫ composition of the vehicle (penetration enhancement)
    ▫ wetting of the skin by the vehicle (addition of surfactant)
    ▫ solubility of the drug in the vehicle
    ▫ viscosity of the vehicle
    ▫ alteration of the vehicle after application on the skin (evaporation)
    ▫ alterations of the skin by the vehicle (hydration enhancement; occlusion)
    ▫ spreading on the skin (area, layer thickness)

across the horny layer occurs by passive diffusion, the distribution of the drug between the formulation and the skin is a very important parameter and with that also the factors affecting the distribution behavior (section 7.5).

Other important considerations are possible metabolic conversion of the drug in the skin and how the active ingredients bind to skin proteins and other tissue components. Cutaneous application of pharmaceutical preparations may be considered for three therapeutic aims:

1. The drug should remain on the skin surface or penetrate only superficially, such as antiseptic agents or sunscreens.
2. The drug should exert a local or regional effect in the skin or in deeper tissues; this refers to most formulations for skin application.
3. Application of a drug should be at such a (high) dose that a systemic effect is obtained. This can be achieved only for a few semi-solid drug formulations (e.g., hormone preparations). Transdermal patches are most effective for achieving this purpose (section 16.4).

It is the aim of the formulation development to find the proper base and additives as well as adequate production technologies that lead to sufficient release of active ingredient from the formulation and, if so required, ensure skin penetration. Because of the complex composition of most dermatological formulations, it is not possible to give a simple recipe to achieve this; this can only be elaborated individueally during the development process.

Actives are absorbed from semi-solid preparations far more easily via mucosal tissue (e.g., in vagina or nose), than across the skin, since the former lack a horny layer but instead possess a readily permeable epithelium with mucus secreting beaker cells.

15.6.2   Area of Application and Vehicle Effects of Nonmedicated Dermal Formulation

Depending on the secretory condition of the skin, in particular of the sebaceous glands, several skin types and conditions may be distinguished. Extreme forms include the oily-moist skin condition (seborrhea), characterized by enhanced sebum production and perspiration and the disorders connected with it (acne vulgaris, rosacea, seborrhoic eczema, and others), and the dry low-fat skin (sebostasis) resulting from a defect in the barrier function and a disturbed hydro-lipid film. Pronounced sebostasis can be an accompanying symptom of certain skin diseases and also occurs more often in elderly people.

For the sebostatic skin, lipid-rich formulations such as ointments or lipophilic creams are favored. Seborrhoic skin is adequately treated with compresses, shake lotions, hydrogels, or other hydrophilic basis.

More frequently occurring than these two extreme skin conditions are the moderate types in between, those described as "tending to the seborrhoic type" and "tending to the sebostatic type"; these are treated with hydrophilic creams.

The preferential base type for application on a diseased skin is determined by the acuteness of the dermatosis, unless other criteria need to be given priority. Roughly speaking, the guiding principle is "moist on moist." That implies, for instance, that an acute oozing dermatosis is treated with moist compresses. On the other side, chronic dermatoses, accompanied by a thickening of the horny layer (hyperkeratosis), are treated with greasy ointments, or bases belonging to the water-emulsifying hydrophobic ointments.

This type of base has a skin-softening and macerating effect based on its (partially) occlusive properties. The hydration effect that comes along with this property enhances skin penetration of the active ingredient. Sometimes this is called as "effect in the deep."

Table 15-5 classifies a variety of dermal basis according to their preferred use on the diseased skin and the intrinsic effect of the vehicle. It should be kept in mind, however, that this classification only has an orienting character and does not take into consideration any special galenic features of the vehicle.

Table 15-5 Classification of Dermatics According to Depth Action, Flow Direction, Vehicle Activity, and Disease Stage

Type of base	Properties of the base		Effect of base on the skin (Vehicle effect)						Severity of Skin Disease
	Water content	Lipid content	Drug penetration	Antiexsudative	Drying	Cooling	Hydrating	Macerating	
Moist dressing Topical liquid Shake lotion O/W-emulsion W/O-emulsion O/W cream W/O cream Paste Hydrophobic ointment Occlusion bandage									Acute, oosing Subacute Subchronic Chronic Chronic, hyperkeratotic

15.6.3   Penetration Enhancement

Because of the excellent barrier properties of the intact horny layer, only substances with certain properties will succeed in overcoming this barrier. These properties include, among others, low molecular mass (<500 Dalton), moderate lipophilicity (octanol-water distribution coefficient between 10 and 1,000) and moderate melting point (<200°C), in combination with sufficient solubility.

Even when a substance possesses such properties, the amount of active substance that is actually penetrating is commonly quite low. This often calls for measures to enhance penetration in and transport across the barrier (*Stratum corneum*) in order to achieve better drug action.

15.6.3.1   Super-saturation

Super-saturation is a measure that improves skin penetration without interfering with the structure of the *Stratum corneum*. The mechanism of this penetration enhancement is simply based on increasing the thermodynamic activity of the drug in the vehicle. This increases the concentration gradient and promotes the uptake of the active agent in the *Stratum corneum* and, in accordance with Fick's law of diffusion, the transport across the barrier.

Super-saturated systems arise when, for instance, the water phase of vehicle evaporates after application. If a water-soluble active is present, loss of aqeous phase causes its concentration to increase to above saturation. Super-saturated systems are, by definition, thermodynamically unstable. They are therefore likely to recrystallize, resulting in loss of the desired effect. That is why special measures are required to stabilize the supersaturation for an adequate amount of time. This may be achieved, for example, by addition of a polymer to inhibit nucleation that, in turn, will temporarily delay recrystallization.

15.6.3.2   Water as Penetration Enhancer

Improved hydration of the *Stratum corneum* is the simplest measure to enhance penetration of many active ingredients by affecting the barrier. The accommodation of water molecules loosens the compact structure of the horny layer and makes it more permeable. The water content of the *Stratum corneum* can be increased by water released from the vehicle. Substantially more effective, however, is the application of (partially) occlusive preparations, which inhibit the transepidermal water loss and thus accomplish hydration of the *Stratum corneum*.

Table 15-6 summarizes the basic effects of vehicles on the water content of the *Stratum corneum* and drug penetration.

Table 15-6 Influence of Different Vehicles on the Hydration of the skin Barrier and Its Permeability

Vehicle	Effect on Hydration	Effect on Skin Permeability
Occlusive Bandages	Complete Inhibition of water loss, effectuate maximal hydration	very strong increase
hydrophobic ointments, lipophilic gels	largely inhibit water loss, may cause complete hydration	strong increase
water-emulsifying ointments	inhibit water loss, strong hydration increase	strong increase
lipohilic creams	reduce water loss	increase
hydrophilic creams	enhance hydration can release water, slight hydration enhancement	small increase

15.6.3.3   Penetration Enhancers

A variety of excipients have the capacity to promote drug transport across the skin barrier, based on different mechanisms. The most important are:

- Extraction of lipids from the *Stratum corneum*
- Alteration of the distribution coefficient vehicle/skin
- Structural perturbation of the intercellular lipid bilayers
- Displacing bound water
- Loosening of the keratin structure in the corneocytes
- Delamination of the *Stratum corneum*

Penetration enhancers can be classified in different groups. Solvents such as alcohols, alkyl-methyl sulfoxides, and polyols mainly enhance the solubility of the drug in the skin barrier and thus promote the distribution into the horny layer. Apart from that, some solvents, such as DMSO or ethanol, are able to extract epidermal lipids and enhance in this way the permeability of the horny layer. Oleic acid, ε-laurocapram (Azone®) and isopropylmyristate are typical examples of penetration enhancers, which intercalate in the epidermal lipid double layers and thus perturb their dense packing. This leads to a more fluid structure and an increase on the diffusion velocity. Ionic surfactants, decyl-methyl sulfoxide, DMSO, urea, and salicylic acid interact with the keratin in the corneocytes. This loosens the compact protein structure and increases the diffusion coefficient, in particular for substances that favor the intracellular route.

Traditionally, urea and salicylic acid will be found in a variety of dermatological formulations for improving penetration, due to their keratolytic action. Hyaluronidase may also act as a drug penetration enhancer because it degrades hyaluronic acid enzymatically. Hyaluronic acid is a mucopolysaccharide made up of glucuronic acid and N-acetylglucosamine, and together with chondroitine sulfate, it forms the main constituent of connective tissue.

Table 15-7 lists a number of substances that facilitate in particular the diffusion along the intercellular path, which is mainly followed by most active agents. These penetration enhancers can be divided in two groups: those that affect the lipid part of the intercellular lipid film (non-polar route) and those that affect the hydrophilic part (polar route).

As can be concluded from Fig. 15-24, the deployment of penetration enhancers may substantially improve the penetration of actives—for example, corticosteroids such as fluocinolonacetonid.

Penetration enhancers should meet the following criteria: They should be nonallergenic and display at most low irritation potential. Besides, their effect on the barrier function of the skin should be fully reversible. However, penetration enhancers often constitute as much as 10% to 50% of the total mass of a preparation. Since their mechanism of action involves intensive interaction with the lipids or the corneocytes of the *Stratum corneum*, their application brings along limitations with respect to local tolerance. Significant skin irritation is frequently observed.

Table 15-7 Examples of Penetration Enhancers and the Transport Route They Affect

	Penetration Enhancement via the Enhancer	
	Polar Route	Nonpolar Route
oleic acid	X	
terpenes	X	
glycolipids	X	
medium-chain triglycerides	X	
synthetic waxes (isopropylmyristate)	X	
branched-chain fatty alcohols (e.g., octyldodecanol; Eutanol®G)	X	X
urea	X	
propylene glycol	X	
ε-laurocaprame (Azone®)	X	X
dimethyl sulfoxide	X	X

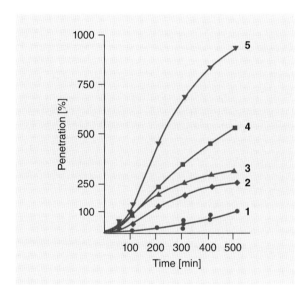

Fig. 15-24 Comparison of percutaneous penetration of fluocinolonacetonide from different solvents: 1 ethanol, 2 tetrahydrofurfuryl alcohol, 3 dimethylacetamide, 4 propylene glycol, 5 dimethyl sulfoxide.

15.6.3.4 Physical Measures to Achieve Penetration Enhancement

The entry of an active ingredient in the skin may be promoted by hydration of the horny layer as well as by the addition of penetration enhancers, which transiently affect the barrier properties of the skin. In most cases, neither method by itself will be sufficient to allow transport of therapeutically relevant amounts of drug in case the drug is ionized, has a high molecular weight or low intrinsic activity. In these cases, technologies based on physical effects have proven to be highly efficient. Nonetheless, such methods will bring about at least temporary damage of the skin.

Phonophoresis (or *Sonophoresis*) exploits the energy of ultrasound to improve drug penetration. The ultrasonic waves induce cavitation in the skin, that is, the formation and subsequent collapse of gas bubbles in a fluid. This causes the formation of holes in the corneocytes, enlargement of the intercellular space, and perturbation of the structure of the intercellular lipid film. Besides, the tissue warms up by several degrees, leading to a general increase in the diffusion velocity and in the fluidity of the *Stratum corneum* lipids, which, in turn, brings about penetration enhancement.

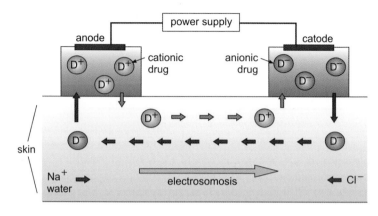

Fig. 15-25 Principle of iontophoresis.

Iontophoresis is based on the application of a low voltage on the skin promoting the electrophoretic transport of mainly charged molecules into the skin. For that purpose, an electrode is placed on the skin with a charge identical to that of the penetrating ion. A counter electrode is placed randomly elsewhere on the body. When applying a voltage, the drug ions are repelled from the identically charged working electrode and pushed into the skin (Fig. 15-25). This simple electrostatic repulsion is the main mechanism responsible for the penetration enhancement of ionized active agents. The number of iontophoretically transported ions is directly proportional to the electrical current. Thus, the amount of delivered drug can be controlled by the strength of the current. Besides, the flow of an electric current through the skin enhances its permeability while the occurrence of the electro-osmosis effect additionally promotes the penetration of noncharged molecules. Electro-osmosis arises upon applying a voltage and inducing a flow of fluid in electrolyte solutions, including body fluids. This flow transports all molecules dissolved in the fluid, also allowing improvement of the penetration of neutral and extremely polar substances that otherwise are not able to penetrate the skin markedly.

Electroporation, also known as electro-mesotherapy, is likewise based on the application of an electric current on the skin. Contrary to electrophoresis, which uses low-voltage currents, in this case (very) short pulses (10 μs to 100 ms) of high voltage are employed. This causes the induction of transient hydrophilic pores in the skin barrier, which are permeable even to large hydrophilic molecules.

The application of *microneedles* derives from attempts to improve the transport of drugs through the skin barrier by means of minimally invasive techniques. To achieve the desired effect, such systems should penetrate over at least the thickness of the horny layer (10 to 20 μm). The manufacturing of such fine structures is achieved with the aid of micro-production techniques. Current developments in this field focus on the concept of microneedle arrays. In such devices, a multitude of needles measuring 10 to 600 μm long and 10 to 50 μm wide are arranged together in small, patch-like units. The individual needles can be either massive or hollow and are connected to a drug reservoir. Another method is to form dissolving microneedles from a hydrogel (e.g., carboxymethylcellulose, amylopectin and albumin) (Fig. 15-26). Microneedle arrays pierce the upper epidermis to enhance the permeability of the skin and facilitate the delivery of active ingredients without reaching the pain receptors in the dermis. The method has no limitations with respect to the polarity and molecular mass of the applied active substances.

15.6.3.5   Formulation Concepts with Colloidal Carriers
Penetration enhancement via special formulation concepts is mostly based on the deployment of colloidal carriers. Such submicron particles presumably transport entrapped drug molecules into the skin. This group of carrier systems includes microemulsions (section 20.5), liposomes and transfersomes (section 20.3), as well as nanoemulsions, lipid nanoparticles, and nanostructured lipid carriers (section 20.6). Most studies on such systems indicate a partial localization of the carrier in the *Stratum corneum* or the upper skin layers.

Electroosmosis

The reason for the effect of electroosmosis is that a liquid is electrically neutral in its volume (i.e., inside), but an electrochemical double layer forms on the surface. This layer is about a nanometer thick (depends on the ions dissolved in the liquid). The water is therefore not electrically neutral at the surface. If an electric field is applied parallel to the surface, a force acts on the water causing a flow from the anode to the cathode. This is only possible with insulating surfaces like in the skin; metals and other electrical conductors would short-circuit a field parallel to the surface.

Since the force acts only on a very thin liquid layer, electroosmosis can only be observed in thin capillaries (some nanometers up to a maximum of a few micrometers). In the case of thicker liquid layers or columns, the effects of the water volume (ion conduction, electrolysis, electrophoresis) are dominating.

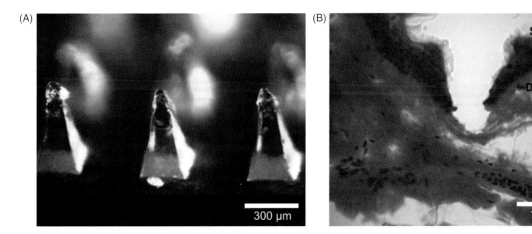

Fig. 15-26 Function of a microneedle device: (A) Microneedles made of a hydrogel; (B) cross-sectional image of stained skin at a site of microneedle penetration. (SC: Stratum corneum, VE: viable epidermis, D: dermis (from Lee et al. 2008). Reproduced with permission from Elsevier.

Generally, it is believed that these vehicles do not reach the viable skin. Nonetheless, several studies claim positive effects of these carrier systems with respect to epidermal and dermal drug uptake. The efficiency of colloidal carrier systems can be enhanced by combination with physical methods.

15.6.3.6 Prodrug Systems

Active agents often lack the molecular prerequisites, in particular *lipophilicity*, required to enter or cross the skin in therapeutically relevant concentrations. Derivation, or alterations in the chemical structure, e.g., formation of a more lipophilic ester, may improve the conditions for skin penetration and result in higher permeation rates. Until recently, this principle was applied, for example, with estradiol, metronizadol, 5-amino-levulinic acid, and glucocorticoids. The active agent is converted into a more lipophilic ester derivative, which, as such, is therapeutically inactive but better able to pass the *Stratum corneum*. After having crossed the horny layer, endogenous enzymes cleave the ester bond and thus convert the inactive prodrug into the active drug.

15.6.4 Biopharmaceutical Characterization of Dermal Preparations

To characterize the biopharmaceutical properties of dermatical preparations, suitable tests to demonstrate release, penetration and permeation of the active ingredients are used. These, in turn, are subdivided into *in-vitro*, *ex-vivo* and *in-vivo* models when studies are performed on animal or human skin.

15.6.4.1 Release Models

Basically, all release models consist of a donor compartment (containing the test product) and an receptor compartment. The two compartments may be separated by a selectively permeable membrane, preventing the intermixing of donor and receptor, without impeding the diffusion of the active ingredient. Typical separating membranes for release studies are made from various materials and have different pore sizes. Examples are membrane filters, silicon membranes and siliconized dialysis membranes.

Release studies do not take into account the interaction of the formulation with the skin, which ultimately is highly significant for the action of cutaneously applied drugs. They merely provide primary information on the influence of formulation factors such as concentration, solubility, and distribution of the drug in the carrier. In addition, they serve as an instrument for quality assessment. Ph. Eur. says that it is not mandatory to use suitable tests to

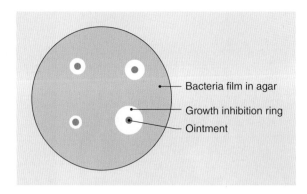

Fig. 15-27   Agar plate test.

demonstrate the desired release of an active substance from semi-solid preparations for cutaneous application. Suitable testmethods are described in the USP.

15.6.4.2   Gel Diffusion Method
This simple method without a separating membrane may be used to test the release of active ingredients that either are colored as such or can be detected by means of a color reaction, display fluorescence or possess antibiotic activity. The test preparation is placed in holes that are punched out of an agar or gelatin gel that serves as a diffusion medium. After an appropriate time interval, diffusion will cause a ring of active ingredient around the hole, which is detectable by its color or fluorescence or by the inhibition of bacterial growth when the gel contains bacteria. The diameter of the ring is a measure of the drug release (Fig. 15-27).

15.6.4.3   Membrane Methods
The standard method for release studies with a separation membrane involves a Franz diffusion cell (Fig. 15-28). This method is also mentioned as "Vertical Diffusion Cell Apparatus" in USP <1724> (see chapter monographs on dosage forms). The diffusion cell consists of a jacketed thermostated glass vessel containing the continuously stirred receptor fluid, which is in direct contact with the lower side of a membrane.

After applying the test formulation on top of the membrane it can be covered, for example, by a glass plate, to prevent evaporation. Test aliquots can be easily drawn from the receptor fluid via a sampling port at the side of the receptor chamber.

Another automatable alternative is the so-called Enhancer™ cell. It consists of a 200-mL paddle-stirred release vessel, containing the receptor fluid, in which a test cell is mounted sealed with a drug permeable membrane.

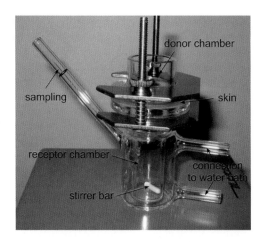

Fig. 15-28   Franz cell: device for testing drug release, penetration, and permeation from dermal preparations in vitro.

15.6.4.4 Evaluation of Results

The release of active agents from topical preparations may be approached under certain boundary conditions mathematically. For *suspension ointments*, equation 15-1 (square root rule, according to Higuchi) applies:

$$Q = \sqrt{2 \cdot c_0 \cdot D \cdot c_s \cdot t} \tag{15-1}$$

| Q | = released quantity of drug per unit surface area
| c_0 | = concentration of non-dissolved particles at time 0 (starting concentration)
| c_s | = saturation concentration of dissolved particles in the ointment
| D | = diffusion coefficient of the drug in the ointment
| t | = time

Accordingly, under constant conditions (c_0, c_S, D), the amount of released drug is proportional to the square root of the time.

$$Q = f(\sqrt{t}) \tag{15-2}$$

The diffusion coefficient D of an active substance in a particular ointment base can be calculated as follows:

$$D = \frac{s^2 \cdot \pi}{q^2 \cdot c_0 \cdot t} \tag{15-3}$$

| s | = amount of substance traveled across a cross section of 1 cm^2
| c_0 | = starting concentration (mg/cm^3)
| t | = time(s)

A boundary condition for the equation to apply is a finely dispersed distribution of the suspended agent with a particle size smaller than the layer thickness of the ointment. The concentration of the suspended substance should be substantially higher than that of the dissolved substance ($c_0 \gg c_s$). Furthermore, the drug taken up by the organism should be carried off rapidly in order for the concentration gradient to remain as high as possible (sink conditions). Favorable drug release rates from suspension ointments are achievable when the active agent slightly dissolves in the base and does not form associates with it and when the pH value permits a high concentration of nondissociated drug.

For *solution ointments*, respective equations have been derived. Prerequisite for their application is that the drug is molecularly dispersed and uniformly distributed and that exclusively the drug diffuses out of the base and none of its constituents penetrates the skin and vice versa. When the ointment layer has a sufficient layer thickness and the percentage of release drug is ≤30%, the following equation applies:

$$Q = 2 \cdot c_0 \sqrt{\frac{D \cdot t}{\pi}} \tag{15-4}$$

| Q = released amount of drug at the ointment/skin per unit interfacial area
| c_0 = starting concentration
| D = Diffusion coefficient of the drug in the ointment
| t = time after application

This simple equation indicates that the release of active ingredient is directly proportional to the initial concentration of the drug. Of essential importance is the diffusion coefficient of the drug, which is affected by various factors such as temperature, viscosity, and molecular size.

Also for *emulsion ointments* and creams, equation 15-5 exists to help us comprehend the release of active substance. Under the presumption that the drug is dissolved and distributed in both phases and the dispersed phase consists of small globules and the volume of the internal phase is small, the following equation may be derived:

$$D_e = \frac{D_1}{V_1 + k \cdot V_2} \left[1 + 3 \cdot V_2 \frac{k \cdot D_2 - D_1}{k \cdot D_2 + 2 \cdot D_1} \right] \tag{15-5}$$

|D_e = effective diffusion coefficient of the system
|D_1 = diffusion coefficient of the drug in the exterior phase
|D_2 = diffusion coefficient of the drug in the internal phase
|V_1 = volume fraction of the exterior phase
|V_2 = volume fraction of the internal phase
|k = distribution coefficient

The complexity of a heterogeneous system like an emulsion allows application of equation 15-5 only under very limited conditions. Nonetheless, the equation reveals the factors that need to be taken into account when designing a semi-solid formulation. Clearly, the effective diffusion coefficient D_e is predominantly determined by the individual diffusion coefficients D_1 and D_2 in the two phases as well as by the distribution coefficient. D_1 and D_2 are, in turn, affected by factors such as viscosity and temperature. When D_1 and D_2 have approximately identical values, the distribution coefficient k becomes the main factor determining the release. When the distribution coefficient favors the accumulation of the drug in the external phase, this will also favor the release rate. Conversely, a value of k favoring accumulation in the interior phase will result in release inhibition.

15.6.4.5   Permeation Models

Because interactions of active agents with the skin are of utmost importance for the activity of cutaneously applied drugs, methods need to be at hand to investigate the transport of drugs through the skin (permeation) before any further conclusions may be drawn. The Franz cell or modifications thereof have established themselves as a standard method for this purpose (see above).

The practical implementation of this method allows variations with respect to the nature of the used skin and the amount of applied test material. Using human skin is regarded as the gold standard. Animal skin is also used, although the permeability of most animal skin, for example that of rodents, is higher than that of human skin. Results obtained with pigskin bear good resemblance to those obtained with human skin.

Furthermore, the thickness of the skin may vary. We distinguish Stratum corneum isolates (heat-separated or trypsinized skin) and full thickness skin (thickness 0.5 to 1 mm).

The disadvantage of both animal and human skin is that the results depend on the natural donor-to-donor variation of the permeability. Better standardization may be attained with 3D-tissue-engineered skin equivalents. The permeability of such artificial skin is, however, clearly higher than that of human skin.

An additional variation in permeation experiments is possible with respect to the amount of applied product. We speak of infinite-dose experiments when at least 50 mg/cm^2 product is applied and the loss of volatile constituents is prevented by covering the donor compartment. The large excess of applied drug ensures the presence of a nearly constant concentration in the donor compartment for an extended period of time, so that after an initial lag period a steady state equilibrium is established. This facilitates the calculation of the permeation rate and makes it possible to compare different formulations. In finite-dose experiments maximally 5 mg/cm^2 of product are applied, without cover. When correctly conducted, the test product shows the same changes due to the evaporation of volatile components as would be the case under real application conditions. Furthermore, the permeation process leads to depletion of the active agent in the vehicle, as it is not present in large excess in this case.

Finite dose tests thus provide a better insight in application-related aspects of the drug permeation.

A simple in vivo permeation test method is the difference method in which a defined amount of a preparation is applied on a skin area of defined size. After a certain incubation time, the remaining preparation is scraped and rinsed off the skin and the amount of drug in the removed preparation is determined. By subtracting this from the total amount applied, the amount of drug that has diffused into the skin can simply be calculated. Obviously, no additional information is obtained in this way (e.g., concerning the depth of penetration).

Recently, more and more minimally invasive *in vivo* studies on human volunteers are conducted in which aliquots of the permeated drug are extracted by means of a micro-dialysis system from the epidermis just below the application site. By means of such investigations, not only the effect of formulation parameters may be evaluated but also the effect of the skin condition or blood flow.

15.6.4.6 Penetration Models

Distinct from the release and permeation models, the use of penetration models aims at the modeling of the penetration kinetics of the active agent in the various skin layers. For the assessment of extent and rate of penetration in the *Stratum corneum*, the tape-stripping test is deployed. After application of the test preparation on the skin, the horny layer is stripped off layer by layer after appropriate time intervals by means of adhesive tape (e.g., Tesafilm[®] or Scotch tape[®]). To this end, the adhesive tape is applied repeatedly with defined pressure to the remaining superficial layer of the *Stratum corneum*. As the whole horny layer is stripped off, for each time point another area of the same skin is required. The individual strips are assessed for the amount of drug, and from this data a concentration-depth profile is revealed. The tape stripping method may be applied *in vivo* as well as *ex vivo*.

To determine the penetration profile in the deeper skin layers, the skin has to be cut horizontally in thin sections at different times after application of the test sample and each layer analyzed for drug content. For obvious reasons, penetration profiles for viable epidermis and dermis are nearly exclusively determined based on *ex vivo* experiments.

Modern spectroscopic techniques in combination with confocal microscopy, such as confocal Raman spectral imaging, allow for a selective number of active agents a spatially resolved *in vivo* quantification and thus to obtain penetration profiles noninvasively.

For *in vitro* penetration studies, multilayer membrane models are available. In these models, the receptor phase consists of multiple stacked membranes that may vary largely in polarity and may be adjusted to the scope of the study. These membranes consist, for instance, of a collodium matrix and may vary in type and amount of membrane lipids (e.g., dodecanol). To mimic also the hydrophilic properties of the skin barrier (e.g., the natural moisturizing substances that are found in the corneocytes), hydrophilic additives such as glycerol of propylene glycol may be incorporated in the matrix, dependent on the test requirements. Following application of the drug preparation and a certain period necessary for the drug to penetrate in the stack of membranes, the latter can be simply separated again and analyzed for drug content so as to yield the corresponding drug penetration profile.

15.6.4.7 *In vivo* Methods to Determine Bioavailability

It is rarely feasible to assess and evaluate the bioavailability of an active agent based on analysis of blood or urine samples, because of the typical poor absorption following topical application. Besides, such assessments obviously are especially indicative for products that should show transdermal activity. For certain groups of active ingredients, simple *in vivo* methods are available to characterize their dermal bioavailability.

15.6.4.8 Vasoconstriction Method

The skin-blanching test is a suitable method to assess the activity of corticosteroids by exploiting their vaso-constrictive effect. Peripheral blood flow as measured by laser-Doppler velocimetry may be exploited as a quantitative measure of hyperemic substances such as nicotinic acid esters and thus assess their dermato-pharmacokinetic properties.

15.6.4.9 Provocation Test on Small Skin Surfaces

This method evaluates the reduction of an artificially elicited inflammation in the skin based on a scoring system. The erythema is predominantly provoked by nicotinic acid esters or croton oil. The test is suitable for the assessment of the anti-inflammation medications action of dermal preparations.

Laser-Doppler velocimetry uses the Doppler shift in a laser beam for measuring the velocity of particles in fluids (blood cells in blood plasma) and works without pre-calibration. It is also known as laser Doppler anemometry.

15.7   Testing of Semi-Solid Preparations

Testing of semi-solid preparations is important during the development process as well as in the context of quality control. After production, the properties of the preparation should be consistent with the product specifications and should not change beyond acceptable limits during storage. When testing semi-solid preparations, relevant results are obtained only after a certain time following production, because the preparations may still undergo changes after completion of the manufacturing process. Particularly, the formation of matrix structures may take several days.

For the testing of semi-solid preparations, a variety of test methods are available. These involve for instance analytical verification of the amounts of active ingredient and certain excipients (e.g., preservatives or anti-oxidants) or the microbial examination (bacterial, yeast and mold count, or, when applicable, sterility and in addition, in the context of development, the efficacy of the chosen preservative). Besides, certain tests for ground substances (e.g., fat tests, melting, and solidification behavior, see section 5.3) may, in part, also be applied to the complete basis. This section discusses the typical tests for final and in-process controls of semi-solid preparations. Methods for biopharmaceutical characterization, including drug release, may be found in section 6.4 of this chapter.

15.7.1   In-Process Controls

In-process controls are an essential instrument in the surveillance of validated manufacturing processes and complete the quality control of the final product. The cGMP guidelines define in-process control as production-associated investigations for the surveillance (in-process testing) and, when applicable, steering (in-process control) of the process, in order to ensure that the product matches its specifications. In the industrial manufacturing of licensed products, in-process controls are obligatory. Many countries require them when unlicensed preparations such as contemporaneous and stock preparations are prepared in the pharmacy.

The methods used should be selected in such a way that they also allow conclusions with respect to the quality of the final product. When contemporaneous preparations are tested, however, in-process testing should be nondisturbing and require only a negligible amount of test sample. Ideally, they should be easy to perform and not interrupt the production process. To avoid contamination, the tests should involve minimal handling. Simple in-process tests for semi-solid preparations may be found, for example, in the DAC/NRF. They include:

- Back weighing of, for example, the weighing boat in case of small quantities of drug after transferring from a carrier (paper, weighing boat, etc.) into the mortar in order to determine the exact amount of drug that has been actually transferred to the mortar
- Clarity, opalescence, turbidity, (lack of) color of fluids and gels
- Color of a trituration or a semi-solid preparation
- Uniform appearance of a suspension-like trituration, a semi-solid preparation, or powder
- Agglomerates, aggregates, lumps in suspensions, semi-solid preparations, and powders
- Particle size and shape, characterization and crystallinity by optical microscopy
- pH value by spotting on a narrow range indicator paper or rod in case of gels
- Temperature by touching the container, liquid thermometer, or infrared laser thermometer
- Complete melting of solid lipids leading to a transparent liquid phase

15.7.2   Macroscopic Appearance, Organoleptic Tests

Macroscopic examination of a final preparation (uniformity, color, shine, structure, consistency) is not only meaningful to gain a first impression when compounding a product but also useful in case of large-scale production. Homogeneity may be assessed by examining very thin smears of the preparation—for instance, on dark shiny paper or between two glass plates. Alterations in smell or discoloration (if possible as compared to a control sample) mostly indicate the occurrence of chemical reactions or microbial decay, particularly upon storage. Rarely are they indications for production failures. Organoleptically assessable properties of contemporaneous preparations are introduced in the corresponding monographs, allowing an orienting test of the required quality.

15.7.3 Rheologic Properties

Because the semi-solid state is characterized by its rheological properties, tests of such properties during the developmental stage (setting the desired properties, validation of storage stability) as well as for quality control purposes, are of the utmost importance. Because semi-solid preparations are complex rheo-dynamic systems and thus the apparent viscosity of these depends on the applied shear intensity as well as on the shear exposure time. Therefore, all rheometric tests have to be performed strictly following a given test protocol. In particular, it is mandatory for reproducible results to be obtained that the history of the preparation (temperature during melting, storage conditions and time, resting time between sample preparation and measurement, preshearing) are normalized and the prescribed conditions during the measurement (e.g., temperature) are strictly adhered to. As the matrix structures that are responsible for the spreading properties are not always completely built up immediately after the production, it is recommended to allow a resting interval of (depending on the product) at least 12 hours following the production before examining a semi-solid preparation.

For a comprehensive characterization of semi-solid preparations it is required to conduct rheological measurements in rotational mode at defined shear rate and stress (section 3.12.5.1). These measurements and their interpretation are relatively complex; therefore, such measurements are predominantly performed during product development. For quality control purposes, often more simple methods are applied, although these mostly do not produce absolute values. For all practical purposes, well-reproducible information can be obtained this way in a short time. For example, they can reveal differences between batches or alterations during storage. Rotational rheological measurements on semi-solid preparations are typically performed with cone-plate or plate-plate measuring geometries (see section 3.12.5.1). The rheograms thus produced yield, for example, information about yield stress, apparent viscosity during increasing or decreasing shear stress (so-called upward and downward flow curve), and thixotropic effects (Fig. 15-29).

Measuring errors may occur due to insufficient adhesion of the sample to the measuring system or when the sample is pulled apart from the measuring gap due to centrifugal forces to

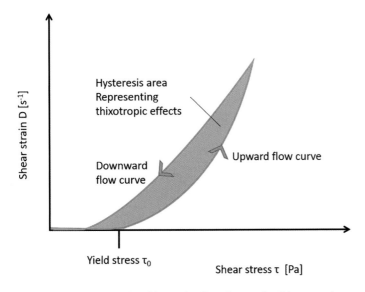

Fig. 15-29 Rheogram to characterize thixotropic effects in a semi-solid preparation.

at high shear rate. The results obtained by the rotational rheological examination characterize the preparation at the onset of (flow point; yield stress) as well as during the flow process (e.g., during a conveying through pipes or upon application).

When required, information about the visco-elastic properties at rest may be obtained by rheological tests in oscillation mode. The sample is then exposed to a very weak, sinusoidally oscillating deformation that is too small to induce flow. A further assay method is the *creep and recovery test*, which is also used in quality control. With this method, a defined shear stress is applied for a particular period of time and the resulting deformation and recovery is monitored. After a certain time interval the strain is relieved and the elastic recovery of the sample is recorded. In this way, *creep curves* are obtained that provide, similar to the oscillation measurements, information on the visco-elastic properties of the product.

Finally, for a simple rheological characterization, *rotating spindle viscosimeters* (relative viscometers) may be deployed. In such a device, a stirring element with a preset rotation velocity is made to rotate in a test vessel containing the sample. The force required for that is determined as torque and is proportional to the viscosity. A calibration curve will yield the correlation between torque and viscosity. Because the measuring geometry (e.g., the width of the shear gap) is not defined precisely, this procedure only allows relative measurements. For the characterization of semi-solid preparations, often a T-bar spindle is used, which during the measurement travels on a helical path deeper and deeper through the preparation. In this way, the measuring system continuously meets always fresh, nonsheared material. Unlike in common rotational viscosimeters, where the sample experiences mechanical strain during the application into the measuring gap, using T-bar spindle with a Helipath® measurement is done on unstrained material. This method produces, however, no absolute values, and is thus only suitable for comparative measurements.

The term *consistency* describes the ointment-like soft properties of semi-solid preparations but is not defined exactly. Consequently, testing the consistency of semi-solid preparations reveals only relative values.

Ph. Eur. describes a measurement of consistency by penetrometry. The penetrometer (Fig. 15-30) expresses consistency as the distance in tenths of a millimeter that a test cone under fixed conditions of temperature, pre-shear intensity and time travels down perpendicularly in a test sample of the material. To adapt the penetrometer to the properties of the test material, different types of the cone may be deployed (e.g., the microcone). Penetrometry can be conducted either on mechanically unstressed material or on a sample that is presheared under defined conditions.

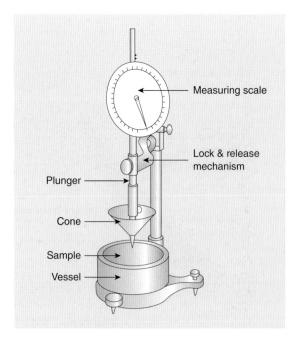

Fig. 15-30 Penetrometer according to Ph. Eur.

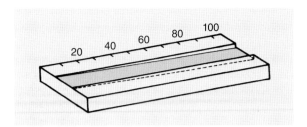

Fig. 15-31 Grindometer.

The consistency of semi-solid preparations may also be characterized by determining their spreading capacity (not to confuse with the spontaneous spreading of a fluid on a surface) by means of an *extensometer*. A defined volume of the preparation (e.g., 0.5 mL) is placed in the center of a glass plate, covered with a second plate and then strained with a defined weight (e.g., 200 g, exerting a force F). After a certain time (e.g., 3 minutes) the average diameter of the area of the squashed sample A is determined. Spreading values of typical creams range from 500 to 4,000 mm^2.

Operating principle of an extensometer:

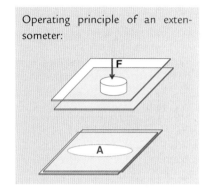

15.7.4 Particle Size

A grindometer (Fig. 15-31) can provide a very quick indication of the high end of the particle size distribution in preparations with suspended active ingredients. It consists of a steel block with a channel of varying depth machined into it, starting at an appropriate depth for the type of suspension to be measured, and becoming shallower at the other side of the steel block (e.g., from 0 to 30 μm or from 0 to 100 μm). The depth at each position can be read on a scale along the grooves. The suspension to be tested is applied to the deep end of the groove, and scraped towards the shallow end with a flat metal scraper. At the point where the particle size of the suspended material exceeds the depth of the groove, drag marks are formed. From the calibration scale, the size of the corresponding particles can be read.

Precise information with respect to particle size, size distribution, and shape, as well as homogeneity of particle distribution in suspension ointments and creams, can, however, only be obtained by means of microscopy (section 3.4.2). Microscopy is also suitable to test preparations with dissolved active substances for the absence of solid particles. Optical microscopy (cf. Ph. Eur. 2.9.37, section 3.3.1.2) may be applied for particles with a size >1 μm. Computer-assisted image analysis simplifies the evaluation and documentation of microscopic investigations.

To facilitate particle size analysis, it may be meaningful to melt or dissolve the base prior to measurement, provided that this does not alter particle size. Suspended crystals can be recognized by means of polarization microscopy. An approximation of particle size in the context of quality control is a shortened test that measures in each of 10 randomly chosen microscope fields of 0.5 mm^2 the largest dimension of the largest observed particle. The 10 values thus obtained are averaged. The pharmacopeia provides only for semi-solid ophthalmological formulations concrete instructions for maximal particle size (section 15.4.1). It also indicates, however, that in all cases measures have to be taken to ensure a suitable and controlled particle size with regard to the intended use.

15.7.5 Thermo-Resistance

Numerous lipophilic components of semi-solid preparations melt and change their state of matter from solid to fluid in the temperature range between 0 and 40°C. The water phase of creams freezes at temperature below 0°C. Because of such phase transitions the consistency of the preparation alters and during crystallization interfacial films may be sheared off—for example, when ice crystals are formed. When preparations contain nonionic macrogol derivatives as emulsifiers, polarity may change due to approaching the phase inversion temperature (PIT).

In summary, these processes may cause a dramatic deterioration of the stability of the preparation. Particularly repeated temperature changes act destabilizing. That makes testing of stability against temperature changes immensely important during product development. Temperature cycling studies involve storing the preparation at alternating high and low temperatures in a closed container (e.g., 24 hours at 40°C, followed by 24 hours at 4°C or 12 hours at 50°C, followed by 12 hours at −10°C). The samples are tested after fixed time intervals predominantly for changes in their physical attributes (e.g., consistency and homogeneity). As part of accelerated stability testing, such thermal stress conditions provide general information concerning stability and behavior of the preparation under various storage conditions within a few weeks.

A modification of the regular temperature cycling test is a temperature-dependent mechanic-dynamic test. It involves the rheological examination of the preparation in the oscillation mode while varying temperature (−10°C → 50°C → −10°C; at a heating/cooling rate of 3°C/min). Already, after three cycles, the first indications of temperature stability may be obtained.

Supplementary to the stress data from temperature cycling tests, temperature stability of preparation semi-solid drug products is assessed under accelerated isothermic stress conditions (e.g., at 40°C and −10°C). In contrast to other pharmaceutical formulations, in case of semi-solid preparations it is in most cases not possible to draw direct conclusions from such studies about their behavior at room temperature. A prediction of stability, for instance, based on the Arrhenius equation (section 25.2.2.4), will fail because state of matter and structure of the preparation will change substantially when common stress conditions are applied. Reliable conclusions concerning shelf life can, therefore, only be drawn from appropriate long-term testing at room temperature or, when applicable, at other relevant temperature ranges.

15.7.6   Determination of Emulsion Type

For the verification of the emulsion type of a cream, preferentially electric conductivity is assessed. In this test system, preparations with a continuous aqueous phase yield distinctly higher electrical conductivity than preparations in which water serves as the dispersed phase. A phase inversion during production or during storage (possibly temperature-induced) is indicated by a steep alteration in electric conductivity. In some cases, measuring a temperature-dependent conductivity may provide some hints of problems concerning storage stability. Other methods, such as staining with lipophilic and hydrophilic dyes or a test on miscibility with aqueous or lipophilic fluids, will only provide qualitative information on the emulsion type of the preparation. For many preparations, an unambiguous assignment to either the O/W or W/O type is not possible especially when systems with an extremely complex structure like bi- or tri-coherent systems (amphiphilc creams) are tested.

15.7.7   Water Absorption Capacity

Determination of water-absorption capacity serves the characterization of lipophilic absorption bases. The test for water uptake capacity as described in the Pharmacopeia (e.g., for wool fat, or wool alcohols) involves the assessment of the amount of water that at room temperature can be maximally incorporated in 10 g of base, before visible water droplets remain. Maximal water uptake is expressed by the *water index*. This is defined as the maximal amount of water in grams that can be retained by 100 g of water-free base at a certain temperature (commonly 15° to 20°C), either permanently or for a defined time period (commonly 24 hours), following a manual incorporation procedure. The amount of water taken up is quantitatively assessed by differential weighing or by determining the water content. The water uptake capacity is altered when an aqueous solution is incorporated instead of pure water. In most cases dissolved substances lower the water index. Water index and water content (which is expressed as a percentage) are not identical. The water index is related to the water-free base, whereas water content relates to the hydrous emulsion ointment.

15.7.8   Water Content

To determine water content of a cream the pharmacopeia prescribes distillation (e.g., wool alcohol ointment, cold cream, hydrous wool fat). Alternatively, for semi-solid preparations loss on drying may be determined. The latter method is, however, not suitable when volatile active or excipients are present (e.g., essential oil, phenols). Besides, to employ this method it is essential that the preparation is spread out in a thin layer, if required after mixing with sand (white or slightly grayish grains of silica with a particle size between 150 μm and 300 μm), in order to ensure that the disperse water phase can evaporate quantitatively. Furthermore, without spreading the lipid phase might splash during evaporation of water, comparable to the behavior of butter during heating in a pan. Another option is to determine water content by titration—for example, using the Karl Fischer method (section 3.8.2.2).

15.7.9   Further Tests

By determining density of a preparation conclusions might be drawn with respect to possible air inclusions. For semi-solid preparations special pycnometers are available with a hemispherical shaped sample vessel. In case of preparations with sufficient fluidity, the oscillating U-tube method may be deployed. This method is based on the Mass-Spring Model where the *eigenfrequency* of U-shaped sample container is influenced by the sample's mass. Evaluation of the refractory index may be used for testing transparent dermatics such as gels. Additionally, pH assessment of hydrophilic creams and gels (e.g., to ensure adequate neutralization during manufacturing of carbomer gels or as an indicator of hydrolytic processes) is commonly performed. After a defined dilution with water, a pH meter provided with a specially modified combination electrode suitable for use in emulsions and creams can be used. An approximate indication of the pH value may be obtained by spotting on narrow range pH indicator paper or rod. For creams, this method is rarely accurate.

15.8   Special Semi-Solid Preparations for Cutaneous Application

15.8.1   Skin Protection Products

A frequent cause of skin disorders, in particular eczemas, is the prolonged and repeated exposure to skin damaging agents, such as occurring in certain professional activities (e.g., food production, hair care, metal processing, construction). Substances attacking the upper skin layers, especially those that may extract epidermal lipids (surfactants, organic solvents), may cause loss of skin barrier function. This will result in enhanced transepidermal water loss and thus to dryness of the skin, causing it to become rough and scaled and diminishing its resistance to permeating noxious substances. Upon prolonged exposure to water, the horny layer may swell and undergo drastic changes in its physical properties. The tear strength of the skin diminishes and the intercellular coherence will loosen. The swelling ultimately leads to desiccation as the absorbed water evaporates again. Additional water can no longer be bound effectively because the natural moisturizing substances are washed out. Irritants and allergens thus penetrate more easily into the deeper skin layers across the damaged barrier.

Traditionally, noxious compounds are categorized according to their chemical structure in two groups:

1. Hydrophilic compounds (e.g., water, aqueous solutions, acids and bases, alcohols)
2. Lipophilic compounds (e.g., organic solvents such as chlorinated hydrocarbons or mineral oil, oil colors, and lacquers)

Skin protection products are preparations that are applied on the skin prior to the contact with hazardous substances (e.g., from the workplace), and whose protective action for this application has been proven. The action of such products is based on prevention or reduction of the contact between the noxious agent and the skin. Additionally, they facilitate cleaning of the contaminated skin so that the use of aggressive cleaning agents that may also damage the barrier function can be avoided. Skin protection products must be adjusted to the nature of the noxious agent. Both hydrophilic (water-soluble) and lipophilic (water insoluble) preparations are deployed.

As a rule of thumb, hydrophilic influences are attenuated by lipophilic preparations and lipophilic influences by application of hydrophilic preparations. Protection from aqueous systems is provided by the use of hydrophobic basis such as soft paraffin, silicon oil, lipogels, lipophilic absorption bases, and lipophilic creams, whereas in case of lipophilic noxious substances, a more hydrophilic base (e.g., hydrophilic creams) is used.

Nonetheless, it has been demonstrated that this general rule does not always apply, so that the suitability of skin protection product needs to be validated for each purpose of application. Skin protection products rather often contain silicon oil, which is ascribed protection properties against hydrophilic as well as lipophilic influences. Predominantly dimethylsiloxans (e.g., Dimeticon 350), are used with amphiphilic creams (base cream DAC) or hydrophilic creams as the most preferred vehicles. To achieve a skin protective effect toward minor aggressive influences, such as those occurring during housework, concentrations of 2% to 5% suffice. For optimal protection from severe noxious chemicals in the occupational field, higher amounts of silicon oil, varying from 10 to 30%, are required, which should not be processed into washable preparations. Silicon oil does not negatively affect physiological functions of the skin, especially transepidermal water loss. Therefore, no risk of occlusion of the skin occurs when using such preparations. Moreover, silicon oils possess good heat-conductance properties, which make them also suitable for application on large skin areas (e.g., for treatment of decubitus).

Special skin protection products are, for example, those containing tannins or adstringent inorganic salts such as aluminum chloride, which reduce perspiration and softening of the skin brought about by carrying rubber gloves. Some preparations also contain buffer systems in order to protect the skin from acids and bases. Sun and UV protection agents are also counted among the special skin protection products (see below).

Besides protection from the noxious substances listed above, protection from caustic substances, as, for example, occur in the cement and galvanization industry, is required. For this purpose, products have proven their efficacy, which consist of polyethylene glycol (macrogol) and inorganic hydrogels to which plastisizers (e.g., glycerol) are added. After drying, they leave an elastic film on the skin (liquid glove), which protects the skin from the caustic noxes.

15.8.2   Sunscreen Products

The protection of the skin from excessive solar radiation serves to protect the skin from sunburn and to prevent the occurrence of chronic damage like the induction of skin cancer and their precursors, as well as premature skin aging (photo aging). The fraction of the sunlight responsible for these phenomena lies in the UV region. The UV radiation of the sun is classified in several ranges, which differently affect the skin:

- UV-A radiation ($\lambda \approx 320–400$ nm): This range of the UV spectrum has an immediate but only transient tanning effect. UV-A radiation penetrates the skin down to the dermis and has only minor acute effects. Only at very high intensities does it lead to erythemata. However, it is considered to increase formation of free radicals and thus to induce the degradation of collagen and elastin, the most serious causes of light-induced skin aging. In addition, UV-A radiation may elicit light dermatoses such as photoallergic or phototoxic dermatitis. The formation of reactive oxygen species is considered an important factor in the etiology of skin tumors. UV-A radiation is immunosuppressive.
- UV-B radiation ($\lambda =$ ca. 280–320 nm, maximum at 307–308 nm): it penetrates only the epidermis, leading to sustained tanning, and after excessive exposure it causes acute skin damage (dermatitis solaris, sunburn). UV-B radiation produces photoproducts in the DNA of skin cells (e.g., cyclobutane-pyrimidine dimers (CPD) by

cross-linking of neighboring thymine bases. The absorption of the radiation also leads to the formation of free radicals that are engaged in secondary photochemical reactions. The most severe late effect of a high UV-B burden is the development of malignant neoplasmata (basaliomes, melanomas).

□ UV-C radiation ($\lambda < 280$ nm): this wavelength range has a very strongly erythema-inducing action. However, Solar UVC is practically completely absorbed by ozone in the stratosphere, so that under normal conditions it does not reach the earth. UV-C radiation can be artificially produced and be used for disinfection of e.g., air and water (ultraviolet germicidal irradiation (UVGI)). UVC also arises during welding processes.

UV-B radiation induces cell proliferation in the basal layer of the epidermis. As a result, the outermost layer of the epidermis, the horny layer, thickens imperceptibly. This hyperkeratosis enhances the natural light protection function of the skin. A further protection mechanism of the skin that is activated by UV-B radiation is the production of the pigment melanin, which is responsible for the tanning process. This natural, slow adaptation to sunlight exposure is nowadays not always sufficient, such as when traveling in regions with intense solar radiation. In addition, various medical preparations (e.g., retinoids, tetracyclins, St. John's wort or neuroleptics) as well as certain cosmetic treatments (e.g., use of peeling preparations) may lead to increased light sensitivity. When excessive exposure to sunlight is not avoidable, sunscreens are an adequate additional means to protect the skin. According to the legislation on cosmetics, sunscreen products are preparations intended to be placed externally in contact with the human skin with the exclusive or predominant aim to protect from UV radiation by absorbing, scattering, or reflecting it. In U.S.A. these products are considered to be drugs and are regulated by the Drug and Cosmetic Act.

Sunscreen products can be effective in preventing sunburn. Scientific findings also suggest that sunscreen products can prevent the damage linked to photo-aging and that they can protect against induced photoimmunosuppression. Model studies demonstrate that regular UV protection, particularly in childhood and adolescence, later in life plays an important role in the prevention of skin cancer.

In order to have these preventive characteristics, sunscreen products need to protect against both UVB and UVA radiation.

Assessment of UV-B protection (sun protection factor SPF) may be performed with an *in vivo* test according to the European COLIPA (International Sun Protection Factor Test Method) or the FDA (Labeling and effectiveness testing; sunscreen drug products for over-the-counter human use). Strictly speaking, the SPF indicates, depending on the test method, how many times longer the skin can be exposed to UV-B radiation after application of a certain amount of the product (2 mg/cm^2) than without that before developing a sunburn. Reference method for the determination of the UVA protection factor is an *in vivo* method for the assessment of the direct pigmentation threshold (Persistent Pigment Darkening, PPD, method). It is presumed that adequate UV-A protection is attained when the UV-A protection factor amounts to at least one-third of the sun protection factor. As in vivo methods raise ethical concerns, the ambition is to employ as soon as possible a validated *in vitro* test method to quantify UV-A as well as UV-B protection.

Such methods are based on the measurement of UV light transmitted through a thin film of the formulation, which is mounted on a suitable substrate. UV filter substances need to be approved and are listed in a "positive list" of the EU cosmetic directive and the corresponding FDA regulation. Among the UV filters deployed in sun protection products, distinction is made between organic (chemical) and mineral (physical) filters. In addition, corresponding to their absorption spectrum, UV-B, UV-A, and broad-spectrum filters are distinguished.

Among the organic compounds, currently 16 UV-B filters, 4 UV-A filters, and 6 broad-spectrum filters are approved. Physical filters that are approved for cosmetics in Europe are the nanopigments zinc oxide and titanium dioxide. To achieve the required protection level in the UV-B and UV-A range, sunscreen products contain combinations of different filter substances (Fig. 15-32).

Organic UV filters are very effective, but not always without problems. They may, for example, lead to allergic or phototoxic reactions and may cause adverse effects following absorption. As alternatives, mineral filter substances are under consideration. These exploit the

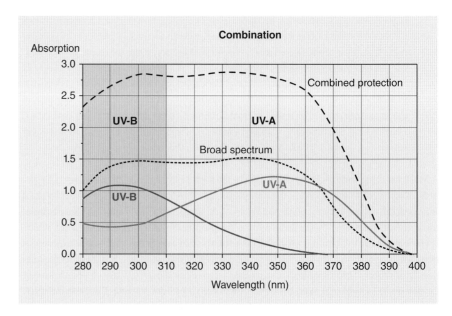

Fig. 15-32   Individual and combined absorption spectra of UV filters. By combination of a UV-A and a UV-B filter absorption in the entire UV range can be obtained, comparable to the effect of a broadband filter.

reflection, scattering, or refractive action of inorganic pigments such as zinc oxide and titanium dioxide. "Normal" pigments with particle sizes of about 200 to 250 nm are deployed in the medical applications—for example, in paste-like products to attain "total" sun protection. They protect on the basis of reflection, scattering, and absorption in the entire UV-A, UV-B, and UV-C range and may therefore be considered broad-band filters, but with minor protective activity. In addition, they intensely scatter visible light and thus produce a cosmetically unfavorable whitening effect. Therefore, sunscreen products contain nanopigments with a far smaller particle size (e.g., ultrafine titanium dioxide <30 nm). These are more effective sunscreens and invisible on the skin because they do not scatter visible light (Fig. 15-33).

The activity of nanopigments is particularly based on the ability to absorb in the entire UV range of the solar spectrum; they are true broad-spectrum filters. The ratio UV-A/UV-B protection performance strongly depends on the nature and size of the particles. Their

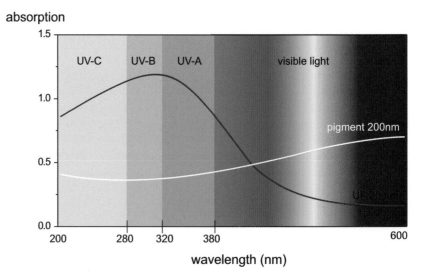

Fig. 15-33   Absorption behavior of ultra-fine titanium dioxide (UF) that has an absorption maximum in the UV-B range as compared to "normal" TiO_2 that scatters in the visible range of the solar spectrum.

processing is quite challenging because the micro-fine character should be unconditionally retained in the formulation. If not, they will lose the properties of a nanopigment and may display, for example, a whitening effect, like the traditional pigments.

Nanopigments are well tolerated on the skin and particularly used for application on sensitive skin and in sunscreen products for children. In addition to UV filters, sunscreen products also contain several secondary active ingredients. The selection of these substances is primarily based on the observation that (1) many skin-damaging effects of UV radiation are mediated by free radicals; (2) UV irradiation leads to skin dryness and irritation; and (3) UV irradiation overstresses the skin's intrinsic repair systems. Accordingly, the complementary secondary additives may be distinguished in moisturizers (e.g., glycerol, hyaluronic acid), antioxidants and radical scavengers (e.g., tocopherol, polyphenols), skin-soothing agents (e.g., bisabolol) and anti-inflammatory substances (e.g., dexpanthenol), as well as DNA repair enzymes (photolyase). A decisive condition for their deployment is that the activity of the preparation has been proven with appropriate test methods.

The base for sunscreen products includes mainly fluid emulsions or creams in which both lipophilic and hydrophilic active agents can be processed and which, in addition to their UV protective activity also contain skin care components. Most widely used are formulations of the O/W type because of their more favorable sensory attributes compared to W/O formulations. The O/W preparations can be fluid emulsions, creams, and sprays (e.g., PIT emulsions).

The type of formulation may affect the applied quantity of sunscreen product (semi-solid creams > thin-fluid spray) and thereby the value of the actual achieved sun protection. Because the combination of UV-A radiation and certain emulsifiers and lipid components together with a certain predisposition may cause a special form of polymorph light dermatosis (Mallorca acne), alternative preparations not containing emulsifiers or lipids are available. Examples are hydrogels, which, however, hardly display any skin care properties and act slightly dehydrating. Hydro-dispersion gels are preparations with a hydrophilic continuous phase and a lipophilic dispersed phase. The lipid content of these emulsions usually lies between 2% and 20%, while the stabilization of the disperse state is not achieved by traditional emulsifiers (surfactants) but rather by a thickening of the continuous phase, ideally with interfacially active macromolecules. In contrast to the hydrogels, in these emulsions not only oil-soluble UV filters, but also lipid-replenishing and water-repelling components can be incorporated. Also, emulsions where mineral UV filters (TiO_2; ZnO) are used as particulate emulsifiers are emulsifier-free; in this case, these compounds simultaneously serve as emulsion stabilizers and UV filters.

Further sunscreen products are marketed as oils and lipogels, in which exclusively lipid-soluble or lipid-dispersible UV filters can be processed; this usually results in relatively low protection levels. An advantage is, though, that preservatives are not required for these water-free formulations. Sticks, such as those based on beeswax, hard paraffin, or ceresin, are predominantly used for lip protection purposes. An additional requirement of contemporary sunscreen products is that they should be adequately waterproof in order to ensure also proper protection during swimming or sports. Products with a lipophilic external phase and in particular those containing silicon oil possess an essentially higher water resistance than hydrophilic preparations. In O/W formulations, water resistance can be promoted by the use of water-insoluble UV filters, reduction of the amount of hydrophilic emulsifiers as well as by the addition of film-forming polymers (alkylated PVP, acrylate polymers with hydrophobic side chains). Encapsulation of UV filters in liposomes may likewise improve water resistance.

15.9   Requirements of Semi-Solid Preparations Not for Dermal Application

Semi-solid preparations intended for applications other than on the skin in part have to fulfill requirements beyond those dealt with in this chapter. That applies, in particular, to sterile eye preparations. For those, as well as for semi-solid preparations for vaginal, rectal, ear, or nasal application, the pharmacopeia is covered in more detail in other chapters.

Semi-solid rectal and vaginal preparations are ointments, creams or gels that are often packaged in single-dose containers provided with a suitable applicator. Normally, they serve the purpose of local treatment (e.g., in case of anal fissures or vaginal mycoses). As a rule, preparations for vaginal application have a hydrophilic character; in most cases they are hydrophilic creams, more rarely hydrogels. Among the rectal preparations we find lipophilic as well as hydrophilic creams or water-emulsifying ointments.

Semi-solid ear preparations are meant for application to the external auditory meatus, if necessary they may be delivered by means of a tampon impregnated with the preparation or in the form of impregnated gauze. In that way, they provide a certain protection against foreign material penetrating into the middle ear in case of eardrum defects. The base of such preparations should not elicit local irritation, and in case of aqueous preparations, they should contain a preservative. Preparations intended for application in the injured ear, especially in case of eardrum perforations or prior to surgical intervention, have to be sterile, free from preservatives, and supplied in a single-dose container. The container should be fitted with a suitable applicator. In practice, semi-solid preparations for the ear play only a minor role.

Semi-solid nasal preparations serve as local treatment in the nasal cavity. Nasal preparations should be as far as possible nonirritating and should not adversely affect the functions of the nasal mucosa and its cilia. Such preparations are hydrophobic ointments, water-emulsifying ointments, hydrophobic creams, or hydrogels, packaged in tubes with a suitable applicator. Hydrophilic creams are not suitable for intra-nasal application. Hydrophobic preparations are only in certain instances suited for nasal application; particularly because of the risk of lipid pneumonia due to aspiration of lipophilic components they may cause problems. Although nasal ointments must be soft in order to allow adequate distribution along the mucosa, nevertheless they should have a sufficiently solid consistency to prevent aspiration of one or more of the components. Lipophilic creams and water-emulsifying ointments for nasal application in most cases contain wool alcohols as emulsifiers. As alternatives to lipophilic bases, hydrogels may be deployed which more clearly comply with the physiological conditions of nasal mucosa. To achieve optimal physiological tolerance hydrophilic nasal gels and aqueous nose drops should be euhydric (pH as close as possible to physiological pH) and approximately isotonic. To adjust tonicity mostly glycerol is used and as gelling agents preferentially hypromellose. Aqueous semi-solid nasal preparations in multiple-dose containers must contain a suitable antimicrobial preservative. Also, creams should be adequately preserved because the risk of contamination with this type of application is very high.

15.9.1   Semi-Solid Eye Preparations

Semi-solid eye preparations are sterile ointments, creams, or gels, which are applied to the conjunctiva or to the eyelids. Compared to liquid preparations they show prolonged action, but since they cause a foreign-body sensation and hinder vision, they are preferentially used overnight or in combination with an eye bandage. They should not cause irritation and should possess adequate adherence to the eye as well as spreadability and smoothness. The Ph. Eur. limits the particle size of preparations with dispersed solid particles in order to exclude irritation. It may be tested microscopically: In a quantity of the preparation containing at least 10 µg of suspended active substance, no particles with a size >90 µm, maximally 2 particles of >50 µm and maximally 20 particles of >25 µm should be present. Therefore, during the production of ocular suspension ointments not only adequately comminuted active substances should be used, but also special care should be taken to avoid changes in particle size and recrystallization phenomena (section 15.3.1.2). During storage of ocular suspension ointments, particle size needs to be assessed regularly. According to Ph. Eur., semi-solid eye preparations should be packed in small, sterilized, collapsible tubes fitted or provided with an application nozzle and containing not more than 10 g of product or in single-dose containers. Packaging in tubes ensures that contamination during application is minimal because of the small cross-sectional area of the tube orifice, while at the same time it provides protection from light. Aluminum tubes should be lined internally with an appropriate lacquer and be free from metal splinters. When multiple-dose containers are used, the aqueous phase should contain a preservative, especially in case of hydrogels and, if applicable, also lipophilic creams. Frequently used preservatives are cetrimide and benzalkonium chloride. Preparations containing a preservative shall be assessed for the efficacy of antimicrobial preservation (Ph. Eur. 5.1.3). Semi-solid eye preparations preferably display a certain degree of hydrophilicity, thus ensuring proper interaction with the tear fluid and adequate distribution in the conjunctival sac. Optimally, a base with a yield stress of < 0.5 Pa and a melting range of 32° to 33°C (temperature of the cornea or conjunctiva) is used. Of the commonly used bases for eye ointments, only very few meet the requirements listed above. Most often, hydrocarbon gels are used (three parts soft paraffin and two parts liquid paraffin to adjust consistency), either as such or with a W/O emulsifier (e.g., cholesterol, wool fat). These water-free bases may be dry-heat sterilized at 160°C. By using sterile aqueous solutions of active ingredient and aseptically processing this into the base, lipophilic creams are produced that are also suitable for ocular application. Bases of the O/W type, on the other hand, are less suitable for this purpose because they contain hydrophilic emulsifiers, which often give rise to irritations in the eye. Therefore, predominantly hydrogels are used as hydrophilic semi-solid bases. Good physiological compatibility is observed for cellulose ethers (e.g., hypromellose), polyvinyl alcohol, and povidone. In licensed medicinal products, carbomers are almost exclusively used as gelling agent. In addition to their good tolerance, carbomers are muco-adhesive and may thus prolong the precorneal residence time. Carbomers are deployed both as a vehicle and as an active ingredient for the treatment of dry eyes. Furthermore, small quantities of lipids (e.g., medium-chain triglycerides) may also be emulsified in carbomer gels (hydrodispersion gels). This lipid fraction is released following application and substitutes the lipid layer of the tear film. In addition to sterility, the Ph. Eur. requires that semi-solid eye preparations do not cause undue local irritation. To achieve that, hydrophilic eye gels should be made isotonic and isohydric, or if justified euhydric (see section 22.2.1.6). As carbomer gels are sensitive to the addition of electrolytes, isotonicity is usually achieved by addition of glycerol.

Terminal sterilization of semi-solid eye preparations is only rarely possible. Mostly, they are prepared under aseptic conditions in order to ensure proper microbiological quality. Therefore, it can be done only in a correspondingly suitable and properly equipped clean working area (e.g., a laminar airflow work station) and should proceed according to standardized operation procedures. The starting materials have to be sterilized by means of suitable procedures. Ointment bases consisting of mainly hydrocarbons, such as cholesterol-containing soft paraffin, may be sterilized by dry heat. Certain bases may sterile filtered using heatable pressure-filtration devices. For the production of eye creams, the active ingredients are dissolved in the water phase. Analogous to the manufacturing of eye drops, the aqueous drug solution is filtered to remove microbial and particulate contaminants and then incorporated under aseptic conditions in the sterile base. When extemporaneous eye creams have to be prepared, this can be done using the syringe-to-syringe technique, where sterile base and aqueous solution are mixed by cycling back and forth from one to the other of two connected syringes. For the production of suspension eye ointments, sufficiently small particle size may be attained by using sterile micronized active substances. Compounding of unlicensed suspension eye ointments of sufficient quality is hardly feasible and should only be pursued in exceptional situations and after a suitable level of risk assessment is undertaken.

Further Reading

Alexander, A., Dwivedi, S., Ajazuddin, Giri T. K., Saraf, S., Saraf, S., et al. "Approaches for Breaking the Barriers of Drug Permeation through Transdermal Drug Delivery." *J Control Release* 164 (1) (November 28, 2012): 26–40.

Ashtikar, M., Nagarsekar, K., Fahr, A. "Transdermal Delivery from Liposomal Formulations—Evolution of the Technology over the Last Three Decades." *Journal of Controlled Release* 242 (2016): 126–140.

Cross, S., Roberts, M. "Physical enhancement of transdermal drug application: is delivery technology keeping up with pharmaceutical development?" *Curr. Drug. Del.* 1 (1) (2004): 81–92.

Elias, P. M. "Epidermal lipids, barrier
   function, and desquamation." *J. Invest.
   Dermatol.* 80 (1983): 44–49.
Hwa, C., Bauer, E. A., Cohen, D. E. "Skin
   biology." *Dermatologic therapy* 24 (5)
   (2011): 464–470.
Lee, J. W., Park, J. H., Prausnitz M. R.
   "Dissolving microneedles for
   transdermal drug delivery." *Biomaterials*
   29 (13) (May 2008): 2113–2124.
Loraschi, A., Marelli, R., Crema, F.,
   Lecchini, S., Cosentino, M. "An unusual
   systemic reaction associated with

topical salicylic acid in a paediatric
   patient." *Br. J. Clin. Pharmacol.* 66 (1)
   (July 2008): 152–153.
Naik, A., Kalia, Y. N., Guy, R. H.
   "Transdermal Drug Delivery:
   Overcoming the Skin's Barrier
   Function." *Pharm Sci Technolo Today* 9 (3)
   (September 2000): 318–326.
Williams, A. C., Barry, B. W. "Skin
   absorption enhancers." *Critical Reviews in
   Therapeutic Drug Carrier Systems* 9 (1992):
   305–353.

Patches/Plasters

16

16.1 General Considerations

Patches are flexible adhesive preparations intended for external use. Inscriptions from ancient Egypt (the Ebers papyrus and in particular the Edwin Smith papyrus) indicate that they were already being applied around 2000 BC and thus represent the oldest medical formulation ever. Patch cooking—that is, the preparation of lead plaster by saponification of triglycerides with lead (II) oxide (lead salts of the fatty acids released during the hydrolytic cleavage of fat)—was a privilege of the pharmacist. In numerous old pharmacopeias lead plasters were described as the base substance for drug-containing patches (lat.: *emplastra*) but nowadays these are considered obsolete. Currently, plasters are made of rubber or are based on co-polymers of acrylic acid and their esters or on silicone polymers, which form a sticky mass. This strongly adhesive material is transferred onto a backing layer consisting for example of a fabric or foil. Patches that are not produced in rolls are provided with a protective liner that covers the sticky material. Plasters and patches are produced almost exclusivley at the industrial scale. They need to have strong adhesive capacity but at the same time should be easily removable from the skin without pain and without leaving a residue.

Simple adhesive patches, which merely consist of a backing and an adhesive layer, serve to keep bandages or medical devices like cannulas or catheters in place. For covering small wounds, patches with a wound coating (adhesive bandages) are often used. Plaster sprays packed in pressurized gas containers (wound sprays) are described in section 23.2.1. Medicated plasters and cutaneous patches that are described in the monograph (Semi-Solid Preparations for Cutaneous Application) contain active ingredients incorporated in the adhesive mass and are intended for local or regional therapy.

Transdermal patches, which are described in a separate monograph of the pharmacopeia, are placed on the intact skin and release the active ingredient in a controlled manner and for prolonged periods of time in order to bring about a systemic effect.

16.2 Structure

The basic structure of all three types of patches (drug-free, medicated, and transdermal) involves multiple characteristic layers. The functionally most important of these is the adhesive layer; this is placed on a backing layer and protected by an easily removable protective liner.

Voigt's Pharmaceutical Technology, First Edition. Alfred Fahr.
© 2018 John Wiley & Sons Ltd. Published 2018 by John Wiley & Sons Ltd.

16.2.1   Adhesive Material

The adhesive mass is composed of matrix components, which provide the adhesive film with solidity and elasticity and a variety of further excipients. In the medical/pharmaceutical field, adhesive material is usually based on rubber and acrylates, while silicones are used more rarely. As the matrix substance for rubber adhesives (polyisobutylene adhesives), natural, modified, or synthetic rubber is used. The stickiness is acquired by carefully adjusted additions of various resins (e.g., colophonium and derivatives). Natural resins used for this purpose are gradually being replaced by synthetic resins. In addition, plasticizers are added, such as wool fat, plant oils, liquid paraffin, or waxes (beeswax, carnauba wax) in order to attain a smooth and soft adhesive mass with adequate adhesive properties. Furthermore, additional filling substances are required for proper adjustment of the consistency; these are in most cases also responsible for the color of the adhesive mass, for which purpose mostly zinc oxide, often also titanium dioxide, chalk, talcum, barium sulfate, or kaolin are used. To enhance stability, the addition of antioxidants is required. The product is manufactured by grinding the mixture of components, which then is melted and thoroughly kneaded with petroleum ether.

Rubber/resin plasters have a high, yet temperature-dependent, adhesive potential. At low temperatures, adhesiveness clearly diminishes and already at body temperature the adhesive mass softens considerably, so that upon removal residues may be left behind on the skin. At temperatures above 60°C, the adhesive mass tends to disintegrate. In addition, often allergic reactions are observed with this material.

Meanwhile, polyacrylate plasters have largely replaced polyisobutylene adhesives. The former are obtained by co-polymerization of acrylic acid, acrylic acid esters and other functional monomers, for example, poly(acrylamid-co-iso-octylacrylate). The polyacrylates should contain only small proportions of monomers and oligomers, as these may elicit irritations and allergies. The adhesive potential of polyacrylates is smaller than that of rubber adhesives, but has the clear advantage that it remains stable over a wide range of temperatures (−40° to 70°C). This type of plaster is very well tolerated on the skin and can painlessly be removed from hairy skin while leaving no residue. Due to their thermo-stability, they can be steam-sterilized and show very high storage stability.

Further alternatives are silicone adhesives that are produced by condensation of poly-dimethyl- or poly-dimethyl-diphenyl-siloxane and a resin (three-dimensional silicate), which is end-blocked with a large number of terminal trimethyl-siloxy groups. An example of such silicone adhesives is poly(trimethylsilyl)silicate[α-hydro-ω-hydroxypolydimethylsiloxan]. As opposed to other adhesive substances, which show increasing adhesiveness over time, silicone adhesives offer optimal, constant adhesive power for the entire duration of use and allow easy removal. Because of their minor interaction with tissues they are maximally biocompatible and, in addition, they offer the advantage of very high permeability with respect to active ingredients.

16.2.2   Carrier Substances

The carrier on which the adhesive substance is applied (backing) is chosen in accordance with the aim of the application. Materials used for this purpose include cotton, spun rayon, or water-resistant cellulose acetate (acetate silk), fleece of synthetic or semi-synthetic cellulose fibers as well as mixtures of those. For the production of transparent fixing plasters, mostly polyethylene, polyester, polyurethane, or polyethylene terephthalate (Pegoterate) foil is used. More recently, composite materials made of open-pore cotton lint and micro-perforated carrier foil or composite foils are under consideration as carrier materials. Carrier foil may be perforated in order to facilitate permeation of air and water. Fabrics should be stretchable, but dense, in order to prevent break-through of the adhesive material. The adhesion force between carrier and adhesive must be sufficiently strong to ensure that no residues are left upon removal from the skin or that the upper surface becomes sticky upon uncoiling the plaster roll.

16.2.3 Protective (Release) Liner

When required, the adhesive material may be covered with an anti-adhesive protective liner consisting of silicone paper, siliconized polyethylene foil, polypropylene, polyester, or polyethylene terephthalate. This coating foil is commonly provided with a strip-off aid (liner) in order to allow easy removal without touching the adhesive layer.

Currently the protective liner is often used as a basis for the manufacturing of the patch instead of the backing layer because the release liner can be made of sturdy material, while the backing layer is very often quite thin and flexible so as to adjust to the movement of the skin.

16.3 Medicated Plasters and Cutaneous Patches

Medicated plasters and cutaneous patches which in the Ph.Eur. are described in the Monograph "Semi-solid preparations for cutaneous application," contain active ingredients incorporated in the adhesive material which are intended for local or regional therapy. Typical areas of application are circulation enhancing drugs for treatment of rheumatism (rheuma patches) or salicylic acid for the softening of cornified skin areas (corn plasters). Also patches containing local anesthetics (e.g., EMLA® Plaster) or anti-inflammatory agents (e.g., Flector® pain patch) or patches for relief of neuropathic pain (e.g., Qutenza® cutaneous patch) are available. Such patches are available in a size ready for application or need to be cut to size prior to application. Their structure is similar to that of transdermal matrix patches (section 16.4.3). Both the traditional rubber adhesive and, in more up-to-date formulations, often highly concentrated hydrogels on a polyacrylate basis serve as the drug-containing adhesive substance. Thus, medicated patches may be considered as semi-solid formulations that are mounted on a carrier layer. This allows on the one hand an improvement of the residence time of the application on the site of administration (*substantivity*) as well as the amount of preparation applied. On the other hand, penetration may be enhanced by using an occlusive backing sheet such as the EMLA® plaster. When using the capsaicin-containing patches Qutenza® sealing of the application site and "clean" handling are important aspects because the active ingredient (the "hot" substance of hot chili peppers) is extremely irritating, so any unintended contact with the skin and even more so with mucosal tissue (eye, mouth, nose) should be avoided.

16.4 Transdermal Patches

16.4.1 General Considerations

Transdermal patches (Transdermal Therapeutic Systems, TTS) are applied to the unbroken skin in order to deliver the active substance to the systemic circulation after passing through the skin barrier (section 15.6.1). To this end transdermal patches contain a reservoir of active ingredient and are applied by the patient on the designated skin area (e.g., behind the ear or on the chest) with the aid of an adhesive layer. There, a certain amount of drug per unit time is delivered to the skin for a prolonged period of time in a controlled manner. Sufficient permeation ability of the active ingredient is essential to attain an effective plasma concentration. A further prerequisite for the proper functioning of the control mechanism of the system is that the release rate of the drug from the patch is lower than the permeation rate through the skin. The application interval of transdermal patches varies and amounts to 24, 72, or occasionally 96 hours or even up to 1 week. By virtue of the gradual, uniform release of the active ingredient within this time span, peaks in plasma levels can be minimized and concomitant side effects mitigated. A further advantage of transdermal patches is that the gastrointestinal tract and thus the hepatic first-pass metabolism are bypassed, so that the required dose often is lower than for an oral formulation.

Also, the option of immediate interruption of the administration of the drug to the body by simply removing the patch is an advantage. Obviously, an active agent that has already penetrated the skin will then still reach the systemic circulation. Disadvantages to be taken into account are: potential occurrence of skin irritations and allergic reactions and the lag-time in the onset of activity following application. Furthermore, the number of active ingredients that can be applied to attain a sufficiently high plasma concentration with this type of formulation is quite limited. Currently, the following active ingredients are available in transdermal patches: scopolamine (motion sickness), glycerol trinitrate (angina pectoris), estradiol (+ norethisterone acetate) and testosterone (hormone therapy), norelgestromin + ethinyl estradiol (contraception), nicotine (smoking withdrawal), fentanyl and buprenorphine (pain therapy), rivastigmine (dementia), oxybutynin (urinary incontinence), and rotigotine (Parkinson). A number of others are under development or are in the phase of clinical testing. Extensive research on permeation enhancers (section 15.6.3) to enlarge the number of drugs applicable to transdermal patch delivery have not yet led to great success. This is to be ascribed in particular to the fact that penetration enhancers strongly affect the skin barrier and thus may give rise to irritations when, as required for transdermal patches, they are in contact with the skin for prolonged periods of time.

The detailed construction of transdermal patches is diverse, although all are characterized by a multilayered structure. Between an occlusive backing layer and a protection foil (release liner) that is removed prior to application on the skin, a drug-containing layer, an adhesive layer and a release-control layer are to be found. Sometimes multiple functions are accommodated in one and the same layer, so that the simplest variant may contain only three layers.

16.4.2   Membrane Systems

First-generation transdermal patches were membrane systems (also known as reservoir systems), with a structure as depicted in Fig. 16-1.

- □ The backing layer is a foil that is impermeable to both water vapor and the active ingredient, and seals off the drug reservoir towards the outside. It consists for example of polyethylene terephthalate / aluminum foil / polypropylene- or polyvinylchloride or polyethylene laminate. The backing layer provides the occlusion conditions that lead to hydration of the skin and an often several-fold increase in permeation rate.
- □ The drug, dissolved or suspended in a fluid or solid medium, is accommodated in the drug reservoir.
- □ Release control is accounted for by a polymer membrane which may be non-porous, micro-porous or semi-permeable (made for example of polypropylene or cellulose acetate or an ethylene/vinyl acetate co-polymer).
- □ The adhesive layer consists of a suitable pressure-sensitive adhesive, most often based on polyacrylate, that serves to make the patch adhere firmly to the skin.
- □ The drug-impermeable protective layer (release liner) has to be removed before application.

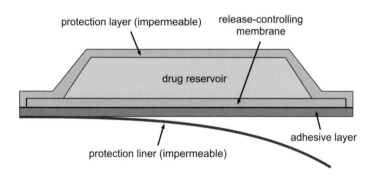

Fig. 16-1 Schematic representation of a transdermal membrane/reservoir type patch.

For a nonporous controlled-release membrane with adhesive layer the release rate from the reservoir, after reaching the dynamic equilibrium, follows from the mathematical relationship:

$$\frac{dQ}{dt} = \frac{c_r}{1/P_m + 1/P_a} \tag{16-1}$$

| Q = quantity of drug released at time t per surface area ($g \cdot cm^{-2}$)
| c_r = drug concentration in the reservoir ($g \cdot cm^{-3}$)
| P_m = permeability coefficient of the membrane ($cm \cdot s^{-1}$)
| P_a = permeability coefficient of the adhesive layer ($cm \cdot s^{-1}$)

The permeability coefficient of a drug depends on the distribution coefficient between membrane and environment, the diffusion coefficient, and membrane thickness:

$$P_m = \frac{K_{m/r} \cdot D_m}{h_m} \quad \text{and} \quad P_a = \frac{K_{m/a} \cdot D_a}{h_a} \tag{16-2}$$

| K_m/r = partition coefficient membrane/reservoir
| K_m/a = partition coefficient membrane/adhesive layer
| D_m = diffusion coefficient membrane ($cm^2 \cdot s^{-1}$)
| D_a = diffusion coefficient adhesive layer ($cm^2 \cdot s^{-1}$)
| h_m = thickness of the membrane (cm),
| h_a = thickness of the adhesive layer (cm)

If one substitutes P_m and P_a in equation 16-1 by the values in equations in 16-2, we obtain

$$\frac{dQ}{dt} = \frac{K_{m/r} \cdot K_{a/m} \cdot D_m \cdot D_a \cdot C_r}{K_{m/r} \cdot D_m \cdot h_a + K_{a/m} \cdot D_a \cdot h_m} \tag{16-3}$$

For porous membranes with an adhesive layer, the porosity ε is included in the membrane diffusion coefficient and the tortuosity τ (ratio of the length of the curved pore versus the distance between the ends of the pore) in the membrane thickness. Under sink conditions, this system allows to obtain zero-order release kinetics, as long as the concentration of dissolved drug in the reservoir remains constant. The clear advantage of the highly precise control of the amount of drug release per unit time obtained with this type of transdermal patch is opposed by the disadvantage that mechanical damage of the control element may lead to spontaneous drug release (dose dumping). Besides, with opiate-containing pain patches, the active ingredient may be removed relatively easily from the reservoir for abusive purposes. During prolonged storage, particularly at elevated temperatures, the drug equilibrates between drug reservoir, control membrane, and adhesive layer. This will result in increased initial release. The resulting enhanced drug release immediately following application may be quite desirable to more rapidly attain dynamic equilibrium and saturate the binding sites in the skin. The extent of this effect may be calculated, so that in the adhesive layer, a defined initial dose may be supplied.

Examples of membrane systems are Estragest® (estradiol/nor-ethisterone) and Nitroderm® (glycerol trinitrate).

16.4.3 Matrix Systems

In patches of this type, the drug reservoir consists of a hydrophilic or lipophilic matrix that contains the major part of the drug homogeneously dispersed in the form of solid particles, while only a small fraction is molecularly dispersed (Fig. 16-2). When under sink conditions

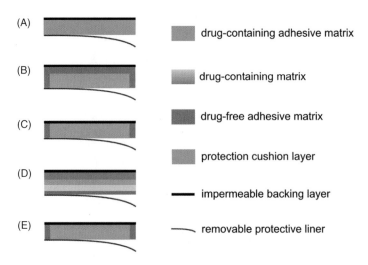

Fig. 16-2 Schematic representation of a transdermal matrix plaster. A: monolithic matrix system (drug-in-adhesive type) B: matrix system with additional adhesive rim C: matrix system with overplastering D: multiple-layered matrix system E: matrix system with absorbent pad

the stationary state has been reached, the release rate is determined by the diffusion of the drug in the matrix, as expressed by the following equation:

$$Q = \sqrt{D_p \cdot t \cdot C_p \cdot 2 \cdot (C_0 - C_p)} \quad \text{and at } C_0 \gg C_p$$
$$\frac{Q}{\sqrt{t}} = \sqrt{2 \cdot D_p \cdot C_p \cdot C_0} \tag{16-4}$$

| Q = quantity of drug released at time t per surface area ($g \cdot cm^{-2}$)
| D_p = diffusion coefficient of the polymer matrix ($cm^2 \cdot s^{-1}$)
| t = release time (s)
| C_p = saturation concentration in the polymer matrix ($g \cdot cm^{-3}$)
| C_0 = drug concentration in the polymer matrix ($g \cdot cm^{-3}$)

Although the equation indicates that with this release principle the release follows the Higuchi square root equation typical of matrix systems, approximate zero-order kinetics may be obtained in case only a small fraction of the drug contained in the matrix is released from the matrix. This minor disadvantage inherent to the matrix type is more than compensated by the notion that these systems are known as particularly safe. Because the drug is homogeneously embedded in the release-controlling matrix, there is no risk of dose dumping as observed with reservoir patches.

The great majority of commercially available transdermal patches are matrix patches. Their production is relatively simple and they are more comfortable for patients to wear because they are thinner than reservoir patches. Structurally, several subtypes of matrix patches can be distinguished (Fig. 16-2).

The most widely used patches are the monolithic matrix systems (drug-in-adhesive type). They are characterized by a simple triple-layered structure consisting of an impermeable backing layer (outer covering), the drug-containing adhesive matrix and the release liner. The adhesive drug-containing matrix functions simultaneously as adhesive and as release control mechanism. In matrix systems with an additional adhesive rim the adhesion of the patches is improved by a drug-free adhesive layer along the circumference of the drug-containing matrix.

Matrix systems with *overplastering* have a nonocclusive coating foil (backing layer) carrying at the skin-facing site a drug-free adhesive layer. The drug-containing matrix is placed centrally on this layer, separated from the adhesive layer by an additional occlusive separation layer. In this way, deterioration of the adhesive power resulting from occlusion-determined water uptake during multiday usage is prevented. Nonocclusive backing layers are rarely used because for most drugs enhancement of penetration by skin hydration is required.

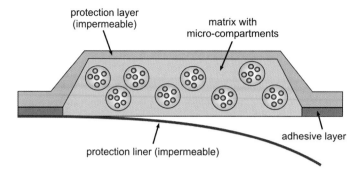

Fig. 16-3   Schematic representation of a transdermal plaster, type micro-reservoir system.

In multilayer matrix systems, the drug is present in more than one layer, either suspended in an adhesive matrix or bound to a carrier. The quantities of embedded active ingredient gradually increase from layer to layer in the direction of the backing layer. In this way, the normally decreasing release rate during prolonged use will be partially compensated, ensuring an approximately constant release over the entire usage period.

Padded matrix systems carry an additional absorbent pad between the backing layer and the drug-containing matrix. Besides a mechanical cushion function this padded layer may serve several other purposes. When it is not separated from the matrix by an occlusive barrier layer, it may be impregnated with a drug solution during manufacturing or it may serve to absorb moisture in order to retain the adhesive power of the plaster.

16.4.4   Micro-Reservoir Systems

In this transdermal patch type a solid polymer matrix contains numerous drug-containing micro-compartments (≤ 100 µm) that may be seen as micro-reservoirs (micro-sealed drug delivery systems, MDD principle). This formulation type is characterized by release mechanisms based on the reservoir as well as on the matrix principle; they are known as hybrid systems. Fig. 16-3 shows the schematic structure of a micro-reservoir system. When required, the release pattern can be further modified by an additional porous membrane. In the Nitrodisc® plaster, a suspension consisting of a glycerol nitrate/lactose trituration is dispersed in an aqueous solution of 40% polyethylene glycol 400 fortified with the penetration enhancer isopropyl palmitate. The dispersion is processed into a viscous silicone elastomer by means of a high-energy dispersion technique, which results in a solid matrix upon addition of a polymerization catalyst. The micro-compartments in the matrix contain the drug particles in a polymer solution. Drug release can be controlled via the dissolution process inside the micro-compartments, as well as via the distribution or diffusion coefficients in the matrix. Whether the release of drug from an MDD system is distribution- or matrix-controlled depends on the ratio of the solubility of the drug in fluid micro-compartment to that in the polymer matrix.

Pharmacopeial Dissolution Tests for Transdermal Patches _____

USP ⟨724⟩ Drug Release
The paddle and vessel assembly described in Ph. Eur. 2.9.3 ("Dissolution Test for Solid Dosage Forms"), USP 711 ("Dissolution") and JP 6.10 ("Dissolution Test") can also be used for testing of transdermal patches. The Ph. Eur. describes three variations of this test. Two of them can also be found in the USP, which additionally includes a further method. In accordance with the conditions on the skin surface, in all cases the temperature of the release medium is maintained at $32° \pm 0.5°C$.

Ph. Eur. 2.9.4: Disk Assembly Method, USP: Apparatus 5 (Paddle over Disk). The patch (in case of matrix patches mostly just a piece of it) is attached with the release surface facing up on a disk assembly. The latter is specified by the Ph. Eur. as a 125 µm mesh stainless steel net, whereas the USP allows also the use of other appropriate devices, which hold the patches in a flat position. The disk assembly with the mounted patch is placed at the bottom of the vessel with the release surface facing upwards, 25 mm below and parallel to the bottom side of the stirring blade. The paddle is rotated, for example, at 100 rpm and samples are withdrawn at predetermined intervals (USP: at least three test time points).

Ph. Eur. 2.9.4: Cell Method. In this case, the patch is fixed, with its releasing surface uppermost, on the disk-shaped support of the extraction cell and is fixed by a ring-shaped cover, which limits the release area to a defined size. If necessary, a membrane is placed between the patch and the cover to isolate the patch from the medium that may modify or adversely affect the physicochemical properties of the patch. The extraction cell is placed in the vessel, with the releasing surface facing upwards, 25 mm below and parallel to the bottom side of the stirring blade. Like in the abovementioned method, the paddle is rotated, for example, at 100 rpm and samples are withdrawn at predetermined intervals.

Ph. Eur. 2.9.4: Rotating Cylinder Method, USP: Apparatus 6 (Cylinder). In this test method, the paddle and shaft are replaced with a stainless steel cylinder stirring element (diameter 4.444 cm). The patch is mounted onto the lateral surface of the cylinder with the release surface uppermost. To this end, the adhesive side of the patch is covered with a piece of suitable inert porous membrane that is at least 1 cm larger on all sides than the patch and fixed to the cylinder using a suitable adhesive or a double-sided adhesive tape. In contrast to the Ph. Eur., the USP allows but does not request the coverage of the patch by a membrane or a nylon net. The cylinder prepared in this way is immersed in the dissolution medium and rotated, for example, at 100 rpm. At determined intervals, samples of the dissolution medium are withdrawn (USP: at least three test time points).

USP: Apparatus 7 (Reciprocating Holder). Apparatus 7, described in USP ⟨724⟩, consists of a set of preferably transparent solution containers, a set of sample holders, and a motor and drive assembly to reciprocate the system vertically and to automatically index the system horizontally to a different row of vessels, if desired. The solution cylinders are partially immersed in a water bath to maintain a temperature of $32° \pm 0.5°C$ inside the containers. Sample holders for transdermal systems are designed as an angled disk (sample fixed to the bottom of the disk) or as a cylinder (sample fixed to the lateral surface of the cylinder). The patch with the release side facing the medium may be attached to the holder by an adhesive, a double-face adhesive tape, a membrane, or a nylon net. The sample holders are reciprocated at a frequency of about 30 cycles per minute with an amplitude of about 2 cm. At each sampling time point (at least three), the solution containers are removed, and before analysis a sufficient volume of solvent is added to correct for evaporation losses.

16.5   Storage Stability and Storage Conditions

Patches, in particular those with rubber adhesive material, are subject to gradual aging, caused by oxidation and depolymerization reactions and resulting in brittleness and loss of adhesiveness. Added antioxidants may prolong shelf life. Also, the presence of short-chain fatty acids may have an unfavorable influence. The large number of double bonds in natural rubber favors radical reactions with oxygen, which, especially during exposure to light, catalyzes oxidation. These reactions cause natural rubber to be more susceptible to aging than the synthetic version. The latter is also less sensitive to "rubber poisons" like Fe, Cu, and Mn ions and rubber-disrupting bacteria. Rubber plasters should be protected from light and moisture and stored at temperatures between 15° and 25°C.

By contrast, polyacrylate patches and likewise those with silicon adhesives, are much less sensitive to aging processes so that in most cases it is not necessary to meet special storage conditions.

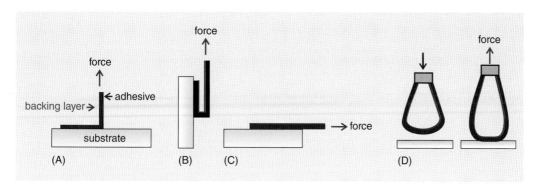

Fig. 16-4 Schematic representation of various methods to evaluate adhesiveness of transdermal patches: (A) 90° peeling test; (B) 180° peeling test; (C) shear force test; (D) loop-tack test.

16.6   Testing

The main components used in the manufacturing of patches are pressure-sensitive adhesives. Ideally, by exerting slight pressure they should spread easily on the skin surface at room temperature, thereby developing sufficient adhesive power. They should therefore display appropriate adhesive power and cohesive strength. Equally important is that appropriate adhesion is already achieved upon short contact time and gentle pressure, so-called *tack*. Nonetheless, it should be peeled off without causing appreciable injury to the skin or detachment of the preparation from the outer covering due to insufficient adhesiveness between reservoir and backing layer. Although adhesive behavior is an extraordinarily important property of patches, no test method is currently described in a pharmacopeia.

Adhesiveness may be assessed by measuring the force required to remove a plaster strip under and angle of 90° or 180° from a steel plate (peeling adhesiveness). Instant adhesiveness may be tested by briefly lowering a plaster loop on the test plate and measuring the force required to tear it off at an angle of 90° (Fig. 16-4). The internal cohesiveness of the plaster material may be tested by applying tensile stress parallel to the plaster surface (shear adhesiveness). The further a plaster adhering to the test plate is displaced under tensile stress, the weaker is the cohesiveness of the material.

Further parameters to be tested include tear strength and stretch ability, as well as the residue-free unrolling of the adhesive material in case of pressure-sensitive adhesives.

Furthermore, fiber density of fabrics, water resistance and air and water vapor permeability may be tested. For medicated patches the Ph. Eur. demands, like for all single-dose preparations, the test on uniformity of the dosage units. Likewise, microbiological quality should be tested since patches are considered to belong to the category of low-germ preparations. Indications of the durability of patches may be obtained by accelerated aging using aggravated conditions of heat, oxygen, and UV radiation.

Further Reading

EMA 23 October 2014 EMA/CHMP/QWP/ 608924/2014: Guideline on quality of transdermal patches. http://www.ema. europa.eu/docs/en_GB/document_ library/Scientific_guideline/2014/12/ WC500179071.pdf

Pastore, M., Kalia, Y. N., Horstmann, M., Roberts, M. S. "Transdermal patches: history, development and pharmacology." *Brit. J. Pharmacol.* 172 (9) (2015): 2179–2209.

Liquid Dosage Forms

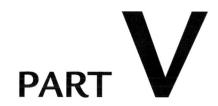

PART **V**

Solutions

17

17.1 Formulations

As a rule, solutions (*solutiones*) are liquid preparations containing drugs, usually dissolved in water- or mainly water-containing fluids. They may be applied either internally or externally. From a technological point of view, solutions are homogeneous, liquid or solid two- or multiple-component systems. The pharmacopeia distinguishes monographs on "Liquid Preparations for Oral Use" and "Liquid Preparations for Dermal Use." In addition, the monograph "Liquid Preparations for Oromucosal Use" refers to solutions for gargling or rinsing the oral cavity, solutions or droplets for application on the gingiva (gums) or in the oral cavity. In most cases, these are aqueous solutions, commercially available as ready-to-use preparations or as concentrates and, when applicable, provided with an appropriate application device. They are characterized by a (near) neutral pH and are, mainly intended to achieve local activity. Generally, solutions, except those containing colloidally dispersed drugs, should be fully transparent. Highly viscous solutions of bulking agents or mucous substances are designated as mucilage (*mucilagines*).

Distinction is made between real solutions with an ion-disperse or molecularly dispersed distribution with particle sizes below 1 nm, and colloidal solutions (lyosols) with particle sizes varying between 1 nm and 1 mm. Thermo-stable active ingredients are preferentially dissolved in warm solvent. In principle, stability should always be a factor to be taken into account when using solutions, because a large number of active ingredients are unstable with respect to light and under bacterial, hydrolytic or oxidative influences (section 25.3 and 25.4). The basic principles of solubility, dissolution rate and solubility improvement (section 3.9), as well as further physicochemical properties of active ingredients which affect absorption behavior, are discussed elsewhere (section 7.6).

Because many drug formulations in the form of solutions are subject to special requirements (solutions for injection or infusion, eye drops, preparations for rinsing etc.), their special requirements are discussed in the corresponding sections of this book.

Commonly, also nasal drops (*rhinoguttae*), ear drops (*otoguttae*), and syrups (*sirupi*) come in the form of solutions. Syrups are liquid preparations of sweet-tasting mono- or disaccharides (mostly sucrose). They may contain pharmaceutical ingredients or plant extracts as additives. For reasons of stability syrups commonly have a sugar content of at least 45%. They are utilized as taste improvers. Simple syrup (*sirupus simplex*) serves as a basis for drug-containing syrups. Syrups are prepared by dissolving sucrose in hot water while stirring. The solution is maintained at boiling temperature for maximally 120 seconds (to avoid inversion of the sugar) and freed from foam. Then the solution is adjusted to the required mass by adding (nearly) boiling water. The hot solution is filled in sterile dry flasks. The flasks should be filled completely and immediately sealed. Syrups containing plant extracts and fruit juices have

Voigt's Pharmaceutical Technology, First Edition. Alfred Fahr.
© 2018 John Wiley & Sons Ltd. Published 2018 by John Wiley & Sons Ltd.

a certain pharmaceutical relevance. Due to the high sugar concentration near the saturation concentration, syrups have a strong osmotic activity and are not susceptible to bacterial decay.

Some older and largely obsolete solution formulations, which are nonetheless still found in some pharmacopeias, include:

- Aromatic waters (*aquae aromaticae*) are manufactured by dissolving aromatic oils in water, often under heat application. Higher aromatic oil concentrations can be reached by addition of nonionic surfactants. They are mostly used as flavor enhancer vehicles.
- Medicinal alcohols (*spirituosa medicata*) contain active ingredients dissolved in ethanol or in ethanol-containing fluids and are produced by mixing, dissolution or distillation (e.g., spirit of camphor).
- Medicinal oils (*olea medicata*) are mostly poorly stable solutions of active ingredients in fatty oils, but also include oily extracts and suspensions (e.g., zinc oil NRF, vitamin A solution).
- Medicinal "wines" (*vina medicata*) are used as basis material for the preparation of medicinal preparations (e.g., liqueur wines, pepsin wine).
- Elixirs (*elixiera medicinalia*) are sweetened solutions based on water/alcohol mixtures.
- *Liquors* are liquids the manufacturing of which involves a chemical reaction (e.g., aluminum acetate-tartrate solution).

Exercise (tutorial)

You are requested to prepare 1,000 mL of a 70% (V/V) ethanol-water mixture. The instructions of an actual pharmacopeia require that, to prepare a total weight amount of 1,000 g, 665 g ethanol 96% (V/V) should be diluted with water to 1,000 g. You mistakenly add too much water. A relative density assay of the mixture yields a value $d_{20/20} = 0.895$. How much ethanol 96% (V/V) should be added to obtain an ethanol-water mixture with the required relative density of 0.885–0.889?

17.1.1 Density Calculation ρ_{20} from the Relative Density $d_{20/20}$ According to "Relative Density" of the Ph. Eur. 2.2.5

The conversion of relative and absolute density (section 3.6.1) follows from equation 17-1:

$$d_{20}^{20} = 1.00180 \, \frac{cm^3}{g} \cdot \rho_{20} \qquad (17\text{-}1)$$

The conversion factor 1.00180 mL/g is the inverse value of density $\rho = 0.9982$ g/mL of water at 20°C.

$$\rho_{20} = \frac{d_{20}^{20}}{1.00180 \frac{cm^3}{g}} = \frac{0.895}{1.00180 \frac{cm^3}{g}} = 0.8934 \frac{g}{cm^3}$$

$$(17\text{-}2)$$

$$m = 100 \, cm^3 \cdot 0.8934 \frac{g}{cm^3} = 893.4 \, g$$

17.1.2 Determining True Ethanol Concentration of a Prepared Dilution

The true ethanol concentration of a prepared dilution can be determined with the help of an ethanol-water table (see Table 17-1), according to Ph. Eur. The prepared ethanol-water mixture has an ethanol content of 66.8% (V/V) or 59.0% (m/m).

Table 17-1 Ph. Eur. 2.9.10 Ethanol Content and Ethanol Tables

Important parameters from the ethanol table

Density ρ_{20} (g/cm^3)	Ethanol Content in Percent (V/V)	Ethanol Content in Percent (m/m)
0.7893	100	100
0.8074	96	93.8
0.8292	90	85.7
0.8855	70	62.4
0.8933	66.8	59.0

17.1.3   Calculation of the Amount of Ethanol to Be Added

Due to the volume contraction occurring during mixing of ethanol and water, dilutions may only be calculated based on mass content of ethanol. The most simple calculation method is the construction of a dilution cross according to the following scheme (equation 17.3).

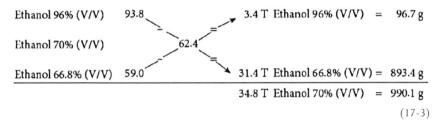

$$(17\text{-}3)$$

In the attempt to prepare 1,000 mL ethanol, 70% (V/V) 893.4 g ethanol 66.8% (V/V) were obtained. The concentration of the mixture should be adjusted to the required value by addition of ethanol 96% (V/V).

In order to obtain 70% ethanol (V/V), 31.4 parts (mass) of ethanol 66.8% (V/V) have to be mixed with 3.4 parts (mass) ethanol 96% (V/V) in order to obtain 34.8 parts (mass) ethanol 70% (V/V). The total mass then amounts to 990.1 g. The total volume may be calculated from the ethanol table:

$$V \,(\text{Ethanol } 70\% \,(V/V)) = \frac{990.1\ \text{g}}{0.8855\ \dfrac{\text{g}}{\text{cm}^3}} = 1118\ \text{cm}^3 \tag{17-4}$$

17.1.4   Mixtures

During preparation of solutions, volume contractions may occur that have to be taken into consideration. By means of a practical example, ethanol dilutions may be calculated.

Similar to ethanol, also isopropyl alcohol (2-propanol) shows a volume contraction upon mixing with water. Instructions for the preparation of isopropanol-water mixtures can be found in many specialized books. Table 17-2 simplifies the preparation of isopropanol-water mixtures. The pharmaceutical term "mixture" (*mixtura*) is used for solutions (rarely suspensions) intended for internal use and taken orally in spoon-size doses. Mixtures for external applications are known as shake lotions (e.g., zinc oxide shake lotion) or lotion (*lotiones*) (e.g., suntan lotion).

Shake lotions

Separate into parts with time and must be shaken into suspension before use.

17.2   Preparation

It is not easy to provide generally applicable rules for the preparation of solutions because, as described above, this type of formulation may vary substantially. A basic prerequisite is the solubility of the solid components in the solvent to be used. This information may be

Table 17-2 Preparation of Isopropanol-Water Mixtures According Pharmacopeias

Concentration Isopropyl Alcohol (V/V, in %)	Mass (g) Isopropyl Alcohol 100%, to Be Completed with Water to 1000.0 g	Relative Density d_{20}^{20}
100	100.0	0.7863
90	86.36	0.8194
80	74.04	0.8496
70	62.80	0.8765
60	52.28	0.9024
50	42.39	0.9274
40	33.18	0.9478

found in the pharmacopeias, and follows the principle *similia similibus solventur* (similar solutes dissolve in similar solvents).

The components of the formulation are weighed separately and consecutively dissolved in the order of increasing quantities in the required mass or volume amount of solvent. Poorly soluble substances are dissolved first. Stirring, swinging, shaking, and heating accelerate the dissolution process. Heating requires thermostability of all components and may lead to evaporation. Evaporated solvent needs to be replenished after cooling. After completion of the cooling process the solution should be checked for recrystallization of dissolved components. Volatile substances such as aromatic oils are generally added last in order to minimize evaporation. As a rule, fine crystalline substances dissolve better than fine powders, which tend to clump.

Incompatibilities between formulation components occurring during the dissolution process have to be taken into account. Often precipitation occurs, especially in case of highly concentrated substances. Therefore, it may be necessary to dissolve each component separately in part of the solvent and subsequently mix the solutions obtained. When hydrophilic and lipophilic substances are processed in solvent mixtures (e.g., ethanol-water), the lipophilic substances are dissolved in the nonpolar solvent and the hydrophilic substances in the hydrophilic solvent. Subsequently, the two solutions are mixed by adding the alcoholic to the aqueous solution. Ready-to-use solutions may need to be filtered.

For a definition of relative terms of solubility see p. 92

Water solubility of selected organic compounds

Compound	Formula	Amount of water (in ml) required to dissolve 1 g of substance
Benzoic acid	C_6H_5COOH	275
Benzyl alcohol	$C_6H_5CH_2OH$	25
Phenol	C_6H_5OH	15
Chloroform	$CHCl_3$	200
Carbon tetrachloride	CCl_4	2000

Large-scale industrial manufacturing is performed in temperature-controlled tanks with stirring devices. Solid components are weighed in fluids are led into the tanks via pipelines. Solutions made in pharmacy conditions should be prepared in transparent containers in order to detect precipitates, undissolved material, and dissolution delay. Only when no complications are to be expected may the solution be produced directly in the dispensing container. Ready-to-use solutions need to be tested organoleptically for clarity and absence of foreign particles. When the occurrence of turbidity cannot be avoided (e.g., in case of processing of plant extracts), the dispensing bottle is provided with the advice "shake before use" in order to prevent dosing errors. During storage of solutions, no precipitates or crystal formation should occur. Any turbidity might also indicate bacterial contamination.

Other frequently used solvents, besides water and ethanol, are glycerol and fatty oils. Glycerol is partly used as pure solvent, but can also be deployed as co-solvent, viscosity enhancer, and as preservative. Besides solvents, excipients such as dissolution enhancers, stabilizers, buffer substances, viscosity enhancers, and antimicrobial or antioxidative agents may be present. In connection with production at the industrial scale, aspects such as large-scale manageability, safety, and environmental protection play a decisive role.

As compared to solid formulations the storage life of solutions is most often limited. This is predominantly due to the high dispersion grade of the active ingredient in the solution and the enhanced reactivity and risk of incompatibilities resulting from that. All aqueous solutions, with the exception of syrups, are ideal nutritional substrates for bacteria and thus have only limited durability. Suitable preservatives for solutions are ethanol and 1,2-propylene glycol (>15%), glycerol (>30%), sorbitol (>70%), benzoic acid/sodium benzoate, sorbic acid/potassium sorbate, or alkyl-4-hydroxy benzoate. It should be kept in mind that many excipients, such as for example benzyl alcohol, ethanol or propylene glycol are not suited for use by children. Propylene glycol not only has laxative effects, it may also lead to accumulation in the body of children younger than 4 years of age. This is due to the still-low alcohol and aldehyde dehydrogenase activity in such children. Likewise, benzoic acid may accumulate in children below the age of 2, as the conjugation to hippuric acid has not fully developed yet at that age. That also applies to benzyl alcohol, which in the body is oxidized to benzoic acid. Caution is urged for newborns and small children with respect to the use of macrogol ricinoleate, because upon repeated administration, there is a risk of allergic reactions. Herbal oils may be oxidized under the influence of light or oxygen and the presence of heavy metal ions; this can be prevented by the addition of antioxidants. Unpleasant smell, taste, and color of solutions may be concealed by addition of smell and taste correcting agents such as sugars and approved sugar substituents or coloring substances; this is of particular importance in the pediatric setting. Undesired taste can be concealed either by the same (e.g., sour by lemon) or by the opposite (e.g., bitter by vanilla) taste group. Also, viscosity-enhancing substances may contribute to taste improvement because they decrease diffusion rate and thus cause fewer taste molecules to reach their receptor per unit of time.

> Especially children have to be accustomed to e.g. bitter tasting material. A study showed for example, that children have to experience 11 times the same bitter substances before they get accustomed to it.

17.3 Delivery Containers and Dosage

In order to ascertain microbiological quality of liquid preparations during packaging, storage, and marketing, appropriate measures need to be taken. Solutions are mostly filled in tightly sealed brown flasks with screw cap. According to the pharmacopeia, proof should be provided that the nominal volume can be taken from the container. One of the big advantages of solutions as opposed to solid formulations is the simple accurate adjustment of the dosage to individual requirements. Nonetheless, the exact dosage of solutions by the patient may present a special problem. The pharmacopeia prescribes for multiple-dose containers that dosing should be performed by means of a suitable dosing device. Thus, the nomenclature of solutions may already indicate the type of application and dosage. *Guttae* are solutions that are to be dosed drop-wise, and often are taken either diluted in water or on sugar. In order to guarantee dosage accuracy, they are provided in containers with a dropper insert, to be distinguished in edge and center droppers. The latter (vertical droppers) may be recognized by an air channel on the side and are to be kept vertical during drop formation. They have a higher dosing accuracy than edge droppers. The latter, also called horizontal or universal droppers, are to be held in a slanted manner with the notch downward. They should be considered a dosing aid rather than an accurate dosing device. This dropper type is therefore preferentially used for preparations with a broad therapeutic window and little risk of side effects. Particularly for officinal preparations, it has to be taken into account that many additives such as sorbic acid, 4-hydroxy benzoic acid esters, or benzoic acid may lead to lowering of surface tension and thus to changes in drop size and number.

Spoon-wise or pipette-administered solutions are considered to belong to the category mixtures, syrups, and juices. Since household spoons may vary considerable in size and shape, patients should be provided with a special measuring spoon, in case of juices also measuring cups or dosage pipettes and syringes should be included. The latter provide a higher dosing accuracy. According to the pharmacopeia, the volume of such appliances should measure 5 mL or a multiple thereof.

Especially for children up to six or seven years of age, peroral liquid formulations are the most predominant peroral drug formulations because they are easy to dose and swallow. Particularly in pediatrics drop-wise administered solutions are suited as child-friendly formulations; they may already be administered to newly born and their dosage can easily be adjusted to body weight and surface.

Dry syrups for children are applied for active substances such as antibiotics, as their stability in dissolved form is limited. Before administration, they are dissolved by gradually adding the solvent while shaking.

For infants, one option is a preloaded single dose that can be directly inserted and emptied in the child's mouth via a beaker provided with an attachable silicon nipple and an adjustable outlet opening. A narrow opening gives a slow outflow, which is beneficial to local therapy in the oral cavity, while for preparations that have to be swallowed a larger opening can be chosen. Because of their security and high accuracy, dosage syringes exploiting the sucking reflex are highly recommended to deliver a liquid formulation to infants. A general advantage of the dosage syringe as compared to dosage spoons is that the graduation on the syringe can be kept in sight during dosing so that overdosing rarely occurs. High acceptance by children is obtained with the dose-sipping technology, which uses a straw filled with a single-dose of pellets that is stuck into a fluid and emptied by sucking.

Flasks containing a drug solution are often provided with a special pressure-twist cap for children's safety. The need to simultaneously twist and press hard to uncap the bottle requires a complex action and prevents children from opening such caps.

17.4   Biopharmaceutical Aspects

A number of drug formulations are solutions (drops, syrups, etc.). From a biopharmaceutical point of view an aqueous drug solution presents an advantage because it will facilitate rapid absorption in the gastrointestinal tract. But also in this case absorption depends on several factors. Obviously, absorption differences may be expected between molecularly dispersed and colloidally dispersed solutions. Furthermore, pH value, degree of ionization, and osmotic pressure are additional critical factors affecting the absorption process. Besides these physico-chemical properties of the solution and the dissolved substance, excipients play an important role. In many cases, addition of ethanol improves absorption: in the stomach active ingredients will precipitate very finely from glycerol or ethanol based solutions and in addition, ethanol has an absorption-enhancing effect by itself. On the other hand, an increase in viscosity will diminish the absorption rate, because it slows down the mobility of the molecules to the area of absorption. Likewise, in case of macromolecular substances, complex formation between active ingredient and excipient may cause a delay in absorption, but may in many cases also lead to improvement of the absorption process. With oily solutions, which are taken perorally only in small volumes and to ascertain better intake, often in the form of gelatin capsules, only slow absorption is possible. When an oily solution is processed into an emulsion, again totally different conditions prevail. In such cases, phase volume ratios, degree of dispersion, and drug distribution have an essential additional influence on drug release. Often, high absorption rates are to be expected when a poorly water-soluble active agent is applied as an aqueous solubilizate instead of as an aqueous solution.

When a poorly soluble drug after application and determined by the stomach acid conditions, precipitates, the microcrystalline precipitate will, in most cases, rapidly dissolve and be absorbed.

17.5   Testing

Depending on the application, solutions must pass the following tests according to the actual Ph. Eur:

- Uniformity of mass (for single-dose solutions)
- Dosage and uniformity of delivered dose of drops for peroral use
- Deliverable mass or volume
- Uniformity of dosage units from metered-dose containers
- When applicable, sterility (for cutaneous application)

The Ph. Eur. gives the following specifications with respect to dosage for liquid preparations for peroral administration:

- Maximal drop release rate 2 drops/second in order to ensure countability.
- The calculated drop mass of 10 doses may deviate maximally $\pm 15\%$ from the mass declaration.
- The mass of individual doses may deviate not more than $\pm 10\%$ from the mean of 10 independent measurements.
- When the dose is given as number of drops, the Ph. Eur. requires that the number of drops per mL or per g of preparation is given.

Furthermore, a large number of physical methods may be applied to secure the quality of solutions, such as determination of ethanol or water content, refractory index, relative density, pH value, surface tension, conductivity, viscosity, and so on.

17.6 Liquid Preparations for Nasal Administration

Liquid preparations for nasal administration (*nasalia*) are classified into nasal drops and nasal rinsing solutions (nasal washes) for local, rarely for systemic (e.g., neostigmine) action. Likewise, nasal sprays may represent solutions (see Appendix A, 24). Nasal drops may be hydrophilic or hydrophobic solutions, emulsions, or suspensions in single-dose as well as multidose containers intended for administration into the nasal cavity. Nasal washes are generally isotonic aqueous solutions to clean the nasal cavity, which in case of injuries or prior to surgery should be sterile.

Irritations of the mucosal tissue and effects on the function of the cilia should be avoided. Therefore, aqueous nasal preparations should be approximately isotonic. Hyper-osmolarity may therapeutically be desirable; the occurrence of hypo-osmolarity can be practically excluded because in the nasal cavity dilution effects are barely to be expected. For the same reason weak buffers (e.g., phosphate, Tris) in the pH range between 6.8 and 8.3 (euhydric) can be used. Citrate buffers are toxic to ciliated epithelia, boric acid is not approved for nasal preparations. Viscosity-enhancing substances may be applied, but effects on the mobility of the cilia should be excluded. Emulsifiers are usually not well tolerated by the nasal mucosa. Preservation, particularly for multidose containers, may be necessary in order to exclude bacterial recontamination. When benzalkonium is applied for this purpose, cilia function may be affected when the preparation is acidic. Prolonged use may induce swelling of the nasal mucosa. An appropriate warning advice for benzalkonium chloride should be provided. Oily preparations (paraffin, fatty oils) bring along the risk of aspiration and lipid pneumonia and should not be used in children. Potential interactions of the oily components with the plastic components of the packaging material should be taken into account.

Nasal washes should be tested for sterility (when required), microbiological quality and appropriate preservation, particle size of suspensions, and the deliverable nominal volume. Nasal drops in multidose containers have to be tested for mass variability and content uniformity.

17.7 Liquid Preparations for Application in the Ear

The Ph. Eur. defines liquid *auricularia* as ear drops and ear washes usually with local action. Ear drops are based on solutions, suspensions or emulsions, mostly in multidose containers and are delivered drop-wise at body temperature to the auditory meatus or placed in the auditory meatus by means of a tampon impregnated with the liquid. Ear washes are aqueous solutions of physiological pH and serve to cleanse the external auditory meatus.

In case of application on an injured ear (e.g., eardrum perforation) and prior to surgery care should be taken that only single-dose containers are used and that the preparation is sterile and contains no preservatives.

Preparations to apply in the middle ear (tympanum) are employed as instillations or as intratympanal injection and in a formal sense do not represent *auricularia*. The liquid basic ingredients (water, glycerol, fatty oils) for the preparation of ear drops and washing fluids should not exert any pressure on the eardrum. Water-based preparations bring along the risk of bacterial or fungal contamination, particularly due to maceration of the skin when the auditory canal is closed off by a tamponade. For that reason preference is given to glycerol, propylene glycol, low-molecular weight macrogols or alcohol, provided that the eardrum is intact. In addition, these substances may have anti-swelling, osmotic, and to some extent antimicrobial effects. Oily preparations (e.g., refined castor oil) are to be deployed only on intact eardrums. As compared to the nasal mucosa the auditory canal is rather insensitive to deviations in isotonicity or pH. Hypotonic solutions may pass the eardrum.

Relevant tests of formulations intended for application in the ear correspond to those used for liquid preparations for intranasal application.

Further Reading

Illum, L. "Nasal drug delivery—recent developments and future prospects." *Journal of controlled release* 161 (2) (2012): 254–263.

Plontke, S. K., Salt, A. N. "Simulation of application strategies for local drug delivery to the inner ear." *ORL* 68 (6) (2006): 386–392.

Emulsions

18

18.1 General Introduction

Emulsions are coarsely dispersed or colloidal systems consisting of two or more immiscible liquids. Taking into account the possible presence of liquid crystalline phases (see section 15.3.5) the International Union of Pure and Applied Chemistry (IUPAC) has proposed the following definition: "In an emulsion liquid droplets and/or liquid crystals are dispersed in a liquid." The term *emulsion* derives from the Latin verb *emulgere*, literally "to milk out" and refers to milk as a type of natural emulsion. As a result of different optical refraction of the components of the emulsion it appears milky and nontransparent. Only exceptionally, when both liquids have identical refractive indices, light falling through the emulsion will be refracted identically by the components and hence the emulsion will be transparent. Also microemulsions, which are fundamentally different from real emulsions in terms of composition, structure, and properties, are transparent (see section 20.5).

As for pharmaceutically applied emulsion systems, the greatest variety can be found among the emulsions intended for external administration. Emulsions for external use are usually of the O/W type (*Oil* in *Water*; for definitions see next section) and are often used to treat inflammatory skin diseases (in particular corticoid-containing emulsions). Emulsions are also commonly applied for skin-care purposes and as sunscreen formulations (chapter 15). Such preparations are often emulsions of the W/O type. The transition from emulsions to creams is seamless. The latter consist of emulsion-like systems, but they lack the characteristic fluidity of real emulsions.

Emulsions for peroral administration are relatively rare. As a rule, they are O/W emulsions in which the disperse phase either represents the active agent itself (e.g., paraffin oil or silicone oil emulsions) or serves as carrier for a lipophilic active ingredient. As the direct oral intake of oily substances is often unpleasant and, in addition, the administration of an emulsion helps to mask a bad taste, oral emulsion-type formulations may serve to enhance the acceptance level of such agents by patients. For administration of lipophilic pharmaceuticals in combination with an oily phase may also contribute to improved bioavailability. As the formulation of voluminous fluid emulsions, especially for highly active agents, does not particularly meet the requirements of up-to-date pharmaceuticals, attempts are being made to formulate such highly active ingredients in anhydrous "self-emulsifying" lipid formulations, from which only after administration and upon contact with body fluids, an emulsion system is formed (e.g., Sandimmun®).

Colloidal lipid emulsions of the O/W type play an important role in intensive care medicine, because in the context of parenteral nutrition they offer the possibility to achieve sufficient caloric intake. They are also applied as carrier systems for poorly water-soluble pharmaceutical agents (e.g., etomidate, diazepam, propofol) (section 20.4).

Voigt's Pharmaceutical Technology, First Edition. Alfred Fahr.
© 2018 John Wiley & Sons Ltd. Published 2018 by John Wiley & Sons Ltd.

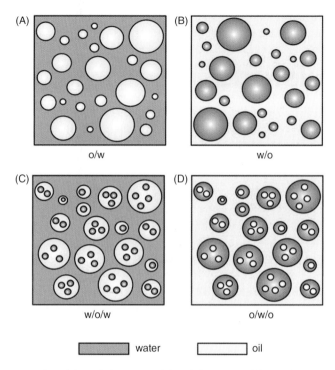

Fig. 18-1 Types of emulsions: (A) O/W emulsion; (B) W/O emulsion; (C) W/O/W emulsion; (D) O/W/O emulsion.

18.2 Emulsion Types

Emulsions consist of two immiscible phases, one of which (disperse phase) is present as droplets in the other (continuous phase). Droplet size has a significant influence on the properties of the emulsion. As a rule, one of the phases has a hydrophilic, the other a lipophilic character. In the pharmaceutical context, the hydrophilic phase usually is water or an aqueous solution, while a mineral, semi-synthetic, or vegetable oil (e.g., paraffin oil, medium-chain triglycerides, soybean or peanut oil) commonly serves as the lipophilic (hydrophobic) phase. Depending on whether the hydrophilic phase is dispersed in the hydrophobic phase or vice versa, the term water-in-oil (W/O) emulsion or oil-in-water (O/W) emulsion is used for such preparations. Conventionally, in these notations W stands for hydrophilic phase and O for lipophilic phase, even when the phases do not consist of water and/or oil. Also multiple emulsions do exist, in which inside the emulsion droplets small droplets of the other phase are present. Depending on the phases involved, such systems are called W/O/W or O/W/O emulsions (Fig. 18-1). The innermost phase of the multiple-emulsion system either has the same (type I) or another (type II) composition as the continuous phase.

Another important type of emulsion-like system is known as 'Microemulsion'. Unlike macro-emulsions microemulsions are thermodynamically stable. See section 20.5 for a detailed description of microemulsions.

> Although of limited to no pharmaceutical use, there are also water-in-water emulsions where both internal and external phases are hydrophilic.
>
> For example: aqueous dispersion of dextran in PEG 400 and gelatin in agar.

18.3 Instability Phenomena and Stabilizing Principles

Based on their dispersed state and the corresponding high interfacial energy, emulsions are thermodynamically unstable systems. During vigorous shaking of the two phases, water and oil, one phase will be dispersed as droplets in the other, but when shaking is interrupted, the two phases will separate rapidly. The droplets will coalesce as soon as they contact each other and the oil phase gradually collects on top of the water phase, until ultimately both phases

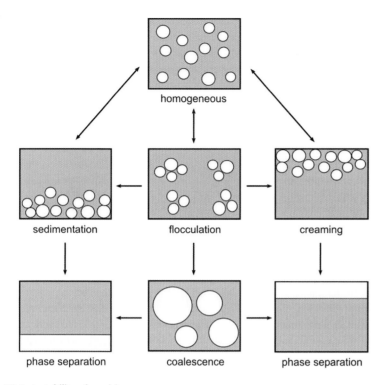

Fig. 18-2 Instability of emulsions.

are fully separated. In this state, water and oil have a minimal contact area (interface) and, as a result, the system has a minimal interfacial energy.

18.3.1   Instability of Emulsions

Even in emulsifier-stabilized emulsions, certain typical instability phenomena are regularly observed (Fig. 18-2). Therefore, during the development of an emulsion system, one of the chief tasks is to prevent such phenomena from occurring. As a rule, the continuous and the disperse phases have different densities, which can cause creaming or sedimentation of the dispersed particles. When the density of the disperse phase is lower than that of the continuous phase, creaming will occur, whereas sedimentation will take place in the opposite case. These phenomena will cause separation of the system into two layers. While the creamed respectively the sedimented layer is enriched in disperse phase, the underlying respectively overlaying layer is deprived of disperse phase. The velocity of this process can be roughly estimated by means of Stokes' sedimentation law (this law is, strictly speaking, only valid for strongly diluted systems):

$$v = \frac{h}{t} = \frac{2}{9} \frac{r^2(\rho_1 - \rho_2) \cdot g}{\eta} \tag{18-1}$$

v   = velocity of the emulsion droplet (traveled distance h per unit of time t)
r   = radius of the emulsion droplet
ρ_1 = density of the continuous phase
ρ_2 = density of the disperse phase
g   = gravitational acceleration
η = viscosity of the continuous phase

From this equation, it can be predicted that the velocity of the creaming (v > 0) or the sedimentation (v < 0) process in the emulsion can be decreased by reducing particle size or minimizing the density difference between the phases, as well as by increasing the viscosity of the continuous phase. Reduction of particle size is a very effective measure, which, however, will also bring about an increase in interfacial energy and will thus have practical limits. When droplet size approaches a size within the colloidal range, the enhanced influence of the Brownian motion will prevent complete creaming or sedimentation of the system. Equalizing the densities of the two phases will be practically feasible only in rare cases and, moreover, can only be exactly achieved for a certain temperature because of the different thermal expansion coefficients of the participating phases. Nonetheless, upon equalizing the densities, creaming and sedimentation of the droplets will come to a complete halt.

The option of increasing the viscosity is frequently applied for stabilization of emulsions intended for oral and, in particular, topical use. When the emulsion is thickened to the extent that it obtains a yield value, the movement of droplets stops completely.

Sedimentation or creaming leads to inhomogeneity in the preparation, but this can be reversed simply by shaking because both number and size of the droplets remain unaltered. When dispensing such preparations, the patient should be informed about the necessity to shake the preparation before use. That also applies to flocculation, during which the emulsion droplets cluster like grapes on a bunch. The increased size of the flocs thus formed will accelerate the sedimentation or creaming process. Sedimentation and creaming as well as the flocculation process will lead to local concentration increase, and thus, to closer mutual proximity of the droplets. This will favor an irreversible process, the coalescence of the droplets, which in extreme cases may lead to complete phase separation (*breaking* or *cracking* of the emulsion). Preparations that have undergone such extreme changes can no longer be used.

Sedimentation, creaming, or flocculation is not necessarily required for coalescence to occur. It may also be observed when emulsion droplets approach one another very closely, until they are ultimately separated from each other by only a thin film of continuous phase. When this film ruptures, the droplets coalesce. Individual droplets in an emulsion are attracted to each other by van der Waals forces, especially when they approach each other very closely (section 19.3.1). Unprotected droplets cannot resist these forces and readily coalesce upon approaching each other. To block this coalescence process effectively it is important to prevent the droplets from coming too close together or to construct a barrier between the droplets. This can, for example, be achieved by bringing on an electric charge (+ or −) on the droplet's surface, which will cause mutual repulsion. Emulsifiers play an essential role for establishing such protective mechanisms.

18.3.2   Stabilizing Principle

In order to preserve the dispersed state achieved and thus obtain a stable emulsion, an emulsifier will be required that will also facilitate the formation of the emulsion. That is why emulsifiers are, besides water and oil phase, essential components of emulsion systems, which are described in the next section.

Definitions from the "Gold Book" (see reference)

Surfactant: A substance which lowers the surface tension of the medium in which it is dissolved, and/or the interfacial tension with other phases, and, accordingly, is positively adsorbed at the liquid/vapour and/or at other interfaces.

Detergent: A surfactant (or a mixture containing one or more surfactants) having cleaning properties in dilute solutions (soaps are surfactants and detergents).

18.4   Surfactants and Emulsifiers

18.4.1   Definition, Characteristics of Amphiphilic Compounds, and Surface Activity

Emulsifiers form a special subgroup of the surfactants. Surfactants are compounds that are capable of diminishing the interfacial or surface tension: they are surface-active agents (section 3.11). The number of surface-active compounds is considerable. In accordance with their specific properties they may be applied as antifoam agents, W/O or O/W emulsifier, wetting agent, detergent or solubilizer.

Surfactants are compounds with a chemical structure containing spatially separated lipophilic and hydrophilic groups. Accordingly, they are also called amphiphiles. Among the hydrophilic groups in surfactants are:

Hydroxyl groups	—OH

Carboxyl groups

$$-C\underset{OH}{\overset{O}{\lVert}}$$

With monovalent cation

$$-C\underset{O^-\ Na^+\ (K^+,\ NH_4^+)}{\overset{O}{\lVert}}$$

Carboxyl groups with divalent cations
$(-COO^-)_2\ Ca^{2+}$ (or Mg^{2+})

Sulfate groups

$$-O-\underset{O}{\overset{O}{\underset{\lVert}{\overset{\lVert}{S}}}}-O^-\ H^+$$

With monovalent cation

$$-O-\underset{O}{\overset{O}{\underset{\lVert}{\overset{\lVert}{S}}}}-O^-\ Na^+$$

Sulfonate groups

$$-CH_2-\underset{O}{\overset{O}{\underset{\lVert}{\overset{\lVert}{S}}}}-O^-\ H^+$$

With monovalent cation

$$-CH_2-\underset{O}{\overset{O}{\underset{\lVert}{\overset{\lVert}{S}}}}-O^-\ Na^+$$

Amino groups

$$-N\underset{H}{\overset{H}{<}}$$

Protonated amino groups

$$-\overset{H}{\underset{H}{N^+}}-H$$

Substituted amino groups

$$-N\underset{R^1}{\overset{H}{<}}\qquad -N\underset{R^1}{\overset{R^2}{<}}\qquad -\overset{R^3}{\underset{R^1}{N^+}}-R^2$$

Polyoxyethylene chains

$$\left(O-CH_2-CH_2\right)_n OH$$

The presence of such polar groups brings about an affinity of the surfactant molecule for polar fluids, in particular water, and thus the hydrophilic character of the molecule.

Lipophilic (hydrophobic) groups are, for example:

Hydrocarbon chains

$$-CH_2-CH_2-CH_2-CH_2-CH_2-CH_3$$

Cyclic hydrocarbons

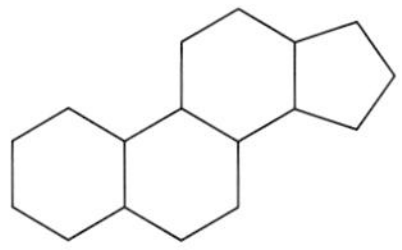

Unsaturated hydrocarbon chains

$$-\underset{H}{\overset{}{C}}=\underset{H}{\overset{}{C}}-$$

This part of the molecule forms the nonpolar moiety. It causes the affinity to organic solvents of low polarity and thus the lipophilic character of the molecule. Surfactants share a certain similarity with both the aqueous and the lipid phase and thus have affinity to both, which explains their tendency to accumulate at interfaces.

Surfactant molecules often have a straight chain-like structure; typical examples are soaps. Schematically the structure of surfactants is often represented by simple symbols, such as a ribbon and a sphere for soap-like surfactants (Fig. 18-3). The ribbon symbolizes the hydrocarbon chain of the molecule and the sphere the carboxyl group. The symmetric hydrocarbon chain represents the nonpolar or neutral moiety of the molecule.

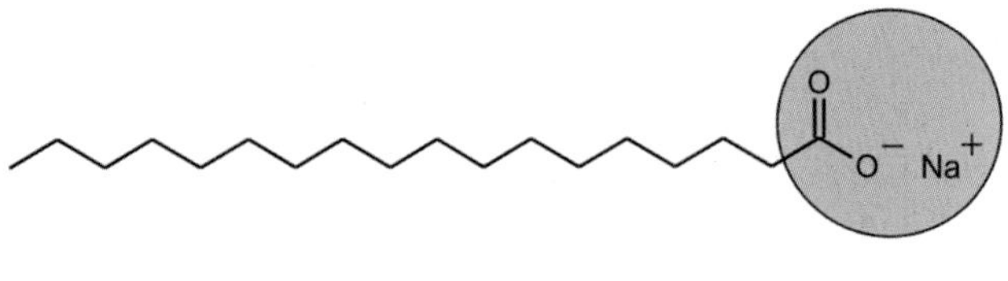

Fig. 18-3 Schematic structure of a soap molecule (sodium stearate), the ribbon-sphere symbolism.

Depending on their charge, surfactants are classified as anionic (negatively charged), cationic (positively charged), ampholytic (carrying positive as well as negatively charged groups), and nonionic (uncharged) compounds (Table 18-1). They may also carry multiple hydrophilic (e.g., block-co-polymers of the poloxamer type) or lipophilic (e.g., phospholipids) groups, as long as the hydrophobic and hydrophilic parts of the molecule remain spatially separated. The surfactants that find application as emulsifiers in the pharmaceutical field are discussed in section 5.4. Pharmaceutically applied surfactants and emulsifiers must meet special requirements. First and for all chemical and physiological compatibility are required. In case of formulations for peroral use taste aspects are furthermore important.

When water-soluble surfactants are added to water, the surfactant molecules accumulate preferentially at the air-water interface. They orient themselves in such a way that the hydrophilic moiety is associated with the aqueous phase while the hydrophobic hydrocarbon chain is turned toward the air.

The adsorption of the surfactant molecules at the air-liquid interface brings about a lowering of the surface tension. When a sufficient amount of surfactant is added to the water, a new interface is formed: water/surfactant/air (Fig. 18-4).

The addition of hydrophilic surfactants to water will cause a rapid decline of the surface tension, but soon a minimal value is reached that cannot be lowered further by addition of more surfactant (the critical micelle concentration of the surfactant is reached). From then

Table 18-1   Examples of Emulsifiers

Substance Class	Emulsion Type	Example
anionic		
alkali soaps	O/W	sodium palmitate
alkyl sulfates	O/W	sodium lauryl sulfate
		sodium cetyl stearyl sulfate
alkyl sulfonates	O/W	sodium lauryl sulfonate
cationic		
quaternary ammonium compounds	O/W	cetrimide
pyridinium compounds	O/W	cetyl pyridinium chloride
ampholytic		
certain phospholipids	O/W, W/O	lecithin
nonionic		
fatty alcohols	W/O	cetyl alcohol
sterols	W/O	cholesterol
		wool alcohols
glycerol fatty acid esters	W/O	glycerol monostearate
sorbitan fatty acid esters	W/O	sorbitan lauric acid ester (Span 20)
macrogol fatty acid esters	O/W	macrogol stearate
macrogol sorbitan fatty acid esters	O/W	macrogol sorbitan oleate (Tween 80)
macrogol glycerol fatty acid esters	O/W	macrogol glycerol monostearate
macrogol fatty alcohol ethers	O/W	macrogol lauryl ether
polyoxypropylene-polyoxyethylene – block-co-polymers	O/W	poloxamer 188

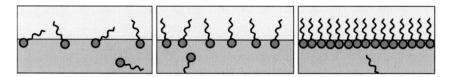

Fig. 18-4 Spatial arrangement of surfactants at the water surface (with increasing concentration).

on, the surfactant molecules associate as micelles (section 3.7.7). The surfactant molecules at the interface as well as those in the micelles are in dynamic equilibrium with single molecules in the bulk solution. Micelle formation will only occur when the surfactant can reach a sufficiently high concentration in the aqueous phase. Therefore, for example, fatty alcohols will not form micelles in water. Also, the solubility of several hydrophilic surfactants at room temperature is insufficient to reach the critical micelle concentration. Commonly, these substances, often containing long saturated alkyl chains, display a strongly temperature-dependent dissolution behavior. Above a certain critical temperature (the Krafft point) solubility sharply increases, allowing the formation of micelles.

In the same way surfactants concentrate and orient themselves at the air/water interface, surface-active substances arrange themselves at the oil/water interface. The presence of the emulsifier during the formation of emulsions diminishes the interfacial tension between the two phases. The surfactant molecules adsorb at the interface and orient themselves parallel to each other in such a way that the hydrophilic groups point towards the aqueous phase and the hydrophobic groups towards the oil phase. The parallel arrangement of the surfactant molecules perpendicular to the plane of the interface brings about a highly ordered state. At that point a monomolecular adsorption layer is attained at the interface. This layer is also known as adsorption film or emulsifier film. The film gives rise to a new interface, at which now a low interfacial tension prevails.

> As example: Stearyl alcohol has a water solubility of 1.1 ng/ml. Stearyl alcohol is a weak W/O surfactant and is mainly used as a cosurfactant.

18.4.2   HLB Value

The HLB (Hydrophilic-Lipophilic Balance) value offers the opportunity to characterize surfactants according to their amphiphilic properties and to classify them according to their application purpose. Originally, the HLB system was developed with regard to the cosmetic industry. Nowadays it serves as a tool for the food and petroleum industries, as well as in detergent manufacturing and all other areas where interfacial activity plays a role.

W. C. Griffin coined the term *HLB* in 1954 for nonionic surfactants. He assigned a dimensionless number to each surfactant that could be calculated from the stoichiometric ratio between the lipophilic and the hydrophilic moieties of the molecule. Thus, the HLB value provides information on the hydrophile/lipophile equilibrium resulting from the size and strength of the lipophilic and hydrophilic groups. A lipophilic substance is assigned a smaller HLB value, a hydrophilic substance a larger value. It follows that by the introduction of hydrophilic groups in a nonionic surfactant, the ratio of the lipophilic and the hydrophilic parts of the molecule change in favor of the latter, resulting in a surfactant with a higher HLB value. In this way, *W/O* emulsifiers can, for example, be converted into O/W emulsifiers with well-defined HLB values.

Example

Span 60® = sorbitan monostearate, HLB value 4.7; Tween 60® = polyoxyethylene sorbitan monostearate, HLB value 14.9.

The HLB system is based on a numeric scale of 1 to 20 (Fig. 18-5). The borderline between predominantly lipophilic substances and predominantly hydrophilic substances lies at a HLB

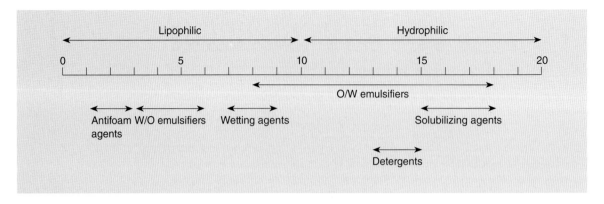

Fig. 18-5 HLB system.

value of approximately 10. Accordingly, a fictitious compound that is 100% hydrophilic has a HLB value of 20. As a consequence, macrogol sorbitan laurate, with a HLB value of 16.7, has a hydrophilic share of 84% relative to the entire molecule. Although HLB values do not represent analytical data in a strict sense, they allow drawing significant conclusions on the behavior of amphiphilic substances at interfaces.

Although initially the HLB system was developed empirically, later an equation was derived that allows calculation of an approximate HLB value from the molecular mass of the hydrophobic share (M_o) and the total molecular mass of the surfactant (M):

$$HLB = 20(1 - M_o/M) \tag{18-2}$$

Often, the HLB value is calculated directly from the chemical formula, in which certain values are assigned to the hydrophilic and hydrophobic properties of the individual chemical groups (see Table 18-2), derived from coalescence measurements:

$$HLB = 7 + \Sigma \text{ hydrophilic group numbers } + \Sigma \text{ lipophilic group numbers} \tag{18-3}$$

Hydrophilic groups are assigned a positive value, hydrophobic groups a negative value. The formula will, however, not permit application in case of unsaturated stereo-isomeric and structurally isomeric compounds.

In addition to the calculation methods described above, there are multiple physicochemical methods to derive HLB values, but there are limits to their general applicability. HLB values for a particular surfactant determined by different methods may differ from each other.

The definition of the HLB value is in principle valid only for non-ionic surfactants, but also then only with certain restrictions. It does not apply for example to surfactants containing propylene oxide, butylene oxide, nitrogen, phosphorus or sulfur, and so on. Ionic surfactants do not obey the principles set out in the foregoing. Therefore, the HLB values of such surfactants are determined experimentally and then fitted in accordance with the Griffin-HLB-system. For example, the HLB value of pure sodium lauryl sulfate is 40, which obviously does not mean that the hydrophilic share of the molecule amounts to 200%, but merely says that this detergents, in comparison with others, has an "apparent" HLB value of 40.

Essential for the practical application of the HLB system is the *algebraic additivity* of the HLB values. By mixing several surfactants, their HLB values are additive, so that by combining nonionic emulsifiers with high and with low HLB values, and taking into consideration the mixing ratios (by mass), the required HLB value can be set. This principle can, however, only be practically applied provided that the two surfactants under consideration are mutually compatible.

Table 18-2 Examples for HLB group numbers

Group	Group Number
Hydrophilic group	
Ester	2.4
Carboxylic group	2.1
Free hydroxyl group	1.9
Ether oxygen	1.3
Hydroxyl group (Sorbitan)	0.5
Lipophilic group	
-CH$_3$	−0.475
=CH$_2$	−0.475
=CH-	−0.475

Example

A mixture of 40% sorbitan monooleate (Span® 80) (HLB-value = 4.3) and 60% poly-oxyethylene (20) sorbitan monostearate (Tween 60®) (HLB-value = 14.9) shows a HLB-value of 10.7:

$$\left(\frac{40}{100} \cdot 4.3 = 1.72; \frac{60}{100} 14.9 = 8.94; 1.72 + 8.94 = 10.66 \right). \tag{18-4}$$

18.4.3 "Required" HLB Value

Although the HLB value of an emulsifier as such gives some insight in its function at an interface, it does not tell us how suitable it will be as an emulsifying agent for a particular lipid phase. Each substance to be emulsified has assigned a "required" HLB value. This is defined as the HLB value that an emulsifier (or a mixture of emulsifiers) should have to be capable of forming a stable and optimally dispersed emulsion from a particular lipid phase and water. The assessment of the required HLB value for a particular lipid phase is performed empirically. For lipidic phases in O/W emulsions, its value is <20; for example, for stearic acid 17, cetyl alcohol 15, liquid paraffin 10, white wax 9, and soft paraffin 7. Also for the required HLB, the principle of algebraic additivity applies. From the individual values of the components of an oil phase and their proportions therein the required HLB value of the mixture is obtained by (weighted) summation. Generally speaking, the most stable emulsions are obtained when the required HLB values of the components of a lipid phase coincide with the apparent HLB value of the emulsifier (or mixture of emulsifiers).

18.4.4 Mechanism of Action of Emulsifiers

The function of emulsifiers is to facilitate the fragmentation of the phase to be dispersed and to protect the emulsion droplets thus formed from recoalescence. This involves various mechanisms that often act in combination. Since the details of the mechanism of action of the emulsifying activity have not yet been fully elucidated, it is still not possible to accurately predict the stability of an emulsion system. Therefore, often one will have to revert to semiempirical approaches.

Emulsifiers significantly reduce the interfacial tension at the water/oil interface. In this way they facilitate the dispersion and reduce the driving force towards phase separation by lowering the interfacial energy. This mechanism by itself is insufficient to produce a stable emulsion, because the phase-separated state still represents an energetically more favorable situation. In practice, emulsions with very low interfacial tension may even be particularly prone to coalesce (for example within the range of the phase inversion temperature, see below). Therefore, additional factors must be responsible for the emulsion-stabilizing action. The prevention of coalescence is predominantly brought about by energetic barriers that are formed by the adsorption of emulsifier molecules. These barriers should be sufficiently high not to be overcome by the kinetic energy of the droplets (Fig. 18-6). On account of the Brownian motion and the sedimentation and creaming processes, some of the emulsion droplets are in rapid motion, which is even enhanced at elevated temperature, partly because of decreased viscosity. When the barrier is sufficiently high, the emulsion is still thermodynamically unstable, but it is kinetically stabilized. Such a situation is called meta-stable. In case of pharmaceutical emulsions, this situation should be maintained all through the storage and application period.

18.4.4.1 Stabilization

Energy barriers may be generated in different ways (Fig. 18-7). An important option is the introduction of charge. Even emulsion droplets without emulsifier usually have a slight negative charge due to the adsorption of ions from the water phase. However, this is not sufficient to lead to stabilization. A considerably stronger charge may be obtained by accumulation of ionic emulsifier molecules at the interface between water and oil.

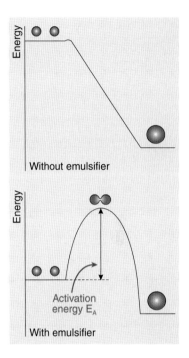

Fig. 18-6 Effect of emulsifiers on the tendency of an emulsion to coalesce.

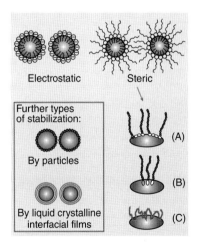

Fig. 18-7 Stabilization principles for emulsions. Steric stabilization may be achieved by: (A) adsorbed block copolymers; (B) nonionic surfactants with polyoxyethylene chains; or (C) amphiphilic macromolecules.

A relation between electrolyte concentration and critical coagulation concentration of emulsion droplets is given by the Schulze-Hardy rule that states that the critical coagulation concentration is inversely proportional to the sixth power of the ionic concentration.

The critical coagulation concentration is the point at which flocculation occurs.

Identically charged emulsion droplets will not contact each other (electrostatic repulsion) and thus will not coalesce. The interaction of charged emulsion droplets is described by the DLVO theory (section 19.3.1). As a result of the attraction of counter ions from the water phase an electrical double layer is formed around the droplet. Addition of electrolytes to electrostatically stabilized emulsions may lead to shielding of the charge around the droplets and thus lower their stability. This phenomenon may, for example, lead to stability problems with colloidal lipid emulsions for parenteral nutrition when electrolytes are added. For that reason, phospholipid-stabilized colloidal lipid emulsions are rather made isotonic with glycerol than sodium chloride.

In many cases, emulsions are stabilized with nonionic surfactants; in this case, the formation of an electric field around the emulsion droplets plays only a minor role. The stabilizing action may then be attributed to the occurrence of steric effects. With respect to steric stabilization, there are essentially two mechanisms:

1. When two emulsion droplets carrying, for instance, hydrated polyoxyethylene chains anchored on their surface approach one another, at a certain distance mutual penetration of the macrogol chains starts to occur. As a result, the chains experience a limitation in their mobility, implying that the system will undergo a loss of entropy. This situation is thermodynamically unfavorable for the system and it may be counteracted by forcing the droplets apart.

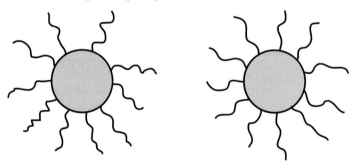

No interaction between sterically-stabilized emulsion droplets

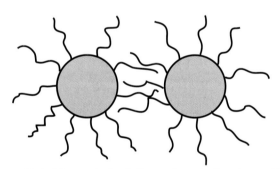

Chain interpenetration is thermodynamically unfavourable

2. In addition, as a result of the locally increased concentration of the polymer chains an osmotic pressure arises within the range of approach. This, in turn, causes a water flow driving the droplets apart.

For highest stability, a gap-free emulsifier film around the emulsified droplet is necessary.

For example; a stable O/W emulsion is formed when emulsified using a mixture of sodium cetyl sulfate and cholesterol, which forms a tight emulsifier film around the oil droplet. However, replacing the cholesterol fraction with oleyl alcohol, which due to its unique shape cannot form a tight film together with sodium cetyl sulfate, will result in an O/W emulsion with poor stability.

Such steric effects may also explain the stabilization with certain macromolecules. It is assumed that the stabilization of W/O emulsions is based on similar effects, which in this case are mediated by the lipophilic chains of the emulsifiers in the oil phase. An important role is also attributed to the structure of the emulsifier film, which should cover the interface completely. When there are gaps in the emulsifier film—for instance, when the available amount of emulsifier is insufficient—droplets may interact at incompletely coated sites and thus, coalesce. The grade of dispersion decreases until the interfacial area has become small enough to allow complete coverage with the available emulsifier molecules. Many emulsifiers produce very stable films that cover the spherical droplets of the disperse phase as a flexible or rigid layer. When droplets of the disperse phase contact each other incidentally, such films provide additional protection from coalescence. Examples of such substances are the protein emulsifiers. Protein-based emulsifiers such as casein or egg yolk are often applied in the food industry. It occurs occasionally that emulsion droplets stick together with their emulsifier film and thus form flocs, which, due to their larger mass, undergo accelerated sedimentation or creaming.

Exclusive use of charged emulsifiers (e.g., soaps, cetyl stearyl sulfate) may give rise to rather porous films because tight packing in the film will be prevented by the mutual electrostatic repulsion of the charged head groups. In order to attain, besides the charge stabilization, a densely packed interfacial film, a second, uncharged surfactant may be applied. Such mixed surfactant systems often produce particularly stable emulsions (see below). In addition to sufficient strength, also elasticity is required of the emulsifier film in order to be able to compensate for deformations occurring during stirring or pouring. Also, the film needs to be able to regenerate. When the film is damaged, emulsifier molecules from the bulk solution should immediately fill up the gap.

18.4.5   Mixed Emulsifier Systems, Complex Emulsifiers

In practice, mixtures of multiple emulsifiers often prove to be more efficient stabilizers than single-component systems. Many pharmaceutically applied emulsifiers are not even chemically pure substances themselves (e.g., cetyl stearyl sulfate, lecithin). By using a mixture of two emulsifiers of the same type (e.g., O/W type or W/O type) emulsifying activity may be enhanced. However, also examples have been reported of mixtures of two emulsifiers impeding the emulsification process (e.g., lecithin and casein). The use of two emulsifiers of different type may cause serious problems. When an emulsifier is added to an emulsion containing an emulsifier of a different type, the emulsion will often break. There are, however, some combinations of an O/W and a W/O emulsifier that perform better than the individual substances by forming a kind of complex in the interface of emulsion droplets. These combinations lower the interfacial tension more efficiently than either one of the individual components by itself and produce optimal occupancy of the interfacial film. As a result, such emulsions are particularly stable.

The mechanism of action of such complex emulsifiers can be explained as follows. The two emulsifiers of opposite type form a film such that the lipophilic groups orient themselves toward the oil phase and the hydrophilic groups to the water phase. In this way, the two emulsifiers intercalate such that the hydrophilic groups are anchored through hydrogen bonds, and the lipophilic groups bind by means of *van der Waals* forces. As a result of the complex formation the water-binding capacity increases and strong hydration films are formed, while viscosity increases. This may lead to gel formation. The very strong films thus formed are responsible for the high stability of such emulsion systems. Complex emulsifiers play a special role in the production of creams (chapter 15). Particularly stable complexes are formed from sodium cetylsulfate and cholesterol (1:1) (reduction of σ by approximately $60 \cdot 10^{-3}$ N · m^{-1} as compared to $22 \cdot 10^{-3}$ N · m^{-1} for the same amount of sodium cetyl sulfate alone). The number of combination options is very high because of the substantial number of surface-active substances. Up to now, favorable emulsifier combinations can be designed only by empirical means. Examples of complex emulsifiers are emulsifying cetostearyl alcohol Type A and B (Ph. Eur.), and nonionic emulsifying wax (Table 18-3).

Table 18-3 Examples of Complex Emulsifiers

Example	W/O Emulsifier	O/W Emulsifier
emulsifying cetostearyl alcohol (Type A) Ph. Eur.	cetostearyl alcohol (minimum 80%)	sodium cetostearyl sulfate (min 7%)
emulsifying cetostearyl alcohol (Type B) Ph. Eur.	cetostearyl alcohol (minimum 80%)	sodium lauril sulfate (min. 7%)
non-ionic emulsifying wax BP	cetostearyl alcohol 80%	cetomacrogol 1000 20%

Typical components of an emulsion other than surfactants:

Oil phase:

Mineral oils, vegetable oils, animal/plant waxes, silicone oil, etc.

Typically in O/W emulsions, the oil phase should be able to dissolve the active pharmaceutical ingredient.

Aqueous phase:

Mainly consists of water, but, depending on application of the formulation other ingredients such as glycerol, low molecular weight polyethylene glycol, propylene glycol etc. might be added to the aqueous phase.

Preservatives:

Parabens, benzoic acid, etc.

Antioxidants:

Ascorbic acid, tocopherol, butylated hydroxyanisol, propyl gallate etc.

Buffers:

Commonly, buffers are not used in emulsions as increased electrolyte concentration might lead to charge shielding and hence results in decreased pharmaceutical stability (except in sterically stabilized emulsions). However, a buffer might be required to modulate tonicity, solubility of ionic components or enhancement of chemical stability.

Depending on the application of emulsion other potential ingredients in a pharmaceutical emulsion include humectants, flavours, sweetening agents etc.

The ability to form complexes is strictly specific. Changes in the molecule (branching of chains, salt formation, steric effects) may prevent the formation of stable adducts. Also in other cases, when no real complex formation occurs, mixtures from W/O and O/W emulsifiers may be advantageous. For example, combinations of sorbitan esters and polysorbates often produce emulsions of higher stability than upon applying a single individual member of this surfactant family with the same HLB value. An additional advantage is in this case the possibility to distribute any excess of components of the emulsifier system between the water and the oil phase.

18.4.6   Stabilization with a Third Phase

Under certain conditions (for example when sufficient amounts of emulsifier are available) it may occur that around emulsion droplets multiple emulsifier layers with a liquid-crystalline structure build-up (Fig. 18.7). Such layers bring along additional mechanical stabilization of the droplet and are of particular relevance in the area of semi-solid preparations. Emulsion systems, which are stabilized by ultrafine solid particles, are called Pickering emulsions. In the pharmaceutical field, however, these are of minor importance so far. The particles cover the emulsion droplets as a continuous layer and thus prevent coalescence of the droplets in a mechanical manner (Fig. 18.7). Such "insoluble emulsifiers" are, for example, bentonite, coal powder, aluminum hydroxide, and magnesium hydroxide as well as modified silica particles. It is assumed that during the emulsion formation with metal soaps the emulsifier precipitates at the interface and that subsequently such surface-active compounds act as particulate emulsifiers. Stabilization of emulsions by particulate solid substances requires that these possess an amphiphilic character and are wetted by both the lipophilic and the hydrophilic phase. Nonetheless, one of the phases will have essentially better wetting properties than the other. Wettability is characterized by the contact angle θ in the contact range between particle and oil/water interface (Fig. 18-8). The wettability decisively affects the position of a solid amphiphilic particle between the oil and the water phase. If the contact angle θ is >90° and $\cos\theta$ henceforth is negative, the particle will be wetted better by oil (particle a in Fig. 18-8); in case θ is <90°, $\cos\theta$ is positive and the particle will be wetted better by water (particle b). The phase that is wetting the particle and in which it penetrates for the greater part will be the external phase. Since the solid particles fully surround their emulsion droplets, the latter can be in contact with each other only via their coating.

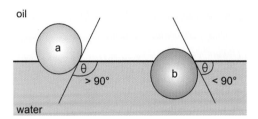

Fig. 18-8   Dependence of the value of the contact angle on the position of an amphiphilic particle at the oil/water interface.

18.4.7   Stabilization by Thickening Agents

As already indicated, the stability of an emulsion can also be enhanced mechanically by the application of thickeners that strongly restrict the mobility of the emulsion droplets. In this way, creaming, sedimentation, or coalescence processes will be prevented. In principle, the droplets of the disperse phase may be retained within the continuous phase merely by the high viscosity of the latter. Typical thickeners are mucilaginous substances, which are highly swellable due to their strong hydration. Among the most frequently used thickeners are tragacanth, gelatin, agar, and many semi-synthetic cellulose ethers as well as weakly cross-linked polyacrylic acids and polyvinyl-pyrrolidone. In addition to their thickening properties, many macromolecules used for this purpose (e.g., cellulose ethers, gelatin, gum arabic) display a certain surface activity, and thus, do not merely act by virtue of an increase in viscosity. Addition of certain polymeric excipients in suitable concentrations may lead to steric stabilization (see above).

In combination with conventional emulsifiers thickeners are valuable excipients that can reduce expenses on low-molecular weight emulsifiers. Especially with respect to tolerability of the formulations, this can be an additional advantage, as low-molecular weight emulsifiers, in particular at high concentration, can cause irritation, for instance, on the skin. When larger amounts of added thickeners give rise to gelation of the continuous phase, semi-solid emulsions are formed.

> When at rest, the thixotropic nature of some thickening agents allows the external phase to acquire a high viscosity, which retards aggregation of the dispersed phase. However, upon application of only a weak force, e.g. pouring of the emulsion out of a container, the viscosity of the external phase already drops down thus allowing the emulsion to flow.

18.5   Emulsion Type

18.5.1   General Considerations

The type of an emulsion (O/W or W/O) is determined by a number of factors, of which in general the characteristics of the applied emulsifier are most important. Additional factors are temperature, the volume ratio between the phases, viscosities, the nature of the oil phase, the nature and concentrations of ions and other additives, as well as the preparation conditions.

As a rule of thumb (the so-called Bancroft rule) the phase in an emulsion system in which the emulsifier dissolves preferentially or is enriched becomes the continuous phase of the emulsion. (Example: alkali soaps dissolve in water and are O/W emulsifiers; multivalent salts of fatty acids accumulate in oil and are W/O emulsifiers. Exception: lecithin, despite its lipid solubility, is as a rule an O/W emulsifier.) The Bancroft rule clearly is in accordance with the HLB concept: Substances that are designated as W/O emulsifiers (lipophilic) on the HLB scale usually form W/O systems, while those classified as O/W emulsifiers (hydrophilic) form O/W emulsions.

These observations are confirmed by geometric considerations on the emulsifier molecules at the water/oil interface. In case of hydrophilic, water-soluble emulsifiers, the hydrophilic part, due to its steric arrangement and/or as a result of its hydration, occupies much space and is space-filling, while the lipophilic moiety takes relatively little space. Thus, the emulsifier molecule takes on a cone-shaped geometry, which forces the emulsifier film into a curved shape (Fig. 18-9). The opposite situation is seen with lipophilic emulsifiers—for instance, soaps with two acyl chains and a bivalent counter cation. The double acyl chain requires

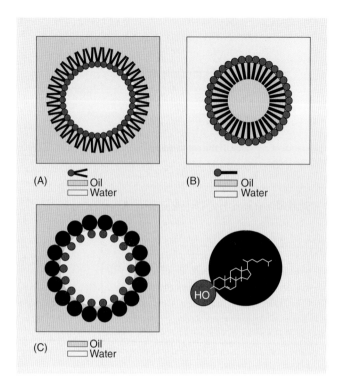

Fig. 18-9   Formation of the emulsifier film: (A) W/O-emulsions (emulsifier: alkaline earth metal or metal soaps); (B) O/W emulsions (emulsifier: alkali soaps); (C) W/O-emulsions (emulsifier: cholesterol).

much more space, while, in addition, alkaline earth metal salts of soaps have a low tendency to dissociate, which moderates the hydration of the carboxyl groups. This leads to bending of the interface around the water droplet. With the theory based on spatial considerations it becomes conceivable that cholesterol must be a W/O emulsifier. The spatial requirements of the bulky steroid skeleton at the interface only allows for an arrangement as depicted in Fig. 18-9 C. Although this geometric theory provides a very illustrative representation of the situation during the formation of emulsions, it will not precisely describe the situation on the formed emulsion droplets as the interfaces in most emulsion systems are practically planar taking into consideration the dimensions of the emulsifier molecules.

The volume ratio of the two phases may influence the emulsion type in the sense that for instance, dependent on the concentration ratios, either a W/O or an O/W emulsion is formed. This does not imply, however, that the volume ratio always has a decisive influence. There are, for example, emulsion systems that contain up to 90% internal phase. Mayonnaise represents a well-known example of such a system from the field of food science. Remarkably, when we assume the presence of rigid equally sized emulsion droplets, a phase fraction of more than 74 vol. % would not be possible as by then the droplets would fill the entire continuous phase (Fig. 18-10 A). The explanation of the much higher values observed in reality lies in the incorrectness of the assumption of equal size. The droplets in an emulsion are as a rule not equal in size but rather poly-disperse, so that the space between the droplets can be used more efficiently (Fig. 18-10 B). When the droplets are deformed even closer packing of the droplets is possible (Fig. 18-10 C).

18.5.2   Phase Inversion and Phase Inversion Temperature

The preparation of stable emulsions requires insight in the mechanisms of emulsion formation and a fundamental characterization of the potential of emulsifiers and emulsifier mixtures.

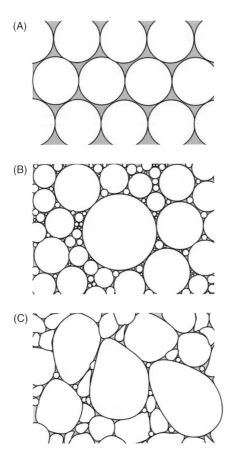

(A)

(B)

(C)

Fig. 18-10   Phase conditions in emulsion systems.

When a hydrophilic surfactant is added to an oil phase, initially a W/O emulsion will be formed upon emulsification, which subsequently, by gradual translocation of the surfactant into the water phase, will convert into an O/W emulsion (phase inversion possibly via a mixed emulsion). An emulsion that is prepared in this way is characterized by the presence of very fine droplets.

When, on the other hand, the surfactant is added to the aqueous phase, there will be no translocation of the surfactant and no phase inversion. This will lead to the formation of a coarse emulsion that can be improved only by vigorous mechanical treatment. In the former case, the formation of a W/O emulsion is due mainly to solubilization of a small amount of water in the oil phase. By simply estimating the water solubilization capacity of the oil phase (amount of water taken up without lasting turbidity) the most favorable emulsifying conditions can be determined. It has been demonstrated that oil-emulsifier mixtures with the highest water solubilization capacity yield emulsions with the finest droplet size. This approach offers an alternative to the HLB procedure because there is a direct relationship between the maximal amount of water that can be solubilized in oil and the HLB value of the surfactant. The phase inversion proceeds rapidly. It can be monitored by viscosity assays, but even better by conductivity measurements.

Temperature changes can alter the polarity of particularly non-ionic emulsifiers and can therefore bring about a phase inversion. Non-ionic emulsifiers, in particular those that carry polyoxyethylene chains, become more lipophilic at higher temperature because their polar chains can no longer interact so well with water. As a result, their HLB value decreases and can therefore at higher temperatures shift to a value in the range of W/O emulsions. O/W emulsions that have been prepared by using such emulsifiers can therefore alter their phase status at that particular temperature. For such emulsions, a typical phase inversion temperature (PIT) can be determined as a characteristic value. This value can be applied to determine the mixing ratio and concentration of the emulsifiers necessary for emulsion formation and stability. For an O/W emulsion, the PIT should be 20° to 60°C above the storage temperature to guarantee product stability. In addition, the PIT can be utilized for emulsion preparation as at the PIT the surface tension is low so that relatively little mechanic force suffices to obtain a fine-disperse emulsion system (PIT emulsification).

It has to be noted that, in principle, the HLB value (including the required HLB), as well as the PIT value as much as all other up to now proposed characteristics, suffer from significant shortcomings. In spite of intense scientific efforts, no generally valid method yet exists that can exactly and reliably predict the stability of an emulsion system.

18.6   Chemical and Microbiological Stability

In addition to the physical stability of an emulsion, that is, the potential to maintain for prolonged periods of time, the homogeneous distribution of the dispersed phase as obtained by the mechanical forces applied during the emulsifying process, the chemical and microbial stability should be guaranteed as well.

Chemical stability is challenged by the condition that emulsified oils are more susceptible to autoxidation than oils in the absence of water. In addition, hydrolytic processes that can lead to partial saponification of the oil are favored by the dispersed state bringing along a substantial increase of the water-oil interface. Also, the stability of the formulated pharmaceuticals often diminishes. Air (especially oxygen), can be incorporated accidentally during the emulsification process and can influence the chemical stability of the oil phase and the incorporated pharmaceuticals. In case unfavorable interactions occur between the emulsifier and the pharmaceutical or additional components, the emulsion may lose its therapeutic potential and as a result of diminished emulsifier activity coalescence may occur. This may happen for instance when an anionic emulsifier is processed together with a cationic drug.

Because of their high water content emulsions are often an excellent nutritional substrate for microorganisms (section 25.5.1). That applies in particular to O/W emulsions. By addition of preservatives that are active in the aqueous phase (section 25.5.3), microbial spoilage can be prevented. It should be taken into consideration that transfer of the preservative into the lipid phase may gradually diminish its concentration in the aqueous phase. In order to assure proper preservation, the concentration of the preservative might have to be adjusted in such cases. In principle, refrigerated storage and tight sealing will prolong the shelf life of the emulsion.

18.7   Preparation Technology

The preparation of emulsions can be approached in different ways:

18.7.1   Suspension (or "Continental") Method

The emulsifier is turned into a suspension by carefully dispersing it in the phase in which it is not soluble (the internal phase). The external phase (in which the emulsifier is soluble or at least wettable) is added to this suspension (if necessary in portions). During the addition of the external phase, a phase reversal occurs, which can lead to the formation of very small particles. As in the suspension, the emulsifier is finely dispersed and can only slowly be extracted by the added phase it is recommended to first prepare a primary emulsion with part of the external phase and let this stand for a while before processing it with the rest of the external phase. This method is, for instance, applied when using gum arabic or gum tragacanth for the preparation of O/W emulsions.

18.7.2   Dissolution (or "English") Method

The emulsifier is dissolved in the external phase, after which the internal phase is emulsified into it. Generally, one will proceed in such a way that the disperse phase is introduced portion-wise into the dispersion medium containing the emulsifier. In this case, no phase inversion will occur so that the dispersion will take place solely by mechanical force.

18.7.3 Emulsification Equipment

During the emulsifying process a hydromechanic material distribution is achieved by supplying energy opposing the interfacial forces between the phases, thus forming new interfaces.

The choice of equipment for the preparation of emulsions depends on the one hand on the size of the starting sample and on the other hand on the viscosity of the emulsion and the surface tension between the phases. For the preparation of relatively fluid emulsions, other equipment is needed than for the preparation of creams. Important considerations are the emulsifying potential of the emulsifier and what level of dispersion one wants to achieve. The lower the surface tension, the easier finely dispersed emulsions can be prepared. Only in case of very low surface tensions can acceptable fluid emulsions be prepared by exclusively manual treatment, for instance by means of a mortar and pestle, or by simple shaking in a large-volume flask. Usually, emulsions thus prepared are coarsely disperse. The use of stirring equipment or shaking machines usually leads to higher levels of dispersion. As a rule, mechanical homogenization is recommended in order to achieve a higher dispersion level and thus a higher stability. High-speed stirring equipment, for example rod stirrers, devices with stirring arms and blenders, will result in effective dispersion of the internal phase. Baffles positioned in the stirring device may further enhance the efficiency of the dispersion process. Centrifugal stirrers produce strong currents that cause sudden changes in flow directions. Thus, occurring shock effects cause a further reduction of the size of the internal phase particles. Useful devices for nonindustrial use are mixing beakers or rods (kitchen machines). With the Ultra-Turrax devices, very finely dispersed emulsions can be obtained (see section 24.7.2.6). Such equipment, which is also applied in the industrial setting, can bring the disperse phase down to in the lower μm range.

Depending on the required dispersion level, industry employs, in addition to such rotor-stator equipment, colloid mills, or specially constructed high-pressure homogenizers. These are devices in which a preemulsified mixture is aspirated from a vessel and pressed through narrow adjustable gaps under very high pressure (gap homogenizers, Fig. 18-11). The gaps are in part formed in such a way that the channels through which the emulsion is squeezed are placed in an angular arrangement, which gives rise to an even stronger dispersion of the inner phase. Homogenizing equipment designed according to these or similar principles and used for large-scale production can produce several thousands of liters emulsion with colloidal particle sizes.

Also, by means of ultrasound very fine-disperse emulsions can be prepared, but this approach is limited to small-scale production.

For each combination of emulsion composition and emulsifying equipment there are optimal process conditions (e.g., with respect to dispersion intensity and duration). For example, during the first few seconds of the emulsifying process the diameter of the droplets strongly decreases and then gradually levels off until a limit value is attained. Continuation of the emulsifying process will, from then on, not yield further improvement of the emulsion quality.

> The power density in a gap homogenizer can reach quite impressive values: up to 10^{13} W/m^3 can be achieved. This value is about the power density of a nuclear power plant, of course only realized here in a volume of some cubic micrometres.
>
> This high power density can nevertheless cause structural changes in the particle matrix besides its size reduction action.

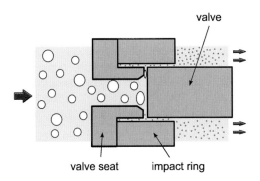

Fig. 18-11 Homogenizing valve.

Upon too forceful mechanical challenges with high-intensity emulsifier equipment it may occur that product quality deteriorates again. For the sake of stability care should be taken that temperature does not increase too strongly. In general, a moderate temperature increase facilitates emulsion formation. When an emulsion is subjected to homogenization processes, often an increase in viscosity is observed. The emulsion droplets behave then like solid particles, which show increased friction between them when the surface area increases.

18.8   Testing

The characterization of an emulsion comprises in the first place the assessment of its particle size and size distribution and, when applicable, also the surface charge of the droplets, verification of the emulsion type, the viscosity of the emulsion and, during the development process also its creaming, sedimentation. and coalescence tendency.

18.8.1   Particle Size and Dispersion Grade

Because particle size is an essential characteristic of a liquid emulsion system, this parameter should be assessed in the context of quality control. Besides, particle size assessment is an important instrument in the development and stability testing. In stable emulsions, the dispersion grade remains unaltered. Changes in this parameter indicate failing stability.

For routine measurements, particularly of O/W emulsions, light scattering techniques are preferred, such as laser diffraction; for colloidal emulsions also photon correlation spectroscopy is used (section 3.4.3.2). In special cases, a single-particle counting technique such as the light-blockage or impulse procedure may be deployed. Alternatively, particle size may be investigated microscopically—for example, by applying a counting chamber—but this is a time-consuming procedure unless an automatic image analysis system is available. Care should be taken that the preparation of the sample does not cause changes in grade of dispersion. Not only average diameter but also size distribution should be assessed, which with modern analytical methods can be done without additional expenditure of time or money.

18.8.2   Creaming and Coalescence

The following procedures serve to characterize the emulsion, particularly with respect to its stability. At the same time they provide useful information concerning the suitability of the used emulsifiers as well as the manufacturing procedure and equipment.

In case of coarsely disperse or unstable systems, it is sometimes possible to draw already certain conclusions concerning stability by simple visual observation during standing at room temperature. For that purpose, for example, the time may be measured until the onset of decay of an emulsion in a graduated cylinder, using the separation of a fixed amount of water, oil, or cream layer as instability criterion. One may also determine the separated amount *versus* time and derive a stability constant from that correlation.

Properly formulated, relatively stable emulsion systems cannot be assessed this way. For these systems, accelerated stability tests must be used in the course of the development process.

The disintegration process of the emulsion may be accelerated by an increase in temperature, which at the same time reduces viscosity and thus enhances the mobility of the disperse phase, which may also contribute to accelerated sedimentation or creaming. Besides, the collision probability of the droplets will be increased by the Brownian motion. Testing may be performed either in a water bath or in a thermostated cabinet. In addition to the options to measure creaming velocity, as described in the foregoing, also regular assessment of particle size may provide an indication of beginning instability. Nonetheless, extrapolation of the findings of storage studies at elevated temperature to the situation at room temperature should only be done with the greatest possible care because, besides the desired conditions, also other parameters of the emulsion system may be affected by a temperature rise, such as the polarity of nonionic emulsifiers or the distribution of certain components of the system between the phases. In the end, the exact storage stability can only be determined by prolonged storage at normal conditions. Also the impact of cold, potentially leading to freezing out of the aqueous phase, may under certain circumstances be used as a stress factor in accelerated stability tests. Particularly, repeated freezing and thawing is of interest in this connection.

The assessment of emulsion stability by means of the method of accelerated creaming involves the measurement of the extent of separation of the internal from the external phase or the change in particle size under the influence of a constant centrifugation velocity. But also in this case, comparison with normal conditions may be tricky. Stability assessment of W/O emulsions may also be performed by determining electric conductivity. The essential parameter in this case is not the absolute value of conductivity of the emulsion but, rather, the extent to which it changes during coalescence. Two platinum electrodes connected to a conductivity assay device are immersed in the emulsion in a position close to the bottom of the container. The time elapsing until a change in conductivity is detected is recorded. This procedure allows the detection of structural changes in the emulsion well before visual evidence of a beginning coalescence becomes manifest.

18.8.3 Emulsion Type

For the determination of the emulsion type several methods are available. It is recommended to deploy different methods as the use of only one method may bring along erroneous results. Particularly in case of methods relying on the addition of further phase components, it is important to take care that no changes in the phase state occur as a result of the addition.

A first indication with respect to the phase state may be given by a *rinsing test*: Only O/W emulsions can be easily rinsed off the skin with water. It is a common experience that removal of a W/O emulsion from the skin or another object with pure water is very difficult.

In the *color method*, a few drops of an aqueous dye solution (e.g., methylene blue) are added to a sample of the emulsion. When the emulsion rapidly, homogeneously, and intensely takes on the color of the dye, we are dealing with an O/W emulsion in whose external phase the dye can rapidly distribute. A comparable staining may be achieved for W/O emulsions by means of a few drops of an oily dye solution (e.g., Sudan-III). The staining method may be particularly well evaluated by microscopy.

The *dilution method* is based on the fact that emulsions can only be diluted with the external phase. When a small amount of water is added to an emulsion sample and this distributes rapidly so that, if necessary after shaking or stirring, a homogeneous emulsion is obtained again, we are apparently dealing with an emulsion of the O/W type. On the other hand, when the same emulsion is diluted with oil, this accumulates on the emulsion. The opposite behavior will be observed for emulsions of the W/O type.

In the *ring test*, a drop of the emulsion is placed on a piece of filter paper. After a short time, O/W emulsions show an aqueous ring around the droplet.

The most reliable assessment of the emulsion type is provided, however, by a *conductivity assay*. Upon immersing the electrodes of a conductometer in the emulsion sample, only an O/W emulsion will show a clear response on the amperometer, because only water as external phase will allow a current to flow. The traces of electrolyte required for this will be found in any water phase. In case of a W/O emulsion, the oil phase acts as an insulator so that no amperometer response will be detected.

Further Reading

Collins-Gold, L., Lyons, R., Bartholow, L. "Parenteral emulsions for drug delivery." *Adv Drug Del Rev.* 5 (3) (1990): 189–208.

Washington, C. "Stability of lipid emulsions for drug delivery." *Adv Drug Del Rev.* 120 (2–3) (1996): 131–145.

IUPAC. Compendium of Chemical Terminology, 2nd ed. (the "Gold Book"). Compiled by A. D. McNaught and A. Wilkinson. Blackwell Scientific Publications, Oxford (1997).

Suspensions

19

19.1 General Introduction

As emulsions, suspensions consist of a dispersed phase and a dispersion medium, the continuous phase. In suspensions, however, the dispersed phase consists of solid substances, which are practically insoluble or at best poorly soluble in the dispersion medium. Substances that are partly soluble in the dispersion medium are much less suitable for the preparation of suspensions because the suspension may become too coarse because of crystal growth (Chapter 19.6). Water-soluble drugs may only be processed into a suspension with lipophilic dispersion media. Formulation of suspensions can facilitate to process poorly soluble active pharmaceutical ingredients into a liquid drug formulation or to achieve a slow dissolution process creating a depot effect.

Suspensions are used for different pharmaceutical applications and can be administered internally (e.g., as oral suspension) as well as externally (e.g., as cutaneous suspension). Suspensions for external use containing an aqueous dispersion medium are often called shake lotions. An example is the zinc oxide shake lotion (*Lotio alba aquosa* DAC), which consists of a mixture of zinc oxide and talcum in a glycerol-containing water phase. Following administration onto the skin, a dehydrated layer is formed upon drying that has a desiccating effect ("liquid powder"). Due to the zinc oxide, the formulation has an anti-inflammatory and slightly astringent effect. The zinc oxide lotion may be used as a base for other active ingredients. Also, poorly soluble drugs such as nystatin or finely distributed light protection pigments are applied dermally in the form of suspensions.

However, suspensions are much more commonly used for systemic drug delivery. Typical examples of suspensions for oral administration are suspensions of acid-binding inorganic drugs and antibiotics, the latter being widely applied in pediatrics. Suspensions also provide an attractive alternative for the formulation of active ingredients with bad taste because undissolved substances do not contribute to the taste of the formulation. A special type of suspension is the *dry suspension*, which is a powder or granule formulation that is converted into a suspension just prior to administration by the addition of water. Such formulations can be used for drugs with insufficient chemical stability or in cases where the liquid suspension has a tendency of caking (formation of a sediment, which is difficult or even impossible to redisperse, see Chapter 19.3).

Parenteral suspensions are mostly used to achieve a depot effect (e.g., insulin or corticosteroid suspensions). Suspensions are also used in eye drop formulations, in pressurized-gas aerosols for inhalation and as filling material in soft gelatin capsules. In addition, several nonfluid drug formulations have a suspension character, for example suspension ointments or suppositories with dispersed solid active ingredient.

Pharmaceutically applied suspensions are mostly coarse disperse systems. As a rule, the suspended particles have diameters larger than 1 µm (i.e., larger than in colloidal systems),

Voigt's Pharmaceutical Technology, First Edition. Alfred Fahr.
© 2018 John Wiley & Sons Ltd. Published 2018 by John Wiley & Sons Ltd.

and may even be as large as 100 μm. For certain applications (e.g., eye drops or parenteral formulations) very strict requirements apply with respect to particle size in order to prevent unwanted side effects such as local irritations due to the presence of the solid particles. In special cases also nano-particulate suspensions are used (Chapter 20.6). The mass fraction of solid material in pharmaceutical suspensions varies, depending on the administration route, between 0.5% and 50%.

Suspensions are, like emulsions, thermodynamically unstable and the development of pharmaceutically acceptable suspensions is often a challenging process. As sedimentation (section 19.3) of the solid particles usually cannot completely be excluded, the pharmacopeias allow sediment formation as long as the sediment can readily be redispersed and the suspension remains homogeneous for a sufficiently long time to ensure accurate dosing.

19.2 Manufacturing Technology

Prior to manufacturing the final suspension, the solid components of the dispersed phase are ground to the desired particle size and, when applicable, classified. For manual production, the solid substances are ground with a small amount of the dispersion medium to obtain a homogeneous, paste-like starting material. In this way, the solid particles become homogeneously wetted by the dispersion medium and the formation of aggregates is avoided. When necessary, the starting material may be submitted to a three-roll mill device to improve the dispersion procedure. Subsequently, the dispersion medium is added stepwise. When the dispersion medium consists of more than one fluid, the initial grinding is done with the fluid with the highest viscosity or providing the best wetting properties for the particles to be dispersed. When using mechanical dispersion devices such high-shear mixers (e.g., Ultra-Turrax, see 24.7.2), which are also applied in industrial manufacturing, the dispersed phase is usually gradually processed into the liquid phase. In case of unsatisfactory dispersion of the solid material in the dispersion medium, the suspension can be subsequently homogenized resulting in deagglomeration of secondary particles and yielding fine and uniform distributions of the dispersed phase. In the industry, colloid mills (section 2.1.4.7) are often deployed to achieve this purpose.

19.3 Physicochemical Aspects

For pharmaceutical suspensions, the homogeneity obtained directly after the manufacturing process should ideally remain unaltered during storage and administration. However, suspensions are thermodynamically unstable systems due to the high interfacial energy. In addition, instability often arises from the density difference of the dispersed particles and the dispersion medium, as well as from interactions between the dispersed particles. Although such instabilities can often be slowed down, in most cases they cannot be fully suppressed. Common instabilities in suspensions are summarized in Fig. 19-1 and the corresponding physicochemical aspects are discussed in the following sections.

19.3.1 The DLVO Theory

By using model systems, colloid scientists have tried to describe the interactions between dispersed particles on the basis of van der Waals attractive forces and electrostatic repulsive forces. The DLVO theory, developed by Derjaguin, Landau, Verwey, and Overbeek, is most frequently used as a model to explain aggregation and flocculation processes in colloidal dispersions. The theory was originally developed for colloidal dispersions containing charged particles, but similar considerations are nowadays also applied for sterically stabilized systems.

It should be kept in mind that these model systems generally deviate from the suspensions used in pharmaceutical practice. In the model systems, the suspended particles are assumed to be spherical and to have the same particle size (monodisperse systems). Moreover, the

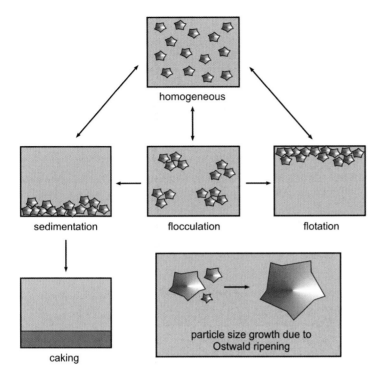

Fig. 19-1 Instability phenomena in suspensions.

Forces of attraction between two particles mainly originate from van der Waals attractive forces whereas repulsive forces are the result of electrostatic repulsion between the particles.

Events occurring at specific points on the graph as the two particles in a suspension approach each other,

1. Secondary minimum: loose aggregates are formed which remain loose (flocculated) as long as E_A is sufficiently high.
2. Energy maximum: particles would experience high repulsive forces.
3. Primary minimum: if the particles are able to overcome the energy barrier, they experience strong attractive forces leading to irreversible coagulation.

concentration of solid material is low (~2%) and the continuous phase consists exclusively of water.

In contrast, both particle size and shape varies usually in pharmaceutical suspensions (polydisperse and heterogeneous dispersions). The concentration of suspended solid material is usually much higher and can be up to 50% in pharmaceutical suspensions. Furthermore, the dispersion medium does not consist solely of water in most cases but contains other additives. Nonetheless, the DLVO theory provides useful information for the development of pharmaceutical suspensions as well as emulsions.

The DLVO theory considers the interaction potential between two particles as a function of the distance between them (Fig. 19-2). The total potential energy (E_T) between two particles is the sum of the attractive potential energy (E_A) and the electrostatic repulsive energy (E_R):

$$E_T = E_A + E_R \qquad (19\text{-}1)$$

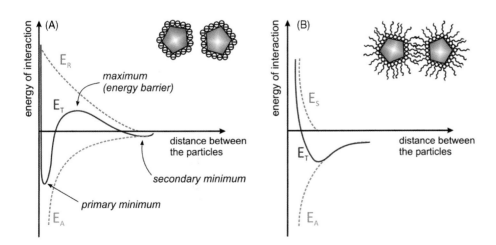

Fig. 19-2 Potential profiles between two particles in case of (A) electrostatic and (B) steric stabilization.

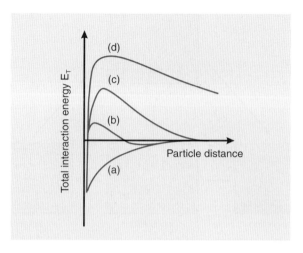

Fig. 19-3 Different profiles of the total potentials of electrostatically stabilized particles according to the DLVO theory as, e.g., triggered by electrolyte addition. Decreasing electrolyte concentration from curve (a) to curve (d).

The terms flocculation and coagulation in connection with a pharmaceutical suspension are used to express an increase in particle size by aggregation.

However, it should be taken into account that flocculation is a readily reversible process occurring at secondary minima on the DLVO-graph whereas coagulation is an irreversible process occurring at the primary minima.

When two particles come closer to each other, both repulsive (E_R) and attractive (E_A) forces between the particles increase. These result in characteristic potential profiles (Fig. 19-2), the shape of the profiles depending on the properties of the suspensions (e.g., particle size and surface charge, composition of the dispersion medium). The profile of the total interaction potential (E_T) provides some characteristic and practically important sections of interparticulate interactions in dependence on the distance between them (Fig. 19-2).

Considering electrostatic stabilization (Fig. 19-2 A), the attractive energy slightly outweighs the repulsive energy ($E_T < 0$) at longer distances between the particles and the potential profile passes a (secondary) energy minimum. At sufficient predominance of attractive energy (i.e., depth of this minimum), flocculation may occur where the loosely packed agglomerates can be readily redispersed. When the particles are moving closer to each other, repulsive forces arising from electrical charges on the particle surface become predominant (first energy maximum in the potential profile). Thus, energy must be spent to overcome this energy barrier (electrostatic stabilization). By forcing the particles closer to each other, a primary energy minimum is reached, resulting in particle aggregation. This energy minimum is usually so deep that aggregation is irreversible (e.g., the aggregates cannot be re-dispersed by shaking).

Depending on the composition and properties of the suspensions, the potential profiles can have other shapes (Fig. 19-3). Compared to curve (b), which corresponds to the potential profile just discussed, the repulsive forces between the particles in the suspension represented by curve (a) are insufficient and rapid and irreversible particle aggregation can be expected. For the suspensions described by curve (c) and (d), strong repulsive forces prevent the particles coming closer to each other even over longer distances. When the repulsive energy barrier is larger than the kinetic energy of the particles, a stable dispersion with respect to particle aggregation is generally obtained. The potential profile of a suspension will change when the repulsive potential in electrostatically stabilized dispersions is modified by addition of electrolytes (section 19.3.3).

19.3.2   Wettability of the Disperse Phase and Flotation

Powdered substances may be easy or very difficult to disperse in a liquid. This is caused by differences in wettability (section 3.11.2). Solid, insoluble particles can bind variable amounts of water on their surface (lyosorption), and this determines the degree of wettability of a substance. Wettability depends on the chemical characteristics of the two phases. Only when the solid material can be sufficiently wetted with the dispersion medium will a homogeneous suspension of low viscosity be obtained.

Hydrophilic powders, often oxygen-containing inorganic compounds, such as oxides, sulfates, and carbonates (zinc oxide, barium sulfate, calcium carbonate), usually have a good wettability with hydrophilic liquids, as they have a small wetting angle with hydrophilic liquids like water. Consequently, a solvation shell of solvent molecules surrounds each suspended particle. These prevent clustering of individual particles into aggregates, thus favoring the formation of a finely dispersed suspension.

Poorly water-wettable substances (large wetting angles), that is, hydrophobic substances such as many poorly water-soluble active ingredients, have a stronger affinity for air than for water (aerophilicity). In the presence of water, they form agglomerates with air inclusions. Although the dispersed substances have a higher density than water, air inclusions or even air bubbles sticking on the particle surface may result in accumulation of the solid suspended material partially or entirely on the top of the dispersion medium (flotation). This may seriously hamper the formation of a homogeneous suspension. The term *flotation* originates from the ore dressing where the fine ore particles were made hydrophobic by chemical means, thus decreasing their wettability with water. This resulted in agglomeration with large air inclusions and flotation and facilitated their separation from other sedimenting compounds.

> Flotation often results in inhomogeneity and can be reduced by inclusion of appropriate wetting agents. Wetting agents have HLB values in the range of 7–9.
>   For example Span 20, Tween 61.

19.3.3   Surfactants and Peptizers as Dispersion Agents

Addition of an amphiphilic compound to a hydrophilic dispersion medium leads to a reduction in surface tension between the dispersed hydrophobic solid particles and the dispersion medium and results in an essential improvement of the wettability of the particles. The surfactant molecules are adsorbed on the particle surface as an interfacial film, which promotes the formation of a closed solvation shell. This prevents or at least diminishes formation of particle agglomerates with air inclusions and thus flotation. The required surfactant concentration to achieve sufficient wetting has to be determined experimentally. It is dependent on the interfacial area and thus on the particle size and the concentration of the solid material. Optimal interfacial coverage may be determined by rheological measurements. An insufficient or too large amount of surfactant can result in strong interparticulate adhesion that, in turn, leads to a significant change in flow behavior. Meaningful information may also be obtained by sedimentation tests. Similarly as in emulsion systems, surfactants show orientation effects depending on the surfaces (liquid/solid in this case, section 18.4.1). Unlike in emulsions, however, the relevant groups of the surfactant molecule cannot penetrate into the solid particle. Therefore, the surfactant merely adsorbs at the particle surface.

> By definition, peptizers are chemicals which prevent coagulation in suspensions. Most common peptizers employed in suspensions are multivalent electrolytes.

Ionic surfactants will also provide the particle surface with an electrical charge. However, suspension particles often carry an electric surface charge that cannot be solely attributed to surfactant adsorption. The electric charge of the particle interface may be a consequence of dissociation of functional groups (e.g., carboxyl groups) at the particle surface. In case of inorganic particles, surface charges may arise from isomorphic substitution (incorporation of foreign ions) or by adsorption of ions from the dispersion medium. A well-known example is the adsorption of silver or halide ions onto the surface of the silver-halide particles formed upon the precipitation process. When a dissociation process is involved in the formation of surface charges, the surface charges depend on pH and thus also suspension properties and stability.

Surface-bound groups or ions, which provide, for example, a negative charge of the surface (potential-determining ions) will attract positively charged ions (so-called counter ions) from the dispersion medium in order to restore electro-neutrality. In this way, electrical double layers arise, and the properties and formation of these electrical double layers can be explained by different theoretical models.

According to Stern, the layer close to the particle surface determining the negative charge of the particle is covered by a fixed layer of counter ions (the Stern layer, Fig. 19-4). This layer, however, in which an approximately linear potential gradient occurs, usually does not provide sufficient counter ions to compensate fully for the surface charge, which may even be amplified by specific adsorption of ions with identical charge. Further charge compensation is reached by a diffuse layer of counter ions, which extends out into the liquid phase. There is a diffuse distribution of both positive and negative ions due to Brownian motion. As

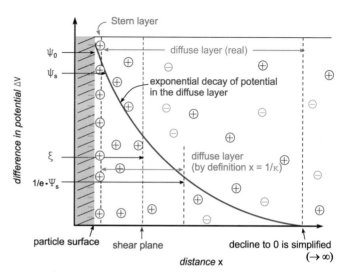

Fig. 19-4 **Potential pattern around a charged particle (ζ: Zeta potential; ψ_S: Stern potential; ψ_0: Nernst potential).**

Upon close inspection of the particle surface, the Stern layer in Fig. 19-4 can be considered as composed of two planes: the inner and outer Helmholtz planes (HP). The inner HP consists for example of ions adsorbed to the particle surface by physicochemical interactions. These interactions can be quite strong and may even lead to a higher potential close to the surface of the particle due to adsorption of dehydrated negative ions to a negative surface overriding the electrical repulsion. The outer HP is more or less identical to the visualized Stern layer as drawn in Fig. 19-4.

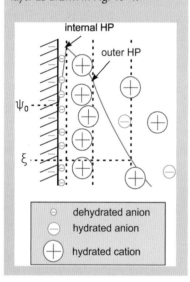

electrostatic attraction between the charged surface and the counter ions in the diffuse layer declines with increasing distance, the concentration of the counter ions decreases likewise until finally neutrality is reached in the neutral zone where negative and positive ions perfectly counter-balance each other. Within the diffuse layer the electric potential around the particles declines exponentially. The thickness of the diffuse layer is an important parameter to characterize the stability of electrostatically stabilized dispersions. However, because of the exponential drop in potential and the difficulty to define the point of neutrality as the ultimate border of the layer, the thickness of the diffuse layer is difficult to determine. For that reason, it is common practice to use the term $1/\kappa$, which marks the distance from the particle surface at which the potential is reduced by $1/\mathrm{e}$-fold the Stern potential, as a measure of the thickness of the diffuse layer.

The real charge of the particle (Nernst potential) is given by the potential difference between the particle surface and the neutral zone (Fig. 19.4). Similarly as the Stern-potential it cannot be determined experimentally. The zeta potential (ζ) has practical importance as it can be determined experimentally. The zeta potential is defined as the potential difference between the neutral zone and the shear plane around the particle, which arises by the stripping off a large part of the diffuse layer due to the movement of the particle. The zeta potential depends on the Nernst potential and the electrolyte concentration in the dispersion medium. It can be assessed in good approximation by measuring the electrophoretic mobility of the particles. An increased surface charge density (increased Nernst potential) at unchanged electrolyte concentration in the dispersion medium will result in an increased zeta potential. The zeta potential provides a relatively accurate measure of the surface charge density and enables to estimate the electrostatic repulsion between the dispersed particles. Generally, stability of a dispersion increases with increasing value of the zeta potential.

For electrostatically stabilized pharmaceutical suspensions, the value of the zeta potential should be at least 50 mV (positive or negative) in order to prevent agglomeration and aggregation. Also, the adsorption of strongly charged ions (peptizers), for example, ions of the water-soluble salts potassium tartrate, sodium oxalate, calcium citrate, and sodium pyro-phosphate, may alter the particle charge. Stabilization by addition of ions (peptization) is, however, not simple. Only with addition of peptizers in appropriate (mostly very low) concentration may a stabilizing effect be expected, which will still be sensitive to external influences. By exceeding the optimum concentration of peptizer, flocculation or aggregation rather than stabilization may occur. This correlates with the high electrolyte sensitivity of the electric potential, which should always be taken into consideration, not just in the case of added peptizers.

At very low electrolyte concentration in the dispersion medium, the concentration of counter ions around a dispersed particle, and thus neutralization of the particle charge by the counter ions, is quite low. As a consequence, the potential curve declines gradually over a rather long distance and the thickness of the diffuse layer is considerable (Curve (d) in Fig. 19-3). Increasing the electrolyte concentration in the dispersion medium leads to a decrease of the thickness of the diffuse layer, as the particle charge can be neutralized (shielded) more efficiently by the higher concentration of counter ions. The steeper decline of the potential curve, at the same position of the plane of shear, results in a lower zeta potential (curves (c), (b), and (a) in Fig. 19-3), and thus in a decrease of suspension stability. A stronger decline in the potential can also be observed when multivalent ions are used instead of monovalent ions (more efficient shielding provided by the multivalent ions). The possibility of influencing the potential pattern around the particles by adding suitable excipients to the dispersion medium triggers controlled flocculation, which may prevent the formation of compacted sediments (caking, section 19.3.4).

Upon addition of nonionic surfactants or surface-active macromolecules, the mechanism of steric stabilization becomes relevant (section 18.4.4.1). Well-hydrated chains of the stabilizer reaching into the dispersion medium prevent particles from coming too close to each other and thus particle aggregation. In contrast to electrostatic repulsion, which is often still effective over rather long distances, steric repulsion is only observed when polymeric chains on the particle surface of two particles start to penetrate each other. Therefore, repulsive potential in steric stabilization is characterized by a sudden onset at a distinct distance from the particle surface (Fig. 19-2 B). Often, additional stabilizing effects by charges are also present in dispersion stabilized with non-ionic surfactants or surface-active polymers. The combination of steric and electrostatic stabilization is also known as *electrosteric* stabilization.

19.3.4 Sedimentation Behavior

An ideal pharmaceutical suspension should not show any tendency of sedimentation, even over prolonged time of storage. In reality, this is difficult to achieve, and is, in practice, rarely sought.

Indicators to evaluate the sedimentation rate can be derived from Stokes' law of sedimentation (cf. 18.3). Despite the prerequisites to apply Stokes' law (smooth spherical particles, laminar flow around the particles, no mutual influence between the particles during the sedimentation) are not fully met in most pharmaceutical suspensions, it is still useful to obtain important information to facilitate options for stabilization against sedimentation. Because the particle size appears as its square in the equation of Stokes law, the sedimentation rate can be reduced distinctly by decreasing particle size. Particles undergoing Brownian motion (diameters $\ll 1$ μm) will not completely sediment within considerable periods of time when the density difference between the particles and the dispersion medium is not too large. Theoretically, micronized or nano-sized solids would be most suited for the production of suspensions, especially as a reduction of particle size will also result in enhancement of activity. However, since such extensive size reduction of solids requires special equipment and extremely fine particles have a strong aggregation tendency, a compromise between particle size and sedimentation rate is usually necessary.

From Stokes' law it may furthermore be derived that the sedimentation rate can be reduced by diminishing the density difference between the dispersed particles and the dispersion medium. Also, by increasing the viscosity of the dispersion medium by, for example, thickeners, the sedimentation rate can be reduced. An increased viscosity will at the same time also improve the adhesive properties of the formulation, which is an important consideration for topically applied suspensions. No sedimentation will occur at all when the two phases have identical densities or when, such as in case of thixotropic bentonite gels, the external phase forms gel structures that are destroyed just before use by shaking (gel-sol conversion). An essential effect on the sedimentation rate has also the concentration of the dispersed phase (phase volume ratio). Sedimentation rate declines with increasing particle concentration.

Depending on the flocculation tendency of the dispersed particles, two different sedimentation behaviors can be distinguished:

1. *Deflocculated suspensions*: In deflocculated suspensions, there are no distinct particle-particle interactions. As pharmaceutical suspensions usually contain suspended particles with different sizes, the largest particles will sediment first, according to Stokes'

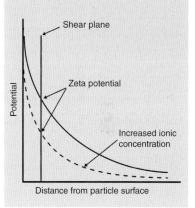

The zeta potential is (among other factors) affected not only by ion/ionic concentration but also by the valency of the counter ions.

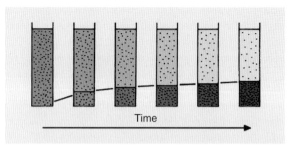

Fig. 19-5   Sedimentation behavior of deflocculated suspensions.

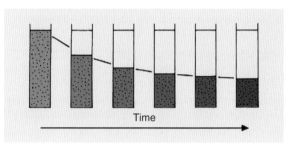

Fig. 19-6   Sedimentation behavior of flocculated suspensions.

> Typically, deflocculated suspensions are characterized by the formation of a cake which is harder to redisperse than flocculated suspensions.

law, and form the lowest layer of the sediment. On top of this (to some extent also in between), the finer particles are deposited, in the order of decreasing size. The volume of the sediment will thus increase with time and ultimately reach its maximum when all particles have sedimented. Simultaneously the particle concentration in the supernatant decreases with time but the supernatant remains turbid for prolonged periods of time as the smallest particles will sediment only very slowly. These ultra-fine particles will have a negligible influence on the volume of the sediment. They just accommodate themselves in the packing gaps between the larger particles (Fig. 19-5).

2. *Flocculated suspensions:* When individual particles agglomerate by flocculation (formation of loose agglomerates, flocs), sedimentation will occur much more rapidly due to the larger size of the flocs compared to the size of the original particles. Moreover, the flocs contain particles of all sizes and the flocs sediment more or less with the same rate forming a very loose, coherent sediment. The sediment volume becomes smaller with time and the supernatant appears clear just from the beginning of sedimentation (Fig. 19-6).

The properties of the sediment may vary largely. The sediment volume is determined by aggregation and flocculation of the primary particles and depends on the geometric arrangement of the particles in the sediment with respect to each other. Addition of surface-active substances may reduce the sediment volume by reducing the flocculation tendency often resulting in tightly packed sediments. The use of amphiphilic substances is therefore not always recommended. As tightly packed sediments have a rather strong tendency to caking (formation of a tight sediment that cannot be redispersed), loose sediments with a large sediment volumes are generally easier to redisperse than tightly packed sediments and therefore are often desirable.

19.4   Stabilization by Macromolecular and Viscosity-Enhancing Additives

As sedimentation usually cannot be suppressed completely in suspensions, the major aim during development of pharmaceutical suspensions is to slow down the sedimentation rate and other processes that might affect the homogeneity of the suspension such as aggregation, flotation, and flocculation. This can be done, in addition to particle size reduction, by increasing the viscosity of the suspension. However, care should be taken that an adequate flow capacity of the suspension is still retained (particularly in oral suspensions).

To increase the viscosity of aqueous suspension media, macromolecular excipients such as tragacanth, pectin, methyl cellulose, hydroxy-ethyl cellulose, carmellose sodium, hydroxyl-alkylated starch derivatives, sodium alginate, polyacrylic acid (carbomers), and dextran are frequently used. Type and amount of the stabilizer need to be determined empirically in each individual case. Macromolecules may also affect the stability of suspensions by other mechanisms. Low polymer concentrations may sensitize the system with respect to salts and may cause destabilization. This may be caused by bridge formation by the binding of individual macromolecules on the particle surface by interactions through specific functional groups or, alternatively, by ionic macromolecules functioning as counter ions resulting in a reduction of the surface charge.

At higher concentrations, the polymers adsorbed at the particle surface result in steric stabilization, as a close contact between the particles is prevented (Figure 19-2), thus counteracting flocculation and aggregation.

Examples of inorganic stabilizers are clay minerals such as bentonite (Veegum®), which swell in water and form, depending on concentration, viscous fluids or thixotropic gels. Similarly, colloidal silica (Aerosil®) forms a thixotropic gel, mainly by hydrogen bonds and van der Waals forces. Colloidal silica is generally also suitable as thickener in oily suspensions. However, aluminum monostearate is preferred for stabilization of parenteral oily suspensions. At adequate concentration, aluminum monostearate rigidifies the oil in such a way that it becomes a gel in the rest state but shaking results in liquefaction and thus in an injectable formulation.

In case of systems without yield value, sedimentation cannot be suppressed completely. Conditions are more favorable for systems having a yield value and thus requiring a shear force (e.g., shaking) to cause flow. By increasing the concentration of solid material in the suspension, a system with a yield value may be obtained. In any case, applicability (e.g., sufficient flowability) and homogeneity to ensure exact dosing of the suspension must be fulfilled.

19.5 Caking

As already discussed, sedimentation cannot be completely suppressed in most pharmaceutical suspension formulations and sediment formation is thus acceptable for pharmaceutical suspensions. A prerequisite for accurate dosing is that the sediment can be readily redispersed by shaking resulting in a homogeneous suspension. Moreover, the suspension should remain sufficiently stable to enable that the correct dose can be withdrawn.

Ensuring easy redispersion of the sediment may, however, be challenging, as polymeric thickeners may result in formation of a tightly packed sediment, causing *caking*. Among the different stabilizing excipients, particularly acacia (gum arabic) is known for its tendency to induce caking in suspension formulations. Caking in suspension can, however, have other reasons. It can be, for example, induced by crystal growth. Particle growth (also called Ostwald ripening; see the next section) can occur when the suspended material is partially soluble in the dispersion medium. Ostwald ripening may strongly impede the ability to redisperse the sediment by shaking. Likewise, a reduction of particle charge and thus stronger adhesion forces, together with the loss of the solvate shells, may result in changes of packing density of the sediment and thus caking.

Caking occurs particularly in deflocculated suspensions as quite densely packed sediments are usually formed in such suspensions. To some extent, repulsion forces between the particles may be outbalanced by gravitational forces of the superimposed particle layers in the sediment. In contrast, rather loose and readily redispersible sediments are usually observed in flocculated suspensions. Flocculated suspensions can be obtained by addition of surfactants or electrolytes such as aluminum salts. The concept of *controlled flocculation* is often used to obtain pharmaceutical suspensions with adequate properties concerning sedimentation rate, ease of redispersion of the sediment, and homogeneity, although this affects the appearance of the suspension.

19.6   Ostwald Ripening

When the dispersed phase is soluble in the dispersion medium to some extent, redissolution processes may not only result in caking of the sediment but also in changes in the particle size. According to Ostwald's law (section 3.9.7.2), the solubility of small particles is higher than that of larger particles. As a result, a higher saturation concentration around smaller particles will be observed compared to larger particles. This will result in a concentration gradient of dissolved compound within the dispersion medium and gradually lead to diffusion of dissolved material from the small particles to the larger ones followed by recrystallization. Thus, large particles will grow at the expense of the smaller particles until, theoretically, the thermodynamically most favorable state (one single large "particle") is reached. The higher the solubility of the suspended material in the dispersion medium and the larger the differences in particle size, the faster this phenomenon, *Ostwald ripening*, proceeds. Ostwald ripening can be suppressed by using a suitable non-solvent, extremely poorly soluble compounds as dispersed materials and by minimizing the differences in particle size. In addition, the adsorption of macromolecules on the particle surface may hinder Ostwald ripening.

19.7   Testing of Pharmaceutical Suspensions

19.7.1   Sedimentation Behavior

19.7.1.1   Sedimentation Rate and Sediment Volume

Sedimentation processes can be well assessed and quantified by using graduated measuring cylinders. The sediment volume can be conveniently determined this way in dependence on time. To also evaluate the sediment volume at different time points during sedimentation, the suspension ratio (SR), which relates the sediment volume to the total volume of the suspension, can be applied:

$$SR_t = SV/TV \qquad (19\text{-}2)$$

SR_t = suspension ratio at time point t
SV = sediment volume of the suspension
TV = total volume of the suspension

An assessment of the SR is only feasible at high concentrations of solid material in the suspensions, formation of clear sedimentation layers, and lack of caking. For flocculated suspension, the SR should be as close as possible to 1.

To evaluate the sedimentation rate, the half-settling time can be used, which is defined as the time where the volume (or height) of the sediment is half (deflocculated suspensions) or double (flocculated suspensions) of the final sediment volume (Fig. 19-7).

19.7.1.2   Ease of Redispersion of the Sediment by Shaking

The suspension containing a sediment is submitted to standardized movements—for example, by tilting the container by 90° at defined velocity. Either the time or the number of movements that are required to completely redisperse the sediment is measured.

19.7.2   Particle Size, Dispersity, and Other Tests

The particle size, as an important quality parameter, can be determined by methods described in section 3.4. Most commonly used are light-scattering methods, but also the particle counters (Coulter counter or light blockage), wet sieving, and sedimentation methods are applied.

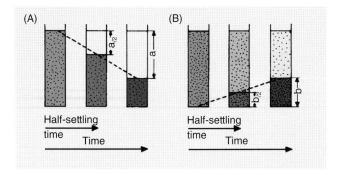

Fig. 19-7 Determination of half-settling time for (A) flocculated and (B) deflocculated suspensions.

Moreover, microscopic techniques providing also information about the particle shape and flocculation state can be applied.

Assessment of the density of the suspension provides information on possible air inclusions between the dispersed particles. During development, assessment of the zeta potential of the particles provides useful information on their expected behaviors (e.g., aggregation tendency) and stability. Rheological measurements will provide essential information about the applicability of the suspensions (e.g., flowability). For cutaneous suspensions, such as the above-mentioned *Lotio alba*, which is intended to form a dry film of solids on the skin after administration, evaluation of adhesiveness is relevant.

Finally, quality assessment of suspensions includes quantitative assays of the drug content in samples, which are withdrawn immediately after redispersion to ensure correct dosing of the suspension.

Further Reading

Gallardo, V., Ruiz, M., Delgado. A. "Pharmaceutical suspensions and their applications" in: Nielloud, F., Marti-Mestres, G., eds. *Pharmaceutical emulsions and suspensions:* Marcel Dekker Inc. New York (2000): 409–464.

Sushma, G., Kumar, K. M., Ajay, B., Ruchi, T. "Advancements and patents in pharmaceutical suspension technologies." *J Biol & Scient Opinion.* 1 (4) (2013): 372–380.

Micro- and Nanodispersed Systems

20

Technology always develops from the primitive through the complex to the simple.

Antoine de Saint Exupéry

20.1 General Introduction

Micro- and nanodispersed systems have acquired an important position in pharmaceutical formulation science especially with regard to the formulation of challenging modern active pharmaceutical ingredients (API). These are, for example, drugs with poor solubility and chemical stability, which require adequate formulation to enable the production of an efficient medicine. Micro- and nanoparticles may also be used as parenteral depot formulations (section 21.6.2) or to obtain a site-specific drug delivery (drug targeting, section 20.2). Colloidal emulsions and suspensions share several properties with other systems that have been presented in preceding chapters. However, they possess some peculiarities with respect to administration and/or production procedures and are thus discussed in this chapter in more detail.

20.2 Tissue-Specific Drug Administration (Drug Targeting)

It was the opera *Der Freischütz* by Carl Maria von Weber, which inspired the German physician and scientist Paul Ehrlich (1854–1915) to develop his famous "magic bullet" concept. A "magic bullet" carries a drug directly to the site of the disease without affecting the healthy tissues. Ever since, this idea has been an important motivation in pharmaceutical formulation research. Nonetheless, in spite of considerable research efforts in this field, implementation of the ultimate goal (to develop a formulation that efficiently uses the drug at the target tissue but avoiding side effects at the same time) still appears to lay in the far future.

The task to achieve the goal of drug targeting presents indeed a tremendous challenge. An ideal drug carrier should protect the associated drug against influences of the biological environment in the body over the whole time between administration and transport to the target tissue, while the drug should be completely released at the site of action (diseased organ or cells). Moreover, it would be desirable that such a carrier system directly delivers the drug into the cell. This is of special importance for biologicals, such as peptides and proteins, which cannot pass cell membranes passively.

Similarly unsolved is the question of how the carrier system will "find" the target site. The simple and straightforward strategy of attachment of a cell-specific antibody on the carrier surface facilitating specific binding to the target cells upon long-enough circulation in

Voigt's Pharmaceutical Technology, First Edition. Alfred Fahr.
© 2018 John Wiley & Sons Ltd. Published 2018 by John Wiley & Sons Ltd.

the blood stream has not yet resulted in marketable products. One of the biggest challenges in this regard is the nonspecific, rapid recognition of such carriers by the immune system and consequently effective removal of the drug-carrier complex before it can reach the target site.

Another hurdle, in addition to all the barriers of the numerous cell membranes that the drug has to cross (e.g., diazepam has to pass many membranes on its way from the gastro-intestinal tract to the site of action in the central nervous system) is the structural complexity of the targeted carrier-drug complex (or the drug itself) impeding a simple and straightforward formulation development process. Such complex structures readily provoke an immune response, which will counteract the desired therapeutic effect (except, of course, in case that an immune-stimulating effect is desired).

All these challenges culminate currently in the development of carrier systems for gene therapy (so-called vectors), where a polar active ingredient with high molecular weight (DNA or RNA) must specifically be transported into a specific cell or in case of DNA even into the cell nucleus.

Although these considerable challenges will still require intensive research efforts for many years, at least some of the above-discussed issues could be addressed by the development of innovative, modern drug formulations.

20.3   Liposomes

20.3.1   Structure and Composition

Liposomes are vesicular structures that are composed of phospholipid bilayers enclosing an internal aqueous compartment (Fig. 20-1). Based on their morphology, one distinguishes unilamellar (one phospholipid bilayer) and oligolamellar (several phospholipid bilayers) liposomes. Larger-sized liposomes can enclose several smaller ones (multivesicular liposomes). Furthermore, liposomes may be distinguished by their size. Smaller liposomes (diameters between about 25 and 200 nm) mainly consist of only one bilayer (small and large unilamellar vesicles; SUV and LUV), while larger vesicles (between about 100 nm up to >1 μm) often consist of several bilayers (multilamellar large vesicles, MLV).

The main component of liposomes is commonly lecithin (phosphatidylcholine) isolated, for example, from egg or soybeans. Phosphatidylcholine is composed of two fatty acid chains esterified to a glycerol molecule. The remaining hydroxyl group of glycerol forms a phosphate

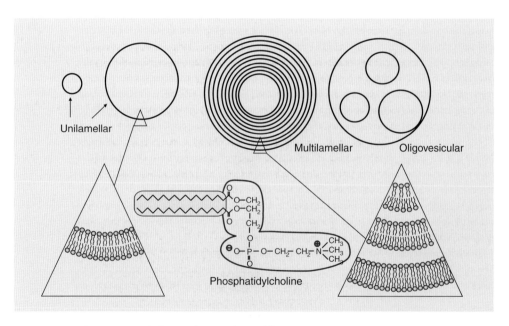

Fig. 20-1 Morphology and composition of liposomes.

ester, which, in turn, is coupled with a choline molecule. There are, however, many other phospholipids, carrying other polar head-groups (e.g., ethanolamine or glycerol) and/or have another fatty acid composition (degree of saturation and chain length), which can be used for liposome preparation. This variety of building blocks provides a large variety in liposome properties—for example, with respect to membrane fluidity (flexibility) and surface charge (polarity). Often, additional lipid molecules are added. Frequently, cholesterol, which is an essential component of biological membranes is added, to stabilize the liposomal bilayer and to minimize drug leakage. Oxidation of unsaturated acyl chains may be prevented by the addition of α-tocopherol, a radical scavenger. Although the acyl ester bonds are susceptible to hydrolysis, hydrolysis rates are practically negligible at or below room temperature at pH values between 6 and 7.

Due to their composition of physiological lipids, their resemblance to biological membranes and their capacity to encapsulate active ingredients, liposomes present a very interesting and promising carrier for drug delivery. Hydrophilic drugs can be encapsulated in the aqueous space(s) within the liposomes or between the bilayers in case of MLV. Lipophilic or amphiphilic drugs, on the other hand, are incorporated in the lipid bilayers.

20.3.2 Preparation

Liposomes are formed by the dispersion of phospholipids in an aqueous medium (e.g., buffer solutions). By simple shaking or stirring, large (>1 μm) multilamellar vesicles are formed. Through subsequent size reduction (e.g., by extrusion, ultrasound, high-pressure homogenization), liposomes with diameters between about 25 and several 100 nm can be obtained. A frequently used technique is membrane extrusion (also called filter extrusion), which involves the extrusion of the vesicle suspension through a filter membrane of defined pore size in the nm-size range (e.g., the Nuclepore® filter, section 2.3.2.1). Extrusion results in rather homogeneous liposome suspensions in a gentle manner, whereas size and lamellarity (e.g., number of bilayers) depend on the pore size of the used filter membranes. There are, however, several alternative preparation methods and the preparation method can be adjusted to the specific requirements of the final preparation and the excipients.

Water-insoluble active ingredients are commonly incorporated in the liposomes by adding them to the organic solvent in which the phospholipids are dissolved. In this way, they become embedded in or associated with the lipid bilayer. Hydrophilic drugs can easily be encapsulated by dissolving them in the suspension buffer. A major disadvantage of this approach is that only a usually very small fraction of the solution is encapsulated in the liposomes, the remainder staying behind in nonencapsulated, free form in the surrounding medium. The nonencapsulated drug may be removed (and recovered if so desired) by size exclusion chromatography (SEC) or dialysis, if required. However, special manufacturing procedures have been developed to improve the encapsulation efficiency of hydrophilic water-soluble substances. A particularly interesting example is the extremely efficient encapsulation of the cytostatic drug doxorubicin in small unilamellar vesicles (Doxil®; Caelyx®). The intra-liposomal accumulation of the drug is driven by a pH gradient across the liposomal membrane. This gradient is formed by the encapsulation of ammonium sulfate in the liposomes. NH_3 molecules, which are in equilibrium with the NH_4^+ ions, readily permeate the liposome bilayer, resulting in a drop of pH within the liposome and thus a pH gradient across the liposomal bilayer. Upon addition of a doxorubicin solution, the neutral form of the drug ($R-NH_2$) permeates the bilayer into the liposomal core, where it becomes protonated ($R-NH_3^+$) and precipitates under formation of a semicrystalline structure, which is stabilized by the sulfate ions. This complex is not able to escape from the liposome, and a very high doxorubicin encapsulation in the liposomes can be attained. The gradient method can also be applied to other active ingredients and may yield extremely high encapsulation efficiencies of up to more than 90%.

Liposome suspensions commonly have a limited lifetime (maximally 1–1.5 years) in contrast to their freeze-dried preparations, which often can be kept for much longer times. In order to avoid aggregation during redispersion of a freeze-dried formulation, excipients such as lactose, sucrose, or trehalose are added to the liposome suspension prior to lyophilization as cryoprotectants (section 5.3.3.4). Freeze-drying is more suitable for liposome formulations of lipophilic drugs, which are incorporated into the lipid membrane, as for of those with encapsulated water-soluble drugs because the risk of drug leakage from the carrier upon resuspension is much lower in case of a lipid-bound drug.

20.3.3   Applications

Liposomes with sizes between about 50 and 200 nm can be administered intravenously and may thus be used for solubilization of poorly water-soluble drugs to obtain an applicable aqueous formulation (Table 20-1). The first approved medicine based on this principle was Ambisome®, an injectable liposome formulation of the fungicide amphotericin B. Ambisome®, which is used to treat systemic fungal infections, is tolerated considerably better than the conventional micellar formulation of this drug. Another example of an approved liposome formulation of a poorly water-soluble drug is Visudyne®, a liposome-associated porphyrin used for the treatment of macular degeneration, a serious eye disorder.

An important promise of liposomes used as an intravenous drug carrier is the potential of drug targeting. This might be implemented, at least partly, for several preparations containing a liposome-encapsulated cytostatic drug. Caelyx® (the first approved liposomal drug) and DaunoXome® are liposome formulations of the cytostatic drugs doxorubicin and daunorubicin, which deliver the drug much more efficiently to the tumor tissue than conventional formulations. Since conventional liposomes distribute rapidly in the organism following intravenous administration and are predominantly taken up by liver and spleen, modified liposome formulations have been designed to optimize the body distribution profile.

The main reason for the rapid elimination of liposomes from the blood circulation is the recognition of the liposomes as "foreign particles" by the immune system. That causes certain plasma proteins to bind to the liposomal surface (opsonization), which, in turn, facilitates their subsequent uptake by macrophages. In order to circumvent this effect, the liposome surface may be modified by coating with hydrophilic macromolecules, which prevent binding of the opsonizing proteins and thus the uptake by immune cells such as macrophages (stealth effect). Most commonly, PEG-modified phospholipids are incorporated in the liposome bilayer for this purpose.

An important function of liposomes as a drug carrier system is the protection of the encapsulated drug against enzymatic degradation during circulation in the blood or elsewhere in the body. However, the phospholipids of the liposome membrane are susceptible to the same metabolic degradation processes as the body's own cell membrane lipids.

Specially designed liposomes can be used as parenteral depot formulation. DepotCyte®, for example, contains relatively large (>1 μm) multivesicular liposomes encapsulating individual small vesicles in a foam-like structure. This special structure is stabilized by the incorporation of triolein in the lipid bilayers. Following intrathecal administration, these liposomes release the encapsulated drug cytarabin over a period of about 14 days.

Antigen-carrying phospholipid vesicles (also called virosomes) are used in some vaccine formulations (e.g., HAVpur®).

Table 20-1   Examples of Intravenously Applicable Liposome Preparations

Product	Drug	Application	Formulation	Composition
AmBisome®	amphotericin B	antimycotic	Powder (infusion)	DSPG, hydrogenated PC, cholesterol
Visudyne®	verteporfin	photodynamic therapy	Powder (infusion)	DMPC, egg PC
Caelyx®	doxorubicin	cystostatic	Liquid concentrate (infusion)	DSPE-mPEG, hydrogenated soy PC, cholesterol
DaunoXome®	daunorubicin	cytostatic	Liquid concentrate (infusion)	DSPC, cholesterol

DSPG: distearoylphosphatidylglycerol; PC: phosphatidylcholine; DMPC: dimyristoylphosphatidylcholine; DSPE: distearoylphosphatidylethanolamine; MPEG: methyl-polyethyleneglycol; DSPC: distearoylphosphatidylcholine

20.3.4   Perspectives

Extensive research efforts are focused on surface modification—for example, with antibodies or antibody fragments to improve the targeting potential of liposomes. Furthermore, liposomes are increasingly investigated as potential carrier system for DNA for gene therapy.

While liposome formulations are widely used in cosmetics, their application as dermal drug formulation has not yet been widely implemented. Among others, this may be because conventional liposomes cannot penetrate the skin barrier intact. Current research is directed on the development of highly deformable vesicles (*transferosomes, invasomes*), which may be capable of squeezing through the narrow intracellular spaces of the stratum corneum, the uppermost layer of the skin. To obtain vesicles with more flexible membranes, destabilizing agents (e.g., micelle-forming surfactants) are added to the membrane-forming phospholipids.

20.4   Colloidal Fat Emulsions

Colloidal O/W fat emulsions are probably the oldest formulation of colloidal drug carriers for intravenous administration. First development approaches date back to the early twentieth century and colloidal fat emulsions have now been in the clinic for more than 50 years in Europe (e.g., Lipofundin®, Intralipid®). In most clinically used parenteral emulsions, the oil phase itself represents the active ingredient.

In intensive care, colloidal fat emulsions are used for parenteral nutrition, where the oil serves as energy source and supply of essential fatty acids (section 21.14.4). However, drug-containing fat emulsions, where the emulsion droplets serve to solubilize lipophilic drugs (e.g., diazepam, etomidate, propofol) or lipid-soluble vitamins, have also been in the clinic for many years (e.g., Diazepam-Lipuro®, Disoprivan®, Lipotalon®, Vitalipid®). Recently, colloidal emulsions of squalene have been introduced as adjuvants in vaccine formulations.

20.4.1   Structure and Composition

The oil phase in fat emulsions for parenteral nutrition is selected on nutritional and physiological aspects. Soybean oil, but also olive oil and fish oil, semi-synthetic triglyceride oils such as medium-chain triglycerides, are most frequently used for this purpose. In drug-containing emulsions, soybean oil is usually selected as oil phase, sometimes in combination with medium-chain triglycerides or partially acetylated glycerides. In accordance with the high demands on physiological tolerance of formulations intended for parenteral administration, phospholipids, particularly egg lecithin, are used as emulsifier. In order not to disturb the electrostatic stabilization of the emulsion droplets, glycerol is added as isotonizing agent instead of electrolytes such as sodium chloride. Some formulations also contain small quantities of α-tocopherol or sodium oleate to improve the chemical and physical stability.

The average droplet size must be distinctly below 1 µm, and only a few droplets may have a size in the lower µm-size range to assure that the droplets will not cause serious side effects (e.g., embolism) by clogging the smallest capillaries. As a rule, the mean droplet size is within the range of 200 to 450 nm, and the proportion of droplets being larger than 5 µm is limited to <0.05%. These emulsions are quite stable.

In order to meet these quality requirements, colloidal fat emulsions are manufactured by high-pressure homogenization (section 18.7.3) after initial pre-dispersion of the two phases by a high-speed mixer. As always, a certain excess of the emulsifying phospholipid has to be used, a small number of liposomes is usually also present in addition to the oil droplets. For drug incorporation, the drug is usually dissolved in the oil phase prior to emulsification. After intravenous administration, the active ingredient is typically rapidly released from the emulsion droplets. Only drugs with a very high affinity to the oil phase may circulate for extended periods of time in the blood stream. Care has to be taken to choose only compatible drugs, as there is a risk of coalescence of the emulsion droplets.

20.5   Microemulsions

Microemulsion definition: "Micro" means here in a historic context "very small." A still good definition is: a microemulsion is a system of water, oil and an amphiphile, which is a optically isotropic and thermodynamically stable liquid solution (Danielsson & Lindman 1981). The size range for microemulsions differs in the literature: 5–50 nm; 5–100 nm. Occasionally, just an upper size limit of 200 nm is given.

Similarly as emulsions, microemulsions consist at least of a hydrophilic, a lipophilic and an amphiphilic substance. However, microemulsions differ from conventional emulsions with respect to their structure, visual appearance and stability. Microemulsions are transparent to opalescent, moderately viscous, optically isotropic and thermodynamically stable systems. Conventional emulsions, on the other hand, are only kinetically stable (i.e., for a limited period). Microemulsions can be considered as a transition stage between micellar solutions and conventional emulsions. Their structure, which strongly depends on the composition of the microemulsion, has not yet been fully elucidated. Structures consisting of very small droplets (predominantly < 100 nm), of highly oil-swollen micelles (Fig. 20-2) or of a bicontinuous structure of hydrophilic and hydrophobic domains are discussed. These domains cannot be described as different phases according to the Gibbs definition, implying that microemulsions represent single-phase systems. They are usually prepared from both a surfactant and a co-surfactant in addition to water and oil. When chosen adequately, surfactant and co-surfactant arrange in such a way that the interfacial tension becomes close to zero (Chapter 3.9). The surface tension is so low that the contribution to the interfacial energy, despite the enormous surface area of the large number of very small droplets, is overcompensated by the increase in entropy during mixing. That is the reason that microemulsions can form spontaneously upon, for example, dilution of a suitable concentrated surfactant/oil mixture with water.

Microemulsions have been used for decades in oil and wax production. Due to their favorable dissolution and solubilization ability for both hydrophilic and hydrophobic substances, they have also found strong interest for pharmaceutical applications. Their naturally high surfactant content (15%–25%) limits, however, their use in pharmaceutical formulations to the peroral and topical administration. During development of microemulsions, care should be taken to the fact that incorporated active ingredients may accumulate between the surfactant molecules thus influencing microemulsion formation and stability. It is, therefore, of uppermost importance to take the physicochemical characteristics of the drug into account in the development of microemulsion formulations.

Currently, the microemulsion technique is, for example, used for oral administration of the extremely poorly water-soluble immune-suppressive cyclosporine (Sandimmun® Neoral). This strongly lipophilic drug is dissolved in a mixture of mono-, di- and triglycerides from corn oil (oil phase), ethoxylated hydrogenated castor oil (surfactant), ethanol (co-surfactant) and α-tocopherol (anti-oxidant). This oily concentrate is filled into soft capsules or used as such to prepare a diluted solution. After ingestion of the capsule (or dilution of the concentrate in water), a microemulsion forms spontaneously. By using this microemulsion formulation, the bioavailability of cyclosporine could be improved considerably.

For topical formulations, the special microemulsion structure and composition enhance drug penetration into the upper layers of the skin. In spite of the proven penetration-enhancing effect of microemulsions, this formulation concept has still not been reached broad application for dermal drug delivery.

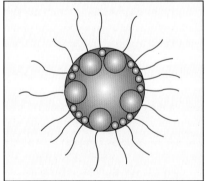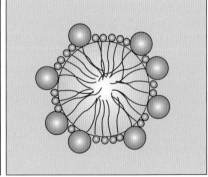

Fig. 20-2   Schematic presentation of W/O (left) and O/W (right) microemulsions.

20.6 Nanoparticles as Drug Carriers

Nanoparticles are usually solid colloidal particles with sizes mostly between 15 and 300 nm. More specifically, a distinction can be made between nanocapsules and nanospheres (Fig. 20-3). Nanoencapsulation can be understood as a coating of colloidal emulsion droplets or solid nanoparticles with a solid coating. On the other hand, nanospheres are colloidal particles in which the active ingredient is embedded in a matrix or adsorbed at the surface.

As carrier materials, mostly natural (e.g., gelatin, albumin, polysaccharides) or synthetic polymers (e.g., polycyanoacrylates, poly(lactic-co-glycolic acid) (PLGA)) are used. By proper polymer selection, the release of active ingredient can be influenced. As a rule, drug release occurs by diffusion and/or by degradation (erosion) of the carrier material.

Nanoparticles are currently being developed as therapeutics and diagnostics, for example, as contrast agent for imaging procedures in computed tomography or magnetic resonance tomography. In the area of drug delivery, nanoparticles are predominantly investigated as drug carriers and depot formulations mostly for innovative drugs based on peptides, proteins and nucleic acids, as well as for antibiotics, cytostatics and hormones. Nanoparticles are mostly intended for parenteral administration. Important prerequisites for parenteral formulations are biodegradability of the particles and adequate particle size. Such particles are under investigation for potential passive or active targeting purposes (Chapter 28), where the nanoparticle surface can be modified according to the targeting purpose.

A large variety of procedures have been developed for the production of nanoparticles depending on the nature of the polymer, the solubility of the drug and the desired structure of the particle. The particles may, for example, be formed directly by polymerization of mono- or oligomers in water or in an emulsion (O/W and W/O). Nanocapsules can be prepared by surface polymerization and condensation of monomers on the dispersed droplets. For the production of nanoparticles from preformed synthetic or natural polymers, physical methods are commonly used. For example, the polymer may be dissolved in an organic, water-immiscible solvent followed by emulsification in water by ultrasound or high-pressure homogenization and subsequent removal of the organic solvent (solvent evaporation method). Upon evaporation or extraction of the organic solvent, the polymer precipitates as fine particles. Polymer nanoparticles may also be produced by precipitation methods, for example by injecting a solution of PLGA in an organic water-miscible solvent into the water phase (solvent shifting method). The nanoprecipitation method to prepare drug-loaded polymer nanoparticles requires two miscible solvents in one of which both the polymer and the drug are soluble while neither one is soluble in the other solvent. When the drug/polymer solution is added dropwise to the non-solvent, instantaneous desolvation of the polymer occurs, resulting in the precipitation of the polymer under simultaneous entrapment of the drug in the polymer particles thus formed. Drug loading can be done during (most commonly) or after

Nanoparticle definition by IUPAC: Particle of any shape with dimensions between 1 nm and 100 nm.

Definition by the European Commission, 18th of October 2011:

A natural, incidental or manufactured material containing particles, in an unbound state or as an aggregate or agglomerate and where, for 50% or more of the particles in the number size distribution, one or more external dimensions is in the size range 1 nm–100 nm.

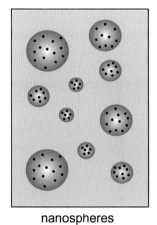

nanospheres

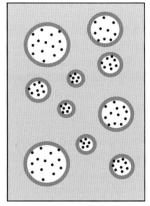

nanocapsules
(with oily core)

Fig. 20-3 Nanospheres and nanocapsules.

nanoparticle preparation by adsorption of the drug on the nanoparticle surface. Often, the nanoparticles are stabilized by addition of surfactants or polymers. After nanoparticle preparation, further processing steps such as nanoparticle purification by ultra-filtration and/or freeze-drying are applied in order to ensure storage stability of these formulations.

Although polymeric nanoparticles possess a great potential as drug carriers and have been intensively investigated for this purpose, nanoparticle based formulations have not yet been established on the market. Currently, only one medicine based on nanoparticle technology, which has been approved a few years ago, is available. Abraxane® presents an associate of the cytostatic drug paclitaxel with human albumin in the form of nanoparticles. It is manufactured by emulsifying a solution of paclitaxel in a water-immiscible solvent in an aqueous albumin solution by high-pressure homogenization, followed by evaporation of the water-immiscible solvent. The formed nanoparticles are stored as freeze-dried powder and are reconstituted in isotonic sodium chloride solution prior administration.

As an alternative to the above described polymeric nanoparticles, nanoparticles based on solid lipids such as fats or waxes are investigated as potential drug carriers (solid lipid nano-particles, SLN). Also for this type of nanoparticles, several preparation methods have been described. Most frequently, the molten lipid is emulsified in the water phase by high-pressure homogenization in the presence of amphiphilic stabilizers at elevated temperatures. The colloidal emulsion thus obtained is then submitted to cooling for recrystallizing the lipid nanoparticles. In addition to parenteral and peroral administration, solid lipid nanoparticles are also promising for dermal drug delivery. Up to now, however, no medicinal product based on this technology has reached the market.

> **Polymers for nanoparticles:**
>
> Natural:
>
> > For example: polysaccharides, proteins (albumin, gelatin)
>
> Synthetic:
>
> > For example: polylactic acid, poly(lactic-co-glycolic acid), polycaprolactone
>
> Semisynthetic:
>
> > For example: ethylcellulose

20.7 Drug Nanoparticles (Drug Nanocrystals)

The nanoparticulate systems presented so far in this chapter all have a carrier structure to which the active ingredients are bound or incorporated. It is, however, also possible to process a solid compound, e.g., a drug, into nanoparticles without adding any carrier material. Such particles must be prevented from agglomeration and aggregation by adding stabilizers such as surfactants or polymers, which adsorb on the nanoparticle surface. Drug nanoparticles may be obtained by nanoprecipitation (comparable to the precipitation of polymer nanoparticles described in section 20.6) or special size-reduction techniques. Most of the commercially available products based on nanocrystals are manufactured by the latter procedure. In addition to high-pressure homogenization (section 18.7.3), wet milling (stirred media mill Fig. 20-4) is frequently used. In this method, a suspension of micronized material is introduced into the milling chamber together with very small (e.g., 500 μm) spherical milling beads. The suspension and milling beads are kept in motion by the rotating milling device resulting in subsequent size reduction of the drug crystals down to the nm-size range. However, the increase of the total particle surface area leads to an enormous increase in surface energy. As a result, the particles have a strong tendency to agglomerate and grow in size, for example by Ostwald ripening processes. A proper choice of suitable stabilizers is thus of uppermost importance. Often polymeric stabilizers (e.g., cellulose ethers or polyvinylpyrrolidone) in combination with ionic surfactants (e.g., sodium lauryl sulfate or sodium dioctylsulfosuccinate) are used. However, for parenteral preparations nonionic stabilizers such as polysorbates have to be applied.

The *nanonization* technique is especially interesting for practically water-insoluble drugs, which are challenging to formulate by other ways to reach a sufficient bioavailability. This applies particularly for drugs, which cannot be processed together with polymers, surfactants or lipids due to their poor solubility properties. The transformation of a solid drug into nanoparticles results, for example, in an oral formulation, in a distinctly enhanced dissolution rate according to the Noyes-Whitney/Nernst-Brunner equation (Chapter 3.7). In addition, in accordance with the Ostwald-Freundlich relation, also a higher solubility can be expected for the nanocrystals. The latter is, however, only relevant with respect to improvement of bioavailability for very small particles (mid and lower nm-size range).

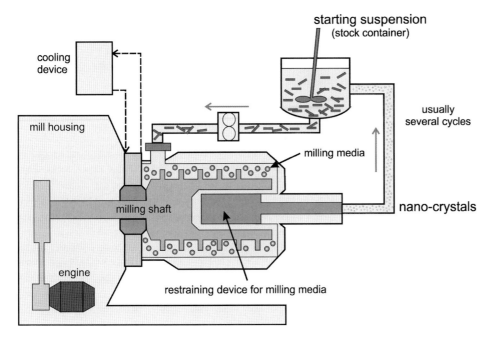

Fig. 20-4   Particle size reduction in a stirred media mill.

During the last few years, some medicines based on nanocrystal technology of poorly water-soluble drugs have reached the market (Table 20-2). In most cases, the nano-suspensions are processed into a dried form from which peroral formulations such as tablets or capsules can be produced. However, also liquid preparations are available. Further examples of nanoparticulate drugs are the nanosized pigments of zinc oxide or titanium dioxide that are applied as physical sun blockers. Finally, iron oxide suspensions stabilized with hydrophilic polymers (commonly dextran) are used as contrast agents for magnetic resonance tomography. These particles are so small (<200 nm) that they can safely be administered intravenously.

20.8   Microparticulate Systems

The range of possible applications and varieties of pharmaceutically used microparticulate systems is tremendous. Microparticles are usually defined as spherical particles in the μm-size range consisting of either a continuous matrix, in which the active ingredient is dissolved or dispersed (microspheres) or a liquid (occasionally also solid) core that is surrounded by a solid coating (microcapsules). In some cases, several small particles can be incorporated into a bigger one. The matrix and coating mostly consists of polymers, but also waxes may be applied. Particle sizes vary between 0.5 and 500 μm and are adjusted to the desired administration route. The rationale for the use of microparticles in pharmaceutical formulations includes taste and odor masking, formulation of oils as freely flowing powders, protection of volatile substances (e.g., essential oils) against evaporation, protection of drugs against physiological degradation processes or protection of the organism against undesired drug effects (e.g., irritation of the stomach), or to achieve retarded drug release. The terminology of

Table 20-2   Examples of Approved Medicines Based on Nanoparticulate Active Agents

Product	Drug	Application	Formulation
Rapamune®	Sirolimus	Immune suppression	Tablet
Emend®	Aprepitant	Anti-emetic	Capsule
Xeplion®	Paliperidone	Schizophrenia	Parenteral depot formulation (suspension)

the underlying processes is not always uniform. The incorporation of drugs into microparticulate formulations is, for example, often generally called *microencapsulation*, even when no defined core-coat structure is involved. The term *microparticles* most commonly refers to *microspheres*.

20.8.1 Microspheres (Microparticles)

Microspheres based on biodegradable polymers are well established as parenteral depot formulations especially for peptide drugs (e.g., Decapeptyl® N, Enantone® Depot, Sandostatin LAR®), but also for low-molecular weight drugs like risperidone (Risperdal® Consta®). They have in the meanwhile gained a substantial market potential. Due to the erosion of the polymer matrix in contact with physiological fluids combined with diffusion processes, the drug is released at the site of action in a controlled manner over a period of weeks to even months. Currently, exclusively polylactic acid (PLA), co-polymers of lactic acid and glycolic acid (polylactic-coglycolic acid, PLGA) as well as a star-shaped branched polymer with PLGA chains connected to a central glucose molecule, are used for this purpose.

20.8.1.1 Microsphere Preparations

The manufacturing of drug-containing microparticles may be accomplished by spray drying, coacervation or solvent extraction and evaporation from emulsions. In the latter methods, a solution of the drug and the polymer in an organic solvent is initially dispersed in an aqueous medium. Subsequently, the solvent is removed from the emulsion droplets resulting in precipitation of the polymer and formation of solid particles. Removal of the organic solvent may be achieved by applying a vacuum (evaporation) or by extraction into the aqueous phase, usually by dilution. Subsequently, the particles are separated from the aqueous medium and dried. Care should be taken to remove all residues of the organic solvent. When the active ingredient is insoluble in the organic polymer solution, it may be suspended or emulsified in it. This procedure is particularly suitable for the incorporation of hydrophilic peptides. For this, an aqueous peptide solution is first emulsified in the organic phase to form a W/O emulsion, which is subsequently emulsified in the aqueous external phase. The resulting W/O/W emulsion is further processed as described above.

Moreover, spray drying is also used to obtain microparticles. Active ingredients may be incorporated in the particles by processing the drug together with the polymer solution. Alternatively, the active ingredient may be added in the form of a suspension or emulsion. Essential oils, for example, are transformed into a dry powder, protecting the oil against evaporation, this way. By appropriate selection of the matrix material, the release rate of the drug can be adjusted depending on the requirements. Rapid drug release is obtained when using readily water-soluble polymers, whereas microparticles with a matrix of insoluble or poorly soluble polymers will release the drug more slowly.

20.8.2 Microcapsules

Traditionally, microencapsulation refers to a coating of finely dispersed liquid droplets or solid particles with coating materials such as gelatin and other natural or synthetic polymers. The thickness of the capsule wall is controlled by the manufacturing procedure, such as the amount of added coating polymer in relation to the material to be encapsulated. The amount of coating material is usually between 2% and 30% of the total capsule mass. Depending on the requirements, the coating can be nonpermeable, semipermeable, or permeable.

The microencapsulation technique had been revolutionary in several technical domains. Microencapsulation has made it possible to produce, for example, carbonless copy paper. The lower side of the upper sheet is here impregnated with a nearly colorless microencapsulated ink and the upper side of the lower sheet is coated with an acidic compound. By applying a pressure on the paper, such as upon writing, the microcapsules break and release the ink, which becomes colored in contact with the acid on the lower sheet. Other examples are microencapsulated flavoring agents as food additives or microencapsulated glues, which only become sticky upon applying a pressure.

The possibility to encapsulate individual solid particles or liquid droplets has also stimulated pharmaceutical formulation scientists. By microencapsulation, liquids can be converted into freely flowing powders while incompatibilities and instabilities can be circumvented. Other applications are taste masking and the already mentioned depot formulations.

20.8.2.1 Microencapsulation Processes

Microcapsules can be produced by means of coacervation. This stands for segregation in solutions of strongly solvatized macromolecules into two fluid phases, one enriched with the polymer and the other depleted of it. Generally, two types of coacervation can be distinguished. In case of *simple coacervation*, phase separation is induced by salting-out (e.g., with ammonium sulfate), temperature or pH changes or addition of ethanol. When two oppositely charged polymers (e.g., gelatin with a positive charge and gum arabic with a negative charge) are mixed, phase separation is obtained by charge neutralization. In this case, the process is called *complex coacervation*.

The microencapsulation procedure is initiated by dispersing the particles (or liquid droplets) of the material to be encapsulated in the solution of the wall material (Fig. 20-5A). Subsequently, the coacervation process is induced as described above. The polymer-rich phase forms droplets of the wall material (Fig. 20-5B) that precipitates on the surface of the dispersed particles (or droplets) until a continuous coating is formed (Fig. 20-5C). During this process, agglomeration of the particles (or droplets) is prevented by constant stirring. Afterward, the coating must be hardened by addition of other excipients such as cross-linking agents or additional physical treatments such as cooling (Fig. 20-5D). Finally, the formed and hardened microcapsules are separated from the liquid and dried. An example of (simple) coacervation induced by electrolyte addition is the phase separation of an aqueous solution of highly solvatized cellulose acetate-phthalate ions (CAP) upon gradual addition of di-sodium phosphate and sodium sulfate. The polymer precipitates as a soft gel coating on the surface of the dispersed drug particles. By further increasing the electrolyte concentration, the coating hardens.

The processes involved are represented by the phase diagram shown in Fig. 20-6. Phase diagrams are useful tools to optimize microencapsulation procedures. Four zones can be distinguished: In zone I, the macromolecules are only partly dissolved and the solution appears turbid. By addition of Na_2HPO_4, the macromolecules transform entirely into a sol and the solution becomes clear (zone II). In zone III, there is equilibrium between the sol and the gel phase of the macromolecules (coacervate). Zone IV represents a miscibility gap where

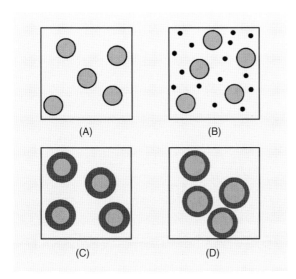

Fig. 20-5 Phases of the microencapsulation procedure (see text for details).

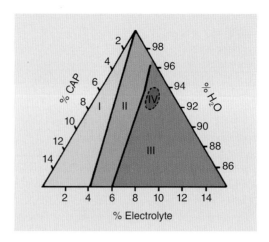

Fig. 20-6   Phase diagram for coacervation of CAP in the presence of electrolytes.

the ratio between electrolyte concentration and CAP concentration is optimal with respect to coacervation.

Drug particles dispersed in liquids can also be coated by other methods. Microencapsulation of water-soluble substances can, for example, be performed by using an organic solvent as dispersion fluid. Also, melting coating materials (e.g., solid lipids), can be used by processing them in an inert fluid. Finally, monomers dissolved in a liquid may be polymerized in the presence of a catalyst, followed by adsorption onto the particles to be coated (interfacial polymerization).

Microcapsules may also be produced by physical or mechanical coating procedures, e.g., in a fluidized bed device working according to the Wurster principle or with a Hüttlin Kugelcoater® (section 10.6.4). In these techniques, the solid particles in the fluidized bed are coated by subsequent spraying a solution containing the coating material whereupon the solvent rapidly evaporates in the hot air stream.

Further Reading

Danielsson, I., Lindman, B. "The definition of microemulsion." *Colloids and Surfaces* 3(4) (1981): 391–392.

Duncan, R. "Polymer therapeutics as nanomedicines: new perspectives." *Curr Opin Biotechnol* 22(4) (2011): 492–501.

Tan, M. L., Choong, P. F., Dass, C. R. "Recent developments in liposomes, microparticles and nanoparticles for protein and peptide drug delivery." *Peptides* 31(1) (2010):184–193.

Parenteral Formulations

21

21.1 General Introduction

The first medical injections in humans were performed already 1656, but it was the development of a syringe (1852), and in particular the ampoule that lead to the widespread use of this form of application. The glass ampoule was described for the first time by the pharmacist *Stanislas Limousin* in France and in Germany by *Louis Friedländer* simultaneously in the year 1886.

This way of application is known as parenteral administration (Gr. $\pi\alpha\rho\alpha$ ἔντερον, para enteron = beside the intestine), as opposed to enteral administration via the gastro-intestinal tract. Because systemic administration of a drug via for example the skin also bypasses the gastrointestinal tract, this should also be considered a parenteral application. However, according to the pharmacopeia only the formulations discussed in the following sections are defined as parenteral formulations.

Parenteral therapy offers significant advantages compared to enteral. The mere selection of the site of administration largely determines the onset and length of the drug action. When rapid drug action is required, the intravenous route is used. When a drug after peroral ingestion is inactivated in the stomach, is poorly absorbed or leads to stomach irritation, it may be directly introduced into the bloodstream. This is, for example, the case with most of the biotechnologically produced product and thus, these products need to be administered parenterally. Parenteral administration is also indicated in case the patient is unconscious. Also with preparations for injection it is possible to control the action of the drug. Drug formulations for injection with a depot action can be produced according to several principles (section 21.7). Solutions for infusion are furthermore used to restore plasma volume in case of severe blood loss or to provide a patient for a prolonged period of time with parenteral nutrition.

These advantages stand opposite a number of disadvantages. Despite the mass production of solutions in ampoules, injection therapy still is quite expensive as compared to other forms of treatment. In addition, only medical staff should administer drugs directly into the bloodstream. Beyond that, although often not justified, many individuals have a severe phobia toward receiving injections. Table 21-1 lists a number of types of administration routes for injections and infusions.

Preparations for injection are sterile solutions, suspensions or emulsions that are injected into the body for therapeutic or diagnostic purposes. They may be injected in the bloodstream, in tissues and or directly into organs. For the injection (Lat. *inicere*, to throw in), a needle is penetrating a physical barrier, such as skin. In contrast to infusions (Lat. *infundere*, to pour in; *infundibilia*), the parenteral administration via injection is often performed manually. There is somewhat an overlap of definitions when using infusion respectively syringe pumps for administration. Parenterals can be further defined by the container size. Small-volume parenterals (SVPs) are parenteral products in a container of maximum 100 mL nominal

Voigt's Pharmaceutical Technology, First Edition. Alfred Fahr.
© 2018 John Wiley & Sons Ltd. Published 2018 by John Wiley & Sons Ltd.

Table 21-1 Routes of Administration of Preparations for Injection and Infusion

Type of Injection	Description	Remarks
intravenous (i.v.)	in a vein (often in the crook of the arm or underarm vein)	Most rapid onset of action due to introduction directly in the bloodstream. Larger amounts of fluid (infusions) can serve to replenish blood pool, rectification of disturbances in electrolyte and water balance or as parenteral nutrition, or to administer certain pharmaceuticals (intravenous drip infusion). A special form of i.v. injection is the administration of hypertonic solutions for the eradication of varices.
intraarterial (i.a.)	in an artery	Rarely, must be performed while applying pressure.
intramuscular (i.m.) (often intragluteal)	in muscle (e.g., gluteal muscle)	When applying aqueous solutions, relatively rapid absorption; with oily solutions depot action.
subcutaneous (s.c.)	in subcutaneous tissue	Possibly slower absorption than after i.m. injection; also infusions are administered along this route (subcutaneous drip infusion). Patients may perform self-administration by s.c. injections.
intracutaneous (i.c.)	in cuticle (immediately underneath the epidermis)	For diagnostic purposes, application of local anesthetics
intrathecal (intralumbal)	between upper lumbar vertebra in the cerebrospinal fluid	For lumbar anesthesia; withdrawal of cerebrospinal fluid
intraperitoneal (i.p.)	in abdominal cavity	
intrapleural	in thoracic cavity	
intraneural	in a nerve	
perineural	in nervous connective tissue	
Intracardial	in the heart	
peridural (epidural)	in the epidural space	For peridural anesthesia
Intraarticular	in the joint	
Intravitreal	in the vitreous body (back of the eye)	

volume, whereas large-volume parenterals (LVP) exceed 100 mL. SVPs and LVPs differ in some requirements, such as allowed limits for subvisible particulates (Ph. Eur. 2.9.19).

Injection and infusion preparations are liquid preparations, or can be prepared as liquid from sterile powders or concentrates by dilution (reconstitution) with an appropriate diluent. Also, implants, emulsions, suspensions or gels may be administered parenterally.

21.2 Requirements of Solutions for Injection and Infusion

An adequate efficacy and safety of parenterally administered medication are guaranteed only when the following qualifications are met:

- Sufficient stability of the active ingredient during storage and administration
- Correct Accurate drug content and identity
- Use of appropriate containers that ensure maintenance of sterility (container closure integrity), allow adequate and correct withdrawal, dosing and administration and exclude adverse interactions between drug and container material
- Adequate safety and tolerability, implying:
  - Absence of microorganisms (sterility)
  - Maximum number of pyrogens and endotoxins (depending on the route of administration and volume administered)
  - Physiological tolerance of the formulation, including solvent and excipients

- Adequate tonicity (preferably, isotonicity)
- Adequate solution pH (preferably, isohydricity, i.e., pH 7.4)
- Essentially free of visible particles and compliant to limits for sub-visible particles

In principle, these requirements equally apply to injection and infusion solutions. Their fulfillment should be strived at in all possible cases. Because for injection fluids, only small volumes are administered, some deviations from physiological blood pH or osmolarity of the preparation will not or at least not significantly be relevant with respect to pain. Precise adjustment of isohydricity and isotonicity of injection fluids is therefore not absolute warranted and is often difficult to accomplish as the stability of the product may require a different pH and deviations from isotonicity. The absolute absence of pyrogens and particulates in injection fluids is practically not achievable, but nonetheless, always desirable and should be minimized.

Although there is great similarity between infusion and injection fluids, one should be aware that both formulations have their own specific features.

> **Not all parenteral formulations need be isotonic with blood:**
> Intravenous injections: Isotonic
> Subcutaneous: Isotonicity not essential
> Intramuscular: Isotonicity not essential
> Intrathecal: Isotonic
> Intraoccular: Isotonic

21.3 Container Closure Systems and Devices for Parenteral Applications

21.3.1 Ampoules

Properties and production of traditional ampoules, as well as of ampoules for injection, ready-to-use syringes, flasks and infusion bags, are described in section 27.3.4. Opening an ampoule by scratching with an ampoule file has become an obsolete procedure. Instead, nowadays either score ring or one-point-cut (OPC) ampoules are used. With the score ring ampoule an enamel ring consisting of inorganic salts is burnt in the neck of the ampoule causing a strain in the glass by virtue of a difference in expansion coefficient, which permits the tip to be easily snapped off. The OPC ampoule has a preformed scratch at the neck, which allows the tip to be snapped off by simply pressing the point mark with one thumb. Care should be taken to prevent small glass particles from entering the injection fluid. This may occur particularly with ampoules of low-quality glass. Ampoules for powdered material (dry ampoules) and for oily substances usually have a wide tip opening. Finally, special glass ampoules are used for infusion solutions (large dual-tip ampoules).

Nowadays, novel products developed as parenteral products are rarely—respectively never—developed as ampoules, given the potential risk of particulate contamination of solution content during the opening, also for OPC.

21.3.2 Glass Vials, Rubber Stoppers, and Aluminum Crimp Cap

The most common container closure system (CCS) for parenteral products is nowadays the glass vial, closed with a rubber stopper and an aluminum crimp cap. The glass vial consists of type 1 glass and can have different dimensions (2–100 mL). The rubber stopper is preferably latex-free and consists today in many cases of bromo- or chlorobutyl rubber and has defined dimensions and elasticity that allow introduction into the glass vial. Finally, the stopper and vial is closed using an aluminum crimp cap that also serves as closure.

21.3.3 Cartridges and Ready-to-Use Syringes

Injection technology has produced numerous developments, some of which will be presented here. "Cartridges" are or have to be placed in an injection device before use. On the other hand, ready-to-use syringes are, as the word says, "ready to use." Syringes are, in many cases, made of glass, and increasingly of plastic. Syringes can contain an embedded (glued in) needle or a luer-type lock. The needle or luer lock is generally protected by a rubber (rigid needle shield, RNS). Injection using a syringe can be performed manually, by pushing the plunger rod and thus, the backside rubber stopper and thus, expelling the injection solution, that is, initiating the injection. Syringes may also be included into a device (e.g., pen or autoinjector) to facilitate the injection process for a patient or healthcare provider.

21.3.4   Needle-Free Injection

Needle-free injections have also been evaluated in the past, using so-called jet, pressure or spray injectors for subcutaneous, intramuscular, or intradermal administration of parenteral preparations.

The injection is performed without the use of a cannula by means of high pressure or a tensioned spring or gas-driven with a compressed gas (N_2, CO_2, He). Advantages over needle injections are: possibly painless; needle phobia excluded, and avoidance of needle injuries, particularly by nursing personnel.

Disadvantages are the significantly smaller injection volume, potential product incompatibility, possible dose variability and variability in pharmacokinetics as well as the higher price. Besides for treatment of diabetes, thrombosis prophylaxis and local anesthesia such injectors may be particularly interesting for high-throughput vaccinations.

Fluid preparations in the form of solutions or suspensions (insulin, somatostatin) have been mostly administered with so-called DCJIs (disposable cartridge jet injectors), that is, high-pressure injectors with exchangeable single-use ampoules (maximally 1–3 mL). The latter also contain the injector head and the discharge nozzle (Fig. 21-1A).

Powder injectors (also named solid jet injectors) are for example provided with a pressurized container filled with compressed gas (Fig. 21-1A). When the pressure container is opened, the gas expands and accelerates the powder particles to a high velocity (600 m/s), which then can permeate 50–100 μm into the skin (Fig. 21-2A). Ideally, the particles are spherical, mechanically stable and have a size of 30 to 50 μm. Most often sugar-based powders or vaccine-loaded gold particles are used. While with needle injection the preparation is injected at a single spot, the powder injector delivers a dose of about 30 mg at an area of ∼2 cm^2 in the hypodermis, the DCJI in different skin depth areas (epidermis, dermis and hypodermis). Particles accelerated by spring systems (Fig. 21-1B) may not reach the same skin depth due to the spring, as during the actuation the pressure will drop (according to the law of Hooke).

The powder injector principle is already used in clinical studies—for example, immunization by using gold microparticles coated with DNA encoding for viral or bacterial antigens.

A similar technological principle is applied in the liquid jet injectors. A high-speed jet (100–200 m/s) punctures and penetrates the skin (Fig. 21-1B). This technology is used for immunization and also for the delivery of insulin.

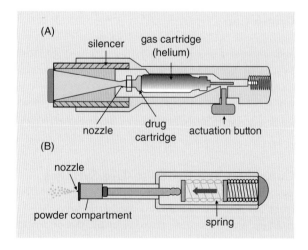

Fig. 21-1 Principle of a needle-less injection system: (A) gas-driven injector; (B) mechanically driven injector.

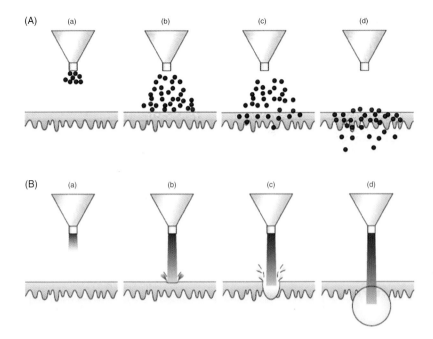

Fig. 21-2 **(A) Drug delivery of a needleless injection system: gas-driven injector: (a) ejection of particles, (b) impact of particles on skin, (c) permeation through stratum corneum, (d) permeation into epidermis; (B) Liquid jet injector (a) formation of liquid, (b) initiation of skin hole formation, (c) progress of hole formation, (d) deposition of drug at the terminal of the hole in a spherical pattern.** Reproduced with permission from Arora *et al.* 2008, Elsevier.

21.4   Preparation of Solutions

21.4.1   Solvents

21.4.1.1   Water for Injection (WFI) as a Solvent for Parenteral Preparations

For most parenteral drugs, water is the main if not only solvent or dispersion agent, and in case of infusion preparations, it is administered to the body in large quantities. It is therefore of eminent importance as an excipient for the production of parenteral preparations. In section 5.2.1 we elaborately discussed production procedures and quality parameters.

21.4.1.2   Nonaqueous Solutions

Organic solvents serve as basic substance for injection solutions under these conditions:

- ▢ The active ingredient is insufficiently soluble in water.
- ▢ The active ingredient readily decomposes in water and the product should be not dried.
- ▢ Depot action is required.

> **Examples of some non-aqueous water-miscible solvents employed for parenteral formulations:**
> polyethylene glycol 400, dioxolanes, dimethyl acetamide, glycerine, ethanol

21.4.1.3   Fatty Oils

A large number of active ingredients are processed as oily solutions or suspensions for injection purposes. The individual pharmacopeias prescribe various vegetable oils for such preparations. Peanut oil, olive oil, almond oil, sunflower oil, soybean oil, and sesame oil are the most commonly products in this connection. In several occasions, castor oil has shown favorable dissolution capacity for active ingredients. These oils are physiologically inert and are well tolerated, provided that they are well purified and possess low acid and peroxide content. When necessary, free fatty acids can be removed by alcohol extraction. Because intravenous administration could lead to a lung embolism due to immiscibility with blood plasma, applications are limited to intramuscular of subcutaneous injection preparations. Oily solutions or suspensions remain at the site of administration for prolonged periods and may release the active ingredients only slowly so that activity might last for up to a few months.

21.4.1.4   Synthetic Fatty Acid Esters

A disadvantage of fatty oils is that at low temperatures they solidify and have to be warmed before use under winter conditions. This is especially relevant for veterinary and army applications and in case of calamities. Ethyl oleate, on the other hand, remains fluid. It has significantly lower viscosity, resulting in better ability to handle and inject with smaller needles and often, more rapid absorption. A further advantage is the well-defined chemical composition. Because several drugs may be prone to oxidation, the use of N_2 is recommended, as well as the addition of antioxidants and protection from light.

Rubber materials and many polymers can be affected by organic solvents. Ethyl oleate specifically serves as a solvent for sex hormones (steroids). For the same purpose, oleyl oleate, isopropyl myristate, isopropyl palmitate, benzyl benzoate, and neutral oil (Miglyol® 812) are used. Thorough toxicological assessments are required prior use. Medium-chain triglycerides are distinguished by adequate dissolving properties for many drugs, low viscosity, and high chemical stability (e.g., during hot-air sterilization).

When it appears that a drug does not dissolve at adequate concentrations in either an aqueous or an oily liquid, the use of solution enhancers may become necessary (section 3.9.9).

21.4.2   Basic Ingredients of Solutions

Solutions for injection and infusion are commonly prepared by compounding the active ingredient (by weight or volume), additions of excipients as solid compounds or stock solutions and the use of solvent (e.g., water for injection). Thus, concentration is given as m/V. The density of the formulation should be individually measured and assessed. Aqueous solutions with a low concentration of dissolved ingredient have a density of close to ~1 g/cm³. Therefore, we can fill up the solution to the required concentration with pure water in weight (1 mL = 1 g). For highly concentrated ingredients (e.g., glucose 40%) density will strongly deviate from 1 g/cm³. In that case, we will have to fill up exactly to the required volume in order to obtain the desired concentration. For example, 100 g 50% glucose solution takes a volume of only 85 mL. To minimize particulates and reduce potential microbiological bioburden, the solutions are sterile filtered (section 4.2.8). In cases where terminal sterilization is applicable, parenteral products must the terminally sterilized (e.g., using dry heat or autoclaving, or alternatively chemical sterilization or irradiation). When a product cannot be terminally sterilized, for example due to degradation of the active ingredient—which is the case for protein drugs—the sterile filtration is performed in aseptic environment in order to ensure sterility of the final drug product.

21.4.3   Isotonic Solutions

21.4.3.1   Introduction

Injection and infusion solutions as well as eye drops should to be adjusted osmotically close to the tonicity of blood, tissue and tear fluid (identical osmotic pressure). Blood and tissue fluid possess identical osmotic pressure. Injection of hypertonic or hypotonic liquid will likely not change the injection sensation because the excess of blood volume will rapidly dilute the hyperosmotic fluid, however nonisotonic infusions also have been reported to possibly cause damage to blood vessel walls and erythrocytes. When hypotonic solutions are introduced in the bloodstream, water is transported into the erythrocytes across their semipermeable cell membrane. This will result in a volume increase and enhanced intracellular pressure. Already a 0.4% NaCl solution suffices to cause this phenomenon. When sufficient amounts of a 0.3% NaCl solution are administered, the pressure in the red blood cells may increase to an extent that they could burst (hemolysis), which would result in release of hemoglobin into the plasma. The opposite effect is brought about by hypertonic solutions (higher osmotic pressure than blood), which may cause shrinkage of the erythrocytes due to water loss. The result is plasmolysis. Administration of an isotonic solution results in fluid exchange in an equilibrium situation. An isotonic (with blood) NaCl solution (0.9%) has an osmotic pressure equivalent to 0.686 MPa, 6.86 bar) which approximately equals that of

---

Typical excipients for solutions for parenteral applications include:

Antimicrobials (typical concentrations used) e.g. Benzyl alcohol (0.5-10%), methylparaben (0.01-0.18%), propylparaben (0.005-0.035%), butylparaben (0.015%), thiomersal (0.001-0.02%) etc.
NOTE: According to the actual Ph. Eur, no preservatives should be included if volume of injection exceeds 15 ml unless use of preservatives is justified.

Antioxidants: (typical concentrations used) Ascorbic acid (0.02-0.1%), sodium bisulfite (0.1-0.15%), tocopherol (0.05-0.075%)

Emulsifiers: phospholipids, Tweens, Spans, sodium deoxycholate etc.

Buffers: Acetate, phosphate, benzoate, citrate, bicarbonate etc.

Tonicity modifiers: Glycerin, lactose, mannitol, dextrose, sodium chloride, sorbitol etc.

Chelating agents: Sodium salts of ethylenediaminetetraacetic acid (sodium EDTA)

blood (0.662 MPa, 6.62 bar) and will therefore not cause any change in the erythrocytes following i.v. administration.

Hypotonic solutions can also be adjusted to isotonicity with body fluids by addition of suitable substances, assuming product stability is still warranted.

21.4.3.2   Osmotic Pressure and Freezing Point Depression

When isotonizing a drug solution its osmotic pressure is equalized with that of blood. The osmotic pressure of a solution represents its tendency to pull the solvent (in most cases water) across a semi-permeable membrane (of a cell for instance). The solution thus experiences a volume increase that will put pressure on the enclosing wall material. The counter pressure that is capable of stopping the solvent flow equals the osmotic pressure. This could for instance be the hydrostatic pressure building up in a standpipe above the solution. Like freezing point depression and boiling point elevation, osmotic pressure is a colligative term, that is, it depends on the number of osmotically active particles in the solution but not on their physical nature. According to J. H. van't Hoff (1887), the osmotic pressure π can be calculated as follows:

$$\pi = \frac{N}{V} \cdot R \cdot T = c \cdot R \cdot T \tag{21-1}$$

N/V concentration c (mol/L) (N = number of moles, V = volume) | R = gas constant
T = absolute temperature

This relation applies exactly to ideal, that is, strongly diluted solutions in which intermolecular interactions may be ignored. For electrolytes the number of osmotically active particles per volume is determined by the number of ions into which a molecule of the electrolyte dissociates and, if the electrolyte dissociates only partially, also on the dissociation coefficient α. Both effects are taken into account by the van't Hoff factor (i).

$$i = 1 + \alpha\,(n - 1) \tag{21-2}$$

n = number of ions into which one molecule of the electrolyte dissociates
($n = 2$ for binary, $n = 3$ for tertiary electrolytes).

From this follows the calculation of the osmotic pressure:

$$\pi = i \cdot c \cdot R \cdot T \tag{21-3}$$

Because the direct experimental assessment of the osmotic pressure is cumbersome, the osmotic properties of a solution are most often determined by means of the freezing point depression, which, as a colligative property, is directly proportional to the osmotic pressure.

The freezing point depression is obtained from the molal concentration c of the active particles and the cryoscopic constant K of the solvent (for water $K_f = 1.86$ K $\cdot$ kg$\cdot$ mol^{-1})

$$\Delta T = K \cdot c \qquad \text{or} \qquad \Delta T = K \cdot m \cdot n/M \cdot L \tag{21-4}$$

| ΔT = freezing point depression referred to pure solvent (K)
| K = cryoscopic constant (K $\cdot$ kg mol^{-1})
| c = molal concentration of the dissolved osmotically active particles with c =
        mol/kg (as opposed to the molar concentration, the molal concentration is
        volume independent because following a change in temperature or
        concentration volume may change as well.
| m = mass of the dissolved substances (g)
| M = molecular mass of the dissolved compound (g/mol)
| n – number of ions into which the substance dissociates upon dissolution
| L = mass of the solvent (kg)

In addition to the ionicity n, also in this case the ionization degree α needs to be taken into account, for example by means of the van't Hoff factor i. Like for the osmotic pressure, also the freezing point depression deviations from this rule are observed when the solution can no longer be considered ideal. The osmolality (symbol: osm; unit: mol) characterizes the mass quantity of the osmotically active particles. The concentration of the osmotically active particles is designated as osmolarity (mol/L) or osmolality (mol/kg). The osmolality of an aqueous solution is the ratio between the freezing point depression of the solution and the cryoscopy constant of water.

$$\frac{osm}{m} = \frac{\Delta T}{1.86 K \cdot kg \cdot mol^{-1}} \tag{21-5}$$

For practical purposes, an adequate approximation of the iso-osmotic concentration of solutions containing nonelectrolyte solutes can be made based on the freezing point depression of plasma (0.52 K) and the known molecular mass of the solute (see Example: "Calculation of the Amount of NaCl Required to Prepare a Solution Isotonic with Blood"). Due to intermolecular or interionic interactions an exact calculation of the osmotic pressure or the freezing point depression is fraught with uncertainties. For weak electrolytes, it often fails because the concentration-dependent degree of dissociation is not known. Particularly in case of weak electrolytes, experimental determination is therefore to be preferred (see below).

A solution with the same osmotic pressure or freezing point depression as the reference system (e.g., serum, plasma, tissue, tear fluid) is designated iso-osmotic resp. iso-cryoscopic. Such a solution will in most cases also be isotonic, that is, physiologically, it will be osmotically inactive and tolerated without irritation. Nonetheless, it should be taken into account that some pharmaceutical substances, even in iso-osmotic concentrations, may lead to hemolytic reactions following i.v. administration. In these cases, osmotic pressure and tonicity are not equivalent; such iso-osmotic resp. iso-cryoscopic solutions behave as if they were hypotonic with respect to blood. This deviating behavior is caused by the partial permeability of biological membranes, which are not ideally semi-permeable and therefore allow not merely permeation of water but also of substances such as ammonium chloride, ethanol or urea. Also micelle-forming ingredients or partially ionizing salts yield lower values than calculated.

Example

Calculation of the Amount of NaCl Required for the Preparation of a Solution Isotonic with Blood

By converting equation 21-4, we can calculate the mass of a substance required to produce a certain freezing point depression:

$$m = \frac{\Delta T \cdot M \cdot L}{K \cdot n} \tag{21-6}$$

| m = amount of substance required for desired freezing point depression (g)
| ΔT = desired freezing point depression (K)
| M = molecular mass of the dissolved substance (mol/g)
| L = mass of the solvent (kg)
| K = cryoscopy constant of the solvent (K · kg mol^{-1})
| n = ionicity (number of ions into which one molecule of the substance dissociates)

With $\Delta T = 0.52$ K (freezing point depression of blood plasma) and K = 1.86 K· kg mol^{-1} we obtain:

$$m = \frac{0.52 K}{1.86 K \cdot kg \cdot mol^{-1}} \cdot \frac{M \cdot L}{n} = 0.28 \frac{mol}{kg} \cdot \frac{M \cdot L}{n}$$

For an iso-osmotic sodium chloride solution ($M_{NaCl} = 58.45$ g/mol) we find for L = 1 kg solvent a required amount of salt to be weighed of 0.818 g for 100 g solvent. This value approximates the 0.9% NaCl solution designated as isotonic with blood, but nonetheless already reveals a certain deviation from the ideal situation.

21.4.3.3 Determination of Freezing Point Depression

In order to assess the freezing point depression of a solution we have to determine the freezing temperatures of the pure solvent and of the solution. For routine assessments the freezing point depression of pharmaceutical solutions is performed with an electronic osmometer (semi-micro-osmometer, Fig. 21-3). This allows a quick assessment on minute amounts of solution/solvent. In this device the fluid to be assessed is cooled in the cooling block down to below its freezing point but without allowing it to rigidify. Only after reaching a particular undercooled temperature crystallization is induced by a mechanical trigger. The released crystallization heat leads to a raise in temperature to a maximal value that is recorded as the rigidification point (Fig. 21-4). In case of a pure solvent the temperature of the rigidifying fluid rises until the melting point and remains at this value till all fluid has solidified (plateau value) and subsequently decreases again. In case of a solution the maximum temperature recorded as freezing temperature is maintained only for a very short time. This is due to the condition that only crystals of the pure solvent separate off, which causes the solution to become more and more concentrated and the freezing point to decrease.

Assessment of freezing point depression by means of the Beckmann apparatus (Fig. 21-5) is based on the same principle as described above. Technically, this instrument is simpler, but substantially more time-consuming. The Beckmann thermometer has a graduation in 0.01 K so as to allow very precise readings, but only in a small temperature range.

When a more conventional thermometer with a wider temperature range is used instead, the instrument will also allow assessment of the rigidification point of other substances.

21.4.3.4 Calculation of the Amount of Excipient to Be Added to Attain Isotonicity

This assay is based on Freezing Point Depression phenomenon. To calculate the amount of a substance (e.g., excipient) that is required to equalize tonicity, we measure the freezing point depression of the hypotonic drug solution (ΔT_A value) and subtract this value from 0.52 K (ΔT value of serum or tear fluid). The difference represents the ΔT deficit that has to be compensated by addition of a suitable additive. The ΔT_A values (Table 21-2) that are mostly maintained for 1% solutions of pharmaceuticals may be found in relevant

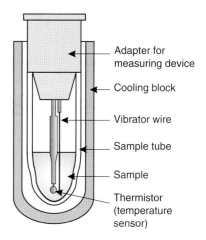

Fig. 21-3 Semi-micro-osmometer (measuring head).

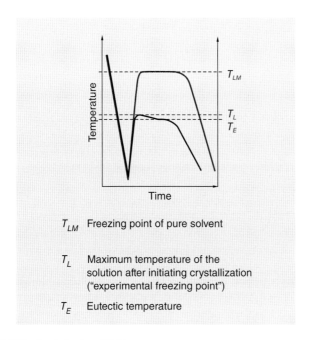

T_{LM} Freezing point of pure solvent

T_L Maximum temperature of the solution after initiating crystallization ("experimental freezing point")

T_E Eutectic temperature

Fig. 21-4 Rigidification behavior of fluids.

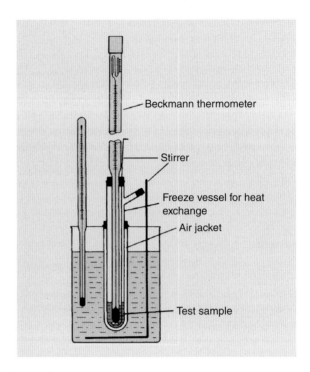

Fig. 21-5 Beckmann thermometer.

handbooks (such as DAC). When the prescription contains multiple ingredients, the sum of the ΔT_A values applies. When the calculation is performed according to equation 21-7 the required amount of the excipient to attain isotonicity is obtained in percent values.

$$\text{Excipient}(\%) = \frac{0.52K - n(\Delta T_A)}{\Delta T_H} \tag{21-7}$$

| n = drug content of the solution (%)
| ΔT_A = freezing point depression of a 1% solution of the active ingredient (K)
| ΔT_H = freezing point depression of a 1% solution of the isotonizing agent
        (for NaCl = 0.58 K, for KNO_3 = 0.32 K)
| 0.52 K = freezing point depression of blood serum

Example

The assignment is to make 50 mL of a solution containing 1 g of procaine hydrochloride isotonic with the help of sodium chloride. The concentration of drug solution is calculated as 2%, the ΔT_A value of the 1% solution is 0.12 (Table 21-2) and the ΔT_H value for NaCl as isotonizing agent amounts to 0.58K. Substituting these values in equation 21-7 yields:

$$\text{NaCl}(\%) = \frac{0.52K - 2 \cdot 0.12K}{0.58K} = 0.483\% \tag{21-8}$$

To make 50 mL of the procaine solution isotonic with blood 0.24 g of NaCl are required.

21.4.3.5   Assessment by Making Use of the Sodium Chloride Equivalent

The sodium chloride equivalent (E value) indicates the amount of NaCl (g) that, when dissolved in water, yields a solution with the same osmotic activity as a solution of 1 g of the drug under consideration in the same amount of water. The E values of a large number of pharmaceutical ingredients may be found in pharmaceutical handbooks. For the calculation, the

Table 21-2   Δ*T*A Values of Active Agents and Excipients at 1 g/100 mL in K

Active Agent	ΔT_A
atropine sulfate	0.074
benzylpenicillin sodium	0.100
boric acid	0.283
calcium chloride dihydrate	0.300
calcium chloride hexahydrate	0.219
cocaine hydrochloride	0.090
diacetyl tannin-protein-silver	0.096
diethazine hydrochloride	0.110
dihydrostreptomycin sulfate	0.034
ephedrine hydrochloride	0.165
epinephrine bitartrate	0.100
fluorescein sodium	0.182
homatropine hydrobromide	0.097
potassium chloride	0.439
potassium iodide	0.210
potassium nitrate	0.324
lidocaine hydrochloride	0.130
narcotin hydrochloride	0.079
sodium acetate	0.260
sodium chloride	0.576
sodium citrate	0.178
sodium bicarbonate	0.380
sodium iodide	0.248
sodium tetraborate	0.241
neostigmine bromide	0.120
oxytetracyclin hydrochloride	0.075
papaverine hydrochloride	0.061
physostigmine salicylate	0.090
pilocarpine hydrochloride	0.130
procaine hydrochloride	0.122
scopolamine hydrobromide	0.069
silver nitrate	0.190
streptomycin sulfate	0.034
sodium salts of sulfonamides (average)	0.135
tetracaine hydrochloride	0.124
tolazoline hydrochloride	0.180
zinc sulfate	0.083

amount (mass) of the required pharmaceutical is multiplied by the E value from Table 21-3. In case of more than one pharmaceutical, the NaCl equivalent of each individual substance is calculated. The sum of the sodium equivalents of the individual pharmaceuticals is then subtracted from the quantity of sodium chloride theoretically required for the total volume. The result is the amount of NaCl that must be added to the formulation to obtain an isotonic solution.

Table 21-3   Sodium Chloride Equivalents and Isotonicity Factors of Some Drugs

Drug	NaCl Equivalents (*E*)	Isotonicity Factors (*I*)
ascorbic acid	0.18	19
benzylpenicillin potassium	0.16	17
clonidine hydrochloride	0.22	23
ethylmorphine hydrochloride	0.15	16
histamine hydrochloride	0.40	43
morphine hydrochloride	0.16	15
sodium iodide	0.30	38
pilocarpine hydrochloride	0.22	23
procaine hydrochloride	0.21	23
streptomycin sulfate	0.06	6
tolazoline hydrochloride	0.31	33

Ph. Eur. 2.2.35 Osmolality _____

USP ⟨785⟩ Osmolality and Osmolarity

JP 2.47 Osmolarity determination

The osmotic concentration can be defined in two ways, one being mass-based concentration (osmolality, osmol/kg) and the other, volume-based concentration (osmolarity, osmol/L). The Ph. Eur. describes only osmolality, USP mentions both and gives instructions for conversion and the JP prefers to express; the osmotic concentration as osmolarity. The osmotic concentration is assessed according to all pharmacopeias by determining the freezing point depression by means of an osmometer. This consists of a sample cell, a cooling appliance (commonly a Peltier module), a temperature measurement device (thermistor), and a mixing mechanism to trigger the crystallization process.

For calibration, the pharmacopeias present seven standard solutions (NaCl solutions of varying concentration). Water can also be used as a standard solution (0 mosmol/kg). As a rule, a dual-point calibration is performed with two different standard solutions just covering the expected osmotic concentration of a sample solution.

An alternative version of this method, which is also based on the use of E values, calculates the volume of water (V) in which to dissolve the required amount of pharmaceutical substance in order to obtain an isotonic preparation.

$$V = m \cdot E \cdot V' \tag{21-9}$$

| V = volume of water required to dissolve the pharmaceutical substance (mL)
| m = mass of the required pharmaceutical (g)
| E = sodium chloride equivalent of the pharmaceutical (g^{-1})
| V' = volume of an isotonic aqueous NaCl solution containing 1 g of NaCl (111.1 mL).

This isotonic solution is completed to the desired final volume with an isotonic solution of an excipient (usually 0.9% NaCl in water). Because V' represents a constant, further calculation simplification may be obtained by using the isotonicity factor I as the product of E· 111.1 mL. This leads to:

$$V = m \cdot I \tag{21-10}$$

Also, isotonicity factors may be found listed in handbooks.

Example

How to isotonize 50 mL of a solution containing 1 g of procaine hydrochloride with the help of sodium chloride? The E value for procaine hydrochloride is 0.21 (Table 21-3)—that is, 1 g of procaine is equivalent to 0.21 g of NaCl (the amount of NaCl in 50 mL of a 0.9% NaCl solution is 0.45 g), yielding a difference of 0.24 g NaCl. This is the amount that has to be added to the procaine solution in order to obtain an isotonic solution.

One may also obtain information on required amounts of isotonizing additives manually from tonicity curves or nomograms. Nomograms graphically represent the relation between molality and freezing point depression. As these are pre–Information Age procedures, we will not go into detail of these procedures.

21.4.4   Isohydric Solutions

The pH of body fluids is in the weakly alkaline range, around 7.4. Physiological buffer systems (e.g., phosphate) provide sufficient buffer capacity close to pH 7.4. Proteins like albumins in the blood show buffering capacity and pKas as well. The numerous amino groups of proteins are predominantly responsible for this phenomenon.

When an injection fluid with a pH value deviating from that of blood is introduced into the bloodstream, it will be rapidly diluted and buffered by the plasma. Depending on the buffer capacity of the injected or infused solution and administered volume and speed, compatibility may differ.

Also i.v. injections with more extreme pH values (e.g., pH 3, corresponding to 0.001 M HCl or pH 11, corresponding to 0.001 M NaOH) are tolerated under normal conditions. Although pH values of infusion solutions should preferably be analogue to blood values prior to administration (isohydricity), any addition of acid or base is usually not recommendable to products that have been developed and produced at any different pH, as this pH change may adversely impact product stability. Isohydric conditions are not considered an essential requirement. pH values <3.5 or >9.5 have been reported to cause damage to the endothelium and a pain sensation for subcutaneous products; however, in general controlled clinical studies are lacking. The buffer capacity of parenteral preparations, that is, the basicity or acidity that can be titrated, is at least as important as the pH value as such. An isotonic NaCl solution that can show a pH value of 5 due to the dissolved CO_2 from the air can be infused without objections because the protons thus added are very few in number and are therefore rapidly neutralized by the blood fluid. A 5% sodium bicarbonate solution of pH 8.4, on the other hand, that is, deviating less from the isohydric pH value than the NaCl solution, has a substantial buffer capacity. As much as 12 mL 1 M HCl will be required to adjust 200 mL of such a solution to pH 7.4. This explains that—in particular, for solutions with a high buffer capacity—it is important to understand and assess the potential clinical impact and relevance of the formulation on biological buffer systems and homeostatic regulation mechanisms of an already weakened organism. Often buffer systems are applied for formulations, such as histidine, citrate, acetate, or phosphate buffers (mixtures of dihydrogen phosphate and monohydrogen phosphate), depending on the target pH (but commercial formulations should not be changed by hospital pharmacists).

21.4.5 Stabilization

Injection fluids containing *oxidation-sensitive pharmaceutical agents* may require special stabilization measures. Since chemical reactions proceed at a higher speed at elevated temperature it is essential that the drugs are protected from heat such as steam or heat sterilization. Some excipients may carry peroxides or metals into the formulation, thus, increasing oxidation of the active ingredient.

In order to avoid oxidation reactions, oxygen should be minimized or excluded, which can be achieved by gassing with an inert gas. This procedure may be required at all stages of the preparation—that is, during weighing, dissolving, and filtration. Suitable gases are, in particular, nitrogen. These gases are obtained in adequate purity from pressurized flasks and, after filter sterilization used for the creation of a protective atmosphere during the filling stage (section 25.4.2).

Nitrogen gassing alone often appears not to provide sufficient protection from oxidation. In such cases, the drug solution is fortified with an antioxidative stabilizer having a stronger negative redox potential than the drug itself. The following substances have been employed as antioxidants, although their individual use needs to be closely evaluated: methionine cysteine, ascorbic acid, α-tocopherol and 2-butyl-4-hydroxy-anisol and others (see section 5.6.1). Since oxidation is catalyzed by heavy metal ions that are already active at concentrations below conventional chemical impurity limits, *heavy metal scavengers* such as EDTA (Titriplex®) also have been employed, yet, these may also pose challenges for safety in some cases.

To avoid the enhancing *influence of light* on oxidation processes, in many cases it is necessary to evaluate the impact of light during production and storage. In some cases, special protection from light may be required. Previously, containers made of brown glass have been used to protect light-sensitive drugs from decaying. For optimal stabilization, it may be required to prepare and store the preparation in absence of a buffer substance at a pH value that guarantees maximal stability (section 25.4.2).

Preparations that do not tolerate heat sterilization, autoclaving, chemical sterilization or irradiation, must be prepared aseptically using sterile filters. *Drugs susceptible to hydrolysis* are filled into adequate containers, dried (e.g., lyophilized) in these containers and reconstituted before use. Lyophilization may increase the wettability and thus, solution behavior of some active ingredients.

In certain cases preservative agents may have to be added to injection fluids to prevent bacterial contamination. That applies for example to parenteral preparations in multidose containers in order to ensure that the preparation maintains sterility also after repeated withdrawal of single doses. In most cases, when the active ingredient itself possesses antimicrobial activity, there is no need for additional preservation measures (see section 25.5.2).

Addition of preservatives is not suggested when the volume of a single dose exceeds 15 mL (with a few exceptions) or when it concerns an application which excludes this on medical grounds. The latter includes intrathecal, epidural, intra- or retro-ocular administration. Antimicrobial efficacy of a preservative must be demonstrated as regulated by the pharmacopeias.

For elaborate substantiations concerning stability and stabilization of pharmaceutical substances and formulations, see chapter 25.

21.4.6   Sterilization

Parenteral preparation should preferably undergo terminal sterilization. With aqueous solutions, emulsions, and suspensions, this can be performed by autoclaving at $\geq 121°C$ for at least 15 minutes, heat sterilization, chemical sterilization (e.g., using ethylene oxide), or irradiation. In some cases, sterilization conditions must be adapted, such as in case of oily solutions and suspensions by means of hot air at 160° to 180°C. In case of thermolabile substances, aseptic production using sterile filtration is warranted (see section 4.2.8).

21.4.7   Pyrogens

21.4.7.1   General Introduction

As long as 100 years ago, after intravenous administration of large doses of a proven sterile solution, occasionally severe symptoms were observed such as high fever, shivering, discomfort, shortness of breath, circulatory insufficiency and head and joint aching. Such hyperthermic conditions often lead to leukopenia (shortness of white blood cells), followed by leukocytosis (increase in white blood cell count). Under unfavorable conditions, such infusion incidents may even lead to death.

Substances that can trigger hyperthermia following parenteral application are called pyrogens (from Greek: $\pi \tilde{v} \rho$ (pyr) = fire (pyromaniac!) or fever; pyrogen: fever-inducing). Pyrogens stimulate phagocytosing cells to release interleukins, TNF-α and prostaglandins, which, via the hypothalamus, induce an elevation of body temperature. One special group of pyrogens are the *endotoxins*. Because of their biological and physicochemical properties, they are of particular importance (Table 21-4).

Endotoxins are cell wall constituents of Gram-negative bacteria (*E. coli*, *salmonellae*, *pseudomonads*). Endotoxins induce fever already at extremely low (ng) quantities. Besides endotoxins, numerous other pyrogenic substances are known, both from living organisms (Gram-negative and -positive bacteria, viruses, fungi) and nonliving material (zinc compounds derived from rubber or polymer seals, iron and copper ions, drugs such as plant alkaloids, steroids, polynucleotides with CpG motifs).

The essential and most pyrogenic moiety of the endotoxin complex is a phosphorylated polysaccharide tightly connected to a lipid component. The other components of the integral

Table 21-4 Structure of Endotoxins

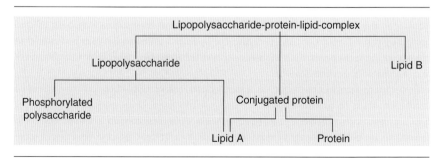

complex, comprising a second lipid moiety and a proteinaceous structure, can be easily split off from the complex and usually have no physiological activity. In exceptional cases, also the protein moiety may display pyrogenic properties. Because the endotoxins are of a size in the macromolecular range, they cannot be removed from a solution by a sterilizing-grade filter. Boiling and even dry air sterilization at 180°C does not lead to destruction of the endotoxins. Complete degradation can only be achieved by autoclaving for several hours or by heat treatment for 1 hour at 200°C or for 30 minutes at 250°C. However, this is obviously not compatible with the stability of most active substances and excipients. Some specific filters, e.g., with positive surface charge (e.g., Zeta Plus®), can partly remove the negatively charged endotoxins from solutions. (Beware that the filter will become saturated and may gradually lose its effectiveness!). In view of their molecular mass (>10 kDa), endotoxins may be reduced by ultrafiltration. For products that need to be manufactured aseptically, using a sterilizing-grade filter, endotoxin limits of raw material and equipment are be warranted, and measures such as de-pyrogenation, must be taken and validated for all material in use and contact with product solution.

From the foregoing it may have become clear that effective removal of endotoxins is not an easy task. Pyrogenic impurities may occur in distilled water after prolonged storage, in active as well as excipients ingredients, adsorbed to containers used for production and storage of parenteral solutions and not in the least in syringes, cannulas, and infusion tubing. Therefore, adequate measures must be taken. The production of pyrogen-free parenteral products (i.e., insurance of maximum limits depending on route of administration and administration volume) is required, and it must be ascertained that they remain nonpyrogenic up to the time point of their application. Only when from a pharmaceutical and medical point of view everything possible has been done to exclude the formation of pyrogenic agents and to completely remove any pyrogen already present, can the occurrence of hyperthermia and any further undesired effects of the parenteral application of a pharmaceutical preparation be excluded.

The Ph. Eur. requires that parenteral products comply with requirements for pyrogen and endotoxin limits. The term *pyrogen-free* should not be understood in an absolute way. It merely indicates that, when tested in a biological test (rabbit test), a certain dose will not cause an increase in body temperature. Today, the rabbit pyrogen test is mostly avoided, as this would require animal testing. Preferably the limulus amebocyte lysate (LAL) test is performed, which is able to detect bacterial endotoxin reliably. Obviously, the risk of hyperthermia is correspondingly higher when using infusion solutions (large volumes). Limits for endotoxin units are thus dependent on amount of volume administered as well as administration route.

An unconditional requirement that nonetheless remains is that also the personnel in the clinic maintains the corresponding safety measures by careful cleaning of all supplies such as syringes, cannulas and infusion necessities and ensuring that proper and adequate sterilization procedures are conducted.

21.4.7.2   Pyrogen-Free Water

In the production of pyrogen-free solutions multiple aspects require attention.

Distilled water that has been stored for prolonged periods of time commonly contains a multiplicity of germs and is therefore not free from pyrogens. Even when produced entirely in accordance with the rules or after repeated distillation, distilled water may merely be considered pyrogen-poor. For obvious reasons, water that is intended for injection should meet exceptional requirements. It is general experience that, when distilled water is processed into injection or infusion solutions immediately following distillation and when these solutions are steam-sterilized, biological testing for pyrogens yields a permissible result.

A common procedure to make a solution pyrogen-free is ultrafiltration. Furthermore, pyrogenic substances may be effectively removed from aqueous solutions by means of special adsorption filters. The endotoxins adsorb to the filter material. Obviously, the binding capacity is limited so that pyrogens may end up in the filtrate once the adsorption capacity of the filter is exceeded. It will be equally obvious that removal of pyrogens from weakly contaminated solutions is more secure than from heavily contaminated solutions.

Removal of pyrogens may also be accomplished by means of aluminum oxide columns or by filtration over activated charcoal. Also by γ-radiation (Cobalt 60) pyrogen depletion may be achieved. However, irrespective of the applied procedure, it will always remain necessary to check the final product for the absence of pyrogens.

For the testing fluids on bacterial endotoxins, pyrogen-free water is required to prepare and dilute the necessary reactants. This is obtained by triple-distillation, paying care that during distillation no droplets are transferred from the distillation vessel into the distillate. Obviously, the endotoxin test of this water must give a negative result.

21.4.7.3   Freeing Drugs and Excipients from Pyrogens

Only active ingredients and excipients of the highest purity grade may be used for the production of injection and infusion solutions. Decisive for solution quality are furthermore the storage conditions. Dust and moisture are often the source of pyrogenicity; therefore all ingredients have to be stored in tightly sealed containers and under dry conditions. Particularly substances of biological origin bring along the risk of being contaminated with pyrogenic material. Examples are antibiotics, gum arabic, glucose, fructose, sodium citrate and lactate, dextran, heparin, liver extracts and insulin. Guaranteed elimination of pyrogens in actives and excipients would be for example 1-hour heating at 200°C. However, only few substances (e.g., NaCl) will tolerate such treatment without being destroyed. If such substances are found to be unacceptably contaminated with pyrogens, they cannot be used for pharmaceutical manufacture and either destroyed or returned to the manufacturer in case he is responsible for the impurity.

21.4.7.4   Pyrogen Elimination from Containers and Stopper Materials

Before subjecting containers and materials involved in the production and storage of solutions for injection or infusion to a pyrogen elimination procedure, the objects and materials are thoroughly cleaned. Whenever possible, pyrogen elimination is accomplished by means of dry heat.

21.4.7.5   Testing

A pyrogen test is performed with the *rabbit test*, or bacterial endotoxins—constituting a majority of pyrogens—via the *limulus test* or the *monocyte activation test*.

In the rabbit test, the solution to be tested is injected in an ear vein of a rabbit and body temperature is rectally monitored. This test includes all types of pyrogens, not only the endotoxins.

The limulus-amebocyte-lysate-test (LAL test, Pyrogel®, Pyrotell®) is up to 100-fold more sensitive than the rabbit test and an *in vitro* test. It only detects endotoxins and no other pyrogens. The test can be performed within 90 min. It is to be noted that the LAL test may be sensitive to disturbances by other substances. Although the LAL test is not considered an animal test, it is brought to mind that the lysate is obtained from the hemolymph of the horseshoe crab (*limulus polyphemus* or *tachypleus tridentatus*). The horseshoe crab is a living fossil and has a primitive immune system that is localized in the granules of the amebocytes. The latter are a cellular component of the blue-colored blood of the crab. These amebocytes agglutinate with endotoxins. A lysate that is obtained from these cells also reacts with endotoxins, which leads to gel formation that reveals the presence of endotoxins. With approval of the relevant authority, the LAL replaces the rabbit pyrogen testing. As is common practice for biological products, the lysate sensitivity needs to be determined for each individual batch. The LAL test is standardized against a reference pyrogen, the Reference Standard Endotoxin (RSE), which is represented by *E. coli* endotoxin EC-6. One endotoxin unit (EU) is defined as 0.1 ng of EC-6. Recently, the LAL test has been reported to possibly report false negative values due to endotoxin masking or *low endotoxin recovery*. This can be caused by specific active ingredients or certain combinations of formulation excipients. Other reference standards and further optimization of the LAL test are being developed. Also, recombinant Factor C is now mentioned by the Ph. Eur. for endotoxin testing.

The monocyte-activation test (MAT, for example PyroDetect®) is based on the *in vitro* activation of human monocytes by pyrogens, which is accompanied by the release of pro-inflammatory cytokines (e.g., TNF-α, IL-1β, IL-6), which may be quantified by ELISA or RIA. These cytokines play a role in the pathogenesis of fever. The MAT was accepted in 2010 by the Eur. Ph. as an alternative to the rabbit test along with a product specific validation. At present various new methods are under development. A bacterial phage is able to immobilize lipopolysaccharide selectively and quantitatively to a solid phase (microtiter plate). The test matrix and with that numerous potentially interfering factors are removed by washing. The LPS then activates the zymogen form of the recombinant factor C. The reaction involving the conversion of a fluorogenic substrate can then be quantified fluorimetrically (EndoLISA®).

Ph. Eur. 2.6.8 Pyrogens

Ph. Eur. 2.6.14 Bacterial endotoxins
Ph. Eur. 2.6.30 Monocyte-activation test
Ph. Eur. 5.1.10 Guidelines for using the test for bacterial endotoxins
USP ⟨85⟩ Bacterial endotoxins test
USP ⟨151⟩ Pyrogen test
JP 4.01 Bacterial endotoxins test
JP 4.04 Pyrogen test
JP G4 Microorganisms—Decision of limit for bacterial endotoxins

The testing for pyrogenic substances is the topic of four chapters in the Eur. Ph., two chapters in the USP and three chapters in the JP. Three different test systems can be employed for the detection and quantification of pyrogenic substances. The rabbit test and the monocyte-activation test are able to detect a variety of different substances with pyrogenic properties whereas the bacterial endotoxin test is specific for lipopolysaccharides of Gram-negative bacterial origin, which are the most important types of pyrogens in pharmaceutical preparations.

Test for pyrogens

The test for pyrogens according to Ph. Eur. 2.6.8 (Pyrogens), USP ⟨151⟩ Pyrogen test and JP 4.04 (Pyrogen test) is based on the measurement of the body temperature increase arising from an intravenous injection of a (sterilized) solution in a rabbit. The test is performed with a group of three animals whose rectal temperature is measured up to 3 hours following the injection and at intervals of maximally 30 minutes. For each animal, the difference between the maximally measured temperature and the initial temperature is determined. The USP considers the test as "passed" (negative) if no rabbit shows an individual rise in temperature of 0.5° or more. The criterion of Ph. Eur. and JP is the sum of the temperature rises of the three animals tested. It must not exceed a value of 1.15°C to pass the test according to Ph. Eur. or must be $\leq 1.3°C$ in case of JP. If these limits are exceeded, it is permitted to repeat the test and make the evaluation with specified criteria based on the extended number of animals.

Test for bacterial endotoxins

The test for bacterial endotoxins describes an in vitro method exploiting a lysate from the hemolymph of the horseshoe crab. In the absence of evidence to the contrary, the test for bacterial endotoxins is preferred over the test for pyrogens, since it is usually considered to provide equal or better protection to the patient. The pharmacopeias describe six methods to implement the test, based on three different principles: gel formation, turbidity assessment (turbidimetry) and the color reaction of a chromogenic peptide. The gel formation method can be performed as a limit test (Ph. Eur. method A) or, quantitatively, by evaluation of a four-step geometric dilution series (Ph. Eur. method B). In both cases, the reaction mixture consisting of test solution and lysate is incubated, in accordance with the manufacturer's recommendations, protected from vibrations for a fixed period of time (commonly 60 minutes at 37°C). When at the end of the incubation period a solid gel is formed which stays in the test tube upon turning it upside down, the test is considered positive (failed). The turbidimetric and chromogenic methods are based on the photometric assessment of the reaction process. In the former case turbidity is measured and in the latter case light absorption of a chromophore is determined which is released from a synthetic chromogenic substrate by the reaction of endotoxins with the lysate. Both procedures may be performed either as a kinetic (Ph. Eur. method C kinetic-turbidimetric and

D kinetic-chromogenic) or as an end point (Ph. Eur. method E end-point-turbidimetric and F end-point-chromogenic) assay. In the end-point methods turbidity and absorption are assayed respectively after a fixed period of time. The limit test according to the gel-clot technique serves as a reference because it should always be employed when the test for bacterial endotoxins is prescribed without specification of the assay method. Before using any lysate solution, it is mandatory to check with a four-step dilution series whether the lysate sensitivity determined in one's own lab is not lower than 0.5 times and not higher than two times the value given by the manufacturer. Furthermore, it is required to perform a negative control test with pyrogen-free water as well as to exclude by means of a "test for interfering factors" that the test is either positively or negatively influenced by the product to be tested. When evidence of the presence of interfering substances is obtained, these must be removed by means of appropriate treatment, or by reducing their concentration by dilution of the test solution. The maximally permitted dilution before reaching the lower detection limit (Maximum Valid Dilution, MVD) may be calculated as the product of the endotoxin limit and the concentration of the test solution, divided by the labeled lysate sensitivity λ. The endotoxin limit is obtained as the ratio between the threshold pyrogenic dose of endotoxin per kg of body weight and per hour (K) and the recommended maximal dose of the product per kg body weight and per hour (M):

$$MVD = \frac{\text{Endotoxin limit} \times \text{Concentration of test solution}}{\lambda} \qquad (21\text{-}11)$$

$$\text{Endotoxin limit} = \frac{K}{M} \qquad (21\text{-}12)$$

For intravenous preparations K amounts to 5.0, for intravenous radioactive drugs 2.5 and for preparations for intrathecal administration 0.2 IU of endotoxin per kg body mass and per hour.

Monocyte-activation test

The underlying principle of the "Monocyte-activation test" (MAT) is the detection or quantification of pro-inflammatory cytokines (e.g., TNF-α, IL-1β, IL-6) involved in the pathogenesis of fever. Since exogenous pyrogens stimulate the secretion of these endogenous mediators, their presence may be detected by the MAT method. The test includes is sensitive to all substances with pyrogenic activity and is not limited to bacterial endotoxins. After product-specific validation it may replace the rabbit test. The sample to be tested is mixed with human monocytes or monocytic cells (fresh peripheral heparinized blood, peripheral blood mononuclear cells or a human mononuclear cell line) and incubated under cell culture conditions at 37°C in a humidified atmosphere containing 5% CO_2. To eliminate interfering factors, the sample is diluted before the test. The maximally permissible dilution (MVD) is calculated in a similar way as for the test for bacterial endotoxins (equation 21-11), while substituting the limit of detection (LOD) for λ. LOD may be obtained from a blank test, performed in quadruplicate, with the help of the calibration curve. The analytical method is not further specified in the Ph. Eur. Commonly, the concentration of IL-1β or IL-6 is determined following a 16- or 24-hour incubation.

The test may be implemented as a quantitative test (method A), as a semi-quantitative test (method B) or as a reference lot comparison test (method C). For method A, a calibration curve is calculated from the values obtained from with four dilution steps of an endotoxin standard. Each one of the dilutions is incubated with cells from four individual donors or with cells from 1 passage of a human monocytic cell line and subsequently subjected to a cytokine assay. From the test solution a three-step dilution series is prepared in a concentration ratio 1:2:4. At the end of the incubation time, the raw data (in quadruplicate) are converted by means of the calibration curve into endotoxin equivalents. The endotoxin concentration of the test sample is obtained as the mean value of the results from the three dilution steps after correction for the dilution factors. The presence of interfering factors in the test sample may be excluded when the value of a sample that is spiked with endotoxin standard, after subtraction of the result for an identical nonspiked sample, is within 50% to 200% of the spiked concentration.

In the semi-quantitative method B the test signal at the detection limit (mean ($n = 4$) of the blank signal + 3 × standard deviation) is taken as the decision criterion between positive and negative test signals. Only one conclusion is possible in that case, that is, the pyrogen content of the product is either above or below the permitted limit.

Method C is used when in the test on interfering factors the recovered amount of spiked endotoxin is outside the 50% to 200% range of the spiked concentration. In this case, the samples are not compared with dilutions of an endotoxin standard but rather with a validated reference batch of the product.

21.5   Suspensions for Injection

Suspensions for injection can be distinguished in aqueous and oily preparations. All requirements listed in chapter 19 that are demanded of suspensions should be fulfilled. In accordance with those, special attention may be paid to Stokes' law on particle size and the density of the suspension agent. Particle size also deserves attention from another point of view. By means of well-balanced mixtures of particles of different crystal size (or solubility) a preparation may be obtained in which initial dose and depot dose are combined (e.g., hormone preparations). In such preparations, particle size should not exceed 40 μm and are limited to subcutaneous or intramuscular administration. Such suspensions represent the principle of prolongation of activity. For additional possibilities to achieve prolonged drug action of parenteral formulations see section 21.7.

Suspensions for injection contain, in addition to excipients, which reduce sedimentation (mucilages) or facilitate resuspension of a sediment (surfactants, peptizer), often also isotonization agents, buffer substances, preservatives etc. The optimal zeta potential is −50 mV; at this value an easily redispersible flaky system with a loosely packed, voluminous sediment may be obtained. By producing a rigid thixotropic gel with the aid of suitable viscosity enhancers (aluminum stearate) any sedimentation may be prevented. Such preparations may still be administered by means of a syringe provided that they are shaken immediately before application. When an active ingredient is not stable in aqueous environment, it may be filled as a dry powder in injection containers (e.g., lyophilisate), together with relevant excipients. In these cases an injectable suspension is obtained by addition of water for injection shortly prior administration.

21.6   Parenteral Depot Drug Formulations

Parenterally applicable preparations with prolonged action have been available for quite some time. But in more recent years, they have clearly gained considerable attention.

These formulations are predominantly administered intramuscularly, more rarely subcutaneously. The problems encountered in the development of depot formulations are as complex and multifaceted as those experienced for peroral formulations. A variety of principles, applied either individually or in combination, has been mobilized to help fulfill these purposes (Table 21-5). Additional pharmacological methods have already been introduced in section 12.2. In the following paragraphs the most important chemical, pharmacological and technological principles will be discussed.

21.6.1   Chemical Methods

These are based on the reduction of water solubility of the drug. In this connection, quite often use is made of the influence of salt formation on drug activity. Intramuscular injections of benzylpenicillin-G sodium will lead within 30 min to high blood levels, which, however, drop rapidly. By using a less soluble procaine salt therapeutically active blood levels may be sustained for 12 to 24 hours. When this salt is combined with additional substances and when solutions of high viscosity are used, further prolongation of drug activity may be achieved. Further improvement of drug circulation time may be obtained by applying oily suspensions

Table 21-5   Principles Applied to Prolong Drug Activity of Injection Preparations

Principle	Method	Examples
pharmacological interference with a second active ingredient	occlusion by vasoconstrictors, inhibition of metabolism	epinephrine with local anesthetics
chemical modification of the active ingredient	use of poorly soluble salts, esters, complexes; pro-drug formation	procaine penicillin, protamine insulin, protamine zinc insulin, vitamin B_{12} zinc tannate complex, fatty acid and polyphosphoric acid esters of steroid alcohols, vitamin B_{12} as hydroxyl cobalamine for sustained release
pharmaceutical-technological modification of the active ingredient and/or the injection vehicle	variation of particle size/shape, choice of vehicle (e.g., oily rather than aqueous solution), use of aqueous or oily suspensions, addition of viscosity enhancing substances to water (mucilages) or oil (aluminum stearate), addition of adsorbents and complex builders, use of solutions from which the active ingredient precipitates in a microcrystalline form in the tissues, use of implants, formation of polymer embeddings as microparticles	diphtheria and tetanus toxoid adsorbed to aluminum hydroxide or aluminum phosphate gel, vitamin B12 as hydroxyl cobalamine for sustained release, adsorbed vaccines (e.g., binding to highly disperse aluminum oxide), binding of vaccines to antigens, polyphlorctine phosphate as complex builder with ACTH, poly-hydroxy fatty acid embeddings

of penicillin-G procaine, which consists of particles (<5 μm) suspended in peanut oil to which 2% aluminum stearate is added. In order to achieve a rapid onset of the drug effect, a dose of water-soluble penicillin-G sodium is added to such depot penicillin formulations. By replacing procaine by other nitrogen bases, functional penicillin levels may even prevail for more than one week.

Sustained-release formulations of steroids are preferentially prepared from esters dispersed in an oily solution. Particularly steroid hormones have been investigated elaborately; they are applied as esters of a multitude of organic acids. The esters as such are inactive. Only following uptake by the body, esterases catalyze the release of the active steroid with its free hydroxyl groups. Depending on the nature of the acid moiety the hydrolysis proceeds with different velocities. By mixing esters of different acids in one preparation, instant and depot effect may be combined. When acids with two or more carboxyl functions are used, while only one is used for esterification with the steroid, the remaining free carboxyl group(s) (or free OH groups) may be used to couple for example a phosphate group so as to enhance water solubility (e.g., disodium salt of prednisolone-21-phosphate).

21.6.2   Pharmaceutical-Technological Methods

Because absorption from aqueous solutions usually proceeds relatively rapidly, it is common practice to apply *oily solutions* as a vehicle when retarded absorption is required. A similar effect may be achieved with other nonaqueous solvents. Release depends on the solvent/water *distribution coefficient* of the active ingredient as well as of the *viscosity* of the solution. In case of aqueous solutions, release and diffusion of the active ingredient are substantially decreased by addition of viscosity-enhancing macromolecules, while in case of oily solutions, aluminum stearate (~2%) is added to achieve this purpose. Nonetheless, care should be taken that the solutions remain suitable for injection purposes (easy flow through syringe needle) ("Gels for the production of injection preparations"). Also because of intensified pain sensation limits are set to viscosity enhancement. For example, hyaluronic acid is applied as a viscoelastic gel to smoothen wrinkles.

In situ systems are fluid preparations, mostly based on polymers, which only after introduction into the body form a biodegradable semi-solid or solid depot (*in situ* gel formation). Such solutions may be sterilized by filtration; they are readily parenterally applicable and cause less discomfort. A disadvantage is that the form of the depot is not controllable after injection. Until the onset of gelation a rapid, often rapid unwanted release of active ingredient may occur. To effectuate gelation, various formulation components or physical effects are required, which may provoke tissue damage.

Dependent on the way they are formed, various *in situ* systems may be distinguished. Thermoplastic pastes (PLGA, poly-ortho-ester) need to be warmed to above body temperature (37° to 60°C) in order to fluidize the preparation before administration and will solidify upon cooling down to 37°C. Thermo-gelation polymer solutions, on the other hand, (e.g., Poloxamer) have low viscosity and only upon injection will undergo a sol/gel transition. Based on this principle ReGel®, consisting of an ABA triblock copolymer (PLGA-PEG-PLGA) may form a depot application of interleukin-2 or paclitaxel.

InGell Gamma Hydrogel (PCLA-PEG-PCLA) encapsulates poorly soluble substances in micelles, which only at the injection site at body temperature form a gelatinized depot. In all cases, gel formation follows immediately after injection; release of active ingredient occurs subsequently by erosion.

Furthermore, radical or ionogenic (alginate + calcium, chitosan + phosphate) reactions may cause chemical or physical cross-linking immediately after application to form a depot.

However, this brings along a higher risk of tissue toxicity due to chemical reactions. Besides, a pH change may be responsible for chitosan, dissolved in an acidic medium, to gelatinize upon injection in the (neutral) body fluid. Glycerol monostearate and glycerol monolinoleate in aqueous media will form *in situ* cubic phases in which pharmaceutical substances may be embedded.

Alternatively, the precipitation of biodegradable polymers may be exploited to form a depot. To that end, the polymers are dissolved in a biocompatible organic solvent, from which, upon contact with the aqueous body fluids, the polymer will precipitate or viscosity will increase due to diffusion of the organic solvent (Atrigel®).

Very often, aqueous and oily suspensions containing poorly soluble active ingredients are employed to achieve a reduction of the absorption rate. The magnitude of this effect may in addition be manipulated by a proper choice of the particle size. As may be expected, in case of aqueous suspensions larger particles will result in more prolonged therapeutic effect. By contrast, in oily dispersion agents a similar effect is often attainable with micronized particles. Clearly, small particles in an oily dispersion medium do not experience the favorable (as compared to larger particles) release conditions that apply for an aqueous dispersion (more specifically, the intensified contact with the tissue fluid); this results in a reduction of the release and absorption rates. Occasionally, W/O emulsions serve as depot vehicles for water-soluble drugs. An interesting pharmaceutical formulation is represented by aqueous crystal suspensions, which are in particular widely applied in the area of hormone therapy. Such formulations represent aqueous injectable suspensions containing hormone crystals of variable size. Predominantly, hormone esters are used in such preparations (acetic, propionic, butyric, benzoic).

Furthermore, adsorbents and complex builders frequently find application in this connection. As an example, we present the complexes made of insulin with protamine and metals, such as zinc. Vitamin B_{12} suspended in oil and converted to an aluminum monostearate gel likewise represents a proper depot effect. In depot formulations often water-soluble macromolecular compounds (dextran, polyvinylpyrrolidone, gelatin and sodium carboxymethylcellulose) are used. Their release-prolonging effect is at least in part accounted for by viscosity enhancement, but it is likely that complex formation plays a role as well. These macromolecules find especially application in slow-release preparations of antibiotics, antihistaminic drugs, anesthetics, hypnotics and adrenal hormones.

In many cases a drug only becomes poorly absorbable once in the body. When a poorly water-soluble drug is dissolved in an organic solvent that is miscible with water, the substance will precipitate upon intramuscular injection of this solution due to dilution with tissue fluid and will then be poorly absorbed by the body.

The depot formulations for parenteral administration also enclose implants. These are solid, sterile, mostly cylindrically shaped objects, individually wrapped in a sterile package,

During the last decade, we have also seen the emergence of biopharmaceuticals, which are covalently coupled to macromolecules such as polyethylene glycols.

For example: Plegridy® (Biogen, USA) is a PEGylated interferon beta for subcutaneous injection, approved for the treatment of multiple sclerosis. PEGylated interferon is injected once every two weeks which compares favourably with the conventional therapy requiring 2–3 times weekly administration of interferon beta. A major drawback of such a strategy is that the active pharmaceutical ingredient needs to be reapproved by the regulatory authorities for example via the 'New Drug Application' procedure for the US-FDA.

which are inserted subcutaneously via an incision in the skin and release their active ingredient over a period of several weeks or months (e.g., Profact Depot®, Zoladex®). Implants may merely consist of an active substance, but more commonly this is compressed together with excipients or embedded in a polymer matrix, for example by means of melt extrusion, or coated with a polymer membrane. Especially hormonal preparations (ovulation inhibitor, prostaglandins) and antibiotics are administered in this way. Since the polymeric carrier materials, such as silicones, are not biodegradable, the empty vehicle has to be removed. This procedure can be circumvented by using biodegradable polymers (e.g., poly-lactate).

Biodegradable microparticles (e.g., Decapeptyl®Depot, Enantone® Depot) constitute multiple small depot units, which can be applied easily and without causing discomfort (section 20.8.1). Further possibilities to establish a depot effect are offered by the application of nanoparticles (section 20.6) and liposomes (section 20.3).

21.7   Implantable Therapeutic Systems

Subcutaneously or intraperitoneally implantable osmotic miniature pumps (controlled release pumps, Alzet®, Alza Corp. Palo Alto/USA) for pharmacological investigations in small laboratory animals have found widespread application in basic research (Fig. 21-6). After application, water from the interstitial fluid can flow at a controlled rate across a semipermeable rigid membrane in the system. An osmotically active substance attracts the water and thus compresses a reservoir consisting of an impermeable flexible membrane which contains (a solution, suspension or emulsion of) the active ingredient. The compression of the reservoir causes the drug to exit through the delivery portal. The rates of water influx and drug release are constant as long as there is an excess of osmotically active substance. The pump may be refilled with needle and syringe. The mini-pumps have a capacity of 200 μL and a constant release rate of 1 μL/h with a life span of 1 or 2 weeks. Comparable osmotic systems with a higher capacity (2 mL), release rate (up to 10 μL/hour) and life span (up to 4 weeks) are available.

A further development of the Alzet® pump for application in human medicine is the DUROS® system that is applied subcutaneously and is based on the same osmotic principle. A variation is represented by the combination with a miniaturized catheter, which allows direct delivery to the target tissue. The Viadur™ implant system containing leuprorelin acetate as the active ingredient is available on the U.S. market as a system for palliative treatment of prostate carcinoma. The reservoir consists of a titanium alloy and contains the drug dissolved in DMSO, separated by an elastomeric seal of tablets with osmotically active and swellable excipients (NaCl, sodium carboxymethylcellulose, Povidone). Influx of water is controlled via a semi-permeable polyurethane membrane, while the release of drug is controlled via an outlet made of polyethylene. The drug is continuously released with zero-order kinetics in a period of 12 months.

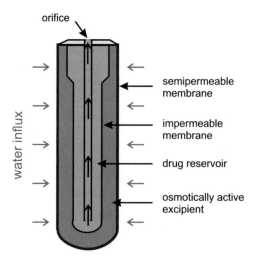

Fig. 21-6 Controlled release pump by Alzet®.

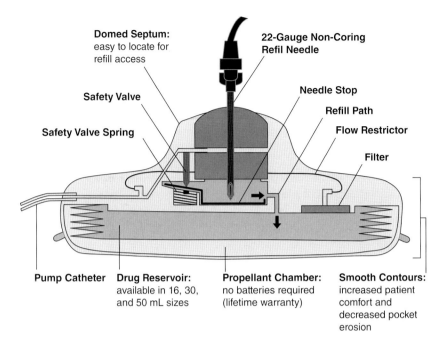

Fig. 21-7 Codman Model 3000 Constant flow implantable infusion controlled release pump (shown in refill modus). Reproduced with permission from Macmillan Publishers Ltd: Spinal Cord, Ethans et al. 2005.

In the United States, also other implantable pumps, operating via a propellant gas (e.g., Freon), have already been approved for human therapeutic applications. With release rates of up to 3 mL/d they find application for delivery of cytostatics and morphin in cancer therapy.

21.8 Therapeutic Systems (TS) for Infusion Therapy

Also therapeutic systems for long-term infusion therapy have been designed, such as for instance the SynchroMed Infusion System, InfusAid® Pump or Codman pump (Fig. 21-7). The active ingredient is contained in a pressurized reservoir (maximally 60 mL solution) and is programmed for continuous intravenous delivery for 24 hours via a tubing. The system may be carried inconspicuously attached to the under or upper arm. It is predominantly in use for anticoagulation treatment, antibiotic therapy in chronic renal and urinary tract infections, as well as for cytostatic therapy (e.g., Travenol®). There is also considerable interest in portable TS for insulin delivery. Worldwide, the number of such devices has increased substantially within just a few years. Whereas for pumps with constant flow rates dosage may only be adjusted by changing the concentration in the reservoir, programmable infusion pumps allow programmed external control of time and dose.

TS with a closed control cycle are under development. They will include sensors, a computer, and a feedback system. Although not yet available in ready-to-use form, the future development of such systems is certainly conceivable. Implantation of glucose sensors coupled with a TS that delivers insulin to the organism according to need may conceivably become a reality in the not so distant future. Such developments would have a revolutionary effect on the treatment of diabetes.

21.9 Biopharmaceutical Aspects

Whereas in case of i.v. injections (introduction directly into the bloodstream) there is obviously no absorption phase, and thus, bioavailability is 100%, for other administration routes (in particular i.m and s.c) the active ingredient first has to cross the capillary walls in order to arrive from a localized tissue region in the vascular system. The capillary system allows an exchange between blood and tissue and is highly permeable to the vast majority of pharmaceutical substances. The pore radius of peripheral capillaries in humans is approximately 2 to 4 nm and thus essentially larger than that of membrane pores. Capillary walls may be considered highly porous lipid membranes with a much weaker barrier function than the epithelial layers of the gastrointestinal tract (section 7.1). This implies that the absorption of drugs from the subcutaneous or muscle tissue proceeds more readily than via the epithelial layer. Nonetheless, biopharmaceutical problems may occur that are based on structural diversity and functional changes of the capillary wall whose permeability in individual organs and tissues strongly varies and, in addition, diminishes with age.

Lipid-soluble substances permeate the capillary wall rapidly, while the permeation of lipid-insoluble compounds will depend on the pores discussed (section 7.5.1). For lipid-soluble substances, the permeation rate depends on the diffusion coefficients, concentration gradient, and lipid-water distribution coefficient and ionization grade.

The absorption process depends, furthermore, on the blood flow in the capillaries and the condition of the intercellular matrix that predominantly consists of hyaluronic acid. Upon subcutaneous injection, especially of larger volumes, an induration at the injection site can be observed. Addition of hyaluronidase to the injection fluid will cause this to spread over a much wider capillary area. A comparable effect may be achieved by adjusting the administration technique: Intramuscular injection involves a larger muscle area, making an enhanced diffusion surface available.

21.10   Special Infusion and Injection Solutions

21.10.1   Ringer Solution

For a long time, insufficiency of blood volume was corrected by infusion of a 0.9% solution of sodium chloride; more recently, Ringer solution serves as well as an important therapy for short-term volume deficits. Besides NaCl, it contains KCl and $CaCl_2$, while in some modifications also $NaHCO_3$ or sodium acetate is added (Ringer acetate solution) or, alternatively, sodium lactate (Hartmann solution). Solutions without $NaHCO_3$ can be heat sterilized; autoclaving of Na-bicarbonate solutions is only possible after gassing with CO_2. Non-gassed solutions must be aseptically manufactured using sterilizing grade filters.

21.10.2   Sodium Bicarbonate and Other Neutralizing Solutions

Steam sterilization of such solutions is not possible without taking certain measures since carbon dioxide may be released. An increase in pH may be the result as well as the production of physiologically dubious sodium carbonate and the formation of calcium carbonate precipitates (Ca^{2+} ions may arise from the glass container or as an impurity of the $NaHCO_3$. The escape of CO_2 (and the resulting pH increase) may also occur during preparation of $NaHCO_3$ solutions; it can be avoided by careful stirring during the dissolution process. More up-to-date preparation instructions will require gassing with CO_2 to allow autoclaving. Such solutions may be kept in storage for up to 4 weeks, during which pH will hardly change. Because of the pressure conditions during heat sterilization the containers should be filled to minimally 80% and maximally 90% and flasks should be placed upside down in the autoclave. For the sake of safety the autoclave should not be opened before the contents have cooled down to room temperature. Most common are an isotonic 1.4% solution and a 4% solution of $NaHCO_3$.

- *Biogenic carbonates.* Instead of the cumbersome handling of bicarbonates, occasionally sodium acetate or lactate is used as biogenic carbonate for the treatment of mild acidosis. In the citric acid cycle this is metabolized to CO_2.

- *Biogenic hydrochloric acid.* For the treatment of alkalosis, isotonic solutions fortified with ammonium chloride are used (section 21.4.3.2). While the ammonia moiety of this compound is metabolized in the urea cycle, the remaining HCl may serve to neutralize the alkalosis.

21.10.3 Sugar Solutions

21.10.3.1 Glucose (Dextrose, *Saccharum Amylaceum*)

The steam sterilization of glucose solutions leads to a yellowish to yellow-brown coloration of the solution (polymerization of the degradation product hydroxymethylfurfural), which is considered physiologically harmless. The coloration increases with the sugar concentration. Since purity of the glucose plays a role, it is recommended to use a specially purified product. The coloration is also affected by the length of the heat treatment; shortening of the cooling phase may be achieved with autoclaves equipped with a special cooling device. The degradation reaction is pH-dependent; at pH 3.5, the sugar is maximally stable. Therefore, degradation and thus coloration can be minimized by addition of HCl or by intensive CO_2 gassing. A weak yellowish discoloration is permissible. The solution pH of 3.5 is typically considered not a concern and is well tolerated, given the solution is unbuffered.

21.10.3.2 Fructose

Discoloration occurs to a lower extent than with glucose; the special measures described above for glucose are required for fructose only at concentrations of over 20%.

Caveat: Application in patients suffering from hereditary fructose intolerance may experience severe side effects.

21.10.3.3 Mannitol and Sorbitol

Solutions of these sugar alcohols may be sterilized without special precautions.

21.11 Solutions for Electrolyte Therapy

21.11.1 Principles of the Electrolyte Infusion Therapy

60% of the weight of the human body is accounted for by water. That means that an adult person of 80 kg carries about 50 L of water. We distinguish water that is inside cells (intracellular water, 56-70%) and extracellular water, which can be subdivided in intravascular fluid in the blood and lymph circulation ($\sim$3 L) and the interstitial water between the cells. Between the circulatory water and the water in the interstitial space fluid and ion exchange occurs by diffusion. The entrance of electrolytes in the cells is facilitated by membrane-bound transport systems. This presents an adequate means to control the electrolyte compositions of the cellular fluid and the extracellular space, which are by no means identical. The most predominant cation in the intracellular fluid is potassium, next to smaller amounts of magnesium. The dominating anions are phosphate, mono-, di- and tri-phosphates of adenosine (AMP, ADP, ATP) and hexose monophosphate and in addition to that sulfate ions. In the extracellular fluid sodium dominates as a cation while chloride and bicarbonate are the most abundant anions. Minor differences are observed between the Na^+ and Cl^- concentrations of the intravascular and the interstitial fluids. For all practical purposes the latter might therefore be considered as one single functional compartment. Table 21-6 present the electrolyte composition of blood plasma.

When in earlier times a traumatic event led to blood loss exclusively physiological NaCl or Ringer solutions were used to replenish the blood volume. Although this could often successfully prevent shock conditions and the subsequent potentially catastrophic reactions, it took insufficiently into account that the blood volume represents only about 4% of the total volume of body fluid and that every minute 73% of the water present in blood exchanges with

Table 21-6 Electrolyte Content of Blood Plasma

Ion	Normal value (mmol/L)
Na^+	142
K^+	5
Ca^{2+}	2.5
Mg^{2+}	0.85
Cl^-	103
HCO_3^-	27
HPO_4^{2-}	0.67
SO_4^{2-}	0.35
Proteins	16

the extravascular space. A decisive step in the introduction of therapeutic electrolyte solutions was the recognition that parenterally administered solutions also reach the intercellular space and that, thanks to clinical-physiological procedures, it became possible to determine disturbances in the water/electrolyte balance of the organism with great precision.

Such disturbances can be treated effectively with specifically composed infusion solutions. A clinically identified deviation of an ion concentration from the normal valued may thus be neutralized by a substitution therapy with electrolyte infusion solutions. A disturbed ion balance, which is often accompanied by changes in pH and may bring about severe clinical symptoms, can thus readily be normalized. An excess of anions (particularly Cl-), disturbs the acid-base equilibrium and leads to acidosis, while an excess of cations ($Na+$, K^+, Mg^{2+}) causes alkalosis. In the electrolyte therapy it is important to ascertain that the patient receives the required ions in the correct amounts and ratios. Replacing one compound for another, for instance a sodium salt by the corresponding potassium salt, is therefore not allowed without taking special additional measures. Physiological-chemically, potassium and sodium are pronounced antagonists. That also applies to potassium *vs.* magnesium and calcium ions.

Like all infusion solutions, therapeutic electrolyte solutions should first and for all be isotonic. Often it may be advantageous however to prepare electrolyte solutions that are hypertonic. Isotonicity should therefore not be considered a generally valid requirement of electrolyte solutions.

Electrolyte solutions are therapeutically employed for:

    □ Protection against a physiological water deficit
    □ Protection against a physiological electrolyte deficit
    □ Compensation of disturbances in the acid-base equilibrium
    □ Starting of recovery of impaired kidney function

Electrolyte therapy may become imperative in case of disturbances in the water-electrolyte balance, which may be caused by a variety of events, including accidents, burns, surgical interventions, and pathological changes of endocrine organs, in particular the adrenal cortex.

21.11.2   Calculating the Concentration of Electrolyte Solutions

The electrolyte balance of body fluids presents the foundation of electrolyte therapy. For proper application of this treatment, knowledge of the quantitative ratios of the ions involved is indispensable (Table 21-6). Of secondary concern is the exact nature of the salts furnishing these anions and cations. Expressing electrolyte concentrations in mg/100 mL may lead to incorrect conclusions with respect to the properties of the electrolytes as in physiological processes the number of charged and noncharged particles is determinant. The internationally agreed unit for the ion concentration is the quantity per volume expressed in mol/l in accordance with the SI system. The expression of ion concentrations in equivalents (eq) per liter, as was common practice in earlier times, is no longer permitted.

Because electrolyte solutions are prepared by weighing the relevant salts, the required amounts are calculated based on the relative molecular and atomic masses, taking into account the stoichiometric composition of the electrolytes.

21.12   Blood Preparations

Parenteral administration of blood or blood derivatives is performed in case of heavy blood losses, erythrocyte and/or leukocyte deficiency and blood disorders.

Blood substitution may be accomplished by transfusion of blood directly from donor to patient, but more common is the application of full blood or serum in stored form, almost exclusively provided by blood banks. The donor blood is processed into a durable product by addition of stabilizing agents. The commonly used stabilizer solution CPDA-1 contains citric acid/ sodium citrate, glucose, sodium bicarbonate and adenine. Clotting is prevented by the sodium citrate (through formation of calcium citrate), glucose and adenine prolong the viability of the red cells. Such stabilized full blood preparations may be kept for up to five weeks.

The aging of blood mainly concerns the leukocytes, followed by the erythrocytes. It has become apparent that for effective blood replacement therapy, the cellular components of the blood usually play a subordinate role. Therefore, instead of the infusion of full blood preparations, the replacement of individual serum components may be sufficient in many cases.

Plasma is commonly obtained by means of plasmapheresis. The full blood of the donor is centrifuged in order to separate cellular components. The cells are reinfused in the donor thus avoiding that the donor must replenish these, a process that would take several weeks. With modern equipment, blood withdrawal and plasma reinfusion occur in a continuous process where cells and plasma are separated by filtration rather than by centrifugation. The body compensates much more rapidly for the protein loss represented by the plasma withdrawal.

The plasma thus obtained is frozen or further processed. Besides fresh frozen human plasma, dried plasma (dissolved in sterile solution, for infusion) and preserved serum preparations are used in the clinic. The latter mainly serves to restore blood volume. It contains full plasma without fibrinogen.

The preparation of clinically relevant plasma components such as albumin, immunoglobulins, fibrinogen, pro-thrombin complex and concentrates of blood clotting factors (factors VII and IX), the method of preference is the cold-precipitation procedure according to Cohn. In this procedure, different plasma fractions are precipitated by stepwise addition of ethanol to cooled plasma at progressive pH values and the fractions subjected to further purification by chromatographic methods (mostly gel-exclusion chromatography). Ethanol concentrations of >20% will effectively inactivate HIV particles.

The ultimate products are often freeze-dried preparations that may be kept for several years at temperatures of 2° to 8°C, provided that they are filled under appropriate conditions in *vacuo* or in a dry inert-gas atmosphere. Albumin is most commonly employed as a 4% to 5% solution intended for blood volume correction and as a 15% to 25% solution for protein substitution.

A special position is taken by preparations with specific immunoglobulins obtained from the plasma of immunized individuals and meant to serve for passive immunization instead of immune sera (see section 21.17). Such products are employed for therapeutic and prophylactic purpose, for example with reference to measles, rubella, mumps and poliomyelitis. They can only be administered i.m. Only after a special pretreatment (inactivation of parts of the peptide) and in low concentration i.v. administration of such preparations is permitted.

For the patient, the risk of infection during the transfusion is minimized by testing potential blood donors for HIV and, if need be, also by pasteurizing the preparation. The exclusion of HIV infections has required significant efforts. The donors have to meet high demands, which have led to exclusion of individuals bringing on an enhanced risk level.

A problem is that antibodies in blood cannot be detected within 4 weeks following infection. This implies that it is not possible to determine whether the donor was infected in the weeks before the donation. If he was, his blood might already be infectious. To minimize the risk of infections, whenever possible, preference is given to autologous blood. For the treatment of hemophilia patients, preferentially clotting factors prepared by gene technology are deployed.

> CPDA is an abbreviation for: citrate phosphate dextrose adenine.

> Plasma fractionation started with the need to obtain blood serum products as therapy for wounded soldiers in World War II. E.J. Cohn from Harvard was in the 1940s one of the leaders on this task by developing the "Cohn fractionation process," still the basis of today's methods.

21.13 Plasma Substitutes and Plasma Expanders

21.13.1 General Introduction

The body will compensate for blood losses of less than 10% of total blood. When larger losses occur, the body will need blood substitutes to replenish the plasma. This may be necessary in case of a hemorrhagic shock, such as from a traumatic insult (burning, internal injuries) and during prolonged diarrhea or vomiting.

Due to the transfer of large amounts of plasma fluid into the tissues, the amount of fluid in the circulatory system diminishes, causing an increase in blood viscosity, which, in turn, may result in serious circulatory problems.

The most appropriate method to replenish the blood circulation is the transfusion of preserved whole blood. This is particularly essential in case of heavy blood losses. Blood substitute solutions are administered to patients when blood loss is less serious, or in the context of emergency assistance to fill up the circulation just to the extent that it will allow the injured individual to be transported to the hospital. They are infused in amounts of 500 to 1,000 mL. When no better option is available, even a simple physiological NaCl solution (or an electrolyte solution) might be sufficient to temporarily replenish blood volume, but due to rapid excretion by the kidneys the administered fluid will remain in the circulation only briefly, necessitating more suitable measures at a (not much) later stage. Solutions containing macromolecules will have a longer vascular circulation time because macromolecules diffuse only slowly (or not at all) and in addition are able to retain large amounts of water by hydration.

Essential properties determining the suitability of a substance as plasma substitute is, besides the chemical structure, the molecular mass that should exceed 20 kDa. Colloids with a lower molecular mass leave the blood circulation quite rapidly and are excreted. An excessively high molecular mass might, on the other hand, bring along the risk of prolonged storage in the organism.

Blood possesses an osmotic pressure (at body temperature 0.65–0.8 MPa or 6.5–8 bar), which is determined by the integral collection of dissolved molecules and ions. It is composed of the actual osmotic pressure resulting from the electrolytes and the *oncotic* (colloid-chemical) pressure ($P_{tot} = P_{\text{van't Hoff}} + P_{colloid}$). The latter is accounted for by the water-attracting force of the colloids. Since the vascular wall is only permeable to truly dissolved substances and not to colloids, it is this force that has to be overcome when lymph plasma permeates the capillary wall. Whereas the oncotic pressure in normal blood from a quantitative point of view is negligible (3–4 kPa of 0.03–0.04 bar), it becomes quite appreciable when blood substitutes are employed. Plasma expanders are colloidal solutions with an oncotic pressure higher than that of blood. Plasma substitutes are iso-oncotic—that is, they have the same oncotic pressure as blood plasma. As macromolecules mainly hydroxyethyl starch and to a lesser extent also gelatin and dextran are applied.

21.13.2   Gelatin

In earlier times, it was common to liquefy gelatin solutions by heating prior to infusion. Instead, nowadays depolymerized and cross-linked gelatin derivatives are produced, which at room temperature still form liquid sols. The solutions of gelatin derivatives contain in addition certain electrolytes.

Cross-linking is accomplished at the amino groups of basic amino acids (lysine, histidine), as well as at the terminal amino groups of amino acids. They are predominantly eliminated via the kidneys. For the rest, protein derivatives are degraded by peptidases. Modified fluid gelatin (MFG) or gelatin polysuccinate (35 kDa) is cross-linked with succinic acid hydride and is applied in a Ca-containing NaCl solution (Gelafundin®) or in Ringer acetate solution (Gelafusal®, Thomaegelin®). Oxypolygelatin (Gelifundol®, 20–27 kDa) is a product that is cross-linked with guanidinium. The gelatin fragments are cross-linked with each other through di-isocyanate by means of ureate bridges. Attempts have been made to obtain products by hydrolysis of gelatin, which in solution pass into the gel state only at lower temperatures. Better results were obtained by treating gelatin with glyoxal. This blocks the amino and guanidino groups in the molecule by a condensation reaction and leads via subsequent oxidation with hydrogen peroxide to an increase in the number of carboxyl groups. As blood substitution fluids, 5% solutions of this product made isotonic with NaCl, are prepared, which even at low temperature do not gelatinize.

21.13.3 Dextran

Dextran is a polysaccharide made of glucose units, glycosidically connected to each other via α-1,6 bonds. In current use, in dextran preparations over 90% of the chemical bonds are of the α-1,6 type; the remainder are α-1,3 and α-1,4 bonds.

Electron-microscopic studies have revealed that dextran molecules form elongated branched strands. They are formed in sucrose-containing media by the enzyme dextran-sucrase that is produced by several strains of the Gram-positive bacterium *Leuconostoc*. Depending on the strain, during uncontrolled synthesis branched and nonbranched high molecular weight dextran is obtained with a molar mass of several millions. In this form, the molecule is not suitable for clinical use. Under controlled conditions or by post-hoc acid hydrolysis dextrans of the desired molar mass can be obtained. Partially hydrolyzed dextran is fractionally precipitated from the aqueous preparation by addition of an organic solvent such as methanol. As plasma substitutes 10% or 6% dextran solutions of dextran 40 (kDa) and dextran 70 (kDa) are used, respectively, in 0.9% NaCl. The numbers represent average molecular weights. The half-life in blood is 3 to 4 hours for the lower and 6 to 8 hours for the higher molecular mass. In general, the production of dextran solutions proceeds without problems. Solutions can be readily sterilized at 120°C. When stored at 4°C, sterilized dextran solutions are stable for as long as 10 years.

21.13.4 Hydroxyethyl Starch

Hydroxyethyl starch (HES) is a hydroxy-ethylated amylopectine hydrolysate mostly derived from waxy corn or potato starch and has been in use since the 1960s. By chemical modification rapid cleavage of the polysaccharide by serum α-amylase can be prevented and the degradation as well as the elimination via stool and urine retarded. HES species of various average molecular sizes are employed: 70,000 (6%), 200,000 (3%, 6%, and 10%) and 450,000 (6%ig), (HAES-steril®, Hemohes®, Plasmasteril®, Rheohes®, Sera-HAES®). The substitution grade amounts to ~0.5 for low and intermediate molecular weight and 0.7 for high-molecular-weight species. The HES molecule has a more or less spherical shape due to its highly branched structure. That is why, despite its high molecular weight, HES solutions show relatively low viscosity. The half-life in blood lies between 8 and 12 hours. In humans some accumulation in liver, spleen, kidney, skeletal muscle, lymph nodes and skin has been observed. The accumulation in skin may cause significant and prolonged (up to several years) itchy irritation. The latest evaluation of risks and benefits of HES preparations indicated that the use of HES brings along relatively high risk of complications and that the benefits no longer outweigh the risks. In none of the studies was a survival benefit found for patients treated with HES, relative to patients treated with crystalloid infusion solutions, while in addition HES-treatment revealed a risk of kidney damage. Currently, the FDA recommends that the use of HES in products be suspended, particularly in critically ill patients.

21.14 Preparations for Parenteral Nutrition

21.14.1 General Introduction

When normal food intake is not possible (following surgery, in case of carcinomas or neonatal disorders), parenteral nutrition becomes a necessity. It is required to maintain vital functions and the concomitant delivery of essential fatty acids keeps also the protein metabolism in balance. Although the body has substantial spare supplies of fat and protein at its disposal, which can be addressed during periods of nutritional insufficiency, (spare) supplies of water, glucose, and potassium are limited. Even after a relatively short interruption of food (and water) intake, artificial administration of these substances becomes necessary. This can be established either by tube feeding or by parenteral infusion. Often, full-fledged nutritional support is required, sometimes for weeks—in many cases, even for months. Recent trends in research concern the effect of nutritional elements on the modulation of immune and inflammation reactions as part of nutritional strategies (pharmacological nutrition, immune-nutrition). It is generally assumed that arginine, glutamine, and polyunsaturated fatty acids of the Ω-3 and Ω-6 family possess such immune-modulating activity. Parenteral administration is usually performed by intravenous infusion. When the patient receives an integral mixture of nutrients, we speak of a TPN (total parenteral nutrition) regime. When all components are administered as a mixture by means of a single infusion, it is called an AIO (all in one) regime. Parenteral nutrition is based on the supply of carbohydrates, amino acids, and fats.

21.14.2   Carbohydrates

Sugars serve as a quick energy supply and are commonly administered as a 5% glucose solution (Glucosteril®). The caloric supply that can be achieved in this way is moderate (838 kJ/L or 200 kcal/L). Because of the risk of vascular damage, substantially more concentrated glucose solutions (>10%) can only be administered via the central vein. If amino acids are present, glucose is replaced by mannitol or sorbitol (see next section). Substitution of sugars by sugar substitutes is expensive and offers few advantages, as they possess even lower metabolic capacity than glucose. The use of fructose and sorbitol brings along the risk of intolerance (and thus malabsorption). Xylitol may cause the formation of oxalate and thus of kidney stones.

21.14.3   Amino Acids

Severe protein insufficiency (blood loss, burns, surgery, starvation) can be corrected by infusion of amino acid preparations (L-amino acids, 5%–15%). Further components of such preparations are sorbitol as energy supplier (also ethanol is used), often also vitamins and categorical an electrolyte supply. The pH of such solutions is adjusted to ~6.0. Higher pH values decrease their stability. In order to minimize (oxidative) disintegration of individual amino acids during heat sterilization, which is generally performed at 120°C in a steam sterilizer, solutions for amino acid infusion are produced under inert gas saturation conditions. Since the presence of reducing sugars in amino acid mixtures causes coloration upon sterilization (Maillard reaction), mannitol or sorbitol replace glucose in such preparations. By the same token, the amino acids used should be of high purity; tryptophan is particularly prone to oxidize in the presence of impurities. The stability of amino acid solutions is affected by light in presence of oxygen. Amino acid preparations are administered by prolonged intravenous drip infusion (Alvesin®, Aminofusin®).

21.14.4   Fat

Intravenously infused fat emulsions are particularly suited to provide the patient with high energy values. A prerequisite for physiological tolerance of such fat emulsions is that the applied oil is of adequate purity and that the droplet size of the lipid phase of these O/W emulsions is ≤ 1 μm. Special attention needs to be paid to the dispersion grade in view of stability during autoclavation as well as during storage (see section 19.6). The fat component consists of vegetable oil, especially soybean and cottonseed oil. Occasionally, also synthetic saturated medium-chain glycerides (Miglyol®812) are applied.

The fat content in the emulsions varies from 10% to 30%. As emulsifiers, lecithins are used, which are obtained today exclusively from egg yolk, as there was in earlier years a gossypol contamination of cottonseed oil concomitantly used with soybean lecithins, which was falsely attributed to soybean lecithin. Antioxidants enhance the stability of such preparations. Water-for-injection serves as a solvent, and glycerol is often added for isotonicity. Homogenization is performed in the first step by high-shear mixing (e.g., Ultra-turrax device) and in a second step by high-pressure homogenization (see section 18.7.3). The usual size of the emulsion droplets is about 300 nm. Fat emulsions for infusion may be autoclaved without loss of quality. Before application in the clinical setting, the emulsions need to be tested for the compliance to sterility and endotoxin limits. The most common commercial preparations are Lipofundin MCT®, Lipovenös ®, and Intralipid®.

21.14.5   Production

Preparations for parenteral nutrition are commercially available as so-called standard or combination solutions that are adapted to the average requirements of an adult individual. They contain amino acids, carbohydrates and electrolytes in dual-compartment bags. The triple-compartment bags also contain a fat component. Immediately prior to applying the infusion, the separation walls between the compartments are perforated and their contents mixed.

Instabilities and the need to adjust the dosage to the requirements of the individual patient nonetheless often call for individual production of the preparation, which should proceed under aseptic conditions in a laminar flow cabinet. In a closed system, the required volumes of the separate infusion solutions and fat emulsion are pumped into the mixing bag. Fully automatized systems operate with a computer-controlled dosing mode and a recording system fully complying with GMP regulations. The mixing bags are mostly made of ethyl-vinyl-acetate devoid of plasticizers. Due to the complex composition of the TPN preparations, numerous potential stability hazards and incompatibilities must be taken into account during production, as these may lead to precipitations, sorption phenomena, and phase separations. The order in which the individual components are added plays a decisive role:

To avoid the formation of precipitates of insoluble salts such as for example phosphates of alkaline earth metal ions, calcium and magnesium are first prediluted in the amino acid solution and then mixed with phosphates, which are dissolved in the sugar solution in order to avoid the occurrence of locally high concentrations. Multivalent cations, high electrolyte concentrations and acidic glucose solutions may cause a lowering of the zeta potential of the fat droplets at the infusion site, which may cause destabilization of the emulsion. That is why fat emulsions usually are added as the last component to the system. Chemical changes or degradation of the components (e.g., lipid peroxidation, Maillard reaction involving amino acids and glucose, decomposition of vitamins) as well as ad-, ab-, and desorption phenomena involving the container material (insulin, vitamin A, plasticizers) all have to be taken into account. Important nutritional components can be inactivated, and toxic and reactive products such as radicals may be formed.

As a rule, TPN preparations are not used as carriers for medicines, as these will often interact with one or more of the many components of these complex systems. Virtually all pharmaceutics are administered separate in time.

21.15   Radiopharmaceuticals

21.15.1   General Introduction

Radiopharmaceuticals, also known as nuclear pharmaceuticals or radioactive pharmaceuticals, are applied in nuclear medicine for diagnostic and therapeutic purposes. The most important among the radiopharmaceuticals are intravenously administered injection solutions. To these, the same general requirements apply that are demanded from injection and infusion solutions. The principle of a radiopharmaceutical application involves the administration of a radioactive tracer to a patient and subsequent evaluation of the radioactivity delivered at the target site. The term *tracer* emphasizes that the doses administered here represent extremely small quantities of material. We should not expect here any pharmacological effect but are rather focusing on organ specificity. Most radiopharmaceuticals are diagnostics. They should produce radioactive radiation with sufficient penetration capacity to allow its detection outside the body. Most and for all, γ-emitters are applied with an energy within the appropriate range. γ-rays represent nonparticulate electromagnetic radiation. β-radiation, on the other hand, consists of high-energy electrons and, as a consequence of its particulate character, has a relatively low penetration range. Apart from certain diagnostic applications, it is mainly employed for therapeutic aims. Furthermore, β-radiation is applied in *in vitro* diagnostics.

The most relevant consideration in the selection of diagnostic radionuclides is that the radiation burden for the patient should be minimal. That is why, as a rule, radionuclides with a short physical half-life and radiotracers with a short biological half-life are used. Further, biokinetic parameters that have to be taken into account are the uptake in the target organ, body distribution, degradation, and formation of radiolabeled fragments and elimination from the body. An important parameter is the effective half-life, which is derived from the values of biological and physical half-life.

Only exceptionally the available radionuclides by itself display satisfactory affinity for the target organ. In general, the radionuclide first needs to be converted to a radiotracer that, based on its molecular size and geometry and its chemical and physical properties, will be enriched in the target organ.

For the manufacturing of a radiopharmaceutical the pure nonradioactive chemical substance is subjected to neutron radiation in a nuclear reactor or bombarded with charged particles, usually protons, in a cyclotron. Radioactive materials that emit α-particles (nuclei of helium) are pharmaceutically not interesting because the radioactive toxicity of the elements concerned is too high.

21.15.2   Production

The demand for a minimal physical half-life requires that the applied radionuclides be produced directly on the spot. This has become possible by virtue of the development of radionuclide generators. The principle of such generators is the mother–daughter relationship between certain nuclides, allowing a relatively rapid establishment of an equilibrium situation.

The generator contains the mother nuclide fixed in a nonexchangeable manner to an adsorbent column. The daughter nuclide, which represents the medically relevant species, is periodically collected from the column by elution. The currently most frequently used radionuclide ^{99m}Tc has ideal properties for (nuclear) medical investigations. It produces a pure γ-radiation and has a physical half-life of 6 hours. To achieve satisfactory organotropism, ^{99m}Tc is converted into a variety of complexes. For the preparation of such complexes, prefabricated kits are available containing all substances necessary for the formation of the complex in lyophilized form. Shortly before the application, the desired tracer is produced by adding the corresponding short-lived radionuclide. The radio tracer is present in a highly diluted solution, which therefore is extremely susceptible to any changes, in particular of pH. To counter this effect, commonly the same compound (but not radioactive) is added in higher concentration as a partner to improve stability and to minimize the radiolytic process and any adsorption of the tracer to the container material. For the production of colloidal solutions stabilizers such as gelatin, polyvinylpyrrolidone, dextran, or mannitol are employed.

When dealing with radioactive materials, it is of the highest importance to stick to the corresponding legal regulations. For personal protection, the cumulative dose is recorded with a dosimeter. A contamination monitor is used to check hands and fingers for traces of radioactivity after finishing working with radiochemicals.

Multidose containers (glass vials) that are meant to contain injection fluids must have normalized dimensions in order to permit standardized intensity measurements in the ionization chamber to obtain an exact amount.

During transport and storage, the vials should be kept in a lead container. Expiration date (and hour when applicable) should be clearly quoted.

21.15.3   Preservation

Since the radioactive radiation of the active ingredient may bring about radiolytic decay of an added preservative, such addition to a radioactive injection solution is in general not meaningful. An exception is benzyl alcohol, which is most frequently used as a preservative for radioactive solutions, since it is relatively resistant to destruction by radioactive radiation. An additional advantage of this preservative is that it may be used at relatively high concentrations of up to 1%. Since injection solutions are commonly prepared in small volumes, such concentration makes accurate dosing of the preservative easier.

The radiolysis product formed from benzyl alcohol by oxidation is benzoic acid, which by itself has bacteriostatic properties, but is poorly soluble (precipitation). As an alternative, phenylethyl alcohol is used (0.3%–0.6%). Some pharmacopeias strongly reject the use of preservatives in therapeutic injection fluids; for diagnostic preparations, the addition of preservatives is generally approved of.

21.15.4 Testing

Obviously, radioactive injection solutions must meet the corresponding requirements of the pharmacopeias. The required *Testing for Sterility* comes with difficulties in case of radioactive injection solutions. The short physical half-life of many radionuclides is hardly compatible with the 7 days demanded by the corresponding methods described in the pharmacopeias. Some pharmacopeias allow the distribution and application of the preparations before completion of the sterility test. A meaningful measure to test for microbial contamination of short-lived radionuclides is a daily check of a sample of culture medium, inoculated with the substance to be tested, for microbial growth. In this way, the test results can be made available before distribution and application of the solution. An additional problem is the small number of vials in one batch, which does not allow sometimes significant variation.

Because of the complications of the sterility test, alternative approaches are developed. One approach is the so-called "Validation of growth-based rapid microbiological methods (RMM) for sterility testing for cellular and gene therapy products" (see draft guidance for industry by FDA, 2008). Especially for cell therapy this "rapid MM" will grow in importance, as these products are obviously maximally stable for 24 hours at room temperature.

The checking the proper functioning of the sterilizing method being used might also be a kind of approach, but is no substitution for the test just mentioned. The approaches make for example use of indicator tape adhered on the surface of the container. This indicator changes color at given temperatures. This allows us to conclude whether the solution has been exposed to the required temperature.

A limulus test is used to perform the pyrogen test for radioactive preparations. Other required tests include those for radiochemical purity (i.e., the proportion of the radioactivity that is present in the form of the radioactive substance to be used) and the purity of the radionuclide itself.

21.16 Solutions for Hemodialysis and Peritoneal Dialysis

Hemodialysis solutions are used in the artificial kidney. This is a device based on the principle of dialyzing the patient's blood in a closed system of semipermeable membranes against the hemodialysis solution. The blood is drawn from an artery and guided via a system of flexible tubes into the dialyzer consisting of numerous hollow fibers with a semipermeable wall. These are washed around by a counter flow of rinsing fluid that is kept at a constant temperature. The cleansing fluid (dialysate) carries off the toxic small molecular weight components that pass through the membranes and is collected as waste. The cleansed remainder of the blood is reinfused into the patient. The magnitude of the dialysis effect depends on several factors: the effective surface and pore diameter of the membrane, the circulation velocity of the blood and cleansing fluid, the concentration gradient between blood and dialysate and the temperature of the dialysis fluid.

The composition of the hemodialysis solution should simulate normal blood values as closely as possible and represent a total osmolarity between 290 and 400 mosm/L. From a logistic point of view, supplying the dialysis centers with ready-to-use hemodialysis solutions is not meaningful. Therefore, the pharmacist of the center prepares a concentrated solution that is diluted to the required concentration with "water for hemodialysis solutions" shortly prior to use. The water is especially tested for the absence of aluminum ions, as these are suspected of causing neurotoxic effects. For home dialysis, drinking water may also be used, provided that account is taken of the ions in the water. Intensive filtration can remove contaminations and yield a germ-poor or germ-free filtrate. Dilution of the concentrate is in the clinical setting achieved by means of mixing equipment using "water for the dilution of concentrated hemodialysis solutions." When required, the hemodialysis solution thus prepared may be modified by addition of supplements.

Dialysis solutions of similar composition are used for *peritoneal dialysis*. This procedure is deployed in the same way in case of uremic conditions or intoxications to eliminate urophanic or toxic substances from blood via the peritoneum that functions as a semi-permeable membrane. Since these solutions are infused into the peritoneal cavity (and withdrawn after a certain time interval), they belong to the infusion solutions and hence must be sterilized in the autoclave, in contrast to the extracorporeal cleansing solutions used in the artificial kidney.

Example

The standard approval of an acetate-hemodialysis concentrate prescribes the following composition for ready-to-use solutions:

Na^+	120–155 mmol/L
K^+	0–4.5 mmol/L
Ca^{2+}	0–2.5 mmol/L
Mg^{2+}	0–2.5 mmol/L
Cl^-	90–130 mmol/L
acetate	25–45 mmol/L
glucose	0–6 g/L

21.17   Immune Sera and Vaccines

Immune sera and vaccines serve to achieve *immunization*. Immunity is the result of the battle of an organism with an antigenic substance (infectious agent, snake venom), ultimately leading to the formation of antibodies. Passive immunization is achieved by means of a serum obtained from a living creature that in the past was exposed to an antigen and had formed antibodies against it. Immune sera are preparations containing immunoglobulins (*heterologous antibodies*) from the serum of animals and provide immediate protection against the antigen. These sera may be available in liquid or freeze-dried form. The protective effect is limited in time and does not protect against a second challenge with the antigen.

This type of immunization represents primarily a therapeutic intervention. It is applied in case of botulism, various gangrene forms and venom poisoning (snakes, scorpions). As from then on these foreign antibodies may themselves act as antigens, it cannot be excluded that upon repeated immunization the species-foreign, mostly animal protein may cause an allergic or immunogenic reaction. That is why, whenever possible, more and more use is made of specific immunoglobulins isolated from the serum of immunized humans (section 21.12).

We speak of *active immunization* when modified antigens in the form of killed or attenuated bacteria, viruses or toxoids (= toxins converted by formaldehyde or heat treatment) are injected, leading to homologous antibody production. As the antibodies have to be produced in the body, immune protection does not arise immediately, but once acquired it may last for up to 10 years. Protection may be prolonged by secondary immunization. This method is applied as a prophylactic protection against many infectious diseases.

Vaccines for human use are commonly distinguished in:
- Bacterial vaccines, produced by culturing suitable strains on a fluid or solid substrate. They come in liquid or freeze-dried form and contain inactivated bacteria (dead vaccine) or live bacteria (live vaccine).

- Toxoid vaccines, usually of bacterial origin and adsorbed to a carrier such as aluminum hydroxide or aluminum or calcium phosphate. These carriers are often adjuvants, that is, they amplify the antigenic activity of the toxoid.
- Viral vaccines, consisting of live or inactivated virus or immunizing subunits thereof; they are obtained from animals, eggs, cell culture, and tissues.

Immune sera and vaccines in single-dose packaging can be preserved; those in multiple-dose packaging need to be preserved.

As preservatives mostly phenol (maximal concentration 0.25%) and phenol derivatives are used, but also thiomersal and benzalkonium salts are in use. Because they are biological products, immune sera and vaccines are often prone to decomposition and in most cases need to be protected from light and stored in the refrigerator at 2° to 8°C, but protected from freezing. Their shelf life varies with the biological origin and the type of preparation. In most cases, they can be kept for 2 to 5 years. Some vaccines, such as, for example, against yellow fever, hepatitis B, and rubella live vaccine, are so unstable that during transport uninterrupted cooling (*cold chain*) needs to be guaranteed.

21.18   Formulation of Biologics

21.18.1   Requirements

Increasingly, biologics are available to treat severe diseases, including cancer and autoimmune diseases. These include recombinantly produced proteins, such as monoclonal antibodies, fusion proteins and other proteins, chemically or synthetically produced peptides, conjugates of peptides or proteins with small molecules, including antibody-drug conjugates, and others. All these substances require parenteral administration in order to lead to systemic effects in patients, given they are digested or otherwise deactivated if administered by nonparenteral (e.g., oral) routes.

Biologics intended for parenteral administration need to comply to requirements for parenteral products, mentioned elsewhere (see sections 3.13), including sterility, limits to pyrogens/endotoxins, limits for subvisible particulate matter, being essentially free of visible particles, and preferably, targeting isotonicity and isohydric pH.

> According to definition of the US-FDA, biologics include a wide variety of products such as vaccines, blood and blood components, allergenics, somatic cells, gene therapy, tissues and recombinant therapeutic proteins. Typically, from a regulator's perspective biologics and conventional drug products have a separate set of guidelines in order to accommodate the complexities associated with biologics.

21.18.2   Stability of Proteins

Peptides and proteins can degrade via chemical and physical degradation pathways. Chemical degradation is constituted by chemical modifications of the primary sequence of a peptide or protein. Examples include fragmentation, oxidation, deamidation, or disulfide exchange. Physical degradation involves changes in the structure of the active ingredient, and this includes denaturation (unfolding), adsorption, aggregation (oligomerization) or precipitation (formation of macroscopically visible aggregates, and particles). The tendency of a peptide or protein to show chemical degradation is determined by its primary sequence, and whether susceptible amino acid residues are surface exposed, and thus, if they are easily attacked in their formulation.

21.18.3   Dosage Forms, Primary Packaging, and Routes of Administration

Biologics are typically developed as liquid or dried dosage form. Considering the size of a protein, that is, a 150 kDa monocloncal antibody would typically show a diameter of ca 10 nm, solutions containing these would be considered a colloidal solution. Solutions containing a protein are mostly based on Water for Injection (WFI) as solvent, given that organic solvents in most cases lead to protein denaturation or other protein instabilities. Dried dosage forms are mostly based on freeze-drying. Spray-drying or other drying techniques are less preferred for parenteral biologics dosage forms, given the need and challenge related to filling sterile powder into primary packaging such as vials. However, when inhalative administration is desired, for example, for local treatment in the lungs, drying by spray-drying can also be considered, next to nebulization of a liquid dosage form.

All different kinds of primary packaging are considerable for biologics; however, mostly glass vials, rubber stoppers, and aluminum crimp caps are used, followed by glass syringes, or any other kind of injection device (e.g., autoinjectors, pens, injection pumps). Only in few cases, primary packaging out of plastic is used, given that plastic containers are often insufficiently gas right and that proteins and peptides are often easily oxidized. Furthermore, plastic containers might leach undesired compounds into the parenteral product, that may be a safety concern for patients, or that may themselves degrade proteins or peptides.

Different routes of parenteral administration are considerable for proteins and peptides. In many cases, these products are administered intravenously (i.v.), subcutaneously (s.c.), and sometimes intramuscularly (i.m.), intradermally (i.d.), intravitreally (i.v.t.), or intrathecally. Different considerations need to be made for different routes of administration. For example, the injection volume for subcutenously and intravitreal formulations is typically quite limited, thus requiring very highly concentrated protein formulations for proteins requiring a high dose. This can lead to significant challenges related to product viscosity and ability to manufacture and administer these drugs. In another example, proteins for intrathecal administration need to consider tighter limits for pyrogens and endotoxins, and the choice of excipients in this case is also very limited, given possible regulatory and safety concerns for direct administration into the central nervous system.

21.18.4   Formulation, Choice of Excipients, and Storage Conditions

Formulations for biologics usually contain an aqueous buffer, in order to maintain the target pH over the intended shelf life. The pH is one of, if not the most important, formulation parameters for peptide and protein stability. Apart from the buffer, one or more stabilizers are required in the formulation, to ensure sufficient stability and tonicity. Typically, surfactants, such as polysorbate 20, polysorbate 80, or Poloxamer 188 are used in sufficient amount (0.001%–0.1% w/v) to stabilize the protein or peptide against surface-induced degradation reactions. Sugars, sugar alcohols, amino acids, or salts can be used to ensure product tonicity, to slightly improve product stability or provide sufficient structure and texture for a freeze-dried cake. Sugars may include saccharose (sucrose) or trehalose. Reducing sugars like lactose need to be avoided, as these may react with primary amino groups in a peptide or protein, like a side chain lysine residue (Maillard reaction). Sugar alcohols like mannitol are sometimes used to provide elegance of the freeze-dried cake, yet, are poor protein stabilizers and have some other challenges. Amino acids can add to tonicity, may help to reduce viscosity in some protein formulations, or (e.g., methionine or tryptophan) can help to reduce or mitigate protein oxidation.

The storage of biologics drug products is typically refrigerated (2°–8°C). In some cases, products cannot be frozen, and related product labeling would in these cases contain a mention "do not freeze." Light can also lead to peptide and protein instability, and in most cases, these products should be protected from direct light and long-term exposure. Product labels in these cases contain the claim "protect from light" or "protect from direct sunlight." In few cases, light sensitivity is extreme, so that these products need protection from light even during patient administration.

21.18.5   Drug Product Manufacturing

Biologic drug products need to be sterile. Although parenteral products are preferably manufactured by terminal sterilization (autoclave, heat sterilization, gas sterilization, or ionizing radiation), these methods of sterilization are generally not applicable for peptide or protein drugs as they would degrade during processing. The preferred method of sterilization of biologics drug products is aseptic manufacturing in combination with the use of sterilizing-grade filtration. When filtration cannot be used, aseptic compounding must be explored.

Biologics require some specific consideration for processing and manufacturing, given their sensitivity. For example, rotary piston pumps that are traditionally used for filling sterile drugs in most cases lead to protein aggregation and particle formation, and thus, peristaltic pumps are a better choice. Protein, peptides, and some excipients such as surfactants or some preservatives may also interact with various surfaces during processing, including disposable tubing. Careful selection of processing materials is key to ensure product quality when manufacturing biologics.

21.18.6   Drug Product Control Strategy

Comprehensive product and method understanding is required to set up adequate characterization and control strategies for biologics. All requirements for the parenteral products must be carefully evaluated for product release and stability, including sterility, pH, osmolality, particulates, endotoxins/pyrogens, extractable volume, and so on. Additionally, product concentration, biological activity, and a panel of different purity endpoints need to be assessed. For peptides and proteins, this includes evaluation size (aggregates, oligomers), charge heterogeneity and oxidation state.

Biologic products are parenteral products. All requirements for parenteral products must be fulfilled also for related biologics products. However, many approaches cannot be directly applied for biologics.

21.19   Cytostatic Drugs

Cytostatic drug are substances that inhibit cell growth or division and are deployed as chemotherapeutic anti-cancer agents. Due to their oncogenic, mutagenic, and teratogenic potential, their production entails special requirements with respect to personal protection, such as availability of appropriate instructions, wearing protective equipment, and implementation according to up-to-date technical standards, extending beyond the requirements of the common pharmacy work rules. That is why the production of ready-to-use cytostatic formulations mostly occurs in central production facilities of specialized pharmacies on an individual patient basis (unit-dose service) and only by skilled and properly instructed personnel.

Most cytostatics are administered intravenously; only rarely is the peroral, subcutaneous or intrathecal route chosen. As a rule, cytostatics for intravenous administration are commercially available in the form of concentrates or lyophilisates. Because of their limited stability, a solution is prepared only shortly before use for each individual patient, either for a bolus injection or for an infusion. Preparation involves the dissolution of the dry substance in the prescribed solvent and dosing the dissolved substance into a carrier solution into a syringe or an infusion bag. Carrier solutions are most commonly 0.9% NaCl or 5% glucose, depending on the cytostatic. Chloride-containing solutions promote, for example, the stability of melphalan, bendamustine, and cis-platinum.

Cytostatics need to be kept and handled in a closed system, preferentially by using needle-free systems, to avoid contaminations. They must be taken from, dissolved, and mixed via special transition systems or pressure release devices (Cyto-Set®, Securmix®, PhaSeal®). Aerosol-tight membranes and filters (e.g., Extra-Spike®) further enhance safety. In order to prevent a pressure build-up forcing the cannula to detach from a syringe, a Luer-lock connecting system can be used.

The production follows either volume-oriented by measuring out with a single-use syringe or mass-oriented by weighing. Dosing of cytostatics is done according to body surface area (norm dose in mg/m^2) or body weight (mg/kg) in order to ensure comparable drug exposure for all patients and to allow direct comparison between species (animal vs. human) so that preclinical results obtained with animals may be extrapolated more accurately to human use.

Since sterilization in the final container is not possible, the manufacturing proceeds under aseptic conditions using sterilizing-grade filters in laminar-flow safety cabinets provided with air filters that can be easily replaced with a minimal risk of contamination. At the same time, the use of such a cabinet meets the requirement by law that the production of cytostatic drug formulations be performed in a closed system for the protection of the manufacturer. In view of the risk of microbial contamination, solutions should be administered to patients as soon as possible, but no more than 24 hours at 2° to 8°C after their conversion to the final formulation. In the United States, microbiological stability after opening has received significantly more attention after a number of deaths have occurred only few years ago. Microbiological stability after opening is the United States needs to be tested for each given product. A sterility test is in general not possible, as it concerns individually prepared formulations. Absence of germs in the final product should be guaranteed by process validation of the aseptic production in the clinical facility, microbiological tests of equipment, workspaces, and personnel. It also helps to identify sterility problems if one runs the production process once by using culture media instead of the drug solution (media fills).

Transparent, shatterproof, and fluid-tight polymer containers are the preferred packaging material. They should allow visual inspection for precipitates and particles and be absolutely tight after the insertion of the drug solutions. PVC is not optimally suitable because it contains the softener phthalate, which might dissolve in case of a lipophilic drug dissolved in a solvent containing a solubilizer (e.g., paclitaxel in Cremophor EL) and might also adsorb the cytostatic. In addition, the oxygen permeability of PVC facilitates oxidative decomposition of cytostatics (e.g., photolysis of doxorubicin). Because of the risk of shattering, only in (substantiated) exceptional cases, such as incompatibilities, may glass containers be used. Filled syringes are mostly provided with Luer-lock screw caps. Furthermore, ready-to-use preparations may be sealed individually in fluid-tight foil in order to prevent manipulation or contamination from the environment in case the primary package might not be perfectly fluid-tight. For continuous application of cytostatics for a longer period (i.v., i.a., s.c., epidural), portable pumps have been developed (Infusor, Ultraflow, Surefuser) that allow ambulant therapy and permit patient mobility. A syringe containing the cytostatic preparation is connected to the drug portal of the pump, and in this way the preparation is transferred to the reservoir of the pump.

21.20   Testing

21.20.1   Tightness of Container Closure Systems

The tightness of container closure systems needs to be ensured before a product is to be used with a given container closure system, well prior to first human use.

Minute, often macroscopically not visible, cracks or fissures, especially located at the capped area vials, represent a safety hazard for the patient with respect to contamination of solutions for injection. To date, testing for leaks in the primary packaging has been accomplished by placing the unit dose containers (e.g., vials, syringes) under vacuum in a dye bath (methylene blue). Upon subsequent relief of the vacuum, any capillary cracks will allow the dye solution to enter the ampoules and stain the fluid inside. Unit doses containing a colored drug and immersed in a water bath will release part of the drug under vacuum conditions if any cracks are present. This will readily show up in the surrounding water.

Today, probabilistic testing like dye ingress testing is less preferred, and deterministic container closure integrity tests like helium leakage, or gas heapspace analysis are preferred.

21.20.2   Nondissolved Impurities and Contamination with Particles

Visual observation is applied in case of undissolved impurities, and in particular has been used to visualize suspended matter and glass splinters. Even a fully appropriate production procedure cannot guarantee the complete absence of particles in solutions or lyophilisates for injection and infusion. Sources of contamination are manifold. Endogenous impurities are formed in originally perfectly clear solutions as a result of the formation of molecular aggregates during aging, super-saturation, polymerization, and interaction processes. On the other hand, exogenous impurities commonly arise during the production process. They can originate from the equipment, filter materials, primary packaging material, and the environment (airborne particles). With glass vials, glass particulates may also be sometimes present. They often withstand intensive purification procedures. Ampoules are generally considered an obsolete unit dose container, as, upon opening the ampoule, glass splinters may end up in the product solution. Phase contrast microscopy revealed that in every ampoule, glass particles with a size of up to 100 μm occur. Precipitates and suspended material will only arise during application of the solution by manipulation of the medical personnel. As a result of the addition of further active ingredients by the physician incompatibilities may arise that could lead to the formation of precipitates.

However, there appears to be no consensus opinion concerning the potential risks that a patient runs upon injection with a solution containing suspended material. It is interesting to note that in animal experiments, no adverse effects were observed after i.v. injection of a solution containing suspended glass splinters originating from ampoules. Nonetheless, in the lungs of patients who had received large volumes of infusion fluids for an extended period of time, numerous insoluble components were found that supposedly originated from the infusion fluid. It remains unlikely that it will be easy to prove a causal relationship between the presence of larger particles in the organism and long-term effects caused by it.

In the Ph. Eur. and USP, the following methods are described to test contamination by particles:

- *Sub-visible* may be assessed by measuring light obscuration. Furthermore, a *microscopic method* is described.
- *Visible particulate contaminations* are evaluated by visual inspection against a dull-white or black background during defined illumination of the probe. This test is not suited for radioactive drugs.

Most pharmacopeias require visual testing. In visual inspection, the probabilistic detection limit is around 70 to 150 μm, depending on the light source conditions, inspection time, operator training, and other factors. For the assessment of absence of particles also semi-or fully automated inspection systems have been developed that do not depend on the human eye. They are based on different principles. Internationally obligatory assay methods are lacking. In the method involving assessment of transmission, a light beam traverses an ampoule and is projected on a sensor system. The vial is rotated and subsequently rotation is terminated. Particulate contaminations in the solution remain in motion for a while, causing a moving shadow to fall on the sensor. The changes in light intensity are determined and evaluated. The method is error prone because of its sensitivity to air bubbles that can cause false interpretations. The system has to be optimized accordingly in order to avoid erroneous measurements. The level of filling of the vials may be assessed simultaneously.

Ph. Eur. 2.9.19 Particle contamination—Nonvisible particles ⎯⎯⎯⎯⎯⎯⎯⎯⎯⎯⎯

USP ⟨788⟩ Particulate matter in injections
USP ⟨1788⟩ Methods for the determination of particulate matter in injections and ophthalmic solutions
USP ⟨787⟩ Subvisible particulate matter in therapeutic protein injections
USP ⟨1787⟩ Measurement of subvisible particulate matter in therapeutic protein injections
JP 6.07 Insoluble particulate matter test for injections
Particulate matter in injections and parenteral infusions consists of extraneous mobile undissolved particles, other than gas bubbles, unintentionally present in the solutions. The pharmacopeias describe two methods to assess particulate contaminations of injection and infusion solutions. Both are based on particle counting, one by means of light absorption

and the other by microscopy. Both tests are performed under laminar flow conditions to prevent creation of additional contaminations. The glassware and equipment is rinsed with particle-free (0.22 μm filtered) water immediately before use.

Light Obscuration Particle Count Test

The principle of this method is that suspended particles in the sample fluid flowing between a light source and a sensor produce changes in the signal that are correlated to the particle dimension (section 3.4.3.4). For parenterals having a volume of 25 mL or more, single units are tested, which are drawn using an appropriate sampling plan. For parenterals less than 25 mL in volume, the contents of 10 or more units are combined in a cleaned container to obtain a volume of not less than 25 mL. From each test solution, four 5-mL sample aliquots are withdrawn and analyzed by counting the number of particles equal to or greater than 10 mm and 25 mm. As the first measurement could be inaccurate, the result obtained for the first sample aliquot is disregarded and from the other aliquots the mean number of particles is calculated.

The preparation meets the requirements when the following maximally allowed particle counts are not exceeded:

Nominal Volume	Tolerated Average Particle Count (Particle Size)	
	($\geq$ 10 μm)	($\geq$ 25 μm)
> 100 mL (Ph. Eur., USP), $\geq$ 100 mL (JP)	$\leq$ 25 per mL	$\leq$ 3 per mL
$\leq$ 100 mL (Ph. Eur., USP), < 100 mL (JP)	$\leq$ 6,000 per container	$\leq$ 600 per container

Microscopic Particle Count Test

When methods based on light blockade cannot be used because the preparation is insufficiently transparent, is too viscous, or forms gas bubbles while flowing through the detector, microscopic particle count should be carried out. The preparation is filtered through a black or dark-gray membrane filter. For parenterals having a volume of 25 mL or more, single units are tested, which are drawn using an appropriate sampling plan. For parenterals less than 25 mL in volume, the contents of 10 or more units are combined in a cleaned container to obtain a volume of not less than 25 mL. After drying, the filter is placed under a binocular microscope, which in addition to the episcopic brightfield illuminator internal to the microscope is equipped with an external, focusable auxiliary illuminator that can be adjusted to give reflected oblique illumination at an angle of 10° to 20°. The entire filter membrane or a representative portion of it is scanned for particles at 100x magnification. By comparing with circular 10- and 25-μm marks on an ocular micrometer, the size of the particles is estimated and the number of particles in both size categories is determined.

The preparation meets the requirements when the following maximally allowed particle counts are not exceeded:

Nominal Volume	Tolerated Average Particle Count (particle size)	
	($\geq$ 10 μm)	($\geq$ 25 μm)
> 100 mL (Ph. Eur., USP), $\geq$ 100 mL (JP)	$\leq$ 12 per mL	$\leq$ 2 per mL
$\leq$ 100 mL (Ph. Eur., USP), < 100 mL (JP)	$\leq$ 3,000 per container	$\leq$ 300 per container

The USP includes two chapters dedicated to subvisible particulate matter in therapeutic protein injections (⟨787⟩, ⟨1787⟩). Chapter ⟨787⟩ specifically addresses therapeutic protein injections and related preparations and can be used as an alternative to the general chapter ⟨788⟩. It allows the use of smaller sample volumes and smaller test aliquots, as well as sample-handling instructions that take into account the issues associated with the analysis of these materials.

The light obscuration method has some technical limitations when used for analyzing certain particle types, such as those that have low contrast in the product medium and/or may change shape/size during analysis, as is typical for inherent particles in therapeutic protein injections. These inherent particles are known and expected, arising from the association of protein molecules that can be present in a continuum of sizes, ranging from nanometers (dimers) to hundreds of micrometers (multimers and visible particles). Protein aggregates inherent in therapeutic protein products may consist of a heterogeneous population, and therefore, size alone does not adequately describe them. Chapter ⟨1787⟩ therefore describes a variety of additional methods for characterization of particle size and size distribution, particle morphology and chemical composition, including infrared and Raman microspectroscopy, electron microscopy with electron energy loss spectroscopy, time-of-flight secondary ion, mass spectrometry, and others.

21.20.3 Additional Tests

Additional tests for parenteral dosage form concern the *quantitative contents* of each unit dose container and are meant to ensure that these do contain the prescribed quantities of solution, suspension, emulsion, or dry material (nominal content and additional volume (overfill). Both excess volume and minimal volume depend on the nominal content, as well as on the nature of the unit dose container content, and may be found in representative tables.

In case of oily solutions or suspensions for injection, a test for material texture is required (mostly done by rheology). It serves to guarantee that such preparations are sufficiently fluid to permit injection. A common criterion is the time required for a fixed volume of the preparation to flow out from a perpendicularly positioned syringe with standardized nozzle. In modern testing, injectability is tested using an apparatus simulating the injection at a constant volume per time and measuring the required injection force the injection to break loose, or for constant flow (glide force).

A test for *homogeneity* is done for suspensions that have to appear homogeneous for a fixed amount of time following shaking.

Sterility is tested microbiologically, applying a prescribed culture medium. The required number of containers to be tested of each batch varies in different pharmacopeias. The designation "sterile" is only justified under the test conditions for sterility (see section 4.4.2 and Ph. Eur. 2.6.1); no growth of microorganisms was detected. In cases where no sterility test is conducted, information concerning the sterilization method is required (e.g., steam-sterilized; hot-air sterilized; bacterium-free filtered, etc.). When required, a "Test for satisfactory preservation" should be performed (Ph. Eur. 5.1.3).

Pyrogenic contamination is tested by the limulus test, the monocyte activation test, or, occasionally, the rabbit test (see section 21.4.7.5).

Ph. Eur. 2.9.20 Particle contamination—Visible particles _____

USP ⟨790⟩ Visible particulates in injections

JP 6.06 Foreign insoluble matter test for injections

All products intended for parenteral administration must be visually inspected for the presence of particulate matter. Examples of such particulate matter include, but are not limited to, fibers, glass, metal, elastomeric materials, and precipitates. All units of a produced batch are inspected and must be free from visible particulates when examined without magnification against a black background and against a white background. The intensity of illumination at the viewing point is required by Ph. Eur. and USP to be between 2,000 and 3,750 lux and by JP to be 1000 lux. A higher illumination intensity is recommended for the examination of colored solutions or products in plastic containers (JP: 8,000 to 10,000 lux). Ph. Eur. describes a special viewing station to be used for this purpose. This consists of a vertical rear panel which surface is divided in a matt black and a non-glare white area, and an adjustable white-light source. After gently swirling, the container is inspected for about 5 seconds in front of the white and another 5 seconds in front of the black panel.

This test is performed as a 100% manufacturing inspection, as mentioned above. In addition, according to USP, a representative sample is inspected subsequently for batch release testing. Sampling for this purpose is done following the rules for acceptance sampling in accordance to ANSI/ASQ Z1.4 or ISO 2859-1 at inspection level II with an acceptance quality limit (AQL) of 0.65%.

Ph. Eur. 2.9.17 Test for extractable volume of parenteral preparations —————

USP ⟨697⟩ Container content for injections

JP 6.05 Test for extractable volume of parenteral preparations

Preparations for single-dose injection and for infusions need to be filled with volume to sufficient to permit administration of the nominal volume declared on the label. The same applies for multiple-dose containers labeled to yield a specific number of doses of a stated volume. As compared to the nominal volume, a single-dose vessel should not contain a volume that is so large that application of the entire contents might present a risk for the patient. Except for infusion preparations, the testing usually proceeds in such a way that the total volume is withdrawn with one syringe (for multiple-dose containers with several syringes) and, without emptying the needle, transferred into a graduated cylinder or a tared beaker. Because there will always be some residual fluid left behind in the syringe, the described procedure does not measure the withdrawable but, more accurately, the applicable volume.

Further Reading ————————————————————————

Arora, A., Prausnitz, M. R., and Mitragotri, S. "Micro-scale Devices for Transdermal Drug Delivery." *International Journal of Pharmaceutics* 364(2) (2008): 227–236.

Ethans, K. D., Schryvers, O. I., Nance, P. W., and Casey, A. R. "Intrathecal Drug Therapy Using the Codman Model 3000 Constant Flow Implantable Infusion Pumps: Experience with 17 Cases." *Spinal Cord* 43(4) (Apr 2005): 214–218.

Kale, T. R., and Momin, M. "Needle Free Injection Technology—An Overview." *INNOVATIONS in Pharmacy* 5(1) (2014): 10.

Ophthalmic Preparations

22

22.1 General Introduction

Eye preparations (ophthalmica) include eye drops (*guttae opthalmicae*), semi-solid preparations for application in the eye, powders for eye drops (section 15.9.1) as well as eye wash (collyria). In addition, a number of rarely used special application forms (lamellae, eye sprays) as well as ophthalmic inserts as sustained release forms belong to this category. All of them are intended for application upon the eyeball and/or to the conjunctiva or for insertion in the conjunctival sac. Preparations for intraocular injection are administered retrobulbar (behind the eyeball), intravitreal (in the *corpus vitreum*) or subconjunctival (underneath the conjunctiva) and are discussed in chapter 21. Care products for contact lenses, which, despite their widespread use, have not yet found their way into the pharmacopeias, are nonetheless treated as equal to ophthalmics because of identical microbiological requirements.

Eye preparations are intended for diagnostic and therapeutic purposes. Their pharmacological action is usually local and limited to the eye or surrounding tissues. Nonetheless, it should be taken into account that they may display systemic effects. For example, parasympathomimetics may cause cardiovascular side effects.

The following drug classes are used predominantly in ophthalmology:

- Pupil-widening drugs (mydriatics): atropine, scopolamine, phenylephrine, and epinephrine
- Pupil-narrowing drugs (miotics): pilocarpine, physostigmine, neostigmine, beta-blockers
- Anti-infective agents: antibiotics (e.g., chloramphenicol, tyrothricine) and virostatics
- Local anesthetics (cocaine, tetracaine)
- Anti-inflammatory drugs (zinc sulfate, corticosteroids)
- Anti-allergic drugs (sodium cromoglycate)

The eye represents one of the most sensitive organs of the human body and is a potential portal of entry for microorganisms. It is therefore justified to demand high quality from ophthalmic pharmaceutics. Eye drops not only need to display adequate activity, they also should be physiologically tolerated (i.e., not cause pain or irritation), and must be stable and sterile.

Voigt's Pharmaceutical Technology, First Edition. Alfred Fahr.
© 2018 John Wiley & Sons Ltd. Published 2018 by John Wiley & Sons Ltd.

22.2   Eye Drops

22.2.1   Aqueous Solutions

22.2.1.1   Requirements

The following parameters need to be taken into consideration in the production of well-tolerated preparations:

- Sterility
- Clarity (practically free from foreign particles); (practically clear in case of eye droplet solutions)
- Preservation
- Tonicity
- Stability

In addition to that, optimal pH values (buffering) and viscosity are important parameters.

22.2.1.2   Sterility

The application of microbiologically contaminated eye droplets has repeatedly led to serious incidents. Several cases are known where the application of solutions containing microorganisms resulted in severe irritations often leading to partial loss of vision or permanent eye damage. Contamination may result from the active ingredients or excipients, or be caused by nonaseptic handling or failing final sterilization as well as by recontamination during application. Pathogenic organisms may remain viable even in solutions containing silver compounds or antibiotics, which for a long time were considered autosterile. Especially critical are the bacteria *Pseudomonas aeruginosa*, which contain an enzyme that degrades the collagen of the cornea, *Escherichia coli*, *Pyocyaneus* and representatives of the *Subtilis* group. Among the lower fungi, predominantly *Aspergillus fumigatus* is often responsible for the occurrence of infections. Also viruses (specifically adenoviruses) may lead to pathological eye conditions (keratoconjunctivitis). The intact horny layer represents an adequate barrier against microorganisms. It may, however, also act as an effective substratum for microorganisms to grow.

All modern pharmacopeias require sterility from ophthalmics. The manufacturing of eye droplets should fully respect the basic rules of aseptic procedures; special attention should be paid to the use of water for injections, sterilized container and sealing materials. In view of the required absence of germs, eye droplets are dispensed in volumes of maximally 10 mL.

22.2.1.3   Clarity (Absence of Foreign Particles)

The requirement of solutions to be practically free or clear from particles should prevent potential mechanical irritation by solid materials. Therefore solutions are sterile filtered before filling them into final containers. An optimal solution of the filter problem of eye preparations (but also for other small volumes) is the combination of a traditional syringe with an additional filter device (Fig. 22-1). By applying the adequate membrane filter, all possible filtration options can be exploited. Dosing syringes in combination with a filter device, which allow sterile filtration and dosing in one single step by manipulation of a lever, have already proven their usefulness.

Filter manufacturers offer for this purpose, sterilized and contamination-proof packed polymer filtration devices for single use. For larger volumes the regular pressure-filtration devices for the production of solutions for injection and infusion are available (section 4.2.8).

22.2.1.4   Preservation

With the exception of preparations intended for use in injured eyes or surgical procedures, which are manufactured as single-dose formulations or, by virtue of their very composition, have an inherent antimicrobial activity, eye droplets must be preserved. Eye droplets without antimicrobial excipients in multidose preparations may only be supplied in containers that exclude microbial contamination of the content after opening. The excipients used for preservation should fulfill the requirements presented in section 25.5.3, with special

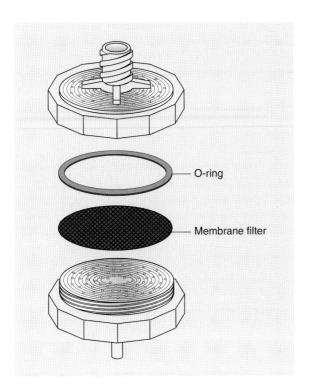

Fig. 22-1   Filtration unit.

attention for the effectiveness against problem germs (*P. aeruginosa*). Among the extensive collection of pharmaceutically used preservatives are the following substances with proven effectiveness: thiomersal (0.002%), alkonium and benzalkonium salts (0.002–0.01%), combined with sodium EDTA (0.1%), chlorhexidine (0.005%–0.01%), chlorobutanol (0.5%), and benzyl alcohol (0.5%–1%). Benzalkonium chloride possesses surface-active properties, which shorten the break-up time of the tear film and the residence time of active ingredients by emulsification of lipid components. The lowering of surface tension may enhance corneal permeation and decompaction of the upper layer of the corneal epithelium. For chlorhexidine and thiomersal, minor changes in the epithelium are observed. These aspects should be taken into consideration in the case of long-term administration.

When selecting the preservative and its concentration, compatibility with the active ingredients, excipients, and with the packaging and sealing materials as well as the pH value of the preparation should all be taken into account. Whenever applicable, adsorption-mediated losses should be compensated by increasing the concentration of the preservative. Because the concentration of preservative in prescribed formulations is usually very low, in most cases stock solutions are prepared that are subsequently, adequately diluted in order to ensure exact dosing. The name of each preservative used in a preparation is to be indicated on the label. Benzalkonium chloride has been previously related to observed allergies and irritations, as well as to coloration of soft contact lenses.

22.2.1.5   Tonicity

As a result of the electrolyte and colloid content, tear fluid has an osmotic value that equals that of blood and tissue fluid. It amounts to 0.65–0.8 MPa (6.5–8 bar), corresponding to a freezing point depression with respect to water of $\Delta T = 0.52$ K or of a 0.9% NaCl solution.

With respect to tonicity, the eye has a quite high tolerance in which no or only minor, but acceptable, physiological effects occur. Solutions within a tonicity range of $\Delta T = 0.4$–0.8 K, corresponding to NaCl concentrations of 0.7–1.45%, are tolerated without discomfort and do not cause tear flow, which results in washing out of the drug.

Hypertonic solutions are better tolerated than hypotonic solutions. Eye preparations are applied in quite small quantities (one drop); therefore, an approximate adjustment to isotonicity will usually suffice. Solutions used in the injured or surgically operated eye require isotonicity. Isotonicity is commonly achieved by the addition of NaCl, occasionally also by KNO_3 (particularly when silver ions are present in the solution) or boric acid. Alternatively, the procedure via freezing point depression to determine the amount of excipient needed to achieve isotonicity and provides the corresponding values for active and other ingredients often used in ophthalmology. In addition, the E *value method* (use of the sodium chloride equivalent) is often applied in practice. Both procedures are extensively discussed in section 21.4.3.

22.2.1.6   pH Value

The buffer capacity of the eye is lower than that of blood because in the eye the hemoglobin/oxy-hemoglobin buffer system is lacking. The buffer capacity of the eye is mainly accounted for by carbonate, phosphate and protein. While the pH of the eye is mostly around that of blood (7.4), escaping carbon dioxide may cause it to rise to values of 8-9. For the pH tolerance range of the unimpaired eye, variable values may be found in literature. At the usual drop-wise administration, unbuffered solutions in a pH range of 7.3 to 9.7 are experienced as fully pain-free. Ranges from 5.5 to 11.4 are still considered acceptable. Eye drops may be buffered for a variety of reasons, for instance to optimize the therapeutic activity (e.g., oxytetracycline) or to achieve adequate solubility (e.g., chloramphenicol).

To achieve a complete irritation-free preparation adjustment to isohydric conditions (pH 7.4) is desirable but in most cases not practically feasible. Solubility and stability of the drug (frequently also of the excipients) and the efficacy optimum play a significant role in this type of formulation, were the physiological effect (tolerance) comes only second. These aspects are, however, only rarely optimal at physiological pH values. The most favorable pH value represents a compromise between all factors listed. It is designated as the euhydric value; for example, most alkaloid salts used in ophthalmic formulations show maximal stability in a pH range 2–4, which is absolutely nonphysiologic. For the ophthalmologically relevant local anesthetics (maximal stability at pH 2.5–4.5) conditions are equally unfavorable. This is worsened by the fact that increasing pH values bring along higher therapeutic effect due to a better cornea penetration. In consideration of physiological adjustment, pH values of such solutions are set at 5.5-6.5.

For finished dosage forms a double-chamber system is available (e.g., Timpilo®). During storage, drug solution (pH 3.5) and buffer solution (pH 9.0) are separated, which secures shelf life. Immediately before application, the two solutions are mixed, yielding a buffered drug solution of pH 6.6 with improved biopharmaceutical properties.

pH adjustment proceeds by addition of acid, base, or buffer. As a buffer solution, sodium acetate/acetic acid buffer (acid range) and phosphate buffer (neutral range) are predominantly used. When the pH value required for stability reasons lies outside the acceptable physiological range, the use of a buffer system would be limited and instead use acid or alkali for pH adjustment. Solutions prepared in this way have practically no buffer capacity and are therefore more easily adjusted to physiological values by the tear fluid than buffered solutions. Isotonic and eu-hydric conditions are to some extent related when it comes to physiological compatibility: When a solution is approximately isotonic, it will still be tolerated without irritation at an unfavorable pH value.

22.2.1.7   Viscosity

The disadvantage of aqueous eye drops is that they are squeezed out of the conjunctival sac by movements of the eyelid, causing a reduction of the exposure time. By increasing the viscosity, better distribution of the active ingredient and a longer exposure time may be achieved. Furthermore, such preparations have lubricating properties and diminish irritations. That is why they are particularly useful in the treatment of keratoconjunctivitis. Commonly used viscosity enhancers are cellulose ethers (e.g., methylcellulose, hypromellose), polyacrylic acid and polyvinylpyrrolidone. Particularly 1%–2% of low-molecular weight poly(vinyl alcohol) (PVA) has proven its usefulness in this respect.

The viscosity of these preparations should remain below 25 mPa · s in order to avoid blocking of the tear duct (*ductus lacrimalis*). Commonly used solutions have viscosity values between 2 and 15 mPa · s. Filter sterilization is still possible up to viscosity values of ~10 mPa · s. It has to be taken into account that the rheologic behavior of polymer solutions is not only important in the resting state of the eye, but in particular during eyelid movements, when shear velocities of 10,000 to 40,000 s^{-1} may occur. As the viscosity of ideal viscous solutions is independent of shear stress, obstruction of eyelid movement may be observed with sufficiently thickened preparations. The same holds true for gels with plastic rheologic properties with high yield strength. Solutions with pseudo-plastic rheologic properties display a shear dilution effect during eye blinking and do not affect the eyelid movement. Anionic thickeners, such as carmellose and hyaluronic acid may interact with cations in the tear fluid, which may lead to an irreversible decrease in viscosity. In situ gel-forming systems are low viscous, droplet-forming solutions. Upon contact with the tear fluid they undergo a solution-gel conversion due to pH change (cellulose acetate phthalate-latex), temperature increase (poloxamer 127) or increased electrolyte concentration (gellan gum).

In addition, some of these polymers, such as polyacrylic acids, chitosan or hyaluronic acid (Fermavisc®), display muco-adhesive properties. The gel adsorbs tightly to the mucus via various physical and chemical mechanisms, involving mutual penetration of the macro-molecules of the gel and the mucus layer (inter-penetration phase). The results are longer exposure times and higher bioavailability.

Viscosity-enhancing effects are also employed in artificial tear fluid, during insertion of contact lenses or measuring instrumentation (e.g., for intraocular pressure measurement) because of their lubricating properties. They result in hydration of the cornea surface as well as lubrication of the corneal epithelium on the inside of the eyelid.

22.2.2   Oily Solutions

The importance of oily solutions has strongly declined in favor of aqueous solutions. Although they display extended contact time at the cornea and are not readily washed out, their major disadvantage is obscuration of vision. Drug absorption from lipid vehicles proceeds more slowly, which may bring about a depot effect. When using oxidation- or hydrolysis-sensitive active ingredients, employing oily base vehicles might enhance stability. Isotonicity and isohydricity do not play a role in the case of oily preparations. Although oily media do not form a substratum for the growth of microorganisms, they may harbor spores. Therefore, sterilization may be required, but no preservation. Highly purified and peroxide-poor vegetable oils of low acidity are preferentially used, especially peanut oil and castor oil, or medium-chain triglycerides that have favorable viscosity properties.

22.2.3   Suspensions

Suspension preparations are required when the active ingredient (e.g., corticosteroids) is insufficiently soluble in the vehicle or when aiming at a depot effect. A major requirement of aqueous as well as oily suspensions is particle size limitation. Micronized powders may in principle be used to exclude eye irritation and ensure medicinal action. Most pharmacopeias require a maximal particle size of 25 μm for applications in the eye. Large particles may cause irritations, while smaller (<3 μm) are washed out too rapidly. Because storage of industrially produced products may give rise to crystal growth, the development phase calls for special attention for particle size stability. Stabilization may be promoted by addition of viscosity enhancers (section 19.4). Despite such stabilization measures, it is not always possible to produce nonsedimenting preparations. In such cases, it is important to concentrate on the ability of the preparation to redisperse on shaking. Homogeneity of the redispersed suspensions should remain at least for the duration of the application to enable the correct dose to be delivered. Alternative stabilization measures include the use of peptizers and wetting agents.

22.2.4   Containers and Storage

Eye drops may be filled in single-dose or multiple-dose containers. Single-dose containers contain a single drug dose for one-time use. Routinely used containers include polymer ampoules (Opthiole®, Flexiole®) or small polymer ampoule flasks (bottle pack). It should be demonstrated that the nominal content can be withdrawn from the single-dose container. Multiple-dose containers are mostly brown-colored hydrolysis-resistant glass flasks with an externally oriented drop-tip made of chlorobutyl or bromobutyl rubber, squeeze or bottle pack® flasks are made of polyethylene and polypropylene. A small cover cap serves to protect the drop-tip during storage. The solution is introduced directly into the conjunctival sac by simply turning the container upside-down or gently pressing the drop-tip. The geometry of the tip affects the drop size and the force required to build the drop. Primary polymeric packaging materials may adsorb preservatives and may present problems when using steam sterilization. Similar problems may be encountered with sealing materials. They should have little capacity to adsorb active ingredients and excipients and not release any foreign material in the drug solution. Furthermore, they need to be sterilizable without influence on their elastic properties.

For multidose containers the period post-opening of the container after which the contents must not be used should be specified. In general, for eye drops a limit is set to the ultimate date before which it may still be used. According to the Ph. Eur. this period does not exceed 4 weeks after opening the container. From the point of view of drug activity, it may be recommendable to store the container cooled and to maintain a shorter usage time than indicated. Unpreserved eye drops should be used at the latest 24 hours after opening. Multi-dose containers are often provided with shrink tubing or a fracture ring to guarantee original sealing.

The COMOD (continuous mono dose) container is meant to avoid preservatives in multidose containers, while keeping eye drops sterile for up to 12 weeks. The preparation is contained in a flexible bag and is delivered in exact doses by means of an air-free pump, not allowing air to flow into the bag. Instead, the pressure compensation is established via a gap between the container wall and the bag inside it. The negative pressure arising in the bag folds up the bag, thus preventing the entry of any microorganisms. In addition, all parts of the device coming into contact with the product are coated with a silver layer, thus exploiting the antimicrobial and oligodynamic effect of silver. Also the ABAK (Thea Holding) system offers protection against contamination without the use of preservatives. It filters the solution upon applying pressure and drop formation through a filter membrane (0.2 μm pore size) while, upon releasing the pressure, air and solution are reabsorbed and sterile filtered again.

Both single- and multiple-dose containers made of polyethylene or polypropylene can be produced by the blow-fill seal technology (section 27.3.3.2). Under sterile and pyrogen-free conditions the extruded granules forming the polymer tubing are blown into the desired shape in one single process step and then, after cooling, filled with the sterile content material and sealed by fusion.

22.3   Eye Lotions

Eye lotions, also known as eye water (*collyria*), are sterile aqueous solutions intended for use in rinsing or bathing the eye or for impregnating eye dressings. They are employed in the treatment of chemical injuries and burns (first aid), but also as disinfecting rinsing solutions. Eye washes have to be produced according to the principles maintained for eye drops and need to have the same microbial purity. Multidose preparations do not contain more than 200 mL eye lotion per container.

Whenever possible, eye washes need to be stored refrigerated and protected from light and in germ-tight sealed containers. They should be used within 4 weeks after opening.

22.4   Ocular Therapeutic Systems

Ophthalmic inserts are sterile, solid or semi-solid preparations designed to be inserted in the conjunctival sac. They consist of a matrix, containing an embedded drug reservoir. The release rate of the active ingredient, which is usually soluble in physiological fluids, is membrane-controlled. Ophthalmic inserts are individually packaged in a sterile container. On the label the total quantity of active substance per insert and the dose released per unit

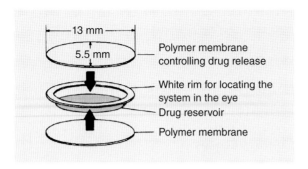

Fig. 22-2   Schematic representation of the TS Ocusert®.

time are indicated. Biologically degradable and nondegradable systems are distinguished. Soluble ophthalmic drug inserts (SODI) consist of thin soluble polymer films (e.g., acrylamide, N-vinylpyrrolidone, ethyl acrylate co-polymers), which soften within 15 seconds in the conjunctival sac and dissolve within a few hours while releasing the active ingredient (e.g., dexamethasone, gentamicine). Bioadhesive ophthalmic drug inserts (BODI) have in addition, bioadhesive properties to prevent the insert from releasing from the eye.

The first application of a therapeutic system (TS) in ophthalmology was Ocusert®, which was applied in the chronic treatment of glaucoma. This system is still available as Ocusert® Pilo-20 or Pilo-40 in the United States and the United Kingdom. The ellipsoid, flexible and transparent system is applied in the lower eyelid pocket and contains the active ingredient pilocarpine in an alginic acid membrane (drug reservoir). The drug lowers the intraocular pressure. The membrane controlling the drug release consists of ethylene vinyl acetate co-polymer. A white rim of titanium dioxide serves to position the insert in the eye (Fig. 22-2).

In the treatment of glaucoma Ocusert® P 20 releases 20 µg/h and Ocusert® P 40 40 µg/h pilocarpine in the tear fluid for a period of minimally 7 days after a brief initial burst of a larger dose. The total dose delivered is 3.4 and 6.7 mg for the two Ocusert® types, respectively. In order to keep the rate of the diffusion-controlled drug release at a constant level, the reservoir needs to contain an excess of drug. The Ocuserts contain a total amount of 5.0 and 11.0 mg pilocarpine, respectively. To achieve the same therapeutic effect with pilocarpine eye drops 2%, 4x daily, 28 mg of the drug are required in a period of 7 days. Furthermore, the reduced total drug dose effectuated by using the Ocusert® device also brings along a reduction of side effects. Unfortunately, this innovative system ultimately was not able to gain acceptance in the market, mainly because of high costs and the occurrence of adhesions with the cornea and application problems in elderly patients. By embedding pilocarpine in a poly(vinyl alcohol) film, a novel system with an eightfold enhanced bioavailability compared to eye drops could be achieved (new ophthalmic delivery system, NODS®). Also lyophilizates have recently been tested, but up to now they have produced retarded release properties only to a limited extent.

Ocular iontophoresis is a technique to enhance delivery of ionized and unionized drug moieties to the ocular tissue with the help of electrical potential. Due to the non-invasive nature of this technique it is gaining a lot of attention. For example, dexamethasone phosphate is delivered using the EyeGate® II (EyeGate Pharma, USA) iontophoresis device in the treatment of corneal graft rejection.

Eye implants, on the other hand, are inserted into the eye by minimally invasive surgery, but they have to be removed again in the case of insufficient biodegradability. They release drugs for extended periods of time, for example Vitrasert®, which releases ganciclovir intravitreally for as long as 5 to 8 months to treat CMV retinitis in HIV patients. Fluocinolone acetonide (Medidur®) in the form of an implant is used to treat diabetic macula edema for up to 36 months.

By binding active ingredients to ion exchange resins penetration of the active substance into the eye can be retarded and better local compatibility may be accomplished. This is for instance achieved with BetopticS® for the drug betaxolol by ionic binding to amberlite suspended in polyacrylic acid. By exchange with Na^+ ions in the tear fluid betaxolol is released.

Also liposomes, nanoparticles and microemulsions (see chapter 20) are employed to achieve an extended constant drug release and improved bioavailability in the eye.

Furthermore, contact lenses with controlled drug release, as well as drug-loaded punctum plugs of silicone are quite promising. Punctal plugs block the tear ducts (*puncta*) and thus reduce drainage of tear fluid for periods of 3 to 6 months in patients suffering from dry eyes.

22.5   Maintenance Solutions for Contact Lenses

22.5.1   Contact Lenses

The preferred materials for contact lenses are hydrophilic polymers, in particular copolymers of hydroxyethylmethacrylate (HEMA) and N-vinylpyrrolidone (NVP) or methacrylic acid (MA). Instead of HEMA methyl methacrylate (MMA) may be used for the polymerization. Hard lenses, nowadays known as form-stable lenses, are made of copolymers of MMA with fluorine- and/or silicone-containing methacrylates. They have low water content and are less flexible. With the newer materials this is less pronounced than for the PMMA lenses used before. That is why these lenses are known as *hard-flexible lenses*. The wearing comfort has substantially increased by this development. Some vision defects can only be corrected with hard lenses, while the risk of contamination with viruses, bacteria, and fungi is lower. The soft hydrophilic lenses are made of HEMA copolymers; they may be considered as fluid-enriched gels with an elastic character. They are quite comfortable to wear, have a high mechanical strength (flexibility), high water content, and high oxygen permeability. Their properties can be controlled by the specific nature of the copolymers used. The use of glycerol methacrylate provides the lenses with a high water uptake capacity, which allows them to bind more tear fluid than hard lenses.

Lack of tear fluid may lead to disturbed oxygen transport into the cornea. In addition, contact lenses with high water content tend to accumulate depositions. It is important to remove these depositions (lipids, mucins, proteins), as these substances form a nutritional source for microorganisms, which may develop a biofilm on the lens surface. Risk factors for the development of eye disorders are insufficient cleaning and disinfection of the lenses. Since likewise lens storage containers may get contaminated with bacteria, effective disinfection and cleaning measures of those are mandatory as well.

Hygienic systems for contact lenses should provide effective antimicrobial activity, but must not be toxic, as traces of it may come in contact with the eyes. They should have minimal effect on the properties of the contact lenses. Similar microbial purity requirements apply as for eye lotions. Also, solutions for lens maintenance may become microbially contaminated by sucking up microorganisms from the air. Finger contact with the bottle opening, leaving the bottle without capping, and contact of the bottle opening with contaminated surfaces are further causes of contamination. Solutions for various applications are available—for example: rinsing fluid, detergent cleaner, enzyme cleaner, disinfection agent, storage solutions.

22.5.2   Cleaning

Mechanical surface cleaning is done by rubbing the lens between two fingers and rinsing with rinsing solution (isotonic sodium chloride). This should be done on a daily basis after wearing the lenses. Detergent cleaners remove loosely attached deposits and tissue debris by desorption and solubilization, including microorganisms, and should effectively eliminate lipids, mucins, and proteins. Tough deposits, in particular bound proteins, require an enzyme cleaner (proteases, lipases, and glucosidases) that removes any proteins, lipids, and mucins remaining after detergent cleaning, by enzymatic degradation. Complex-forming agents (EDTA, citrate) eliminate inorganic and organic deposits by chelation or complex formation.

It is important to stick to the indicated cleaning times in order to prevent incorporation of foreign substances, particularly in porous lenses. In the case of enzyme cleaning, only suitable solvents are to be used (most commonly isotonic NaCl, peroxide solution) in order to maintain the optimum pH for enzyme activity.

The strict requirements prescribed for ophthalmic drug preparations obviously apply equally to the maintenance liquids for contact lenses.

22.5.2.1   Disinfecting Agents

Disinfection involves the destruction of microorganisms by attacking their cell walls and/or inhibiting protein synthesis. Contact lenses may be disinfected by physical or chemical means. Two types of chemical disinfection can be applied: chemical solutions and hydrogen peroxide. The antimicrobial action of hydrogen peroxide is based on the oxidative destruction of essential cell components by highly reactive oxygen species arising from the peroxide. Obviously, preservation of such preparations is therefore not required. The hydrogen peroxide should, under no circumstance end up in the eye, but can easily be inactivated by a redox reaction producing water and oxygen. For that purpose, tablets containing 0.3 mg catalase are available; in the instruction leaflet, the degradative process is commonly referred to with the term *neutralization*.

Chemical disinfection is carried out with polymers such as polyaminopropyl biguanide (Dymed), Tris Chem, and polyquats. Benzalkonium chloride and thiomersal are only suited for form-stable lenses because these compounds tend to adsorb to highly porous, hydrophilic soft lens materials. Mixtures of preparations (e.g., chlorhexidine with quaternary ammonium bases) are to be avoided, as this may lead to the *mixed solution syndrome* because of interactions of the components. This may involve severe keratopathies.

Among the physical disinfection procedures, heating is the most widely applied. Others include microwave treatment, ultrasound, UV radiation, and stationary (sound) waves.

22.5.2.2   Combined Solutions

Combined solutions are a cleaning and storage solution in one. Disinfection is established by substances that are well tolerated in the eye. The cleaning power of these substances is not high; therefore, the lenses have to be cleaned additionally by other means (protein elimination or surface cleaning). Wetting solutions for form-stable lenses contain detergents and viscosity-enhancing or moisture-binding components, such as macrogols, PVA, or PVP. They are meant to reduce the "foreign-body sensation" during insertion of the lenses.

22.5.3   Contact Lenses as Drug Carriers

Before the administration of an ophthalmic preparation, contact lenses should be removed because oily and semisolid preparations may cause the lenses to adhere, restrict their mobility on the cornea, bring about color changes of the lens material (e.g., by rifampicin or physostigmine) or adsorb drug molecules, which are subsequently desorbed again in an uncontrolled manner. The uptake of pharmaceutics by lenses may also be exploited for the transport of active ingredients or nanoparticles in the eye. Drugs may be introduced by soaking the lenses in a solution of the drug or by direct instillation in the lens. They will be released between the lens and the cornea over a period of up to several hours without being washed away. Because the release profile is difficult to control, with high variability, current research aims at the incorporation of nanoparticles into the lens for additional and improved control of release. In that case, the nanoparticles control the actual release mechanism.

22.6   Biopharmaceutical Aspects

Ophthalmic preparations are used mainly for therapeutic purposes in the anterior area of the eye (i.e., the cornea, conjunctiva, iris, lens and ciliary bodies). Diagnostic use includes, for example, the visualization of cornea defects by means of fluorescein-Na (Fig. 22-3).

Of extraordinary importance are ophthalmics in the treatment of glaucoma where they reduce the enhanced intraocular pressure. Additional drugs frequently used for the treatment of eye disorders are anti-inflammatory drugs, antibiotics, antivirals and local anesthetics. The preferred application site for ophthalmic formulations is the conjunctival sac, which

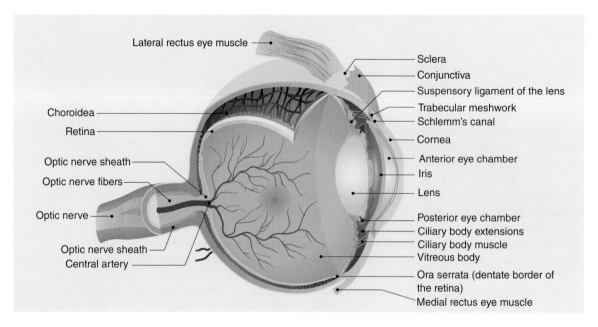

Fig. 22-3   Cross section of the eye.

is formed by the space between the conjunctiva and the cornea and contains approximately 30 μL of tear fluid. It can accommodate no more than a droplet of fluid or a very small amount of ointment. Per minute the tear glands produce about 1 to 2 μL fluid, allowing the tear film (ca.7 μL) to be continuously renewed. At the same time, per minute maximally 50 μL fluid is drained via the tear ducts to the lower nose opening (*meatus nasi inferior*). Due to the continuous renewal, a considerable decline in drug concentration is observed within 8 to 10 minutes following the administration of an aqueous eye drop preparation. This implies that only about 10% to 30% of the administered dose is effectively used. Substances that are meant to activate inside the eye chamber will have to permeate across the cornea into the aqueous humour.

The cornea is built up by three anatomical layers and consists of a hydrophilic stroma, lined by a multi-layered epithelium one side and a single endothelial layer on the other. The two border layers have a lipophilic character. With respect to drug permeation, which proceeds via passive diffusion, the epithelium, wetted by a tear film, presents the main diffusion barrier. Transcorneal drug transport is subject to well-known dependence on the lipid–water distribution coefficient. Although transport across the cornea is of minor magnitude, therapeutically active concentrations may be obtained in the aqueous humour that are higher than after systemic i.v. injection. A transfer in the vitreous body is nearly excluded. Substances with molecular weights < 500 g/mol diffuse more easily than larger molecules such as bacitracin.

The bioavailability of a drug in an aqueous drop formulation can be influenced only to a limited extent by enhancing viscosity. Nonetheless, preparations with enhanced viscosity may promote that the drug is less rapidly washed out by tear flow and a better-tolerated formulation. In this way, patient compliance is enhanced. Inserts, on the other hand, bring along a considerable depot effect. Addition of detergents to aqueous eye drops may be necessary to improve the solubility of problematic drugs or wettability in case of suspension eye drops, but thorough testing of physiological compatibility is mandatory. Also keep in mind that detergents may alter drop volume, which may lead to erroneous dosing. Besides, inclusion of micelles will lower the active concentration of drugs and preservation agents. Surface-active substances (e.g., benzalkonium chloride), intravitreal injections and damaged cornea epithelium resulting from injuries or surgical intervention promote drug transport into the posterior areas of the eye.

The residence time of ophthalmics may be prolonged by suppression of the eyelid movements or closing off the tear duct by applying light pressure with a fingertip on the nose bone in the corner of the eye (naso-lacrimal occlusion). At the same time, this reduces the risk of systemic side effects. Due to a targeted affinity for certain tissues a drug may give rise to depot formation such as, for instance, atropine, which tends to accumulate in the iris and from there undergoes sustained release.

22.7   Testing

The following tests may be conducted on fluid eye preparations:

- Testing for clarity or absence of particles; only the presence of very few single fibers is permitted but no nondissolved particles
- Testing for sterility according to the instructions of the pharmacopeia
- Testing for tonicity by determining freeze point depression *versus* pure water
- Testing for particle size of suspensions by microscopic measurement (see section 3.4.2)
- Withdrawable mass or volume (for single-dose containers)
- Testing for satisfactory preservation

Powders for eye drops or eye lotions in single-dose containers need to be tested for uniformity of content and mass. Eye inserts are to be tested for uniformity of content.

Further Reading

Ali, Y., Lehmussaaril, K. "Industrial perspective in ocular drug delivery." *Adv Drug Del Rev* 58(11) (2006): 1258–1268.

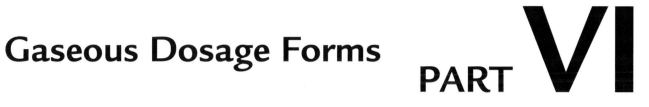

Gaseous Dosage Forms

PART **VI**

Inhalation Dosage Forms

23

23.1 Inhalants

Around the year 800 BC, the priestess Pythia of the Delphi oracle breathed intoxicating vapors escaping from a crevice in the Apollo temple, causing her to enter in a hypnotic trance. This allowed her to whisper her famous prophecies. However, such predictions came to an end in 391 AD, when the Roman emperor Theodosius closed all oracle sites. The treatment of respiratory disorders by inhalation dates back even earlier. In the Ebers papyrus (1554 BC), reference can be found to inhalations. The inhalation of cromones was practiced in Assyria at about 650 BC. An inhalation device was already described by Hippocrates (460–377 BC). He used an apparatus consisting of a pot provided with a lid, which had an opening to insert a hollow cane. Vapor from the pot could thus be inhaled while oral blister formation was prevented by means of moist sponges. In the pot he boiled herbs and resins in vinegar and oil (Sanders 2011). We speak in general of inhalants when an active ingredient, either dissolved in water droplets or as a dry suspension mixed with air, is administered to the organism via the respiratory tract. Preparations for inhalation are liquid or solid formulations that are introduced into the respiratory tract as a vapor, aerosol or powder with the purpose to achieve a local or systemic effect. The Ph. Eur. for example distinguishes the following preparations for inhalation:

- Liquid preparations for inhalation
- Liquids for nebulization
- Preparations in pressurized-gas dosage inhalers
- Powders for inhalation

Inhalable gases for anesthetic purposes are not included in this chapter.

23.1.1 Preparations for Inhalation

Liquid preparations may be added to hot water and then inhaled as a vapor. Even this simple system (used for at least centuries) may produce some particles in the lower μm size range, which may reach the lower pulmonary tract. A similar particle size distribution may be produced during hot showering, which could lead to intoxication when poor-quality water is used (Zhou et al. 2007). Better-defined inhalable aerosols can for example be produced by means of pressurized gases or ultrasonic vibrations. Inhalation powders are administered by means of powder inhalers.

23.1.2 Aerosols

When a drug formulation is nongaseous and cannot easily be inhaled upon evaporation, it may be administered as an aerosol. An aerosol is a disperse system consisting of air containing

Voigt's Pharmaceutical Technology, First Edition. Alfred Fahr.
© 2018 John Wiley & Sons Ltd. Published 2018 by John Wiley & Sons Ltd.

finely dispersed solid (dust aerosols) or liquid (mist aerosols, mist) particles. Smoke contains solid and gaseous components while vapor contains liquid and gaseous components. Aerosols are applied on the nasal mucosa, in the mouth, the pharynx or the airways (larynx, trachea, bronchi, alveoli by inhalation). They are predominantly used in allergic, chronically obstructive, or inflammatory airway disorders (allergic rhinitis, bronchial asthma, chronic bronchitis and mucoviscidosis (cystic fibrosis)). Two parameters are decisive for the drug to reach the target tissue in the lung and to achieve the desired therapeutic result: particle size and the velocity at which the droplets or particles are introduced in the branched bronchial spaces. When the particles are too large, they are deposited in the upper airways. When they are too small, they will not be retained in the lung but rather exhaled again. When the introduction velocity is too high, the majority of the particles will collide with the walls of pharynx, larynx, and trachea. Often, in automated devices, the inhalation device is not activated when a certain minimal inhalation velocity is not reached.

Successful inhalation therapy critically depends on detailed knowledge of the geometry of the respiratory tract. The airway system is a highly branched structure called the pulmonary tree (Fig. 23-1). From the trachea downward, each airway segment divides into two subsequently smaller segments. In this model, a total of 24 airway segments are thus formed (Fig. 23-1). Ultimately, as many as about 300 million alveoli terminate the respiratory system, representing a surface of about 130 m^2 in young adults and about 100 m^2 at old age (Colebatch and Ng, 1992). All the dimensional aspects of this system (length of airway segment, ratio of diameters) have been carefully adjusted by evolution to assure a complete exchange of air in each breath taken. Airflow is turbulent in the tracheal part, but gradually (*transition flow*) becomes laminar from the medium-sized bronchi toward the smallest airways—that is, under conditions of quiet breathing. During exercise, laminar flow is restricted to the smallest airways only).

23.1.3   Deposition Mechanisms

The following deposition mechanisms of particles from the airflow are distinguished (Fig. 23-2):

- *Impaction (collision deposition, inertial impaction)*. This is the deposition of large and fast particles that do not follow the directional changes of the airflow, but rather, advance linearly as a result of inertness and centrifugal force. This leads to deposition at

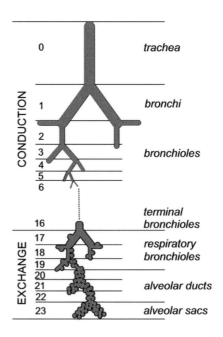

Fig. 23-1 Model of the pulmonary tree (modified from Weibel 1963). Numbers indicate the branch generation.

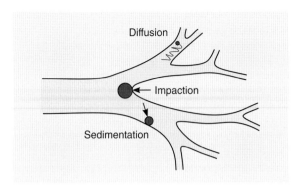

Fig. 23-2 Deposition mechanism.

bifurcations or constrictions. Particles with an aerodynamic diameter of >10 μm are predominantly deposited in the mouth and pharyngeal/laryngeal area or in the upper bronchial branches as a result of impaction. For sprays intended for nose, mouth, and pharyngeal area, the aerodynamic diameter should therefore measure >30 μm in order to avoid delivery to the lungs. The optimal aerodynamic particle-size range for preparations intended for application in the small airways of the lung lies between 0.5 and 5 μm.

- *Sedimentation*. Particles in the size range 1 to 5 μm are deposited predominantly by sedimentation under the influence of gravity. This occurs in the peripheral lung areas, the bronchioles, alveolar ducts, and alveoli, and is therefore the preferred mechanism for aerosol deposition.

- *Diffusion*. Aerosol particles below 0.5 μm are propelled by collisions with the gas molecules (Brownian motion). When the particles move collectively, we speak of diffusion. The smaller the particles are, the more effective the deposition by diffusion will be. By contrast, particles below 1 μm remain floating and thus are exhaled for the greater part when, after administering the puff, breath is not held long enough. Since pharmaceutical aerosols are only rarely mono-disperse, in practice all depositing mechanisms occur simultaneously. That is why generally only part of the aerosol will reach the desired site of the respiratory tract.

In addition to the most crucial factor deciding on successful deposition (i.e., particle size), other factors like particle velocity, inhalation technique, residence time, and respiratory tract geometry play an important role as well. For example, slower inhalation may promote penetration of larger particles in the deeper regions of the lung while prolonged breath-holding following administration favors particle deposition by sedimentation and diffusion. By contrast, fast airflow enhances the deposition of aerosol in the oropharynx region and upper airways and reduces the amount of drug deposited in the deeper regions. Very slow airflow reduces the chances of particle impaction, reducing thereby the deposition in the upper airway and enhancing deposition in the deeper regions. Therefore, patients should be advised to breathe slowly and deeply and hold their breath when inhaling a medication.

23.1.4   Aerosol Application

The factors mentioned above give rise to the following requirements of aerosol application systems:

- Maximization of the particle fraction with size <5 μm
- Constant dosing, high dosing accuracy
- No hygroscopic growth of particles (adsorption of water on the surface) during air flow from pharynx to respiratory bronchioles due to lung humidity and temperature (99.5% relative humidity and 37°C in the bronchioles)
- No effect of inhalation technique and storage on particle size and distribution
- Simple and safe to use, portable, eco-friendly, low cost

Aerodynamic Diameter

The International Commission on Radiological Protection Task Group on Lung Dynamics (1964) defined aerodynamic diameter as the diameter of a unity density sphere with the same settling velocity as the particle in question. Larger particles with a lower density (due to porous structure for example) may therefore have a similar aerodynamic diameter as a smaller particle with a higher density.

The following procedures can be distinguished in aerosol production:
- Metered dose aerosols containing a gas propellant
- Nebulization of an aqueous solution of the active ingredient
- Dry nebulization of a powdery active ingredient

The break-up of the medication form into an aerosol occurs by dispersion during spraying of fluids or by nebulization of solids (whirling up of powder sediments, mechanical processing of solid materials). Other processes to produce aerosols, such as condensation (cooling below vapor saturation or chemical reactions between gaseous phases) are of minor importance for pharmaceutical preparations.

- *Pressurized metered dose inhaler (pMDI)*. The active ingredient is contained in a pressurized gas container, either as a suspension or dissolved in the propellant gas; the substance escapes as an aerosol from the container by opening a valve.
- *Nebulization of an active ingredient dissolved or suspended in water*. Jet- or ultrasound-operated nebulizers are employed to release liquid droplets of a drug solution or suspension suitable for inhalation.
- *Dry nebulization of powdered drugs: dry powder inhaler, DPI*. With this device, a powdered drug is released and dispersed as a result of the inhalation.

23.2   Pressurized Metered Dose Inhalers (pMDI, MDI)

Owing to the development of suitable propellant gases, containers, and dosing devices, it has become possible to achieve fine nebulization and atomization of fluids, emulsions, and suspensions. The dosing aerosols meet the requirements of constant dosing, high dosing accuracy, and a virtual lack of effects on the particle spectrum by external influences and inhalation technique. The first aerosol generator was developed in 1956 by an engineer whose 13-year-old daughter was suffering from asthma. She asked her father why she could not take her medicine like she used her hair spray, rather than by means of the cumbersome and fragile balloon inhaler.

In the aerosol generator the active ingredient is contained within a pressure-tight container together with a liquid with a boiling point below room temperature and the propellant gas. In the container a positive pressure prevails. By opening the valve, the drug in the form of a solution or a finely dispersed suspension is forced out. In the process, the solvent evaporates explosively and the active ingredient is dispersed. The aerosol cloud leaves the valve at a very high initial velocity (30–50 m/s or 108–180 km/h) and consists of propellant droplets and drug particles coated by propellant. These primary particles are relatively large (30–50 μm) but become rapidly smaller due to evaporation of the propellant gas. Because of the evaporation and the volume expansion of the propellant the aerosol cloud cools down rapidly.

These propellant-driven dosing aerosols present two major problems, which are responsible for therapeutic failures in many, particularly elderly, patients and children:

1. Due to the size of the particles, a large proportion of the dose is deposited in the oral-pharyngeal space, which may cause side effects. Especially with glucocorticoids, the risk of mouth sores is considerable.
2. The high velocity of the aerosol requires synchronization of the release of the spray burst and inhalation by the patient. In particular for elderly patients and children, this often turns out to be a difficult task. Improper synchronization may again cause deposition of the material in the oral-pharyngeal space. The cold stimulus may furthermore trigger a cough reflex, or in asthma patients it may lead to an exacerbation of the condition. Thus, application of the dosing aerosol requires elaborate consultation and briefing of the patient, as many patients (see section 23.6) are using the device incorrectly, thus potentially affecting the therapeutic effect.

The aerosol device needs to be shaken well before use in order to homogenize the suspension inside. The patient exhales thoroughly, encircles the mouth piece with his lips and inhales slowly and deeply. While doing so, he releases the spray valve and continues to inhale deeply. Subsequently, he holds his breath for at least 10 seconds in order to prolong the residence time of the particles in the respiratory tract. Then he may exhale normally. The spray mouthpiece and the outlet opening need to be cleaned regularly with warm water. For the inhalation of corticosteroid-containing preparations, the application of a spacer is recommended. After use, the patient should rinse his mouth with water.

23.2.1   Application Examples

Drugs taken in aerosol form are generally absorbed extremely rapidly due to the large total surface area of the lungs. Sprays in pressurized containers are also used in cosmetics and for a variety of other domestic and industrial purposes.

Inhalation aerosols are predominantly employed for topical treatment of bronchial disorders. They exert a local effect on the airway mucosa or on the bronchial muscles (anti-asthmatic aerosols). For acute treatment of bronchial obstruction, $\beta 2$-mimetic or anti-cholinergic drugs are employed. Anti-inflammatory therapy of *asthma bronchiale* is effectuated by inhalation steroids such as beclomethasone and budenoside. Inhalation may also be used to bring about a systemic effect, facilitated by the large internal surface area of the lungs being in close apposition to the lung capillaries, which facilitates the diffusion of substances to the blood circulation. Pulmonary absorption may be exploited for drugs that are liable to degradation in the gastrointestinal tract or are poorly absorbed there. Thus far, this approach has been rarely taken, but it may gain acceptance in the future, especially for delivery of peptides and nucleic acids. With drugs like ergotamine tartrate, insulin, and octyl nitrite, systemic effects upon inhalation have already been reported.

Aerosols for cutaneous application include liquid bandages that serve to protect the injured skin against external influences by the formation of an elastic membrane. The membrane must be formed within maximally 30 seconds and be permeable to water vapor in order to ensure normal regeneration of the injured tissue underneath the bandage. They are either water-washable (polyvinylpyrrolidone, cellulose derivatives) or not washable (acrylic resins) and may contain antibiotics or antiseptic agents. Especially wounds that are difficult to dress with traditional bandages (in the neck, face, head, armpit and anal area) are suited for aerosol dressing. Special surgical preparations contain esters of 2-cyanoacrylic acid, which polymerize rapidly in presence of moisture and produce hemostatic films that cause wound edges to stick together.

Authentic dermatological aerosols include antiseptic, anti-mycotic, anti-inflammatory, anti-pruritic and anti-allergic preparations, as well as agents for the treatment of burns. Aerosols are specifically suitable to apply solutions, suspensions, foams, ointments, and powders on the skin. A special group of aerosols serves to be applied in body cavities, such as the mouth and the pharyngeal area (infections), the rectum (itching, hemorrhoids), and vagina (contraceptives).

Finally, aerosols are employed for local surface anesthesia, diagnostic purposes, and disinfection of air, operating areas, and surgical instruments.

23.2.2   Containers

Aerosol containers contain pressurized fluids and obviously need to sustain this pressure (around 7 bar at 25°C for HFA 134). They should therefore withstand pressures of 10 to 13 bar at about 55°C. The most frequently used material for containers is aluminum, as it is lightweight and less prone to corrosion than most other metals. Seamless aerosol containers are produced by an impact extrusion process, which assures safety against leakage, incompatibility, and corrosion. Epoxy, phenolic or vinyl resin coatings are applied to minimize the interaction between the aluminum and the formulation. Tin-plated steel is an alternative option, as it is also lightweight and inexpensive. Both sides of the tin are electroplated with steel layers. This layered system is coated by an epoxy coating. The best material would be stainless steel because of its noncorrosiveness and sturdiness, but this is a quite expensive solution. As plastics are permeable to air (oxygen!) and to the pressurized vapor inside, this material is rarely used, except for nonpharmaceutical applications. Glass is only used as MDI container in the development stage for easier control of stability and homogeneity.

23.2.3   Valve Systems

The valve system consists of the valve case, which is positioned on the valve plate and contains the mechanical device, the feed tube, that reaches into the spray fluid, and the spray nozzle (Fig. 23-3). The valve system needs to meet special requirements. Tightness and precise functioning are of decisive importance for aerosol generators. The material as such and the required tightness should not be affected by the contents. Synthetic polymers (nylon, low-pressure polyethylene) are the materials of preference; the spring that is used in many systems is preferentially made of stainless steel. By pressing the valve with a finger, a channel is opened, causing the propellant to push the drug solution through the feed tube into the nozzle, which brings about atomization. It is important that the valve promptly closes again automatically after use. The fineness of the sprayed material is essentially determined by the diameter of the valve opening, the pressure, and the anatomy of the spray nozzle. A polymer cap protects the valve against damage and prevents unintentional spraying.

For a proper aerosol therapy, the delivery of a fixed dosage should be guaranteed. For that purpose, special valves equipped with a dosing chamber are required, which deliver the exact dose in this chamber at each spray burst.

In Fig. 23-4, one version (out of several available) of such a metered dose valve systems is schematically depicted: In the resting position, the spray fluid (note: being under high

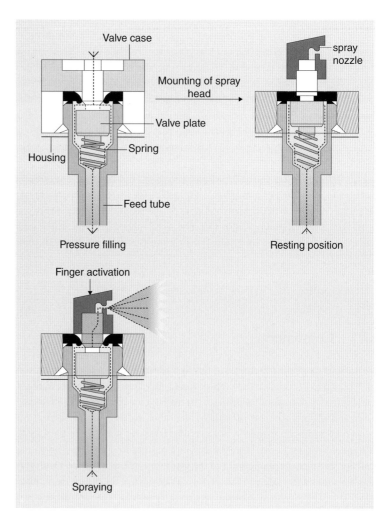

Fig. 23-3 Valve system.

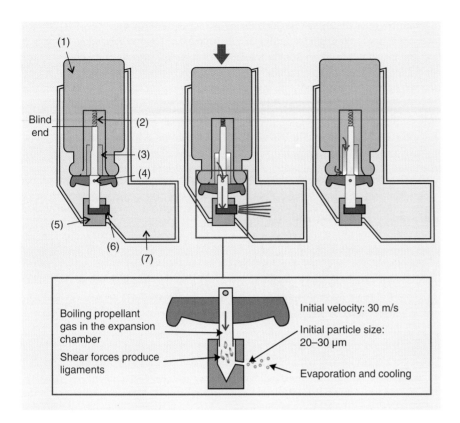

Fig. 23-4 Metered dose system: (6) nozzle orifice, (7) mouthpiece. The other numbers are explained in the text.

pressure) in the stock container (1) is connected with the actual dosing chamber (3). A spring (2) keeps the valve stem (a thin tube, represented in white) in the resting position. Upon triggering the spray burst by pressing up the actuator (5) or pressing down the container (fat green arrow) against the actuator (5), first the dosing chamber is closed off from the stock spray solution by the bulge on the valve shaft. As a result of the further sliding of the shaft, the hole (4) in the shaft that is initially positioned outside now becomes immersed in the metering chamber (3). Thus, the spray fluid in the dosing chamber can exit through the hole in the valve head and enter the orifice (6) via the hollow valve shaft from where it is released. Upon releasing the finger, the spring (2) pushes the valve shaft again in the resting position and the dosing chamber is filled again from the stock container.

What precisely happens in the valve head? As soon as the highly pressurized fluid in the dosing chamber enters the expansion chamber, the fluid begins to boil explosively because of the ambient pressure prevailing there. Thus, the vapor produced pushes the remaining boiling fluid in the direction of the valve hole. While the fluid is on its way there, shear forces induce the formation of fluid ligaments, which in turn are fragmented to small droplets when exiting the orifice (see Fig. 23-4 for details).

23.2.4   Accessories for the Improvement of Application

The use of the conventional propellant-driven dosing aerosols does not come without problems. To overcome these, a number of improvements have been developed. Extension pieces (spacers) are tube-like hollow bodies with a volume of between 50 and 900 mL, which can be placed on the mouthpiece and thus increase the distance to the mouth. Furthermore, a back-pressure valve may be added to the mouthpiece of the spacer. Inside the spacer, the velocity of the aerosol diminishes, as does the impaction rate in the oral-pharyngeal cavity. The cold stimulus lessens and the coordination between triggering the spray burst and inhalation becomes less critical. A disadvantage of these auxiliary pieces is their physical size and the potential electrostatic deposition of drug in the spacer.

Breath-triggered dosing valves release the aerosol when the inhaled airflow releases a lock mechanism due to the arising negative pressure (Autohaler®). Before inhalation, the drug is dosed by manipulating a lever. It is the inhalation that causes the release of the dose from the container. This eliminates the need for synchronization between inhalation and inducing the dose release.

A computer-controlled auxiliary device (SmartMist®, Aradigm Corp.), into which the conventional MDI may be inserted, permits dose release only when the required breathing frequency has been attained. The device records the number of delivered doses and the dose frequency and can be programmed such that the dose can be delivered only at minimal intervals. Compliance and evaluation of clinical data are significantly improved in this way.

23.2.5   Propellants

General Introduction

A prerequisite of the use of a propellant is that it is physiologically harmless upon intentional as well as unintentional inhalation. It must also be tolerated well by the skin, while compounds formed upon heating should be nontoxic. A tolerance criterion is the maximal accepted concentration (MAC). The MAC value indicates the number of ppm (volume parts per million, or cm^3/m^3) of a gaseous substance that is tolerated, without presenting a health risk, on the skin or mucosal tissue or by breathing during an 8-hour/day and a 5-day/week exposure. Propellants must have a high vapor pressure at room temperature and should neither interact with the active ingredients nor with the container or valve materials. They should be neither inflammable nor explosive. In order to warrant maintenance of the internal pressure and satisfactory spraying properties, propellants need to possess a certain degree of solubility in the drug solution. They are distinguished in compressed and liquefied gases.

23.2.5.1   Compressed Gases

The main representatives of this group are nitrogen, carbon dioxide, and nitrogen dioxide. The disadvantage of compressed gases is the steady decrease of pressure in the container throughout the use of the aerosol device. In fact, the pressure inside the container is proportional to the filling ratio of the container. As the generated particle size is also a function of the remaining pressure in the container, this fact also adds to the disadvantages of using compressed gases.

Molecular Nitrogen (N_2)

Major advantages of this gas are that it is inert, tasteless, inexpensive, and easy to fill in containers. Unfavorable characteristics are its practical insolubility in the used solvents, the fact that fine nebulization is barely possible, and that during spraying the container should be held perpendicular in order to avoid immediate release of the gas. Nitrogen is used for pressurized gas packaging of ointments and pastes.

Carbon Dioxide

Also carbon dioxide is a relatively inert, tasteless, and inexpensive gas. An additional advantage is its solubility in a variety of solvents, including water and ethanol. This brings along a less strong pressure drop during usage as for nitrogen. The spray effect is better than for nitrogen. Because of a relatively low dissolution rate the filling process is more time consuming.

23.2.5.2   Liquefied Gases

These are fluids with a very low boiling point, which at room temperature are in the gas phase, while inside the aerosol container they are partly fluid due to the pressure conditions. Liquid and gas phase are in equilibrium inside the container. During a spray burst, part of the gas escapes and is immediately supplemented by the phase transition from liquid to gas. In this way, the application of such compounds (fluorohydrocarbons, lower hydrocarbons) guarantees a constant internal pressure in the container until it is empty. All gases have a critical temperature above which the gas can no longer be liquefied, but rather, prevails in a supercritical condition. Then, pressure increases so strongly that, for example, CO_2, with a critical temperature of 31°C, cannot be used as a liquefied gas.

Short-Chain Hydrocarbons

n-Propane (boiling point −42°C; pressure at room temperature ∼0.8 MPa) and n-butane (b.p. 0.5°C; pressure at R.T. ∼0.25 MPa) are physiologically inert and inexpensive. A disadvantage is their flammability and the risk of explosion. However, in mixtures with fluorinated hydrocarbons, they have proven their usefulness, as in these combinations they no longer show the aforementioned disadvantages.

Chlorofluorocarbons (CFC) and Hydrochlorofluorocarbons (HCFC)

The ideal propellant is non-flammable and readily miscible with aliphatic and aromatic hydrocarbons designed for aerosolization. The formerly extensively used CFCs (chlorofluorocarbons) and HCFCs (hydrochlorofluorocarbons) no longer play a role as a propellant gas because of their detrimental ecological effects. They diffuse undamaged into the stratosphere where, under the influence of intense sunlight, radical degradation products are formed. These gradually destroy the ozone layer surrounding the earth serving to provide protection from UV radiation. Moreover, HCFCs contribute substantially to the greenhouse effect. The Montreal protocols (1987, amended in 1992) have led to an almost complete abolition of the use of CFCs and HCFCs. Although globally the consumption of HCFCs for inhalants has been reduced by one third, this is much less than initially anticipated. There are several reasons for that discrepancy, among them the growth of the health care systems in developing countries. This has led to an increase in the demand for inhalers, which at the local level are often produced as aerosols.

23.2.6 Hydrofluoroalkanes (HFA, HFC)

These compounds are employed as substitutes for HCFCs, and since 2006 they represent the most widely used propellant in inhalation aerosols. Although as a result of the substitution of the chlorine they do not contribute to the destruction of the ozone layer, they still contribute to the greenhouse effect. The physicochemical properties of these compounds differ significantly from those of the HCFCs, bringing along the necessity of intensive developmental efforts, in particular for the valve systems. Currently, the hydrofluorocarbons (HFA, HFCs), Apaflurane (heptafluoropropane, HFA227) and Norflurane (tetrafluoroethane, HFA 134a, HFC 134a) are used as propellants, although for most drugs they have very poor solvent capacities. That is why co-solvents are added such as ethanol in case of corticosteroids (concentration ∼8 %). Besides, for drug suspensions additives such as oleic acid, sorbitan trioleate or lecithin are added, serving as suspension stabilizers and valve lubricants. A further advantage is the small size of the obtained particles, in comparison to HCFCs, and the accompanying reduction in discharge velocity, causing less impaction in the pharyngeal space. In 2016, at the 28th meeting of the Parties to the Montreal Protocol, negotiators from 197 nations agreed upon another amendment of the Montreal Protocol in Kigali (Rwanda). As per agreement, these countries are expected to reduce the manufacture and use of Hydrofluoroalkanes (HFAs) by roughly 80–85% of their respective baselines, by 2045. US, Japan, and Europe will start phasing out HFAs in 2019, China in 2024 and the remaining countries in 2028. This calls for new propellants and may further influence the importance of powder inhalers.

23.2.7 Dimethyl Ether

As a result of these considerations, currently short-chain hydrocarbons are gaining importance again despite their flammability. An already tested potential substitute is dimethyl ether. This compound is environmentally less burdensome because of its rapid degradation, and it is partially miscible with water. A major drawback is its flammability, which can be reduced by addition of water.

23.2.8   Multiple-Phase Aerosols

23.2.8.1   Two-Phase Aerosol

When the liquefied or gaseous propellant is miscible with the drug solution or when the drug is dissolvable in the liquefied propellant, we are dealing with a two-phase aerosol (gas phase, drug in propellant) (Fig. 23-5A). The fineness of the atomized preparation is determined by the mixing ratio of propellant:drug solution and the solubility of the propellant in the drug solution. In two-phase aerosols, the fraction of the propellant that is in the fluid phase will push the fluid phase, containing the dissolved or suspended drug, through the valve.

Rapid evaporation results in a several hundredfold volume increase and very fine atomization. The proportion of active ingredient amounts to 5% to 15%. For reasons of miscibility, only organic solvents are suitable for the production of aerosol solutions; particularly, ethanol or ethanol-water mixtures have proven their suitability in this connection. When suspensions are used, particles measure between 2 and 5 μm in diameter. Apart from that, all usual criteria concerning this type of formulation apply (sedimentation, creaming, particle size increase). Addition of a stabilizer may be required (lecithin or oleic acid as wetting agents).

23.2.8.2   Three-Phase Aerosols

When the drug solution is not or only slightly soluble in the propellant, we are dealing with a three-phase aerosol (gas phase, drug solution, fluid propellant). In case the density of the liquefied propellant is higher than that of the drug solution (e.g., hydrofluoroalkanes), the fluid fraction of the propellant forms the bottom phase (Fig. 23-5C). In this case, the feed tube should not reach all the way to the bottom of the container. Lighter hydrocarbons will float on top of the drug solution (Fig. 23-5B). In the latter case, very fine atomization will not be achieved. Because in case of three-phase systems the propellant only serves to generate pressure and has no influence on the atomization process at the moment of ejection from the container, special spray nozzles with a mechanical swirling facility have been designed.

23.2.8.3   Powder Aerosols

Powder aerosols often contain antibiotics or anti-mycotics and are widely applied as body or foot sprays. Formulating such sprays does not proceed without various difficulties. The solid materials, including the necessary excipients, must be reduced to particle sizes of <30–40 μm and homogeneously distributed in a fluid that is miscible with the

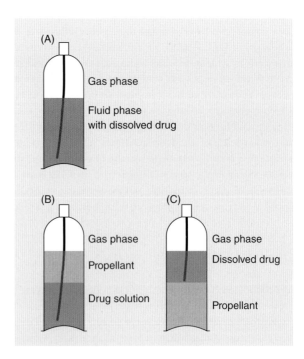

Fig. 23-5 Two- and three-phase aerosols.

propellant. In general, the concentration of solid substance amounts to maximally 10% to 15% so as to avoid obstruction of the valve. Concomitantly, the propellant fraction is quite high in powder aerosols (~90%). Nonetheless, the proportion of solid substance may be enhanced by further reduction of particle size (<10 μm). At higher proportions of solid material, often glass or metal spheres are added to improve the capacity to be stirred up.

23.2.8.4   Foam Aerosols

Generally speaking, foam aerosols consist of an O/W emulsion. The dispersed phase is formed by a fluid propellant dissolved in a lipid component (vegetable oil or liquid paraffin). Anionic or nonionic detergents serve as emulsifiers. Isopropyl myristate and –palmitate improve spreadability. During the release from a special valve, which has to be highly corrosion-resistant because of the presence of water in the filling material, the emulsion is inflated by the propellant dissolved in the internal phase. Dependent on the composition, stable and unstable aqueous foams are distinguished. Facilitated by the propellant concentration, which in usually is essentially lower in foam aerosols than in other aerosol preparations, (3% to 12%) and by the appropriate choice of emulsifier, all conceivable favorable foam properties may be achieved. Because the mechanism does not involve atomization of a solution into very fine particles, the designation "foam aerosol" is strictly speaking incorrect; nonetheless, it is commonly used. Further insight into foam drug delivery systems can be found in Shinde et al. 2013.

23.2.9   Filling and Sealing of Containers

Pressurized gases must be filled under pressure. In case of liquefied gases two procedures are in use: cold filling and pressure filling. In the cold filling procedure the undercooled (−60°C) propellant and the material to be sprayed are introduced as a liquid into the container, which is subsequently sealed off. In the pressure filling procedure, first a concentrate of drug in a propellant is filled into the container at ambient pressure and temperature, then the container is closed off with the valve head and ultimately, additional propellant is filled through the valve at higher pressure. In an alternative procedure (under-the-cap filling) the container is filled with the drug solution and, after lifting up the valve and removal of air, the undercooled propellant is forced inside under pressure and the container is sealed by placing the valve in position again.

23.2.10   Double-Chamber Pressurized Gas Containers

The internal space of these containers is separated into two chambers by means of a flexible impermeable bag (high-pressure polyethylene or aluminum foil). The bag is filled with the drug solution, and then pressurized air or nitrogen is pressed into the container via a hole at the bottom that can be closed off by a rubber stopper. When the valve is opened, the pressure of the propellant on the bag forces the drug solution out of the bag (to the spray head). Depending on the valve and spray nozzle system, the device produces a spray mist, a fluid jet, or a strand of ointment. As a result of content depletion, the volume of the bag diminishes and the operational pressure drops so that, when the bag finally is completely empty, only a slight residual pressure remains. Such double-chamber containers have the advantage that there is no risk of incompatibility between the filling substance, the container and/or the propellant. Nonetheless, they are not likely to replace the fluid-gas aerosols because they cannot compete with the fineness and consistency of the sprayed particles that can be obtained with the latter. Another disadvantage is the relatively high cost due to high material input and complexity of the filling technology. Besides, they are not suited for application of powders and foams.

23.3   Nebulizers

Nebulization of active substances that are dissolved or suspended in water may be achieved by compressed air or ultrasound. The resulting particle spectrum is superior to propellant-driven or powder aerosols with in terms of respirability. However, because of the low drug concentration, inhalation times of as long as 10 to 20 minutes are required. As a matter of fact, this type of inhalation is suited particularly for treatment of severe asthma and, due to the simple inhalation technique, also suited for children and patients experiencing problems with breathing coordination. Available devices include stationary equipment as well as small devices for portable use. Obviously, the latter will still be larger than MDIs or DPIs. Hygienic handling is mandatory in order to reduce the otherwise high risk of contamination. The mouthpiece as well as the spray nozzle needs to be cleaned after each use. The applicability is limited to microbiologically clean, isotonic and pH-neutral aqueous drug solutions or suspensions.

23.3.1   Jet Nebulizers

> Venturi effect (Bernoulli principle): fluid (for example air) flows through a narrowing tube. The velocity of the fluid increases, due to the conservation of energy law the pressure has to decrease at this place.

The first devices for inhalation were based on the principle of nebulization (atomization) and have been available since about 1850 (Nikander and Sanders 2010). In nebulization, a powerful air stream passes along the open end of a capillary tube through which the drug solution is drawn up (also the principle of the perfume atomizer, see Fig. 23-6). In manually operated glass nebulizers, the airflow is generated by pressing a rubber ball or by pumping, but creating an insufficient airflow for producing small particles. Modern stationary devices for aerosol therapy operate by means of compressed air and can produce a particle profile with over 50% of particles within the optimal size range of 1 to 5 μm. Compressed air is accelerated via a nozzle and drags along the drug solution through capillaries (Venturi's application of the Bernoulli Effect; see Fig. 23-6), which, as a result, becomes nebulized. In addition, a collision plate right behind the nozzle serves to further diminish particle size. This principle was used in 1849 by Auphan, who projected a fine stream of water against a room wall, filling the room with a fine mist and allow patients to inhale there. By virtue of the presence of blocking structures in the airflow, currently available devices ensure that only the smallest particles escape, while the larger ones flow back into the reservoir to be nebulized once more. During inhalation, massive evaporation occurs, which causes the production of a cold aerosol and the concentration of the active ingredient.

23.3.2   Ultrasonic Nebulizers

A piezo crystal is induced to vibrate by means of a high-frequency alternating current. The vibrations are transferred to the drug solution via a suitable transfer medium and release ultrafine fluid droplets from the solution, while warming it up. Currently available devices

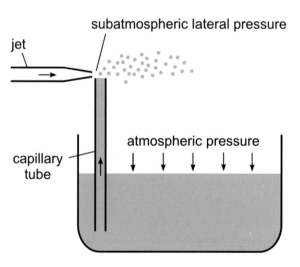

Fig. 23-6 Nebulization (Atomization) of a liquid using the Venturi-Bernoulli principle.

(e.g., Omron®, e-flow®) are essentially portable. Nonetheless, these systems are not suited for suspensions, as the particles therein may clog narrow channels within the device.

23.3.3 Multiple-Dose Jet Nebulizers

The operation of this system (Respimat® Softhaler) is started by manually twisting the housing part, causing a spring inside the device to become tightly tensioned, building up a pressure of up to 250 bar. A capillary tube leads the drug solution from the exchangeable cartridge (4 mL) into the dosing chamber (15 μL). Upon pressing the pressure release button the energy released from the spring forces the drug solution from the dosing chamber via a special nozzle (dual-jet impact nozzle). As a result, an ultrafine mist is generated (particle size predominantly <5.8 μm). Additional advantages of this system are the relatively long spraying time (1.2 s vs. 0.2 for dosing aerosols), the lower escape velocity (0.8 m/s vs. 6 to 30 m/s for dosing aerosols) and the lower impact velocity in the pharyngeal space. This leads to an approximately threefold higher lung deposition.

23.4 Powder Inhalers (Dry Powder Inhalers DPI)

23.4.1 General Introduction

Powder inhalers release the aerosol by means of the inhalation process; the energy required for the dispersion is obtained through the inspiration flow. This type of aerosol generation demands special requirements of the powder processing. To produce respirable particle sizes the powder must be micronized. The extreme pulverization of the particles brings along a substantial increase in surface area and surface energy of the particles. That results in the formation of agglomerates that have poor flow properties and are not respirable. Therefore they must be de-agglomerated. For that purpose, powder inhalers are equipped with special construction parts (ventilator, turbulence channels, baffle plates). Also, the energy required for this purpose is derived from the inhaled airflow. These conditions create some disadvantages for the powder inhaler:

- ▫ The respiratory flow generated by the patient must be sufficient to produce a respirable particle spectrum, which might be a problem for patients suffering from asthma.
- ▫ The powder loses its finely disperse character upon attracting moisture and hence it must be protected from that by thorough packaging.

Dosing improvement may be obtained by taking the following measures:

- ▫ Interactive powder mixtures contain an inert and considerably coarser carrier substance to which the micronized active substance adheres (Fig. 23-7). As a result, the mutual attraction forces between the micronized particles are replaced by the essentially weaker bonds with the carrier material. During inhalation, the carrier particles remain in the oral-pharyngeal cavity, while the drug particles are detached during

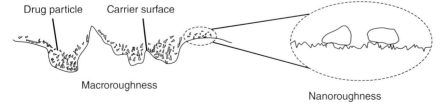

Fig. 23-7 Surface roughness of carrier particles at different length scales. From Ali Nokhodchi and Gary Martin, ed., *Pulmonary Drug Delivery: Advances and Challenges*, Wiley Series on Advances in Pharmaceutical Technology (Chichester, West Sussex: John Wiley & Sons, 2015).

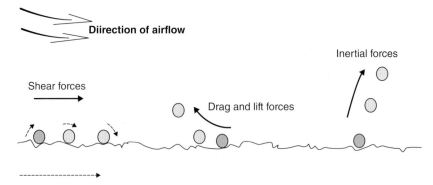

Fig. 23-8 Mechanisms of drug detachment from carrier surface. From Ali Nokhodchi and Gary Martin, ed., *Pulmonary Drug Delivery: Advances and Challenges*, Wiley Series on Advances in Pharmaceutical Technology (Chichester, West Sussex: John Wiley & Sons, 2015).

the first fly-phase as a result of different mechanisms and thus allowed to reach into the desired part of the respiratory tract. A suitable excipient to achieve this is α-lactose monohydrate, which has a smooth-surface crystal structure. By contrast, the surface of β-lactose crystals is much less smoothly structured. This causes the adhered drug particles to be much less readily released in the pharyngeal space upon leaving the nozzle (see Fig. 23-8 for mechanisms of drug detachment). If the surface of the carrier is too rough, a pretreatment of the carrier with micronized carrier might close the microclefts on the course surface. Adherence of drug particles will then be not so strong.

□ Controlled (weak) agglomeration converts the micronized drug into larger units. These larger units do not tend to agglomerate among each other and disintegrate to the original size upon dosing (Turbohaler®, Astra Zeneca, Fig. 23-10).

Electromechanical (i.e., battery-driven impellers), which are activated via the inhaled air and inhalation velocity, improve the available dose as well as dosing accuracy (Spiros®, Dura).

The first DPI was patented in 1852, but had no commercial success. The first successful DPI was the Fisons Spinhaler® in 1971. This device delivered sodium cromolyn in single hard gelatin capsules. There are many devices from different companies available for the administration of a powder (Fig. 23-9).

DPIs can be classified by dose type into four categories: single-unit dose (medication form filled in replaceable capsules); single-use disposable; multi-unit dose (medication form in factory metered and sealed doses packaged within the device) and multi-dose reservoir (medication form in bulk, device uses a mechanism to meter individual doses upon actuation).

23.4.2   Single-Dose Systems

Single-unit dose inhalers contain only one dose of active drug that is contained in a hard gelatin capsule. When using the device, the capsule is punched and the powder is inhaled while the powder is dispersed inside the inhaler. Depending on the particular device, we distinguish spinning impeller (Spinhaler®) pressure drop, shear forces, grids and turbulence channels as dispersion tools inside the devices. Different active ingredients require different carriers. The dose fraction of the powder that actually leaves the capsule is quite variable (30-60%) which accordingly affects dose accuracy.

Disposable single dose inhalers offer, beside favourable hygienic conditions, also the elimination of potential performance failures caused by poor maintenance or damage after falling. Yet another advantage is the avoidance of moisture due to inadvertent exhalation into the inhaler, often occurring during use by children. There are about ten disposable dry power inhalers for general purpose on the market.

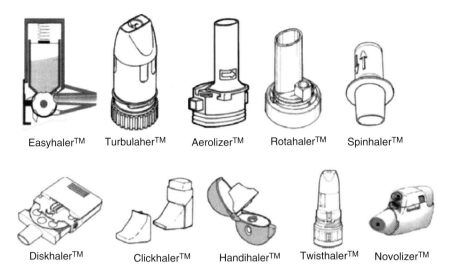

Easyhaler™   Turbulaher™   Aerolizer™   Rotahaler™   Spinhaler™

Diskhaler™   Clickhaler™   Handihaler™   Twisthaler™   Novolizer™

Fig. 23-9   Some common DPI devices. From Ali Nokhodchi and Gary Martin, ed., *Pulmonary Drug Delivery: Advances and Challenges*, Wiley Series on Advances in Pharmaceutical Technology (Chichester, West Sussex: John Wiley & Sons, 2015).

23.4.2.1   Single-Dosed Multiple-Dose Systems

Reusable Systems

In this case, the powder inhaler can be charged with several single doses separately packaged in capsules (InhalatorM®) or blisters (Diskhaler®). After emptying, capsules or blisters are discarded.

Non-Reusable Systems

The powder inhaler Diskus® or Accuhaler® (Fig. 23-10) contains a blister strip with 60 single doses that is rolled up inside the inhaler. The strip is transported via a transport mechanism which also removes the upper part of each individual blister and moves the dose in front of the air channel. The emptied part of the blister is rolled up again. The number of remaining

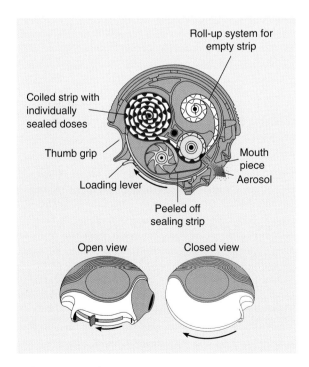

Fig. 23-10   Diskus® or Accuhaler® (GlaxoSmithKline).

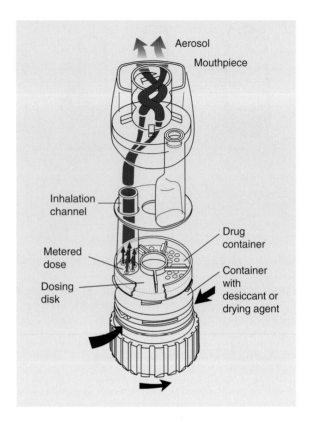

Fig. 23-11   Turbohaler or Turbuhaler (Astra Zeneca).

doses can be read from a counting device. After all blisters have been emptied the entire device is discarded.

23.4.3   Multiple-Dose Systems

The powder inhaler contains an amount of powder sufficient for 200 single doses in a reservoir. By pressing the upper part, one single powder dose is deposited via a dosing wheel in the inhalation channel (Easyhaler) or is dosed by one hence-and-forth turn of the dosing wheel at the bottom side of the inhaler and transported into the turbulence channel (Turbohaler, Fig. 23-11).

23.4.4   Active Dry-Powder Inhalers

The MicroDose® DPI uses a piezo vibrator to de-aggregate the drug powder in an aluminum blister. This vibrator is triggered via a sensor sensing the patient's starting of inhalation measuring the airflow through the device. The high-frequency vibration also creates jets in the blister to bring powder through small holes in the top of the blister, upon which the powder is inhaled. A similar technology is implemented in the Oriel Therapeutics DPI®. The big advantage of these devices is that aerosol generation is independent of the airflow created by the user. Especially for patients with reduced airflow (e.g., asthma patients), this will allow controlled de-aggregation of the powder mixture.

23.4.5   Thermal Vaporization

Alexza Pharmaceuticals has developed the Staccato® System, which integrates chemical and electronic components. In this system a steel surface that can be heated is coated with a film of a pure, heat-stable drug (5–10 mg). A rapid temperature increase of the plate (approx. 400°C for 200 msec) triggered by the patient's inhalation causes the drug to evaporate and thus produces a homogeneous aerosol with defined particle size (about 2 μm) that can be easily inhaled and is deposited in the alveoli (Dinh et al. 2011). No specific hand-breathing coordination is necessary.

23.5 Microbiological Requirements

Aerosols must possess high microbiological purity. Sterility is required for preparations applied in surgery or ophthalmology as well as for wound dressings. Sterilization of aerosols is quite complicated, but two methods are commonly used:

1. The individual components (i.e., the container, valve, and active ingredients) are individually and separately sterilized and the container is filled under aseptic conditions.
2. Alternatively, the container may be filled under the cleanest possible conditions and subsequently the entire preparation is sterilized, for example by γ-radiation.

When choosing the sterilization method, the type of sealing and the materials used for protective casings as well as the resistance of the lacquer and of the active ingredient have to be taken into account.

23.6 (In)competence of Using an Inhaler

Many studies (e.g., Price et al. 2013) have noted that a high percentage of patients have problems adopting the correct inhaler technique and therefore suffer from incorrect medication. This is true for both DPIs and MDIs. Each of these systems requires a certain level of physical skill, manipulation, dexterity, hand strength, lung capacity, and/or handling or coordination in order to ensure correct inhaler use. Several studies demonstrate that these requirements are often not met. The error list in the cited publication (Price et al. 2013) contains 55 points starting with "failure to remove the cap" via "inhalation through the nose," ending with "failure to replace cap after second inhalation." The authors cite another study, indicating that under the applied conditions, only 5% of the patients used a MDI correctly. In a review of 21 studies, the error rate was between 14 and 90% with an average of 50% (Braido et al. 2016). The solution of this problem would be better education, but it is apparently not so easy to do this, as the problem exists since the first introduction of MDIs and DPIs many decades ago.

23.7 Biopharmaceutical Considerations

Particles deposited in the respiratory tract by inhalation are cleared either physically from the lung, adsorbed into blood/lymphatic system or degraded (Fig. 23-12).

The defense mechanism for removing airborne (pollutant) particles is called mucociliary clearance (MCC). MCC clears the conducting airways of its own secreted mucus, together with substances trapped in it, by means of the mucociliary escalator (Houtmeyers et al. 1999). Coughing serves as a back-up system. When particles larger than 10 μm are inhaled, coughing is provoked. This occurs within 24 hours after inhalation. Since in asthmatic patients, coughing is the main clearing mechanism, as MCC is impaired, this also calls for particle sizes less than 10 μm mandatory for such patients. If the inhaled drug has poor solubility, it is most probably cleared by alveolar macrophages. Biochemical degradation may also occur for drugs, as cytochrome P-450 enzymes are expressed in lung epithelia, as well as phase II metabolic enzymes such as esterases and peptidases.

A 39 year old man with a 5 year history of asthma opened his spinhaler to inspect it. He sucked at the capsule to check if its contents were moist. That caused the capsule and propeller to come off the spindle so that he accidentally aspirated them. He attended an emergency ward, where his chest X-ray was found normal. Over the next three months, however, he developed dyspnoea and pain in his chest. He also noticed a whistling noise from his chest, which became more pronounced when he was lying on his right side. Upon renewed examination, it appeared that....an occasional whistling wheeze was heard on that side. His chest X-ray was again normal. The spindle was removed by rigid bronchoscopy from its lodged position in the right intermediary bronchus just beyond the orifice to the upper right lobe (Polosa and Finnert (1991)).

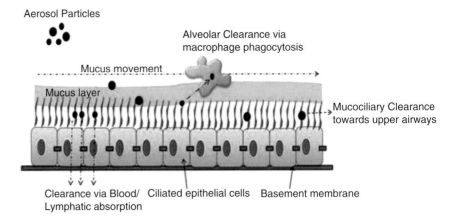

Aerosol Particles

Fig. 23-12 Clearance mechanisms for particles in the respiratory tract after inhalation. From Ali Nokhodchi and Gary Martin, ed., *Pulmonary Drug Delivery: Advances and Challenges*, Wiley Series on Advances in Pharmaceutical Technology (Chichester, West Sussex: John Wiley & Sons, 2015).

23.8   Tests and Legal Provisions

Preparations in pressurized containers and intended for inhalation are formally subject to extensive testing. The test requirements extend to the individual components, as well as the content and the final product. In particular, for containers, the emphasis lies on tests for tightness and contamination with foreign particles.

The containers are tested for resistance to internal pressure (minimally 1 MPa = 10 bar), quality, and continuity of the internal lacquer layer and for the valves (bore size, shape retention, functionality, tightness). With respect to stability of the active ingredient, it has to be kept in mind that oxygen dissolves quite well in HFCs and HFAs, which calls for an input control.

The filled containers need to be tested for internal pressure resistance, shock resistance, and tightness. Several tests concern flammability of the final product, spray tests ensure functionality and in further tests pressure retention, dosing, and fineness of the spray are checked. Upon falling from a height of 2.5 m, the pressure container should not show any damage. Finally, tests for physiological compatibility (irritation of skin as well as nasal, pharyngeal, and eye mucosa), are required.

Safety measures apply to prevent fire and explosion damage by spray cans during transport and storage. In addition, in relevant cases special warnings and instructions need to be clearly visible on the containers. For example:

- For containers under pressure, do not heat above 50°C (at that temperature a pressure of 11 bar builds up in the container with HFA134a; the critical temperature is 122°C).
- Do not damage or use force to open.
- Protect against direct sun radiation.
- Discard only when completely empty.
- Do not expose container (even if empty) to fire (explosion hazard).
- Do not spray in open fire or on a hot surface (formation of toxic products).

The potential of the Twin-impinger and the cascade impactor to simulate the physiology of the respiratory tract is limited but suffices for development and registration purposes. A lung cast made by 3D-printing fed by a digital reference model of a real lung (Schmidt et al. 2004) is a much better simulator. Deposition analysis using such casts is not only restricted to basic science, as new reports indicate (Nordlund et al. 2017).

The Ph. Eur. requires testing of the size of the aerosol particles (Aerodynamic Assessment Ph. Eur. 2.9.18, section 3.4.7), dose uniformity and the number of puffs per container. In addition to the glass impinger (Device A of the Ph. Eur., see 3.4.7), the cascade impactor is used particularly in industry for development (Fig. 3.22), as this allows simulation of the physiology of the respiratory tract to some extent. Further pharmacopeia requirements for all inhalation devices can be found in the Appendix (section 18).

Further Reading

Braido, F., Chrystyn, H., Baiardini, I., Bosnic-Anticevich, S., et al. "Trying, But Failing—The Role of Inhaler Technique and Mode of Delivery in Respiratory Medication Adherence." *The Journal of Allergy and Clinical Immunology: In Practice* 4 (5) (2016): 823–832.

Colebatch, H., and Ng, C. "Estimating Alveolar Surface Area During Life." *Respir Physiol* 88 (1–2) (1992): 163–170.

Dinh, K., Myers, D. J., Glazer, M., Shmidt, T., Devereaux, C., Simis, K., et al. "In vitro aerosol characterization of Staccato® loxapine." *International Journal of Pharmaceutics* 403 (1) (2011): 101–108.

Giraud, V., and Roche, N. "Misuse of Corticosteroid Metered-Dose Inhaler Is Associated with Decreased Asthma Stability." *Eur Respir J* 19 (2) (2002): 246–251.

Hickey, A. H. *Pharmaceutical Inhalation Aerosol Technology*, 2nd ed. New York: Marcel Dekker, Inc., 2004.

Hickey, A. J., Martonen, T. B. "Behavior of hygroscopic pharmaceutical aerosols and the influence of hydrophobic additives." *Pharmaceutical research* 10 (1) (1993): 1–7.

Houtmeyers, E., Gosselink, R., Gayan-Ramirez, G., and Decramer, M. "Regulation of Mucociliary Clearance in Health and Disease." *Eur Respir J* 13 (5) (1999): 1177–1188.

Ibrahim, M., Verma, R., and Garcia-Contreras, L. "Inhalation Drug Delivery Devices: Technology Update." *Medical Devices* (Auckland, NZ) 8 (2015): 131.

Nikander, K., and Sanders, M. "The Early Evolution of Nebulizers." *Medicamundi* 54 (2010): 47–53.

Nokhodchi, A., and Martin, G., eds. Pulmonary Drug Delivery: Advances and Challenges. Wiley Series on Advances in Pharmaceutical Technology. Chichester, West Sussex: John Wiley & Sons, 2015.

Nordlund, M., Belka, M., Kuczaj, A. K., Lizal, F., Jedelsky, J., Elcner, J., et al. "Multicomponent aerosol particle deposition in a realistic cast of the human upper respiratory tract." *Inhal Toxicol* 29 (3) (2017): 113–125.

Polosa, R., Finnerty, J. "Inhalation of the propeller from a spinhaler" *Eur Respir J* 4 (2) (1991): 236–237.

Price, D., Bosnic-Anticevich, S., Briggs, A., Chrystyn, H., et al. "Inhaler Competence in Asthma: Common Errors, Barriers to Use and Recommended Solutions." *Respir Med* 107 (1) (2013): 37–46.

Sanders, M. "Pulmonary Drug Delivery: An Historical Overview." In: Smyth, H. D. C., and Hickey, S. J., eds. *Controlled Pulmonary Drug Delivery*. New York: Springer New York 2011: 51–73.

Schmidt, A., Zidowitz, S., Kriete, A., Denhard, T., Krass, S., Peitgen, H. O. "A digital reference model of the human bronchial tree." *Comput Med Imaging Graph* 28 (4) (2004): 203–211.

Shinde, N. G., Aloorkar, N. H., Bangar, B. N., Deshmukh, S. M., Shirke, M. V., Kale, B. B. "Pharmaceutical Foam Drug Delivery System: General Considerations." *Indo American Journal of Pharmaceutical Research* 3 (12) (2013): 1322–1327.

Stein, S. W., Sheth, P., Hodson, P. D., Myrdal, P. B. "Advances in metered dose inhaler technology: Hardware Development." *AAPS PharmSciTech* 15 (2) (2014): 326–338.

Weibel, E. R. *Morphometry of the Human Lung*. Berlin: Springer Verlag, 1963.

Zhou, Y., Benson, J. M., Irvin, C., Irshad, H., and Cheng, Y-S. "Particle Size Distribution and Inhalation Dose of Shower Water under Selected Operating Conditions." *Inhalation Toxicol* 19 (4) (2007): 333–342.

General Aspects of Dosage Forms

PART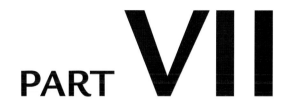

Herbal Drug Preparations (Extracts, Tinctures, and Aqueous Preparations)

24

24.1 General Introduction

Since ancient times, herbal and animal preparations and drug formulations extracted thereof have benefited the health of both man and animal. Even though in modern pharmacotherapy the use of chemically and pharmacologically well-defined drugs has become common practice, extensive use is still made of crude preparations of vegetable or animal origin. In addition to partially purified pharmaceutically active components and chemically pure substances derived from it, extracts, tinctures, and extractions of the crude material are used for the preparation of drug formulations. Many of those preparations can be considered obsolete, however, because preservability of active ingredients and stability of formulations of the drug cannot be guaranteed. Although in practice crude dry material plays an important role in the preparation of herbal teas, application in the form of dry powders (*pulveres normati, pulveres titrati*) is rare. Powdered herbal medicines are also marketed as components of prefabricated tablets, capsules, or dragées. Furthermore, dried herbal preparations are applied in the manufacturing of the following drug formulations: infusions, decoctions, macerates, tinctures, extracts, aromatic waters, spirits, medicinal wines, syrups, and ointments. These products are used either as such or as intermediates in the production of further pharmaceutical preparations.

The production of up-to-date dosage forms containing active ingredients from herbal or animal material requires full compliance with the following demands:

- The assurance of obtaining the active ingredients as much as possible in unchanged form from high-quality and uniform starting material in accordance with the pharmacopeia.
- Achieving high yields.
- Ensuring prolonged preservation of the concentration of active ingredient (stability of the active ingredients during the production process and storage) by selecting adequate production technologies and appropriate dosage forms.
- Creation of a dosage form that can be produced with established and validated production techniques.

As the production of herbal drug preparations involves several processes that are quite different from those used for other formulations, a general overview of the production process for herbal drug preparations is shown in Fig. 24-1.

> **GACP = Good Agricultural and Collection Practice.** These WHO guidelines are primarily intended to provide general technical guidance on obtaining medicinal plant materials of good quality for the sustainable production of herbal products classified as medicines.

Voigt's Pharmaceutical Technology, First Edition. Alfred Fahr.
© 2018 John Wiley & Sons Ltd. Published 2018 by John Wiley & Sons Ltd.

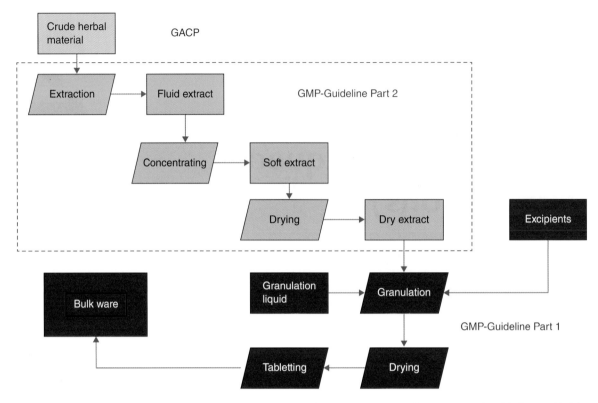

Fig. 24-1 Process outline for herbal drug preparations (Information kindly provided by Dr. Tegtmeier, Germany); GACP = Good Agricultural and Collection Practice.

24.2 Crude Herbal Material as a Starting Substance for Dosage Forms

The starting material for the fabrication of herbal dosage forms may include both fresh and dried (parts of) plants as well as crude plant products such as resins or lattices. A requirement for the production of high-quality dosage forms is optimal quality of the starting material, as specified in the corresponding monographs of the pharmacopeias. In some cases, the pharmacopeias provide storage instructions of individual products. In the Ph. Eur., relevant commentaries may be found in the comprehensive "General Monographs" on medicinal products of herbal origin. Special storage regulations apply to herbal material containing aromatic oils. These should, for example, not be kept in powdered form for prolonged periods of time. Storage in metal containers or in special polymer bags may help to prevent such oils from evaporation. For industrially applied herbal material containing aromatic oils, container types and storage conditions are defined in detail in the corresponding approval documents.

24.3 Pretreatment of the Material

During harvesting of cultured plants or the collection of wild-growing plants as well as during the drying process, a variety of impurities may be introduced, which have to be removed before further processing. Visual inspection and handpicking on the conveyor belt is still considered the best method to recognize and remove adulterations, erroneous replacements, and contaminations with foreign components. Any contaminating metal parts are separated by a metal separator.

The raw material always contains a certain amount of naturally occurring nonpathogenic and/or pathogenic microorganisms and pest insects (bark lice, beetles, mots) as well as their larvae and eggs. Germ reduction and disinfesting (killing of pest insects) are advised from a hygienic as well as an economic point of view in order to avoid losses during storage (see Tables 25.6 to 25.8). In the past, ethylene oxide was used for this purpose, but since 1990

Container types for crude herbal material. In the CTD it is the relevant chapter 3.2.S.6 "Container closure system". The individual character of the plant material defines the type of the material for the bag or container. Key points for the selection of components for the "Container closure system" are:

- Fresh or dried plant material
- Dimension of volatile compounds
- Protection against oxygen of air
- Protection against humidity of air

Some examples should illustrate this diversity: gunnysack for coffee, steel container for fruits, polyethylene bags for dried leaves and paper bags for dried rhizomes.

it is no longer allowed because of the potential accumulation of carcinogenic residues in the material that may thus arise. Likewise, in some countries (e.g., Germany), the use of ionizing radiation is prohibited for treatment of herbal pharmaceutics. Alternative procedures such as alcohol vapors may bring along the risk of introducing changes in the material. CO_2 pressure treatment (pressure expansion (PEX) procedure) is used but it is technically complex: during a short-term pressure treatment (10–30 bar) followed by quick pressure release, beetles and their larvae are effectively killed, but the killing of insect eggs requires a higher pressure or a longer exposure time. A further alternative is the so-called cold disinfesting procedure. The herbal material is shock-frozen in a cold chamber with liquid nitrogen down to −100°C (peripheral temperature of the material −60°C) so that the core temperature reaches a value of −20°C or below). The advantages of this procedure are that 100% of all insects, including all developmental stages (egg, larva, pupa), are killed, that it is ecologically acceptable and that it operates by physical means at normal pressure. However, this procedure has to be checked for suitability for each specific herbal material.

24.4 Principles for Enzyme Elimination

24.4.1 General Introduction

While enzymatic processes in the living plant are indispensable for the synthesis of therapeutically useful products, during drying and storage of herbal products they are likely to have a deteriorating effect on quality. Obviously, this applies in particular to enzymatic reactions leading to partial or complete inactivation of pharmacologically active compounds. All measures aiming at inhibition of such enzymatic processes will contribute to stabilization of the herbal material. Aqueous preparations and expressed juices have to be stabilized. Most enzymes are highly sensitive to elevated temperatures (>60°C) and to alcohols. This offers several options to inactivate the enzyme. Often, the special properties of the enzyme are exploited to inactivate it.

24.4.2 Inactivation

24.4.2.1 Water Elimination
Since the presence of water is essential for enzyme activity, drying of plant material represents a meaningful measure to prevent enzyme-mediated loss of quality.

When water is eliminated by heating, a fast heating rate should ensure that the optimum temperature of the enzyme is quickly passed.

24.4.2.2 Changing pH Value
Enzyme activity can be reduced or eliminated by bringing a preparation to a suitable pH value. This may, however, bring about irreversible (chemical) changes of the herbal compounds, which clearly puts a limit to the use of this approach.

24.4.2.3 Precipitation and Removal of Enzymes
In the isolation of natural compounds, widespread use is made of the precipitation of proteins and enzymes. Precipitation can be achieved for example by means of ammonium sulfate (e.g., in the isolation of pure glycosides) or with water-miscible organic solvents.

24.4.3 Irreversible Impairment

Enzymes may be impaired by protein denaturation or by damaging or eliminating essential cofactors:
- *Heat.* The optimum temperature of plant enzymes lies in general around room temperature. By heating to 60°C or above, most proteins in aqueous solution, including enzymes, will be irreversibly damaged.
- *Ethanol.* Even cold ethanol has a denaturing effect on enzymes. At boiling temperature (78°C) or with ethanol vapor, this effect is even enhanced.

24.5   Herbal Preparations as Multiple Component Systems

Plants are always mixtures of numerous substances. That also applies to the pharmaceutically employed parts of plants and to the extracts obtained from them, as well as to herbal medicinal products. Although extraction procedures result in a selection of the desired herbal substances, the extracts obtained still contain a multitude of chemical compounds. In the following sections, these are briefly presented in different categories:

- *Active substances.* The active substances can be distinguished in major and minor active substances. In particular, alkaloids and glycosides are synthesized by plants in numerous chemical varieties, which calls for a subdivision (major vs. minor alkaloids and major vs. minor glycosides).
- *Excipients.* These are compounds that might influence the therapeutic effect of the major and minor active substance (e.g., saponin, which accelerates absorption).
- *Ballast substances.* These are substances that unavoidably end up in the final formulation during the production process but are fully inactive by themselves. Their presence is undesirable and may under certain circumstances even negatively affect therapeutic activity. More common is, however, that they merely affect color, odor, and/or smell of the formulation or cause turbidity. Often, they influence stability of the preparation, while they frequently disturb analytical assessment of the active ingredient. Ballast substances include chlorophyll, proteins, fats, mucins, and resins, for example.
- *Structural substances.* While the substances referred to above may end up in the final formulation, cell wall material such as cellulose will stay behind in the plant residue.

24.6   Directions for the Conversion of Plant Components into a Drug Formulation

Herbal drug formulations can be produced by either pressing or extraction procedures.

24.6.1   Pressing Procedures

With pressing procedures, pressed juices are obtained. As starting material, finely minced fresh plant material is used, such as artichoke flower buds or purple coneflower leaves. Fruit juices are used for the production of officinal syrups. Pressed juices are aqueous solutions and contain all water-soluble components in the same ratio as the starting material. Only insoluble substances will stay behind in the residue. Besides screw presses, for the production of pressed juices most commonly hydraulic presses are used. The pressed juice is subjected to decanting, centrifugation, and filtration, particularly to remove protein components. Subsequently, it undergoes uperization (ultra-short heat treatment) to reduce germ count. In this procedure, the juice is heated for a few seconds under pressure up to 150°C and subsequently filled at approximately 70°C in germ-free containers which are then immediately passed through a cooling tunnel. In this way, the temperature burden is kept at a minimum.

24.6.2   Extraction Procedure

Extraction procedures are very important for the production of herbal drug formulations.

Minced fresh (parts of) plants or dried plant materials are treated with a liquid (for example a water/ethanol mixture). Which type of extraction procedure and what extraction agent (extraction fluid, *menstruum*) is used depends predominantly on the solubility and the stability of the compounds of interest. Although a pressed juice and a primary fluid extract containing the extracted compounds are both multicomponent systems, they differ significantly. Whereas in the former all compounds of the pressed juice are present in the same ratio as in the cell sap, amounts, and type of the extracted components in the extract depend on the type and composition of the extraction fluid. Thus, certain compounds present in the pressed juice may be lacking in the extract and *vice versa*. For the production of appropriate dosage forms mostly ethanol-water mixtures are used as extraction fluid.

24.6.3   Degree of Fragmentation of the Herbal Material

A prerequisite for the collection of plant contents is the appropriate fragmentation of the starting material. With diminishing dimensions of the fragments the surface area increases and thus the extent of interaction with the extraction fluid. Powdered plant material has a very large surface area and contains, in addition and dependent on the degree of pulverization, numerous damaged cells whose contents can be taken directly up by the extraction fluid. Nonetheless, extreme pulverization is not necessarily meaningful because it may create problems when separating the extract from the residue. Besides, active substances may become too tightly adsorbed to the residue. Understandably, the efficiency of extraction of active substances from herbal material depends on the anatomic structure of the plant material. Diffusion of active ingredient will be largely limited when the outer layers of the plant material are poorly permeable to water. This concerns in particular epidermal structures with a thick cuticle and cork cells. Therefore, proper fragmentation of wood, bark, seeds, fruits, roots, and root stock is essential. This applies as well to material containing lipophilic active substances (e.g., aromatic oils) that are stored in excretory cells and excretion reservoirs with most often poorly permeable walls, localized in the deeper layers of the tissues. On the other hand, aromatic oils in glandular scales or hairs are easily accessible. In case of leaves, extraction conditions are more favorable. The stored intact or fragmented (but not powdered!) starting material is further fragmented to an extent as required by the pharmacopeia for each individual drug formulation.

24.6.4   Solubility and Stability of Relevant Substances in Plant Material

From a technological point of view solubility and stability of herbal compounds are essential properties that need to be taken into account when formulating medicines. Because many compounds of herbal origin are soluble in water or ethanol, preferentially these solvents are used as extraction fluids.

Lipophilic solvents
Lipid-soluble natural substances can be extracted with organic solvents. Oily extracts or balms are obtained by extraction with fatty oils and melted fats. An example is *Hyperici oleum* (St. John's Wort oil) that is obtained by extraction of soluble components with olive oil.

Water
Water has considerable extraction power for therapeutically used hydrophilic herbal substances, but it also accommodates considerable amounts of ballast material. A further disadvantage of water is that it facilitates enzymatic or nonenzymatic hydrolysis, possibly leading to rapid degradation of active ingredients. Aqueous solutions are furthermore liable to be infested by microorganisms. Occasionally there is a risk that the plant material swells up to such an extent that active ingredients remain tightly associated with the material.

Ethanol
Ethanol does not produce swelling of the cell walls and stabilizes dissolved active substances. Furthermore, ethanol precipitates proteins and thus inhibits enzyme activity.

In most cases mixtures of solvents are used as extraction fluid, particularly water-ethanol mixtures. Optimal yields of active substances, with only minor amounts of ballast material, are often obtained with ethanol concentrations between 30 and 70% (V/V).

Alkaloids

Alkaloids and other nitrogen-containing organic bases are in general soluble in lipophilic solvents whereas their salts dissolve readily in hydrophilic solvents. In plants, alkaloids are most often present as salts of organic acids (tartrates, citrates).

- □ Alkaloid salts can be extracted directly from the plant with a hydrophilic solvent (water, ethanol). To convert alkaloid salts into a drug formulation generally ethanol-water mixtures are used.
- □ Upon addition of alkali, the alkaloids are converted to the base form. Extraction then proceeds with lipophilic solvents (e.g., ether, toluene).
- □ When the alkaloid in the plant is bound to tannins or similar plant acids whose salts are poorly or not at all water-soluble, addition of excess acid (hydrochloric acid, tartaric acid, citric acid, and lactic acid) will convert it to a water- or ethanol-soluble salt.

Due to the heterogeneous chemical structures of the alkaloids it is not feasible to make firm general statements on their stability.

Glycosides

Glycosides are in general readily soluble in water and ethanol, but most often insoluble in solvents such as ether or hexane. Dilute acids and alkali, enzymes and often even merely warming of an aqueous solution will suffice to cleave the glycoside.

Saponins

Saponins resemble glycosides in that they are colloidally soluble and have a glycosidic character. Particularly spirostanols can be precipitated by cholesterol.

Tannins

Tannins are readily soluble in water, acetone, and acetic acid but to a lesser extent in ether and hexane. In aqueous solution, tannins can associate and partially form colloidal solutions. Exposure to alkali, acids, air, or oxygen may lead to degradation.

Bitter compounds

The solubility of bitter compounds varies largely, due to their heterogeneous chemical structures. Some are readily soluble in water, others in organic solvents, of which ethanol is the most frequently used.

Aromatic oils

These are readily soluble in absolute ethanol, ether, and hexane as well as in fatty oils. Solubility in water is low. In dilute ethanol, oxygen-containing compounds (carboxylic acids, ketones, aldehydes) dissolve better than in terpene hydrocarbons. Under the influence of light, air and heat chemical changes may readily occur, especially polymerization processes.

Ballast compounds

Aqueous extracts of plants may contain sugars, mucins, amines, vitamins, organic acids and inorganic salts as well as protein degradation products since all of these are readily water-soluble. Ethanolic extracts contain resins and chlorophyll, but to some extent also organic acid, inorganic salts, and sugars.

24.7 Principles of Plant Extraction

24.7.1 Extraction Phases

In the extraction process, we distinguish in principle two phases: the wash-out phase and the extraction phase (Fig. 24-2).

Examples of chemical constituents
1. Alkaloids: Strychnine, ipecac, catharanthus, periwinkle
2. Glycosides: Ginseng, digitalis, aloe
3. Tannins: Tea, catechu
4. Resins: Tolu balsam, benzoin
5. Aromatic oils: Clove, cinnamom

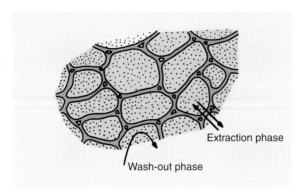

Fig. 24-2 Wash-out and extraction phase.

24.7.1.1   Wash-Out Phase

Immediately upon mixing the extraction fluid with the material to be extracted, the plant cells, damaged or destroyed as they are by the fragmentation procedure, become accessible to the solvent. Thus, the cell components are easily taken up or washed out by the solvent. This implies that in this first phase of the extraction part of the active substances will be transferred to the solvent nearly instantaneously. The finer the powdered material, the greater the importance of the wash-out phase becomes.

24.7.1.2   Extraction Phase

The subsequently following processes are more complicated, because the solvent will first have to penetrate the still intact cells in order to reach and dissolve the active substances located there. The shriveled up and shrunken cell walls in the extraction material first have to be converted to a state that will allow penetration of the solvent into the cell interior. That occurs by uptake of solvent molecules by the cell wall causing the latter to swell up and undergo a volume increase. The ability of the cellulose skeleton to bind solvent molecules causes the skeleton to loosen up in such a way that interfibrillar spaces are formed, which allow the solvent to enter the cell interior. These swelling processes are predominantly brought about by water. It is also for this reason that alcohol-water mixtures are favorable extraction fluids in the production of pharmaceutical herbal preparations. During the drying process the protoplasm of cells in fresh plants shrinks substantially. In the dried state it merely forms a thin sheet. The molecules of the cell content are then mostly present in crystalline or amorphous form. Also this dried protoplasm swells up upon the entrance of solvent molecules in the intracellular space and the individual components dissolve in accordance to their solubility. The molecularly dissolved substances travel by diffusion across the interfibrillar space driven by the concentration gradient between the solution in the cell and the surrounding extraction fluid. This continues until concentrations inside and outside the cells are in equilibrium. The extent to which colloids penetrate the cell membrane depends on the pore diameter. The processes described are in principle involved in all extraction processes discussed below. Specific attention will be paid to individual special processes.

24.7.2   Maceration and Maceration-Derived Extraction Procedures

24.7.2.1   Maceration

Maceration (from Latin: *macerare* = to soften) is the most simple extraction procedure (in most cases minced or coarsely powdered). The fragmented plant material is incubated with the extraction fluid. The primary mixture is protected from direct sunlight to prevent light-catalyzed reactions and color changes, and allowed to stand under periodic shaking. The maceration time varies; individual pharmacopeias advise 4 to 10 days. Empirically, an incubation period of about 5 days suffices to complete the processes underlying the wash-out and extraction phases discussed above. As a rule, by that time concentration equilibrium will have been reached between the compounds still in the cell interior and those already in the extraction fluid, provided that the mixture is repetitively shaken (about three times per day). The latter treatment ensures faster equalization of the concentrations of the compounds of interest between the cells and the extraction fluid. Nonetheless, maceration never results in complete extraction. In the traditional procedure the macerated mixture is filtered over a cloth and the residue is pressed. For that purpose tincture presses (spindle presses) or hydraulic presses are used. The maceration filtrate and the fluid from the pressing procedure are combined and brought to the prescribed volume by washing the residue with extraction fluid. The washing procedure serves to collect remaining extracted substances and to compensate for losses occurring during cloth filtration and pressing step. The combined extract is stored refrigerated and subsequently filtered.

24.7.2.2   Remaceration

Sometimes the plant material is macerated twice with the same solvent (i.e., first with half of the solvent and subsequently with the other half). This procedure hardly yields better results. The procedure is considered somewhat more favorable when the plant material is first extracted with 20% of the extraction solvent, followed by extraction with the remainder.

24.7.2.3   Digestion

The term *digestion* is used when maceration is performed at elevated temperature (30° to 50°C). This increases the yield of extracted active substances. However, during the subsequent cooling to room temperature the solubility of the extracted substances decreases. This may cause the occurrence of turbidity and precipitation. Infusions and decoctions may be considered special forms of digestion.

24.7.2.4   Shaking Maceration

Although intense shaking by means of a mechanical shaker will not increase the extraction efficacy, it will lead faster to equilibrium and thus to shorter extraction times. In individual cases it was reported to establish equilibrium within 10 to 30 minutes.

24.7.2.5   Turbo-Extraction (Whirl Extraction)

In this procedure, the material is mixed with the extraction fluid and then treated with a high-speed (~10.000 rpm) mixer provided with rotating knives. The intense whirling of the extraction fluid and the plant material tremendously accelerates the dissolution and extraction processes so that extraction times of merely 5 to 10 minutes may suffice. The procedure is particularly useful to extract small amounts of material. The rotating knives provide for further fragmentation of the plant material. Care should be taken to exclude loss of fluid by properly covering the container. Temperature should not rise above 40°C during extraction. Turbo-extraction yields extracts of comparable if not higher quality than the maceration or percolation (section 24.7.3) procedure.

Microwave assisted extraction is one of the novel techniques which is used to improve the kinetics of the extraction process. It is often used in combination with conventional extraction methods. Some popular methodologies include microwave-assisted pressurized extraction and solvent free microwave-assisted extraction.

24.7.2.6   Ultra-Turrax Extraction

In the Utra-turrax device (Fig. 24-3), the product is sucked into a whirl chamber in which adjustable high-frequency shear, mechanical impact, and collision effects, combined with hydrodynamic potential gradients and highly effective turbulent fluid movements, act together, thus ensuring economically efficient degradation of materials of herbal as well as animal origin. Ultra-turrax devices are commercially available in a variety of sizes. The smallest are operated in a test-tube size glass vessel; instruments for the industrial scale can process volumes of up to 10,000 liters.

24.7.2.7   Ultrasound Extraction

Treatment of an extraction mixture with regular sound may already affect the extraction yield. For obvious reasons, such a procedure has little practical value because of the noise annoyance connected with it. Much more favorable is the application of ultrasound. The human ear perceives sound between 16 and 20 kHz. Sound waves with frequencies beyond the audible range

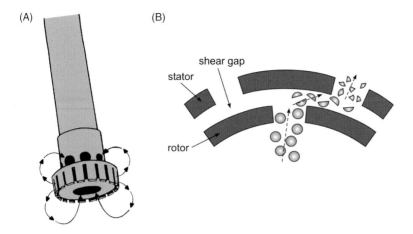

(A) (B)

shear gap

stator

rotor

Fig. 24-3 (A) Ultra-turrax; (B) mode of operation.

are called ultrasound. Modern equipment can generate ultrasonic waves with frequencies up to 1 GHz. With ultrasound, plant extracts can be produced in 5 to 15 minutes. Nonetheless, in each individual case it has to be confirmed that the active substances do not undergo chemical changes. High yields of active substance do not unconditionally reflect the efficiency of the procedure. Natural substances in their extraction fluid and obtained by means of ultrasound often appear to be quite susceptible to hydrolytic and oxidative processes.

24.7.3 Percolation and Percolation-Derived Extraction Procedures

24.7.3.1 Percolation

Percolation (Latin: *percolare* = to seep through) is performed in a vertically positioned cylindrical or conical vessel (percolator) with appropriate in- and outlet (Fig. 24-4). Extraction fluid is continuously introduced from the top and slowly flows through the coarsely powdered material to be extracted. By constant renewal of the solvent, in practice a multistep maceration is ensured. Whereas in the simple maceration process exhaustive extraction is not achievable, since ultimately equilibrium is established between extraction fluid and intracellular solution, the constant renewal of solvent during percolation causes a constant shift in the equilibrium, thus theoretically allowing complete extraction. In practice, up to 95% of the extractable substances can be collected. The procedure is less suitable for strongly swelling or highly voluminous material. Forced percolation can be accomplished by applying negative pressure (at the bottom part; evacolation) or positive pressure (on top; diacolation).

Prolonged extraction times ensure good yields of active substance. Before filling the percolator, the material is well moisturized with extraction fluid and allowed to swell in order to facilitate penetration of extraction fluid in the cell structures during percolation. When pre-moisturizing is performed in the percolator, the latter may become clogged. Filling the percolator is not an easy task. On the one hand, no empty spaces should remain in the filling material, since these would lead to discontinuities in the liquid flow and cause a reduction in extraction efficiency. On the other hand, when the filling is too compact, the solvent flow may become too slow or even come to a complete halt. After feeding in the extraction solvent as prescribed by the pharmacopeia, the first drop is awaited and then the stopcock is closed. When the solvent stands 1 to 2 cm above the material in the percolator, the stopcock is opened again. In the meantime, after-swelling and maceration take place. Only then will the actual percolation start. The flow rate is adjusted in such a way that per unit of time, equal numbers of drops enter and leave the percolator. It is essential that the volume of the emerging extract equals the volume of added solvent and that the volume per unit of time is adjusted to the selected percolation method.

After completion of the percolation process, the solid material is pressed and the collected fluid is added to the percolate and the volume is adjusted to the desired concentration.

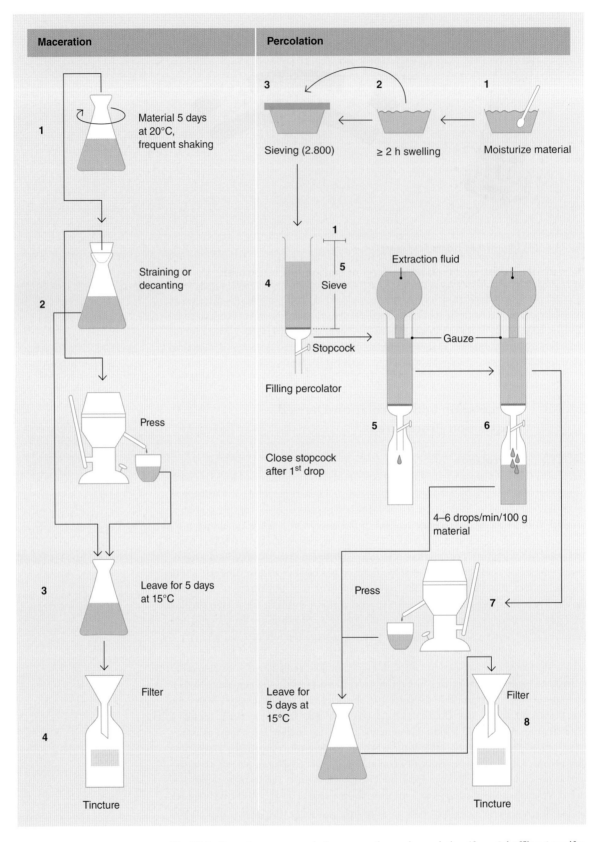

Maceration

1 — Material 5 days at 20°C, frequent shaking

2 — Straining or decanting

Press

3 — Leave for 5 days at 15°C

4 — Filter

Tincture

Percolation

3 — Sieving (2.800)   2 — ≥ 2 h swelling   1 — Moisturize material

1
5
Sieve

4 — Filling percolator

Close stopcock after 1ˢᵗ drop

Stopcock

Extraction fluid

Gauze

5   6

4–6 drops/min/100 g material

Press   7

Leave for 5 days at 15°C

Filter   8

Tincture

Fig. 24-4 Operation sequence during maceration and percolation (from Schöffling Arzneiformenlehre, 6th ed. 2015).

To obtain a dry extract, the extracted solution is evaporated. After production of a fluid extract, this is left standing for several days, and subsequently the fluid is decanted and filtered. Advantages of the percolation procedure include high yields of active substances, rich extracts and thus optimal exploitation of the plant material, as well as relatively short production times. On the other hand, it requires continuous attention and surveillance.

24.7.3.2   Repercolation

In some pharmacopeias, mention is made of a procedure to obtain fluid extracts from plant material containing aromatic oils. In this procedure, the plant material is divided in three portions. The first portion is percolated and the percolate is collected into two fractions, a pre-fraction and an after-fraction. A second part of the material is then percolated with the after-fraction and once more a pre- and an after-fraction are collected. The latter is again used to percolate the third portion of material. The three combined pre-fractions together constitute the percolate.

24.7.3.3   Soxhlet Procedure (Fig. 24.5)

The material to be extracted is placed in a paper or cardboard extraction insert, which, in turn, is positioned inside a continuously operating cylindrical glass extraction column. This column is mounted in between a distillation flask and a reflux condenser and connected to the flask by a siphon tube. The flask contains the solvent, which evaporates upon heating and travels through the steam connection to the return condenser where it condenses. From there, it drips on the plant material and extracts the substance(s) of interest. The solution accumulates in the column, and after reaching a maximum level, it is automatically siphoned

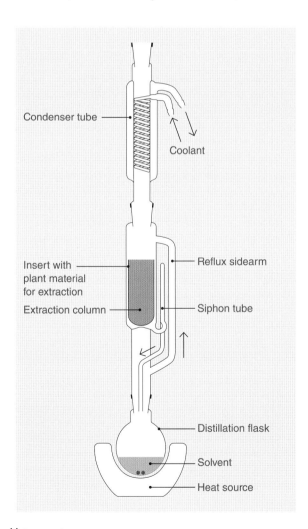

Fig. 24-5 Soxhlet apparatus.

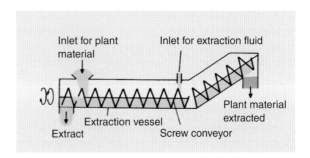

Fig. 24-6 Counter-current extraction apparatus.

back into the distillation flask. The fluid in the flask becomes more and more enriched in extracted substances, while the pure solvent continuously evaporates. A clear advantage of this method is that it consumes very little solvent, while, in addition, the material is continuously extracted with pure solvent, which allows a steady renewal of the concentration gradient and thus more efficient extraction. A disadvantage is that the procedure requires several hours and thus brings along high energy consumption. Furthermore, the plant material in the middle part of the apparatus, directly connected to the distillation flask, is heating up. The extent to which this occurs depends on the duration of the extraction procedure, but particularly on the boiling point of the solvent. It may thus challenge the stability of temperature-sensitive substances (glycosides, alkaloids). Finally, the extracted compounds accumulating in the flask are exposed to heat for a prolonged period of time. All this explains why the Soxhlet equipment, which is frequently used in the laboratory setting for research purposes, has barely found application in the large-scale production of herbal pharmaceutics.

24.7.3.4   Counter-Current Extraction

A continuously operating extraction procedure used in the industrial setting is the counter-current extraction (Fig. 24-6). Via a dosing facility the plant material is introduced into the extraction trough in which it is slowly transported by a screw conveyor with adjustable rotating speed against a stream of extraction fluid. The latter enters the trough from the back side via a dosing valve and exits at the other side via a sieve as an extract. The extracted plant material is carried off at the end of the trough. Any adsorbed fluid can be recovered by pressing or centrifugation. In some special facilities, the extraction trough is provided with a jacket, allowing heating or cooling. Attempts to formulate the physical rules of the extraction processes are gaining increasing attention. This will contribute to further technological development and optimization of methodology.

24.7.3.5   Extraction with Super-Critical Gases

Gases have only limited dissolving capacity. This can be substantially enhanced, however, by compression of the gas, which opens the way to use such compressed gases for the extraction of natural substances.

Under appropriate conditions of pressure and temperature, gases may be liquefied. However, above the so-called critical temperature, this is no longer possible, even at the highest possible pressure. The pressure corresponding to the critical temperature is the critical pressure.

When above the critical temperature pressure is increased above the critical pressure, a super-critical phase of the gas comes into existence. This brings along an increase in density and the di-electric constant of the gas. As a result, the dissolving capacity of the gas increases but might be reduced again by lowering the pressure.

Suitable gases are CO_2, NH_3, N_2O, and noble gases. Most often CO_2 is used as it is nontoxic, nonflammable, and inexpensive. Super-critical operational temperatures range between 35° and 40°C and pressures between 7.3 and 35 MPa. Under these conditions, CO_2 has the density of a liquid but the viscosity of a gas, which considerably facilitates penetration into the plant material.

Super-critical CO_2 readily extracts lipophilic organic substances with relatively low polarity (esters, ethers, lactones) already at pressures between 7 and 10 MPa. Compounds with strongly polar functional groups (−OH, −COOH) hamper extractability but benzene derivatives with three phenolic OH groups or with one COOH group and two OH groups can still be extracted, in contrast to substances carrying one COOH group and three or more OH groups. By the same token, strongly polar substances like sugars and amino acids are not extractable. In case of substances with strongly differing polarity fractionation is possible by means of changing pressure.

Extraction with super-critical gases (fluid extraction) has not yet established itself as an accepted method in the production of herbal pharmaceutics because of the unfortunate lack of acceptance up to now by the approving authorities. Otherwise, it might offer an interesting alternative for the extraction of active substances from medicinal plants like chamomile, valerian, and *Papaver somniferum*. When not used for the production of a medical formulation, the advantages of this extraction principle are avidly applied. For example, for the isolation of fats and oils (soy oil, cocoa butter) as well as for the decaffeination of coffee beans extraction with super-critical carbon dioxide is already a routine procedure.

24.8 Dosage Forms

24.8.1 Aqueous Plant Extracts

24.8.1.1 General Introduction
Aqueous extracts of plant material are among the oldest pharmaceutical preparations. Often such preparations are quickly and strongly contaminated by microorganisms and, in addition, many pharmacologically active substances show severely limited stability in aqueous solutions. For these reasons, aqueous plant extracts should either be immediately further processed (for instance, to a dry extract or a preserved dosage form) or consumed immediately after preparation (e.g., a medicinal tea).

When not prescribed otherwise, aqueous extracts are prepared from 1 part of herbal material and 10 parts of water. For preparations that are only available on prescription special provisions apply.

24.8.1.2 Infusions, Decoctions, and Macerates
Infusions (Hot Infusions, *infusa*)
In these procedures, the extraction material, after appropriate fragmentation, is kneaded with a small quantity of water and allowed to stand for a prescribed period of time before being dashed with boiling water. The mixture is kept in a hot water bath for 5 minutes under repeated stirring. After cooling down to about 30°C the mixture is filtered through a cloth filter. In order to attain the prescribed content, it may be required to wash the residue with cold water followed by gentle pressing. For extraction of aromatic oils or glycosides ethanol is commonly used as a solvent (usually 70% V/V). By addition of organic acids most tannin-bound alkaloids are converted to their water-soluble form. For the sake of better taste often citric acid is added.

Decoctions
The material is fragmented according to prescribed size and is dependent on pharmacopeia instructions—steeped with either cold or 90°C water and then left for 30 minutes under occasional stirring.

Macerates (*macerata*)
After prescribed fragmentation the material is dashed with water of room temperature and left to stand at room temperature for 30 minutes under occasional stirring. Subsequently, it is cloth-filtered and adjusted to the desired concentration by washing the residue with water. Extracts from mucilage containing plant materials (e.g., roots of the marshmallow plant (*Althea*

officinalis), linseed (*Linum usitatissimum*)) are obtained similarly but without heat challenge since that would lead to agglutination of the product.

24.8.2   Tinctures

24.8.2.1   General Introduction

The term tincture (*tinctura*) is derived from the Latin word *tingere* = to wet, moisturize. In ancient Greece, the term was used for dyes. After Avicenna reported on tinctures in connection with medicine, Paracelsus introduced the term in the therapeutic context. Since the seventeenth century, tinctures are included in the pharmacopeias (Dispensatorium of Valerius Cordius, 1666). Over the centuries, the meaning of the term tincture has undergone several changes, particularly manifested as a narrowing of its definition. Nowadays we understand tinctures in general as ethanolic extracts from herbal or animal material. They are preferentially produced with 70% ethanol, while the ratio of material to extraction fluid is most commonly maintained at 1:5 or 1:10. The ethanol content of the tinctures obtained in this way varies depending on the amount of remaining extraction fluid in the residue material.

Tinctures may be produced by maceration, percolation or turbo-extraction methods. Tinctures may be further diluted with extraction fluid.

Turbidities or precipitations in tinctures may have various causes. Upon cold storage solubility of certain compounds may be exceeded, which may lead to precipitation. The same may occur by loss of ethanol due to evaporation. Also chemical modifications by for instance hydrolytic or oxidative processes may cause turbidity or sediments. Exposure to light may accelerate such processes, representing an important reason to store tinctures in brown glass vessels. Temperature-induced turbidities disappear upon warming to room temperature. Therefore, such turbidities should not be removed by filtration. Not only the filtration process as such will remove active substance, but also adsorption to the filter material may cause its partial depletion. According to the requirements of the Ph. Eur., tinctures should be clear, and filtration should be performed only at room temperature.

24.8.2.2   Sensory, Identity, and Purity Tests

Although sensory testing of tinctures for color, smell, and taste, as described in the pharmacopeias, may help to characterize them, it has to be kept in mind that such information not only is subject to individual interpretation, but also substantial differences are observed between tinctures as such. Depending on origin, harvest time, drying procedure, storage conditions, and so on, even the starting material is already subject to variations, which will inevitably lead to differences in organoleptically observable properties. Also, color, shade, and smell of a tincture might change during storage. For example, gradual decomposition of chlorophyll causes its green color to turn brown.

Accurate assays of active substances and purity tests are nowadays performed with chromatographic procedures. Among these, thin-layer chromatography is quite suitable for the pharmacy laboratory, whereas in industrial labs mainly high-performance liquid chromatography (HPLC) and gas chromatography (GC) are employed. In general, the analytical procedures include identification and purity tests and quantitative content assays. Among the commonly performed purity assessments are assays for limit values for aflatoxins, pesticides, and heavy metals, as well as screening for microbiological quality.

24.8.2.3   Determination of Dry Residue (Ph. Eur. 2.8.16)

The dry residue provides information on the quality of herbal extracts (tinctures, fluid extracts). The residue that remains after evaporation of the solvent characterizes the extracting capacity of the extraction fluid and gives insight in the efficiency of the extraction procedure.

For this purpose, 2.0 g of fluid extract is accurately weighed in a heat-dried (105°C), sealable weighing flask of defined height and width and the solvent is evaporated by heating on a water bath till dryness. The residue is further dried for 3 hours in a stove at 100° to 105°C. Strict observance of the conditions is absolutely necessary, since shape and size of the weighing flask may already affect the outcome. The weighing vessel must be sealable in order to avoid evaporation of the solvent during weighing as well as attraction of moisture from the air.

Drying at elevated temperature until constant weight is not feasible, since organic substances may volatilize or decompose under loss of weight.

24.8.2.4 Determination of Ethanol Content (Ph. Eur. 2.9.10)

In all pharmacopeias, instructions may be found on the determination of ethanol content in tinctures and fluid extracts. Two general methods are available for this purpose.

1. After removal of the ethanol from the fluid extract or the tincture by means of distillation, the residual alcohol content may be determined by density assessment. This procedure requires only simple equipment so that it can easily be performed in the pharmacy setting.
2. Alternatively, alcohol content may be determined by gas chromatography. This procedure is less time-consuming and can be easily automatized. In larger laboratory facilities, it has been adopted as the standard assay procedure.

24.8.3 Extracts

24.8.3.1 Classification

As also indicated in the Ph. Eur., the classification of extracts is based on two systems: one pharmaco-therapeutic and the other pharmaceutical-technological. In the former, standardized extracts (*extracta normata*), quantified extracts (*extracta quantificata*), and other extracts (*extracta*) are distinguished.

Standardization can only be accomplished when the compound(s) responsible for the pharmacological (therapeutic) effect has/have been identified. In that case the preparation is adjusted to a fixed content of the pharmacologically relevant compound(s), for example by mixing different extract batches or by addition of inert excipients. Examples of such extracts are standardized aloe dry extract (*Aloes extractum siccum normatum*) or standardized and refined extract of milk thistle fruit (*Silybi mariani extractum siccum raffinatum et normatum*).

In case of a quantified extract, adjustment is performed according to different concentration ranges of the active compounds. These may correlate with activity but may also represent maximal limits for safe application. Usually, adjustment occurs by mixing different extract batches. A typical example is the quantified refined ginkgo dry extract (*Ginkgo extractum siccum raffinatum et quantificatum*).

When neither the criteria of a standardized nor those of a quantified extract are fulfilled, we are dealing with an "other extract." The designation "other extract" is a deliberate choice of the European Pharmacopeia Commission and thus is an official designation. The quality of "other extract" is determined by its manufacturing process and the specifications for starting materials (plant material and extraction solvent) and the extract itself. Prominent examples of "other extract" are the dry extracts of melissa leaves (*Melissae folium extractum siccum*) and of willow bark (*Salicis corticis extractum siccum*).

In accordance with the pharmaceutical-technological classification, five types of extracts are commonly distinguished. When extracting herbal material, as a rule, initially a fluid extract is obtained (*extractum fluidum*). In general, one part of herbal material corresponds to one part of fluid extract. When the (mostly ethanolic) extraction medium is partially or completely evaporated, extracts are obtained which can be subdivided according to their properties in:

- Fluid extracts (*extracta fluida*)
- Thin extracts (*extracta tenua*): nowadays, such preparations are obsolete
- Thick-fluid extracts, thick extracts (*extracta spissa*): such preparations are gummy and have very limited flow capacity when cold. Water content usually amounts to up to 30%. This dosage form prevails only as an intermediate in the production of dry extracts. Besides, it may serve to produce fluid formulations with a defined concentration of active ingredient(s). The high water content brings along instability of the dosage form (bacterial decay) and possibly of the active ingredient (chemical decomposition); for that reason rapid further processing is mandatory.

□ Dry extracts (*extracta sicca*): these possess a dry consistency and are usually readily miscible so that further processing is simple (e.g., dry mixtures with excipients for the production of a tableting mixture. In certain cases they have a tendency to be hygroscopic, which will require special measures during further processing. Fluid, thick, and dry extracts are dosage forms that still receive attention in many pharmacopeias. In addition to those, the Ph. Eur. contains a monograph on oily resins:

□ Oily resins (*oleoresina, oleosa*). These lipophilic extracts with a semi-solid consistency consist of a resin dissolved in aromatic or fatty oil.

24.8.3.2   Dry Extracts

For a better understanding, we will describe the sequence of the process steps during the production of dry extracts. Firstly, a thick extract is produced from the initially formed fluid extract by evaporation of the extraction liquid. Since the extraction liquids often consist of mixtures of organic solvents with water (e.g., 30% ethanol V/V), thick extracts will contain only water as a liquid, in addition to the extracted plant constituents. Subsequently, the thick extract is dried, commonly until less than 5% residual moisture is present in the dry extract. This step concludes the production of the dry extract.

24.8.3.3   Production of the Fluid Extract

Fluid extracts (*extracta fluida*) are commonly obtained by percolation, using ethanol/water mixtures with various ethanol concentrations as extraction fluids. In small-scale procedures, mostly glass percolators are used whereas in industry percolators are predominantly made of steel (Fig. 24-7). In really large-scale facilities, individual percolators may be combined into percolator batteries.

Generally, percolation is considered to be terminated when from one part of dry starting material to four parts of extract have been obtained. Although this does not imply

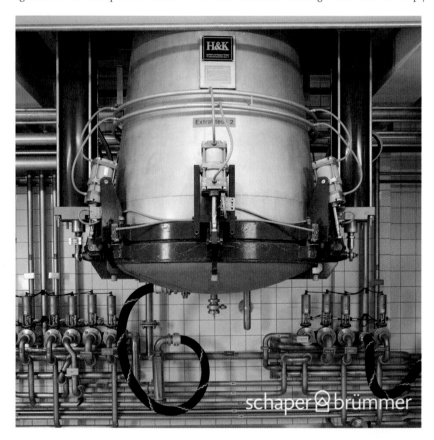

Fig. 24-7 Extraction in industrial scale (Dimension: approx. 6 m, 3 m, 3 m (H, L, W); volume 2 m^3; mode of extraction: maceration or percolation; duration of extraction depending on the type of plant type and extract). Reproduced with permission from Schaper & Brümmer, Germany © 2016.

exhaustive extraction, it usually suffices to extract the major part of the substance to be extracted. Additional percolations would be required to harvest the remaining substance of interest. This would, however, require disproportional time and energy expenditure unless, like in the industrial production, particularly when using percolation batteries, pre- and after-flow were to be used for extraction of the next batch of material.

24.8.3.4   Evaporation of the Extraction Fluid

The extraction fluid may be evaporated in a distillation flask on a water bath of a temperature of maximally 50°C. Removal of the thickened extract is facilitated when using a flat-bottom flask. Excess heating of the gradually thickening product (low water content) should be avoided (not to speak of scorching!). In principle, the evaporation procedure starts with the last percolate in order to avoid the richer initial percolates to become unnecessarily exposed to heat. It is most effective to introduce the fluid extract into the evaporation flask at a rate that precisely compensates for the amount of evaporating solvent.

In a rotary evaporator, a thin film of fluid extract is formed on the wall of the rotating flask, which, due to the substantial increase in surface area thus obtained, greatly facilitates evaporation of the solvent. By regulating the immersion depth of the flask in the water bath, bath temperature, pressure (vacuum), and temperature of the cooling water, optimal conditions may be created.

Thin-layer evaporators as used in the industrial setting constitute evacuated meters-high perpendicularly positioned cylinders along whose inner walls the fluid extract flows downward in a thin layer. In addition, rotating wiper blades serve to promote uniform coating of the cylinder walls with the fluid. At high flow rates and at temperature of 30° to 50°C, concentrates may be obtained within 30 seconds, due to the large surface area of the fluid extract.

Plate evaporators (Fig. 24-9) are suitable for thermostable extracts and allow short process times for the production of thickened extract, where for thermolabile substances the vacuum circulation evaporator is used (Fig. 24-8).

In other evaporator types, surface increase of the fluid extract is accomplished by allowing the extract to flow through cylinders filled with glass wool or a similar large-surface material. The described procedures are particularly suited for extracts containing thermo-labile and foaming substances. Residual moisture may be eliminated by further drying processes. The simplest method to accomplish that is to store the thickened extract in a compartment dryer. However, to achieve a water-free product, prolonged drying periods may be required and/or correspondingly high drying temperatures, even when the material to be dried is spread out in a thin layer. This last step in the entire drying process presents therefore a substantial challenge to thermo-labile compounds. In order to reduce that burden, evacuated drying facilities and (evacuated) roller dryers may be engaged (section 2.4.3.4). An even more gentle approach is to produce a dry extract by freeze drying. Although quite time-consuming, this method avoids heat exposure altogether. Very efficient and gentle is furthermore the spray-drying method, yielding a dry product in a very rapid one-step procedure. A special method to produce extracts in powdered or granulated form allows the production of instant preparations. This method yields an easily wettable and rapidly and completely water-soluble product without clump formation. This typical instant property results from the capillary action of the highly porous dried material which draws up the fluid very rapidly and efficiently. In order to attain the instant effect, a dry extract, which has already been prepared by spray or roller drying is once more moistened. Subsequently, another drying cycle is performed according to a special process in which, for example, a special spray technique or vacuum drying is applied.

As filling material, sucrose, lactose, or dextrins are used at concentrations of 50% to 90%.

Instant extracts of medicinal plants are quite popular as herbal powder infusions. Instant infusions from material containing aromatic oils are not simple to produce because of the volatility of the oils. That is why the aromatic oil is often added to the spray-dried powder in the form of microcapsules.

24.8.3.5   Complications during Evaporation of Extraction Fluids

The concentration of the extract starts with the last percolate. Refilling with additional per-colate fluid should proceed with care in order to avoid excessive foaming. Freshly added portions of the extract will have higher ethanol content than the fluid in the distillation flask;

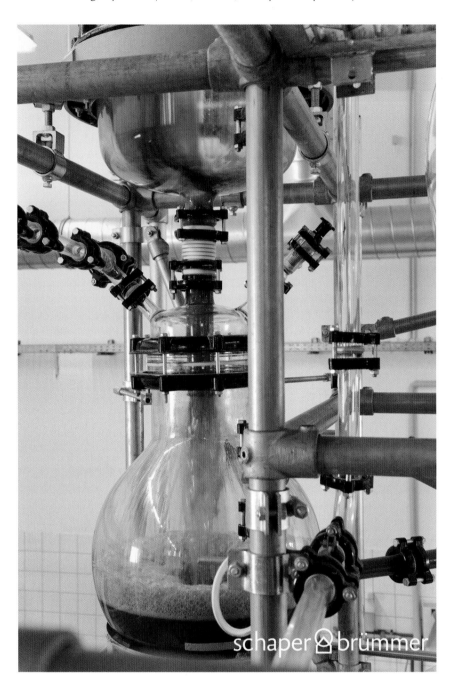

Fig. 24-8 Detail of an evaporation in industrial scale (Dimension of the complete evaporator: approx. 8 m, 2 m, 2 m (H, L, W), Volume 0.5 m³; mode of evaporation: vacuum circulation evaporation; duration of evaporation not more than 24 hours; temperature: 30° to 55°C; vacuum pressure 0.2 to 0.8 bar; concrete process parameter depending on the type of plant constituents). Reproduced with permission from Schaper & Brümmer, Germany © 2016.

these will, therefore, boil at a lower temperature. When refilling proceeds too fast, boiling delay may occur. It is therefore recommended to slowly and continuously add the fluid extract drop by drop from a valve. When foam formation occurs during refilling or concentration, the vacuum may temporarily be released. Exceptionally annoying foaming may occur during concentration of extracts containing saponins or proteins. It may become so intense that further evaporation of the fluid extract becomes impossible. Foam formation intensifies during evaporation because the fluid extract will contain an increasing proportion of water, which enhances the activity of the surface-active constituents. Simply reducing the vacuum cannot always be applied to suppress foam formation because it will simultaneously lead to an

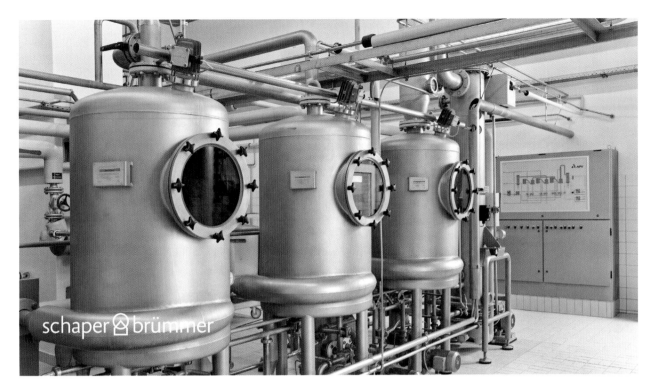

Fig. 24-9 Plate evaporator in industrial scale (Dimension of the complete evaporator: approx. 4 m, 10 m, 2,5 m (H, L, W), Volume 1.5 m^3; mode of evaporation: plate evaporation; duration of evaporation not more than 10 h; temperature: 45° to 100°C; concrete process parameter depending on the type of plant constituents). Reproduced with permission from Schaper & Brümmer, Germany © 2016.

increase in boiling temperature and thus to prolongation of the process. Special glass devices mounted in the distillation facility to serve as so-called foam reducers may be helpful. More favorable may be to the addition of foam-disturbing agents (defoaming agents, anti-frothing agents). These are compounds that often are surface active by themselves but accumulate at the fluid-gas interface and thus strongly reduce the stability of the foam lamellae, which depends on surface tension and surface viscosity (e.g., Span® types). However, the addition of de-foaming agents may bring along new problems. Measures should be taken to avoid that they permanently contaminate the extract. This can be achieved by using octanol, which is distilled off with the ethanol; repeated addition will therefore be necessary. Silicone oils offer special advantages in this connection. They are active already at dilutions of 1:10,000 to 1:20,000. This abolishes the absolute need to remove them from the distillation residue.

To avoid bumping of the fluid while operating under reduced pressure boiling chips could be added in the distillation flask. The small glass pearls that are routinely used for this purpose in the laboratory are not recommendable however, as it may turn out to be quite difficult to remove them from the dried residue.

24.8.3.6   Storage

Generally speaking, extracts need to be stored under protection from moisture and light. Dry extracts are most often hygroscopic. Inadequate storage may therefore easily lead to moist preparations and therefore tight sealing is crucial. While industrial products are commonly packaged in air-tight, (often vacuum-)sealed containers (plate or glass), in the pharmacy glass flasks closed by hollow stoppers filled with a hygroscopic substance (preferentially calcium chloride) are more common. Also, immersing the top of the flask in melted paraffin and the thus-formed coating has proven its usefulness in officinal storage. When dry extracts are stored strictly according to the regulations, they represent quite stable dosage forms. Appropriate inert, nonhygroscopic substances for the dilution of extracts to the desired concentrations of active ingredient are dextrin, sucrose, glucose, lactose, starch, and gum arabic.

24.8.3.7   Testing

The pharmacopeias most often contain a description of extracts (color, taste, smell), an identification test (thin-layer chromatography), an assay for drying losses and when applicable an assay of the drug content. To test drying losses (Ph. Eur. 2.8.17) 0.50 g of powdered dry extract is weighed precisely in a covered weighing glass of defined size and shape, dried at 105°C, and then dried for 3 hours at 100° to 105°C. It is then allowed to cool in a desiccator and subsequently weighed again. Most pharmacopeias put a limit of 3% to 5% on the acceptable residual moisture content (= drying loss).

24.8.3.8   Fluid Extracts

Fluid extracts (*extracta fluida*), are extracts prepared from (dry) plant material with variable concentrations of ethanol (when so required containing certain additions), in such a way that one part of material corresponds to one or two parts of extract. They are in general obtained by means of percolation. Many instructions recommend setting aside the first portion of the extract as a forerun. This forerun consists of 85 parts of fluid extract from 100 parts of dry plant material.

After collecting the after-run by continued percolation, this is concentrated and combined with the forerun fraction, such that ultimately one part fluid extract corresponds to one part dry material. For economic reasons exhaustive extraction is not aimed at because of high costs involved in concentrating large amounts of fluid extract. Therefore percolation is terminated after collection of four after-runs, which ensures extraction of most of the substance of interest present in the material. Other methods skip the collection of after-runs altogether, thus avoiding the necessity to concentrate partial percolates. In such methods, percolation is continued until one or two parts of extraction fluid have been obtained per one part of dry starting material.

24.8.3.9   Extracts

Extracts are preparations of fluid, semi-solid, or solid consistency that are produced by interaction of ethanol-water mixtures or other solvents with plant- or animal-derived material. During the process substances of interest are transferred from the material into the solvent.

The material to be extracted may be subjected to pretreatments like fragmentation, defatting or inactivation of enzyme activities. When so required, the fluid extract is adjusted to the desired concentration by (partial) elimination of extraction fluid. Aromatic oils, which may separate during processing, may be added again at later stages of the procedure. Also, other additives such as stabilizers or preservatives may be added.

In cases where a defined active substance has been identified, the extract may be brought to a consistent concentration of this substance by adding filling agents or by mixing different batches. In such cases, we speak of standardized extracts.

When pharmacological activity is accounted for by a mixture of compounds, each of which contributing to overall activity, *quantified extracts* may be produced. These are adjusted to a certain concentration range of activity-determining substances (active markers), for example, by simply mixing various batches of starting material or extract.

When neither active substances nor excipients have been identified, quality can only be derived from a minimal content of analytical lead substances and by accurate definition of the production process. Such preparations are summarized in the Ph. Eur. under the term "Other Extracts."

When in the production process purification steps are included—for example, to increase the content of active substance or to decrease the content of toxic components—we speak of *refined extracts*. Depending on their consistency and the mass ratio of starting material (drug) and extract, without additives, (Drug-Extract-Relation = DER), the Ph. Eur. distinguishes fluid extracts, tinctures, semi-fluid and thickened extracts, oily resins, and dry extracts.

Fluid Extracts

For fluid extracts the DER usually amounts to 1:1, that is, one part of extract per one part of starting material. Only in case of mucous material should a ratio of 1:2 be maintained, as otherwise the extract would show a gelatinous consistency. For fluid extracts, only ethanol,

---

Label for a marketed Ginkgo bailoba dietary supplement

Each tablet contains:

Gingko bailoba extract (leaf) – 60 mg

   Containing

   Ginkgo flavanoids – 24%

   Ginkolic acid – less than 6 ppm

   Terpenes – 3%

Other Ingredients: microcrystalline cellulose (bulking agent), dicalcium phosphate (bulking agent), silicon dioxide (anti caking agent), magnessium stearate (anti caking agent), hydroxypropylmethylcellulose (glazing agent), glycerine (glazing agent).

ethanol-water mixtures, or water are permitted as extraction fluids. Fluid extracts may also be produced by diluting/dissolving thickened or dry extracts, provided that the latter were prepared with the same extraction fluid (identical ethanol concentration).

Tinctures

For the preparation of tinctures 1 part of starting material is extracted by means of maceration or percolation with 5 or 10 parts ethanol of suitable concentration. The amount of macerate or percolate obtained is determined by the effectiveness of the pressing procedure. Accordingly, DER values amount to 1:4–4.5 or 1:8–9.

Semi-Fluid Extracts, Thick Extracts

Semi-fluid extracts are obtained by gentle concentration of fluid extracts. Defined DER values are not specified, but they have to be stated.

Oily Resins

Oily resins are semi-solid solutions of resins in aromatic or fatty oil. They are obtained from the starting material by solvent extraction and subsequent evaporation of the solvent.

Dry Extracts

Dry extracts are obtained by complete removal of solvent following extraction of the starting material. When, in the corresponding monograph, not otherwise prescribed, water content should not exceed 5% (m/m). A defined DER value is not specified, but has to be stated as

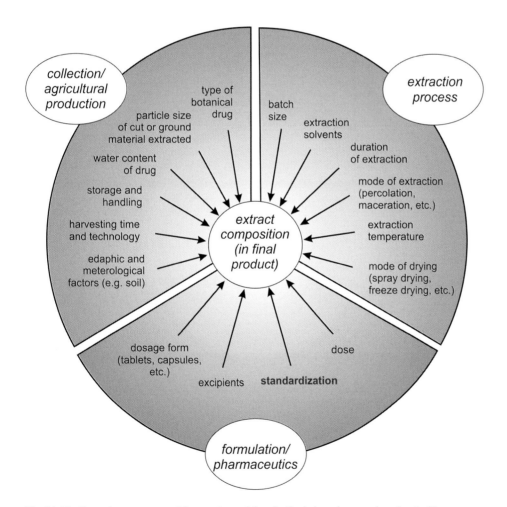

Fig. 24-10 Extraction process and factors determining the final plant drug product. Inspired by a drawing in "Fundamentals of Pharmacognosy and Phytotherapy," Heinrich et al., Churchill Livingstone Elsevier Ltd. 2012.

native DER. Since most dry extracts contain additives, the stated DER value commonly does not refer to the total mass of the dry extract.

The following information should be indicated for extracts:

- The processed starting material (herbal or animal)
- The type of extract (fluid, semi-fluid, dry, tincture)
- For standardized extracts the concentration of active substance(s)
- For quantified extracts, the content of the auxiliary compounds used for quantification
- The mass ratio of starting material (drug) and the total amount of extract obtained from it (without additives) = native DER
- The solvent(s) used for the extraction
- When applicable, a clear indication that fresh, nondried material was used
- When applicable, a clear indication that it concerns a refined extract
- Names and amounts of all added excipients are provided, including stabilizers and preservatives.
- For fluid and semi-fluid extracts and tinctures, the dry residue in %.

Many factors (several of them interacting with each other) are relevant for the correct formulation of a plant-based drug. A schematic diagram representing the multitude of factors involved in the development of an effective herbal medicine is given in Fig. 24-10. This short chapter has discussed only a few of them.

Further Reading

Heinrich, M., Barnes, J., Gibbons, S., and Williamson, E. M. *Fundamentals of Pharmacognosy and Phytotherapy*. Churchill Livingstone Elsevier, 2012.

Khan, J., Alexander, A., Ajazuddin, S., and Saraf, S. "Recent advances and future prospects of phyto-phospholipid complexation technique for improving pharmacokinetic profile of plant actives." *J Control Release* 168 (1) (May 28, 2013): 50–60.

Schöffling, U. "Arzneiformenlehre", 6th ed., Stuttgart: Deutscher Apotheker Verlag, 2015.

Tegtmeier, M. *Extracts and Production of Extracts*. In: Blaschek W. (ed.). Wichtl—Teedrogen und Phytopharmaka, 6. Auflage. Stuttgart: Wissenschaftliche Verlagsgesellschaft, 2016, 27–32.

Stability and Stabilization

25

25.1 General Introduction

In the last decades, questions concerning stability and stabilization of drugs and drug formulations have gained increasing attention. The reason for this is the rapidly increasing introduction of modern, highly pharmacologically active, but often unstable substances, including numerous low-molecular weight compounds but especially raising numbers of peptides and proteins.

The currently available analytical procedures and the ever-increasing demands on quality have contributed to the development of stricter stability criteria and requirements with respect to shelf life. Stability investigations not only form the basis for the specification and assessment of the shelf life, they also are indispensable for the planning and evaluation of biopharmaceutical, preclinical and clinical studies.

Stability studies are therefore an absolute necessity in the early evaluation of the drug substance as well as later in the formulation development of the drug product. Preliminary experiments carried out with a new chemical entity, NCE or new biological entity, NBE in solid or dissolved form are aimed at determining whether they are sufficiently stable to justify further development steps. In addition, they should exclude erroneous interpretation of the results of pharmacological and chemical testing. The next step is screening for an optimal formulation. In this step, it is crucial to establish the stability of the active compound in the presence of excipients and under consideration of the process conditions and, if necessary, to take adequate measures to improve stabilization. Finally, the formulated drug product will have to be subjected to final long term stability testing.

Stability means that the essential characteristics (CQAs = critical quality attributes) of the drug product (drug as well as formulation), when stored under adequate conditions in the defined packaging, do not change at all or only to an acceptable extent.

Quality attributes are established during development and documented in a specification. A specification is a list of analytical tests and corresponding acceptance criteria that define a series of characteristics that the drug product should match in order to guarantee effective and safe application. Essential quality attributes are the content of active substance and degradation products, physical parameters including organoleptically detectable properties, bioburden and toxicological properties as well as therapeutic activity. The acceptance limits of these quality parameters need to be clearly substantiated by the manufacturer and approved by the appropriate authorities. In the process of establishing and justifying the acceptance limits, provisions of pharmacopeias and other officially accepted regulations are taken into consideration as well. All specified quality criteria must not exceed the defined limits of a pharmaceutical product within the entire claimed shelf life.

To account for storage-induced changes, separate acceptance criteria are defined for the release test of the drug product (testing immediately after production) and for end of shelf

Voigt's Pharmaceutical Technology, First Edition. Alfred Fahr.
© 2018 John Wiley & Sons Ltd. Published 2018 by John Wiley & Sons Ltd.

life. The release limits are set sufficiently tight to ensure that the approved, broader shelf life limits are not exceeded, despite unavoidable changes during storage.

For industrially produced finished dosage forms, which are often stored for prolonged periods, manufacturers usually strive for a shelf life of five years. If this cannot be achieved, a shelf life of at least three years is being aimed for. A frequently used method to determine the maximal storage period (in accordance with ICH guideline Q1A(R2), Stability testing of new drug substances and products) is based on the statistical analysis of the temporal change of quantitative quality parameters during long-term studies. Critical parameters include, for example, the concentration of the active ingredient or of degradation products. From such data, the regression line as well as its one-sided 95% confidence range is determined. In the case of decreasing values (e.g., drug substance content), the lower confidence interval is of interest, whereas for increasing values (e.g., degradation products), the upper confidence interval is relevant. The maximum allowable storage period coincides with the point in time when the confidence interval exceeds the value of the corresponding acceptance criterion. Under consistent production conditions, at least 95% of all produced batches should comply with the specified acceptance limits throughout the defined shelf life.

Extemporaneously prepared medicinal products, which are mostly intended for immediate use, should be stable for at least a few months, whenever possible. For those products however, experimentally based predictions on stability are not feasible; nonetheless, legal provisions require a clear statement on the ultimate date of use, commonly expressed as: "use by…" (day/month/year). The German compendium "DAC" provides guidelines for the maximal storage time for various dosage forms, which in absence of exact data may be used to estimate an appropriate expiry date.

In the case of multidose containers, the in-use shelf life after opening the container or after reconstitution of the ready-to-use preparation must additionally be indicated. The same applies to industrially produced finished dosage forms. When required, these should provide such information in the package insert.

The stability of active substances and excipients is related to their chemical structures and their physical properties. External factors, such as temperature, moisture, oxygen and light, may trigger or accelerate reactions leading to quality decline.

The extent to which the above factors are contributing depends largely on the dosage form. Liquid preparations, such as injection and infusion solutions, eye and nasal drops, suspensions and emulsions, extracts, and also highly viscous water-containing systems such as creams and pastes, are usually more susceptible to decomposition than solid dosage forms. For didactic reasons, a distinction is made between physical, chemical, and microbiological changes. In practice, it is often not possible to accurately ascribe instability to one of these categories, because in most cases we are dealing with a complex event to which different mechanisms contribute. For example, when a carmellose-sodium solution becomes microbiologically contaminated, enzymatic activity of bacterial cellulases might lead to chemical decomposition of the polymeric structures, which, in turn, might cause physical changes in terms of lowering of viscosity.

25.2   Methods to Determine Stability

Independent of the character of the degradation process (chemical, physical, or microbiological), it is important to know for how long the drug or the drug formulation will meet the requirements set. To study the stability behavior, the preparation is tested at specified intervals during storage under controlled temperature and moisture conditions, with respect to quality-relevant parameters. Distinction is made between long-term stability studies, which are performed at the inteded storage temperature and humidity, and accelerated stability studies (stress tests), which proceed under enhanced thermal challenge and at elevated air humidity.

Stability studies are performed at the very beginning of the formulation development stage and are later continued during the production stage. Prior to this, the active ingredient itself is stress-tested for stability. In the preformulation phase, stability studies serve to allow selection of the optimal formulation as well as to facilitate the choice of appropriate excipients and the processing methodology. The results of stress tests, which are conducted with the scale-up batches, will provide useful information concerning desirable storage conditions, requirements of packaging materials, and parameters for subsequent long-term studies.

The studies are conducted in parallel with additional stress tests with three representative batches of the final product to be submitted for registration. At that stage, formulation and packaging are identical to those of the future commercial product. With these tests, the final shelf life claim is established and data concerning stability are generated for the marketing authorization dossier. Following approval, the long-term study is usually continued as an ongoing stability test. Based on those results the shelf life, which initially had to be specified conservatively because data from late pull points were still lacking, might be extended. In the post-marketing phase, one produced batch per year is subjected to a follow-up stability test (FUST) in order to recognize suddenly or gradually occurring changes in storage stability.

For routine stability tests in the development and follow-up phase, long-term, intermediate, and accelerated storage conditions are defined by the ICH guideline Q1A(R2). In general these are:

- Long-term: 25°C ± 2°C/60 % r.h. ± 5 % r.h. or: 30°C ± 2°C/65 % r.h. ± 5 % r.h.
- Intermediate: 30°C ± 2°C/65 % r.h. ± 5 % r.h.
- Accelerated: 40°C ± 2°C/75 % r.h. ± 5 % r.h.

Drug formulations that need to be stored refrigerated are tested at 5°C ± 3°C in long-term tests and at 25°C ± 2°C/60% r.h. ± 5% r.h. in accelerated tests.

Ph. Eur. 1.2 Definitions in the General Chapters and Monographs _____

(Temperature Specifications) The Ph. Eur. *distinguishes the following temperature specifications:*

In a deep freeze: −15°C

In a refrigerator: 2° and 8°C

Cold or cool: between 8° and 15°C

Room temperature: between 15° and 25°C

25.2.1 Long-Term Stability Test

In the long-term test, a sufficient number of units of the product is stored in a climatized cabinet or room during a relevant period of time under the required or desired conditions (temperature, light, air, humidity). At appropriate time intervals and at the end of the test, a fixed number of units are withdrawn and predefined quality criteria are tested. The time-points of sample withdrawal are commonly called "pull points". These studies extend over periods of several years. Only long-term studies yield reliable data for the specification and justification of shelf life. Since the test is conducted at one single temperature only, no conclusions can generally be drawn from it concerning the mechanism of decomposition.

25.2.2 Accelerated Stability Tests and Stress Tests

Accelerated stability tests are conducted at elevated temperature and in most cases also at enhanced air humidity. In routine studies, according to ICH guideline Q1A(R2), the purpose of accelerated and stress testing is not to create data for kinetic analyses but to obtain preliminary information in short time. Another purpose is to detect changes that proceed slowly and, thus, might remain hidden in long-term studies within the tested time frame. If stress studies are performed at more than one elevated storage temperature, the laws of reaction kinetics can be applied for prediction purposes, in that the decomposition rates at high temperatures are assessed and extrapolated to that at room temperature. In common stress tests,

Temperature specifications according to USP ⟨659⟩ (Packaging and storage requirements):

Freezer: between −25° and −10°C

Refrigerator: between 2° and 8°C

Cold: ≤8°C

Cool: between 8° and 15°C

Room temperature = Ambient temperature: "temperature prevailing in a working environment"

Controlled room temperature: between 20° and 25°C. Excursions between 15° and 30°C are allowed, provided the mean kinetic temperature does not exceed 25°C. Transient spikes up to 40°C (<24 h) are permitted.

Warm: between 30° and 40°C

Excessive heat: >40°C

Temperature specifications according to JP (General notices):

Standard temperature: 20°C

Ordinary temperature: between 15° and 25°C

Room temperature: between 1° and 30°C

Lukewarm: between 30° and 40°C

Cold place: between 1° and 15°C

the product is stored under isothermal conditions at one temperature or several temperatures in parallel tests. At appropriate time intervals, the concentration of degradation products or of the amount of remaining drug is determined. From these data both the concentration dependence and the temperature dependence of the decomposition rate can be calculated.

Mainly in the preformulation phase of drug product development stability is sometimes tested under nonisothermal conditions. In those studies the temperature is continuously increased during the storage period. This makes it possible to predict the stability based on the results of one single individual test series. However, this method requires substantial investment in equipment and complex data analysis. Thus far, it has mainly been applied for solutions.

Calculation of physical stability based on the results of accelerated tests is only feasible in exceptional cases. Often, however, this type of stress test may provide valuable information concerning the trend of the changes that occur.

25.2.2.1   Determination of Reaction Rate Constants under Isothermal Conditions

The reaction rate (v) of a chemical system is defined as the change in concentration (dc) of the reaction partners as function of time (t)

$$v = dc/dt \tag{25-1}$$

The concentration change can be expressed as either a decrease in the concentration of the starting substances (reactants or educts) or an increase in the concentration of the reaction products.

$$v = \frac{-dc_{react.}}{dt} \quad \text{bzw.} \quad v = \frac{dc_{prod.}}{dt} \tag{25-2}$$

For a reaction of the type $A \rightarrow B + C$ the reaction rate may thus be given by

$$v = -\frac{d[A]}{dt} = k[A] \tag{25-3}$$

(under the condition that B and C do not affect the reaction rate)

$[A]$ = concentration of A (mol $\cdot$ 1^{-1})
k   = reaction rate constant
t   = reaction time

The reaction rate is proportional to the concentration of A. Under isothermic conditions k is a constant that is characteristic of the reaction.

Under the condition that the concentration of A at $t = 0$ equals $[A]_0$ and at time t $[A]_t$, from equation 25-3, the following explicit relation may be obtained by integration:

$$\int_{[A]_0}^{[A]} \frac{d[A]}{[A]} = -k \int_0^t dt$$

$$\ln \frac{[A]}{[A]_0} = -k \cdot t \tag{25-4}$$

$$\ln[A] = -k \cdot t + \ln[A]_0$$

After conversion of ln to $\log_{10}$ we obtain:

$$\lg[A] = -\frac{k}{2.303} t + \lg[A]_0 \tag{25-5}$$

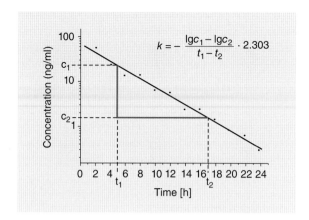

Fig. 25-1   Concentration vs. time diagram for first-order reaction.

As in studies of reaction kinetics, since the decrease in concentration is expressed as the amount of A that has reacted at time t (designated as turnover variable $x = [A]_0 - [A]$), we can formulate:

$$\lg([A]_0 - x) = -\frac{k}{2.303}t + \lg[A]_0$$

$$k = \frac{2.303}{t}\lg\frac{[A]_0}{[A]_0 - x}$$

$$(25\text{-}6)$$

When we plot log $[A]$ or log $([A]_0 - x)$, respectively, (determined by concentration assay) as a function of time in a coordinate system (abscissa $= t$; ordinate $= c$) a straight line is obtained with a slope $= -k/2.303$ and an intercept with the ordinate of log $[A]_0$ (Fig. 25-1).

Instead of the reaction rate constant, a more illustrative unit, the half-life $t_{1/2}$, is often used. The half-life is the amount of time required for half of the starting compounds to react. It is obtained after conversion of equation 25-4 and replacing $[A]$ by $\frac{1}{2}[A]_0$.

$$t = \frac{\ln\frac{[A]}{[A_0]}}{-k} = \frac{\ln\frac{[A_0]}{[A]}}{k}$$

$$t_{1/2} = \frac{\ln\frac{[A_0]}{1/2[A_0]}}{k} = \frac{\ln 2}{k} = \frac{2.303 \cdot \lg 2}{k}$$

$$(25\text{-}7)$$

$$t_{1/2} = \frac{0.693}{k}$$

The derived correlations apply to first-order reactions. Table 25-1 presents in summary the basic rate correlations for different reaction orders, without mathematically deriving them

Table 25-1   Rate Equations for 0, First-, Second-, and Third-Order Reactions

Order	Initial Concentration	Differential Quotient	Integrated Equation ($x = 0$, when $t = 0$)	Half-Life	Equation for Straight Line	Slope
0	a	$\frac{dx}{dt} = k$	$k = \frac{x}{t}$	$t_{1/2} = \frac{a}{2k}$	$x = kt$	k
1	a	$\frac{dx}{dt} = k(a - x)$	$k = \frac{2.303}{t}\lg\frac{a}{a - x}$	$t_{1/2} = \frac{0.693}{k}$	$\lg(a - x) = \lg a - \frac{kt}{2.303}$	$-\frac{k}{2.303}$
2	a = b	$\frac{dx}{dt} = k(a - x)^2$	$k = \frac{1}{t}\left(\frac{1}{a - x} - \frac{1}{a}\right)$	$t_{1/2} = \frac{1}{ak}$	$\frac{1}{a - x} = \frac{1}{a} + kt$	k
2	a ≠ b	$\frac{dx}{dt} = k(a - x)(b - x)$	$k = \frac{2.303}{t(a - b)}\lg\frac{b(a - x)}{a(b - x)}$		$\lg\frac{a - x}{b - x} = \lg\frac{a}{b} + kt\frac{a - b}{2.303}$	$\frac{k(a - b)}{2.303}$
3	a = b = c	$\frac{dx}{dt} = k(a - x)^3$	$k = \frac{1}{2t}\left[\frac{1}{(a - x)^2} - \frac{1}{a^2}\right]$	$t_{1/2} = \frac{3}{2}\cdot\frac{1}{a^2 k}$	$\frac{1}{(a - x)^2} = \frac{1}{a^2} + 2kt$	$2k$

(for simplicity's sake.) These mathematical derivations may be found in relevant textbooks on physical chemistry (see, e.g., Atkins and de Paula 2013).

For many chemical conversions of drug molecules, which do not represent monomolecular reactions, the time rule for first-order reactions still applies. This is the case when one of the reaction partners is present in large excess and whose concentration therefore may be considered constant for the time course of the reaction (e.g., water during the inversion of sucrose), or when the concentration of one of the reaction partners is otherwise kept constant. Such reactions are known as pseudo-first-order reactions. In order to derive from the empirically obtained data (concentration changes as a function of time) the reaction order, and with that also the kinetics applying to this reaction, different procedures may be used, two of which will be discussed below.

25.2.2.2　Substitution Procedure

The experimental data (t and c) are introduced into the integrated equations for the various reaction orders. The mathematical equation in which the k values are constant, taking into account an appropriate error limit, indicates the order of the reaction.

25.2.2.3　Graphical Method

In this method, different functions of the concentration (ordinate) are plotted against time (abscissa). The plot presenting the measured points as a straight line corresponds to the reaction order. From its slope the reaction rate can be calculated. Yet another option is to determine half-life ($t_{1/2}$) values, either by calculation or graphically.

25.2.2.4　Determination of the Dependence of Temperature on Reaction Rate Constant

It is well known that with raising temperature, the reaction rate increases. As a rule of thumb the van 't Hoff correlation applies: A temperature rise of 10 K causes on average a 2-4-fold increase in reaction rate. (Jacobus Henricus van't Hoff, 1852–1911, a Dutch chemist and the first Nobel Prize laureate for chemistry). For stability determination, however, this rule is not sufficiently accurate. An exact relationship between temperature dependence and reaction rate was derived by Arrhenius (Svante August Arrhenius, 1859–1927, Swedish physicist and chemist and Nobel Prize laureate for chemistry, spent a study period at van't Hoff in Amsterdam 1888).

$$k = A \cdot e^{-\frac{E}{R \cdot T}}$$

$$\ln k = \ln A - \frac{E}{R \cdot T}$$

$$\lg k = \lg A - \frac{E}{2.303 \cdot R} \cdot \frac{1}{T} \tag{25-8}$$

$$\lg k = -\frac{E}{2.303 \cdot R} \cdot \frac{1}{T} + \lg A$$

E　=　activation energy ($J \cdot mol^{-1}$)
A　=　collision frequency factor
R　=　universal gas constant
T　=　absolute temperature (K)
k　=　reaction rate constant

To assess temperature dependence on reaction rate, k values are determined at a minimum of three different temperatures. By plotting the logarithm of the rate constants (log k = ordinate) as a function of the reciprocal temperature (1/T = abscissa), a straight line is obtained (Fig. 25-2) with a slope as given in equation 25.9.

$$\frac{\Delta \lg k}{\Delta \left(\frac{1}{T}\right)} = -\frac{E}{2.303 \cdot R} \tag{25-9}$$

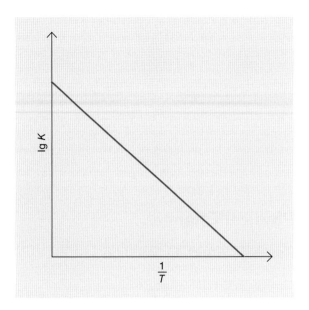

Fig. 25-2   Dependence of reaction rate on temperature.

This expression allows the calculation of the activation energy E, with which the collision factor A can be calculated in turn.

$$\lg A = \lg k + \frac{E}{2.303 \cdot R \cdot T} \tag{25-10}$$

Knowing these two thermodynamic parameters, the reaction rate constant can be obtained for different temperatures. This, in turn, provides a measure for the decomposition of the studied substance.

$$\lg k = -\frac{E}{2.303 \cdot R \cdot T} + \lg A \tag{25-11}$$

Alternatively, E is calculated from a modified version of the Arrhenius equation, based on two different temperatures, T_1 and T_2.

$$\lg k_1 = -\frac{E}{2.303 \cdot R \cdot T_1} + \lg A$$
$$\lg k_2 = -\frac{E}{2.303 \cdot R \cdot T_2} + \lg A \tag{25-12}$$

By subtraction of the two equations, we obtain

$$\lg \frac{k_1}{k_2} = \frac{E}{2.303 \cdot R} \left(\frac{1}{T_2} - \frac{1}{T_1} \right) \tag{25-13}$$

k_1 = reaction rate constant at T_1
k_2 = reaction rate constant at T_2

Finally, the reaction rate constants for specified temperatures of interest may be read directly from the corresponding extrapolation of the straight lines in the graphic presentation $\log k = f(1/T)$. Since, for a prediction of stability the most interesting parameter is not the rate constant, but rather, the time in which a certain quantity of drug decomposes, further calculation is required. For a first-order degradation reaction, the time required for 10% of the drug to decompose (90% remaining) may be obtained from equation 25.14:

$$t_{90\%} = \frac{\ln 1.11}{k} = \frac{0.105}{k} \tag{25-14}$$

Accelerated stability tests are not universally applicable to predict stability. They are only meaningful when decomposition at higher temperatures proceeds according to the same mechanism as at lower temperatures, and the activation energy lies in the range $42-126$ kJ $\cdot$ mol^{-1}. Often, these important criteria are not fulfilled. As kinetic laws strictly apply only to homogeneous systems (e.g., solutions), they are not fully applicable to multiphase systems, such as most drug formulations. In addition, many drug formulations undergo unacceptable physical changes at elevated temperatures—for example, changes in the consistency of ointments and pastes, or alterations of the dispersed state of emulsions and suspensions. In such cases, information on stability and shelf life may only be obtained by means of long-term testing.

25.3   Physical Changes

25.3.1   Processes Affecting Stability

25.3.1.1   Changes in Crystal Structure

Many active substances show polymorphic behavior (section 3.2.1.1), that is, they exist in various crystalline modifications. During storage, polymorph conversions may occur in a pharmaceutical preparation, either as a slow continuous process or induced by changes in environment. Although such changes may not be macroscopically observable (smell, odor, visual appearance), they are often responsible for changes in release and absorption behavior. Examples of the large number of substances that are able to crystallize in different structures, the following are especially noteworthy: steroids (cortisone and prednisolone), spironolactone, furosemide, and ritonavir.

The protease inhibitor ritonavir was launched in 1996, among other dosage forms as a capsule formulation (Norvir®). It contained the poorly soluble, and for this reason, poorly bioavailable drug in an aqueous ethanolic solution. During development, only a single crystal form of the substance was known. When in 1998 the first batches of the product revealed problems in dissolution testing, a so far unknown, more stable and insoluble, polymorphic modification was identified as the cause of the problems. The new crystal form precipitated at a concentration 400 times lower than that in the capsule filling. Since even the tiniest traces of this new modification could act as crystallization nuclei and as this substance had contaminated the whole production area, it was no longer possible to produce any capsules containing the specified amount of dissolved drug. As a consequence, the capsule product was withdrawn from the market (see Datta and Grant 2008).

Another example concerns the Parkinson's drug rotigotin, which is on the market as a transdermal patch under the name Neupro®. The matrix of the patch contains the drug in dissolved form. In this case also, only one crystal form was known when the product was launched to the market. In 2007, it was found that during storage, crystallization occurred in numerous patches, characterized by snowflake-like patterns in the drug-containing layer of the patches. Investigations demonstrated that the phenomenon was caused by the formation of a poorly soluble polymorph modification. The undissolved portions of the drug are no longer bioavailable to a sufficient extent. Therefore, the patch was withdrawn from the market in 2008 and reintroduced in 2012 after a thorough reformulation. These examples painfully demonstrate the enormous importance of polymorphism for the bioavailability and stability of pharmaceutical substances.

25.3.1.2   Alterations in the Distribution State

As a result of density differences, demixing phenomena may occur in liquid multiphase systems, which initially are only observable as microscopic inhomogeneities in particle distribution, but in later stages may also become visible macroscopically as sedimentation or creaming. Well-known examples are the breaking of emulsions and sedimentation phenomena in suspensions. Due to such alterations exact dosing of the active ingredient is hampered.

A size change of dispersed particles can also affect the distribution of the drug and the degree of dispersion of a preparation. Particle growth during storage may occur, for example, in suspension ointments, pastes, and liquid suspensions.

This should be taken into account when the suspended solid has a broad particle size distribution. As a result of the higher solubility of smaller particles (section 3.9.7.2) a higher saturation concentration occurs in their vicinity than around larger particles. Diffusion will tend to equalize this difference, ultimately leading to supersaturation in the vicinity of larger particles and thus to crystal growth. The suspension system gradually becomes depleted of smaller particles, while the larger particles keep growing.

Recrystallization of active ingredients in solution ointments can also occur in supersaturated preparations. Colloidal solutions often show aging phenomena during storage, which manifests as flocculation.

25.3.1.3 Changes in Consistency and Aggregation State

Semi-solid pharmaceutical preparations such as ointments and pastes may display post-hardening during storage, which in extreme cases may lead to solidification and thus to deterioration of applicability. Drug formulations like tablets, film- and sugar-coated tablets and suppositories are also subject to ageing processes, which become unfavorably apparent as prolonged disintegration, dissolution and melting times.

25.3.1.4 Changes of Solubility Behavior

In molecularly dispersed systems (e.g., drug solutions), concentration changes may occur as a result of evaporation of solvent from improperly sealed or gas-permeable containers, or by temperature changes. The solubility of the product may thus be exceeded, leading to precipitation (crystallization) of dissolved substances. Obviously, the risk for such issues is greater in near-saturated solutions.

25.3.1.5 Changes of the Hydration Conditions

The uptake or release of water by a compound has a profound influence on its hydration state and thus on its properties. Prominent examples are dry extracts that can wet and become lumpy or even liquefy due to their pronounced hygroscopicity. Many drugs and excipients are more or less hygroscopic and equilibrate their water content with the ambient air humidity. The prevailing hydrate form of pseudopolymorphic substances also depends on the humidity of the surrounding air.

25.3.2 Measures to Improve Stability

To stabilize physically unstable systems, physical methods and physical stabilizers are employed. For example, sedimentation processes in suspensions may at least be slowed down by reducing particle size, equalizing density of the two phases involved, or adding viscosity-enhancing substances. When sedimentation is preceded by particle growth due to aggregation, the addition of surface-active substances or protective colloids may be beneficial. By the same token, the breaking of emulsions may be eliminated or at least suppressed by homogenization and the addition of suitable emulsifiers at optimal concentrations. Hygroscopicity of substances may be countered by addition of moisture absorbers such as colloidal silicon dioxide, or simply by using water-vapor-tight packaging.

It is not possible to generally define which stabilization measures are optimal. Their selection depends on the nature of the active ingredients, the formulation, and the intended use. In many cases (e.g., changes in gels, post-hardening of tablets), physically generated instabilities may only be eliminated by change of excipients and adaption of the composition.

25.4 Chemical Changes

25.4.1 General Introduction

Chemical reactions affecting shelf life (e.g., hydrolyses, oxidations, reductions, steric conversions, decarboxylations, polymerizations), may proceed in homogeneous systems (e.g., solutions) or in heterogeneous systems (e.g., multiphase systems such as emulsions, suspensions, and ointments). While the former, in so far as they proceed according to straightforward mechanisms, are amenable to kinetic investigation, reactions in multiphase systems are not, or only under certain circumstances. Information on the stability of those systems has to be primarily based on long-term data from real-time studies.

Chemical conversions in homogeneous systems also often represent complex events in which different reaction types may be involved, either consecutively or simultaneously (parallel reactions). An example of a partially resolved complex decomposition mechanism is that of ascorbic acid.

In the presence of oxygen, degradation proceeds according to an aerobic mechanism. In the first oxidation step, the semidehydroascorbate radical anion is formed, which is a potent free radical scavenger. This property represents an essential aspect of the mechanism of action of ascorbic acid as an antioxidant. The radical ion reacts with itself or with other free radicals. In a second, reversible, oxidative step, dehydroascorbic acid is formed, which undergoes an irreversible hydrolytic ring opening under formation of diketogulonic acid. The latter is split into threonic acid and oxalic acid by a yet not fully understood multistep oxidative reaction mechanism. Also, in the absence of oxygen, ascorbic acid is not perfectly stable. In an anaerobic, slowly proceeding reaction it may be decarboxylated to form the final product furfural. Similarly, complex degradation mechanisms are known for other pharmaceutically relevant compounds such as hormones and antibiotics.

25.4.2 Hydrolytic Processes

25.4.2.1 General Introduction

Next to oxidative changes, hydrolytic processes represent the most important degradation reaction pathway. In the following, examples are given of drugs that are susceptible to hydrolytic degradation reactions.

- □ *Esters.* Acetylcholine, esters of acetylsalicylic acid, local anesthetics of the p-aminobenzoic acid ester type (e.g., benzocaine, procaine, oxyprocaine, tetracaine, dimethocaine), cocaine, ester alkaloids (e.g., atropine, hyoscyamine, scopolamine) and others.
- □ *Amides and thioamides.* Nicotinamide, chloramphenicol, barbituric acid derivatives (e.g., barbital, phenobarbital), glutethimide, phenytoine, cinchocaine, lidocaine, penicillin and its derivatives, trimethadone, thiamine, pantothenic acid.
- □ *Ethers, glycosides.* Diphenhydramine, streptomycin, glycosides (e.g., digitalis glycosides, rutin).
- □ *Lactones and lactams.* Penicillin, cycloserine, ascorbic acid, and their derivatives.
- □ Certain *excipients* may also undergo hydrolytic decomposition that will negatively affect the properties of a drug formulation—for example, hydrolysis of polylactides (PLA) or of copolymers of lactic acid and glycolic acid (PLGA). Following administration of preparations based on these biodegradable polymers, polymer hydrolysis is a desirable process that is required not only to release the active ingredient but also for the elimination of the polymer from the body. However, when hydrolysis takes place during storage of the drug product, the release profile of the active ingredient changes in an uncontrolled way. Many PLA or PLGA-based drug formulations therefore need to be stored at 2° to 8°C under rigorous exclusion of moisture, just like the polymer itself.

Hydrolytic degradation reactions proceed more or less according to the same reaction mechanism. In principle, distinction can be made between acid- and base-catalyzed hydrolysis.

Whereas acid-catalyzed hydrolysis represents an equilibrium reaction, base-catalyzed hydrolysis proceeds only in one direction due to the formation of a charge-stabilized acid anion. Acid amides, which, compared to esters, are less electronegative, are more resistant to hydrolytic degradation. Ethers are only susceptible to acid hydrolysis; in alkaline medium, they are stable.

Acid-Catalyzed Hydrolysis of Esters

Base-Catalyzed Hydrolysis of Esters

$$H_2N-\underset{}{\bigcirc}-\overset{\overset{O}{\|}}{C}-O-CH_2-CH_2-N\overset{C_2H_5}{\underset{C_2H_5}{}}$$

$$\downarrow H^+/OH^-$$

$$H_2N-\underset{}{\bigcirc}-COOH \;+\; HOCH_2-CH_2-N\overset{C_2H_5}{\underset{C_2H_5}{}}$$

Fig. 25-3   **pH-dependence of the decomposition of procaine in aqueous solution.**

25.4.2.2   Quantitative Aspects of Influencing Factors and Stabilization Measures

pH Value and pH Adjustment

Hydrolytic degradation processes are strongly pH-dependent. One of the most important stabilization measures for hydrolysis-sensitive systems is proper adjustment of pH. This will be explained by means of an intensely studied ester hydrolysis: the degradation of procaine. In aqueous solution, procaine undergoes hydrolytic cleavage to form p-aminobenzoic acid and diethylaminoethanol. Fig. 25-3 (pH-dependence of the rate of hydrolysis) shows that the decomposition curve has a minimum at pH 3.5—that is, at that pH value, stability is maximal. Adjustment to this pH would therefore guarantee maximal stability of procaine. This approach is, however, only applicable in a few cases as the pH of the stability maximum will often lie outside the physiologically acceptable range or because other important factors such as solubility, activity or decomposition reactions of other components in the formulation will have to be taken into account. It may be concluded that the optimal storage pH in practice represents a compromise between all important relevant aspects of the formulation.

pH adjustment is mostly performed with buffer solutions. When selecting the buffer system, it has to be taken into consideration that buffer substances may give rise to general acid-base catalytic reactions. General catalysis is to be understood as the phenomenon that, in addition to hydroxyl and hydronium ions, salt components of buffers, which according to the Brönstedt theory also represent acids and bases, may have a catalytic effect. General catalysis can be recognized when it is observed that degradation proceeds, under conditions of identical pH and ionic strength, at different rates in solutions containing different salts or salt mixtures (buffers).

A typical example of a hydrolytic degradation by general acid-base catalysis is chloramphenicol. In aqueous solution chloramphenicol is cleaved in dichloroacetic acid and the amino compound 2-amino-1-(4-nitrophenyl)propane-1,3-diol. Whereas hydrochloric acid and citric acid at the same pH show identical reaction rates, in the presence of acetic acid and especially in phosphate buffer, reaction rates are clearly enhanced, as expressed by the $t_{1/2}$ values presented in Table 25-2.

Indiscriminate use of buffers or salt additions should therefore by all means be avoided. Acid amides especially are subject to general acid-base catalysis, while up to now this has not been observed for pharmaceutically applied esters. Furthermore, the deamidation of

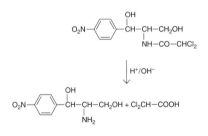

Table 25-2   Effect of Electrolytes on the Degradation Rate of Chloramphenicol

Electrolyte	$t_{1/2}$ (h)
HCl	10.5
$C_6H_8O_7$ (citric acid)	10.5
CH_3COOH (acetic acid)	6.0
HPO_4^{2-}	3.0

Table 25-3 Effect of Dielectric Constant and Ionic Strength of the Reaction Medium on Reaction Rate

	Effect of Increase of	
Type of Reaction	Dielectric Constant	Ionic Strength
dipole-dipole → polar product ion-ion	increase	none
ions of identical sign	increase	increase
ions of opposite sign	decrease	decrease
ion and neutral molecule	increase	none

asparagine and glutamine side chains, which is a common degradation reaction during storage of inadequately stabilized protein and peptide solutions, is subject to a general acid-base catalysis.

25.4.2.3 Temperature

As might be expected, raising the temperature will accelerate the reaction rate. When aqueous systems such as solutions for injection or infusion are thermally challenged, for instance during sterilization, the rate of hydrolysis is not only enhanced by the temperature-induced increase in reaction rate, but also as a result of a change in the dissociation of water. With rising temperature, the ionization of water strongly increases. For example, at 100°C water is over 10-fold more dissociated than at 20°C, causing acid-base-catalyzed reactions to be substantially accelerated by heating.

25.4.2.4 Polarity of the Medium and Ionic Strength

The polarity of the solvent, expressed as its dielectric constant, has an effect on reaction rate and often on the equilibrium state of a reaction. As indicated in Table 25-3, this effect varies with the polarity of the reaction partners. In contrast to earlier assumptions, stabilization of pharmaceuticals will not always be achieved by lowering the polarity of the medium (e.g., by substituting water for alcohol or polyalcohols). With reactions between ions, ionic strength of the solution should always be taken into account.

25.4.3 Oxidative Processes

25.4.3.1 General Introduction

Besides hydrolysis, above all, oxidative processes determine the decomposition of drugs and drug formulations. Oxidation-sensitive drugs include, in particular, the following categories of compounds:

- Phenols: resorcinol, hydroquinone, naphthols, epinephrine, physostigmine and others
- Olefins: polyenes (e.g., carotenes, vitamin A), unsaturated fatty acids and their derivatives, essential oils (e.g., terpenes)
- Endiols: ascorbic acid
- Ethers: diethylether, polyethylene glycols
- Hydroxymethylketones: prednisolone and its derivatives
- Amines: morphine, atropine

Alkaloids especially (e.g., morphine, apomorphine, physostigmine and reserpine), are prone to oxidative decomposition.

As a result of oxidative reactions, degradation products are formed that are typically less active than the parent molecule and additionally may be (more) toxic. The degradation products formed, either directly or by subsequent reactions, may lead to changes in perceptible properties such as taste, smell and appearance. For example, aqueous solutions of apomorphine rapidly turn green under the influence of light and oxygen. Many details of oxidative degradation reactions are still largely unknown. Many cases concern radical autoxidation reactions. The extent to which an oxidation process proceeds is expressed by the Nernst redox potential. For oxidative drug degradation reactions, which often involve proton transfer, this may be described as follows:

$$E = E_0 + \frac{R \cdot T}{n \cdot F} \ln \frac{[Ox] \cdot [H^+]^m}{[Red]} \qquad (25\text{-}15)$$

After conversion of R and F to numerical values, the following equation is found for the redox potential E, at 25°C (T = 298 K)

$$E = E_0 + \frac{0.059}{n} \lg \frac{[Ox] \cdot [H^+]^m}{[Red]} \qquad (25\text{-}16)$$

E = redox potential (*V*)
E_0 = standard redox potential (*V*) (concentration-independent term)
R = universal gas constant
n = number of transferred electrons
m = number of involved protons
T = absolute temperature (K)
F = Faraday's constant

Equation 25.16 reveals, that the redox potential depends on the concentrations of the reaction partners, temperature and, most of all, on the proton concentration, that is, pH, of the solution.

25.4.3.2   Fat Deterioration

For several reasons, deterioration of fats has to be prevented in medicinal products. Fats and oils are important bases and excipients of pharmaceutical products and their impeccable quality is an essential prerequisite for drug stability. The degradation products formed during spoilage of fats do not only result in the organoleptically clearly perceptible rancidness, which by itself already necessitates rejection, but may also cause quality loss by uncontrolled reactions with active ingredients and/or excipients. Furthermore, the primary, as well as secondary cleavage products formed during fat deterioration are by no means physiologically inert. They may for example cause sensitization and pathological effects in the skin. Knowledge about the chemical reactions occurring during fat deterioration is also important for the understanding of stability issues of active substances with a polyene structure (e.g., vitamin A, carotenes), which by virtue of their chemical structure share certain aspects of their degradation processes with fats.

Fat deterioration involves a complex sequence of chemical conversions, mainly hydrolyses and oxidations. Microbiological and biochemical processes may also induce deterioration of fats (see Table 25-4). For both the (purely) chemical and the biological (enzymatic) processes involved, hydrolytic and oxidative events proceed partly consecutively and partly simultaneously.

25.4.3.3   Hydrolytic Degradation

Like all compounds with an ester structure, triglycerides are subject to hydrolytic cleavage in the presence of water, yielding glycerol and free fatty acids as their degradation products. The latter are responsible for the acid value of the fats. Enzymatic hydrolysis by lipases likewise leads to the formation of the mentioned degradation products. Lipases occur in animal as well as plant tissues or may be of microbiological origin. Lipases involved in fat decomposition

Table 25-4 Main Pathways of Fat Spoilage

Chemical Processes	Biological (Enzymatic) Processes
hydrolytic processes (acidification, saponification)	hydrolytic processes (acidification, saponification)
oxidative processes (peroxide formation, turning rancid, turning tallow, etc.)	oxidative (desmolytic) processes (turning ketotic, rancid, tallow; perfume rancidness)

are predominantly of microbiological origin. Molds of the genus penicillium and aspergillus are notorious sources of lipase activity in pharmaceutical products. Optimal conditions for enzymatic hydrolysis are 37°C and a pH value around 7. The more unsaturated the fatty acid in the triglyceride, the faster the hydrolytic cleavage proceeds.

25.4.3.4 Oxidative Decomposition

Oils and fats, in particular those with a high content of unsaturated fatty acids, are furthermore susceptible to oxidative decomposition. The final products thus formed, predominantly ketones, acids and short-chain aldehydes, are characterized by an intense smell and taste. Even minimal (µg range) amounts suffice for rancidness to become discernable. The peroxide value indicates quality-affecting oxidative changes of fats, fatty oils and some other comparable substances. This value indicates the amount of peroxides, expressed as milliequivalents (1 milliequivalent = 0.5 millimole) of active oxygen, present in 1,000 g material. It is mostly determined by iodometric assay. The peroxide value encompasses the amount of oxygen bound as peroxide and is mainly represented by hydroperoxides.

Since peroxides are just labile intermediate products that are subject to further decomposition, the peroxide value only allows preliminary conclusions concerning the degree of degradation of a fat or oil. Upon advanced decomposition of the product, the peroxide value decreases again. Fat decomposition starts with a radical autoxidation (Fig. 25-4).

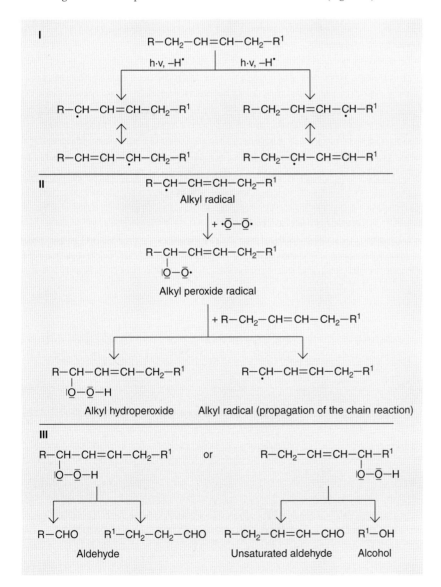

Fig. 25-4 Oxidative fatty acid degradation.

In the initial stage (I), a hydrogen atom is abstracted from a methylene group adjacent to a double bond under the influence of energy (light, heat), thus forming an alkyl radical. In the second stage (II), the oxygen di-radical ·O-O· reacts with the alkyl radical forming alkyl peroxide radicals. These are converted to alkyl peroxides, under the involvement of a second intact fatty acid molecule, while the formed radical continues the chain reaction. Finally, in the third stage (III), the energy-rich alkyl peroxides disintegrate, yielding aldehydes, ketones, acids, hydroxy- and keto acids (tallowing), alcohols, and other degradation products. In this phase also, polymerization and condensation reactions may occur, leading to thickening (viscosity increase) and varnish formation of the product.

25.4.3.5   Enzymatic Oxidative Fat Degradation

Enzymatic oxidation of fatty acids may proceed by two different types of enzymes. In biochemical degradation, lipoxidases originating from vegetable raw material play an important role. These fatty acid-oxidizing enzymes specifically attack unsaturated fatty acids and are still active at lower temperatures.

Another type of oxidative degradation is catalyzed by fungal enzymes (mainly aspergillus and penicillium), quite similar to the reaction sequence of β- oxidation. Among the degradation products are several methyl ketones, responsible for a variety of cheese-like odors (*perfume rancidity*).

25.4.3.6   Influential Parameters and Stabilization Measures

pH Value and Adjustment

For the stabilization of oxidation-sensitive drugs, pH adjustment to the lowest possible value is very important. With increasing pH of a solution the redox potential will decrease, according to the Nernst equation, and thus the oxidation reaction will proceed faster and the conversion will be more complete. For example, the oxidative decomposition of epinephrine (Fig. 25-5), which leads to the formation of adrenochrome and (by this) to coloration of solutions, can be minimized by adjusting pH to 3.0. Lower pH values are not acceptable for physiological reasons and because at pH values <3 the compound racemizes quickly. Evidently, the choice of drug product pH is always a matter of compromise between all factors playing a role in stability.

25.4.3.7   Light and Light Protection

Radical reactions are induced by light, especially shortwave radiation. This necessitates storage of oxidation-sensitive compounds in lightproof containers (e.g., black-colored plastic, porcelain or brown-glass jars). Likewise, exposure to other energy sources such as ultrasound and

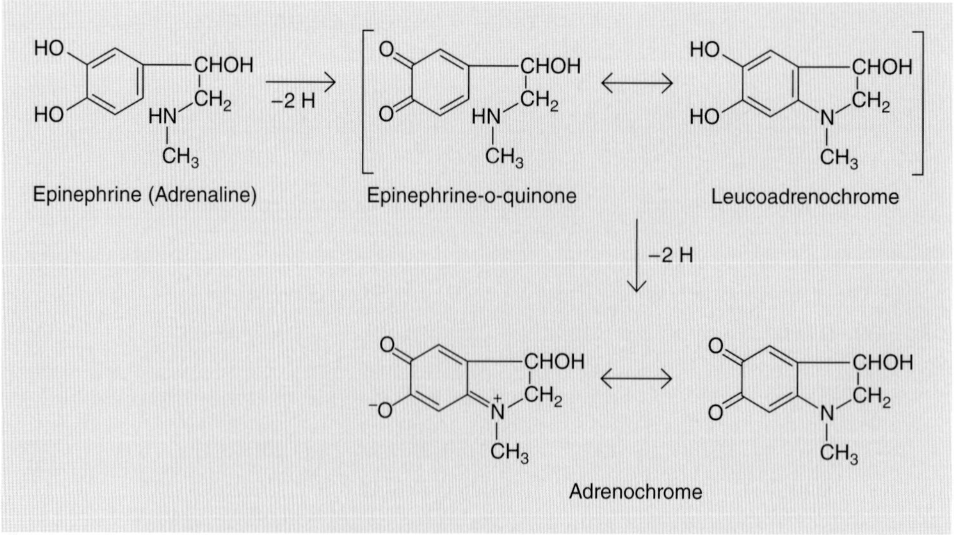

Fig. 25-5 Oxidative degradation of epinephrine.

ionizing radiation, which are used for sterilization purposes, should be avoided for the same reasons as in the case of oxidation-sensitive substances.

25.4.3.8 Atmospheric Oxygen and Its Restriction

With very few exceptions, oxidative degradation reactions depend on the presence of oxygen. Efficient protection is therefore provided by exclusion, or at least minimization, of exposure to air. Table 25-5 lists the most common methods to reduce the oxygen content of aqueous drug solutions. Evidently, exhaustive boiling of water has little effect, as oxygen will reversibly dissolve again upon cooling.

Better results are obtained by providing an inert atmosphere in or above the preparation. Primarily CO_2 and N_2 are applied as protective gases. In principle, CO_2 offers a number of advantages compared to N_2; for instance it has a better solubility in water (CO_2: 1690 mg/L vs. N_2: 18.6 mg/L in water at 20°C) so that it can fairly rapidly displace the air in the solution.

A further advantage of CO_2 is its higher density compared to air, thus facilitating the expulsion of air from the container, such as an injection vial. Unfortunately, CO_2 acidifies aqueous solutions, thus jeopardizing the stability of acid-labile compounds, possibly leading to decomposition or the formation of precipitates. Finally, it should be taken into account that acidic solutions for parenteral administration need to be buffered by the blood, which can be problematic with higher volumes. For all these reasons, the use of CO_2 is generally avoided. If necessary, drug solutions are only to be gassed with CO_2 when it concerns small volumes (a few mL). Fig. 25-6 demonstrates as an example the stabilizing effect of CO_2 gassing on epinephrine degradation.

As a rule, effective, protective gassing begins during the compounding of solutions for injection or infusion. If exclusion of oxygen is necessary, drug and excipient solutions, are prepared under an atmosphere of the protective gas and are also overlaid with it through all subsequent production stages, up to the final filling step. Preparations that are sensitive to stirring and to changing air/liquid interfaces, such as protein solutions, must not be bubbled with gas. In such cases, overlaying the solution with the gas is the only option after the active ingredient has been added. During the filling step, the headspace above the solution in the primary packaging container is gassed. This is performed with a gassing needle, which flushes the empty container (before filling) and the headspace after filling, with an excess of the protective gas.

In order to minimize exposure of compounds susceptible to autoxidation (fats, aromatic oils, and ointments containing such components) to air, they must be stored in tightly sealed containers which are filled to capacity. In addition, the surface area should be kept as small as possible. Because radicals and peroxides act catalytically, already stored residues should not be

Table 25-5 Oxygen Content of Water after different Types of Treatment

Procedure	Oxygen Content (mL/L)
Saturated with O_2	6.4
Distilled from metal or glass equipment	6.0
Distilled, boiled for 5–15 min	2.2
Distilled, saturated with N_2	1.1
Distilled, saturated with CO_2	0.5

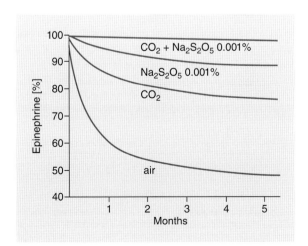

Fig. 25-6 Effectiveness of stabilization measures (protective gas, antioxidants) for epinephrine in a drug product solution (procaine 0.01 g, epinephrine 0.0002 g, water for injection ad 1.0 mL, sterilized).

filled up with fresh substance, nor should containers be used that have not been appropriately cleaned.

25.4.3.9   Heavy Metal Ions

Ions of heavy metals, in particular Cu^{2+}, $Fe^{2+/3+}$ and Mn^{2+}, have a pronounced prooxidative catalytic effect that may manifest at very low concentrations. The origin of such metal ions are in general the ingredients, both actives and excipients, and the processing equipment and containers. Precipitation reactions such as commonly used in inorganic analysis, are incapable to remove all traces of heavy metals. Also, repeated distillation is not suitable for this purpose due to the formation of relatively volatile metal hydrides. Instead, inactivation by complex formation is preferred. Pharmaceutically important heavy metal scavengers include tartaric acid, citric acid, phosphates and polyphosphates and ethylenediaminetetraacetate (EDTA).

Especially the di-sodium salt of EDTA, sodium edetate (Titriplex® III), and Mg-EDTA have proven their anti-catalytic potency. In acid milieu, they form stable metal chelates. In the concentrations applied (0.01% to 0.07 %), the salts of EDTA do not show any adverse effects.

25.4.3.10   Antioxidants

The most effective, but also the most problematic, method to protect oxidation-sensitive systems is the addition of antioxidants. These are substances that are able to inhibit oxidative processes based on their low redox potential, which causes them to be oxidized preferentially to the substances to be protected. In addition, they act as donors of hydrogen atoms, which shift the equilibrium of the redox reaction to the reduced form—that is, the intact drug molecule.

Drug system: $Red \rightleftharpoons Ox + 2\,H$

Antioxidant system: $Red \rightleftharpoons Ox + 2\,H$

The antioxidants used to stabilize aqueous preparations must have a substantially lower redox potential than the drug system to be protected. Antioxidative activity in nonaqueous medium cannot be explained with the redox potential.

Antioxidants with a phenolic character, such as simple diphenols (hydroquinone), are capable of interfering with the radical mechanism of autoxidation if they scavenge formed radicals and convert them to stable products (inhibitors, radical scavengers). The principle of the chain termination mechanism is the transfer of a hydrogen atom to the alkyl peroxide radical. This traps the radicals required for the continuation of the reaction chain. Fig. 25-7 illustrates the antioxidative mechanism of hydroquinone.

The first step is the formation of a semiquinone radical, which further reacts with another alkyl peroxide radical to form a stable product. The activity of the antioxidant is substance-specific and dependent on the medium. Therefore, the optimally suitable antioxidant has to be experimentally determined for each individual system. Keep in mind that antioxidants are consumed while exerting their activity. Chapter 5 includes a list of the most common antioxidants.

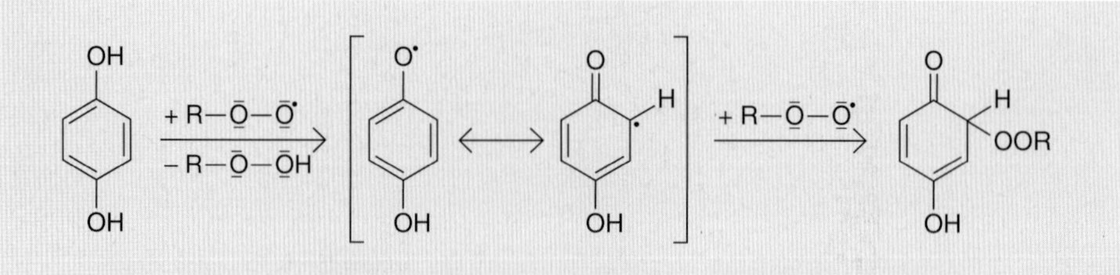

Fig. 25-7 Mechanism of anti-oxidative activity of hydroquinone.

25.4.4 Steric Rearrangements

25.4.4.1 General Introduction

The pharmacological activity of many pharmaceutical substances is connected to their stereo-specific structure. In many cases, only one isomeric form of the active ingredient has significant activity (the eutomer), while the other is barely active (the distomer). Among the steric rearrangements affecting quality of active ingredients, racemizations take a pronounced position. Rearrangements of conformational isomers (confomers) and *cis-trans* isomerizations are of lesser importance. Racemization reactions proceed via a symmetric intermediate stage from which equal portions of the two optic antipodes (together constituting the racemate) are formed. Examples of drugs susceptible to racemization are L-epinephrine, L-hyoscyamine, L-cocaine, and L-methadone. Ergot alkaloids (ergotamine, ergometrine, alkaloids of the ergo-toxin group) may undergo a double stereomeric rearrangement.

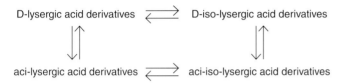

Besides the epimerization, which leads to the pharmacologically poorly active D-iso-lysergic acid derivatives (ergotaminine, ergometrinine etc.), under the influence of acid a rearrangement occurs in the peptide moiety of the alkaloid, which is known as aci-rearrangement.

Like the D-iso-lysergic acid derivatives, the aci dervatives have low activity.

25.4.4.2 Influential Parameters and Stabilization Measures

Racemization processes can be suppressed by adjusting pH to a favorable value because they represent pH-dependent reactions. Nonetheless, it is not possible to make general predictions concerning the correlation between pH and stability. For each pharmaceutical substance, the most favorable pH value has to be determined empirically.

In the case of L-epinephrine, maximal isomeric stability was observed in the pH range 3.5 to 5.5. For optimal pH adjustment, the simultaneously occurring oxidative decomposition and the physiological tolerance must be taken into consideration. The polarity of the solvent also plays a role that should not be underestimated. For example, the epimerization of ergo-tamine to ergotaminine is enhanced by solvents in the following order: acetone < methylene chloride < chloroform < ethanol. Multivalent alcohols, such as glycerol, have a stabilizing effect on the racemization as well as on the aci-rearrangement.

25.4.5 Further Reactions

Besides the decomposition processes described above, decarboxylation and polymerization reactions may also lead to the deterioration of pharmaceutical product quality.

25.4.5.1 Decarboxylations

An example of a decarboxylation reaction is the decomposition of p-amino salicylic acid. At elevated temperatures in particular, this compound is broken down to the toxic aminophenol, which, due to the occurrence of polymerization processes, brings about a yellow coloration of the solution.

Decarboxylations are pH-dependent. Stabilization may be promoted by adjusting the pH to the range in which minimal decomposition occurs and by avoiding exposure to heat. Decarboxylations are particularly important as consecutive reactions of hydrolytic cleavage processes (e.g., acetylsalicylic acid, derivatives of p-aminobenzoic acid, mesazaline).

25.4.5.2   Polymerizations

Polymerizations, as reactions secondary to hydrolytic and autooxidative events, are in many cases responsible for the emergence of colored degradation products. While the exact mechanism of these mostly multistep, complex reactions is not well understood, dimerization products have been identified that arise, for example, during the radical-mediated decomposition of morphine to pseudo-morphine or during the degradation of atropine to belladonnine. The discoloration of glucose solutions can also be traced back to polymerization of cleavage products. Attempts to stabilize such systems must focus on suppression of the primary reactions. Furthermore, protection from light is desirable. In the case of paraformaldehyde formation in solutions of formaldehyde, the conditions are more straightforward. The polymerization of formaldehyde proceeds according to an anionic chain mechanism. The formation of the linear reaction products, which become manifest by the formation of a precipitate, can be largely suppressed by addition of methanol (5% to 15%).

$$H_2C{=}O \xrightarrow{\ +OH^-\ } HO{-}CH_2{-}O^-$$

$$\xrightarrow{\ +n\ H_2C{=}O\ } HO{-}\!\!\left[CH_2{-}O\right]_n\!\!CH_2{-}O^-$$

25.4.6   Stabilization Measures

The specific character and wide variation of (chemical) structures of active substances and their formulations make it impossible to find generally applicable stability-enhancing measures for all drug-containing systems. This implies that for each newly designed drug, formulation-specific stability issues must be dealt with anew. The following measures should therefore be understood, as general suggestions that for each individual case have to be evaluated and further specified.

25.4.6.1   Provisions for Storage Conditions and Limitation of Storage Time

In general, storage at low temperature will improve shelf life of pharmaceutical products because of a lowered degradation rate. That is why all pharmacopeias provide mandatory requirements for the storage temperatures of drugs and drug formulations with poor stability. However, for many drug products storage temperatures below 0 °C have to be strictly avoided, as the physical structure, e.g. the dispersion state of emulsions and suspensions, or the conformation in case of proteins can irreversibly be changed by freeze-thaw cycles.

Several decomposition processes are promoted by light. This applies to many oxidation and polymerization reactions but also hydrolyses and isomerizations often involve photochemical reactions. When applicable, drugs and drug products need to be stored protected from light. Sometimes, only a very limited extension of shelf life can be achieved by specific and general protection measures. In such cases, the product must be prepared shortly before application or reconstituted from a storable form; alternatively, shelf life or in-use time, must be limited.

25.4.6.2   Pharmaceutical Technological Measures

Stabilization may also be achieved by technological measures and procedures. By inclusion in micelles it is possible to suppress hydrolytic degradation processes (section 3.9.9.6). Oxidation-sensitive pharmaceutics, such as vitamin K for example, can be stabilized by formation of inclusion complexes with cyclodextrins. The common encapsulation procedures such as microencapsulation also represent suitable protective measures. Nonetheless, it has to be kept in mind that such measures usually also change the biopharmaceutical properties.

Because degradation reactions occur preferentially in aqueous media, removal of water is a universal stabilization method. Drying procedures can effectively stabilize highly labile pharmaceutical preparations such as fluid and thick-fluid extracts (converting them to dry extracts). Obviously, this goes at the expense of the advantages of the original formulation.

In some cases, as with lyophilizates (e.g., many biopharmaceuticals), bedside preparation of the ready-for-use formulation (i.e., the injectable solution) is performed immediately prior to administration.

25.4.6.3 Stability Compensation by Addition of Overages

Many active substances, like antibiotics and vitamins, display unsatisfactory intrinsic stability, affecting storability and limiting shelf life. When stability-enhancing measures and production technology are insufficient to achieve satisfactory stability, it may be necessary to add an excess (overage) of active ingredient to the formulation to compensate for the predicted loss of activity during storage. However, this procedure is not encouraged unless absolutely necessary (ICH Guideline Q8(R2), EMEA/CHMP/167068/2004). This approach is only justified if it is proved that no increase in overall toxicity can occur, as a result of the larger content of active substance or of its degradation products. Overages may also serve to compensate for drug loss during manufacturing. In such cases, the excess ingredient will not be apparent in the final product. The amount of excess should be as small as possible. Overages have to be reported in the submission dossier and need approval by the authorities. Both the amount of the overage and the reason for this have to be justified.

25.5 Microbial Changes

25.5.1 General Introduction

The ubiquitous occurrence of microorganisms (bacteria, yeasts, molds) presents a serious risk of microbial contamination during the production, packaging, storage, and application of pharmaceutical products. The main sources of contamination are humans, environment (production rooms, air), ingredients, equipment, and primary packaging material.

Depending on the composition and physical conditions, many pharmaceutical products are more or less promoting microbial propagation. In particular, aqueous liquid and semi-solid formulations provide excellent growth conditions for microorganisms. Examples are emulsions, creams, syrups, suspensions, and solutions for parenteral administration. Only the unbound fraction of water is available to facilitate microbial growth. This molecular mobility is expressed in terms of water activity. While bacteria do not proliferate below a water activitiy of 0.9, most molds cease to grow if the water activity falls below 0.8. Besides the available water, the pH is also a critical determinant for microbial growth. Optimal pH conditions range from 6 to 8 for bacteria and from 4 to 6 for molds, but many species can survive in a much broader pH range (1.5–11).

Microorganisms bring about multiple undesirable changes in medical products. In addition to turbidity, foul odor, and fermentation, pathogenic microorganisms can create a direct risk of infections as well as the formation of toxic metabolic products (e.g., pyrogens). Furthermore, bacteria and lower fungi are capable to cause, or at least to trigger or to accelerate, chemical alterations in active ingredients and excipients (*e.g.* rancidity).

Significant measures to reduce the number of microorganisms include avoidance (production hygiene), removal (filtration), and inactivation (physical and chemical procedures) of microorganisms. To maintain the microbiological purity achieved during production and also during storage, the addition of antimicrobial agents (preservation) may be necessary. That applies particularly to sterile multidose preparations. Preparations for which sterility is not mandatory yet still hold potential for microbial growth, must also be preserved.

25.5.2 Microbiological Quality of Pharmaceutical Preparations

Microbiological purity requirements for pharmaceutical preparations and ingredients are listed in Tables 25-6 to 25-8.

Table 25-6 Acceptance Criteria for Microbiological Quality of Nonsterile Dosage Forms (Ph. Eur. 5.1.4, USP ⟨1111⟩, JP G4—Microbial Attributes of Nonsterile Pharmaceutical Products)

Route of administration	TAMC (CFU/g or CFU/mL)	TYMC (CFU/g or CFU/mL)	Specified microorganisms
Non-aqueous preparations for oral use	10^3	10^2	Absence of *Escherichia coli* (1 g or 1 mL)
Aqueous preparations for oral use	10^2	10^1	Absence of *Escherichia coli* (1 g or 1 mL)
Rectal use	10^3	10^2	—
Oromucosal use Gingival use Cutaneous use Nasal use Auricular use	10^2	10^1	Absence of *Staphylococcus aureus* (1 g or 1 mL) Absence of *Pseudomonas aeruginosa* (1 g or 1 mL)
Vaginal use	10^2	10^1	Absence of *Pseudomonas aeruginosa* (1 g or 1 mL) Absence of *Staphylococcus aureus* (1 g or 1 mL) Absence of *Condida albicans* (1 g or 1 mL)
Transdermal patches (acceptance criteria for one patch including adhesive layer and backing)	10^2	10^1	Absence of *Staphylococcus aureus* (1 patch) Absence of *Pseudomonas aeruginosa* (1 patch)
Inhalation use (special requirements apply to liquid preparations for nebulisation)	10^2	10^1	Absence of *Staphylococcus aureus* (1 g or 1 mL) Absence of *Pseudomonas aeruginosa* (1 g or 1 mL) Absence of bile-tolerant gram-negative bacteria (1 g or 1 mL)
Special Ph. Eur. provision for oral dosage forms containing raw materials of natural (animal, vegetal or mineral) origin for which antimicrobial pretreatment is not feasible and for which the competent authority accepts TAMC of the raw material exceeding 10^3 CFU/g or CFU/mL.	10^4	10^2	Not more than 10^2 CFU of bile-tolerant gram-negative bacteria (1 g or 1 mL) Absence of *Salmonella* (1 g or 10 mL) Absence of *Escherichia coli* (1 g or 1 mL) Absence of *Staphylococcus aureus* (1 g or 1 mL)

25.5.3   Preservatives

25.5.3.1   Mechanisms of Action

The potential of certain chemical substances to exert a damaging effect on microorganisms can be traced back to their primary toxicity—that is, a manifestation of their general toxic action on the cell wall or the structures inside the cell. Depending on the prevailing preservative concentration, different stages are distinguished:

□ At very low concentrations, substances are accumulated at or in the cell membrane, leading to changes in permeability of the cytoplasm barrier without causing damage to the cell. Often, an enhanced permeability leads to increased viability of the microorganism.

□ At microbiostatic concentrations (i.e., at concentrations that inhibit the growth of microorganisms), the changes occurring in the cell membrane cause a toxic effect. Reportedly, the permeability increase causes enhanced accumulation of the antimicrobial substance in/at the cell membrane and/or internal structures.

□ At microbiocidal concentrations (i.e., in concentrations leading to cell death), cell membrane permeability is enhanced to such an extent that the preservative penetrating into the cell interior brings about a disorganization of the colloid-physical system of the cell (coagulation, precipitation). In extreme cases, this may even lead to autolysis (release of intracellular components).

Besides the above mechanisms, which apply to all preservatives, additional specific reactions may be involved, such as the inhibition of vital enzyme systems such as by mercury-containing preservatives.

Table 25-7 Recommended Acceptance Criteria for the Microbiological Quality of Herbal Medicinal Products for Oral Use (Ph. Eur. 5.1.8, USP ⟨2023⟩, JP G4—Microbial Attributes of Nonsterile Pharmaceutical Products)

Category	Medicinal Product	TAMC Acceptance Criterion (CFU/g or mL)	TYMC Acceptance Criterion (CFU/g or mL)	Specified Microorganisms Acceptance Criterion (CFU/g or mL) (if absence is required the sample weight is indicated in brackets)			
				Bile-tolerant gram-negative bacteria	Escherichia coli	Enterobacteria and other gram-negative bacteria	Salmonella
A	Herbal medicinal products for the preparation of infusions and decoctions using boiling water	Ph. Eur.: 10^7 (max. accept. count: 50,000,000)	Ph. Eur.: 10^5 (max. accept. count: 500,000)	Ph. Eur.: n.d.	Ph. Eur.: 10^3	Ph. Eur.: n.d.	Ph. Eur.: absence (25 g)
		USP: 10^6	USP: 10^4	USP: 10^2	USP: absence (10 g)	USP: n.d.	USP: absence (10 g)
		JP: 10^7	JP: 10^4	JP: n.d.	JP: 10^2 (sample wt. n.d.)	JP: n.d.	JP: absence (sample wt. n.d.)
B	Herbal medicinal products where the method of processing (e.g., extraction) or pre-treatment reduces the level of organisms to below those stated for this category	Ph. Eur.: 10^4 (max. accept. count: 50,000)	Ph. Eur.: 10^2 (max. accept. count: 500)	Ph. Eur.: 10^2	Ph. Eur.: absence (1 g or mL)	Ph. Eur.: n.d.	Ph. Eur.: absence (25 g or mL)
		USP: n.d.	USP: n.d.	USP: n.d.	USP: n.d.	USP: n.d.	USP: n.d.
		JP: n.d.	JP: n.d.	JP: n.d.	JP: n.d.	JP: n.d.	JP: n.d.
C	Herbal medicinal products where the method of processing (e.g., extraction with low strength ethanol) or pretreatment would not reduce the level of organisms sufficiently to reach the criteria required under B	Ph. Eur.: 10^5 (max. accept. count: 500,000)	Ph. Eur.: 10^4 (max. accept. count: 50,000)	Ph. Eur.: 10^4	Ph. Eur.: absence (1 g or mL)	Ph. Eur.: n.d.	Ph. Eur.: absence (25 g or mL)
		USP: 10^5	USP: 10^3	USP: 10^3	USP: absence (10 g)	USP: n.d.	USP: absence (10 g)
		JP: 10^5	JP: 10^3	JP: n.d.	JP: absence (sample wt. n.d.)	JP: 10^3	JP: absence (sample wt. n.d.)

max. accept. count = maximum acceptable count

n.d. = not defined

When an acceptance criterion for microbiological quality is prescribed, it is interpreted as follows:
- 10^1 CFU: maximum acceptable count = 20
- 10^2 CFU: maximum acceptable count = 200
- 10^3 CFU: maximum acceptable count = 2000, and so forth

Table 25-8 Acceptance Criteria for Microbiological Quality of Nonsterile Substances for Pharmaceutical Use (Ph. Eur. 5.1.4, USP ⟨1111⟩, JP G4—Microbial Attributes of Nonsterile Pharmaceutical Products)

	TAMC (CFU/g or mL)	TYMC (CFU/g or mL)
Substances for pharmaceutical use	10^3	10^2

(TAMC = total aerobic microbial count, TYMC = total combined yeasts/molds count)

The acceptance criteria presented are interpreted as follows:

10^1 CFU: maximum acceptable count: 20

10^2 CFU: maximum acceptable count: 200

10^3 CFU: maximum acceptable count: 2,000, etc.

25.5.3.2   Activity-Affecting Factors

Distribution Behavior

The activity of preservation agents is crucially influenced by their distribution behavior. They need to possess a well-balanced lipophilic/hydrophilic ratio; its hydrophilic property ensures that the substance reaches the cell membrane of the microorganism, while its lipophilic character allows for penetration into and across the membrane barrier. In the case of multiphase systems, a high affinity to the lipophilic phase, characterized by a large distribution coefficient (section 7.6.6), leads to a considerable decrease in concentration of the preservative in the aqueous phase, which jeopardizes its antimicrobial effect. For example: The concentration of chlorocresol in the water phase of a peanut oil/water (1:1) system will decrease from an initial value of 0.1% to as little as 0.0017%, due to its unfavorable distribution coefficient of 117.

pH Value

In case of preservatives that can exist both in an undissociated and in a dissociated form the degree of dissociation strongly depends on the pH (section 7.6.5). Since the noncharged form is the more lipophilic one, the correlation between pH and activity can be explained by a shift in the distribution coefficient. This effect is particularly pronounced for organic acids (e.g., sorbic acid and benzoic acid) and phenolic agents. The rule that the noncharged form (i.e., the more lipophilic) is the most active of the two does not always apply, as it also appears to depend on the microorganism species involved. In full accordance with this rule, phenols display their highest activity against gram-negative bacteria at low pH values, but in contrast to the expected effect, against gram-positive species their highest activity is observed in alkaline (pH 8.5) medium.

Concentration

The correlation between concentration and activity is characterized by the dilution coefficient.

$$\left(\frac{c_1}{c_2}\right)^n = \frac{t_2}{t_1} \tag{25-17}$$

n = dilution coefficient
t_1, t_2 = exposure times required to reduce the microbial count by 99% at the concentrations c_1 and c_2, respectively

The dilution coefficient depends on the chemical structure of the preservative and may vary considerably from $n = 0.5$ for organic mercury compounds, to $n = 6$ for phenols. For the latter, a 50% reduction in concentration leads to a very substantial reduction in activity, expressed as a 64-fold prolongation of the time to kill all microorganisms.

Such losses of preservatives are quite possible for emulsions and therefore practically relevant. They are caused by an unfavorable distribution of the preservative between the hydrophilic phase to be preserved and the lipophilic phase, by sorption of preservatives to elastomeric closures and plastic containers, binding to macromolecular excipients or by inclusion in surfactant micelles.

Temperature

In general, the activity of preserving agents increases with temperature, dependent on the type of agent. The magnitude of this effect is characterized by the temperature coefficient, which is defined as the reduction of the required exposure time caused by a 10 K temperature rise. This activity-enhancing effect is practically exploited in the chemo-thermal treatment.

25.5.3.3   Requirements and Classification

Chemical substances used for microbial stabilization of pharmaceutical products have to meet the following requirements:

- Physiological compatibility: At the concentrations used, no toxic, allergic, or sensibilization effects should occur.

□ Compatibility with active agents, excipients, and packaging materials: No, or only very limited, inactivation may occur by container and closure materials or by inclusion into surfactant micelles (section 3.9.9.6).

□ Chemical stability: A sufficient degree of temperature stability is desirable.

□ Smell and taste: Preservatives intended for preparations for oral application should be tasteless and odorless.

□ Activity profile: Preferably preservatives should be both bacteriocidal and fungicidal or at least should possess bacteriostatic and fungistatic activity. Rapid onset of activity is required as well as a minor pH dependence.

According to their chemical structure the pharmaceutically most commonly applied preservatives are categorized in five groups:

1. Phenol and phenol derivatives
2. Aliphatic and aromatic alcohols
3. Organic mercury compounds
4. Quaternary ammonium compounds
5. Carboxylic acids

The desirable properties of substances to be used as preservatives are described in chapter 5.

25.5.3.4   Tests for Adequate Preservation

Antimicrobial effectiveness testing is a method for characterization of preserved drug products, which is mainly applied in the development of liquid and semi-solid drug products. The test requires the inoculation of the preparation, wherever possible in its final container, with bacteria and fungi. In accordance with the Ph. Eur. and USP, *Pseudomonas aeruginosa*, *Staphylococcus aureus*, *Candida albicans*, and *Aspergillus brasiliensis* serve as test microorganisms. Preparations for oral use should additionally be tested with E. coli and those containing high sugar content with *Zygosaccharomyces rouxii*. The concentration of the microorganisms is adjusted to 10^5–10^6 per mL or gram of the preparation. This high concentration is chosen for methodological reasons and does not reflect realistic values of contamination. The preservative effect in the preparations stored at 25°C is determined by counting the number of colony-forming units (CFU) at distinct time intervals during a 28-day test period. The antimicrobial activity is satisfactory when a microbial count reduction is achieved corresponding to the limit values tabulated in the pharmacopeias. In these tables, distinction is made between: (i) Parenteral preparations and ophthalmics; (ii) Preparations for application in the ear, in the nose or on the skin, and for inhalation; and (iii) Preparations for oral and rectal application, including the oral cavity. For all categories the requirements as to the microbial count reductions to be achieved according to Ph. Eur. are clearly more rigorous than those of the USP. While the Ph. Eur. requires for preserved parenterals, ophthalmics, and topical preparations that the microbial count is reduced by several orders of magnitude within the first 6 hours to 2 days, the first testing time point according to the USP is on the 7th or the 14th day.

Further Reading

Atkins P., and de Paula, J. *Atkins' Physical Chemistry*. Oxford: Oxford University Press, 2014, or the Kindle edition: Atkins, P., and de Paula, J. *Elements of Physical Chemistry* (Kindle edition). Oxford: Oxford University Press, 2013.

Datta, S., Grant, D. J. "Crystal structures of drugs: advances in determination, prediction and engineering." *Nature reviews Drug discovery* 3 (1) (2004): 42–57.

Incompatibilities

26

26.1 General Introduction

In the context of pharmaceutical technology, incompatibilities are understood as interactions between two or more constituents of a pharmaceutical preparation, which affect the pharmaceutical and/or therapeutic quality of a drug product beyond an acceptable level. In other words, incompatibilities are the result of unintentional reactions of components, which either affect the activity, prohibit exact dosing, or have such an unfavorable effect on the physical properties of a formulation that the required quality can no longer be guaranteed. Reactions causing incompatibility may occur between active ingredients, between excipients and between active ingredients and excipients, as well as between components of the preparation and the primary packaging material. But not in all cases are the active ingredients or excipients by themselves the cause of incompatibility. Sometimes, incompatibilities may also be due to (permitted) impurities in the used substances or packaging materials. Examples of this are the occurrence of turbidity in oily solutions when substances containing water of crystallization are employed, the oxidation of phenolic compounds by (per)oxidases present in gum arabic and reductive changes of active ingredients in presence of peroxide-containing macrogols or macrogol derivatives. Such undesirable reactions can be avoided by employing specifically purified products.

From a pharmaceutical-technological point of view, the following incompatibilities can be distinguished:

- physical incompatibilities
- chemical incompatibilities
- physicochemical incompatibilities

There are no strict boundaries between the individual forms of incompatibility. In fact, a clear distinction cannot be made between cause and effect in all cases. The initial cause of an incompatibility that manifests itself by a change in physical properties of a preparation, such as a change in the degree of dispersity of an emulsion, may lie in a chemical reaction with the emulsifier. Likewise, it is difficult to distinguish sharply between incompatibility and instability. An essential difference between the two is the time scale on which the reactions proceed. Incompatibilities are based on rapidly proceeding reactions and therefore occur during or shortly after production or packaging. Instability reactions, on the other hand, are usually slow, and their consequences therefore often appear only after a certain storage time. In the following sections, processes that are determined by components of the drug product—including packaging material that is in direct contact with the formulation—and develop during and immediately following processing, are considered incompatibilities. Changes triggered by factors like air, light, and temperature or based on slowly proceeding reactions are assigned to instability problems (Chapter 25.1).

Voigt's Pharmaceutical Technology, First Edition. Alfred Fahr.
© 2018 John Wiley & Sons Ltd. Published 2018 by John Wiley & Sons Ltd.

The most important causes of incompatibility are ionic interactions between cations and anions, hydrogen bonds between phenols and ethers, as well as hydrophobic interactions between amphiphilic molecules. The most common reaction partners among the excipients are polymers and surfactants.

Additional causes of incompatibilities include redistribution processes and solubility changes.

Incompatibilities may be either manifest or masked. *Manifest incompatibilities* are changes that can be perceived organoleptically—that is, without the help of analytical methods. Among the manifest incompatibilities are changes in solubility and dispersion state (e.g., turbidity, precipitation, coagulation, aggregation), changes in consistency (e.g., solidification, fluidization) as well as color changes and changes in smell and taste (e.g., off-odor, discoloration).

Masked (invisible) incompatibilities cannot be perceived sensorily. They can only be detected by suitable test methods, such as, for instance, the test for efficacy of antimicrobial preservation (microbial challenge test). They are often physicochemical-based interactions (formation of soluble complexes and associates, absorption, and adsorption reactions). Statements concerning compatibility and incompatibility are always concentration-dependent. Two substances that at high concentration are incompatible may be fully compatible at lower concentration. Furthermore, a manifest incompatibility may change into a masked incompatibility by reducing the substance's concentration. Incompatibilities occur mainly in fluid and semi-solid preparations and much more rarely in solid formulations, because the interactions causing the phenomenon most often prevail at the molecular or colloidal level and only exceptionally at the particulate level.

26.2   Ionic Interactions

Ionic interactions are strong and act over a long-range, which is why they are often the cause of incompatibilities in aqueous systems. Widely differing mechanisms may underlie the observed action. In water-free preparations, ionic interactions do not occur.

26.2.1   Cation-Anion Interactions

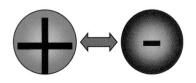

Cation-Anion Interaction

Cation-anion interactions may lead to the formation of salts with a lesser degree of dissociation and consequently reduced hydration and solubility. This reaction is particularly pronounced when organic anions and cations react together—for example, benzalkonium cations or salicylate anions, small multivalent ions, such as sulfate anions or aluminum cations, or polyelectrolytes (electrically charged polymers) such as carmellose-sodium (gelling agent) or polyhexanide (polyhexamethylene-biguanide hydrochloride; an antimicrobial active).

In accordance with this, important reaction partners among the excipients include charged surfactants and anionic gelling agents, while among the active substances salts of acidic and basic drugs play an important role in this connection. The resulting incompatibilities may be manifest and present themselves as precipitations, viscosity lowering and breaking of emulsions. When cationic active substances or preservatives are bound to anionic gelling agents or to micelles of anionic surfactants, this may, depending on the mixing ratio of the two reactants, also only be expressed as a masked incompatibility. In that case, the bioavailability of a drug may be reduced or the effectiveness of a preservative restricted.

26.2.2   Cation-Anion Reactions with Gelling Agents

Many gelling agents and thickening agents in pharmaceutical preparations are organic polyanions such as carbomer or carmellose-Na, or inorganic polyanions such as bentonite (section 15.3.3). When these gelling agents form poorly dissociated salts with organic cations such as benzalkonium chloride, they will become less hydrated and gel formation will be compromised. A reaction with multivalent cations, such as Al^{3+}, may at low concentration

Table 26-1 Examples of Pairs of Substances Whose Interaction May Lead to Precipitation

Cation	Anion
alkaloid hydrochloride alkaloid nitrate	bromide, iodide, acetate, citrate, salicylate, benzoate, tannate
benzalkonium chloride cetyl pyridinium chloride	nitrate, iodide, salicylate, lauryl sulfate-Na, benzyl penicillin-K
phenyl mercuric-acetate, -nitrate, -borate,-	iodide, bromide
ephedrine hydrochloride, codeine phosphate, procaine hydrochloride, tetracaine hydrochloride	lauryl sulfate-Na
calcium-, magnesium-, aluminum ions	sodium-, potassium stearate
calcium ions	tetracycline

also lead to viscosity enhancement, due to cross-linking of the polymer strands, while higher salt concentrations result in precipitation.

When a cationic active substance or preservative interact, its bioavailability or preserving activity, respectively, may be constrained: this is a masked incompatibility.

Inorganic gelling agents of the type of swellable phyllosilicates (e.g., bentonite), have cations embedded in between the layers. In the case of gelling agents, these are monovalent cations, mostly sodium ions. These may be readily exchanged with other cations. Upon significant progression of the reaction, the capacity to build gels is reduced: a manifest incompatibility. When active ingredients or preservatives interact at low concentrations, their availability may be reduced, without the occurrence of any change in consistency.

Silanol groups present at the surface of silica particles are weakly acid and act therefore as cation exchangers, which is why they can reversibly bind cationic substances. Since colloidal silica particles are characterized by a very large specific surface area, the extent of adsorption for some substances is considerable. Binding of cationic surfactants (quats, invert soaps) and cationic dyes (methyl-rosanilinium chloride, fuchsine and ethacridine), has been reported, in connection with a reduced anti-microbial efficacy of these substances. The strongly basic polypeptides tyrothricine and bacitracine are fully inactivated by adsorption to silica.

26.2.3 Reactions with Anionic Surfactants

Anion-active surfactants, such for example cetostearyl sulfate-Na, are often used as hydrophilic emulsifiers and components of a liquid-crystalline gel network in creams. Salt binding with organic cations or (multivalent) inorganic cations changes their hydration status. As a result, the emulsion-stabilizing properties are limited and the typical water-binding capacity of a liquid-crystalline gel matrix is reduced. When this leads to breaking of the emulsion or when water is expelled from the cream, we are dealing with a manifest incompatibility. For example, the reaction of alkali, ammonium, or amine salts of fatty acids with multivalent cations (e.g., Ca^{2+}, Al^{3+}) results in their precipitation, while the emulsion breaks. Organic cations participating in the reaction will experience diminished availability—so that, for example, preservatives will no longer display sufficient activity: a masked incompatibility.

26.2.4 Exceeding the Solubility Product by Addition of Ions of Identical Charge Sign

In the case of preparations in the form of saturated or nearly saturated solutions of a salt, addition of electrolytes that share one ion type with the dissolved compound may cause the solubility product of the salt to be exceeded and thus induce precipitation. For example, when in an eye drop formulation the active ingredient is present as hydrochloride or nitrate, adjustment of tonicity with NaCl or $NaNO_3$ may lead to precipitation of the active ingredient.

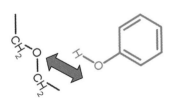

Fig. 26-1 Structural formula of macrogol lauryl ether (Polidocanol 600 = Lauromacrogol 400: $n = 9$).

26.2.5   Nonspecific Interaction with Electrolytes

26.2.5.1   Salting Out

Besides a direct ionic interaction, the addition of salts can also reduce the solubility of other ingredients as a result of changes in the water structure; in that case, we speak of a salting-out phenomenon.

Under those conditions, a large amount of salt competes with the dissolved substance, for example, a macromolecule, for the free water. This causes the hydration of the polymer to decline until it ultimately precipitates; this is a clear case of a manifest incompatibility. This process is not limited to charged polymers but may, in principle, also involve nonionic molecules since no direct ionic interaction with the macromolecule is required. The efficacy of a salt with respect to its salting-out effect is characterized by the *Hofmeister-series* (lyotropic series). Anions and cations with a structure-building effect, such as sulfate anions and ammonium cations, have a particularly strong salting-out activity.

26.2.5.2   Reduction of the Electrostatic Repulsion

In systems where electrostatic repulsion plays a role, addition of electrolytes may lead to incompatibilities. In electrostatically stabilized suspensions, polymer dispersions or emulsions, the addition of electrolytes not only gives rise to a decline in the zeta potential but it also diminishes the range of the electrostatic repulsion force (reduction of the Debye length), causing the preparation to flocculate. Emulsions may subsequently break and polymer dispersions irreversibly coagulate. In the case of charged gelling agents (e.g., polyacrylate), electrostatic repulsion of the dissociated carboxyl groups may lead to stretching of the macromolecule and decisively contributes to gel formation. Addition of electrolyte reduces repulsion of groups of like charge, the polymer transforms into a random-coil conformation and viscosity drops. When the spreading property of a cream is based on a liquid-crystalline matrix containing an anionic surfactant, as in hydrophilic cream, addition of salt brings about a reduction in lateral repulsion of the surfactant molecules. As a result, the matrix shrinks, the water-binding capacity drops, and water exudes from the cream.

26.3   Phenol–Ether Interactions

Phenols and ethers can form hydrogen bonds. The reaction is quite intense when substances with several functional groups, such as polyethers and polyphenols, react with each other.

Important reaction partners participating in this kind of interaction include excipients such as macrogols and their derivatives as well as nonionic gelling agents of the cellulose ether type. Among the active substances, all organic molecules with one or more phenolic hydroxyl groups may be involved.

Active substances or preservatives involved in phenol-ether interactions may be limited in their availability as a result. Reduced bioavailability and insufficient preservation are possible consequences of this example of masked incompatibility.

When one of the reaction partners is a gelling agent, such as hydroxylethylcellulose, its hydration will be diminished, commonly leading to reduced consistency. A reaction with polyphenols such as tannic acid may, at low concentrations, lead to a viscosity increase as a

Phenol-Ether Interactions

result of a slight cross-linking of the polymer strands. At higher concentrations, phenols, and particularly polyphenols often have a tendency to precipitate followed by a loss of consistency.

When macrogol surfactants are among the reaction partners (PEG surfactants, ethoxylated surfactants), reaction with a phenol may reduce emulsion stability as well as the water-binding capacity of the liquid-crystalline matrix of a cream, and with that, affect its spreadability.

26.4   Interactions between Surfactants

Like surfactants, numerous drug compounds or preservatives have an amphiphilic structure. Two examples include ketoprofen-Na and benzalkonium chloride. In preparations containing surfactants, they may become incorporated into micelles or liquid-crystalline associations of surfactants or in interfacial films, as a result of hydrophobic interactions.

This phenomenon will reduce the availability of such active ingredients or preservatives, a typical masked incompatibility.

The effect of such a process will be particularly pronounced when polar amphiphilic substances become accommodated in the interfacial film of W/O emulsions or creams. This will lead to a massive weakening of the interfacial film and, as a consequence, breaking of the emulsion, accompanied by water exudation. An example of such an incompatibility is the addition of polydocanol 600, an anti-itching agent, to a lipophilic cream such as Hydrous Woolfat (Lanolin Cream) or the Lipophilic Base Cream (see Table 15.3).

Incompatibilities occurring upon mixing of dermatological vehicles of different emulsion types (e.g., W/O creams with water-absorbing ointments of the O/W type (section 15.3.2)) are to be similarly evaluated.

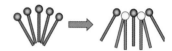

Interactions between Amphiphilic Molecules

26.5   Solubility Changes

26.5.1   Precipitation of Weak Acids or Bases by pH Change

A weak, poorly soluble acid (HA) in water undergoes protolysis as follows:

$$HA + H_2O \leftrightarrow H_3O^+ + A^-$$

The equilibrium constant of this process also represents the dissociation constant K_a.

$$K_a = \frac{[H_3O^+] \cdot [A^-]}{[HA]}$$

$$[A^-] = \frac{[HA] \cdot K_a}{[H_3O^+]}$$
(26-1)

Because the concentration of the nondissociated acid in a saturated solution is constant, solubility (S) equals [HA] + [A$^-$]. By introducing Equation 26-1 and after proper mathematic conversion, we obtain:

$$S = [HA] + \frac{K_a \cdot [HA]}{[H_3O^+]}$$
(26-2)

From this, it appears that with decreasing oxonium ion concentration (i.e., with increasing pH), solubility increases due to the change in dissociation grade. By further conversion, we can finally calculate at which pH value precipitation of the poorly soluble acid occurs.

$$pH = pK_a + \lg \frac{S - [HA]}{[HA]}$$
(26-3)

When considering salts of weak acids, such as, for example, sodium salicylate, sodium benzoate, and benzylpenicillin sodium, their solubility is so high that the poor solubility of the

Table 26-2 pH-Dependence of Solubility of Weak, Poorly Soluble Acids

Acid	pK$_a$ Value	Solubility (g/L) a	Required pH to Obtain a Solubility of			
			a	2a	11a	101a
p-aminosalicylic acid	3.6	1	<2.6	3.6	4.6	5.6
benzoic acid	4.2	3	<3.2	4.2	5.2	6.2
diclofenac	4.0	0.0009	<3.0	4.0	5.0	6.0
ibuprofen	4.5	0.049	<3.5	4.5	5.5	6.5
morphine hydrochloride	9.8	0.2	<8.8	9.8	10.8	11.8
salicylic acid	3.0	2	<2.0	3.0	4.0	5.0
sorbic acid	4.8	1.5	<3.8	4.8	5.8	6.8
theobromine	10.0	0.6	<9.0	10.0	11.0	12.0
theophylline	8.6	5	<7.6	8.6	9.6	–

nondissociated acids is practically negligible. Under such conditions (S ≫ [HA]), Equation 26-3 may be simplified to:

$$pH = pK_a + \lg \frac{S}{[HA]} \qquad (26\text{-}4)$$

In other words, when the pK$_a$ of an acid, its concentration [HA], and its maximal solubility are known, the pH at which the poorly soluble acid precipitates, also called the critical pH, can be calculated and used to predict incompatibility.

As is apparent from Equation 26-4, the critical pH value is a concentration-dependent parameter. When concentration increases by one order of magnitude, the critical pH value increases by one unit. Table 26-2 lists the pH-dependent solubility of a number of weak acids.

Below the indicated pH values, the poorly soluble acids precipitate.

By analogy, the precipitation critical pH values of weak bases (B) can be calculated.

$$pH = pK_a + \lg \frac{[B]}{S - [B]} \qquad (26\text{-}5)$$

Taking into account that, when we are dealing with water-soluble salts (e.g., alkaloid hydrochloride), S ≫ [B], equation 26-5 simplifies to

$$pH = pK_a + \lg \frac{[B]}{S} \qquad (26\text{-}6)$$

Thus, for weak and poorly soluble bases, the occurrence of pH-dependent incompatibilities can also be predicted. From equation 26-6, we may, analogous to weak acids, derive that the critical pH value depends on the concentration of the compound.

When concentration increases by one log the critical precipitation pH value drops by one unit.

Table 26-3 lists pH-dependent solubility of a number of weak, poorly soluble bases. Below the indicated pH values the poorly soluble base will precipitate. pH changes may be brought about by any acidic or alkaline salt or by mixing drug solutions of different pH. To prevent pH-induced precipitation, knowledge about the pH conditions prevailing during the production phase is required.

In general, knowledge of acid and base properties of active, as well as excipients, is a prerequisite when attempting to avoid these type of incompatibilities.

By way of example, Tables 26-4 and 26-5 list a number of acidic or basic active and excipients in 1% aqueous solution.

26.5.2   Precipitation in Solvent Mixtures

In real regular and irregular solutions, solubility depends on the type of solvent. By mixing different solvents, solubility may be either enhanced or decreased. When a drug is present

Table 26-3 pH-Dependent Solubility of Weak and Poorly Soluble Bases

Acid	pK_a Value	Solubility (g/L) a	pH Required to Obtain a Solubility of			
			a	$2a$	$11a$	$101a$
atropine	9.7	1.5	>10.7	9.7	8.7	7.7
dihydrocodeine	8.0	1.3	>9.0	8.0	7.0	–
ephedrine	9.6	50.0	>10.6	9.6	(8.6)	–
codeine	8.0	8.0	>9.0	8.0	(7.0)	–
cocaine	8.4	1.2	>9.4	8.4	7.4	6.4
methadone	9.5	0.1	>10.5	9.5	8.5	7.5
morphine	9.8	0.2	>10.8	9.8	8.8	7.8
narcotine	6.2	0.02	>7.2	6.2	5.2	4.2
papaverine	6.4	0.02	>7.4	6.4	5.4	4.4
pethidine	8.7	3.8	>9.7	8.7	7.7	6.7
procaine	9.0	1.3	>10.0	9.0	8.0	7.0
tetracaine	8.5	0.16	>9.5	8.5	7.5	6.5

Table 26-4 pH Values of Aqueous Solutions of Some Acidic Actives and Excipients (concentration 1%)

Substance	pH Value	Substance	pH Value
ammonium chloride	5.0	methadone hydrochloride	5.0
ascorbic acid	2.5	morphine hydrochloride	4.8
citric acid	2.0	nicotinic acid	3.1
cocaine hydrochloride	4.5	papaverine hydrochloride	4.0
codeine phosphate	5.0	pilocarpine hydrochloride	4.0
caffeine-sodium salicylate	6.2	procaine hydrochloride	5.4
DL-ephedrine hydrochloride	5.4	quinine hydrochloride	6.1
ethyl morphine hydrochloride	5.0	mercury(II) chloride	4.5
isoniazide	6.5	thiamine hydrochloride	2.8

in a preparation dissolved in one solvent, recrystallization may occur when a second, poor solvent is added, due to the fact that the saturation concentration is exceeded. In such a case, particle size of the crystals cannot be controlled. For example, salicylic acid will recrystallize in a suspension ointment, when preparing a concentrated predispersion in a liquid excipient in which it is fairly soluble and when a hydrocarbon (paraffin), in which it is clearly less soluble, is subsequently added. Addition of water to an aqueous-ethanolic herbal drug extract may similarly give rise to precipitations because the solubility of nonpolar extracted substances will be exceeded. The same type of reaction occurs when liquid extracts or tinctures, prepared with different alcohol-water mixtures, are further processed by mixing the extracts. Also, hydrophilic polymers like carmellose-Na often floccculate upon addition of large amounts of water-miscible solvents such as ethanol, likewise by reduction of solubility, accompanied by a clear drop in viscosity. On the other hand, in the case of carmellose-Na, addition of alcohol up to a concentration below the precipitation limit results in a slight enhancement of viscosity, while for methylcellulose, this leads to a considerable increase in viscosity. This is due to an enhanced polymer-polymer interaction, which results in physical cross-linking of the polymer strands.

Table 26-5 pH Values of Active and Excipients That React Acidic or Basic in a 1% Aqueous Solution

Substance	pH Value
barbital-sodium	9.2
di-sodium hydrogen phosphate	8.5
methenamine	8.3
phenobarbital-sodium	8.5
theobromine-sodium salicylate	9.8
theophylline-sodium acetate	9.6

26.5.3 Recrystallization by Formation of Hydrates and Solvates

Hydrates and solvates show a lower solubility than the water-free or solvent-free crystal forms of the same substance. The formation of hydrates and solvates in a suspension or nearly saturated drug solution is subsequently accompanied by recrystallization. For example, prednisolone transforms in a water-containing dermal vehicle into the even more poorly soluble prednisolone-hydrate, while forming long crystal needles. Depending on the size of the formed crystals, these can either be detected only microscopically (masked incompatibility) or cause a scratchy skin feel upon application (manifest incompatibility). The employment of a suspension concentrate in the corresponding water-containing basic material, which after recrystallization is once more homogenized, may solve the problem in such cases.

26.6   Redistribution Processes

In dispersed systems, the dissolved components of a preparation will distribute between the dispersed phase and the dispersion agent, according to their distribution coefficient. As a result of redistribution processes, a distribution equilibrium will be achieved whose position is determined by the distribution coefficient, but independent of whether the substance originally was dissolved in the continuous or the dispersed phase. When this redistribution is not desirable and has a negative influence on quality, it is a masked incompatibility, which may limit availability of an active substance or the activity of a preservation.

In principle, such redistribution processes may occur in coarse, colloidal, as well as in molecularly dispersed systems. Bindings to macromolecules or surfactant associates (colloidal disperse systems) are, in most cases, not counted among the distribution processes in the narrow sense. Corresponding processes in colloidal and molecular disperse systems find their cause in the type of interactions that were already discussed in section 3.9.9.6. The magnitude of redistribution processes not only depends on the distribution coefficient DC but also on the volume ratio ϕ between the phases, as follows:

$$DC = c_1/c_2 \text{ and } \phi = V_1/V_2$$

with

$$c_1 = n_1/V_1 \text{ and } c_2 = n_2/V_2$$

we obtain:

$$n_1 = n_2 \cdot DC \cdot \phi$$
$$|n_1; n_2 = \text{amount of substance in phase 1 and phase 2, respectively}$$
$$|V_1; V_2 = \text{volume of phase 1 and phase 2, respectively}$$

In multiphase preparations such as creams, which besides an oil and a water phase also contain a liquid-crystalline phase, the distribution processes may be quite complex, so that a quantitative prediction will rarely be possible.

26.6.1   Coarsely Dispersed Systems

Emulsions are coarsely dispersed systems in which redistribution events occur most frequently. Suspensions are much more rarely affected by this phenomenon because solubility in the dispersed solid phase is usually poor. Nonetheless, with decreasing degree of crystallinity of the solid (equivalent to increasing amorphous fraction), solubility increases, thus explaining the considerable extent to which certain substances dissolve in amorphous polymers of similar polarity. As long as the substance is soluble in both phases, redistribution just leads to concentration changes (i.e., a masked incompatibility). A typical example is the redistribution of preservatives such as alkyl-4-hydroxy benzoates (parabenes) from the water phase into the oil phase, potentially causing the concentration of the preservative in the aqueous phase to drop below the minimal antimicrobial concentration. In that case, the emulsion is no longer sufficiently protected from microbial growth.

In complex emulsions, redistribution may concern several substances. For example, a co-solvent that was added to the water phase to improve solubility of the active ingredient in this phase may redistribute to the oil phase, causing the solubility of the drug in the water phase to decrease. When, as a result, the concentration exceeds saturation solubility, the substance will precipitate (crystallize) from the now super-saturated solution. Often, crystal formation starts at the oil/water interface. When, thus, large crystals are formed, the reaction may be perceived as a manifest incompatibility.

Redistribution processes may also occur as incompatibilities in soft capsules (section 11.2.2). This may involve transfer of active ingredient and of components of the (fluid) capsule filling into the capsule shell, but also transfer of water and plasticizer (e.g., glycerol) from the capsule shell into the filling material. The change thus brought about in the composition of the capsule shell may lead to softening or brittling of the capsule and thus present a manifest incompatibility.

26.6.2 Colloidally Dispersed Systems

Colloidal solutions are dispersed systems in which colloids are finely dispersed in a continuous phase. In general colloids consist of macromolecules, aggregates, or clusters of several molecules or small solid particles. In special cases concerning surface-active substances, the surfactants aggregate into micelles and/or vesicles, which are also known as association colloids.

Among the colloidally dispersed systems are polymer solutions, surfactant micelles (association colloids) and polymer dispersions (latices). Causes and actions of the interactions with the former have previously been described in this chapter.

Aqueous polymer dispersions are predominantly employed as a coating material in the production of film tablets. They represent nano-dispersed suspensions of mostly amorphous polymers, allowing low-molecular weight substances to redistribute extensively from the aqueous phase into the polymer phase. This is precisely what plasticizers are expected to do.

As a result of this, the glass transition temperature of the polymer drops and its properties, with respect to further processing, change. The resulting film coatings can be sticky and display an enhanced permeability for active ingredients.

The most important incompatibility caused by redistribution processes in colloidal dispersed systems is the inclusion in micelles and other surfactant aggregates. The effect may be exploited to improve solubility of poorly water-soluble drugs (solubilization; see section 3.9.9). When it occurs unintentionally, it represents a masked incompatibility, as it may effect a drugs bioavailability (Chapter 7.4). By the same token, the anti-microbial potency of preservatives and antiseptic agents may be reduced by inclusion in micelles. Because of their pronounced solubilization potential this effect is particularly conspicuous with non-ionic surfactants. In the case of phenolic preservatives, phenol-ether interactions with surfactants carrying macrogol residues additionally contribute to micellar inclusion (Chapter 26-2). For example, nonionic surfactants of the polysorbate type substantially reduce the antimicrobial activity of alkyl-4-hydroxybenzoates (parabenes) and chloroxylenol. Polysorbate 80 in a 5% aqueous solution inactivates methyl- and propyl-4-hydroxybenzoate by 80% and 90%, respectively. Similarly, macrogol stearates in concentrations above the critical micellar concentration inhibit the antibacterial activity of phenolic agents. A substantial increase in concentration of the preservative would be required to ensure effective antibacterial activity (Table 26-6).

Table 26-6 Concentration Enhancement of Phenolic Compounds Required to Maintain Their Antibacterial Activity in Presence of 5% Macrogol Stearates

Antimicrobial Substance	Macrogol Stearate X		
	X = 400	X = 1,000	X = 2,000
		Required enhancement	
o-chloro-m-cresol	8.5-fold	10-fold	7-fold
thymol	39-fold	34-fold	18-fold
o-chloro-m-xylenol	42-fold	45-fold	26-fold

26.6.3   Molecular Dispersed Systems

In molecular dispersed systems, the formation of complexes and inclusion compounds, and the displacement of substances from them, may also be considered to count among distribution processes.

The extent to which complexes and inclusion compounds are formed depends on the binding constants involved as well as on the concentration conditions. The displacement of a substance from a complex or inclusion compound may cause its solubility to be exceeded, followed by its recrystallization. This is a manifest incompatibility, recognized by the occurrence of turbidity or visible crystal formation. On the other hand, formation of a complex or inclusion compound may limit the availability of an active constituent or the activity of a preservative, a typical example of a masked incompatibility.

26.7   Changes in the State of Phase

26.7.1   Eutectic Mixtures

Certain mixtures of active substances are characterized by the occurrence of an eutectic point (Chapter 2.1). Since, by definition, a eutectic mixture has a melting point lying below that of any of the individual components, powders of such mixtures may liquefy upon intense mixing, giving rise to a manifest incompatibility, only occurring in solid formulations. As can be seen in the phase diagram presented in Fig. 26-2, the mixture of propyphenazone and acetylsalicylic acid has a eutectic temperature that is characterized by a defined mixing ratio of the two components. For this example, the composition of the eutectic mixture is 1:1 and the eutectic temperature 55°C. When the eutectic temperature lies around or below room temperature, or the processing temperature, the mixture will liquefy, appearing as being "wet." Table 26-7 lists a number of pharmaceutically relevant eutectic mixtures. A particularly pronounced eutectic mixture is the thymol/camphor system. In the concentration range of 30% to 70% (m/m) thymol, the mixture will be fluid down to a temperature of −15°C. The occurrence of eutectic systems not only refers to their melting point but is also connected to a change in some other physical and physicochemical properties, including, for instance, their solubility, and may thus significantly affect the biopharmaceutical properties.

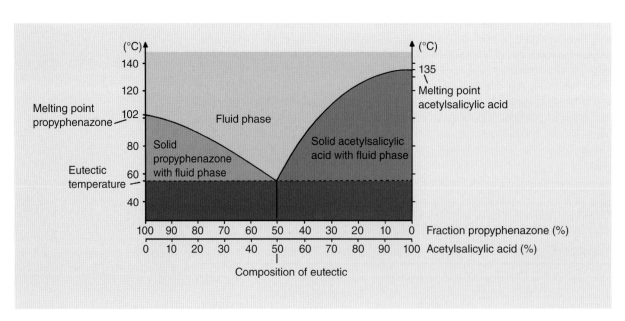

Fig. 26-2   Phase diagram of propyphenazone and acetylsalicylic acid mixtures (formation of an eutectic).

Table 26-7 Eutectic Mixtures

Component I	Component II	Concentration Component I (Mass %)	Eutectic Temperature (°C)
propyphenazone	acetylsalicylic acid	50.0	55.0
propyphenazone	paracetamol (acetaminophen)	35.0	65.0
thymol	urea	95.5	43.0
thymol	salicylic acid	96.2	46.2
thymol	camphor		−15.0
L-methadone	D-methadone	50.0	70.0
lidocaine	prilocaine	50.0	18.0

26.7.2   Gas Formation

Gas formation is a manifest incompatibility and is most often based on a reaction of (bi-) carbonates with acidic active ingredients or excipients. This incompatibility reaction requires at least traces of water, but may also occur in solid formulations such as effervescent tablets.

26.8   Incompatibilities with Primary Packaging Material

Incompatibilities with primary packaging materials are based on adsorption and absorption as well as desorption from the materials. The main effects resulting from these processes are:

- Sorption losses to surfaces (low-dosed drugs, preservatives)
- Transfer of components of the packaging (e.g., polymeric additives, monomers) into the filling material and vice versa from the filling material into the packaging material (migration).
- Permeation and evaporation losses (preservatives, aromatic compounds, solvents).

These initially physical and physicochemical interactions may be followed by subsequent chemical reactions, such as:

- Hydrolytic reactions of active ingredients and preservatives caused by alkali equivalents released from glass with low hydrolytic resistance
- Reactions triggered by migrating additives from polymers and elastomers, such as:
  - Precipitation reactions
  - Catalytic degradation reactions of readily oxidized active substances
  - Corrosion of metallic parts of containers by acid components of the formulation

Incompatibilities with primary packaging material are quite frequently based on migration processes. Because the mass transport involved is based on diffusion processes, such incompatibilities are less likely to occur in solid formulations. In liquids and semi-solid preparations, the probability of such interactions is, however, quite substantial. The risk of affecting the quality of the preparation by such processes largely depends on the route of administration of the medication. Accordingly, Table 26-8 presents the risk of interactions between packaging material and drug formulation with respect to type of application.

26.8.1   Incompatibilities with Glass

Incompatibilities with glass as the primary packaging material are, on the one hand, the result of release of ions from the glass and, on the other hand, the result of adsorption of active ingredients to the glass surface.

Since the surface area of containers is relatively small, adsorption plays only a relevant role in material losses in the case of very low-dose active ingredients or preservatives. When the active ingredient is a protein, binding to the glass surface may lead to denaturation. When

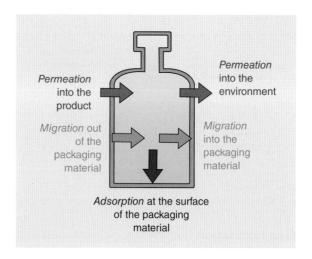

Fig. 26-3 Possible interactions between primary packaging material, preparation and environment.

Table 26-8 Classification of Interactions of Packaging Materials with Different Formulation Types in Accordance with an FDA Guideline for the Pharmaceutical Industry

Relevance in Relation to Route of Administration	Probability of Interactions between Packaging Components and Formulation		
	High	**Intermediate**	**Low**
Highest	parenterals, inhalation aerosols	sterile powders powders for injection powders for inhalation	
High	liquid and semi-solid Eye preparations or preparations for nasal application, transdermal patches		
Low	liquid and semi-solid preparations for application in eye or nose, transdermal plasters	powders for ingestion or topical application	tablets, soft and hard capsules

the binding is reversible, a gradual loss of activity may occur, as little by little, all protein molecules may undergo the adsorption-denaturation reaction. The velocity of this type of reaction may be considerably accelerated as a result of movement of the solution inside the primary container. Furthermore, the dissolution of alkali and alkaline earth ions from the glass matrix may constitute a major cause of incompatibility with glass. The extent of ion release from the glass depends on its hydrolytic resistance (section 27.2.1). Among the consequences of ion release from the glass, alkalinization of aqueous solutions and the concomitant pH-induced incompatibilities or instabilities play an important role. Dissolved Ca^{2+} ions may cause precipitation reactions, for example, in phosphate-buffered solutions.

26.8.2 Incompatibilities with Polymeric Packaging Materials

Polymers employed for primary packaging constitute a very heterogeneous group of materials. In addition to organic polymers, polymer packaging materials contain a variety of additional substances that serve to meet the specific properties required of the material. These additives are able to migrate into the pharmaceutical preparation and may trigger incompatibility reactions. Conversely, active ingredients and excipients (preservative, antioxidant) may migrate into the polymer packaging. As a result of such absorption processes, substantial losses of activity of active ingredients and excipients may occur (Table 26-9). Very frequently, migration of substances into elastomers (e.g., of rubber stoppers or droppers for eye drops) is observed. This often concerns preservatives such as benzalkonium chloride, chlorhexidine, or thiomersal. The resulting decline in concentration of these low-dosed substances represents a masked incompatibility

26.8.3   Incompatibilities with Metal Packaging Materials

Primary packaging materials made of metal are applied as tubes for semi-solid formulations and cans for pressurized-gas containers. The metal involved is most often aluminum and more rarely tin plate. Incompatibilities may result from direct reaction of the contents with the metal (corrosion). The metal cations thus released may, in turn, trigger incompatibility reactions with the preparation (section 27.2.3). To prevent such reactions from occurring, metal primary packaging material is often coated with a protective lacquer layer on the inside (e.g., based on an epoxy resin). Nonetheless, incompatibilities may also occur with this protective layer, including creation of holes in, or even complete dissolution of, the layer, again subsequently giving rise to corrosion.

26.9   Avoidance and Elimination of Incompatibilities

To avoid or eliminate incompatibilities, knowledge of the devaluating processes is a prerequisite. Because most drug formulations are complex multicomponent systems and the reactions involved are not of a readily overseeable complexity, there are no simple and generally applicable rules as to how to eliminate incompatibilities. Based on theoretical considerations, the disturbing factors involved need to be assessed and eliminated on empirical grounds.

pH-mediated incompatibilities can often be eliminated by appropriate pH adjustment. More extensive measures involve exchange of certain components. As a rule, such measures may only be considered for excipients, because neither the type nor amount of active ingredients should be subject to change.

Often, elimination of the incompatibility can be achieved by appropriate choice of suitable excipients. In the case of cation-anion incompatibilities, the replacement of one of the ionic substances by a nonionic equivalent is indicated (anionic emulsifier → nonionic emulsifier; anionic gelling agent → nonionic gelling agent). When a phenolic drug binds to a PEG surfactant or to a cellulose ether, respectively, replacement by an anionic surfactant or gelling agent, respectively, may solve the problem.

In the case of incompatibility between two active ingredients, more extensive galenic measures are necessary. Among others, separate granulation may represent a suitable remedy. When this alone is insufficient to ensure proper spatial separation of the two incompatible components, encapsulation of one may allow common processing of the powders. Separation of incompatible constituents may also be achieved by the production of layered or coated tablets (Chapter 12.5). The compounds involved are then present in the different layers or in the core and coat of the tablet, respectively, possibly even separated by a separation layer.

Such a spatial separation is difficult, if not impossible, to realize with fluid and semi-solid formulations. In such cases, the only way to solve the problem is through separated administration, implying separation in time. When, for example, two active ingredients that need to be administered as an infusion are mutually incompatible, two separate infusion solutions must be prepared, for consecutive administration.

Table 26-9   Loss of Preservatives (%) During the Storage of Solutions in Containers of Polyvinylchloride (PVC) and Polyethylene (PE). Storage time: 12 weeks at 20°C

Compound	Conc. in Percent	PVC	PE
Benzalkonium chloride	0.1	0.2	2.5
Benzyl alcohol	2.0	1.3	15.5
Chlorocresol	0.1	8.3	57.8
Chlorhexidine acetate	0.05	0	2.2

Further Reading

FDA Guidance for Industry: Container Closure Systems for Packaging Human Drugs and Biologics. May 1999. https://www.fda.gov/downloads/drugs/guidances/ucm070551.pdf

Packaging Materials and Technology

27

27.1   General Introduction

Just as many drug substances will not exert their full effect without being transferred into an applicable and bioavailable dosage form, the benefit of a dosage form for its part will be also limited if the packaging does not prevent quality loss over the shelf life and enable proper administration.

The term *packaging* comprises the container, the closure, and the outer encasement, including the information leaflet; in other words, it covers the entire unit as it is stored and brought onto the market. The marketed product is the combination of the content (the pharmaceutical preparation) and the packaging material. Packaging material that is in direct contact with the pharmaceutical preparation is called *primary packaging material*, as opposed to outer encasements such as cardboard boxes, which represent the secondary packaging materials. The packaging, including its labeling, is an essential part of a medicinal product. It has to be taken into account in all quality-relevant considerations, from the development up to and including the market release and must be approved in the context of the authorization procedures.

The packaging of a pharmaceutical product has three fundamental functions:

1. It serves as a container of the pharmaceutical preparation.
2. It preserves the properties of the drug.
3. It ensures safe application, including providing the patient with information on the proper use and preventing improper use.

All components of the packaging that serve to protect the product from environmental influences are commonly designated the container closure system. That includes the primary packaging components (e.g., containers, closures) and in many cases also the secondary packaging material, when this contributes to product protection. Another purpose of the packaging is the prevention of improper use or abuse. This aspect includes, for example, the limitation of the size of the package to a safe total dose or the application of childproof packaging. The latter should prevent or hamper ingestion of pharmaceutics by small children, thus reducing the risk of drug poisoning. Childproof packaging should prevent access of children to the pharmaceutical preparation, while opening and closing should be easy for adults.

Each individual medicine demands specific requirements of proper packaging. This may, for example, include exclusion of microbial contamination, as well as protection from light, oxygen, or moisture. In many cases, it is even required to maintain moisture equilibrium in order to avoid excessive drying—for instance, to stabilize hydrates and to avoid release of unbound water thus promoting the transition from a more to a less hydrated pseudo-polymorph. Also, interactions with the packaging material are quite frequent and vary between preparations. In one case, a hydrophilic surface may have a stabilizing effect, in another case, a hydrophobic material may be advantageous. Because of the complexity of

Voigt's Pharmaceutical Technology, First Edition. Alfred Fahr.
© 2018 John Wiley & Sons Ltd. Published 2018 by John Wiley & Sons Ltd.

all these aspects, packaging engineering has evolved into a scientific discipline within the field of pharmaceutical product development. Nowadays, the selection of suitable packaging materials starts in the early development stages, with the screening of product-packaging interactions, stability studies involving various container types and materials and risk based evaluations of the different options.

A vital point is the selection of suitable container material. In addition to the traditional materials such as metal and glass, nowadays an ever-increasing variety of plastics with optimized properties is available. Due to the development of composite materials that may consist of six or even more individual components, the range of different container materials has reached an extent that can hardly be overseen by nonspecialized professionals. The following sections describe the most important pharmaceutically applied container and closure materials, their structure, properties, and applications as well as the relevant aspects in connection with drug manufacturing.

27.2   Container Materials

27.2.1   Glass

Silicate glasses are amorphous inorganic melt products mainly composed of silicon dioxide, alkali, and alkaline earth metals. Their structure consists of SiO_4 tetrahedrons, interconnected via their corners but building a nonordered random network. Incorporated metal ions serve to create or maintain distance between the silica residues and are known as network modifiers. These ions disrupt the Si-O-Si bonds and turn the bridging oxygen atoms into negatively charged nonbridging oxygen atoms that then are bound only on one side to silicon atoms. This enhances the mobility of the silica matrix and lowers the softening point of the glass. While pure alkali silicate glasses are water-soluble (water glass), addition of Ca^{2+} ions induces the formation of water-insoluble glasses. By melting together quartz sand (SiO_2), sodium carbonate (Na_2CO_3), and lime (CaO) at a temperature above 1200°C, soda-lime-silica glass is obtained. It represents the consumer glassware that is used, for example, in bottles and windowpane. It consists of about 75% SiO_2, 15% Na_2O, and up to 10% CaO.

This glass is unsuitable for the production of containers for aqueous parenteral solutions because it is insufficiently resistant to water. It releases Na^+ ions to and takes up H^+ ions from the water. The glass surface thus acts as an ion exchanger. The withdrawal of H^+ ions causes an increase in pH of the solution. Also, other components of the glass, such as Ca^{2+}, may be exchanged to a minor extent against H^+ ions from the water or against other cations present in the solution. Turbidities occurring in solutions of alkali citrate, tartrate, or phosphate in glass containers can also be attributed to ion exchange (Na^+ in the solution against Ca^{2+} of the glass), causing poorly soluble calcium salts to precipitate.

The dissolution of ions from the glass surface and the formation of soluble silicates cause cracks in the silica matrix at the surface and the exposure of new glass surface to be attacked by the solution. This may cause thin, flexible, and poorly detectable glass fragments to shed from the surface. This process is called delamination and can even be observed to a certain degree in glass of higher hydrolytic resistance. It should be taken into account as a potential source of particulate impurities in infusion and injection fluids and should be minimized by proper selection of the glass quality and the excipients in the solution.

The surface resistance of glass against water, acids, and alkali is enhanced when SiO_2 is partly replaced by boron or aluminum oxide. When, in addition, alkali ions are incorporated into such a network, a fraction of the triple-coordinated boron atoms will shift to a quadruple coordination. The network connectivity increases and, hence, also the chemical resistance. Ion exchange (alkali for H^+) in such glasses is impeded, as it involves the breakage of covalent bonds and reorganization of the network structure, rather than ionic interactions.

The pharmacopeias (Ph. Eur. 3.2.1, USP ⟨660⟩) distinguish three glass types as material for glass containers for the storage of pharmaceutical preparations, based on their hydrolytic resistance, and lay down rules for their application.

Type I glass containers: Containers of neutral (borosilicate) glass with high hydrolytic resistance based on its composition. This type is suitable for most parenteral and non-parenteral preparations.

Type II glass containers: Containers of surface-treated soda-lime-silica glass. By a special surface treatment, it has acquired a high hydrolytic resistance. This type is suited for most aqueous parenteral and nonparenteral preparations with neutral or acidic pH.

Type III glass containers: Containers of soda-lime-silica glass with moderate hydrolytic resistance. This type is suited for nonaqueous parenteral preparations, for powders for parenteral administration, except lyophilizates, and for preparations for nonparenteral application.

While for container types I and III the composition of the melt determines the hydrolytic behavior, type II glass containers owe their hydrolytic resistance to a surface treatment. The composition of the glass is, in this case, the same as for type III, but the inner surface of the container is treated at temperatures of 500° to >600°C with sulfur dioxide or ammonium sulfate (which at those temperatures splits off SO_2). During this process, alkali and alkali earth ions in the glass surface form soluble salts that are subsequently washed out of the silicate matrix with dilute acid. The glass surface is thus partially depleted of ions so that neutral or acidic solutions will no longer have much of a leaching effect. Glass treated in this way should not be autoclaved more than once and is not suitable for multiple use. Repeated heating will bring cations from the deeper layers of the glass to the surface, which will obliterate the treatment effect. Type II glass containers are cheaper than type I and can be manufactured much more easily because of the lower melting point.

A relatively new method for the finishing of glass surfaces is the Plasma Impulse Chemical Vapor Deposition (PICVD) technique. In this technique, the internal surface of the container is coated with an ultra-thin (0.1–0.2 µm) film of SiO_2 that forms an effective diffusion barrier. This layer effectuates a high resistance, also against alkaline solutions and ion-complexing excipients.

Table 27-1 Physical parameters and chemical composition of different glass types according to ASTM E438-92 and Ph. Eur./USP classification

Glass type according to ASTM E438-92	Type I, Class A (low-expansion borosilicate glass) weight %	Type I, Class B (Alumino-borosilicate glass) weight %	Type II (soda-lime glass) weight %
Type of glass container acc. to Ph. Eur. and USP	Type I	Type I	Type III
Brand names (selection)	BORO-8330™ (Schott) W33 (Nipro) Gx®33 (Gerresheimer) Corning® 33 Tubing (Corning)	Fiolax® (Schott) NSV51 (Nipro) Gx® 51-V (Gerresheimer) Corning® 51-V Tubing (Corning)	AR-Glas® (Schott) WG6 (Nipro)
Physical parameters			
Linear coefficient of expansion (cm/cm·°C × 10^{-7})	32-33	49-54	91-93
Annealing point (°C)	557-565	565-570	520-530
Softening point (°C)	807-825	785-789	706-720
Density, annealed (g/cm^3)	2.22-2.23	2.31-2.34	2.50-2.52
Chemical durability Titration equivalent of 0.02N H_2SO_4/10 g of glass (ml)	< 1.0	< 1.0	< 9.5
Approximate amount of constituents			
SiO_2	80-81	72-75	approx. 69
B_2O_3	12.7-13.7	10.5-11.5	< 1
Al_2O_3	2.0-2.6	5.0-6.8	2.8-4.0
BaO	< 0.05	< 0.1	2.0-2.5
CaO	< 0.1	0.4-1.5	5.0-5.5
MgO	< 0.1	< 0.3	3.0-3.5
Na_2O	3.5-4.3	6.5-7	approx. 13
K_2O	< 0.75	1.0-2.4	3.0-3.2
As_2O_2 plus Sb_2O_3	< 0.005	< 0.1	< 0.1
PbO	< 0.1	< 0.1	< 0.1
ZnO	< 0.1	< 0.1	–
All other constituents	< 0.2	< 1.0	< 1.0

Amber glass contains 1% Fe_2O_3 and about 3 to 5% TiO_2 (e.g. Fiolax® amber (Schott), Corning® 51-A Tubing).
Addition of about 0.7 to 1.0% CeO_3 reduces brown discoloration upon gamma sterilization (e.g. Corning® 51-C Tubing).

The pharmacopeias specify three methods to distinguish the types of glass containers. All three are based on the assessment of the amount of alkali hydroxide that is released during a defined autoclaving process in distilled water. With the surface test (Ph. Eur.: Test A) types I and II can be distinguished from type III. The glass grains test (Ph. Eur.: Test B) and the test of the internal surface of the container after hydro fluoric acid treatment (etching test, Ph. Eur.: Test C) serve to distinguish glass type I from types II and III. In the latter two methods, material layers from underneath the treated surface are exposed. In test B, this is achieved by fracture and in test C by etching away the surface layer. In order to distinguish between types I and II, a combination of the surface test and the glass grains test must be performed.

Another important characteristic of glass is the thermal expansion coefficient. This not only has relevance for glass production but characterizes the glass composition and, thus, can be related to different hydrolytic properties these materials.

Even type I glass containers do not guarantee full protection against leaching of ions into the product solution. Under certain circumstances these ions can react with components of the drug product. As an example, barium ions leaching from glass vials could precipitate with sulfate ions from the formulation. A similar interaction can occur between aluminum from the glass and phosphate from the drug product.

Ph. Eur. 3.2.1 Glass containers for pharmaceutical use—Test for hydrolytic resistance

USP ⟨660⟩ Containers – glass
USP ⟨1660⟩ Evaluation of the inner surface durability of glass containers

A. Hydrolytic resistance of the inner surfaces of glass containers (Surface test).

This test serves to distinguish container types I and II from type III. It is performed in accordance with ISO 4802-1. The required test containers are first rinsed with water and then with freshly distilled water. The containers are filled up to 90% of their brimful volume with freshly distilled water and subsequently autoclaved for 60 minutes at 121°C (warming and cooling down times precisely specified). Sealed ampoules are not rinsed but, rather, heated at 50°C for 2 minutes before filling. After autoclaving, the content of the container is homogenized and an aliquot is titrated with 0.01 M HCl against methyl red. The maximally allowed consumption of the HCl solution (titrant) depends on the type of glass and the size of the container. For type III glass containers, it is tenfold larger than for types I and II, and for cylindrical containers it is proportional to the internal surface. As an alternative to the titration method and in conformity with to ISO 4802-2 the Ph. Eur. describes a flame-spectrometric analysis of the test solution after autoclaving.

B. Hydrolytic resistance of glass grains (Glass grains test).

With this test container type I can be distinguished from types II and III, according with ISO 720. The test analyzes the basic matrix of the glass beneath a possibly hydrolytically resistant surface. To that end, at least three glass containers are crushed in a steel mortar and of each of them two samples of glass grains with a particle size of between 300 and 424 μm are taken. After removal of any steel particles with a magnet, the samples are repeatedly washed with acetone and dried. Of each sample, 10 g is mixed with 50 mL of freshly distilled water and then autoclaved for 30 minutes at 121°C. Subsequently, the water is titrated with 0.02 M HCl against methyl red; 1 mL of 0.02 M HCl corresponds to 620 μg of Na_2O. For glass type I, not more than 0.1 mL and for types II and III not more than 0.85 mL of the titrant should be consumed per gram of glass.

C. Determination whether the containers have been surface-treated (Etching test).

Also this test serves to distinguish between container types I and II. A possibly present surface treatment is destroyed by 10-minutes etching of the glass surface with a mixture of one volume hydrofluoric acid (40%) and 9 volumes hydrochloric acid (36%). After the acid mixture is removed and the glass is rinsed six times with water, as described under A, the container is filled with freshly distilled water and autoclaved and the content titrated with 0.01 M HCl. HCl consumption that far exceeds the value obtained with method A is indicative for container type II.

Glass may be colored by adding various metal ions. Dependent on the shade of the color, colored glass absorbs light in different wavelength ranges. Colored glass containers have been employed to protect light-sensitive products during storage and application from light effects.

Most frequently for this purpose, brown glass is used, which owes its color to Fe^{3+} ions. Additionally, any additives to the glass may leach into product solution. For products such as biologics that are sensitive to oxidation, iron is generally not favored in solution, given its propensity to facilitate oxidation. Thus, use of brown glass should be avoided, especially for biologics. A disadvantage of colored glass is, particularly for packaging of injection and infusion solutions, the restricted visibility of the contents of the containers, which will hamper the visual detection of particulate impurities.

For all drugs that are sensitive only in the UV range this disadvantage may be met by using vials and flasks that are coated with UV-absorbing shrink foil, which is transparent for visible light and thus colorless. This option may also be used in case the light absorption of thin-walled brown glass in the 300 to 400 nm range is insufficient.

27.2.2   Plastics

27.2.2.1   General Introduction

Among the various packaging materials, plastics form a group that has gained most importance in recent years. The current trend is characterized by an increasing substitution of glass and metal by plastic packagings and a steadily expanding field of applications for continuously improved plastic materials. The main reason for this is the enormous versatility of synthetic polymers and the possibility to flexibly adjust the properties of the packaging materials made from them to the requirements of the particular products. Their advantages include their low density, high fracture strength, in many cases high chemical inertness, and low price. On the other hand, when the packaging material is maladjusted to the properties of the contents, moisture and oxygen may penetrate in the filling, while low-molecular weight components of the filling may leak out, especially when they are volatile. In addition, polymer components and their additives may pass over into the contents, while conversely components of the content may adsorb to or be absorbed by the polymer material.

Finally, chemical or physical reactions between polymer components and contents could result in precipitates or discoloration and deformation of the container. The contents might be in contact with the polymer for extended periods and under various external conditions (temperature, humidity, light), and thus undesired interactions between the polymer and the active substance are likely to occur over time.

Plastics are solid substances consisting of organic macromolecules made up of one (homopolymers) or several (copolymers) monomers. They might be of purely synthetic or semi-synthetic origin. The physical properties of synthetic polymers are decisively determined by the degree of polymerization, which determines the size of the molecules, and the molecular structure. Two types of polymers are distinguished: thermoplastics and thermosets. Thermoplastics soften upon heating; as a result they become deformable and can be cast into a desired shape. Upon cooling, the material rigidifies and becomes dimensionally stable. The shaping process can be repeated by reheating. Thermosets can be shaped only once. With monomers or low-molecular weight precursors as starting material, the polymer is formed by chemical cross-linking of the molecules, leading to hardening of the material. As compared to thermoplastics, thermosets play only a minor role in packaging technology.

Synthetic polymers consist of structurally more or less homogeneous macromolecules. Variation in polydispersity, type and degree of branching, kind of linkage between the monomers, and the terminal groups bring along a multitude of different structures. These variables also affect the arrangement of the polymer chains with respect to one another, which may result in amorphous or partially crystalline materials. Homopolymers are those that are built up of identical monomeric units. Copolymers, on the other hand, are composed of different monomers. The monomers in a copolymer may be connected to each other alternatingly (A-B-A-B-A-B), randomly (A-B-B-A-B-A-A-B), or block-wise (A-A-A-A-B-B-B-B) (section 5.3.6). We speak of alternating, random, and block copolymers, respectively. Graft copolymers are those in which a main polymer chain (A) carries side chains consisting of one type of copolymer (B).

With respect to their synthesis, condensation polymers and addition polymers are distinguished.

Condensation polymers are formed by *polycondensation*, where monomers link together, eliminating a low molecular weight product, such as HCl, NH_3, or H_2O, in each reaction step. Stepwise formation of intermediates ensues, which may be isolated as such or allowed to further condensate. With progressing reaction time, the degree of condensation of the compound increases. Typical polycondensates are polyesters and some polyamides.

Polyaddition, by contrast, does not involve the elimination of any small reaction product. In this process, low molecular weight polyfunctional compounds associate under rearrangement of certain molecular moieties into macromolecules. Polyurethanes and epoxide resins may be produced by *polyaddition*. But also, most of the general-purpose plastics, like polyethylene, polypropylene, and polyvinyl chloride, are addition polymers. They are synthesized from unsaturated monomers by breaking their C=C π-bonds and linking them by single bonds. During this process, the double bonds in the monomers are converted to single bonds. This process represents a chain reaction comprising an initiation, a propagation, and a termination step. The growth rate and ultimate chain length may be controlled by the applied reaction conditions. When applying polyunsaturated monomers, branched chains are formed.

Polymerizations can be performed with different techniques and may proceed in the gas phase as well as in the fluid or dispersed phase. Polymerization of undiluted liquid monomer is called *bulk polymerization*. In this procedure, the dissipation of the reaction heat is often difficult to control. The same holds true with respect to the homogeneity of the reaction (viscosity increase). Both problems are often reasons to prefer polymerization in a heterogeneous phase. An attractive alternative is *polymerization in solution*, where both the monomer and the formed polymer are dissolved in a solvent. In a modification of this method, the solvent is chosen such that only the monomer is soluble in it while the polymer precipitates as solid. In the *pearl or suspension polymerization*, the polymerization process takes place under vigorous stirring of a monomer or a momoner/solvent mixture in a fluid (commonly aqueous) phase, in which neither the monomers nor the solvent nor the initiator are soluble and, thus, form emulsion droplets (usually >10 μm), inside of which the polymerization takes place. Dispersants or protection colloids are added to ensure that the pearl polymerization product that is formed remains suspended. In case of *emulsion polymerization*, due to the solubility of the initiator in the dispersion medium, the polymerization reaction proceeds inside emulsifier micelles that, during the process, swell up to form emulsifier-stabilized polymer particles. Replenishment of monomers in the dispersion medium is achieved by a continuous diffusive flow from emulsified monomer droplets. These serve as a reservoir from which monomer molecules are released at the same rate at which they are taken up by the micelles. Unlike suspension polymerization, in emulsion polymerization the size of the polymer particles formed is not determined by the size of the original emulsion droplets but by the formulation and process parameters (e.g., concentration of monomers, emulsifier/monomer ratio, concentration of the initiator, temperature, ionic strength). Yet another polymerization method is the gas phase polymerization, which is applied in case of gaseous monomers. It is employed for the production of polyethylene and proceeds under high pressure and temperature.

27.2.2.2   Polymer Additives

The production of polymers requires additives that serve to initiate the polymerization process and control the course of the reaction as desired. These substances include initiators, activators, nucleation inducers, and inhibitors. Usually, also specific additives are necessary to obtain polymers that meet the requirements of their specific application. Since many of these additives are not physiologically safe, it is essential for polymers intended for pharmaceutical and medical as well as food-industrial applications to keep the amount of such additives to an absolute minimum and only select substances with minimal toxicity. This strongly limits the spectrum of polymers suitable for pharmaceutical application. In addition, extensive testing of the selected substances prior to application is a necessity. The most important groups of additives in polymer production and their functions are listed in Table 27-2.

Besides fillers, plasticizers are the most abundantly used additives. They serve to provide the product with the necessary elasticity or plasticity. Distinction is made between intrinsic and

Table 27-2 Polymer Additives

hardeners = initiators	initiate the polymerization or cross-linking process (e.g., peroxides)
accelerators, activators	reduce the energy required for the decomposition of the initiator (e.g., cobalt and vanadium compounds, amines)
nucleation agents	enhance the degree of crystallization in semi-crystalline thermoplastics (e.g., talcum, silica, kaolin, salts of carboxylic acids, pigments, polymers)
inhibitors	retard the cross-linking process, enhance storage stability of monomers (e.g., alkylated phenols, cresols and quinones)
emulsifiers	facilitate polymerization in heterogeneous systems such as emulsion polymerization (e.g., anionic and nonionic emulsifiers)
flow enhancers	facilitate processing by injection molding, extrusion, blow molding, and calendering (e.g., acrylate polymers)
lubricants	diminish sticking of the polymer mass to machine parts during processing (e.g., stearates)
solid lubricants	reduce friction and attrition of machine parts during polymer processing (e.g., molybdenum disulfide)
heat stabilizers	protect polymers against heat during processing and use, in PVC for example by binding released HCl (e.g., sulfur-containing tin compounds)
adhesion enhancers	form connecting layers during lamination or co-extrusion (e.g., polyesters, polyisocyanates, polyisocyanurates)
fillers	□ dilute expensive polymers and make them cheaper (e.g., calcium carbonate, kaolin, barium sulfate) □ improve form stability, rigidity or hardness (quartz, glass pearls)
plasticizers (specifically, extrinsic plasticizers)	enhance plasticity, lower glass transition temperature (e.g., esters of phthalic acid, adipic acid azelaic acid and sebacic acid, phosphate esters, fatty acid esters)
impact resistance enhancers	confer impact resistance to polymers, also in the cold (e.g., elastomers, calcium carbonate)
antioxidants	protect against oxidation: □ primary anti-oxidants: react with chain-forming radicals (e.g., butylhydroxytoluene = BHT) □ secondary anti-oxidants: convert peroxides and hydroperoxides (e.g., phosphites, phosphonates, thio compounds)
UV-stabilizers	convert energy-rich UV radiation to heat (carbon black, hydroxyphenyl benzotriazole, hydroxybenzophenone)
quenchers	can absorb photon energy that has already been transferred to a macromolecule by energy transfer and convert it to heat (e.g., cinnamic acid, nickel chelates)
antistatics	diminish sticking together of foils and rapid pollution with dust (e.g., quaternary ammonium salts, stearyl betaine)
antimicrobial additives	prevent microbial decomposition of plasticizers, pigments, filling material or stabilizers (not to be used for polymers that come in contact with food stuffs or pharmaceutical products)
flame retardants	reduce flammability (e.g., aliphatic and aromatic bromides and chlorides, halogenated alkyl and phenyl phosphates and phosphites)
coloring agents	confer color to a polymer (lipid-soluble dyes, e.g., azo- and anthraquinone dyes or organic or inorganic pigments such as titanium dioxide, carbon black, ultramarine blue, phthalocyanine pigments, rylene (perylene-based) dyes

extrinsic softening. The former is achieved by copolymerization of the main monomer with a co-monomer. In case of extrinsic softening, low-molecular weight substances are added that do not engage in covalent bonds with the macromolecules but are bound by coordination bonds. They act by breaking up the coordination forces between the polymer chains, widening up the molecular network by intercalation, enhancing the mobility of the chain segments and thus lowering the glass transition temperature of the polymer to below room temperature. Commonly applied plasticizers are esters of dicarboxylic acids (phthalic acid, adipic acid, sebacic acid), epoxidized fatty acid esters, and esters of alkyl sulfonic acids. Addition of plasticizers is only required for polymers that at room temperature are in a glassy state. Plasticizers that are readily released from the polymer may also facilitate the migration of other additives. Furthermore, they can substantially affect the permeability of the material to water vapor and gases. When they leach from a polymer packaging material into the pharmaceutical or nutritional product inside it, they may accumulate there to toxic concentrations.

27.2.2.3   Processing Technology

The processing of thermoplastics involves mainly injection molding, extrusion, and extrusion-blow technologies.

In the injection-molding procedure, the raw granules are transferred via a filling funnel into a heated cylinder in which the polymer melts. A piston, which at the same time interrupts flow of raw material, pushes the plastic mass into a cold cast, where the polymer rigidifies. Depending on the type of polymer, the plasticizing or injection temperature amounts to 100° to 300°C for only about 3 seconds. Fully automatic machines produce up to 100,000 units per hour.

In case of extrusion, the material is transported forward in a heated cylinder by a rotating screw press (extruder), compressed, plasticized, and pressed through an orifice. The melting heat is partially supplied from an external source and partially produced by internal friction in the cylinder. Polymer foils can also be produced using this procedure if a wide slot nozzle is used.

Extrusion blow molding is the most important procedure to produce hollow objects. An extruder presses the plastic mass through a ring-shaped die so that a flexible tube is formed. This is pressed against the wall of a hollow cast by means of compressed air, thus forming the properly shaped desired container. In a similar procedure without using a cast, the tube formed by the annular die is inflated to a thin-walled tubular bag that can be cut to yield sheets or roll stock films.

27.2.2.4 Thermoplastics

Polyethylene (PE)

Polyethylene is the most abundantly produced polymer worldwide. It is produced by polymerization of ethane, which yields products with varying properties, depending on the reaction conditions. The most widely used types are low-density polyethylene (LDPE), which, by reference to the process pressure, is also called high-pressure polyethylene, and high-density polyethylene (HDPE), also known as low-pressure polyethylene, again by reference to the pressure conditions during production.

The higher density of HDPE is a result of the higher degree of crystallinity, that is, a larger number of densely packed ordered domains. The highly branched polymer chains of LDPE hamper the formation of crystalline structure, lending the material more amorphous character. The crystalline domains provide mechanical strength and enhance the polymer's heat resistance. Due to light scattering by the crystallites, material containing such domains is less transparent. That is why HDPE is more opaque, but also has higher tensile strength and is more rigid, more abrasion-resistant, and melts at higher temperatures (128°–136°C) than LDPE. It is therefore also called hard polyethylene, while the more flexible LDPE (melting range 105°–115°C) is known as soft polyethylene. For both types of PE, though, softening begins way below the melting range. HDPE is therefore heat-resistant until about 105°C and LDPE only till about 80°C. Polyethylene can therefore not be sterilized by autoclaving. With a glass transition temperature of −100° to −125°C (LDPE) and −70° to −80°C (HDPE), respectively, polyethylene at room temperature is in a rubbery elastic state. All polyethylenes exhibit high chemical stability toward acids, alkali, and nearly all polar solvents. Polyethylene is not biologically degradable, but can be recycled. During combustion, only carbon dioxide and water are formed.

Application: LDPE is mainly used for the production of foils and soft bags, but also for bottles for infusion solutions (e.g., Ecoflac®) or ampoules, produced by the bottle-pack procedure (e.g., Mini-Plasco®). With HDPE, bottles of higher rigidity are obtained, at the expense of lower transparency. Its high permeability for a variety of substances and its high absorption capacity—for example, for preservatives (benzalkonium chloride, benzyl alcohol, 2-phenylethanol) and steroids or alkaloids (scopolamine, pilocarpine)—limit the use of polyethylene.

Polypropylene

Polypropylene is obtained by polymerization of propene. Depending on the type of linkage of the monomers, different stereo isomeric configurations are formed. For industrial use, isotactic polypropylene is important; it is carrying all of its methyl groups on one side of the polymer chain. Because of their regular structure, the polymer chains form helical structures that arrange themselves into crystallites. In between those, amorphous domains are located

$$\left[CH_2\!-\!CH_2 \right]_n$$

Polyethylene (PE) e.g. low-density PE (LDPE): Petrothene®, Lupolen®, high-density PE (HDPE): Alathon®, Hostalen®

Table 27-3 Degree of Crystallinity of Polyethylene

Degree of crystallinity (%)	Density (g/cm³)
LDPE 40–50	0.92–0.93
HDPE 60–80	0.94–0.96

$$\left[CH_2\!-\!CH \right]_n$$
$$\qquad\quad | $$
$$\qquad\quad CH_3$$

Polypropylene (PP) e.g. Hostalen PP®, Novolen®

in which chain segments are accommodated in an irregular convoluted manner. The degree of crystallinity of isotactic polypropylene varies from 45% to 65% (Table 27-3). This pronounced crystalline fraction is responsible for its high rigidity and melting range of about 160° to 166°C. The maximum service temperature of 125°C is significantly higher than that of polyethylene. Short-time heating at 140°C is permissible, which will often allow sterilization by autoclaving. The scattering of light on crystallites and spherulitic supra-structures (103–105 nm) gives the polymer an opaque appearance. Syndiotactic propylene, in which the methyl groups are positioned regularly alternating at either side of the carbon chain, has a crystallinity degree of only 30% and, as a consequence, a relatively low melting point of around 130°C. In atactic polypropylene, the position of the methyl groups is fully irregular; this polymer is therefore completely amorphous. Both types are of minor importance for technical applications. Below the glass transition temperature of about −10°C polypropylene is relatively brittle. This disadvantage can be eliminated by copolymerization of propylene with ethane (intrinsic softening). The density of polypropylene (0.910 g/cm³) is lower than that of polyethylene. With respect to chemical stability, the two polymers are comparable, but polypropylene is slightly more susceptible to strongly oxidizing chemicals.

Application: Because of its limited permeability to water vapor and because it can be autoclaved, propylene is a widely used material for packaging (e.g., bottles).

It is gradually replacing PVC in blister foil. Also with respect to infusion bags, a change is in progress toward polypropylene-based materials (e.g., triple-layered laminar PP/PE/PET foil (Ecobag®)).

Cyclic Olefin Copolymers (COC), Cyclic Olefin Polymers (COP)

By copolymerization of ethene with cyclic olefins, cyclic olefin copolymers are formed and homopolymerization of cyclic olefins leads to cyclic olefin polymers.

Important representatives are ethylene-norbornene copolymers of which several types with different norbornene content are commercially available. COCs are fully amorphous. The glass transition temperature of ethylene-norbornene copolymers increases with increasing norbornene content and varies between 78° and 178°C for the available types. The types with higher transition temperatures can be autoclaved at 121° or even 134°C. COC has a high rigidity and hardness, low density (1.02 g/cm³), and is highly transparent. The polymer is resistant to acids, alkali, alcohols, and some other polar solvents, but not to nonpolar solvents.

Ethylene-norbornene copolymer e.g. Topas®

Application: Because COC can be autoclaved and has glass-like optical properties, it is not only used for foils and blister packaging but also for the production of injection vials and prefillable ready-to-use syringes. However, it does not withstand the temperatures in a depyrogenation tunnel, which is often used to introduce vials into a filling line.

Polystyrene (PS)

Polystyrene is a relatively inexpensive standard polymer. It is made in large quantities by radical polymerization of phenylethene (styrene). Without application of special catalysts, an atactic polymer is formed in which the phenyl residues are positioned along the main chain in random steric order, which prevents crystallization. This atactic, amorphous polystyrene (standard polystyrene, general purpose polystyrene (GPPS)) is crystal clear because of the absence of light-scattering crystallites and has a glass transition temperature of around 100°C. At room temperature, it is in a glassy state, implying that it is hard and susceptible to mechanical impact and tends to form tension cracks. When knocking on it, it makes a crisp rattling sound. Because it softens above the glass transition temperature, it cannot be autoclaved. Due to accelerated aging under warm conditions, the upper temperature limit at which it can be used is 70°C. At temperature between 150° and 260°C, it is processed mainly by injection-molding and extrusion techniques. Polystyrene has a density of 1.05 g/cm³. It is resistant to alkali, dilute weak acids, long-chain alcohols, and fats and oils, but has low resistance to most other organic solvents.

Polystyrene (PS) e.g. Edistir®, Hostyren®, Expanded polystyrene e.g. Styrofoam®

Application: Polystyrene is used on a large scale for the production of cans and bottles, characterized by high transparency and rigidity as well as brittleness.

$$\left[CH_2-CH_2\right]_n$$
$$\quad\quad\; |$$
$$\quad\quad\; Cl$$

Polyvinylchloride (PVC) e.g. Ekadur®, Hostalit®

Polyvinylchloride (PVC)

Polyvinylchloride is an amorphous polymer, produced by polymerization of vinyl chloride. It nearly completely lacks crystallinity due to the predominantly atactic arrangement of the chlorine atoms (irregularly on either side of the carbon chain). Without addition of additives during the polymerization, it is a glass-like material at room temperature (glass transition temperature approximately 80°C), meaning that it is hard and brittle (hard PVC). By addition of plasticizers, the glass transition temperature can be lowered to −40°C, causing the resulting polymer to become soft and rubbery (soft PVC). The plasticizer molecules accommodate themselves between the polymer molecules, diminish the intermolecular interactions, and increase the free volume of the polymer molecules—that is, the empty space between the polymer chains. That is why soft PVC has a lower density (1.20–1.35 g/cm^3) than hard PVC (1.38–1.40 g/cm^3).

At 160° to 180°C, PVC begins to decompose under release of hydrochloric acid, but addition of thermostabilizers will allow processing in the temperature range of 160° to 200°C. Hard PVC will display its desired usage properties only in the glass-like state. It can therefore be applied only below 70°C and is deformed upon autoclaving. Soft PVC, on the other hand, which is particularly used for the production of objects not requiring form-stability (e.g., flexible bags), can be autoclaved at 121°C. Due to its amorphous character, PVC is highly transparent; however, additives mostly have a negative influence on transparency. The polymer is highly resistant to oils, alcohols, and alkali, but not to oxidative acids. Esters, some ketones, or halogenated hydrocarbons cause them to swell or to dissolve.

Application: Polyvinylchloride is still the most abundantly used material for blister foil. Up to the 1990s, it was the only material used for this purpose. Another important application is the infusion bag. Because of its high permeability to water vapor, PVC infusion bags are sealed in a protective foil in order to prevent appreciable water loss during prolonged storage and concomitant increases in concentration of the contents. Certain drugs, such as the monoclonal antibody Infliximab, have been reported as not being compatible with PVC bags. Several preparations of poorly soluble drugs, such as paclitaxel or ciclosporin, contain high concentrations of macrogol ricinoleate as a solubility enhancer. This substance may cause phthalates, added as plasticizers to PVC, to migrate from the material of the bag into the infusion solution. That is why for such preparations another type of material should be chosen for the infusion container. PVC is more transparent than HDPE and may be used as an alternative for polymer bottles when transparency is important. In addition, it has a lower absorption capacity for volatile components in the contents and lower permeability to odorous substances.

$$\quad\quad\quad Cl$$
$$\quad\quad\quad |$$
$$\left[CH_2-C\right]_n$$
$$\quad\quad\quad |$$
$$\quad\quad\quad Cl$$

Polyvinylidene chloride (PVDC) e.g. Saran®

Polyvinylidene Chloride Copolymers (PVDC)

Polyvinylidene chloride consists of a carbon chain in which every second carbon atom is substituted with two chlorine atoms. It is produced by polymerization of 1,1-dichloro ethane. In contrast to PVC, vinylidene homopolymers are partially crystalline (50%–80%) because of their symmetric molecular structure. This property renders it quite hard and brittle material. Already well below its melting temperature of around 200°C it readily decomposes, which hampers its processing. PVDC is therefore practically exclusively employed in the form of copolymers (fraction of VDC 75%–95%). These copolymers are less crystalline (40%–50%), have a lower melting point (140°–175°C), and have a higher glass transition temperature than pure PVDC (T$_g$ of PVDC homopolymer: −11° to −19°C; copolymer 0°–35°C). They become soft at 100° to 120°C and therefore cannot be autoclaved. The high crystallinity and density ($\geq$1.67 g/cm^3) provide PVDC with adequate resistance toward solvents, fats and chemicals as well as with excellent barrier properties. Whereas several polymers combine satisfactory tightness for water vapor with high oxygen permeability, PVDC combines low permeability for both water vapor and oxygen.

Application: Because of its low permeability, PVDC is widely used as a barrier layer in composite films for blister packages. Application as monofilms is limited by the relatively high price of this material.

Polychlorotrifluoroethylene (PCTFE)

Polychlorotrifluoroethylene is a fully halogenated, semicrystalline polymer synthesized from chlorotrifluoroethene. The chlorine atom in the repetitive unit occupies more space than the fluorine atom and disturbs in this way the crystallization. The degree of crystallinity is therefore lower than that of polychlorotrifluoroethylene (PTFE, Teflon®). It varies between 45% and 65% and is determined by the cooling rate of the melt, rapid cooling producing a more amorphous material. The latter is optically clear, whereas a higher crystallization degree lends the polymer an opaque appearance. The melting range lies between 211° and 216°C, rendering the polymer fit for use at temperatures up to 180°C and also suitable for autoclaving.

With a glass transition temperature between 71° and 99°C, it exists in the glass-like state at room temperature. As a result, it has a solid structure and is dimensionally stable. PCTFE is highly resistant to chemicals and solvents. Due to its high fluorine content, it is also very stable toward oxidative agents. Only a few esters and halogenated and aromatic hydrocarbons are able to make it swell. An excellent property of PCTFE is its extremely low permeability for water vapor. It can be processed by extrusion, injection molding, and pressing.

Application: Because of its low water vapor permeability, PCTFE is processed to high-quality composite foils for blister packaging in combination with polymers with low oxygen permeability. This composite foil material approaches the barrier properties of aluminum foil.

Polyethylene Terephthalate (PET)

Polyethylene terephthalate is a polyester made from terephthalic acid (1,4-benzyldicarboxylic acid) and ethylene glycol. As a polymerization catalyst, antimony (III) oxide is often used. Residues of this substance may remain in the polymer and traces may leach from there in the packaged material (especially fluids). Although the minor concentrations thus arising usually stay below the legal limits and are considered safe, alternative production procedures are currently being developed in which titanium instead of antimony is used.

PET is produced in three different crystalline forms: as microcrystalline PET for bottles, as amorphous PET (APET) for thermally shaped cups, and as crystalline PET (CPET) for heat-stable ovenable and microwave-resistant packaging material. APET is formed by rapid cooling of a polymer melt, whereas slow cooling or heating of amorphous material above 140°C (solid-state crystallization) produces polymers with crystallinity degrees of over 70% (CPET). CPET is nontransparent due to light scattering by the spherulites and has a high melting point (>260°C). Compared to APET, CPET is harder and more rigid due to the stronger interactions in the crystalline domains, but it is less resistant to mechanical impact (brittleness). Microcrystalline PET is produced by stretching of amorphous PET foil longitudinally and cross-directionally, followed by subsequent tempering in the temperature range between glass transition and melting. During the production of bottles and hollow objects the stretching process is performed by means of a blow molding procedure. In both cases, the mechanical deformation brings about a parallel orientation of the polymer chains. This, in turn, causes the formation of numerous ordered micro-domains that act as crystallization nuclei for the subsequent solid-phase crystallization process. Because of the large number of crystallites simultaneously growing in this way, these remain much smaller than in case of CPET. The size of the spherulites thus formed remains below the wavelength of visible light. Like amorphous PET, microcrystalline PET is therefore characterized by a high degree of transparence.

By replacing 15% to 34% of the ethylene units by 1,4-cyclohexylene units, glycol-modified polyethylene terephthalate (PETG) is obtained. The voluminous cyclohexylene groups prevent the formation of ordered crystallite structure, giving rise to a glass-clear, fully amorphous and noncrystallizable polymer. PETG has a glass transition temperature of 81°C but no crystalline melting point. In contrast to CPET, PETG cannot be autoclaved.

The density of PET depends on the crystallization degree and is around $1.4 \, g/cm^3$. PET is quite resistant to a large number of organic solvents, except halogenated and aromatic compounds and ketones. It is not resistant to acid and alkali.

Application: Besides for polymer bottles and textile fibers, PET and PETG are particularly used for the production of foils.

Polychlorotrifluoroethylene (PCTFE) e.g. Kel-F®

Polyethylene terephthalate (PET) e.g. Impet®

$$\left[CH_2-CH_2\right]_n \left[CH_2-CH\right]_m$$
$$\qquad\qquad\qquad\qquad |$$
$$\qquad\qquad\qquad\qquad OH$$

Ethylene vinyl alkohol copolymer (EVOH)
e.g. EVAL™

$$\left[CH_2-CH_2\right]_n \left[CH_2-CH\right]$$
$$\qquad\qquad\qquad\qquad |$$
$$\qquad\qquad\qquad\qquad O$$
$$\qquad\qquad\qquad\qquad |$$
$$\qquad\qquad\qquad O=C$$
$$\qquad\qquad\qquad\qquad |$$
$$\qquad\qquad\qquad\qquad CH_3\big]_m$$

Ethylene vinyl acetate copolymer (EVA)
e.g. Greenflex®, Evatane®, Phylon®

Ethylene Vinyl Alcohol Copolymers (EVOH)

Ethylene vinyl alcohol copolymers consist of ethylene and hydroxyethylene units. Commercially available types have an ethylene content of between 24% and 48%. Since vinyl alcohol mainly exists as the tautomeric acetaldehyde, the substance is produced by hydrolysis of ethylene vinyl acetate (EVA), which is obtained by copolymerization of ethylene and vinyl acetate. Independent of the ratio of the two monomers, all EVOH copolymers are semi-crystalline. Their glass transition temperature lies in the range of 55° to 69°C and rises, like the melting point (156°–191°C) with increasing proportion of hydroxyethylene. This is caused by the strong inter- and intramolecular hydrogen bridges between the OH groups, which bring the polymer chains in close contact and thus limit their free mobility. This leads to a condensation of the polymer structure (1.12–1.22 g/cm³) and a concomitant reduction of free volume. This, in turn, results in the application-wise most important property of EVOH copolymers, their extremely low gas permeability. It is the result of a good barrier function of the crystalline domains and the low diffusiveness in the densely packed, at room temperature glass-like structure of the amorphous domains. These barrier properties do not extend to water vapor, however. EVOH is strongly hygroscopic. The interaction of absorbed water molecules with the OH groups of the polymer weakens the hydrogen bonding between the polymer chains and thus enlarges the free volume and chain mobility. Both are essential factors in the diffusion processes in polymers. At high air humidity, the permeability of EVOH will therefore increase also for other gases than water vapor.

Application: Because of its good barrier function toward gases and volatile substances, EVOH is mainly used for foils and coating purposes. It is commonly processed into composite materials, together with other polymers. Such sandwich structures, like, for example, with polypropylene, can be autoclaved, if also the other composit components allow this.

Ethylene Vinyl Acetate Copolymers (EVA)

Ethylene vinyl acetate copolymers are produced by polymerization of ethylene and vinyl acetate (VA). The monomer ratio may be varied in quite a broad range, producing a wide variety of properties and allowing for very different applications. The acetyloxy groups disturb the ordering of the polymer chains, so that crystallinity drops with increasing proportions of this moiety. While EVA types with a VA proportion below 50% are semi-crystalline, types with higher proportions of VA rather are amorphous. EVA copolymers have a low melting point, which further drops with decreasing crystallinity. While a copolymer with 9% VA still has a melting point of 100°C, 40% VA reduces this to a mere 40°C. Amorphous copolymers do not show a melting point. Based on this behavior toward temperature only the higher-melting EVA types with a VA content of 7% to 18% can be used for the production of foil material. Those with a VA proportion of 18% to 40% serve as hot melt adhesives. The glass transition temperature of the polymer increases with increasing VA content from −30°C to 0°C. Therefore, at room temperature EVA exists in the rubber-elastic state and the amorphous types (40% to 90% VA) possess elastomeric properties.

Application: Low-melting types can be applied on foils as hot-seal coatings. Higher-melting copolymers serve as plasticizers-free material for infusion bags. Especially mixing bags for parenteral nutrition are nowadays often made from EVA, because the plasticizers in PVC bags may migrate into fat-containing preparations. Because EVA cannot be autoclaved, application is limited to aseptically prepared drug products without the need of terminal sterilization.

27.2.2.5   Elastomers

General Introduction

In pharmaceutical applications, elastomers are used predominantly for the production of closures for infusion bottles, vials and syringes, as well as for flexible tubes. Elastomers are solid materials, mainly consisting of highly polymerized organic substances, with rubber-elastic behavior. The term covers all products from natural and synthetic rubber and rubber-like substances. Rubber elasticity may be characterized as follows: a relatively minor external tensile force (0.1–1 N/mm²) results in a strong deformation of as much as 800% to

1,000%, accompanied by a ten- to hundredfold strain hardening. The deformation is sustained for a prolonged period of time without a reduction of the accompanying final tension. When releasing the applied force, the object nearly completely regains its original state within fractions of a second (reversible deformation). Permanent deformation (difference between native state and state after tensile loading), is limited to less than 1% (residual shape change).

In the nondeformed state, elastomers are amorphous, while during stretching crystallization phenomena occur. Determinant for the rubber-elastic behavior of a polymer is the presence of long mutually entangled polymer chains, which upon mechanical stress may change their shapes. Tension forces lead to stretching and a parallel alignment of the chain-like macromolecules. The mechanical or heat-induced deformation of raw rubber is only partially reversible (transition to the plastic state due to depolymerization), and leads to stickiness. For this reason, the material is vulcanized with sulfur (hot-air vulcanization) or with disulfur dichloride (cold vulcanization), which leads to the formation of disulfide bridges between the rubber molecules. The formation of intermolecular bridges enlarges the number of cross-links and reduces mobility of the molecular chains. Henceforth, deformation is limited and stronger forces are required to bring it about, but it is reversible. Vulcanization of other polymers is carried out with oxides, peroxides and divalent metal ions (introduction of ether bridges). For synthetic polymers chemical bonding between the macromolecular chains during the polymerization process is accomplished by cross-linking compounds. Addition of carbon black, silicon dioxide, and others, furthermore, bring about strengthening of the physical binding by the formation of crystalline domains.

For pharmaceutical primary packaging materials, predominantly synthetic polymers are employed—in particular, chlorobutyl rubber and bromobutyl rubber. Approximately 90% of the currently used stoppers for vials and prefilled syringes are made of these two materials. Styrene butadiene rubber is mainly used for needle shields of prefilled syringes.

In accordance with its purity requirements, the Ph. Eur. distinguishes two types of rubber stoppers. Those made of synthetic basic elastomers usually meet the requirements for type I. Based on their purity and uniformity, they hardly release leachables into the preparation. With respect to elasticity and fragmentation resistance, however, they are inferior to rubber materials containing natural rubber additives to improve their performance characteristics. The latter have a more complex composition and a higher tendency to release undesired substances. As a rule, stoppers made of these materials only fulfill the less stringent requirements of type II rubber stoppers. They are mainly employed for multidose containers, but their use is becoming more and more restricted. Silicon rubber has a niche position as closure material. It is in particular applied for sealing and tubing material used in manufacturing processes.

Chlorobutyl Rubber and Bromobutyl Rubber

Butyl rubbers (code designation IIR = isobutene isoprene rubber) are copolymers of isobutene and up to about 2.5% isoprene (2-methylbuta-1,3-diene). The proportion of isoprene determines the number of double bonds that remain after polymerization. These can be exploited for the purpose of cross-linking of the polymer chains as well as for derivation by substituting halogenation. By reaction with chlorine or bromine, accompanied by cleavage of hydrogen halogenide, chlorobutyl rubber (CIIR) or bromobutyl rubber (BIIR) is formed. In this way, the properties of the materials can be selectively modified. Following halogenation, cross-linking is mostly achieved by catalysis with zinc oxide, leading to the formation of stable C-C bonds between the polymer chains.

Butyl rubber and its halogen derivatives are only moderately permeable to water vapor and gas and are not affected by dilute acids and bases.

Styrene Butadiene Rubber

Styrene butadiene rubber (SBR) is a copolymer of 1,3-butadiene (ca. 77%) and styrene (ca. 23%). It is nowadays the most frequently applied synthetic rubber. It is harder than chlorobutyl rubber, but has a somewhat lower chemical resistance. Due to its higher gas permeability, e.g. for ethylene oxide, styrene butadiene rubber is often used for needle shields, as

$$\left[CH_2-\underset{\underset{CH_3}{|}}{\overset{\overset{CH_3}{|}}{C}}\right]_m\left[CH_2-\underset{}{\overset{\overset{CH_3}{|}}{C}}=CH-CH_2\right]_n \quad \xrightarrow[-\ HBr]{+\ Br_2}$$

$$\left[CH_2-\underset{\underset{CH_3}{|}}{\overset{\overset{CH_3}{|}}{C}}\right]_m\left[CH_2-\underset{\underset{Br}{|}}{\overset{\overset{CH_2}{\|}}{C}}-CH-CH_2\right]_n$$

$$-CH_2-\underset{\underset{CH_2}{\|}}{CH}-C-CH_2-\underset{\underset{CH_3}{|}}{\overset{\overset{CH_3}{|}}{C}}-CH_2-$$

$$-CH_2-\underset{\underset{CH_3}{|}}{\overset{\overset{CH_3}{|}}{C}}-CH_2-\underset{\underset{Br}{|}}{\overset{\overset{CH_2}{\|}}{C}}-CH-CH_2-$$

$$\xrightarrow[-\ 2\ HBr]{ZnO,\ \Delta}$$

$$-CH_2-CH=C-CH_2-\underset{\underset{CH_3}{|}}{\overset{\overset{CH_3}{|}}{C}}-CH_2-$$

$$-CH_2-\underset{\underset{CH_3}{|}}{C}-CH=C-CH=CH-$$

Bromobutyl rubber (BIIR) (synthesis by cross-linking of brominated isobutene-isoprene copolymers) e.g. West® PH 7025/65, Stelmi 6720

$$\left[CH_2-CH\right]_m\left[CH-CH_2\right]_n\left[CH_2-CH=CH-CH_2\right]_l$$

Styrene butadien rubber (SBR) e.g. Helvoet FM 27

$$-O-\underset{\underset{CH_2}{|}}{\overset{\overset{CH_3}{|}}{Si}}-O-\underset{\underset{CH_3}{|}}{\overset{\overset{CH_3}{|}}{Si}}-O-\underset{\underset{CH_3}{|}}{\overset{\overset{CH_3}{|}}{Si}}-O-\underset{\underset{CH_2}{|}}{\overset{\overset{CH_3}{|}}{Si}}-O-\underset{\underset{CH_3}{|}}{\overset{\overset{CH_3}{|}}{Si}}-O-$$

Stilicone rubber, platinum cured

it enables gas sterilization of staked needle syringes in the assembled state, when the needle is already covered by the needle shield.

Silicone Rubber

Silicon elastomers are formed by cross-linking of linear polysiloxanes that contain a small number of methylvinylsiloxy groups in their molecular chains of dimethylsiloxy units. Polysiloxan chains can cross-link by virtue of the vinyl double bonds that proceeds either by a radical or an addition mechanism. Radical curing (HTC = high temperature cross-linking) is catalyzed by peroxides that are added to the silicone to a concentration of approximately 1%. The peroxide is consumed in the reaction, but its reaction products may persist in the polymer. Later, when the rubber is in use as a primary packaging component they may be released and potentially end up in products that are in direct contact with the elastomer. Addition cured silicones are lacking such by byproducts. Synthesis proceeds by addition of oligomers containing Si-H groups to the double bonds of vinyl-functionalized silicone polymers, with 5-15 ppm platinum added as a catalyst. In spite of their higher price, gaskets and tubes made from platinum cured silicones are preferred in pharmaceutical production. Silicone rubber is resistant to oils and fats and temperature-resistant up to 250°C. Shortcomings are the extremely high permeability for gases and the poor tear-resistance.

27.2.3   Metals

Aluminum and tinplate are the most frequently used metals for pharmaceutical packaging purposes. Stainless steel finds application in bulk storage vessels and containers used during the production process.

27.2.3.1   Stainless Steel

Stainless steel is strongly resistant to many substances and is in nearly all cases the optimal material for surfaces in direct contact with products. In the manufacture of pharmaceutical products chrome-nickel-molybdenum steel with a high corrosion resistance is used. Standard qualities for pharmaceutical applications are the two similar alloys 1.4404 and 1.4435 (both AISI alloy 316L), in addition to the even more resistant alloy 1.4539 (AISI 904L). The relatively high price of these materials and their poor processability prohibit widespread use as disposable packaging material for finished dosage forms.

27.2.3.2   Tinplate

Tinplate is electrolytically tin-coated steel sheet. To prevent direct contact with the pharmaceutical product, an inert lacquer or polymer coating of the material at the inside of the container is required. Often also the outside is coated for printing purposes. The main applications for tin plate in the pharmaceutical packaging domain are aerosol spray cans. Also slip cap and screw cap jars, e.g., for creams, as well as bottles or canisters for light-protected storage of vegetable oils etc. are made of tinplate. Because of its absolute tightness for volatile substances (e.g., essential oils), it also is the typical material for tea storage tins.

27.2.3.3   Aluminum

Aluminum is the most widely used metal for pharmaceutical packaging. It is used for cans, flasks, lids and screw caps, tubing, bags, strips, and blister packaging purposes. To enhance its mechanical sturdiness, it is alloyed with small proportions of silicon, copper, magnesium, manganese or iron. For further processing it is rolled to form sheets. Immediately following the rolling process aluminum is hard and brittle and in this state it is not suitable for many application purposes. It is only through subsequent soft annealing that it obtains its necessary plasticity and ductility. The annealing process makes it possible to adjust the properties of the material to the specific requirements of the application. Because in particular acidic preparations attack the metal surface, under formation of soluble aluminum salts, the inside of aluminum containers is usually protected by a lacquer or polymer coating layer. Aluminum foils are commonly layered with polymers so as to form composite films.

27.3   Containers

Containers for pharmaceutical products should serve a dual purpose: containment of the contents (including protection of the environment against potential impact of the product) and protection of the product against influences of the environment. Secure containment is particularly relevant when the product should be kept away from children or has strongly toxic properties (e.g., cytostatics and other CMR (carcinogenic, mutagenic, toxic for reproduction) agents). The protective function includes, depending on necessity, exclusion from light, moisture, oxygen, biological contamination or mechanical damage. Furthermore, packaging has an identification and information function. Many drug formulations come in multiple-dose packaging of which the part that is in direct contact with the pharmaceutical product is the primary packaging and the outer encasement that is not in contact with the product, is designated as secondary packaging. Tight containment is predominantly taken care of by the primary packaging material, while the secondary packaging mainly serves to protect the product against external influences such as light or mechanical damage, to identify the product and to hold information leaflets, dosing aids, measuring and administration devices. Both the primary and the secondary packaging are integral components of a pharmaceutical product. Stability studies to determine shelf life are basically conducted on the entire product. This implies that the indicated date of expiry only applies for as long as the drug product is stored in the intact and entire original packaging unit.

With respect to primary packaging, distinction is made between single- and multiple-dose containers. The former contain the amounts of the preparation, individually packaged for a single application, while the latter contain a supply for several doses, from which individually measured doses for each single application can be taken (volumetrically like in case of injections or in numbers for tablets, etc.). Multiple-dose containers must be re-sealable. As a rule, the expiry date indicated on the package no longer applies after the packaging has been opened for the first time, because storage conditions are altered upon opening the packaging—for example, by exposure to moisture, oxygen, or microbial contamination. In special types of primary packaging, the application aid is physically connected with the storage container, or it is prefilled with the pharmaceutical preparation. Examples of this type are prefilled syringes, injection pens, eye drop flasks, and inhalers. The in-use shelf life after opening is determined by a separate assessment (in-use-stability test) and has to be indicated on the label. For sterile products, the in-use shelf life (maximum storage time after opening) is—because of concerns related to growth of potential microbiological contaminants—normally no longer than 24 hours at refrigerator temperature, unless the container was opened under aseptic conditions.

27.3.1   Containers for Solid Dosage Forms

27.3.1.1   Jars and Cans

The great majority of solid dosage forms are tablets and capsules. In (Western) Europe, these are only rarely packaged in jars or cans, but rather, are packaged in blister strips for distribution. In the United States, by contrast, prescription drugs are rarely sold in finished packaging, and the pharmacist must repack and distribute the prescribed number of tablets or capsules from a larger storage container. In addition, prescriptions are often dispensed to patients in jars or cans. Thus, they are therefore much more important in the United States than in Europe. In Europe, such types of containers are mainly used to bring powders and granules to the market. A special form concerns dry syrups that are filled in bottles as powders and then reconstituted to a ready-for-use product by addition of water. For the packaging of powders and granules, mostly plastic jars and cans are used, besides glass containers. The latter do not have to meet highest standards with respect to hydrolytic resistance. Soda-lime-silica glasses of a lower hydrolytic quality, such as specified for type III glass containers, may be employed for this purpose.

Plastic jars often consist of polyethylene or polypropylene. It has to be ascertained that no components of the filling material (e.g., preservatives, essential oils) are absorbed or adsorbed by the container material and thus withdrawn from the preparation. In case of hygroscopic or moisture-sensitive preparations, both container and its closure system should be sufficiently impermeable for water vapor. To improve sealing tightness before opening, glass and plastic jars are often sealed with an aluminum foil disk underneath the screw cap. This is commonly done by induction sealing, a noncontact heating process. The sealing insert inside the cap consists of a cardboard disc, bonded by a wax layer to an aluminum foil. This, in turn, is coated with a low-melting polymer. After screwing on the cap, a high-frequency electromagnetic

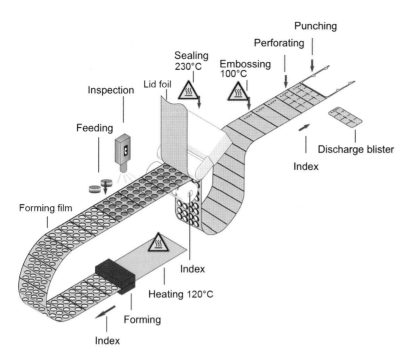

Fig. 27-1 Schematic presentation of the thermo blister-forming process (continuous procedure). Reproduced with permission from Uhlmann © 2016.

field is applied that creates an eddy current in the aluminum foil that heats it up. This causes the wax to melt and to be absorbed by the cardboard disc, which then detaches from the foil. Simultaneously, the polymer layer melts and hermetically seals the foil to the lip of the jar. When the container is uncapped, the cardboard disc, detached from the aluminum foil, remains inside the cap while the foil sticks tightly to the lip and can be removed by means of a tab.

27.3.1.2 Foil Packages

Blister packages are already in use for more than 50 years, predominantly for solid single-dose formulations. They allow withdrawal of single units without affecting the protection of the remaining doses against microbial contamination and environmental influences. In addition to that, they provide the opportunity to package multiple different formulations according to a predetermined dosing scheme and thus facilitate patient compliance to the dosing scheme (e.g., contraceptives). In Europe, 85% of the solid formulations are marketed in blister packages, as compared to 20% in the United States. Blister packages consist, as a rule, of a polymer foil with thermoformed cavities or aluminum foil with similar cold-formed cavities, covered by a flat aluminum foil. To withdraw the dose, either the sealed unit is pushed out from the blister, causing the sealing foil to tear, or, in case of mechanically sensitive dosage forms (e.g., oral lyophilisates), the coating foil is torn away from the cavity. Strip packages are distinct from blister packages in that the individual doses are sealed in between two not pre-shaped foil sheets.

In the blister-forming process the shaping of the packaging material, the filling and the sealing are performed in a continuous sequence of consecutive steps in one single machine. After unwinding from the roll the thermoforming foil passes through a heating station where it is brought to the temperature required for deformation. Foils based on PVC are deep-drawn at 120° to 145°C, whereas polypropylene is formed in the softened state at 150°C, just below its melting range. Aluminum foil is shaped at room temperature. The deep-drawing step is achieved by applying negative pressure or by using a stamp device. When applicable, the cooling process starts as soon as the foil contacts the deep-drawing mold. Especially for polypropylene foils active cooling is necessary. Subsequently the cavities are filled with the units to be packaged and covered by a layer of sealing foil, which is heat welded with the deep-draw foil.

This welding process can be accomplished either continuously by sealing rollers or time-pulsed by sealing plates. Although the continuous process is faster it requires higher temperatures (200° to 300°C), while the pulsed procedure proceeds at 140° to 200°C and is gentler on materials. In the final step the foil is perforated and punched out in the desired shape.

There is a large variety of different foil materials available and its selection is to be adapted to the specific requirements of the product to be packaged. From an economic point of view the primary material of choice for deep-draw foil is hard PVC. It is easily processed on all common types of machines and has good chemical resistance. PVC is a purely amorphous polymer. Above its glass transition temperature of about 80°C, it undergoes a transition to a rubbery state and by vacuum thermoforming it can be brought to a new shape in which it is fixed upon cooling. The only limitation in the use of PVC is the high permeability for water vapor.

Polypropylene (PP) shares the low price with PVC, but has threefold lower water vapor permeability and a higher chemical resistance. It is progressively used as an alternative to PVC. Disadvantages are its extremely high permeability for oxygen and, more importantly, its different thermic behavior. The latter calls for precise temperature control during processing and may, in combination with its higher rigidity and potential shrinkage after processing, lead to tensions in the blisters.

In contrast to PVC, PP is a semi-crystalline material. With a glass transition temperature of about −10°C, PP is already at room temperature in a rubber-elastic state. However, the clearly stronger secondary valence forces in the crystalline domains make forming more difficult. Only upon heating to a temperature just below the crystallite melting range does it soften adequately for a deep-draw process. While amorphous polymers are slowly softening after exceeding the glass transition temperature and are formable in a wide temperature range, semi-crystalline polymers have a quite narrow melting range. This particularly applies to PP (melting range 160°–166°C), which seriously complicates temperature control during the deep-draw process as compared to PVC.

In the permeation of gases or vapors through a polymer foil, three process steps can be distinguished:

1. Absorption of the molecules or atoms in the surface layers
2. Diffusion through the polymer
3. Desorption at the opposite polymer surface

Thus, permeability is determined by the solubility and the diffusion capacity of the permeating substance in the polymer. Diffusion is limited to the less densely packed amorphous domains of the polymer and thus drops with increasing degree of crystallinity. Within the amorphous domains the diffusion rate drops abruptly at the transition from the rubber-elastic to the glass-like state. Thus, it is an advantage when the glass transition temperature is higher than room temperature. As the first step of the permeation process is the absorption of the permeating agent, its solubility in the polymer determines the permeability in such a way that low affinity between the permeating molecules and the polymer chains causes high barrier properties. Although strongly hydrophobic polymers like PP retain water vapor quite well, they are fairly permeable to gases such as oxygen. In addition to that, in case of PP the packing density of the chains is reduced by the space requirement of the methyl groups. Furthermore, the glass transition temperature lies below room temperature. Together these factors lead to an extremely high oxygen transmission rate (OTR). Coating with for instance PVDC may counteract this. PVDC is a polymer with very effective barrier properties, particularly manifested by a very low oxygen permeability. This is due to the high degree of crystallinity of the material. For economic reasons PVDC is not used as a mono-foil, but rather as a composite layer on a carrier foil made of cheaper material like PVC. Such composite foils made of different polymers can be produced by lamination (bonding together two foil sheets or ribbons) or by coextrusion.

Whereas PVDC possesses excellent barrier properties for oxygen as well as water vapor, polymers with higher polarity, resulting from ester (PETG) or particularly hydroxyl (EVOH) groups, combine low oxygen permeability with high water vapor permeability. In particular EVOH thus accomplishes similarly low OTR values as PVDC. In order to achieve at the same time satisfactory moisture retention capacity, these materials are combined with less water-vapor permeable polymers so as to form multilayer foils.

A transparent foil material with minimal water vapor permeability is PCTFE, commercially available under the brand names Aclar or Vaposhield. PCTFE is a better barrier to water vapor than PVDC, but it offers little protection against oxygen. It is used as composite material in combination with PVC or other polymers. A composite of PCTFE and EVOH combines excellent moisture protection with minimal oxygen permeability. Thus, it closely approaches aluminum foil as fully impermeable material, but offers in addition full transparency. A disadvantage of all PCTFE-containing foils is their relatively high price.

A halogen-free alternative among the polymer foils is COC. Combined with PP, it reduces the latter's water vapor permeability, without a clear improvement of its oxygen tightness, however. By combination with EVOH, a synergistic effect can be achieved, allowing the production of a fluorine- and chlorine-free foil with extremely low MVTR (moisture vapor transmission rate) and OTR (oxygen transmission rate) values.

Full impermeability toward water vapor, gas, and light is offered by Alu-Alu blisters. These foils commonly have a thickness of 45 μm. The side that is in contact with the product is coated with PVC (alternatively PE), applied by a hot-sealing procedure, while the outer side is laminated with oriented polyamide (oPA). The latter is obtained by biaxial stretching of PA foil, which provides improved mechanical strength (tear resistance, elastic modulus). The oPA layer has a mechanical support function and is intended to prevent ruptures in the aluminum foil. In contrast to polymer blisters, aluminum blisters are produced by cold forming by means of stamp devices. Because the material does not allow molding at 90° angles, the indentations are shallower and have a larger diameter. This causes higher material consumption and longer production time, which renders aluminum blisters one of the most expensive packaging variants.

In recent years, moisture-absorbing blister foils have been developed for the packaging of highly moisture-sensitive agents. These contain zeolite (molecular sieve) or calcium oxide particles, embedded in a PE or PP layer (Activ-Blister®, Formpack Dessiflex™ Plus). Also, plastic jars can be equipped with an internal layer of this material (Activ-Vial®).

During deep-drawing, the foil distends, which brings along a reduction in thickness, particularly at strongly curved areas. This, in turn, leads to a deterioration of the barrier function. Composite foils bear the risk that the thinner barrier layers tear and lose integrity, although the thicker support layer gives the impression of a sufficient total strength of the film.

The coating foil of blister packages usually consists of aluminum, which at the product-contact side is coated with a hot-seal lacquer. The latter is bonded, by applying pressure and heat, to the upper product-contact layer of the deep-draw foil. The aluminum layer of the sealing foil commonly has a thickness of 25 μm. Thinner foils may contain micro-cracks, which may affect impermeability. This is mostly caused by organic impurities in the molten aluminum or mechanical stress during the rolling process. The rolling creates tensions in the material that make the foil hard and brittle. In Europe, such hard-aluminum foils are the most widely used sealing material for push-through blister packs. The brittleness allows the foil to tear easily upon applying force and thus facilitates pushing out the formulation. By soft annealing after the rolling process these tensions are released and the aluminum becomes soft and flexible again. Soft aluminum is often used for childproof push-through packaging, as the flexibility of the metal requires a stronger force to break through the foil. On the other hand, this limits its suitability for relatively unstable pharmaceutical formulations such as soft capsules. With "peel-off-push-through" packaging, first a paper layer has to be torn away before the product can be pushed out of the aluminum foil.

27.3.1.3 Foil Packaging for Rectal and Vaginal Suppositories

Due to their low melting temperature and their soft character, suppositories impose special requirements on packaging. At the pharmacy level, sometimes small numbers of extemporaneously prepared suppositories for prompt use are packaged unwrapped in plastic boxes. This, however, brings along the risk that already during transport unavoidable mechanical impact causes chipping or breakage of individual units. Particularly, preparations based on hydrogels easily stick to one another during densely packed storage. This also applies for fat-based preparations upon exposure to heat and in extreme cases may even go at the expense of their essential shape.

A range of rectal and vaginal products are commercially available in plastic or more often aluminum strip packaging. This type of packaging allows separation of individual units and thus prevents them from sticking together. It does, however, fail to provide mechanical protection or to preserve their shape upon exposure to heat. That is why, to date, molded dosage forms for rectal or vaginal application are marketed in more or less rigid-walled, thermoshaped suppository shells with preformed cavities that precisely fit the enclosed units. The molten mass is poured directly into these disposable shells, which do not need any lubrication. They can be obtained preformed as reel packaging, which then only have to be filled, sealed and cooled to solidify the content. Alternatively, the deep drawing and sealing of two reel-fed sheets occurs consecutively, together with the filling of the cavities and the closing, in a single machine. Because in this case, the packaging process is inextricably linked with the formulation of the pharmaceutical agent, this process is represented in detail in section 13.7. In the same manner also small single-dose liquid preparations can be filled. In that case no solidification step is required after sealing. As sheet material, polymer or aluminum/PE is used. The aluminum foil usually has a thickness of 25 μm and, in order to allow a hot-sealing procedure, it is coated with a 25 or 40 μm polyethylene layer (LDPE). In the latter case, the stronger sealing layer allows opening the package by pulling apart the two fused foil sheets (peel packaging). Packages with a thin sealing layer are opened by tearing apart the foil, starting at a prefabricated incision. The most commonly used polymer foils are made of PVC or the combinations thereof, with PE and PVDC/PE. In these cases PVC serves as the protection layer and makes up the major part of the foil thickness. For the packaging of rectal and vaginal suppositories relatively stronger foils with a thickness of 130 to 160 μm are employed. They are opened by tearing or the sealing seam. In case of fluid contents, a higher rigidity is required, which is obtained with foil thicknesses of 200 to 300 μm. These are opened by pulling or snapping off the foil at a preformed site. Disposable PVC/PE casting molds for rectal and vaginal formulations are also commercially available for extemporaneous preparations. Sealing is performed either with hot air or by self-adhesive sealing tape.

27.3.2 Containers for Semi-Solid Pharmaceuticals

27.3.2.1 Tubes
Tubes are standard packaging materials for creams, ointments, pastes, and other semi-solid dosage forms, body care products and cosmetics. They can be emptied easily and nearly completely and largely protect the product during withdrawal from contamination by contact with fingers or dirty instruments. They can be made from metal, plastics, or combinations thereof. Metal tubes consist of tinplate or aluminum and are produced by a single-step extrusion procedure. The inner wall is coated with a layer consisting of vinyl, acryl, or epoxy resin to avoid direct contact between metal and contents.

Plastic tubes, on the other hand, are manufactured in a two-step procedure. First a hollow sleeve is fabricated, which is subsequently connected to the conical threaded part. In case of single-layer tubes, mostly made of LDPE, the seamless sleeve is extruded by means of an annular gap nozzle. The inner wall of the tube is subsequently provided with a coating to reduce water-vapor permeability. Laminated tubes are often composed of 6 to 10 layers, one of those made of aluminum. Strips of the laminated foil are wound around a cylinder and inductively fused in the overlapping area. The threaded moiety is formed by an injection-molding procedure and in the same procedure connected with the prefabricated tube sleeve.

27.3.3 Containers for Liquid Medical Products

27.3.3.1 Bottles
Bottles for liquid drug products can be made of glass, plastics or metal. Glass bottles for parenteral solutions should be made of glass types I or II; containers for oral or other

nonparenteral preparations are permitted to have a lower hydrolytic resistance. There are two fundamentally different techniques for production of glass containers. While ampoules, syringes, and cartridges are formed from glass tubing, bottles are only made by molding. In the production of vials, both methods can be applied. In the following section on glass bottles, the molding technique is explained. The manufacture of tubing glass containers is described in section 27.3.4 (Containers for Parenteral Preparations).

Glass Bottles

Glass bottles are almost exclusively produced by means of hollow molds in a two-step process. In the first step, a hollow preliminary work piece, the parison, is made from a solid cylinder of glass melt (gob). In the blow and blow process this is done by means of compressed air that inflates the viscous gob uniformly against the inner wall of a parison mold. In the press and blow procedure, on the other hand, the gob is not blown, but rather pressed by a plunger upon which the glass mass is distributed in the space between the plunger and the mold. In the second step, the preblown or prepressed parison is transferred to another hollow mold representing the final shape of the product. In this final mold the parison is blown into its final shape by compressed air. The shape of the parison determines the later distribution of the glass in the final product and in this way has a decisive influence on the strength of wall and bottom. As the distribution of the glass mass in the parison can be controlled more accurately by pressing than by blowing, the press and blow procedure allows the production of thinner-walled containers.

Plastic Bottles

Similar to the blow procedure for glass bottles also the production of plastic bottles proceeds by a multistep blow-molding procedure. Dependent on the size of the bottle and the properties of the polymer material, three procedures may be followed: injection-blow molding, extrusion-blow molding and stretch-blow molding. Injection-blow molding is predominantly applied in the production of small bottles with volumes of less than 50 mL as well as for polymer vials. Polymer granules are melted in an extruder and the fluid mass is injected under pressure into a preliminary mold, thereby shaping a slender hollow cylinder, which has the length but not yet the width of the ultimate bottle. At one end, however, it already has the final screw thread. The still soft preliminary body thus formed is transferred to a second female tool that coincides in shape and size the ultimate bottle. By blowing in filtered air the preshaped cylinder is inflated until it touches and clings to the inner wall of the cooled mold, where it solidifies and is ejected after opening of the multi-part mold.

Similarly, in the extrusion-blow molding polymer granules are melted in an extruder. The molten mass is pressed to a hose through an annular die without the involvement of any type of mold. By means of co-extrusion of several different polymers through concentric annular dies multilayered bottle walls can be produced. When the required length of the hose has been attained, a multi-part mold encircles the hose segment and squeezes it together at the lower end during closing of the mold parts. At the top of the mold a blowpipe is inserted and subsequently blows up the hose to form the final shape in the closed mold. By extrusion blow molding mainly bottles with a volume of over 100 mL are produced. While both in the injection and in the extrusion blow molding procedure the preliminary product is stretched up in circumferential direction only, in the stretch blow molding stretching occurs both axially and circumferentially. The biaxial orientation of the polymer chains that occurs during this process increases the ordered domains of the polymer and thus strengthens the material. In this way, it is possible to reduce the thickness of the wall and save material as well as weight.

27.3.3.2 Blow-Fill Seal (BFS) Technology

A further development of the extrusion-blow molding procedure is the blow-fill seal technology, also called bottle-pack procedure, in which the filling and sealing steps are integrated in the bottle production process. After the blow-molding of the bottle, filling proceeds either already prior to the ejection from the mold or in a separate station of the machine. As soon as the filling process is terminated and the filling spike has been withdrawn from the neck of the bottle, the opening is sealed with hot polymer by means of a sealing mold. Often an opening tab is formed during this process that needs to be twisted off causing the bottle neck

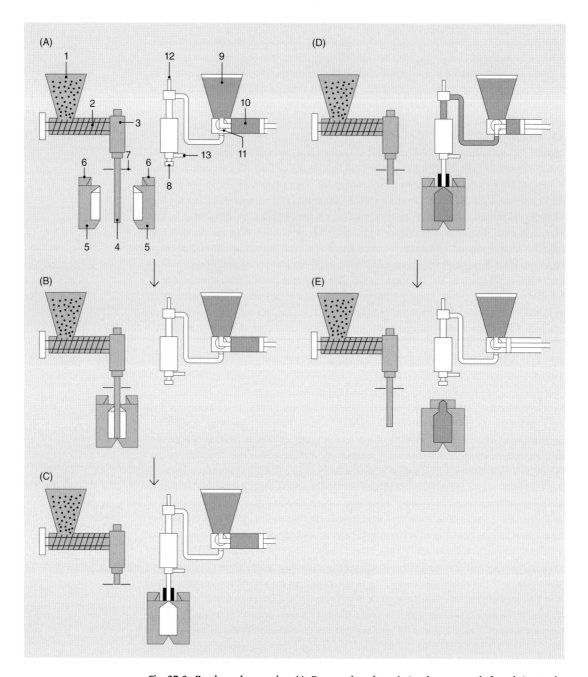

Fig. 27-2 Bottle-pack procedure (A–E: operation phases). 1 polymer granule funnel, 2 extruder screw, 3 hose head, 4 hot polymer hose, 5 flask bottom mold, 6 flask top mold, 7 cutting knife, 8 blow and filling spike, 9 filling funnel, 10 piston dosing pump, 11 three-way valve, 12 compressed air connection, 13 exhaust pipe.

to break at a predetermined site. For infusion containers, a rubber stopper is fused in the neck of the bottle that can be perforated with a cannula. Nowadays the BSF technology is employed for numerous products. With this method, containers with filling volumes ranging from 0.1 mL to 10 l may be produced. The procedure is particularly relevant for the production of single-dose containers for eye, nose or ear drop formulations.

Fig. 27-2 illustrates the process in detail. An extruder is fed with the thermoplastic polymer (e.g., polyethylene) and continuously produces in an extrusion head a polymer hose of appropriate length and strength (Fig. 27-2A). Underneath the extrusion head, a four-part mold is mounted, consisting of two bottom halves and two top halves (jaws), together shaping the main body of the bottle. The two bottom parts close and receive the still-hot polymer hose. A cutting device separates the hose from the extrusion head. A carrier moves the mold to the filling station (Fig. 27-2B), where a filling pipe is positioned into the still-hot hose such that it is placed on the conical neck of the flask mold. The filling pipe consists of three channels, a blow-air channel (to blow up the hose), a filling channel (through which the fluid is filled), and an exhaust channel (through which air and foam (when present) escape. The shaping of the bottle is achieved by a burst of air, which inflates the polymer hose against the mold cavity (Fig. 27-2C). Then a defined volume of filling fluid, measured by a dosing pump, is introduced into the just-formed bottle via the filling channel and simultaneously cools it. Air is expelled from the bottle via the exhaust channel (Fig. 27-2D). After the filling, the filling pipe is withdrawn, making space for the top jaws, which come together by means of two closing cylinders, thus tightly sealing the bottle and forming its top under vacuum (Fig. 27-2E). When the top has obtained sufficient stability, the mold opens and separates the bottom residue from the bottle. The filled flask leaves the machine via a discharge chute. Meanwhile, the extruder has formed another hose segment and a new cycle starts. Several common process steps for container filling, such as washing and sterilization, are not required in this case, as the produced containers are sterile per se. A variety of such BSF machines are commercially available, allowing production of a wide range of container sizes. Commonly used types are able to produce and fill about 2,500 container of 3 to 10 mL each hour, 800 to 900 bottles of 50 to 200 mL content, and about 500 bottles with a volume of 700 to 1,000 mL.

27.3.4 Containers for Parenteral Preparations

27.3.4.1 Ampoules

Ampoules are cylindrically formed flat-bottomed containers made of glass (less often plastics) and equipped with a tip. A shape variant, pulled out at both ends (double-tip ampoules), has become rather obsolete and is only still in use for some peroral (drink ampoules) and cosmetic preparations. Ampoules are single-dose containers, as their content is intended for one single application. They are predominantly employed for injectables, more rarely for oral or topical products. The production process for ampoules differs from that of other glass containers. The starting material is a glass tube that is formed into its desired shape by controlled section-wise heating and stretching while continuously rotated. Prior to use ampoules have to be washed, sterilized and depyrogenized. These preparatory process steps, just like the subsequent filling step, are similar to those described for vials in section 27.3.4.3

After ampoules are filled, they are closed by heat sealing, which is mostly accomplished by a gas flame. The flame is directed to the center of the rotating ampoule's stem. When the glass has softened, the outermost part of the stem is grabbed by a pair of grip jaws and pulled away from the body of the ampoule. In doing so, the tip is constricted and sealed by melting. The disadvantage of gas flames is that, in case of misalignment, contamination of the glass and the solution by soot particles can occur. For this reason alternative melting techniques have been developed, which, however, have not yet found wide application thus far. Fully flameless is the procedure in which a CO_2 laser heats the ampoule by infrared light; the laser wavelength of 10.6 μm is very effectively absorbed by glass. Another technology applies a hot jet of plasma created by an air stream passing an electric arc, which is forced through the opening of a nozzle. At the industrial production scale, fully automatic facilities are employed in which all steps in the production process, starting from cleaning via sterilization, cooling and filling down to sealing of the ampoules are performed inside an isolator ventilated with sterile air. Such facilities operate with multiple filling and sealing stations and achieve performances of up to 24,000 ampoules per hour.

27.3.4.2 Vials and Infusion Bottles

Vials are the currently most frequently used primary packaging container for liquid and freeze-dried injection preparations. Vials may be single- or multiple-dose containers. They serve to contain solutions, suspensions, powder formulations or lyophilisates and have, as a rule, volumes varying from 1 to 100 mL. The production of glass vials proceeds either by the same procedure as applied in ampoule production, however with the opening being shaped by a forming tool, or by means of a blow procedure as described for the production of bottles. (section 27.3.3). Correspondingly, tubular glass vials are distinguished from molded glass vials. Tubular glass vials have a thinner wall and a more uniform strength as well as a more regularly shaped bottom. For that reason they are lighter than molded glass vials and allow more efficient heat exchange between the shelf and the bottom during freeze-drying.

Infusion bottles mostly have a volume of 100 to 1,000 mL. Glass infusion bottles are produced by the blow technique (molded glass), and are therefore relatively heavy and have thick walls. That is why currently more and more often plastic infusion bottles (mostly PE and PP) are used. They are formed, filled, and sealed in one single process (BFS technology, section 27.3.3.2).

The dimensions of glass containers for injections and infusions are standardized (ISO 8362–1: Injection vials made of glass tubing; ISO 8362–4: Injection vials made of molded glass). For infusion bottles, the pharmacopeias require minimally type II glass containers.

For certain applications, it may be useful to siliconize the inside walls of the vials or bottles. To that end, the containers are sprayed with 0.5% to 1.5% aqueous emulsions of polydimethylsiloxane and optionally heated to 200° to 400°C to fix the coating. This process creates a silicone film on the glass surface, of which the lowermost layer is firmly attached to the glass. The overlaying layers are much less tightly bound to the surface and have an oily, mobile character. The silicone film hydrophobizes the hydrophilic glass surface, which allows much better removal of aqueous solutions (pearling) so that the nominal contents can be more completely withdrawn. This effect is most noticeable with suspensions, as suspended particles often strongly adhere to the hydrophilic glass wall. During lyophilization, adhesion of the cake to uncoated glass surfaces often leads to the formation of a ring of material, sticking to the wall during the drying process, from which the rest of the lyophilizate spalls off due to shrinking. By employing siliconized vials, crack-free products with a smooth surface are obtained.

As compared to glass vials, polymer vials are much less widely used. Formerly, they were made of PP, but now they are increasingly produced from cyclic olefin polymers (COP) and cyclic olefin copolymers (COC). Because these are amorphous polymers, vials made of these materials are crystal-clear and optically hardly distinguishable from glass. The COP and COC types used for this purpose have high glass transition temperatures, which allows autoclaving at 121° or 134°C. However, they are not resistant to sterilization and depyrogenation by dry heat. This precludes the possibility to introduce them into an aseptic filling zone via a depyrogenation tunnel, which is well established. Compared to glass containers, COP and COC vials show increased risk for extractables and leachables, and a non-negligible degree of oxygen permeability. Their suitability has to be thoroughly evaluated for drugs (among them also proteins) that are prone to oxidation. If necessary they have to be sealed in an oxygen-tight blister package and an oxygen absorber has to be enclosed.

27.3.4.3   Production of Filled Vials

Cleaning and Depyrogenation

Although prewashed and presterilized, ready-to-use, glass vials recently have become available, the common practice is still to source injection vials as unwashed and nonsterile material and feed them prior to use through a washing machine and a sterilization and depyrogenation tunnel into the aseptic filling area. The cleaning process is performed in automatically operated vial washers, where high-pressure water jets (WFI) were sprayed onto the inner and outer surfaces of the vials. In some machines, cleaning is supported by ultrasound. After drying with compressed air the ampoules are sterilized and depyrogenated by passing them through a dry-heat tunnel (depyrogenation tunnel) where they are exposed to temperatures above 280°C for several minutes. This treatment needs to be validated to not only inactivate microorganisms but also to remove endotoxins.

Filling

Filling of the vials is done by means of metering pumps; these are often peristaltic pumps or valveless piston pumps, which draw the product from a bulk storage tank and transfer it via tubing lines to the filling needles.

Many products are susceptible to oxidation and therefore require an oxygen-excluding filling process. To that end, the head space of the vial is gassed with nitrogen or argon

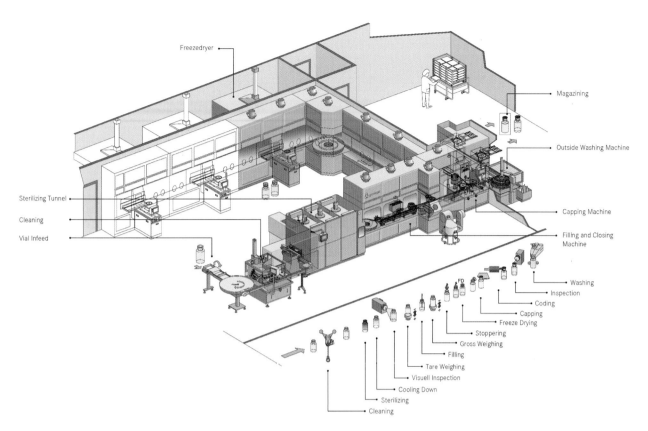

Fig. 27-3 High-speed vial line under isolator with connection to freeze dryer. Reproduced with permission from Groninger & Co. GmbH, Germany.

immediately before and after the filling step through a separated gassing needle. In this way, a residual oxygen content of less than 5%, in most cases even as little as 1%, is achieved.

Vials that are terminally sterilized after stoppering, should be filled up to maximally 90% of their total volume to prevent any risk of bursting. With an increasing amount of aqueous liquid in the vial, the temperature-induced volume expansion of the water (approximately 6% between 20° and 121°C) causes an increasing compression of the gas/vapor in the head space of the container, resulting in a concomitant pressure rise. This pressure relates hyperbolically to the filling volume, causing a steep rise beyond a 90% filling degree, so that bursting of the container can no longer be ruled out [pressure-increase factor = head-space volume / (head-space volume − expansion volume of the fluid)]. The vapor pressure of the water may be ignored in this context because, apart from temporary inequalities during the heating and cooling phase, the vapor pressure in the autoclave chamber is equal to that in the vial.

Because the user will not be able to quantitatively withdraw the injection solution from the vial, since a small fraction will remain attached to the wall, the volume filled in the vial has to be slightly larger than indicated on the label (the nominal volume). The excess amount depends on viscosity, surface tension, hydrophilicity, and nominal volume of the fluid and the properties of the (inner) container surface (siliconization). Smaller vials require a somewhat larger overfill than larger containers. General recommendations for excess volumes in injections containers are given in Table 1 of USP chapter ⟨1151⟩. The excess volumes proposed there range between 0.01 mL for a labeled volume of a mobile liquid of 0.5 mL to 3% of the labeled volume if the latter is ≥ 50 mL and the liquid is viscous.

Vials are sealed with a rubber stopper that is attached to the neck of the container by means of an aluminum crimp cap (Fig. 27-4). Shape and size of stoppers and caps are defined by a series of ISO standards (ISO 8362−2, ISO 8362−3, ISO 8362−5, ISO 8362−6, ISO 8362− 7). The rubber stopper is shaped in such a way that it is thinnest in the center. This site, which is protected by a plastic flip-off cap or a tear-off metal tab, is pierced by the injection needle through which the injection fluid is aspirated. Vials containing a dry substance that is unstable in solution have to be reconstituted by the addition of water for injection, isotonic

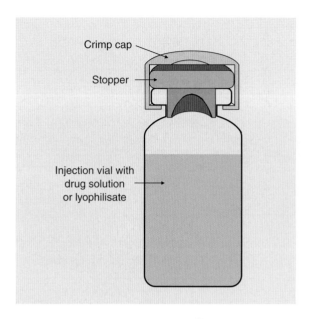

Fig. 27-4 Sealing of a vial with rubber stopper and crimp cap.

NaCl, glucose, or a specific diluent. The fluid to be used is mostly provided in a separate vial or in a prefilled syringe and is added by an injection needle or a needle-free adapter, immediately before administration.

27.3.4.4   Rubber Stoppers

A sealing stopper for parenteral preparations has to meet numerous requirements. It should be optimally adapted to the product in question and its production process (including sterilization) as well as to application conditions. It should, for example, guarantee perfectly tight sealing, impermeability to gases and water vapor (if required), easy mechanical insertion, resistance in a wide temperature range in connection to sterilization and freeze-drying, and it should not absorb components of the product or release stopper material to the product or change the product in any other way. It should allow easy penetration with the defined tools (injection needle, infusion sets or needle-free vial adapter) without punching out stopper material or producing particulate contamination. In case of multiple-dose containers the stopper should perfectly reseal after withdrawing the needle and it should maintain all properties required for proper application, even after repeated perforation.

During storage, but also under the influence of heat-sterilization, there is a risk that polymer additives leach from the rubber stopper into the solution. This may concern vulcanization agents, vulcanization accelerators, activators, plasticizers, antioxidants or other substances. These may have an immediate toxic potential (e.g., pyrogenic effect), affect the stability of the active ingredient, or promote the formation of toxic products by reaction with the active ingredient. Conversely, there is also the possibility that active ingredients are adsorbed to or absorbed by the stopper material. Especially, preservatives are known to migrate readily into rubber materials. Since preservatives are usually present in the product in only low concentration, sorption by the stopper material often suffices to deplete the solution of preservative to such an extent that adequate preservation is no longer guaranteed.

To avoid unwanted interactions between stopper and product rubber stoppers can be coated, for example with high-molecular weight polydimethylsiloxanes. The polymer is sprayed on the stopper and then cross-linked by UV irradiation. Alternatively, the stopper is coated with ethylene-tetrafluoroethylene copolymers (e.g., FluroTec®). In addition to the improved compatibility with the contents, a stopper coating reduces the shedding of particles from the stopper and facilitates insertion of the stopper in the vial. Stoppers used in a lyophilization procedure are usually coated on the top side. After the completion of the lyophilization process, the distance between the shelves is reduced by moving them down in order to push the stoppers entirely into the vial necks. In this process the underside of each shelf is pressed against the stoppers on the next shelf down. A coating on their top sides avoids sticking to the shelves when they are lifted again after the closing step and, thus, prevents the vials from reopening or tipping over.

27.3.4.5 Container Closure Integrity

For primary packaging containers, the adequate design of all related components should be evaluated and ensured by the pharmaceutical manufacturer. In the case of vials, this includes evaluating the fit of the vial with the rubber stopper and aluminum crimp cap. Container closure systems are evaluated for dimensional variances and whether the system would be still suitable in case of related variations. For parenteral products, the container closure system has also to be tested experimentally for container closure integrity—for example, using deterministic methods like volumetric (helium) glass flow.

27.3.4.6 Cylinder Ampoules and Prefilled Syringes

Formulations for injection in containers, which do not necessitate the use of a separate syringe for administration, are becoming increasingly popular.

Cylinder Ampoules

Cylinder ampoules (cartridges, carpules) are glass cylinders that at one end are closed by a sliding cylindrical rubber stopper, which serves as a piston. At the other end, the cylinder is tapered and closed with a septum in the form of a thin rubber disk (Fig. 27-5). By inserting the cylinder in an injection device (e.g., a carpule syringe, an injection pen or an autoinjector device), this disk is penetrated by the rear end of a double-tipped needle. During the injection, the stopper is pushed forward with a plunger, expelling the fluid through the needle. Carpule cylinders require sufficient lubrication, such as by siliconization, to minimize the break-loose and gliding force, and thus stopper movement and functionality, is warranted.

Cylinder ampoules have been in use for a long time, especially for example for the administration of local anesthetics for dental procedures. Wider application of cylinder ampoules has followed the development of the injection pen (e.g., for insulin). Injection pens are pen-shaped devices that allow safe and easy multiple injections from cylinder ampoules. The device permits adjustment of individual doses by means of a setting screw. The inconspicuous appearance and easy operation of the device allow the patient to self-administration of subcutaneous injections even in everyday situations.

Prefilled Syringes

A prefilled syringe consists of a glass or polymer barrel with a rubber stopper inserted to which a plunger rod is mounted or can be screwed in prior to use.

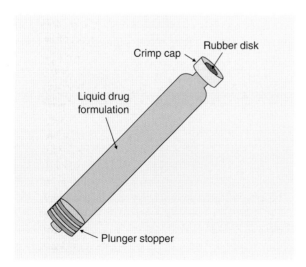

Fig. 27-5 Cylinder ampoule.

The rear end of the syringe barrel is shaped as a finger flange or, alternatively, a plastic device with identical function is attached. The tip has either a Luer-Lock tip onto which prior to use a needle is screwed, or the needle is permanently glued into this end of the cylinder (staked needle). The Luer-Lock tip or the needle is covered with a rubber tip cap or a needle shield, respectively. Often the rubber tip caps on Luer-Lock syringes are shielded by a tamper-evident closure that has to be broken to remove it.

Double-chamber syringes are systems that permit separate storage of two different solutions or a powder and a liquid. Immediately prior to injection, the two components are combined. This may be accomplished for instance by pushing forward a second stopper, which separates the two contents, together with the fluid behind it, until it reaches a linear groove in the cylinder wall through which fluid from the upper chamber can bypass the stopper. The application of double-chamber syringes may be an advantage in case of unstable active substances.

Injection cylinders made of glass require internal coating with silicone oil in order to allow uniform sliding of the piston. The siliconized surface and, even more so, detached silicon oil droplets may interact with the content of the syringe or lead to particulates in solution that require specific analytical methods in order to detect and distinguish them from other, undesired particulate matter.

27.3.4.7   Infusion Bags

For the sake of weight reduction during transport and avoidance of glass breakage, nowadays many infusion solutions are filled into polymer bags. Another advantage of this packaging method is that the content can be emptied without ventilation as the bags collapse upon withdrawal of the liquid. Infusion bags are available in sizes varying from 50 to 3,000 mL. They are mostly made of PVC, PE, or ethylene vinyl acetate copolymers. Many types consist of multiple-layered composite structures of different polymers. PVC is relatively inexpensive and is quite compatible with blood, which renders it suitable for blood bags. Disadvantages are its high water vapor permeability, often bringing along the necessity of sealing it in a protection bag and its strong capacity to absorb numerous drugs (e.g., diazepam, and glycerol trinitrate), that may lead to a rapid drop in drug concentration.

For all infusion bags, weld seams or other connections between different parts are critical sites with respect to potential leakage. For this reason, leak tests, often called *container closure integrity tests*, are necessary to prove tightness of the seals over the whole shelf life and resistance to the thermal stress during the sterilization process. Infusion bags have a withdrawal port ensuring safe connection of an infusion set. Often, they also have a perforable injection port to permit addition of further drug solutions. Particularly bags with 0.9% NaCl or 5% glucose solution, which serve as carrier solutions for added medical ingredients, have a high expansion capacity, allowing injections of 15% to 60% additional fluid, related to the filling volume.

For total parenteral nutrition (TPN) double- and triple-chamber bags are used, which contain glucose and amino acid solutions and a fat emulsion in separated compartments. Before use, the bag is compressed, causing the seal seams between the chambers to rupture and the liquids to mix.

Recent and Future Developments in Pharmaceutical Technology

28

It's hard to make predictions, especially about the future
(Niels Bohr)

I never think about the future, it will come soon enough
(Albert Einstein)

Novel developments in pharmaceutical technology are not only driven by the peculiarities of newly developed active agents, but often come forth from the ambition to circumvent patented technology. For example, scientific ideas developed in companies producing generics may give rise to truly novel drug formulations, which in turn may be adopted by other companies for further development. Novel drug formulations are not only developed in research labs of pharmaceutical companies but academic institutions also contribute their part in this connection. While many developments may just represent follow-ups of known technologies, they will nonetheless incur additional costs to carry them on to a new product. Leaning on a wealth of innovative ideas, such developments will often lead to significant therapeutic improvements.

Recently a research group from Boston (Chertok et al. 2013) published a series of innovative ideas in the *Journal of Molecular Pharmaceutics*. Their futuristic views are based on a 1966 movie by Richard Fleischer called *Fantastic Voyage*, starring Stephen Boyd and Raquel Welch. Five CIA agents have themselves shrunken to microscopic size and are subsequently injected into the blood stream of a communistic defector. Their aim is to remove a blood clot in the defector's brain. The Bostonian authors outline the possibilities of designing a nano-submarine over the course of the next 50 years (Fig. 28-1), setting their hopes on nano-3D printing. They play with the idea of a cruise-missile-like drug carrier that, after introduction into the bloodstream, would automatically find its way to its target, where it would "explode" to deliver its therapeutic cargo precisely at the desired site.

In this final chapter, we will not look that far in the future. Rather, we will limit ourselves to a discussion of current and near-future developments in drug formulation, which will demand shorter development times, and of the technologies required for that purpose, either within reach or already on the market.

28.1 Nano-Systems

28.1.1 Pharmaceutical Nano-Systems

When searching a literature data bank for "nano" and "drug delivery systems," we obtained 155 hits in references before 1990, but in literature just from 2015–2017, as many as

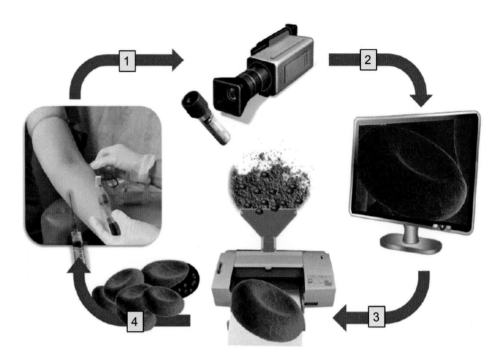

Fig. 28-1   Idea of a future production of drug delivery systems mimicking the structure of a patient's cells: (1) Patient's cell analysis by a 3D high-resolution device from a blood sample; (2) reconstruction of a typical cell and storage of the data in the patient's medical records; (3) with a 3D printer, biocompatible drug-loaded polymer replicas are produced; (4) injection of the delivery system for treatment. Reprinted with permission from Chertok et al. Copyright 2013 American Chemical Society.

13,475 references were found. For the construction of nano-systems, a variety of building blocks may be envisaged, including those that nature provides. For example, liposomes can be constructed from phospholipids (section 20.3), while many polymers may be turned into a nanoparticulate form through controlled procedures (section 20.6).

In addition, the versatile DNA molecule may be used to construct drug delivery systems (origami-DNA). Drugs can be stored inside these nanobots. Aptamers are short DNA strands with a site-specific sequence that may dock on, for example, a tumor cell. This contact leads to a conformational change of the nanobots with subsequent release of the drug (Douglas et al. 2012).

Besides exploitation of physicochemical phenomena such as the enhanced permeation and retention (EPR) effect (section 7.1), attempts are made to improve this passive targeting mechanism by biology-based modifications. To that end, for example, antibodies are coupled to nano-systems in order to improve their target specificity (e.g., tumor cells). It is only fair to conclude that such attempts have been only marginally successful up to now. This should not be taken as a big surprise, however, taking into consideration that in nature, binding of an antibody to a virus, for example, is not meant to guide the virus to its target, but rather, to mark it as a foreign particle to be removed from the blood. Viruses exploit peptides and/or sugars at their surface as synergistic targeting devices, including their intracellular uptake by the target cell. At present, we do not yet fully comprehend the complex individual functions of the surface structures involved in these processes. Other side effects, such as the body's immunological responses to antibodies, are further reasons why early high expectations of antibody-conjugated, nano-scale drug carrier systems have meanwhile been adjusted to a somewhat more modest level.

The proverbial smallness of nano-systems have a drawback in that they interact in many different ways with a wide variety of tissues, often even penetrating into cells. This has initiated a new research area, known as nano-toxicology, which also must be considered from a pharmaceutical point of view. Although side effects are mostly observed in the application of colloidal metallic materials and rarely with liposomal nano-systems, potential safety concerns for the public require that this matter is carefully dealt with.

28.1.2 Other Nano-Systems Used in Pharmaceutics

The nano revolution is also taking place in other areas. For instance, in nano-electronics (but yet officially named micro-electronics), conducting paths with a width of as little as 14 nm have been developed. This allows the construction of complete control circuits with sensor technology and mechanical components at the smallest possible scale (micro-electromechanical/nano-electromechanical systems, MEMS/NEMS), which can be integrated into regular-size drug formulations or even introduced into the body. An example of such a system is a normal-size capsule (Intellicap®, iPill), which, after its ingestion, releases its active ingredient dependent on pH, temperature, pressure, or time, controlled by a corresponding sensor. At the same time, physiological data can be recorded during passage through the intestinal tract, and drug release can be regulated by remote control. Another example is its exploitation in transdermal therapeutic systems. During iontophoresis, the drug transport system can be regulated by a sensor in the skin or even in the blood by means of voltage regulation, in such a way that the drug's concentration in blood remains constant or, in case of chrono-pharmacokinetically operating systems, can be adjusted to demand.

Another application of MEMS/NEMS concerns the use of larger implants, which release their active ingredient by remote control, as described above or, more sophisticatedly, automatically on command of a sensored parameter such as blood glucose concentration. In addition to the obvious drawback of such systems that they need to be recharged with energy and active ingredient occasionally, the sensors also present the problem that the body identifies them as foreign material that might render them useless due to immunological reactions, or as a result of encapsulation by connective tissue.

Continued research efforts will be required to solve this incompatibility issue.

The database DaNa (in English and German) http://www.nanopartikel .info/en/projects/current-projects/ dana-2-0 contains definitions and valid, quality controlled information about nanoparticles as well as actual research activities.

28.2 Carrier Systems in Gene Therapy

Despite the early enthusiasm and perpetual extensive research efforts, introduction of genes into somatic cells in order to restore gene defects or cure diseases is still in its infancy. This cannot only be blamed on imperfection of the gene constructs that somehow has to be inserted properly into the cellular genome. Rather, a lack of adequate carrier systems (vectors) presents an even higher hurdle. Although viruses seem to offer an almost ideal, even targetable, carrier system, up to now our understanding of the way they function is still quite limited, which prevents us from gaining control over their behavior in the body.

In 1992, administration of a modified virus containing an appropriate gene construct to a patient lead to a fatal incident (Limberis 2012). Besides, evolution has effectively adjusted man to viral attacks. Therefore, we will have to gain more understanding of the mechanisms involved in the ultimate elimination of viruses by the immune system and thus learn to cope with this problem.

Alongside the research groups aiming at improvement of such viral vectors, several others rather focus on non-viral gene vectors (Limberis 2012). These are based on polymers and liposomes as well as on inorganic nanoparticles, all carrying a positive surface charge for optimal condensation of the elongated negatively charged DNA strands. Bear in mind that the amount of DNA in a typical dose required for a gene-therapeutic treatment has a total length stretching from the Earth to the moon ($3 \cdot 10^5$ km)! Besides condensation of the DNA, the task of the carrier system is also to help deliver the DNA to the cell nucleus. Up until now, this has been successful under special conditions. Often, "brute-force" methods are able to deliver perhaps only one copy out of the several thousands of DNA fragments internalized by the cell, into the nucleus. For certain types of application one may, for the time being, resort to the *gene gun*. For example, gold nanoparticles, surface-coated with the gene construct, are fired with high velocity into the tissue. A fraction of the particles ends up in the cytoplasm of the cell, and an even (much) smaller fraction makes it to the nucleus, where it may bring about the desired result of the treatment.

28.3   Polymers as Carrier Systems

The number of potential polymers that can be constructed from a much smaller number of building blocks is endless. They may not only be used as matrix systems in various pharmaceutical preparations (transdermal therapeutic systems, or, for example, in tablets), but also for more novel applications.

Two extreme examples are presented here: a hydrophilic/hydrophobic block- copolymer forming micelles confining a lipophilic drug within its core, or micelles of a hydrophilic/ cationic block-copolymer carrying condensed DNA within their core. For quite some time, conjugation of therapeutic proteins with polyethylene glycol (PEG) has been known to enhance the protein's half life in the blood circulation (stealth effect, see 20.3.3) and reduce hypersensitivity, thus bringing about a therapeutic advantage over the unconjugated protein (Duncan 2003). Recent developments in polymer chemistry have led to the construction of polymers that are sensitive to pH, light, or temperature, allowing them to release associated drugs at the target site in response to such (locally prevailing or externally applied) triggers.

28.4   Inhalation Systems

Application of inhalation devices often requires several steps, and for many devices synchronized actions are required from the patient. This gives rise to serious operating errors by more than 40% of the patients, and thus to deficient therapeutic result (chapter 23). In order to improve overall therapeutic efficacy, pharmaceutical companies have started to step into the *connected medical market*. Novartis, in cooperation with an electronic company, is developing a new generation of the Breezhaler™. A module inside the inhaler detects and reports usage, the time when the inhaler is used and additional information. This is sent to an app of the patient's smartphone, which, in turn, sends it to a data cloud, where it is analyzed and made available to the patient and his physician.

28.5   Carrier Systems for Peptide/ Protein Drugs

The design of patient-compatible formulations of peptides and proteins is currently one of the major challenges in pharmaceutical technology. Until now, these substances are mainly administered by injection or occasionally as depot formulation. Despite the evident aimed to develop a nonparenteral formulation, no such leap forward has been made as yet. Despite high expectations, attempts to design an inhalation formulation of insulin (Exubera®) have failed, due to highly variable bioavailability. More application-specific formulations of inhalable insulin may possibly yield better results (e.g., pre-prandial administration). Clinical studies with Afrezza® appear to be promising, which may be attributable to the monomeric form of insulin in this lung-accessible particulate formulation. The intrinsic variability of absorption, including the enzymatic degradation of peptides and proteins via pulmonary or other epithelial (e.g. nasal) passages, may nonetheless lead to promising future developments.

Although systems such as MEMS/NEMS (section 28.1.2) might offer the solution to long-term therapies with this type of active agent, for now it is hard to imagine that this application will be helpful in acute care.

28.6   Individualized Therapeutic Systems

Whereas the production processes in pharmaceutical industry and the approval-associated regulations are currently still geared toward the production of large batches, in the therapeutic domain a trend reversal toward personalized medicinal therapy is emerging (see Rantanen and Khinast 2105).

It is therefore necessary to develop production methods for individualized drug formulations, not only with respect to dose but also with respect to flexible combinations of different drugs (polypills) and for individually adjusted duration of activity, such as retarded action.

Thus, the development of systems allowing finely tuned either stepwise or continuous dosing, and those that permit a combination of active substances, have made most progress.

28.6.1   Systems for Individualized Dosing

Drugs that can be dosed precisely to individual needs are ranked as the most frequently used among the parenteral preparations. Examples are infusion solutions, which may, for instance, be administered by means of perfusors or ambulant infusion pumps, but also include insulin pens, as well as graduated prefilled syringes. Nonetheless, for the administration of peroral drug formulations, further individualization would be welcome (Wening and Breitkreutz 2011), even to the extent of pump-controlled constant-rate administration. For long-term treatment with buccal or orally administered drugs, small, implantable electric drug pumps have been described, inserted in the jaw so as to replace two wisdom teeth.

Especially for solid peroral formulations, dose adjustments, if so desired, are currently made by means of relatively coarse gradations, either by choosing a single one from multiple available drug strengths or by dividing tablets. In this way, dose adjustment merely means either doubling or dividing in halves. Low doses, as commonly required for small children, cannot be measured out in most cases.

In the years to come, a solution may become available in mini-tablet form, taken from a dosing system that automatically releases the required number of units. Another alternative are tablets that can be divided in a large number of small subunits, which can either be taken individually or as multiple fragments of individually determined size. It should be noted that with diminishing fragment size, the accuracy of the drug content decreases. When the individual segments of tablets, with their multiple nicks, have a different number of fracture planes (e.g., terminal segments *vs.* middle segments), this may result in a non-uniform release profile of the active ingredient. The disadvantage of divisible tablets might be overcome by tablet formulations in which drug-containing segments alternate with drug-free segments. The fracture nicks are then positioned in the drug-free segments, thus preventing fragments from having unequal drug content and preventing differences in drug release.

Another innovative system is continuous dosing, which, up to now, is still in the developmental stage. This system has the size of a ballpoint pen with a refillable drug-containing polymer rod inside. This rod can, for instance, be manufactured by melt extrusion. The pen can, accurate to a fraction of a millimeter, measure and cut off the protruding part of the drug, which contains an amount of drug proportional to its length that can be orally ingested.

28.6.2   Individualized Drug Combinations

For many, particularly older, patients the necessity to take several different medicines on a daily basis (polypharmacy) presents a major problem. Different dosing intervals of individual formulations further complicate the intake schedule and enhance the risk of incorrect ingestion and reduce patient compliance. Nowadays, the patient receives from the pharmacy a patient-specific blister package of the drugs, containing the units that have to be taken at a certain time of the day. Obviously, this approach does not reduce the number of units to be taken.

To overcome this problem, production of administration units, in which different patient-specific drugs can be variably combined, is under consideration. One such approach is the still experimental Dome Matrix® technology, in which tablet-shaped entities can be put together according to the construction-kit principle with multiple convex and concave modules. This will permit not only individual combinations of different drugs, but also the variation in release profile by unrestricted combination of initial and maintenance doses. Retention in the stomach can be attained by combining the units into a hollow body, which will float on the stomach contents and thus bring about retarded intestinal passage.

28.6.3   Printing Techniques for the Preparation of Drug Formulations

The examples discussed above demonstrate that economic production of such patient-specific formulations requires a very different methodology than that which currently prevails in pharmaceutical production facilities. A very promising technology developed in the previous decade is the application of two- and three-dimensional digital printing techniques.

Structured, two-dimensional drug-containing layers can be produced by web-fed printing as well as by electronic ink-jet procedures (Kolakovic et al. 2013). In case of orodispersible films, which up to now have been made by molding and spread-plate methodology, attempts have been made to employ printing procedures such as flexography. In this process, a drug/excipient solution is transferred via the raised structures of a flexible polymer plate to a foil-like substrate (e.g., edible sugar foil). Although, in principle, it would be possible to achieve this adaptive dosing approach by individual tailoring of orodispersible films, techniques requiring a printed formulation are usually too rigid for economic production of individual, patient-specific, on-demand dosing. Ink-jet printing is much more suitable for this purpose. This method is already in use to print, with a simple office or home printer, sugar foils of edible ink for the decoration of pastry. Preliminary attempts have produced proof of the suitability of this method to print dissolved drugs or nano-suspensions on films of cellulose ether, starch, or sugar.

On a pilot base, three-dimensional objects, such as coronary stents, have already been coated with pharmacologically active substances by means of this method. For the purpose of diffusion-controlled drug release, it is possible to coat a drug-containing layer—for example, by printing an ethylcellulose film on it.

Three-dimensional printers also offer the possibility to construct complex 3-D structures layer by layer. By combining differently composed layers or by generating drug concentration gradients, it is also possible to design complex release profiles or pulsatile release patterns. For example, matrix tablets with a radial drug gradient and drug-free barrier layers at the top and bottom sides have been produced experimentally, which release 98% of the drug with linear kinetics. Examples of other structures that cannot be produced by conventional methods but have been tentatively produced by print technology are layered tablets of which each individual layer represents a coated tablet with a drug-containing core. In addition to oral formulations, implants and other monolithic entities can be produced by this method. The technology that is most widely used in 3-D printing is based on application of thin layers of powder, consecutively hardened each time by spraying droplets of binding agent with micrometer precision on the solidifying attachment sites. When, after several repeats of this procedure, the final shape and thickness of the object has been obtained, loose powder remnants are removed, which up to that point served to support subsequent layers.

Although only a few reports have been published on printed drug formulations (e.g., Ursan et al. 2013; Sandler and Preis 2016), this method offers an enormous potential for new opportunities. The first drug of this kind already has been approved by the FDA. Spritam is produced by the 3D-ZipDose®-technology. It consists of 25–50 layers with a total thickness of 250 μm rapidly disintegrating when taken orally. On the one hand, it allows the production of structures whose generation by traditional procedures would be utterly impossible; on the other hand, it brings user-oriented production of patient-specific application units within the reach of reality. For the time being, regulatory prerequisites are still standing in the way of such developments, but the first signs of a cautious change in perspective are detectable.

28.7   Carrier Systems and Biotechnology

Carrier systems have to overcome structural barriers in the body without leaving behind permanent damage. It is especially difficult to accomplish this in case of the blood-brain barrier

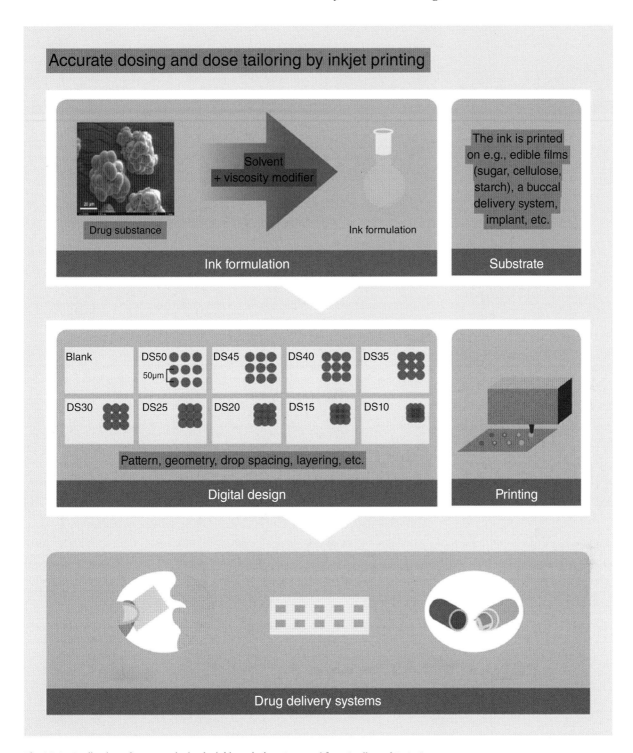

Fig. 28-2   Realization of accurate dosing by inkjet printing. Reprinted from Sandler and Preis. Copyright 2016 with permission from Elsevier, see complete reference at end of chapter.

(BBB). Although literature reports claims of successful delivery of high-molecular weight drugs to the brain by means of nanoparticles, this was most likely mediated by transient openings in the endothelial barrier, which may bring along undesirable influx of other substances into the brain as well. It would appear that this particularly tight barrier cannot be overcome by traditional carrier systems. Possibly, low molecular weight drugs (<400 Da) with few hydrogen bonds (<8) can overcome the BBB, but for larger molecules such as peptides and proteins, the BBB represents a formidable obstacle. A potential solution (besides systems such as MEMS and NEMS) may lie in the exploitation of transport systems located in the endothelial cells lining the blood vessels, responsible for the supply of nutrients to the brain. To that end, the drug must either bear resemblance to the physiological substrate of one of the many transport systems in the brain or it must be hidden, like the Greek soldiers in the Trojan horse, while coupled to an antibody, which by means of receptor-mediated endocytosis may gain access to the brain. Preliminary results of this approach are encouraging (Pardridge 2012).

Let us now turn back to the micro-submarine we referred to earlier in this chapter. Red blood cells or their precursors could be considered a meager version of this submarine. The outer surface of these cells can be modified by special biotechnological techniques, without inducing immunogenicity (Shi et al. 2014). Such erythrocytes may circulate in the bloodstream for several months and then, while circulating, dock to target cells or release a drug that was either encapsulated or even synthesized inside the cells.

This brief survey of intermediate or long-term developments of novel, already existing, or potential future drug formulations, illustrates that pharmaceutical technology will exploit, like it has always done, cutting-edge technologies provided by all scientific disciplines, for the development of new products for the benefit of patients as well as shareholders. These developments often take more time to mature than the original technologies, which is inherent to this field, where drug safety invariably relishes highest priority for the sake of patient protection.

We should look forward, with high expectations, to future innovations in the pharmaceutical field. As Charles H. Duell (United States Commissioner of Patent, 1898–1901) said in 1902: "In my opinion, all previous advances in the various lines of invention will appear totally insignificant when compared with those which the present century will witness. I almost wish that I might live my life over again to see the wonders which are at the threshold."

Further Reading

Chertok, B., et al. "Drug Delivery Interfaces in the 21st Century: From Science Fiction Ideas to Viable Technologies." *Mol Pharm*. 10 (10) (2013): 3531–3543.

Douglas, S. M., Bachelet, I., Church, G. M. "A Logic-Gated Nanorobot for Targeted Transport of Molecular Payloads." *Science* 335 (6070) (2012): 831–834.

Duncan, R. "The Dawning Era of Polymer Therapeutics." *Nat Rev Drug Discov*. 2 (5) (2003): 347–360.

Heinemann, L. "New ways of insulin delivery." *International Journal of Clinical Practice* 66 (175) (2012): 35–39.

Kolakovic, R., et al. "Printing Technologies in Fabrication of Drug Delivery Systems." *Expert Opinion on Drug Delivery* 10 (12) (2013): 1711–1723.

Limberis, M. P. "Phoenix Rising: Gene Therapy Makes a Comeback." *Acta Biochim Biophys* Sin (Shanghai) 44 (8) (2012): 632–640.

Pardridge, W. M. "Drug Transport Across the Blood-Brain Barrier." *J Cereb Blood Flow Metab*. 3 (11) (2012): 1959–1972.

Rantanen, J., and Khinast, J. "The Future of Pharmaceutical Manufacturing Sciences." *Journal of Pharmaceutical Sciences* 104 (11) (2015): 3612–3638.

Sandler, N., and Preis, M. "Printed Drug-Delivery Systems for Improved Patient Treatment." *Trends Pharmacol Sci* 3 (12) (December 2016): 1070–1080.

Shi, J., et al., "Engineered Red Blood Cells as Carriers for Systemic Delivery of a Wide Array of Functional Probes." *Proc Natl Acad Sci U S A*, (2014).

Ursan, I. D., Chiu, L., and Pierce, A. "Three-Dimensional Drug Printing: A Structured Review." *Journal of the American Pharmacists Association* 53 (2) (2013): 136–144.

Wening, K., and J. Breitkreutz, "Oral Drug Delivery in Personalized Medicine: Unmet Needs and Novel Approaches." *International Journal of Pharmaceutics* 404 (1) (2011): 1–9.

Selected Dosage Forms (Compared between Ph. Eur., USP, and JP)

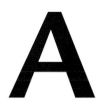

Ph. Eur. 07 Dosage forms

USP ⟨1151⟩ Pharmaceutical dosage forms

JP [2] Monographs for preparations

A dosage form is defined as a combination of drug substance(s) and/or excipient(s) to facilitate dosing, administration, and delivery of the medicine to the patient (USP ⟨1151⟩). Each of three selected main pharmacopeias, Ph. Eur., USP, and USP, contain a general chapter describing the definitions, manufacturing methods, test methods, containers, packaging, and storage for a variety of dosage forms (Ph. Eur. 07 Dosage forms, USP ⟨1151⟩, JP [2]). Table A-1 gives an overview on the terminology of the dosage forms in the different pharmacopeias and which of them correspond.

The classification system applied in the Ph. Eur. is most detailed and consistent and covers not only dosage forms for human use but also those for veterinary use. For this reason, the structure of the following overview was based on the Ph. Eur. chapter 07, Dosage forms. In addition, all relevant information of USP chapter ⟨1151⟩ and JP chapter [2] was included into this Ph. Eur. based framework.

Table A-1 Monographs on dosage forms in Ph. Eur. 07, USP ⟨1151⟩, and JP [2]

Ph. Eur. 07	USP ⟨1151⟩	JP [2]
Premixes for medicated feeding stuffs for veterinary use	–	–
Liquid preparations for oral use • Oral solutions, emulsions and suspensions • Powders and granules for oral solutions and suspensions • Oral drops • Powders for oral drops • Syrups • Powders and granules for syrups	Solutions Emulsions Suspensions	Liquids and solutions for oral administration • Elixirs • Suspensions • Emulsion • Lemonades Syrups Preparations for syrups
Liquid preparations for cutaneous application e.g. • Shampoos • Cutaneous foams	Solutions Emulsions Lotions Suspensions Soaps and shampoos Aerosols • Topical aerosols	Liquids and solutions for cutaneous application • Liniments • Lotions Sprays for cutaneous application • Pump sprays for cutaneous application • Aerosols for cutaneous application

(continued)

Voigt's Pharmaceutical Technology, First Edition. Alfred Fahr.
© 2018 John Wiley & Sons Ltd. Published 2018 by John Wiley & Sons Ltd.

Table A-1   (*Continued*)

Ph. Eur. 07	USP ⟨1151⟩	JP [2]
Veterinary liquid preparations for cutaneous application • Cutaneous foams • Dip concentrates • Pour-on preparations • Shampoos • Spot-on preparations • Sprays • Teat dips • Teat sprays • Udder-washes	Solutions Emulsions Suspensions	–
Granules • Effervescent granules • Coated granules • Gastro-resistant granules • Modified-release granules	Granules e.g. • Effervescent granules	Granules e.g. • Effervescent granules
Semi-solid preparations for cutaneous application • Ointments • Creams • Gels • Pastes • Poultices • Medicated plasters • Cutaneous patches	Ointments Creams Gels Lotions Pastes Tapes	Ointments Creams Gels Patches • Tapes/Plasters • Cataplasms/Gel Patches

Capsules
• Hard capsules
• Soft capsules
• Gastro-resistant capsules
• Modified-release capsules
• Cachets
	Capsules
	• Two-piece or hard-shell capsules
	• One-piece or soft-shell capsules
	• Modified-release capsules
	  ◦ Delayed-release capsules
	  ◦ Extended-release capsules
		Capsules
		• Hard capsules
		• Soft capsules

Chewing gums, medicated	Gums • Melted gums • Directly compressed gums	Tablets for oro-mucosal application: Medicated chewing gums
Parenteral preparations	Injections Implants Solutions Emulsions Suspensions Tablets: Hypodermic tablets	Injections • Parenteral infusions • Implants/Pellets • Prolonged release injections
Powders, oral	Powders	Powders
Powders for cutaneous application	Powders	Solid preparations for cutaneous application • Powders for cutaneous application
Foams, medicated	Foams	–
Sticks	Inserts	–
Tablets • Uncoated tablets • Coated tablets • Gastro-resistant tablets • Modified-release tablets • Effervescent tablets • Soluble tablets • Dispersible tablets • Orodispersible tablets • Chewable tablets • Oral lyophilisates	Tablets • Buccal tablets • Chewable tablets • Effervescent tablets • Hypodermic tablets • Modified-release tablets • Orally disintegrating tablets • Sublingual tablets • Tablets for oral solution • Tablets for oral suspensions • Tablet triturates	Tablets • Orally disintegrating tablets • Chewable tablets • Effervescent tablets • Dispersible tablets • Soluble tablets
Tampons, medicated	–	–
Patches, transdermal	Systems	Preparations for cutaneous application: Patches
Intraruminal devices	–	–

Table A-1 (*Continued*)

Ph. Eur. 07	USP ⟨1151⟩	JP [2]
Pressurized pharmaceutical preparations	Aerosols • Inhalation aerosols (Metered-dose inhalers) • Nasal aerosols • Lingual aerosols • Topical aerosols	Sprays for cutaneous application: Aerosols for cutaneous application
Preparations for irrigation	Irrigations Solutions	–
Eye preparations • Eye drops • Eye lotions • Powders for eye drops and powders for eye lotions • Semi-solid eye preparations • Ophthalmic inserts	Solutions Emulsions Suspensions Gels Ointments Systems	Opththalmic liquids and solutions Ophthalmic ointments
Ear preparations • Ear drops and sprays • Semi-solid ear preparations • Ear powders • Ear washes • Ear tampons	Solutions Emulsions Suspensions	Ear preparations
Preparations for inhalation • Preparations to be converted into vapor • Liquid preparations for nebulization • Pressurized metered-dose preparations for inhalation • Non-pressurized metered-dose preparations for inhalation • Inhalation powders	Solutions Emulsions Suspensions Powders Sprays Inhalation aerosols (Metered-dose inhalers)	Inhalations • Dry powder inhalers • Inhalation liquid preparations • Metered-dose inhalers
Intramammary preparations for veterinary use • Preparations for administration to lactating animals • Preparations for administration to animals at the end of lactation or to non-lactating animals for the treatment or prevention of infection	Solutions Emulsions Suspensions Gels	–
Nasal preparations • Nasal drops and liquid nasal sprays • Nasal powders • Semi-solid nasal preparations • Nasal washes • Nasal sticks	Solutions Emulsions Suspensions Gels Ointments Powders Sprays Nasal aerosols	Nasal preparations • Nasal dry powder inhalers • Nasal liquids and solutions
Rectal preparations • Suppositories • Rectal capsules • Rectal solutions, emulsions and suspensions • Powders and tablets for rectal solutions and suspensions • Semi-solid rectal preparations • Rectal foams • Rectal tampons	Suppositories Solutions Emulsions Suspensions Gels Ointments	Suppositories for rectal application Semi-solid preparations for rectal application Enemas for rectal application
Vaginal preparations • Pessaries • Vaginal tablets • Vaginal capsules • Vaginal solutions, emulsions and suspensions • Tablets for vaginal solutions and suspensions • Semi-solid vaginal preparations • Vaginal foams • Medicated vaginal tampons	Solutions Emulsions Suspensions Gels Ointments Inserts	Tablets for vaginal use Suppositories for vaginal use

(continued)

Table A-1 (*Continued*)

Ph. Eur. 07	USP ⟨1151⟩	JP [2]
Intrauterine preparations for veterinary use • Intrauterine tablets • Intrauterine capsules • Intrauterine solutions, emulsions and suspensions, concentrates for intrauterine solutions • Tablets for intrauterine solutions and suspensions • Semi-solid intrauterine preparations • Intrauterine foams • Intrauterine sticks	Solutions Emulsions Suspensions Ointments Systems	–
Oromucosal preparations • Gargles • Mouthwashes • Gingival solutions • Oromucosal solutions and oromucosal suspensions • Semi-solid oromucosal preparations • Oromucosal drops and sprays, sublingual sprays • Lozenges and pastilles • Compressed lozenges • Sublingual and buccal tablets • Oromucosal capsules • Mucoadhesive preparations • Orodispersible films	Lozenges Tablets Films Solutions Emulsions Suspensions Gels Pastes Sprays Lingual aerosols	Tablets for oro-mucosal application • Troches/Lozenges • Sublingual tablets • Buccal tablets • Mucoadhesive tablets Sprays for oro-mucosal application Semi-solid preparations for oro-mucosal application Preparations for gargle
–	Gases	–
–	Liquids (pure chemical in its liquid state)	–
–	Pellets	–
–	Pills	–
–	Strips	–
–	–	Jellies for oral administration
–	–	Preparations for dialysis • Peritoneal dialysis agents • Hemodialysis agents

1. Ph. Eur. Premixes for medicated feeding stuffs for veterinary use (Praeadmixta ad alimenta medicata ad usum veterinarium)

Premixes for medicated feeding stuffs for veterinary use comprise granules, powders, semi-solid or fluid preparations from which, by mixing with certain types of compound fodder, fodder-associated pharmaceuticals are prepared for application in intensive livestock farming. They consist of active ingredients and carrier substances of which the latter are often not described in monographs of the pharmacopeias (e.g., wheat bran, wheat middlings). Apart from exceptional cases, the content of granulated or pulverized preblends of pharmaceuticals in fodder-associated pharmaceuticals should amount to at least 0.5%. When so required, the product label should provide for example information on the withdrawal period between the last administration of the preparation and collection of the material for human consumption.

Tests

Loss on drying: Apart from exceptional cases, loss on drying of granulated or pulverized preparations is maximally 15% (assessed by drying a 3 g sample for 2 hours at 100°C to 105°C).

2. Ph. Eur. Liquid preparations for oral use (Praeparationes liquidae peroraliae)

USP ⟨2⟩ Oral drug products—product quality tests

JP [2] 1 Preparations for oral administration

Liquid preparations for oral use are solutions, emulsions or suspensions with one or more active ingredients in a suitable vehicle, which are ingested in either diluted or undiluted form. Alternatively, they are prepared immediately prior to use, from concentrated fluid preparations or from powders or granules. Some of them consist of one single liquid active ingredient only. They are marketed in multidose or single-dose containers. According Ph. Eur., liquid preparations for oral ingestion are distinguished in:

- Oral solutions, emulsions and suspensions
- Powders and granules for oral solutions and suspensions
- Oral drops
- Powders for oral drops
- Syrups
- Powders and granules for syrups (oftentimes called "dry syrups")

The classification of liquid preparations for oral use according to USP and JP is shown in Table A-1.

For application, powders and granules are dissolved or dispersed in water or another appropriate liquid (vehicle). When the formulation is ready for use it should meet the specific requirements of the particular preparation. In case of multidose containers, the liquid formulations are administered by means of a suitable measuring device (measuring spoon, measuring cup, syringe, dropper insert).

Emulsions and suspensions may show evidence of phase separation or formation of a sediment, respectively, but they should be readily dispersible by shaking and remain sufficiently stable to enable the correct dose to be delivered.

Liquid preparations for oral use may contain suitable antimicrobial preservatives, antioxidants and other excipients such as dispersing, suspending, thickening, emulsifying, buffering, wetting, solubilizing, stabilizing, flavoring and sweetening agents as well as coloring matter.

The JP describes two dosage forms (elixirs and lemonades) which are neither included in the USP nor in the Ph. Eur. Elixirs are clear, sweetened and aromatic liquid preparations, containing ethanol, and lemonades are sweet and sour, clear liquid preparations, both of them intended for oral administration.

Tests

Ph. Eur.:

- Uniformity of dosage units: Oral solutions, suspensions and emulsions in single-dose containers comply with the test for uniformity of dosage units (Ph. Eur. 2.9.40), or where justified and authorized, with the tests for uniformity of content (Ph. Eur. 2.9.6) or uniformity of mass (Ph. Eur. 2.9.5), as detailed below.
- Uniformity of content: Single dose preparations that are suspensions comply with test B for uniformity of content of single-dose preparations (Ph. Eur. 2.9.6).
- Uniformity of mass: Single dose-preparations that are solutions or emulsions comply with the following test: The contents of 10 containers emptied as completely as possible are weighed individually and the average mass is calculated. Not more than 2 of the individual masses deviate by more than 10% from the average mass and none deviates by more than 20%.
- Dose and uniformity of dose of oral drops: No dose may have a mass deviating by more than 10% from the mean of 10 doses. The calculated mass of 10 doses may deviate maximally 15% from the nominal mass of 10 doses.

◻ Uniformity of mass of delivered doses from multidose containers: Liquid preparations for oral administration in multidose containers, with the exception of oral drops, comply with the test for uniformity of mass of delivered doses from multidose containers (Ph. Eur. 2.9.27).

USP (according to ⟨2⟩ "Oral Drug Products—Product Quality Tests"):

◻ Liquid oral drug products in multiple-dose containers: Deliverable volume ⟨698⟩
◻ Liquid oral drug products containing alcohol: Alcohol determination ⟨611⟩
◻ Aqueous liquid oral drug products: pH ⟨791⟩
◻ Liquid oral drug products (if necessary due to formulation and use): Microbial content
◻ Liquid oral drug products containing an antioxidant: Determination of the antioxidant (at least for batch release)
◻ Liquid oral drug products: Extractables (data should be collected as early in the development process as possible)

JP:

◻ Dissolution, Disintegration: Unless otherwise specified, preparations for syrups other than preparations which are to be used after having been dissolved meet the requirements of Dissolution Test JP 6.10 or Disintegration Test JP 6.09. If ≥90% of the granules are smaller than 500 μm (sieve test according JP 6.03) the Disintegration Test JP 6.09 is not required.

3. Ph. Eur. Liquid preparations for cutaneous application (Praeparationes liquidae ad usum dermicum)

USP ⟨3⟩ Topical and transdermal drug products—Product quality tests

USP ⟨603⟩ Topical aerosols

JP [2] 11 Preparations for cutaneous application

Liquid preparations for cutaneous application comprise solutions, emulsions or suspensions for application on the skin (including the scalp) and/or nails, with the purpose of attaining local or transdermal activity. Besides alcohol-containing solutions (e.g., ethanolic iodine solution), suspensions (shaking mixtures) and emulsions, these also include shampoos and foams for cutaneous application. The latter may also be contained in pressurized containers, which then should meet the Ph. Eur. requirements for "Preparations in pressurized containers" or the USP requirements defined in ⟨603⟩ "Topical Aerosols." Fluid preparations for cutaneous application may contain preservatives, antioxidants and other excipients such as stabilizers, emulsifiers and viscosity enhancers. Certain preparations are called lotions or liniments. Suspensions may contain a sediment; this should be readily resuspendable upon gentle shaking. Emulsions may show signs of phase separation, which should be readily reversed upon gentle shaking. Preparations that are applied on severely damaged skin should be sterile.

Several categories of liquid preparations for cutaneous application can be distinguished. The Ph. Eur. exemplarily mentions shampoos and cutaneous foams. The classification of liquid preparations for cutaneous application according to USP and JP is shown in Table A-1.

Shampoos

Shampoos are liquid viscous preparations for application on the skin of the scalp, followed by washing out with water. They are emulsions, suspensions or solutions containing an active substance commonly in addition to surface-active substances, suitable preservatives, antioxidants and other excipients such as thickeners, buffer substances, stabilizers and coloring agents. In the USP this dosage form can be found in chapter ⟨1151⟩, subchapter "Soaps and shampoos."

Cutaneous foams

Cutaneous foams should meet the requirements listed in the Ph. Eur. monograph "Foams containing active ingredients." In the USP dermatological foams are covered by the chapter ⟨603⟩ "Topical aerosols," along with dermatological sprays.

Tests

Ph. Eur.:
  ▫ Sterility: Where the label indicates that the preparation is sterile, it must comply with the test for sterility (Ph. Eur. 2.6.1).

USP:
Specific tests according to USP ⟨3⟩ "Topical and Transdermal Drug Products—Product Quality Tests":
  ▫ Uniformity of dosage units (single-unit containers) ⟨905⟩
  ▫ Microbial enumeration tests (nonsterile products) ⟨61⟩
  ▫ Tests for specified organisms (nonsterile products) ⟨62⟩
  ▫ Antimicrobial preservative content: Acceptance criteria for antimicrobial preservative content in multidose products should be established based on the levels necessary to pass the antimicrobial effectiveness testing ⟨51⟩
  ▫ Antioxidant content: If antioxidants are present in the drug product, tests of their content should be established
  ▫ Sterility: For sterile products (e.g., application to open wounds or burned areas), sterility of the product should be demonstrated (Sterility Tests ⟨71⟩)
  ▫ pH: When applicable, topically applied drug products should be tested for pH at the time of batch release and at designated storage time points for batch-to-batch monitoring.
  ▫ Particle size: The particle size of the active drug substance(s) in topically applied drug products (suspensions) is usually determined and controlled at the formulation development stage. Topically applied drug products should be examined for evidence of particle size alteration.

Additional tests for topical aerosols (according to ⟨603⟩ "Topical aerosols"):
  ▫ General quality test requirements described in USP chapters Inhalation and nasal drug products—General information and product quality tests ⟨5⟩
  ▫ Minimum fill ⟨755⟩
  ▫ Leak rate ⟨604⟩
  ▫ Delivery rate (only topical aerosols with continuous valve)
  ▫ Delivered amount (only topical aerosols with continuous valve)
  ▫ Pressure test (only topical aerosols with continuous valve)
  ▫ Number of discharges per container (only topical aerosols with dose-metering valve)
  ▫ Delivered-dose uniformity (only topical aerosols with dose-metering valve)

JP:
  ▫ Uniformity of dosage units: Unless otherwise specified, liquids and solutions for cutaneous application in single-dose packages meet the requirements of Uniformity of Dosage Units JP 6.02, except for emulsified or suspended preparations.
  ▫ Uniformity of delivered dose: Unless otherwise specified, metered-dose type sprays show an appropriate uniformity of delivered dose.

4. Ph. Eur. Veterinary liquid preparations for cutaneous application (Praeparationes liquidae veterinariae ad usum dermicum)

Veterinary liquid preparations for cutaneous application are solutions, suspensions or emulsions containing an active ingredient and are used in veterinary medicine to achieve a local or systemic effect.

The monograph includes concentrates of powders, pastes, solutions, or suspensions for the preparation of ready-for-use liquids.

The following preparations are distinguished:

- Cutaneous foams
- Dip concentrates
- Pour-on preparations
- Shampoos
- Spot-on preparations
- Sprays
- Teat dips
- Teat sprays
- Udder-washes

5. Ph. Eur. Granules (Granulata)

USP ⟨2⟩ Oral drug products—product quality tests

JP [2] 1 Preparations for oral administration

Granules are preparations consisting of solid, dry aggregates of powder particles. Granules in accordance with this monograph are formulations for oral administration. Certain types of granules are swallowed as such, others are chewed, more commonly, however, granules are dissolved or dispersed in water or another suitable liquid immediately prior to delivery to the patient.

They are subcategorized in:

- Effervescent granules (Ph. Eur., USP ⟨2⟩, ⟨1151⟩, JP [2])
- Coated granules (Ph. Eur., USP ⟨2⟩)
- Gastro-resistant granules (Ph. Eur.), delayed-release granules (USP ⟨2⟩), enteric-coated granules (JP [2])
- Modified-release granules (Ph. Eur.), extended-release granules (USP ⟨2⟩), JP [2]

The preparations contain one or several active ingredients with or without excipients and in certain cases coloring and flavoring substances. Granules are provided in single-dose or multidose containers. In the latter case, a measuring device is required.

Effervescent granules contain acid substances and carbonates or hydrogen carbonates which react rapidly in the presence of water to release carbon dioxide.

Tests

Ph. Eur.:

- Uniformity of dosage units: Granules in single-dose containers comply with the test for uniformity of dosage units (Ph. Eur. 2.9.40) or alternatively, where justified and authorized, with the tests for uniformity of content of single dose preparations (Ph. Eur. 2.9.6) and/or uniformity of mass (Ph. Eur. 2.9.5).
- Uniformity of content: Granules in single-dose containers with a content of active substance less than 2 mg or 2% of the total mass comply with the test on uniformity of content of single-dose preparations (Ph. Eur. 2.9.6) test B.

- Uniformity of mass: Granules in single-dose containers (except coated granules) comply with the test for uniformity of mass (Ph. Eur. 2.9.5). If the test for uniformity of content is prescribed for all active substances, the test for uniformity of mass is not required.
- Uniformity of mass of delivered doses from multidose containers: Granules in multidose containers comply with the test on uniformity of mass of delivered doses from multidose containers (Ph. Eur. 2.9.27).
- Dissolution: The release of active ingredient from coated granules and gastro-resistant granules as well as from granules with modified drug release is tested according to the dissolution test for solid dosage forms (Ph. Eur. 2.9.3).
- Disintegration: Effervescent granules should completely disintegrate within 5 minutes in 200 mL water of 15°C to 25°C (USP refers to this test in Ph. Eur.).

USP:

Tests that are considered specific to the type of granules include but are not limited to volatile content (⟨731⟩, ⟨921⟩) or powder fineness. Regarding the disintegration for effervescent granules, the USP refers to the Ph. Eur. (see above).

JP:

- Uniformity of dosage units: Unless otherwise specified, granules in single-dose packages meet the requirements of Uniformity of Dosage Units JP 6.02
- Dissolution, Disintegration: Unless otherwise specified, granules comply with Dissolution Test JP 6.10 or Disintegration Test JP 6.09. However, this requirement is not to be applied to effervescent granules, which are dissolved before use. If ≥90% of the granules are smaller than 500 μm (sieve test according JP 6.03) the Disintegration Test JP 6.09 is not required.

6. Ph. Eur. Semi-solid preparations for cutaneous application (Praeparationes molles ad usum dermicum)

USP ⟨3⟩ Topical and transdermal drug products—product quality tests

USP ⟨1724⟩ Semisolid drug products—performance tests

JP [2] 11 Preparations for cutaneous application

Semi-solid preparations for cutaneous application are spreadable systems for local or transdermal delivery of active ingredients. The USP stresses that semi-solid dosage forms may be considered extended-release preparations, and their drug release depends largely on the formulation and manufacturing process (⟨1724⟩).

The following categories are distinguished in the Ph. Eur. (The classification of semi-solid preparations for cutaneous application according to USP and JP is shown in Table A-1):

- Ointments
- Creams
- Gels
- Pastes
- Poultices
- Medicated plasters
- Cutaneous patches

Additionally, USP chapter ⟨1151⟩ also mentions lotions as emulsified liquid dosage forms intended for external application to the skin.

Semi-solid preparations for cutaneous application consist of a simple compound basis in which, usually, one or more active substances are dissolved or dispersed. Also covered by this monograph are drug-containing adhesive plasters (medicated plasters), consisting of a flexible adhesive film containing one or more active substances, spread as a uniform layer. The drug-containing basis may be a single- or multiphase systems with hydrophilic of hydrophobic properties. It may influence the activity of the preparation but may also display a skin-softening respectively -protecting activity by itself. Semi-solid preparations for cutaneous application may contain suitable excipients such as preservatives, antioxidants, stabilizers, emulsifiers, thickeners, and penetration enhancers.

Preparations for application on large open wounds or severely damaged skin are sterile.

Ointments

Ointments consist of a single-phase basis in which solids or liquids may be dispersed. According to USP ⟨1151⟩, ointments usually contain less than 20% water and volatiles, and more than 50% hydrocarbons, waxes, or polyols as the vehicle.

Hydrophobic ointments
Hydrophobic ointments have only limited water-uptake capacity. They are typically prepared from hard, liquid and light liquid paraffins, vegetable oils, animal fats, synthetic glycerides, waxes and liquid polyalkysiloxanes. With particular regard to the first mentioned substances, USP chapter ⟨1151⟩ describes "Hydrocarbon bases" (= "Oleaginous ointment bases") for the preparation of ointments which allow the incorporation of only small amounts of water and are used as occlusive dressings or to provide prolonged contact of the drug substance with the skin.

Water-emulsifying ointments
Water-emulsifying ointments are hydrophobic ointments containing an emulsifier of either the W/O type (wool alcohols, sorbitan esters, monoglycerides, fatty alcohols) or of the O/W type (sulfated fatty alcohols, polysorbates, macrogol cetostearyl ethers, esters of fatty acids with macrogols). USP chapter ⟨1151⟩ describes "Absorption bases" which allow the incorporation of aqueous solutions by formation of semi-solid systems of the W/O type and "Water-removable bases" which can be diluted with water and may be readily washed from the skin in the form of O/W emulsions.

Hydrophilic ointments
Hydrophilic ointments consist of bases that are miscible with water. As a rule, they consist of a mixture of liquid and solid macrogols. They may contain appropriate amounts of water. In USP chapter ⟨1151⟩ the bases for this type of ointments are termed "Water-soluble bases" or "Greaseless ointment bases."

Creams

Creams are multiphase preparations consisting of a lipophilic and an aqueous phase. As detailed in USP chapter ⟨1151⟩, they often contain more than 20% water and volatiles, and/or typically contain less than 50% hydrocarbons, waxes, or polyols as the vehicle for the drug substance. Creams can be formulated as either a water-in-oil emulsion (lipophilic cream) or as an oil-in-water emulsion (hydrophilic cream).

Lipophilic creams
In lipophilic creams the continuous phase is lipophilic. They contain W/O emulsifiers such as wool alcohols, sorbitan esters, and monoglycerides.

Hydrophilic creams

In case of hydrophilic creams the continuous phase is aqueous. They contain O/W emulsifiers such as sodium soaps or trolamine soaps, sulfated fatty alcohols, polysorbates and polyoxyl fatty acid and fatty alcohol esters combined, if necessary, with W/O emulsifiers.

Gels

Gels consist of liquids gelled by means of suitable gelling agents. As outlined in USP ⟨1151⟩, gels can be classed either as single-phase or two-phase systems. Two-phase gels consist of a network of small discrete particles (e.g., aluminum hydroxide gel) and may be thixotropic. They should be shaken before use to ensure homogeneity and should be so labeled. Single-phase gels consist of organic macromolecules uniformly distributed throughout a liquid in such a manner that no apparent boundaries exist between the dispersed macromolecules and the liquid. Single-phase gels made from natural gums (e.g., tragacanth) are also called mucilages. Jellies are types of gels that typically have a higher water content.

Lipophilic gels

Lipophilic gels (oleogels) are in general composed of liquid paraffin with polyethylene or fatty oils gelled with colloidal silica or aluminum or zinc soaps.

Hydrophilic gels

The bases of hydrophilic gels (hydrogels) usually consist of water, glycerol or propylene glycol; these are gelled with suitable gelling agents such as poloxamers, starch, cellulose derivatives, carbomers or magnesium-aluminum silicates.

Pastes

Pastes contain large proportions of solids (20-50%) finely dispersed in the basis. While in the Ph. Eur. "Pastes" represent a subchapter of semi-solid preparations for cutaneous application, in USP chapter ⟨1151⟩ the section "Pastes" includes also dental pastes and orally administered pastes for veterinary use.

Poultices

Poultices consist of a hydrophilic, heat-retentive basis in which solid or liquid active substances are dispersed. They are usually spread thickly on a suitable dressing and heated prior to application on the skin.

Medicated plasters

In case of medicated plasters the basis containing an adhesive agent and one or more active ingredients is spread as a uniform layer on a flexible carrier film. A protective liner, which is removed prior to use, covers the adhesive layer. When removed, the protective liner should not detach the preparation from the carrier film. Medicated plasters are designed to maintain the active substances in close contact with the skin such that these may be absorbed slowly or exert a protective or keratolytic effect. In USP chapter ⟨1151⟩ this dosage form is described in the subchapter "Plasters," where it is mentioned that this term is not preferred and should not be used for new drug product titles.

Cutaneous patches

Cutaneous patches are virtually identical to "Medicated plasters" except for the fact that they are intended to act locally.

Lotions

Lotions (USP <1151>) are not included in the dosage forms listed in Ph. Eur.

Share many characteristics with creams. The distinguishing feature is that they are more fluid than semisolid and thus pourable. Nevertheless, in USP chapter ⟨1724⟩ they are classified as semi-solid dosage forms.

Tests

Ph. Eur.:

- □ Uniformity of dosage units: Semi-solid preparations that are supplied either in in single-dose containers or in metered-dose containers and that are intended to achieve a systemic effect by transdermal delivery of the active substance(s) comply with the test for uniformity of dosage units (Ph. Eur. 2.9.40). When the active substance is dissolved in the base, the preparation is tested for mass variation; when the active substance is suspended, the preparation is tested for content uniformity.
- □ Sterility: Where the label indicates that the preparation is sterile it complies with the test for sterility (Ph. Eur. 2.6.1).
- □ Dissolution: For medicated plasters and cutaneous patches a suitable test may be required to demonstrate the appropriate release of the active substance(s), for example, one of the tests described in "Dissolution test for transdermal patches (Ph. Eur. 2.9.4).

USP:

Specific quality tests for topically applied drug products ⟨3⟩, to be considered on a case-by-case basis:

- □ Uniformity of dosage units (single-unit containers) ⟨905⟩
- □ Water content ⟨921⟩
- □ Microbial enumeration tests (nonsterile products) ⟨61⟩
- □ Tests for specified organisms (nonsterile products) ⟨62⟩
- □ Antimicrobial preservative content: Acceptance criteria for antimicrobial preservative content in multidose products should be established based on the levels necessary to pass the antimicrobial effectiveness testing ⟨51⟩
- □ Antioxidant content: If antioxidants are present in the drug product, tests of their content should be established
- □ Sterility: For sterile products (e.g., application to open wounds or burned areas), sterility of the product should be demonstrated (Sterility Tests ⟨71⟩)
- □ pH: When applicable, topically applied drug products should be tested for pH at the time of batch release and at designated stability time points for batch-to-batch monitoring.
- □ Particle size: The particle size of the active drug substance(s) in topically applied drug products (e.g., pastes) is usually determined and controlled at the formulation development stage. Topically applied drug products should be examined for evidence of particle size alteration.

Specific test for topically applied semi-solid drug products ⟨3⟩ include:

- □ Apparent viscosity
- □ Uniformity in containers

USP ⟨1724⟩ includes detailed descriptions of product performance tests for the assessment of drug release from creams, ointments, lotions, and gels:

- □ Drug release rate determination using vertical diffusion cell apparatus

  The USP describes three models (A, B, and C) of vertical diffusion cells, all of them being modifications of the diffusion cell according to Franz (see Fig. 15.28). The drug product sample and the receptor medium are separated by a synthetic, inert, highly permeable membrane. The experiment is carried out at $32 \pm 1°C$, generally over a 4-6 h time period.

□ Drug release rate determination using immersion cell apparatus

The immersion cell apparatus (enhancer cell), of which two different models (A and B) are described, is composed of a cylindrical sample compartment designed as a circular space (with variable depth in case of model A) within a cylindrical cell body, covered on the upper side by a (usually) synthetic membrane in order to retain the sample in the sample compartment. The membrane is secured to the cell body by a ring. The inner diameter of this ring determines the contact area between the membrane and the receptor medium. The immersion cell can be used with USP Apparatus 2 (⟨711⟩, Dissolution), equipped, most commonly, with 150 or 200 mL vessels. In order to fit into these vessels, the standard paddle has to be replaced by a smaller one. Before starting the test the medium is heated to $32 \pm 0.5°C$ and the immersion cell is placed at the bottom of the vessel with the membrane upside.

□ Drug release determination using USP Apparatus 4 (Flow-through cell)

Apparatus 4, described in ⟨711⟩ (Dissolution), also may be used for the determination of the drug release rate from creams, ointments, lotions, and gels by equipping it with an adapter for semisolid dosage forms. The adapter consists of a cylindrical, cup-shaped sample reservoir (available in different sizes for 400 to 1200 μL product volume). Its opening is covered by a membrane, which is held by a retaining ring, screwed onto the sample reservoir. After loading it with the sample and closing it with the membrane ring the adapter is inserted into the 22.6 mm (internal diameter) flow-through cell with the membrane facing downward. Three spacer ribs on the outside of the ring allow the flowing medium to bypass the adapter. The medium (volume sufficient to achieve sink conditions, typically 50 to 1000 mL) is heated to $32 \pm 0.5°C$ and usually circulated between the cell and a reservoir (closed system), however if appropriate, an open system can be used. Sampling may be performed either manually or automatically from the medium reservoir.

JP:

The sections "Ointments," "Creams," and "Gels" in JP [2] do not contain any reference to a pharmacopial test.

7. Ph. Eur. Capsules (Capsulae)

USP ⟨2⟩ Oral drug products—Product quality tests

USP ⟨1094⟩ Capsules—Dissolution testing and related quality attributes

JP [2] 1 Preparations for oral administration

Capsules according to these monographs are solid single-dose drug preparations intended for oral administration. This definition excludes microcapsules as well as rectal or vaginal capsules. The capsule contains an active substance or a preparation containing such substance enclosed in a hard or soft shell made of gelatin or other substances such as a cellulose derivatives or unleavened bread usually from rice flour capable of being dissolved by the digestive fluids.

The following capsule types are distinguished in the Ph. Eur. (the classification of capsules according to USP and JP is shown in Table A-1):

□ Hard capsules

□ Soft capsules

□ Gastro-resistant capsules

□ Modified-release capsules

□ Cachets

The consistency of the capsule shell can be adjusted by addition of substances such as glycerol or sorbitol. Further excipients may comprise surface-active agents, opaque fillers, antimicrobial preservatives, sweeteners, coloring matter and flavoring substances. The capsules may bear surface markings, such as a printed text. The content of the capsule may be solid, liquid or of paste-like consistency. It consists of one or more active substances with or without excipients such as solvents, diluents, lubricants or disintegrating agents. The contents should not cause deterioration of the shell.

Hard capsules

The shell of hard capsules consists of two prefabricated cylindrical sections, each of with has one rounded, closed end and one open end. The drug preparation is usually filled in a solid form (powder or granules), occasionally as an oily fluid or a paste-like mass into one of the sections that is then closed by slipping the other section over it.

Soft capsules

The shells of these capsules are thicker than those of hard capsules and consist of a single part. They are usually formed, filled and sealed in one operation, but for extemporaneous use the shell may be prefabricated. The shell material may contain an active substance. Liquids may be enclosed directly; solids are usually dissolved or dispersed in a suitable vehicle to give a solution or dispersion of a past-like consistency. Dependent on the nature of the materials and the surfaces in contact partial migration of the constituents from the capsule contents into the shell and vice versa may occur.

Modified-release capsules

Modified-release capsules are either hard or soft capsules with a modified rate, place or time at which the active substance is released (including prolonged-release and delayed-release). This is achieved by application of special excipients or special production processes of either the capsule shell or its contents. The appropriate release characteristics need to be demonstrated by a suitable test.

Gastro-resistant capsules

Gastro-resistant capsules are delayed-release capsules that are resistant to gastric fluid and are intended to release their active substance(s) in the intestinal fluid. They are prepared by filling capsules with granules or particles covered with a gastro-resistant coating or by providing hard or soft capsules with a gastro-resistant shell (enteric capsules). Proper disintegration or release characteristics need to be demonstrated by a suitable test.

Cachets

Cachets consist of two prefabricated flat cylindrical sections made of unleavened bread, which are fitted into each other. They contain a single dose of one or more active substances. To facilitate swallowing, cachets are immersed in water for few seconds prior to administration.

Tests

Ph. Eur.:

- Uniformity of dosage units: Capsules comply with the test for uniformity of dosage units (Ph. Eur. 2.9.40) or, where justified and authorized, with the tests for uniformity of content (Ph. Eur. 2.9.6) and/or uniformity of mass (Ph. Eur. 2.9.5), as described below.
- Uniformity of content: Capsules with a content of active substance less than 2 mg or less than 2% of the fill mass comply with test B for uniformity of content of single dose preparations (Ph. Eur. 2.9.6).

- □ Uniformity of mass: Capsules comply with the test for uniformity of mass of single dose preparations (Ph. Eur. 2.9.5) If the test for uniformity of content is prescribed for all the active substances, the test for uniformity of mass is not required.
- □ Dissolution: Gastro-resistant capsules prepared from granules or particles already covered with a gastro-resistant coating and modified-release capsules are subjected to a suitable test to demonstrate the appropriate release of the active substance(s), for example, the test described in Ph. Eur. 2.9.3 "Dissolution test for solid dosage forms."
- □ Disintegration: Hard capsules, soft capsules, and gastro-resistant capsules comply with the test for disintegration of tablets and capsules (Ph. Eur. 2.9.1). In case of hard and soft capsules the test is performed with water, or, when justified and authorized, with 0.1 M HCl or artificial gastric juice R as liquid medium. Gastro-resistant capsules with a gastro-resistant shell are tested for 2 h in 0.1 M HCl and must not disintegrate or rupture during this period. Subsequently the liquid is replaced by phosphate buffer solution pH 6.8 R (if justified and authorized with added pancreas powder) and the test is continued for 60 minutes.

USP:

The USP includes more than 250 monographs of capsule formulations for different drug substances. Required tests and specification limits are defined individually in each of these monographs. In addition, the general information chapter ⟨1094⟩ provides basic information on dissolution testing, particularly on dissolution procedure development, method validation, and critical quality attributes.

JP:

Uniformity of dosage units: Unless otherwise specified, capsules meet the requirements of Uniformity of Dosage Units JP 6.02

Dissplution, Disintegration: Unless otherwise specified, capsules meet the requirements of Dissolution Test JP 6.10 or Disintegration Test JP 6.09

8. Ph. Eur. Chewing gums, medicated (Masticabilia gummis medicata)

JP [2] 1 Preparations for oro-mucosal application

Medicated chewing gums are solid single-dose preparations, which release the active substance(s) in the saliva by chewing. They are not intended to be swallowed. Medicated chewing gums are used to deliver therapeutic agents for local action in the mouth or for systemic delivery after absorption through the buccal mucosa or from the gastrointestinal tract. The formulation bases are tasteless, masticatory gums that consist of natural or synthetic elastomers. The most widely used is polyisobutylene. Others are polyisoprene, isobutylene-isoprene copolymer, styrene butadiene rubber, polyvinyl acetate, polyethylene, ester gums, or polyterpenes. The gum base is mixed with the active substance(s) and excipients such as fillers, softeners, sweetening agents, flavoring substances, stabilizers, plasticizers and coloring matter and then processed by means of compression, softening or melting to obtain the desired presentation.

Tests

Ph. Eur.:
- □ Uniformity of dosage units: Medicated chewing gums comply with the test for uniformity of dosage units (Ph. Eur. 2.9.40) or, where justified and authorized, with the tests for uniformity of content (Ph. Eur. 2.9.6) and/or uniformity of mass (Ph. Eur. 2.9.5), as described below.
- □ Uniformity of content: Medicated chewing gums with a content of active substance less than 2 mg or less than 2% relative to total mass, comply with the test A for uniformity of content (Ph. Eur. 2.9.6).

◻ Uniformity of mass: Drug-containing chewing gums (except coated drug-containing chewing gums) comply with the test for uniformity of mass (Ph. Eur. 2.9.5). This test is not required if the test on uniformity of content is prescribed for all active substances.

◻ Dissolution test for medicated chewing gums (Ph. Eur. 2.9.25): Two different apparatus are described in the Ph. Eur.:

Apparatus A consists of a 40 ml chewing chamber into which two horizontal pistons plunge from opposite directions. The pistons move with a frequency of 60 cycles per minute synchronically towards each other and can simultaneously rotate around their axis thus simulating the chewing process. A third, vertically positioned piston, the so-called tongue, is pushed into the chewing chamber every time the two horizontal pistons move away from each other. This provides for a longitudinal deformation of the horizontally compressed sample. The chewing chamber is thermostated at 37°C and contains 20 mL buffer solution with a pH of 6.0, approximately corresponding to that in the oral cavity. After an accurately weighed gum sample is placed in the chamber, the equipment is set in motion.

Apparatus B consists of a cylindrical thermostated (37°C) test cell, sealed at the bottom with a flat base chamber that carries the lower chewing surface and of a vertical axis with the upper chewing surface plunging into the upper opening of the cell. The distance between the upper and the lower chewing surface may be set up to 5 mm. In order to prevent the gum from sliding during mastication, the lower surface is designed as a small bowl with a flat bottom and an angled brim. The assembly of the test cell and the base chamber is mounted on a device that performs an up-and-down chewing motion (typically 60 chews per minute). The axis of the upper chewing surface is connected to a revolving device performing a rotary motion of about 20°. After the test cell is filled with 20 mL of buffer solution of pH 6.0 the gum sample is placed on the lower surface and the machine is started.

In both methods at fixed time intervals samples are taken from the dissolution medium to determine the amount of released active substance.

9. Ph. Eur. Parenteral preparations (Parenteralia)

USP ⟨1⟩ Injections and implanted drug products (parenterals)—Product quality tests

JP [2] 3 Preparations for injection

Parenterals are sterile preparations intended for injection, infusion or implantation into the human or animal body. The requirements of the Ph. Eur. monograph "Parenteral preparations" do not necessarily apply to products derived from human blood, to immunological or radiopharmaceutical preparations or certain preparations for veterinary use. In the USP the definitions for sterile preparations for parenteral use generally do not apply in the case of the biologics (special requirements for biologics are detailed in chapter "Biologics" ⟨1041⟩).

Classification according to Ph. Eur.

According to Ph. Eur., the following categories of preparations may be distinguished:

◻ Injections
◻ Infusions
◻ Concentrates for injections or infusions
◻ Powders for injections or infusions
◻ Gels for injections
◻ Implants

Classification according to USP

The USP distinguishes the following categories in chapter $\langle 1 \rangle$ (Injections and implanted drug products (parenterals)—Product quality tests):

- Solutions
- Sterile Powders for Solutions
- Suspensions
- Liposomes
- Sterile Powders for Suspensions
- Emulsions
- Implants
- Drug-Eluting Stents

Classification according to JP

According to JP (chapter [2], Monographs for preparations), the following categories of preparations are distinguished:

- Parenteral infusions
- Implants/Pellets
- Prolonged release injections

Deviating from the Ph. Eur. and JP nomenclature, the USP chapter "Injections" $\langle 1 \rangle$ covers both, preparations to be administered by injection as well as those to be administered by infusion. JP indicates that parenteral infusions are usually injections of not less than 100 mL, intended for intravenous administration.

Parenteral preparations comply with test for sterility. They may require the use of excipients, for example to make the preparation isotonic with respect to blood, to adjust the pH, to increase the solubility, to stabilize the active substances or to ensure sterility. The added excipients should not adversely affect the intended medicinal action nor should they, at the concentration used, cause toxicity or undue local irritation.

For aqueous injections in multidose containers the addition of a suitable preservative is required except when the preparation itself has adequate antimicrobial properties. Also in case of aqueous injections which are prepared using aseptic precautions and which cannot be terminally sterilized the addition of a preservative is recommended. However, antimicrobial preservation is not permitted when the volume of a single dose exceeds 15 mL, which is particularly the case for all infusions. Antimicrobial preservatives must also not be added when for medical reasons addition of a preservative is prohibited, such as in case of epidural, intrathecal, intracisternal or intra- or retro-ocular administration. Suspensions for injection may show sediment that should be readily dispersed upon shaking. Emulsions for injection or infusion should not show any evidence of phase separation. Apart from implants and authorized cases, parenterals must be filled, as far as possible, in containers that are sufficiently transparent to allow the visual inspection of their contents. As a rule, these include ampoules, vials, bottles, cartridges, and prefillable syringes made from glass or plastics as well as plastic bags. The containers have to comply with the requirements specified in the pharmacopeias, for example, in the Ph. Eur. monographs "Materials used for the manufacture of containers" (Ph. Eur. 3.1 and subsections) and "Containers" (Ph. Eur. 3.2 and subsections). The container does not interact physically or chemically with the contents in a way that alters their quality beyond the specified and tolerated limits.

Glass ampoules are sealed containers, that is, they are closed by fusion of the material of the container. They are intended for single use. Vials are glass or plastic containers that are sealed by elastomeric stoppers that ensure a good seal, prevent the access of microorganisms and other contaminants and usually permit the withdrawal of a part or the whole of the contents without the removal of the closure. The plastic materials or the elastomers used to manufacture the closures should permit perforation with a needle with the least possible shedding of particles. Closures for multidose containers are sufficiently elastic to ensure that the puncture is resealed when the needle is withdrawn. The volume of an infusion or of an injection in a single-dose container must be sufficiently large to permit the withdrawal and the administration of the nominal dose using a normal technique (Ph. Eur. 2.9.17).

According to USP ⟨1151⟩ emulsions intended for parenteral administration generally do not contain any preservatives.

Injections

Injections are sterile solutions, emulsions or suspensions. They are prepared by dissolving, emulsifying, or suspending the active substance(s) and any added excipients in water, in a suitable, non-aqueous liquid or in a mixture of these vehicles.

Infusions

Infusions are sterile, aqueous solutions or oil-in-water emulsions. They are usually isotonic with respect to blood and principally intended to be administered in large volume. They do not contain any added antimicrobial preservative.

Concentrates for injections and infusions

Concentrates for injections and infusions are concentrated sterile solutions, which are intended for injection or infusion after dilution to a prescribed volume with a prescribed liquid.

Powders for injections and infusions

Powders for injections and infusions are solid sterile substances, distributed in their final containers, which, when shaken with the prescribed volume of a prescribed sterile liquid, rapidly form either clear and practically particle-free solutions or uniform suspensions. Freeze-dried products for parenteral administration are considered as powders for injections or infusions.

Gels for injections

Gels for injections are sterile gels with a viscosity suitable to guarantee a modified release of the active substance(s) at the site of injection.

Implants

Implants are sterile, solid preparations of a size and shape suitable for parenteral implantation and release of the active substance(s) over an extended period of time. Each dose is provided in a sterile container.

USP chapter ⟨1151⟩ describes several types of implants:

Pellet implants are small, sterile, solid masses composed of a drug substance with or without excipients. They are usually administered by means of a suitable special injector (e.g., trocar) or by surgical incision. Release of the drug substance from pellets is typically controlled by diffusion and dissolution kinetics.

Resorbable microparticles are a type of implant that provides extended release of a drug substance over periods varying from a few weeks to months. They can be administered subcutaneously or intramuscularly for systemic delivery, or they may be deposited in a desired location in the body for site-specific delivery. Injectable resorbable microparticles (or microspheres) generally range from 20 to 100 μm in diameter. They are composed of a drug substance dispersed within a biocompatible, bioresorbable polymeric excipient (matrix). Poly(lactide-co-glycolide) polymers have been used frequently.

Polymer implants can be formed as a single-shaped mass such as a cylinder. The polymer matrix must be biocompatible, but it can be either biodegradable or nonbiodegradable. Shaped polymer implants are administered by means of a suitable special injector. Drug substance release can be controlled by the diffusion of the drug substance from the bulk polymer matrix or by the properties of a rate-limiting polymeric membrane coating.

Drug substance-eluting stents combine the mechanical effect of the stent to maintain arterial patency with the prolonged pharmacologic effect of the incorporated drug substance.

Tests

Ph. Eur.:

- Sterility: Parenteral preparations comply with the test for sterility (Ph. Eur. 2.6.1).
- Bacterial endotoxins/Pyrogens: Preparations for injections and infusions comply with a test for bacterial endotoxins (Ph. Eur. 2.6.14) or, where justified and authorized, with the test for pyrogens (Ph. Eur. 2.6.8) when intended for use in humans. Also concentrates and powders for injections and infusions comply with these requirements after dilution or suspension in a suitable volume of liquid. For preparations for veterinary use a test for bacterial endotoxins/pyrogens is only required when the volume of a single dose is ≥ 15 mL or is equivalent to a dose of ≥ 0.2 mL per kg of body mass.
- Visible particles: Solutions for injection or infusion must be visually clear and practically free from particles.
- Sub-visible particles: Solutions for injection or infusion must comply with the test "Particulate contamination: sub-visible particles" (Ph. Eur. 2.9.19). Radiopharmaceutical preparations and preparations for veterinary use with a nominal content which is ≤ 100 mL and equivalent to a dose of ≤ 1.4 mL per kg of body mass are exempt from these requirements. Higher limits may be appropriate in the case of preparations for subcutaneous or intramuscular injection. Preparations for which the label states that the product is to be used with a final filter are exempt from these requirements, provided that the filter delivers a solution that complies with the test.
- Uniformity of dosage units: Powders for injections or infusions, as well as single-dose suspensions for injection must comply with the test for uniformity of dosage units (Ph. Eur. 2.9.40) or, where justified and authorized, with the test on uniformity of content, as described below (Ph. Eur. 2.9.6) and, in case of powders for injection or infusion, with the test on uniformity of mass (Ph. Eur. 2.9.5).
- Uniformity of content: Powders for injections or infusions, as well as single-dose suspensions for injection with a content of active substance less than 2 mg or 2% of the total mass or with a unit mass ≤ 40 mg must comply with the test A for uniformity of content (Ph. Eur. 2.9.6).
- Uniformity of mass: Powders for injections or infusions must comply with the test for uniformity of mass of single-dose preparations (Ph. Eur. 2.9.5) (Not required if the test on uniformity of content is prescribed for all active substances).

USP:

USP chapter ⟨1⟩ (Injections and implanted drug products (parenterals)—Product quality tests) mentions the following tests for parenterals:

- Universal tests:
  - Identification
  - Assay (specific and stability-indicating test)
  - Impurities
  - Foreign and particulate matter:
    Each final container of all parenteral preparations should be inspected to the extent possible for the presence of observable foreign and particulate matter in its contents. Every container in which the contents show evidence of visible particulates

must be rejected. Large-volume injections for single-dose infusion and small-volume injections, and pharmacy bulk packages are subject to the light obscuration or microscopic procedures and limits set forth in "Particulate matter in injections" ⟨788⟩ unless otherwise specified in the individual monograph.

- ○ Visible Particulates in Injections ⟨790⟩
- ○ Subvisible Particulate Matter in Therapeutic Protein Injections ⟨787⟩
- ○ Particulate Matter in Injections ⟨788⟩
- • Sterility
  - ○ Sterility Tests ⟨71⟩
- • Bacterial endotoxins
  - ○ Bacterial endotoxin test ⟨85⟩
  - ○ Pyrogen test ⟨151⟩
- • Container content
  - ○ Container content for injections ⟨697⟩
- • Packaging systems

  The packaging system should meet the requirements in:
  - ○ Elastomeric closures for injections ⟨381⟩
  - ○ Packaging and storage requirements ⟨659⟩
  - ○ Containers—Glass ⟨660⟩
  - ○ Plastic packaging systems and their materials of construction ⟨661⟩
  - ○ Plastic materials of construction ⟨661.1⟩
  - ○ Plastic packaging systems for pharmaceutical use ⟨661.2⟩
  - ○ Assessment of extractables associated with pharmaceutical packaging/delivery systems ⟨1663⟩
  - ○ Assessment of drug product leachables associated with pharmaceutical packaging/delivery systems ⟨1664⟩
- • Container-closure integrity
  - ○ Package integrity evaluation—Sterile products ⟨1207⟩
  - ○ Package integrity testing in the product life cycle—Test method selection and validation ⟨1207.1⟩
  - ○ Package integrity leak test technologies ⟨1207.2⟩
  - ○ Package seal quality test technologies ⟨1207.3⟩
- □ Specific tests:

  In addition to the universal tests listed above, the following specific tests may be necessary depending on the dosage form:
  - • Uniformity of dosage units
    - ○ Uniformity of dosage units ⟨905⟩
      (applicable to sterile powders for solutions, suspensions, implants, microparticles, and drug-eluting stents)
  - • Antimicrobial preservatives
    - ○ Antimicrobial agents—Content ⟨341⟩
      (applicable to solutions, suspensions, and in situ gels)
  - • Water content
    (applicable to sterile powders for solutions, e.g., freeze-dried products, and microparticles)
    - ○ Water determination ⟨921⟩
    - ○ Loss on drying ⟨731⟩
  - • Aluminum content
    (applicable to injections used in parenteral nutrition therapy for information related to specific labeling requirements)
  - • Particle size
    - ○ Globule size distribution in lipid injectable emulsions ⟨729⟩
      (applicable to emulsions and liposomes)
  - • Biological reactivity
    - ○ Biological reactivity tests, in vivo ⟨88⟩
      (applicable to drug-eluting stents)

JP:

- Bacterial endotoxins/Pyrogens: Unless otherwise specified, Injections and vehicles attached to preparations other than those used exclusively for intracutaneous, subcutaneous or intramuscular administration meet the requirements of Bacterial Endotoxins Test JP 4.01. In the case where the Bacterial Endotoxins Test JP 4.01 is not applicable, Pyrogen Test JP 4.04 may be applied instead.
- Sterility: Unless otherwise specified, injections and vehicles attached to preparations meet the requirements of Sterility Test JP 4.06.
- Material of the container: Containers of Injections meet the requirements of Test for Glass Containers for Injections JP 7.01 or the requirements of Test Methods for Plastic Containers JP 7.02.
- Material of the closure: Unless otherwise specified, rubber stoppers used for glass containers of 100 mL or more of aqueous infusions meet the requirements of Test for Rubber Closure for Aqueous Infusions JP 7.03.
- Foreign and particulate matter: Unless otherwise specified, injections and vehicles attached to preparations meet the requirements of Foreign Insoluble Matter Test for Injections JP 6.06 and of Insoluble Particulate Matter Test for Injections JP 6.07.
- Extractable volume: Unless otherwise specified, the actual volume of injections meets the requirements of test for extractable volume of parenteral preparations JP 6.05.
- Uniformity of dosage units: Unless otherwise specified, injections to be dissolved or suspended before use as well as implants and pellets meet the requirements of Uniformity of Dosage Units JP 6.02.
- Particle size: The maximum size of particles observed in suspensions for injection is usually not larger than 150 µm, and that of particles in emulsions for injection is usually not larger than 7 µm.

10. Ph. Eur. Powders, oral (Pulveres perorales)

USP ⟨2⟩ Oral drug products—product quality tests

JP [2] 1 Preparations for oral administration

Oral powders consist of solid, loose, dry particles of varying degree of fineness containing one or more active substances. They are either swallowed directly or administered in or with water or another suitable liquid. Oral powders are presented as single-dose or multidose preparations; the latter require the provision of a measuring device. Single-dose powders are mostly packaged in sachets or vials. Effervescent powders generally contain acid substances and carbonates or hydrogen carbonates which react rapidly in the presence of water to release carbon dioxide. They are dissolved or dispersed in water before administration.

Tests

Ph. Eur.:

- Uniformity of dosage units: Single-dose oral powders must comply with the test for uniformity of dosage units (Ph. Eur. 2.9.40) or, where justified and authorized, with the test for uniformity of content (Ph. Eur. 2.9.6) and/or uniformity of mass (Ph. Eur. 2.9.5), as described below.
- Uniformity of content: Single-dose oral powders with a content of active substance less than 2 mg or less than 2% of the total mass, must comply with test B for uniformity of content of single-dose preparations (Ph. Eur. 2.9.6).
- Uniformity of mass: Single-dose oral powders must comply with the test on uniformity of mass of single-dose preparations (Ph. Eur. 2.9.5) (Not required if the test on uniformity of content is prescribed for all active substances).

USP:

The following specific tests for powders are listed in USP chapter ⟨2⟩ (Oral drug products—product quality tests):

□ Minimum fill (specifications of ⟨755⟩ that apply to oral powders)
□ Volatile content (⟨731⟩ and ⟨921⟩)

JP:

□ Uniformity of dosage units: Unless otherwise specified, powders in single-dose packages meet the requirements of Uniformity of Dosage Units JP 6.02
□ Dissolution: Unless otherwise specified, powders meet the requirements of Dissolution Test JP 6.10

11. Ph. Eur. Powders for cutaneous application (Pulveres ad usum dermicum)

USP ⟨3⟩ Topical and transdermal drug products—product quality tests

JP [2] 11 Preparations for cutaneous application

Powders for cutaneous application are preparations consisting of solid, loose, dry particles that are free from grittiness and contain one or more active substances, with or without excipients. They are presented as single-dose powders or multidose preparations. Powders specifically intended for use on large open wounds or on severely injured skin must be sterile. Multidose powders for cutaneous application may be dispensed in sifter-top containers, containers equipped with a mechanical spraying device or in pressurized containers.

Tests

Ph. Eur.:

□ Fineness: If prescribed, the fineness of a powder is determined by the sieve test (Ph. Eur. 2.9.35) or another appropriate method.
□ Uniformity of dosage units: Single-dose powders for cutaneous application must comply with the test for uniformity of dosage units (Ph. Eur. 2.9.40) or, where justified and authorized, with the test for uniformity of content (Ph. Eur. 2.9.6) and/or uniformity of mass (Ph. Eur. 2.9.5), as described below.
□ Uniformity of content: Single-dose powders for cutaneous application with a content of active substance of less than 2 mg or 2% of the total mass, must comply with test B for uniformity of content of single-dose preparations (Ph. Eur. 2.9.6).
□ Uniformity of mass: Single-dose powders for cutaneous application must comply with the test for uniformity of mass of single-dose preparations (Ph. Eur. 2.9.5). If the test for uniformity of content is prescribed for all the active substances, the test for uniformity of mass is not required.
□ Sterility: Where the label indicates that the preparation is sterile, it must comply with the test for sterility (Ph. Eur. 2.6.1).

USP:

Specific quality tests for topically applied drug products ⟨3⟩, to be considered on a case-by-case basis:

□ Uniformity of dosage units (single-unit containers) ⟨905⟩
□ Microbial enumeration tests (nonsterile products) ⟨61⟩
□ Tests for specified organisms (nonsterile products) ⟨62⟩
□ Antimicrobial preservative content: Acceptance criteria for antimicrobial preservative content in multidose products should be established based on the levels necessary to pass the antimicrobial effectiveness testing ⟨51⟩

- ▫ Antioxidant content: If antioxidants are present in the drug product, tests of their content should be established
- ▫ Sterility: For sterile products (e.g., application to open wounds or burned areas), sterility of the product should be demonstrated (Sterility Tests ⟨71⟩)
- ▫ Particle size: The particle size of the active drug substance(s) in topically applied drug products is usually determined and controlled at the formulation development stage. Topically applied drug products should be examined for evidence of particle size alteration.

JP:
Uniformity of dosage units: Unless otherwise specified, powders for cutaneous application in single-dose packages meet the requirements of Uniformity of Dosage Units JP 6.02.

12. Ph. Eur. Foams, medicated (Musci medicati)

USP ⟨603⟩ Topical aerosols

JP [2] 11 Preparations for cutaneous application

Medicated foams are preparations consisting of large volumes of gas dispersed in a liquid, generally containing one or more active substances, various excipients and a surface-active substance ensuring foam formation. Usually medicated foams are formed at the time of administration from a liquid preparation in a pressurized container from which the preparation is delivered through a valve that is opened with a push button. The foam is generated by expansion of the gas when the preparation is escaping from the container. Medicated foams are usually intended for application to the skin or mucous membranes. The USP notes in chapter ⟨1151⟩ that they can be formulated to quickly break down into liquid or to remain as foam to ensure prolonged contact. Medicated foams intended for use on large open wounds or severely injured skin must be sterile.

Tests

Ph. Eur.:
  Mediated foams supplied in pressurized containers comply with the requirements of the Ph. Eur. monograph on "Pressurized pharmaceutical preparations."
- ▫ Relative foam density: A tared flat-bottomed dish with a volume of about 60 mL is uniformly filled with foam and excess foam is carefully removed with a slide. The completely filled dish is weighed again, then emptied and refilled with water and weighed once more. The mass ratio of the foam and the same volume of water is the relative foam density.
- ▫ Duration of expansion: The spray nozzle of the pressurized container is connected by means of a plastic tube to the outlet of a 50 ml burette. About 30 mL of foam is introduced into the burette in one single delivery, upon which the stopcock is closed. Immediately following this step, and subsequently at consecutive 10 second intervals, the growing foam volume in the burette is read until the maximum volume is reached. The time required to reach this stage is the expansion time. In none of three subsequent measurements this time should exceed 5 min.
- ▫ When the label indicates that the preparation is sterile, it must comply with the test for sterility (Ph. Eur. 2.6.1).

USP:
See section "Tests-USP" in chapter "3. Ph. Eur. Liquid preparations for cutaneous application."

13. Ph. Eur. Sticks (Styli)

USP ⟨4⟩ Mucosal drug products—product quality testes

Sticks are rod-shaped or conical, solid preparations for local application, for example for insertion into the urethra, vagina, nasal cavity, ear canal or into wounds. They contain one or more active substances that are dissolved or dispersed in a suitable basis which may dissolve or melt at body temperature. Sticks for application into the urethra or into wounds must be sterile.

In USP chapter ⟨1151⟩, solid dosage forms that are inserted into a naturally occurring (nonsurgical) body cavity other than the mouth or rectum are termed inserts.

Tests

Ph. Eur.:

    □ Uniformity of mass of single-dose preparations (Ph. Eur. 2.9.5).
    □ Uniformity of content of single-dose preparations (Ph. Eur. 2.9.6).
    □ Urethral sticks and sticks for insertion into wounds comply with the test for sterility (Ph. Eur. 2.6.1).

USP:
USP chapter ⟨4⟩ (Mucosal drug products—product quality tests) describes general tests for dosage forms administered on membrane surfaces, among others via the otic, nasal, urethral, and vaginal route. However, no product-specific tests for sticks are mentioned there.

14. Ph. Eur. Tablets (Compressi)

USP ⟨2⟩ Oral drug products—product quality tests

JP [2] 1 Preparations for oral administration

Tablets are solid preparations each containing a single dose of one or more active substances. They are obtained by compression of uniform volumes of powders or granules or by other techniques such as extrusion, molding or freeze-drying. As a rule, they are intended for oral application and are either intended to be swallowed whole or after being chewed; some are dissolved or dispersed in water prior to use, while others are retained in the mouth where the active substance is liberated. Tablets that are not used in any of these ways, like for example tablets for implantation or for inhalation solutions or as vaginal tablets do not necessarily need to comply with the descriptions and tests in this monograph. The powders or granules that are compressed into tablets consist of one or more active substances and, when required, excipients such as diluents, binders, disintegrating agents, glidants, lubricants, substances capable of modifying the behavior of the preparation in the digestive tract, coloring matter and flavoring substances. If necessary, the powder particles may be subjected to a pretreatment, for instance granulation. Tablets are flat or convex, may have break-marks, may bear a symbol or other markings and the edges may be beveled. The surface may be covered with a coating. They possess a suitable mechanical strength to withstand handling without breaking or crumbling. The following categories of tablets are distinguished in the Ph. Eur. (the classification of tablets according to USP and JP is shown in Table A-1):

    □ Uncoated tablets
    □ Coated tablets
    □ Gastro-resistant tablets
    □ Modified-release tablets
    □ Effervescent tablets
    □ Soluble tablets

- Dispersible tablets
- Orodispersible tablets
- Chewable tablets
- Oral lyophilisates

Uncoated tablets

The uncoated tablets include single-layer tablets obtained by a single-step compression of particles, and multilayer tablets, obtained by successive compression of particles of different composition. The excipients used are not specifically intended to modify the release of active substance in the digestive fluids. After compression, the tablets do not undergo further treatment. Under a magnifying glass a broken section shows either a uniform texture (single-layer tablets) or a stratified texture (multilayer tablets), but no signs of coating.

Coated tablets

Coated tablets are tablets coated with one or more layers of mixtures of various substances such as natural or synthetic resins, gums, gelatin, inactive and insoluble fillers, sugars, plasticizers, polyols, waxes, authorized coloring matter and sometimes flavoring substances and active substances. The substances used as coatings are usually applied as a solution or suspension in conditions in which evaporation of the vehicle occurs. Tablets with a thin coating are called film-coated tablets; tablets with a thicker, sugar-containing coating are referred to as dragées. Coated tablets have a smooth, often colored surface, which may be polished. Under a magnifying glass a broken section shows a core, surrounded by one or more continuous layers with a different texture.

Chewable tablets

Chewable tablets are intended to be chewed before swallowing.

Gastro-resistant tablets

Gastro-resistant tablets are delayed-release tablets that are resistant to gastric juice and intended to release their active substance(s) in the intestinal fluid. Usually they are prepared by covering tablets with a gastro-resistant coating or from granules or particles already covered with a gastro-resistant coating. Tablets covered with a gastro-resistant coating conform to the definition of "Coated tablets."

Modified–release tablets

Modified-release tablets are coated or uncoated tablets that contain special excipients or are prepared by special procedures designed to modify the rate, the place or the time at which the active substance(s) are released. Modified-release tablets include prolonged-release tablets, delayed-release tablets and pulsatile-release tablets.

Effervescent tablets

Effervescent tablets are uncoated tablets generally containing acid substances and carbonates or hydrogen carbonates, which react rapidly in the presence of water to release carbon dioxide. Prior to use they are dissolved or dispersed in water.

Soluble tablets

Soluble tablets are uncoated or film-coated tablets, which are intended to be dissolved in water prior to administration. The solution thus formed may be slightly opalescent.

Dispersible tablets

Dispersible tablets are uncoated or film-coated tablets, which are intended to be dispersed in water prior to administration, giving a homogeneous dispersion.

Orodispersible tablets

Orodispersible tablets are uncoated tablets that rapidly disperse in the mouth before being swallowed.

Tablets for use in the mouth

Tablets for use in the mouth are usually uncoated tablets. They are formulated to effect a slow release and a local action of the active substance(s) or the release and the absorption of the active substance(s) at a defined part of the mouth. They comply with the requirements of the Ph. Eur. monograph "Oromucosal preparations."

Oral lyophilizates

Oral lyophilizates are freeze-dried solid preparations that either dissolve in the oral cavity or are dispersed in water prior to administration.

Tests

Ph. Eur.:

- Uniformity of dosage units: Tablets comply with the test for uniformity of dosage units (Ph. Eur. 2.9.40) or where justified and authorized, with the tests for uniformity of content (Ph. Eur. 2.9.6) and/or uniformity of mass (Ph. Eur. 2.9.5), as described below.
- Uniformity of content: Tablets with a content of active substance less than 2 mg or less than 2% of the total mass as well as coated tablets other than film coated tablets irrespective of their content of active substance comply with test A for uniformity of content of single dose preparations (Ph. Eur. 2.9.6).
- Uniformity of mass: Tablets comply with the test for uniformity of mass of single dose preparations (Ph. Eur. 2.9.5). If the test for uniformity of content is prescribed for all the active substances, the test for uniformity of mass is not required.
- Dissolution: A suitable test may be carried out to demonstrate the appropriate release of the active substance(s), for example one of the tests described in Ph. Eur. 2.9.3. For modified-release tablets and gastro-resistant tablets produced from gastro-resistant coated granules or particles, the test is obligatory.
- Disintegration: A disintegration test may be not required when a dissolution test is prescribed.

  Under the conditions of the test on "Disintegration of tablets and capsules" (Ph. Eur. 2.9.1) uncoated tablets must have completely disintegrated in water after 15 min.

  Coated tablets, other than film-coated tablets, must have disintegrated within 60 min, film-coated tablets within 30 minutes. If any of the tablets has not disintegrated, the test is repeated on a further 6 tablets, replacing water with 0.1 M HCl. If maximally 2 tablets fail to disintegrate in HCl, the test may be repeated with another 12 tablets. The requirements are met if not fewer than 16 of the 18 tablets tested have disintegrated. In case of tablets covered with a gastro-resistant coating, the test should last for 2 h (or another such time as may be justified and authorized), with 0.1 M HCl as incubation medium. The tablets should not show any signs of disintegration, apart from fragments of the coating, nor any cracks that might allow the escape of contents. The time of resistance to the acid medium varies with the formulation of the tablets.

Typically it amounts to 2 to 3 hours, but even with authorized deviations it should not be less than 1 h. Subsequently the acid is replaced by phosphate buffer pH 6.8 and the incubation is continued for 60 minutes. The tablets fulfill the requirements when all 6 units have disintegrated within this time. Soluble tablets, dispersible tablets and orodispersible tablets disintegrate within 3 minutes in water under the conditions described in Ph. Eur. 2.9.1. For soluble tablets and dispersible tablets the test is performed at 15° to 25°C.

Disintegration of oral lyophilisates is tested by placing each of 6 units in a beaker containing 200 mL of water at 15° to 25°C. They comply with the test if all 6 have disintegrated within 3 minutes.

Also for testing of effervescent tablets, each of 6 tablets is placed in a glass beaker with 200 mL of water of 15°C to 25°C. When the evolution of gas around the tablet or its fragments ceases, the tablet should be dissolved or dispersed without any particle agglomerates remaining. The tablets comply with the test if each of the 6 tablets disintegrates within 5 minutes. The test on disintegration is not applicable to chewing tablets, modified-release tablets and tablets for use in the mouth.

□ Friability of uncoated tablets (Ph. Eur. 2.9.7).

□ Resistance to crushing of tablets (Ph. Eur. 2.9.8).

□ Fineness of dispersion (only for dispersible tablets): all particles of the dispersion should pass a sieve with a nominal mesh aperture of 710 μm.

□ Water: In case of oral lyophilisates water content is tested according to Ph. Eur. 2.5.12.

□ Subdivision of tablets: The subdivision of tablets bearing break-marks is assessed during the development of the product in respect of uniformity of mass of the subdivided parts. 30 randomly selected tablets are manually broken and from all the parts obtained from one tablet one part is taken for the test and all other parts are rejected. Each of the 30 parts is weighed individually and the average is calculated. The tablets fail the test if more than 1 individual mass is outside the limits of 85% to 115% of the average mass or if at least one individual mass is outside the limits of 75% to 125% of the average mass.

USP:

Specific test for tablets include:

□ Volatile content: When the presence of moisture or other volatile material may become critical, the amount of such kind of volatile matter has to be determined by "Loss of drying" (USP ⟨731⟩) or if water is the only volatile constituent by "Water determination" (USP ⟨921⟩). For gas chromatographic quantification of specific residuals solvents and for the definition of limits USP chapter ⟨731⟩ ("Residual solvents") should be consulted.

□ Disintegration: Disintegration is an essential attribute of oral solids, except for those intended to be chewed before being swallowed and for delayed- or extended-release products. A test method for disintegration is described in USP chapter ⟨701⟩ ("Disintegration"). Regarding special test methods for effervescent tablets, disintegrating tablets and soluble tablets the USP refers to the Ph. Eur. Chewable tablets are not required to comply with the disintegration test, however they should undergo dissolution testing, as a product performance test, because they might be swallowed without proper chewing by a patient.

□ Tablet friability: The friability test is applicable to most compressed, uncoated tablets (USP ⟨1216⟩, "Tablet friability")

□ Tablet beaking force: The test for "Tablet breaking force" is described in USP ⟨1217⟩

□ Uniformity of dosage units: Content uniformity is based on the assay of the indivvidual contents of drug substance(s) in a number of dosage units. Weight variation can be used as an altenative unter certain conditions (USP ⟨905⟩, "Uniformity of dosage units").

□ Dispersion fineness: Dispersion fineness is tested in case of disintegrating or dispersible tablets, tablets for oral solution and tablets for oral suspension. The method is described in the section above (Ph. Eur. test "Fineness of dispersion")

JP:

- □ Uniformity of dosage units: Unless otherwise specified, tablets meet the requirements of Uniformity of Dosage Units JP 6.02
- □ Dissplution, Disintegration: Unless otherwise specified, tablets meet the requirements of Dissolution Test JP 6.10 or Disintegration Test JP 6.09. For effervescent tablets from which active substance(s) are dissolved before use and soluble tablets, these tests are not required.

15. Ph. Eur. Tampons, medicated (Tamponae medicatae)

Medicated tampons are solid, single-dose preparations intended to be inserted into the body cavities for a limited period of time. They may consist for instance of cellulose, collagen or silicone impregnated with one or more active substances. Additional requirements may be found in specific corresponding Ph. Eur. monographs, such as "Rectal preparations," "Vaginal preparations," and "Ear preparations."

16. Ph. Eur. Patches, transdermal (Emplastra transcutanea)

USP ⟨3⟩ Topical and transdermal drug products—product quality tests

JP [2] 11 Preparations for cutaneous application

Transdermal patches (transdermal delivery systems) are flexible, multilayered drug-containing systems intended to be adhesively applied to the undamaged skin, in order to deliver the active substance(s) to the systemic circulation after passing through the skin barrier. In general they consist of an outer water-impermeable backing sheet, which is designed to support and protect the preparation. The drug-containing preparation, which may be a single- or multilayer solid or semi-solid matrix, is attached to the backing sheet. If this outer covering sheet is larger than the preparation, the overlapping border is covered by pressure-sensitive adhesives, which assure the adhesion of the preparation to the skin. For the same purpose also the matrix of the preparation may contain adhesive substances.

The release of the active ingredient is either determined by the diffusion-controlling composition and structure of the semi-solid matrix or by a membrane that covers the semi-solid drug reservoir on the side of the skin and controls the drug release. Also this membrane may be covered either fully or at selected sites with pressure-sensitive adhesive substances. At the side of the release surface the transdermal patch is covered with a protective liner consisting of a sheet of plastic or metal material that is removed before application to the skin. Removal of the strip should damage neither the preparation nor the adhesive layer. Normally the patches are individually enclosed in sealed sachets. The label states the total quantity of active substance(s) per patch as well as the dose released per unit time and the area of the releasing surface.

Tests

Ph. Eur.:

- □ Uniformity of dosage units: Transdermal patches must comply with the test for uniformity of dosage units (Ph. Eur. 2.9.40) or, where justified and authorized, with test C for uniformity of content (Ph. Eur. 2.9.6), as described below.
- □ Uniformity of content (Ph. Eur. 2.9.6): Transdermal patches comply with test C for uniformity of content of single-dose preparations.

□ Dissolution: A suitable test may be required to demonstrate the appropriate release of the active substances(s), for example one of the tests described in Ph. Eur. 2.9.4 ("Dissolution test for transdermal patches").

USP:

□ Uniformity of dosage units: USP ⟨905⟩ ("Uniformity of dosage units")

Adhesives in transdermal delivery systems must permit easy removal of the protective liner before use, must adhere properly to the skin during the period of use, ad must permit easy removal of the patch at the end of use. Three types of adhesion tests are described in the USP: peel adhesion test, release liner peel test, and tack test. Acceptance criteria are product-specific. The test should assure that adhesion of each released batch is within the range defined by the product design over the entire product's shelf life.

□ Peel adhesion test: The peel adhesion test measures the force required to remove a transdermal delivery system by peeling it away from a standard substrate with an instrument that allows control of peel angle and peel rate. The peel force is recorded for a minimum of five independent samples.

□ Release liner peel test: The release liner peel test measures the force required to separate the release liner from the adhesive layer of the transdermal delivery system with an instrument that allows control of peel angle and peel rate. The peel force is recorded for a minimum of five independent samples.

□ Tack test: The USP describes two methods of the tack test: the probe tack method and the rolling ball method.

 – Probe tack method: The probe tack method measures the force required to separate the tip of a stainless steel test probe of defined geometry and the transdermal delivery system using a controlled force and specified conditions (i.e., rate, contact time, contact pressure, temperature). This procedure is repeated using a minimum of five independent samples.

 – Rolling ball method: The rolling ball method measures the distance travelled by a defined ball from a ramp (with defined angle and length) on the adhesive layer under defined conditions, as a parameter dependent on the tack properties. This procedure is repeated using a minimum of five independent samples.

□ Leak test: The leak test is an in-process test only for form-fill-seal (reservoir or pouched)-type transdermal delivery systems. Form-fill-seal transdermal delivery systems must be manufactured with zero tolerance for leaks because of their potential for dose dumping if leakage occurs (e.g., in consequence of perforation, cuts, faulty seals, gel splash or misalignment of the layers). The test is carried out as a visual inspection (without pretreatment and after 13.6 kg weight-loading) combined with a wipe test in which a swab is assayed for the drug after the transdermal delivery system and the inside of the primary packaging was wiped).

JP:

□ Uniformity of dosage units: Unless otherwise specified, patches of transdermal systems meet the requirements of Uniformity of Dosage Units JP 6.02.

17. Ph. Eur. Intraruminal devices (Praeparationes intraruminales)

Intraruminal devices are solid preparations for oral application, which release the active substance(s) over periods extending from days to several weeks as a result of prolonged retention in the rumen. Currently available products even provide retention times of as much as 300 days. Release may occur in a continuous or pulsatile manner. Some preparations are intended to float on the surface of the ruminal fluid, while others are intended to settle to remain at the floor of the rumen or reticulum. The release of the active substance(s) may be controlled by erosion, corrosion, diffusion, osmotic pressure, or by means of any other chemical or physical process. A pulsatile pattern can be realized by sequential release from a composite unit consisting of multiple drug reservoirs.

Tests

Ph. Eur.:

  □ Uniformity of dosage units: Constituent tablet units of intraruminal devices comply with the test for uniformity of dosage units (Ph. Eur. 2.9.40) or, where justified and authorized, with the tests for uniformity of content (Ph. Eur. 2.9.6) and/or uniformity of mass (Ph. Eur. 2.9.5), as described below.

  □ Uniformity of content: Constituent tablet units of intraruminal devices with a content of active substance less than 2 mg or less than 2% active ingredient of the total mass, must comply with test A for uniformity of content (Ph. Eur. 2.9.6).

  □ Uniformity of mass: Constituent tablet units of intraruminal devices comply with the test for uniformity of mass (Ph. Eur. 2.9.5). If the test for uniformity of content is prescribed for all the active substances, the test for uniformity of mass is not required.

18. Ph. Eur. Pressurized pharmaceutical preparations (Praeparationes pharmaceuticae in vasis cum pressu)

USP ⟨601⟩ Inhalation and nasal drug products—Aerosols, sprays, and powders—Performance quality tests

USP ⟨603⟩ Topical aerosols

JP [2] 5 Preparations for inhalation

JP [2] 11 Preparations for cutaneous application

Pressurized pharmaceutical preparations are solutions, emulsions or suspensions containing one ore more active substances, which are presented in special containers under pressure of a gas. Upon actuating an appropriate valve the preparation is released in the form of an aerosol (dispersion of solid or liquid particles in a gas) or a liquid or semi-solid jet such as a foam. The pressure for the release is generated by suitable propellants, which are either gases liquefied under pressure or compressed gasses or low-boiling liquids or mixtures thereof. The preparations are intended for local application to the skin or to mucous membranes of various body orifices, or for inhalation. The size of the aerosol particles is adapted to the intended use. The spray characteristics are influenced among others by the type of the spraying device (e.g., dimensions, number and location of orifices). Some valves provide a continuous release, others ("metering dose valves") deliver a defined quantity of product upon each valve actuation. Additional requirements for preparations presented in pressurized containers may be found in other general monographs, for example "Preparations for inhalation," "Liquid preparations for cutaneous application," "Powders for cutaneous application," "Nasal preparations," "Ear preparations" and "Medicated foams."

Tests

Ph. Eur.:
The Ph. Eur. subchapter "Pressurized pharmaceutical preparations" does not describe any tests. Recommendations and instructions for testing may be found in the aforementioned general monographs.

USP:
Test required by the USP for topical aerosols are listed above in subchapter "3. Ph. Eur. Fluid Liquid preparations for cutaneous application." Tests for inhalation and nasal drug products

are detailed in subchapters "22. Ph. Eur. Preparations for inhalation" and "24. Ph. Eur. Nasal preparations."

19. Ph. Eur. Preparations for irrigation (Praeparationes ad irrigationem)

Preparations for irrigation are sterile, aqueous, large-volume preparations intended to be used for irrigation of body cavities, wounds, and surfaces, for example, during surgical procedures. Usually, these are isotonic solutions of one or more active substances, electrolytes or osmotically active substances in water for injection. However, the preparation may also consist of water for injection only. In that case the preparation may be labeled as "Water for irrigation." Preparations for irrigation are supplied in single-dose containers. According to Ph. Eur., the containers and closures comply with the requirements for containers for parenteral preparations but the administration port of the container is incompatible with intravenous administration equipment and does not allow the preparation for irrigation to be administered with such equipment.

Tests

Ph. Eur.:
- Visible particles: Examined in suitable conditions of visibility, preparations for irrigation are clear and practically free from particles.
- Withdrawable content: During the development it must be demonstrated the nominal content can be withdrawn from the container.
- Sterility: Preparations for irrigation comply with the test for sterility (Ph. Eur. 2.6.1).
- Bacterial endotoxins (Ph. Eur. 2.6.14): less than 0.5 I. E. bacterial endotoxins per mL.
- Pyrogens (Ph. Eur. 2.6.8): preparations that do not allow a validated test for bacterial endotoxins comply with the test for pyrogens.

20. Ph. Eur. Eye preparations (Ophthalmica)

USP ⟨4⟩ Mucosal drug products—product quality tests

USP ⟨751⟩ Metal particles in ophthalmic ointments

USP ⟨771⟩ Ophthalmic ointments

JP [2] 6 Preparations for opthalmic application

Eye preparations are sterile, liquid, semi-solid or solid preparations intended for administration upon the eyeball and/or to the conjunctiva, or for insertion in the conjunctival sac. The following categories may be distinguished, according to Ph. Eur. (the classification of eye preparations according to USP and JP is shown in Table A-1):
- Eye drops
- Eye lotions
- Powders for eye drops and powders for eye lotions
- Semi-solid eye preparations
- Ophthalmic inserts

Eye preparations must be prepared using materials and methods designed to ensure sterility and to avoid the introduction of contaminants and growth of microorganisms.

Aqueous eye drops or eye lotions supplied in multidose containers contain a suitable antimicrobial preservative except the preparation itself has adequate antimicrobial properties. If eye drops or eye lotions do not contain antimicrobial preservatives they are supplied in single-dose containers or in multidose containers preventing microbial contamination of the contents after opening. According to Ph. Eur., the label of multidose containers states the period after opening the container after which the contents must not be used (not exceeding 4 weeks unless otherwise justified and authorized). Eye drops or eye lotions intended for use in surgical procedures or eye lotions for first aid-treatment do not contain an antimicrobial preservative and are supplied in single-dose containers. Eye drops and eye lotions may contain excipients, for example, to adjust the tonicity or the viscosity of the preparation, to adjust the pH, to increase the solubility or to stabilize the preparation. Powders for eye drops and powders for eye lotions may additionally contain excipients to facilitate dissolution or dispersion. The excipients should not adversely affect the intended medicinal action of the active ingredient nor cause undue local irritation. The container material should not cause decomposition of the preparation due to release of foreign material into the preparation.

Eye drops

Eye drops are sterile aqueous or oily solutions, emulsions or suspensions of one or more active substances intended for instillation into the eye. Eye drops that are solutions are practically clear and practically free from particles upon visual inspection. Eye drops in the form of suspensions may show sediment that is readily redispersed on shaking. The suspension thus obtained remains sufficiently stable to enable the correct dose to be delivered. Ph. Eur. requests that containers for multidose preparations contain maximally a volume of 10 mL. Multi-dose containers should allow accurate dosing by administration of successive drops.

Eye lotions

Eye lotions are sterile aqueous solutions intended for use in rinsing or bathing the eye or to impregnate eye dressings. Eye lotions are practically clear and practically free from particles upon visual inspection. Ph. Eur. requests that containers for multidose preparations contain maximally a volume of 200 mL and that single-dose containers are provided with the label instruction that the contents are to be used on one occasion only.

Powders for eye drops and powders for eye lotions

Powders for eye drops and powders for eye lotions are sterile powders that are dissolved or suspended in an appropriate liquid vehicle at the time of administration. The obtained solution or suspension complies with the requirements for eye drops or eye lotions, as appropriate.

Semi-solid eye preparations

Semi-solid eye preparations are sterile ointments, creams or gels intended for application to the conjunctiva or the eyelids. They contain one or more active substances dissolved or dispersed in a suitable basis. According to Ph. Eur., they have a homogeneous appearance and comply with the requirements of the Ph. Eur. monograph "Semi-solid preparations for cutaneous application." The basis must be nonirritant to the conjunctiva. Semi-solid eye preparations are packed in small, sterilized collapsible tubes fitted or provided with a sterilized cannula. Ph. Eur. requests that the content must be maximally 10 g. The tubes must be well-closed to prevent microbial contamination. Semi-solid eye preparations may also be packed in single-dose containers. According to Ph. Eur., the label of multidose containers states the period after opening the container after which the contents must not be used (not exceeding 4 weeks unless otherwise justified and authorized).

Ophthalmic inserts

Ophthalmic inserts are sterile, solid or semi-solid preparations designed to be inserted in the conjunctival sac to produce an ocular effect. A reservoir of active substance is embedded in a matrix or bound by a rate-controlling membrane. The release proceeds for a predetermined period of time. Ophthalmic inserts are individually distributed into sterile containers.

Tests

Ph. Eur.:
- Sterility: Eye preparations as well as separately supplied applicators comply with the test for sterility (Ph. Eur. 2.6.1).
- Uniformity of dosage units: Single-dose powders for eye drops and eye lotions as well as ophthalmic inserts comply with the test for uniformity of dosage units (Ph. Eur. 2.9.40) or, where justified and authorized, with the tests on uniformity of content (Ph. Eur. 2.9.6) or in case of single-dose powders with the test on uniformity of mass (Ph. Eur. 2.9.5).
- Uniformity of content: Single-dose powders for eye drops and eye lotions with a content of active substance less than 2 mg or less than 2% of the total mass and ophthalmic inserts, where applicable, comply with the test for uniformity of content (Ph. Eur. 2.9.6) (powders: test B, inserts: test A).
- Uniformity of mass: Single-dose powders for eye drops and eye lotions comply with the test for uniformity of mass (Ph. Eur. 2.9.5). If the test for uniformity of content is prescribed for all the active substances, the test for uniformity of mass is not required.
- Particle size: Eye drops in the form of a suspension and semi-solid eye preparations containing dispersed solid particles comply with the following test: A thin layer of the preparation corresponding to at least 10 µg of solid active substance is scanned under the microscope. Not more than 20 particles have a maximum dimension greater than 25 µm and not more than 2 of these particles have a maximum dimension greater than 50 µm; no particle has a maximum dimension greater than 90 µm.

USP:
USP chapter ⟨4⟩ (Mucosal drug products—product quality tests) mentions the following tests for preparations administered by the ophthalmic route:
- General tests for drug products administered by the ophthalmic route:
  - Foreign and particular matter
  - Sterility
  - Particle size and particle size distribution
  - Antimicrobial preservative
- Product-specific tests for drug products administered by the ophthalmic route:
  - Gels: Minimum fill ⟨755⟩, Topical and transdermal drug products—product quality tests ⟨3⟩
  - Emulsions: Osmolality and osmolarity ⟨785⟩, pH ⟨791⟩, Surface tension, Viscosity—capillary method ⟨911⟩, Viscosity—rotational method ⟨912⟩, Zeta potential
  - Inserts: Bacterial endotoxin test ⟨85⟩
  - Ointments: Minimum fill ⟨755⟩, Topical and transdermal drug products—product quality tests ⟨3⟩
  - Solutions: Particulate matter in ophthalmic solutions ⟨789⟩, pH ⟨791⟩, Viscosity—capillary method ⟨911⟩, Viscosity—rotational method ⟨912⟩, Viscosity—rolling ball method ⟨913⟩, Osmolality and osmolarity ⟨785⟩
  - Suspensions: pH ⟨791⟩, Osmolality and osmolarity ⟨785⟩, Particle size and particle size distribution, Viscosity—capillary method ⟨911⟩, Viscosity—rotational method ⟨912⟩, Viscosity—rolling ball method ⟨913⟩
- Metal particles: USP chapter ⟨751⟩ describes a microscopic test for metal particles in ophthalmic ointment

□ Leakage of tubes: USP chapter ⟨711⟩ describes a test for leakage of tubes filled with ophthalmic ointments. A potential leakage is visually detected by placing 10 tubes on a blotting paper in an oven maintained at a temperature of 60°C for 8 hours.

JP:

□ Sterility: Unless otherwise specified, ophthalmic ointments, liquids and solutions and vehicles attached to the preparations meet the requirements of Sterility Test JP 4.06.

□ Foreign and particulate matter: Unless otherwise specified, ophthalmic liquids and solutions prepared in aqueous solutions or the vehicles attached to the preparations meet the requirements of Foreign Insoluble Matter Test for Ophthalmic Solutions JP 6.11 and of Insoluble Particulate Matter Test for Ophthalmic Solutions JP 6.08.

□ The maximum particle size observed in ophthalmic suspensions and in ophthalmic ointments is usually not larger than 75 μm.

□ Metal particles: Unless otherwise specified, ophthalmic ointments meet the requirements of Test for Metal Particles in Ophthalmic Ointments JP 6.01.

21. Ph. Eur. Ear preparations (Auricularia)

USP ⟨4⟩ Mucosal drug products—product quality tests

JP [2] 7 Preparations for otic application

Ear preparations are liquid, semi-solid or solid preparations, intended for instillation, for spraying, for insufflation for application to the auditory meatus or as an ear wash. The following categories may be distinguished, according to Ph. Eur.:

□ Ear drops and sprays
□ Semi-solid ear preparations
□ Ear powders
□ Ear washes
□ Ear tampons

The preparations may contain excipients to adjust tonicity, pH value or viscosity, to improve stability or solubility or to provide adequate antimicrobial properties. Preparations for application to the injured ear, in particular in case of ear drum perforations, or prior to surgery are sterile, free from antimicrobial preservatives and supplied in single-dose containers. Preparations supplied in multidose containers contain a suitable antimicrobial preservative except where the preparation itself has adequate antimicrobial properties. If necessary, ear preparations are provided with a suitable administration device, which may be designed to avoid the introduction of contaminants.

Ear drops and sprays

Ear drops and ear sprays are solutions, emulsions or suspensions of one or more active substances in appropriate liquids (e.g., water, glycols, fatty oils) suitable for application to the auditory meatus without exerting harmful pressure on the eardrum. They may also be placed in the auditory meatus by means of a tampon impregnated with the liquid. Ear drops are usually supplied in multidose containers fitted with an integral dropper or with a screw cap incorporating a dropper or a plastic teat. Ear sprays are usually supplied in multidose containers, fitted with an appropriate applicator. Sediments that may be found in suspensions should be readily dispersible on shaking. According to Ph. Eur., ear sprays in pressurized containers must comply with the requirements of the Ph. Eur. monograph "Pressurized pharmaceutical preparations."

Semi-solid ear preparations

Semi-solid ear preparations are intended for application to the external auditory meatus. According to Ph. Eur., they are supplied in containers fitted with a suitable applicator and should comply with the requirements of the Ph. Eur. monograph "Semi-solid preparations for cutaneous application."

Ear powders

Ear powders are intended for application into the external auditory meatus. According to Ph. Eur., they comply with the requirements of the Ph. Eur. monograph "Powders for cutaneous application" and are supplied in containers fitted with a suitable application device.

Ear washes

Ear washes are preparations intended for cleansing the external auditory meatus. They are usually aqueous solutions with a pH within physiological limits. When intended for application to injured parts or prior to a surgical operation sterility is required.

Ear tampons

Ear tampons are intended to be inserted into the external auditory meatus. According to Ph. Eur., they comply with the requirements of the Ph. Eur. monograph "Medicated tampons."

Tests

Ph. Eur.:
   □ Uniformity of dosage units: Single-dose ear preparations must comply with the test for uniformity of dosage units (Ph. Eur. 2.9.40) or alternatively, where justified and authorized, with the tests for uniformity of content (Ph. Eur. 2.9.6) and/or uniformity of mass (Ph. Eur. 2.9.5), as described below.
   □ Uniformity of content: Single-dose ear preparations with a content of active substance less than 2 mg or 2% of the total mass comply with test B for uniformity of content of single-dose preparations (Ph. Eur. 2.9.6).
   □ Uniformity of mass: Single-dose ear preparations comply with the test for uniformity of mass of single-dose preparations (Ph. Eur. 2.9.5). If the test for uniformity of content is prescribed for all the active substances, the test for uniformity of mass is not required.
   □ Sterility: Where the label indicates that the ear preparation is sterile, it complies with the test for sterility (Ph. Eur. 2.6.1).

USP:
USP chapter ⟨4⟩ (Mucosal drug products—product quality tests) mentions the following tests for preparations administered by the otic route:
   □ Sterility: Typically, sterility is required where the product is administered to the inner ear or where the eardrum is damaged.
   □ Microbiological examination of nonsterile products: Where sterility is not required, the quantitative enumeration of mesophilic bacteria and fungi that grow under anaerobic conditions (Microbiological examination of nonsterile products: Microbial enumeration tests ⟨61⟩), or the determination of the absence or limited occurrence of specified organisms (Microbiological examination of nonsterile products: Tests for specified microorganisms ⟨62⟩), may be required.
   □ Antimicrobial agents: If the preparation contains an antimicrobial preservative, antimicrobial effectiveness testing ⟨62⟩ and an assay of the antimicrobial agent (Antimicrobial Agents—Content ⟨341⟩) may be required.

JP:
   □ Unless otherwise specified, sterile ear preparations and the vehicles attached to the sterile preparations meet the requirements of Sterility Test ⟨4.06⟩.

22. Ph. Eur. Preparations for inhalation (Inhalanda)

Eur. 2.9.44 Preparations for nebulization: Characterization

USP ⟨5⟩ Inhalation and nasal drug products—general information and product quality tests

USP ⟨601⟩ Inhalation and nasal drug products—Aerosols, sprays, and powders—Performance quality tests

USP ⟨1601⟩ Products for nebulization—characterization tests

JP [2] 5 Preparations for inhalation

Preparations for inhalation are liquid or solid preparations intended for administration as vapors or aerosols to the lung in order to obtain a local or systemic effect. They may contain propellants, cosolvents, diluents, and other excipients. Such substances should not adversely affect the functions of the mucosa of the respiratory tract or its cilia. Suspensions and emulsions should be readily dispersible on shaking and remain sufficiently stable to enable the correct dose to be delivered. Preparations for inhalation are supplied in multidose or single-dose containers, when appropriate, provided with an adequate dosing device. Preparations that are applied as aerosol are administered by of one of the following devices:
- Nebulizer
- Pressurized metered-dose inhaler
- Non-pressurized metered-dose inhaler
- Powder inhalers

Classification according to Ph. Eur.

According to Ph. Eur., the following categories of preparations may de distinguished:
- Preparations to be converted into vapor
- Liquid preparations for nebulization
- Pressurized metered-dose preparations for inhalation
- Non-pressurized metered-dose preparations for inhalation
- Inhalation powders

□ **Preparations to be converted into vapor:** Preparations to be converted into vapor are solutions, suspensions, emulsions or solid preparations usually added to hot water and the vapor generated is inhaled.
□ **Liquid preparations for nebulization:** Liquid preparations for nebulization are solutions, suspensions or emulsions intended to be converted into aerosols by nebulizers driven by high-pressure gases, ultrasonic vibration or other methods. Nebulizers may be breath-triggered or use other means to synchronize or modify the nebulizer operation with the patient's breathing. They allow the dose to be inhaled at an appropriate active-substance delivery rate over an extended period of time, involving consecutive inspirations. The particle size ensures deposition of the preparation in the lungs. Tests on active substance delivery rate and total active substance delivered as well as aerodynamic assessments of nebulized aerosols are performed according to Ph. Eur.

2.9.44 ("Preparations for nebulization: Characterization"). Concentrates are diluted to the prescribed volume with the prescribed liquid prior to administration. When the preparation is in powder form, it is appropriately dissolved before use.

The pH of liquid preparations for nebulization is not lower than 3 and not higher than 10. Liquid preparations supplied in multidose containers may contain an antimicrobial preservative except where the preparation itself has adequate antimicrobial properties. Unpreserved preparations without intrinsic antimicrobial properties supplied in multidose containers must be sterile and the containers must be designed to prevent microbial contamination of the contents during storage and use. Liquid preparations supplied in single-dose containers are sterile and, unless otherwise justified and authorized, free from preservatives.

□ **Pressurized metered-dose preparations for inhalation:** Pressurized metered-dose preparations for inhalation are solutions, suspensions or emulsions. The containers are equipped with a metering valve and are held under pressure with a suitable propellant or a mixture of propellants, which can act also as a solvent. According to Ph. Eur., preparations in pressurized containers must comply with the requirements of the Ph. Eur. monograph "Pressurized pharmaceutical preparations."

The size distribution of the aerosol particles is controlled so that a consistent portion is deposited in the lungs. The determination of the fine-particle characteristics is performed according to Ph. Eur. 2.9.18 ("Preparations for inhalation: Aerodynamic assessment of fine particles").

□ **Non pressurized metered-dose preparations for inhalation:** Non-pressurized metered-dose preparations for inhalation are solutions, suspensions or emulsions for use with inhalers that convert liquids into aerosols using single or multiple liquid jets, ultrasonic vibration or other methods. The volume of liquid to be converted into an aerosol is pre-metered or metered by the inhaler so that the dose delivered from the inhaler can be inhaled with one or more inspirations. Preparations supplied in multidose containers may contain an antimicrobial preservative except where the preparation itself has adequate antimicrobial properties. Unpreserved preparations without intrinsic antimicrobial properties supplied in multidose containers must be sterile and the containers must be designed to prevent microbial contamination of the contents during storage and use. Preparations supplied in single-dose containers are sterile and, unless otherwise justified and authorized, free from preservatives.

The size distribution of the aerosol particles is controlled so that a consistent portion is deposited in the lungs. The determination of the fine-particle characteristics is performed according to Ph. Eur. 2.9.18 ("Preparations for inhalation: Aerodynamic assessment of fine particles"). Alternatively, laser diffraction analysis may be used, when properly validated against Ph. Eur. method 2.9.18 (apparatus C, D or E).

□ **Inhalation powders:** Inhalation powders are supplied in single-dose or multidose containers. The active ingredients may be combined with a suitable carrier. In general, these preparations are administered by means of a powder inhaler. A distinction is made between pre-metered inhalers, which are loaded with powders pre-dispensed in capsules or other suitable dosage forms and inhalers using a powder reservoir, which are equipped with a metering mechanism creating the dose. The size distribution of the aerosol particles is controlled so that a consistent portion is deposited in the lungs. The determination of the fine-particle characteristics is performed according to Ph. Eur. 2.9.18 ("Preparations for inhalation: Aerodynamic assessment of fine particles").

Classification according to USP

The USP distinguishes the following categories in chapter ⟨5⟩ (Inhalation and nasal drug products—General information and product quality tests):

- Inhalation aerosol
- Inhalation solution
- Inhalation suspension
- Solution for inhalation

- Drug for inhalation solution
- Inhalation spray
- Inhalation powder

☐ **Inhalation aerosol:** Inhalation aerosols, also known as MDIs (metered-dose inhalers) are dosage forms consisting of a liquid or solid preparation packaged under pressure and intended for administration as a fine mist. The preparations are characterized by dispersion of the active pharmaceutical ingredient into the airways during oral inspiration for either local or systemic effect. The formulation typically contains drug substance(s) dissolved or suspended in a propellant or a mixture of propellant(s) and cosolvent(s) and possibly other suitable excipients. It delivers a specified amount and quality of therapeutically active ingredient(s) upon activation of an accurately metered valve system.

☐ **Inhalation solution:** Inhalation solutions typically are water-based and are sterile preparations. They are intended for delivery to the lungs by nebulization with an external nebulizer and typically are packaged in single-dose containers. Nebulization involves continuous generation and delivery to the patient of a fine mist of aqueous droplets containing a drug solution by means of ultrasonic energy, Venturi effect, or other appropriate mechanical/electrical means.

☐ **Inhalation suspension:** Inhalation suspensions typically are water-based and are sterile preparations. They are intended for delivery to the lungs by nebulization with an external nebulizer and typically are packaged in single-dose containers. Nebulization involves continuous generation and delivery to the patient of a fine mist of aqueous droplets containing the formulation components by means of ultrasonic energy, Venturi effect, or other appropriate mechanical means.

☐ **Solution for inhalation:** Solutions for inhalation typically are water-based and are sterile preparations. Upon dilution (difference to "Inhalation solutions"), in accordance with labeling, they are intended for delivery to the lungs by nebulization using an external nebulizer. They are typically packaged in single-dose containers. Nebulization involves continuous generation and delivery to the patient of a fine mist of aqueous droplets containing the formulation components by means of ultrasonic energy, Venturi effect, or other appropriate mechanical/electrical means.

☐ **Drug for inhalation solution:** Drugs for inhalation solutions are drug powder formulations that upon the addition of a suitable vehicle, in accordance with labeling, yield solutions conforming in all respects to the inhalation solution requirements.

☐ **Inhalation spray:** Inhalation sprays typically are water-based liquid formulations packaged in a compact container-closure system containing an integral spray pump unit that upon activation delivers an accurately metered amount of fine mist of droplets of the formulation. The droplets can be generated by various means such as mechanical action, power assistance, or energy from the patient's inspiration. These drug products may be unit-dose or multidose presentations. Inhalation sprays may be designed as premetered or device-metered presentations. A premetered unit contains a previously measured amount of liquid formulation in an individual container (e.g., a blister) that is inserted in the device by the patient before use. A device-metered product contains sufficient amount of liquid formulation for a prescribed number of doses in a reservoir, and each dose is delivered as an accurately metered spray by the device.

☐ **Inhalation powder:** Inhalation powders, commonly known as dry powder inhalers (DPIs), dispense powders for inhalation with the use of a device that aerosolizes and delivers an accurately metered amount of active ingredient(s) with consistent physical characteristics alone or with a suitable excipient(s). Current designs include premetered and device-metered DPIs, all of which rely on various energy sources to create and disperse the aerosol during patient inspiration. Premetered DPIs contain previously measured amounts of formulation in individual containers (e.g., capsules or blisters) that are inserted into the device before use. They also may contain premetered dose units as ordered multidose assemblies in the delivery system. Device-metered DPIs have an internal reservoir that contains a sufficient quantity of formulation for multiple doses that are metered by the device itself during actuation by the patient.

Classification according to JP

The JP distinguishes the following categories in chapter [2] (Monographs for preparations):
- Dry powder inhalers
- Inhalation liquid preparations
- Metered-dose inhalers

- ☐ Dry powder inhalers are preparations which deliver a constant respiratory intake, intended for administration as solid particle aerosols.
- ☐ Inhalation liquid preparations are liquid inhalations which are administered by an inhalation device such as operating nebulizers.
- ☐ Metered-dose inhalers are preparations which deliver a constant dose of active substance(s) from the container together with propellant filled in.

Tests

Ph. Eur.:

Tests for metered-dose inhalers and powder inhalers, described in the Ph. Eur. monograph "Preparations for inhalation":

- ☐ Uniformity of delivered dose of metered-dose inhalers: The uniformity of the doses delivered from pressurized metered-dose inhalers and nonpressurized metered-dose inhalers is determined by means of an apparatus which is capable of quantitatively capturing the delivered dose. The apparatus, as described in the Ph. Eur., consists of a collection tube that is tightly connected to the mouthpiece of the inhaler by means of an adaptor. The opposite end of the tube is clamped or screwed to a filter-support base with an open-mesh filter support, accommodating a 25 mm filter disk. The filter-support base is connected to a vacuum source, which is capable, controlled by a flow regulator, to draw an air volume of 28.3 L ($\pm$ 5%) per minute continuously through the apparatus. Ten deliveries from the preparation are collected by the following procedure. The inhaler is prepared as directed in the instructions to the patient and subsequently the number of deliveries that constitute the minimum recommended dose is discharged into the apparatus. The contents of the apparatus are quantitatively collected and the amount of active substance is determined. The procedure is repeated with two further doses and subsequently the inhaler is discharged to waste until one delivery more than half the number of deliveries stated on the label remain. Four doses are collected and analyzed using the procedure described above. Then the inhaler is discharged to waste until three doses remain. These three doses are collected with the apparatus using the abovementioned procedure.

  The preparation complies with the test if 9 out of 10 results lie between 75% and 125% of the average value and all lie between 65% and 135%. If two or three values lie outside the limits of 75% to 125% the test is repeated for two more inhalers. Not more than 3 of the 30 values must lie outside the limits of 75% to 125% and no value must lie outside the limits of 65% to 135%.

- ☐ Uniformity of delivered dose of powder inhalers: The dose collection apparatus closely resembles that for the testing of the metered-dose inhalers. The airstream that is generated by the vacuum pump should be adjusted such that the pressure drop across the inhaler amounts to 4.0 kPa and the flow rate does not exceed 100 L/min. The test flow duration is set so that a volume of 4 L of air is drawn from the mouthpiece of the inhaler. Ten deliveries from the preparation are collected by the following procedure, which slightly differs between pre-dispensed and reservoir systems. The inhaler is connected to the apparatus using an adapter and, air is drawn through the inhaler using the predetermined conditions. This procedure is repeated until the number of deliveries that constitutes the minimum recommended dose has been sampled. The contents of the apparatus are quantitatively collected and the amount of active substance is determined. In case of predispensed inhalers, the procedure is repeated for a further nine doses. For reservoir systems the procedure is repeated for two further doses and subsequently the inhaler is discharged to waste until one delivery more than half the number of deliveries stated on the label remain. Four doses are collected and analyzed using the procedure described above. Then the inhaler is discharged to waste until three doses remain. These three doses are collected with the apparatus using the abovementioned procedure. The preparation complies with the test if 9 out of the 10 results lie between 75% and 125% of the average value and all lie between 65% and 135%. If two or three values lie outside the limits of 75% to 125%, the test is repeated for two more inhalers. Not more than 3 of the 30 values must lie outside the limits of 75% to 125% and no value must lie outside the limits of 65% to 135%. In justified and authorized cases these ranges may be extended but no value should deviate more than ± 50% from the average value.

- □ Fine particle dose: The proportion of fine particles in the dose is determined by means of the method described in Ph. Eur. 2.9.18 ("Preparations for inhalation: Aerodynamic assessment of fine particles"), using apparatus C, D or E.
- □ Number of deliveries per inhaler: The contents of one inhaler are discharged to waste. In case of pressurized metered-dose preparations a minimal time interval of 5 seconds between subsequent actuations of the valve should be maintained. The total number of deliveries so discharged should not be less than the number stated on the label.
- □ Number of deliveries per inhaler for multidose powder inhalers: By means of the apparatus described under "Uniformity of delivered dose of powder inhalers" (see above in this section) and by applying the appropriate pre-selected settings with respect to flow rate and air volume, the number of deliveries required to completely discharge the inhaler is determined. This number should not be less than the number stated on the label.

Tests for nebulizers, described in Ph. Eur. 2.9.44 ("Preparations for nebulization: Characterization") and in USP ⟨1601⟩ ("Products for nebulization—Characterization tests"): Products used for nebulization and intended for pulmonary delivery are characterized using the following tests:

- • Active substance delivery rate and total active substance delivered
- • Aerodynamic assessment of nebulized aerosols

- □ Active substance delivery rate and total active substance delivered: It is essential that breath-enhanced and breath-actuated nebulizers be evaluated by a breathing simulator, as the output of these devices is highly dependent on the inhalation flow rate. Ph. Eur. 2.9.44 and USP ⟨1601⟩ specify different breathing patterns to be used for testing products intended for adults, neonates, infants, and children. A filter, capable of quantitatively collecting the aerosol and enabling recovery of the active substance with an appropriate solvent, is attached to the breath simulator and the mouthpiece of the nebulizer is connected to the other side of the filter. After the breathing simulator is started, the nebulizer is operated for a defined time, usually 60 seconds. This procedure is repeated each time with a fresh filter and filter holder until nebulization ceases. The mass of active substance collected on the filters and filter holders during each time interval is determined, using a suitable method of analysis. In order to calculate the active substance delivery rate, the mass of active substance collected during the first interval is divided by the duration of this interval. The total mass of active substance delivered is determined by summing the mass of active substance collected on all filters and filter holders.
- □ Aerodynamic assessment of nebulized aerosols: The aerosol is characterized in terms of the mass of active substance as a function of aerodynamic diameter, using the cascade impactor "Apparatus E" (Next generation impactor, NGI), described in Ph. Eur. chapter 2.9.18 ("Preparations for inhalation: Aerodynamic assessment of fine particles"). In the USP, this apparatus is referred as "Apparatus 5," described in chapter ⟨601⟩. In order to assure quantitative recovery of active substance, a backup filter must be used in addition to the micro-orifice-collector (MOC) of apparatus E. A pre-separator, however, is not used for testing nebulizer-generated aerosols. Nebulized products need to be size-characterized at flow rates lower than the range that is normally used for powder inhalers and metered-dose inhalers. A flow rate of 15 L/min is recommended

(good approximation to the mid-inhalation flow rate achievable by tidally breathing). As part of the method development, recovery experiments must be performed to validate the method. This includes to determine and to define an appropriate sampling time in such a way as to ensure that the volume of liquid sampled from the nebulizer does not overload the impactor. Once determined, this time must be used in the analytical method for a particular product to ensure that mass fraction data can be compared. The measurements are performed by switching on the flow/compressor for the nebulizer for the predetermined time after a steady flow at 15 L/min has been adjusted and the mouthpiece of the nebulizer has been attached to the induction port of the impactor. After the sampling period, the nebulizer is removed, the impactor is dismantled and the mass of the active substance collected in the induction port, on each stage and on the back-up filter is determined, using a suitable method of analysis. The mass fraction of the active substance deposited on each component of the impactor is calculated and the cumulative fraction of the active substance is plotted versus cut-off diameter. The cut off-diameter at 15 L/min for each stage of the apparatus E can be obtained from a table in Ph. Eur. chapter 2.9.18 or USP chapter ⟨1601⟩.

USP:

The following general quality tests for inhalation drug products are listed in USP chapter ⟨5⟩ (Inhalation and nasal drug products—General information and product quality tests), Performance quality tests are described in chapter ⟨601⟩ (Inhalation and nasal drug products: Aerosols, sprays, and powders—Performance quality tests):

- ▫ Inhalation aerosol:
  - Identification ⟨5⟩
  - Assay ⟨5⟩
  - Impurities and degradation products ⟨5⟩
  - Water content ⟨5⟩
  - Foreign particulate matter ⟨5⟩
  - Leachables ⟨5⟩
  - Spray pattern ⟨5⟩
  - Microbial limit ⟨5⟩
  - Alcohol content (if present) ⟨5⟩
  - Net fill weight ⟨5⟩
  - Leak rate ⟨5⟩
  - Delivered-dose uniformity ⟨601⟩
  - Aerodynamic size distribution ⟨601⟩ (see combined textbox Ph. Eur. 2.9.18/USP ⟨601⟩)

- ▫ Inhalation solution:
  - Identification ⟨5⟩
  - Assay ⟨5⟩
  - Impurities and degradation products ⟨5⟩
  - Content uniformity (premetered) ⟨5⟩
  - Assay for antimicrobial preservative and stabilizing excipients (if present) ⟨5⟩
  - Sterility ⟨5⟩
  - Foreign particulate matter ⟨5⟩
  - pH ⟨5⟩
  - Osmolality ⟨5⟩
  - Leachables ⟨5⟩
  - Net fill weight ⟨5⟩
  - Weight loss ⟨5⟩
  - Aerodynamic size distribution ⟨601⟩ (see combined textbox Ph. Eur. 2.9.18/USP ⟨601⟩)

- ▫ Inhalation suspension:
  - Particle size distribution of the formulation in the immediate container ⟨5⟩
  - For all other general quality attributes, refer to the previous inhalation solution attributes ⟨5⟩

- □ Solution for inhalation:
  - Clarity and color of solution upon dilution in accordance with the labeling ⟨5⟩
  - For all other general quality attributes, refer to the previous inhalation solution attributes ⟨5⟩
- □ Drug for inhalation solution:
  - Water content ⟨5⟩
  - Clarity, color, and completeness of solution within specified time, upon reconstitution ⟨5⟩
  - For all other general quality attributes, refer to the previous inhalation solution attributes upon (re)constitution of the drug product ⟨5⟩
- □ Inhalation spray:
  - Plume geometry ⟨5⟩
  - For all other general quality attributes, refer to the previous inhalation solution attributes ⟨5⟩
  - Delivered-dose uniformity ⟨601⟩
  - Aerodynamic size distribution ⟨601⟩ (see combined textbox Ph. Eur. 2.9.18/USP ⟨601⟩)
- □ Inhalation powder:
  - Identification ⟨5⟩
  - Assay ⟨5⟩
  - Impurities and degradation products ⟨5⟩
  - Content uniformity (premetered) ⟨5⟩
  - Water content ⟨5⟩
  - Foreign particulate matter ⟨5⟩
  - Microbial limit ⟨5⟩
  - Net content (device-metered) ⟨5⟩
  - Residual solvents ⟨5⟩
  - Volatile and semivolatile leachables ⟨5⟩
  - Delivered-dose uniformity ⟨601⟩
  - Aerodynamic size distribution ⟨601⟩ (see combined textbox Ph. Eur. 2.9.18/USP ⟨601⟩)

Tests for nebulizers, described in USP ⟨1601⟩ ("Products for nebulization—Characterization tests"): see above in section "Tests—Ph. Eur."

JP:

- □ Uniformity of delivered dose: Metered-dose inhalers and metered-dose types among dry powder inhalers have an appropriate uniformity of delivered dose of the active substance(s).
- □ Aerodynamic size distribution: The particles of active substance(s) in metered-dose inhalers and in dry powder inhalers have an aerodynamically appropriate size.

23. Ph. Eur. Intramammary preparations for veterinary use (Praeparationes intramammariae ad usum veterinarium)

Intramammary preparations for veterinary use are sterile solutions, emulsions, suspensions or semi-solid preparations, containing one or more active substances. They are intended for introduction into the mammary gland via the teat canal. Two main categories are distinguished:

- □ Preparations for administration to lactating animals
- □ Preparations for administration to animals at the end of lactation or to nonlactating animals for the treatment or prevention of infection

The preparations are supplied in containers for use on one occasion only for introduction in a single teat canal of an animal. If supplied in multidose containers, aqueous preparations contain a suitable antimicrobial preservative, except where the preparation itself has adequate antimicrobial properties.

Tests

□ Efficacy of antimicrobial preservation: During the development of formulations which contain an antimicrobial preservative, the effectiveness of the chosen preservative shall be demonstrated.

□ Deliverable mass or volume: The mean mass or volume does not differ by more than 10% from the nominal value.

□ Sterility: Intramammary preparations for veterinary use comply with the test for sterility (Ph. Eur. 2.6.1).

24. Ph. Eur. Nasal preparations (Nasalia)

USP ⟨4⟩ Mucosal drug products—product quality tests

USP ⟨5⟩ Inhalation and nasal drug products—general information and product quality tests

USP ⟨601⟩ Inhalation and nasal drug products—Aerosols, sprays, and powders—Performance quality tests

JP [2] 8 Preparations for nasal application

Nasal preparations are liquid, semi-solid or solid preparations intended for administration to the nasal cavities to obtain a local or systemic effect.

Classification according to Ph. Eur.

According to Ph. Eur., the following categories of preparations may be distinguished (the classification of nasal preparations according to USP and JP is shown in Table A-1):

□ Nasal drops and liquid nasal sprays

□ Nasal powders

□ Semi-solid nasal preparations

□ Nasal washes

□ Nasal sticks

The preparations are as far as possible nonirritating and do not adversely affect the functions of the nasal mucosal and its cilia. Aqueous nasal preparations are usually isotonic and contain a suitable antimicrobial preservative if they are supplied in multidose containers. If necessary, the containers are provided with a suitable administration device, which may be designed to avoid the introduction of contaminants.

Nasal drops and liquid nasal sprays

Nasal drops and liquid nasal sprays are solutions, emulsions or suspensions intended for instillation or spraying into the nasal cavities. Emulsions may show evidence of phase separation but are easily redispersed on shaking. Suspensions may show a sediment, which is readily dispersible. Nasal drops are usually supplied in multidose containers, provided with a suitable applicator. Nasal sprays are supplied in containers with atomizing devices or in pressurized containers which comply with the requirements of the monograph on "Pressurized pharmaceutical preparations." The size of droplets of the spray is such as to localize their deposition in the nasal cavity.

Nasal powders

Nasal powders are powders intended for insufflation into the nasal cavity. They comply with the requirements of the monograph on "Powders for cutaneous application." The particle size is such as to localize their deposition in the nasal cavity.

Semi-solid nasal preparations

Semi-solid nasal preparations comply with the requirements of the monograph on "Semi-solid preparations for cutaneous application." The containers are adapted to deliver the product to the site of application.

Nasal washes

Nasal washes are generally aqueous isotonic solutions intended to cleanse the nasal cavities. If such preparations are intended to be applied to injured parts or prior to a surgical operation, they must be sterile.

Nasal sticks

Nasal sticks comply with the monograph on "Sticks."

Classification according to USP

USP chapter ⟨5⟩ lists the following categories of nasal drug products:
- **Nasal aerosols:** Drug products for local application into the nasal passages that are packaged under pressure and deliver a specified amount of therapeutically active ingredient(s) upon activation of an accurately metered valve system
- **Nasal sprays:** Nonpressurized, accurately metered, liquid drug dosage forms for local application into the nasal passages that are packaged in containers that upon activation deliver droplets of the formulation
- **Nasal solutions:** Nonpressurized, liquid drug dosage forms for local application into the nasal passages
- **Nasal powders:** Drug powders for local application into the nasal passages with the use of devices that deliver and aerosolize an accurately metered amount of the therapeutically active ingredient(s)

In USP chapter ⟨4⟩ also
- Gels (jellies) and
- Ointments

for administration by the nasal route are mentioned.

Tests

Ph. Eur.:
   Tests for nasal drops in single-dose containers
      □ Uniformity of dosage units: Nasal drops in single-dose containers comply with the test for uniformity of dosage units (Ph. Eur. 2.9.40) or, where justified and authorized, with the test for uniformity of mass or uniformity of content, as described below.
      □ Uniformity of mass: Nasal drops that are solutions comply with the following test. The contents of 10 containers emptied as completely as possible are weighed individually

and the average mass is calculated. Not more than 2 of the individual masses deviate by more than 10% from the average mass, and none deviate by more than 20%.

□ Uniformity of content: Nasal drops that are suspensions or emulsions comply with the test B for uniformity of content of single-dose preparations (Ph. Eur. 2.9.6), carried out on the individual contents of the containers after each of them has been emptied as completely as possible.

Tests for metered-dose nasal sprays

□ Uniformity of dosage units: Metered-dose nasal sprays comply with the test for uniformity of dosage units (Ph. Eur. 2.9.40) or, where justified and authorized, with the test for uniformity of mass or the test for uniformity of delivered dose, shown below. In the case of metered-dose nasal sprays that are solutions each of 10 tested containers is weighed after 5 actuations to waste, then discharged another time to waste and weighed again. The difference between the two masses is calculated for each container and the mass variation is determined. In the case of metered-dose nasal sprays that are suspensions or emulsions the test criterion is the content of active substance. From each of 10 containers the first five doses are discharged to waste and the sixth dose is collected, using an apparatus capable of quantitatively retaining the dose leaving the atomizing device. The active substance retained in the apparatus is collected by successive rinsing and determined from the combined rinses. Finally the content uniformity is calculated from the individual values obtained from the 10 containers.

□ Uniformity of mass: Metered-dose nasal sprays that are solutions comply with the following test, carried out on 10 containers. Each container is weighed after five actuations to waste, then discharged another time to waste and weighed again. The difference between the two masses is calculated. The preparation complies with the test if not more than two of the individual values deviate by more than 25% from the average value, but none of them by more than 35%.

□ Uniformity of delivered dose: Metered-dose nasal sprays that are suspensions or emulsions comply with the following test. The contents of active substance delivered upon the sixth actuation from each of 10 tested containers are determined in the way described above in the section "Uniformity of dosage units." The preparation complies with the test if at least 9 of the 10 contents are within the limits of 75% to 125% of the average content and all contents are between 65% and 135%. If 2 or at most 3 values are outside the 75% to 125% range, but are still within the 65% to 135% range, the test is repeated for 20 more containers. Not more than 3 of the 30 individual contents thus obtained may be outside the 75% to 125% range and none of them outside the 65% to 135% range.

□ Sterility: When the label states that the preparation is sterile, it complies with the test for sterility (Ph. Eur. 2.6.1).

USP:

The following quality tests for nasal drug products are listed in USP chapters ⟨4⟩ (Mucosal drug products) and ⟨5⟩ (Inhalation and nasal drug products—General information and product quality tests). Performance quality tests are described in chapter ⟨601⟩ (Inhalation and nasal drug products: Aerosols, sprays, and powders—Performance quality tests):

□ Nasal aerosol:

- For nasal aerosols USP chapter ⟨5⟩ refers to "Quality tests for inhalation aerosols" (see above in section 22 of the annex)
- Delivered-dose uniformity ⟨601⟩
- Droplet/particle size distribution, Particle size measurement by laser diffractometry ⟨601⟩

□ Nasal spray:

- Identification ⟨5⟩
- Assay ⟨5⟩
- Impurities and degradation products ⟨5⟩
- Assay for preservative and stabilizing excipients (if present) ⟨5⟩
- Content uniformity (premetered) ⟨5⟩

- Particle size distribution (for suspensions) ⟨5⟩
- Foreign particulate matter ⟨5⟩
- Spray pattern ⟨5⟩
- Microbial limit ⟨5⟩
- Leachables ⟨5⟩
- Net fill weight ⟨5⟩
- pH ⟨5⟩
- Osmolality ⟨5⟩
- Viscosity ⟨5⟩
- Sterility (premetered) ⟨5⟩
- Delivered-dose uniformity ⟨601⟩
- Droplet/particle size distribution, Particle size measurement by laser diffractometry ⟨601⟩

□ Nasal powder:

- For nasal powders USP chapter ⟨5⟩ refers to "Quality tests for inhalation powders" (see above in section 22 of the annex) ⟨5⟩
- Delivered-dose uniformity ⟨601⟩
- Droplet/particle size distribution, Particle size measurement by laser diffractometry ⟨601⟩

□ Nasal solution:

- Identification ⟨5⟩
- Assay ⟨5⟩
- Impurities and degradation products ⟨5⟩
- Assay for preservative and stabilizing excipients (if present) ⟨5⟩
- Foreign particulate matter ⟨5⟩
- Microbial limit ⟨5⟩
- Leachables ⟨5⟩
- Net fill weight ⟨5⟩
- pH ⟨5⟩
- Osmolality ⟨5⟩
- Viscosity ⟨5⟩

□ Gels, administered by the nasal route:

- For gels, administered by the nasal route USP chapter ⟨4⟩ refers to "Topical and transdermal drug products—Product quality tests" ⟨3⟩ (see above in section 3 of the annex)

□ Ointments, administered by the nasal route:

- For ointments, administered by the nasal route USP chapter ⟨4⟩ refers to "Topical and transdermal drug products—Product quality tests" ⟨3⟩ (see above in section 3 of the annex)
- Minimum fill ⟨755⟩ ⟨4⟩

JP:

The section "Nasal preparations" in JP [2] does not contain any reference to a pharmacopeial test.

25. Ph. Eur. Rectal preparations (Rectalia)

USP ⟨4⟩ Mucosal drug products—product quality tests

JP [2] 9 Preparations for rectal application

Rectal preparations are intended for rectal use in order to obtain a systemic or local effect, or they may be intended for diagnostic purposes.

According to Ph. Eur., several categories of rectal preparations may be distinguished (the classification of rectal preparations according to USP and JP is shown in Table A-1):

- □ Suppositories
- □ Rectal capsules
- □ Rectal solutions, emulsions and suspensions
- □ Powders and tablets for rectal solutions and suspensions
- □ Semi-solid rectal preparations
- □ Rectal foams
- □ Rectal tampons

Suppositories

Suppositories are solid, single-dose preparations. The shape, volume and consistency are suitable for application into the rectum. The active substance(s) are dispersed or dissolved in a suitable basis that may be soluble or dispersible in water or may melt at body temperature. Excipients such as diluents, absorbents, surface-active agents, lubricants, antimicrobial preservatives and coloring matter may be added if necessary. Suppositories are prepared by compression or molding. Hard fat, macrogols, cocoa butter and various gelatinous mixtures, consisting of, for example, gelatin, water, and glycerol may serve as suitable bases.

Rectal capsules

Rectal capsules are solid, single-dose preparations generally similar to soft capsules, as defined in the monograph "Capsules," except that they may have lubricating coatings. They have an elongated shape, are smooth and have a uniform external appearance.

Rectal solutions, emulsions and suspensions

Rectal solutions, emulsions and suspensions are liquid, single-dose preparations intended for rectal use in order to obtain a systemic or local effect. Emulsions may show evidence of phase separation and suspensions may show a sediment, but they should be readily redispersible upon shaking. To enable the correct dose to be delivered, the redispersed emulsions or suspensions should remain sufficiently stable. Added excipients should neither adversely affect the intended medical action nor cause undue local irritation. Rectal solutions, emulsions and suspensions are supplied in containers containing a volume in the range of 2.5 mL to 2000 mL. The container is adapted to deliver the preparation to the rectum or is accompanied by a suitable applicator.

Powders and tablets for rectal solutions and suspensions

Powders and tablets intended for the preparation of rectal solutions or suspensions are single-dose preparations that are dissolved or dispersed in water or other suitable solvents at the time of administration. The resulting solution or dispersion complies with the requirements for rectal solutions or rectal suspension, as appropriate.

Semi-solid rectal preparations

Semi-solid rectal preparations are ointments, creams or gels. They are often supplied as single-dose preparations in containers provided with a suitable applicator. They comply with the requirements of the monograph "Semi-solid preparations for cutaneous application."

Rectal foams

Rectal foams comply with the requirements of the monograph "Medicated foams."

Rectal tampons

Rectal tampons are solid, single-dose preparations intended to be inserted into the lower part of the rectum for a limited time. They comply with the requirements of the monograph "Medicated tampons."

Tests

Ph. Eur.:

- □ Uniformity of dosage units: Single-dose rectal preparations comply with the test on uniformity of dosage units (Ph. Eur. 2.9.40) or, in case of solid preparations, where justified and authorized, with the test for uniformity of content and/or uniformity of mass, as described below.
- □ Uniformity of content: Solid single-dose rectal preparations with a content of active substance less than 2 mg or 2% of the total mass, must comply with test A (tablets) or test B (suppositories, rectal capsules) for uniformity of content (Ph. Eur. 2.9.6).
- □ Uniformity of mass: Solid single-dose rectal preparations must comply with the test on uniformity of mass (Ph. Eur. 2.9.5). If the test for uniformity of content is prescribed for all active substances, the test for uniformity of mass is not required.
- □ Disintegration: Unless intended for modified release or for prolonged local action, suppositories and rectal capsules comply with the test for disintegration of suppositories and pessaries (Ph. Eur. 2.9.2). The state of the preparation is examined after 30 minutes in case of rectal capsules and suppositories with a fatty base and after 60 minutes in case of suppositories with a water-soluble base.

  Tablets for rectal solutions or suspensions are tested according to Ph. Eur. 2.9.1 ("Disintegration of tablets and capsules"). They must disintegrate within 3 minutes in water at 15° to 25°C.
- □ Dissolution: A suitable test may be required to demonstrate the appropriate release of the active substance(s) from solid single-dose rectal preparations, such as the dissolution test for lipophilic solid dosage forms (Ph. Eur. 2.9.42). Where a dissolution test is prescribed, a disintegration test may not be required.
- □ Softening time of lipophilic suppositories (Ph. Eur. 2.9.22)

USP:

The following quality tests for drug products administered by the rectal route are listed in USP chapter ⟨4⟩:

- □ Foams:
  - Minimum fill ⟨755⟩
  - Physical appearance (of the foam and of the collapsed foam)
  - Relative foam density (determined by weighing a mass of foam (m) and a mass of the same volume of water (e) in a flat-bottom dish. Relative foam density = m/e.)
  - Volume of foam expansion (Estimated by means of a graduated buret to which the dose-actuating device of the foam-generating container is fitted)
- □ Ointments:
  - For ointments, administered by the nasal route USP chapter ⟨4⟩ refers to "Topical and transdermal drug products—Product quality tests" ⟨3⟩ (see above in section 3 of the annex)
  - Minimum fill ⟨755⟩
- □ Suppositories:
  - Softening time of lipophilic suppositories (Time that elapses until a suppository maintained in water at 37°C softens to the extent that it no longer offers resistance when a defined weight is applied)
- □ Solutions:
  - No specific tests
- □ Suspensions:
  - No specific tests

JP:

□ Uniformity of dosage units: Unless otherwise specified, suppositories for rectal application meet the requirements of Uniformity of Dosage Units JP 6.02.

□ Drug release: Suppositories for rectal application show an appropriate release.

26. Ph. Eur. Vaginal preparations (Vaginalia)

USP ⟨4⟩ Mucosal drug products—product quality tests

JP [2] 10 Preparations for vaginal application

Vaginal preparations are liquid, semi-solid or solid preparations intended for administration to the vagina usually in order to obtain a local effect. They contain one or more active substances in a suitable basis. The following categories of vaginal preparations may be distinguished (the classification of vaginal preparations according to USP and JP is shown in Table A-1):

□ Pessaries

□ Vaginal tablets

□ Vaginal capsules

□ Vaginal solutions, emulsions, and suspensions

□ Tablets for vaginal solutions and suspensions

□ Semi-solid vaginal preparations

□ Vaginal foams

□ Medicated vaginal tampons

Pessaries

Pessaries are solid, usually ovoid single-dose preparations, containing one or more active substances. These are dispersed or dissolved in a basis that may be soluble or dispersible in water or may melt at body temperature. Pessaries have a volume and a consistency that is suited for vaginal application. They are commonly produced by means of a molding process. Typical bases are hard fat, macrogols, cocoa butter or various gelatinous mixtures, consisting, for example, of gelatin, water, and glycerol.

Vaginal tablets

Vaginal tablets generally conform to the definition of uncoated or film-coated tablets.

Vaginal capsules

Vaginal capsules (shell pessaries) are generally similar to soft capsules, as defined in the monograph "Capsules," differing only in their shape and size. Usually, they are ovoid and have a uniform external appearance.

Vaginal solutions, emulsions and suspensions

Vaginal solutions, emulsions and suspensions are single-dose, liquid preparations, intended for a local effect, for irrigation for diagnostic purposes. Emulsions may show evidence of phase separation and suspensions may show a sediment, but they should be readily redispersible upon shaking and should remain dispersed for a sufficiently long time to enable a homogenous preparation to be delivered. Any excipients, that may be added, should neither adversely affect the intended medical action nor cause undue local irritation. The container should be adapted to deliver the preparation to the vagina or it should be provided with an appropriate applicator.

Tablets for vaginal solutions and suspensions

Tablets intended for the preparation of vaginal solutions and suspensions are single-dose preparations that are dissolved or dispersed in water at the time of administration. Apart from the test for disintegration, they conform to the definition for "Tablets." After dissolution or dispersion, they comply with the requirements for vaginal solutions or vaginal suspensions, as appropriate.

Semi-solid vaginal preparations

Semi-solid vaginal preparations are ointments, creams or gels. They are often supplied in single-dose containers and provided with a suitable applicator. Semi-solid vaginal preparations comply with the requirements of the monograph "Semi-solid preparations for cutaneous application."

Vaginal foams

Vaginal foams comply with the requirements of the monograph "Medicated foams."

Medicated vaginal tampons

Medicated vaginal tampons are solid single-dose preparations intended to be inserted in the vagina for a limited time. They comply with the requirements of the monograph "Medicated tampons."

Tests

Ph. Eur.:
- Uniformity of dosage units: Single-dose vaginal preparations comply with the test for uniformity of dosage units (Ph. Eur. 2.9.40) or, where justified and authorized, with the test for uniformity of content and/or uniformity of mass, as described below.
- Uniformity of content: Solid single-dose vaginal preparations with a content of active substance less than 2 mg or 2% of the total mass, must comply with test A (vaginal tablets) or test B (pessaries, vaginal capsules) for uniformity of content (Ph. Eur. 2.9.6).
- Uniformity of mass: Solid single-dose vaginal preparations comply with the test for uniformity of mass (Ph. Eur. 2.9.5). If the test for uniformity of content is prescribed for all active substances, the test for uniformity of mass is not required.
- Disintegration: Unless intended for modified release or for prolonged local action, pessaries, vaginal tablets and vaginal capsules comply with the test for disintegration of suppositories and pessaries (Ph. Eur. 2.9.2). The state of the preparation is examined after 30 min in case of vaginal tablets and capsules and after 60 min in case of pessaries.

    Tablets for vaginal solutions or suspensions are tested according to Ph. Eur. 2.9.1 "Disintegration of tablets and capsules." They must disintegrate within 3 min in water at 15-25°C.
- Dissolution: A suitable test may be required to demonstrate the appropriate release of the active substance(s) from solid single-dose vaginal preparations, e.g., one of the tests described in Ph. Eur. chapter 2.9.3 ("Dissolution test for solid dosage forms") or in Ph. Eur. chapter 2.9.43 ("Dissolution test for lipophilic solid dosage forms"). Where a dissolution test is prescribed, a disintegration test may not be required.

USP:
The following quality tests for drug products administered by the vaginal route are listed in USP chapter ⟨4⟩:
- Creams:
  - Minimum fill ⟨755⟩

- For creams, administered by the vaginal route USP chapter ⟨4⟩ refers to "Topical and transdermal drug products—Product quality tests" ⟨3⟩ (see above in section 3 of the annex)
  □ Foams:
  - Minimum fill ⟨755⟩
  - Physical appearance (of the foam and of the collapsed foam)
  - Relative foam density (determined by weighing a mass of foam (m) and a mass of the same volume of water (e) in a flat-bottom dish. Relative foam density = m/e.)
  - Volume of foam expansion (Estimated by means of a graduated buret to which the dose-actuating device of the foam-generating container is fitted)
  □ Gels:
  - Minimum fill ⟨755⟩
  - For gels, administered by the vaginal route USP chapter ⟨4⟩ refers to "Topical and transdermal drug products—Product quality tests" ⟨3⟩ (see above in section 3 of the annex)
  □ Inserts:
  - No specific tests

JP:
  □ Uniformity of dosage units: Unless otherwise specified, tablets and suppositories for vaginal use meet the requirements of Uniformity of Dosage Units JP 6.02.
  □ Drug release: Tablets and suppositories for vaginal use show an appropriate release.

27. Ph. Eur. Intrauterine preparations for veterinary use (Preparationes intra-uterinae ad usum veterinarium)

Intrauterine preparations for veterinary use are liquid, semi-solid or solid preparations intended for the direct administration to the uterus (cervix, cavity or fundus), usually to obtain a local effect. They contain one or more active substances in a suitable basis. The following categories may be distinguished:
  □ Intrauterine tablets
  □ Intrauterine capsules
  □ Intrauterine solutions, emulsions and suspensions, concentrates for intrauterine solutions
  □ Tablets for intrauterine solutions and suspensions
  □ Semi-solid intrauterine preparations
  □ Intrauterine foams
  □ Intrauterine sticks

Intrauterine tablets

In general, intrauterine tablets conform to the definition given in the monograph on "Tablets." For introduction into the uterus a suitable applicator may be used.

Intrauterine capsules

Intrauterine capsules are, in general, similar to soft capsules, differing only in their shape and size. For introduction into the uterus a suitable applicator may be used.

Intrauterine solutions, suspensions and emulsions, concentrates for intrauterine solutions

Intrauterine solutions, suspensions and emulsions as well as concentrates for intrauterine solutions are liquid preparations. Intrauterine emulsions may show evidence of phase separation and suspensions may show a sediment, but they should be readily redispersible upon shaking and should remain dispersed for a sufficiently long time to enable a homogenous preparation to be delivered. Any excipients, that may be added, should neither adversely affect the intended medical action nor cause undue local irritations. The container should be adapted to deliver the preparation to the uterus or it should be provided with an appropriate applicator.

Tablets for intrauterine solutions and suspensions

Tablets intended for the preparation of intrauterine solutions and suspensions are single-dose preparations that are dissolved or dispersed in water at the time of administration. They conform to the definition given in the monograph on "Tablets." After dissolution or dispersion, they comply with the requirements for intrauterine solutions or intrauterine suspensions, as appropriate.

Semi-solid intrauterine preparations

Semi-solid intrauterine preparations are ointments, creams or gels. They comply with the requirements of the monograph on "Semi-solid preparations for cutaneous application." Semi-solid intrauterine preparations are often supplied in single-dose containers with a suitable applicator. The container should be adapted to deliver the preparation to the uterus or it should be provided with an appropriate applicator.

Intrauterine foams

Intrauterine foams must comply with the requirements of the monograph on "Medicated foams." The container is adapted to deliver the preparation to the uterus or may be accompanied by a suitable applicator.

Intrauterine sticks

Intrauterine sticks comply with the requirements of the monograph on "Sticks." Many preparations generate a foam upon contact with physiological fluids.

Tests

Ph. Eur.:
- Uniformity of dosage forms: Single-dose intrauterine preparations for veterinary use comply with the test for uniformity of dosage forms (Ph. Eur. 2.9.40) or, where justified and authorized, with the tests for uniformity of content (Ph. Eur. 2.9.6) and/or uniformity of mass (Ph. Eur. 2.9.5), as described below.
- Uniformity of content: Solid, single-dose intrauterine preparations with a content of less than 2 mg or 2% of the total mass must comply with test A (intrauterine tablets) or test B (intrauterine capsules) for uniformity of content of single-dose preparations (Ph. Eur. 2.9.6).
- Uniformity of mass: Solid single-dose intrauterine preparations for veterinary use comply with the test for uniformity of mass of single-dose preparations (Ph. Eur. 2.9.5). If the test for uniformity of content is prescribed, or justified and authorized, for all the active substances, the test for uniformity of mass is not required.

□ Disintegration: Unless intended for prolonged local action, intrauterine tablets and intrauterine capsules comply with the test for disintegration of suppositories and pessaries (Ph. Eur. 2.9.2). The state of the preparation is examined after 30 min.

Tablets for intrauterine solutions or suspensions are tested according to Ph. Eur. 2.9.1 "Disintegration of tablets and capsules." They must disintegrate within 3 min in water at 15-25°C.

□ Dissolution: A suitable test may be required to demonstrate the appropriate release of the active substance(s) from solid single-dose vaginal preparations, for example, one of the tests described in Ph. Eur. chapter 2.9.3 ("Dissolution Test for Solid Dosage Forms"). Where a dissolution test is prescribed, a disintegration test may not be required. Sterile intrauterine preparations for veterinary use comply with the test for sterility (Ph. Eur. 2.6.1) (This also applies to the separately provided applicators).

28. Ph. Eur. Oromucosal preparations (Praeparationes buccales)

USP ⟨4⟩ Mucosal drug products—product quality tests

JP [2] 1 Preparations for oro-mucosal application

Oromucosal preparations are solid, semi-solid or liquid preparations, containing one or more active substances intended for administration to the oral cavity and/or in the throat to obtain a local or systemic effect. Muco-adhesive preparations are intended to be retained in the oral cavity by adhesion to the mucosal epithelium and may modify systemic drug absorption at the site of application. For many oromucosal preparations, it is likely that some portion of the active substance(s) will be swallowed and may be absorbed via the gastrointestinal tract.

According to Ph. Eur., the following categories of oromucosal preparations may be distinguished (the classification of oromucosal preparations according to USP and JP is shown in Table A-1):

□ Gargles
□ Mouthwashes
□ Gingival solutions
□ Oromucosal solutions and oromucosal suspensions
□ Semi-solid oromucosal preparations (including for example gingival gel gingival paste, oromucosal gel and oromucosal paste)
□ Oromucosal drops and sprays, sublingual sprays (including oropharyngeal sprays)
□ Lozenges and pastilles
□ Compressed lozenges
□ Sublingual and buccal tablets
□ Oromucosal capsules
□ Mucoadhesive preparations
□ Orodispersible films

Gargles

Gargles are aqueous solutions, to the extent possible adjusted to neutral pH, which are intended for gargling to obtain a local effect. They should not be swallowed. Gargles are supplied as ready-to-use solutions or as concentrated solutions to be diluted or they may be prepared from powders or tablets to be dissolved in water before use.

Mouthwashes

Mouthwashes are aqueous solutions, to the extent possible adjusted to neutral pH, which are intended for use in contact with the mucous membrane of the oral cavity. They should not be swallowed. Mouthwashes are supplied as ready-to-use solutions or as concentrated solutions to be diluted or they may be prepared from powders or tablets to be dissolved in water before use.

Gingival solutions

Gingival solutions are intended for administration to the gingivae by means of a suitable applicator.

Oromucosal solutions and oromucosal suspensions

Oromucosal solutions and oromucosal suspensions are liquid preparations intended for administration to the oral cavity by means of a suitable applicator. If suspensions show a sediment, this should be readily dispersible on shaking to give a suspension that remains sufficiently stable to enable the correct dose to be delivered.

Semi-solid oromucosal preparations

Semi-solid oromucosal preparations are hydrophilic gels or pastes intended for administration to the oral cavity or to a specific part of the oral cavity such as the gingivae (gingival gel, gingival paste). They must comply with the requirements of the monograph "Semi-solid preparations for cutaneous use."

Oromucosal drops, oromucosal sprays and sublingual sprays

Oromucosal drops, oromucosal sprays and sublingual sprays are solutions, emulsions or suspensions which are instilled or sprayed into the oral cavity or onto a specific part of the oral cavity (e.g., under the tongue or into the throat) to achieve a local or systemic effect. Emulsions may show evidence of phase separation and suspensions may show a sediment, but they should be readily redispersible upon shaking and should remain dispersed for a sufficiently long time to enable the correct dose to be delivered. Sprays are supplied in containers with atomizing devices or in pressurized containers that comply with the requirements of the monograph "Pressurized pharmaceutical preparations." The size of droplets of the spray is such as to localize their deposition in the oral cavity.

Lozenges and pastilles

Lozenges and pastilles are solid, single-dose preparations intended to be sucked to obtain, usually, a local effect in the oral cavity and the throat. They contain one or more active substances, usually in a flavored and sweetened base and are intended to dissolve or disintegrate slowly in the mouth when sucked.

Lozenges, as defined in the Ph. Eur., are prepared exclusively by molding (in contrast to Compressed lozenges), whereas in the USP the term encompasses both, molded lozenges and compressed lozenges. According to USP (chapter ⟨1151⟩) molded lozenges are also called pastilles, which, however, is mentioned to be an unofficial term, not used in naming pharmacopeial articles. In the terminology of the Ph. Eur. pastilles are soft, flexible preparations and lozenges are hard preparations, both of them prepared by molding.

Compressed lozenges

Compressed lozenges are solid, single-dose preparations intended to be sucked to obtain a local or systemic effect. They are prepared by compression and conform to the general definition of tablets.

Sublingual tablets and buccal tablets

Sublingual tablets and buccal tablets are solid, single-dose preparations to be applied under the tongue or to the buccal cavity, respectively, to obtain a systemic effect. They are prepared by compression of powder mixtures or granules and conform to the general definition of tablets.

Oromucosal capsules

Oromucosal capsules are soft capsules to be chewed or sucked.

Mucoadhesive preparations

Mucoadhesive preparations are mucoadhesive buccal tablets, buccal films or other mucoadhesive solid or semi-solid preparations intended for systemic absorption of one or more active substances through the buccal mucosa over a prolonged period of time. They usually contain hydrophilic polymers, which on wetting with the saliva produce a hydrogel that adheres to the buccal mucosa; in addition buccal films may dissolve. Mucoadhesive buccal tablets are prepared by compression and may be single- or multilayer tablets. Buccal films are single- or multilayer sheets of suitable materials.

Orodispersible films

Orodispersible films are single- or multilayer sheets of suitable materials, to be placed in the mouth where they disperse rapidly

USP chapter ⟨1151⟩ classifies films by the site of application and distinguishes oral films, buccal films, and sublingual films.

Tests

Ph. Eur.:

Tests for uniformity of dosage units, content and mass for single-dose oromucosal preparations:

- ▫ Uniformity of dosage units: Single-dose oromucosal preparations comply with the test for uniformity of dosage units (Ph. Eur. 2.9.40) or, where justified and authorized, with the test for uniformity of content and/or uniformity of mass, as described below.
- ▫ Uniformity of content: Single-dose oromucosal preparations with a content of active substance less than 2 mg or 2% of the total mass must comply with test A (compressed and molded dosage forms) or test B (capsules) for the uniformity of content of single-dose preparations (Ph. Eur. 2.9.6). Oromucosal drops that are suspensions or emulsions comply with the test B for uniformity of content of single-dose preparations (Ph. Eur. 2.9.6), carried out on the individual contents of the containers after each of them has been emptied as completely as possible.
- ▫ Uniformity of mass: Solid single-dose oromucosal preparations must comply with the test for uniformity of mass (Ph. Eur. 2.9.5). If the test for the uniformity of content is prescribed, or justified and authorized, for all active substances, the test for uniformity of mass is not required. Oromucosal drops that are solutions comply with the following test. The contents of 10 containers emptied as completely as possible are weighed individually and the average mass is calculated. Not more than 2 of the individual masses deviate by more than 10% from the average mass and none deviates by more than 20%.

Tests for uniformity of dosage units, content and mass for metered-dose oromucosal sprays and sublingual sprays:

▫ Uniformity of dosage units: Metered-dose oromucosal sprays and sublingual sprays comply with the test for uniformity of dosage units (Ph. Eur. 2.9.40) or, where justified and authorized, with the test for uniformity of mass or the test for uniformity of delivered dose shown below. In the case of metered-dose oromucosal sprays and sublingual sprays that are solutions, each of 10 tested containers is weighed after 5 actuations to waste, then discharged another time to waste and weighed again. The difference between the two masses is calculated for each container and the mass variation is determined. In the case of metered-dose oromucosal sprays and sublingual sprays that are suspensions or emulsions the test criterion is the content of active substance. From each of 10 containers the first five doses are discharged to waste and the sixth dose is collected, using an apparatus capable of quantitatively retaining the dose leaving the atomizing device. The active substance retained in the apparatus is collected by successive rinsing and determined from the combined rinses. Finally the content uniformity is calculated from the individual values obtained from the 10 containers.

▫ Uniformity of mass: Metered-dose oromucosal sprays and sublingual sprays that are solutions comply with the following test, carried out on 10 containers. Each container is weighed after 5 actuations to waste, then discharged another time to waste and weighed again. The difference between the two masses is calculated. The preparation complies with the test if not more than 2 of the individual values deviate by more than 25% from the average value, but none of them by more than 35%.

▫ Uniformity of delivered dose: Metered-dose oromucosal sprays and sublingual sprays that are suspensions or emulsions comply with the following test. The contents of active substance delivered upon the sixth actuation from each of 10 tested containers are determined in the way described above in the section "Uniformity of dosage units." The preparation complies with the test if at least 9 of the 10 contents are within the limits of 75% to 125% of the average content and all contents are between 65% and 135%. If two or maximum three values are outside the 75% to 125% range, but are still within the 65% to 135% range, the test is repeated for 20 more containers. Not more than 3 of the 30 individual contents thus obtained may be outside the 75% to 125% range and none of them outside the 65% to 135% range.

Tests for dissolution and mechanical strength:

▫ Dissolution: For compressed lozenges intended for a systemic effect, sublingual tablets, buccal tablets, mucoadhesive preparations, and orodispersible films, a suitable test is carried out to demonstrate the appropriate release of the active substance(s).

▫ Friability and resistance to crushing: Compressed lozenges, sublingual tablets, buccal tablets, mucoadhesive preparations and orodispersible films should possess suitable mechanical strength to resist handling without crumbling, breaking or damage. This may be demonstrated in case of compressed lozenges, sublingual tablets and buccal tablets by examining the "Friability of uncoated tablets" (Ph. Eur. 2.9.7) and the "Resistance to crushing of tablets" (Ph. Eur. 2.9.8).

USP:

The following quality tests for drug products administered by the oropharyngeal route are listed in USP chapter ⟨4⟩:

▫ Buccal patches:

• For buccal patches USP chapter ⟨4⟩ refers to "Topical and transdermal drug products—Product quality tests" ⟨3⟩ (see above in section 3 of the annex)

▫ Films:

• No specific tests

▫ Gels:

• Minimum fill ⟨755⟩

- For gels, administered by the oropharyngeal route USP chapter ⟨4⟩ refers to "Topical and transdermal drug products—Product quality tests" ⟨3⟩ (see above in section 3 of the annex)

  ◻ Gums:
  - No specific tests

  ◻ Lozenges:
  - No specific tests

  ◻ Ointments:
  - For ointments, administered by the oropharyngeal route USP chapter ⟨4⟩ refers to "Topical and transdermal drug products—Product quality tests" ⟨3⟩ (see above in section 3 of the annex)
  - Minimum fill ⟨755⟩

  ◻ Solutions (Rinses):
  - No specific tests

  ◻ Sprays:
  - For sprays, administered by the oropharyngeal route USP chapter ⟨4⟩ refers to "Inhalation and nasal drug products—general information and product quality tests" ⟨5⟩ (see above in section 24 of the annex)

  ◻ Tablets:
  - For tablets, administered by the oropharyngeal route USP chapter ⟨4⟩ refers to "Oral drug products—product quality tests" ⟨2⟩ (see above in section 14 of the annex)

JP:

  ◻ Tablets for oro-mucosal application:
  - Uniformity of dosage units: Unless otherwise specified, tablets for oro-mucosal application meet the requirements of Uniformity of Dosage Units JP 6.02.
  - Dissolution, Disintegration: Tablets for oro-mucosal application have an appropriate dissolution or disintegration.

  ◻ Sprays for oro-mucosal application:
  - Uniformity of dosage units: Unless otherwise specified, metered-dose types among sprays for oro-mucosal application have an appropriate uniformity of delivered dose.

  ◻ Semi-solid preparations for oro-mucosal application:
  - No specific tests

  ◻ Preparations for gargle:
  - Uniformity of dosage units: Unless otherwise specified, preparations for gargle in single-dose packages meet the requirements of Uniformity of Dosage Units JP 6.02.

Dosage forms listed only in the USP or the JP

In addition to the dosage forms listed above, referring to Ph. Eur., the USP chapter ⟨1151⟩ (Pharmaceutical dosage forms) and the JP chapter [2] (Monographs for preparations) describe several additional types:

USP: Gases

Medical gases are products that are administered directly as a gas. A medical gas has a direct pharmacological action or acts as a diluent for another medical gas. Gases used as excipients for administration of aerosol products, as an adjuvant in packaging, or produced by other dosage forms, are not included in this definition.

USP: Liquids

As a dosage form, a liquid consists of a pure chemical in its liquid state. Examples include mineral oil, isoflurane, and ether. This dosage form term is not applied to solutions.

USP: Pellets

Pellets are dosage forms composed of small, solid particles of uniform shape sometimes called beads (although the use of the term "beads" as a dosage form is not preferred). Typically, pellets are nearly spherical but this is not required. Pellets may be administered by the oral (gastrointestinal) or by the injection route (see also "Pellet implants" above in subchapter "Ph. Eur. Parenteral preparations").

USP: Pills

Pills are drug substance-containing small, spherical, solid bodies intended for oral administration, usually prepared by a wet massing, piping, and molding technique. The pill dosage form has been largely replaced by compressed tablets and by capsules.

USP: Strips

A strip is a dosage form or device in the shape of a long, narrow, thin, absorbent, solid material such as filter paper. Typically it is sterile and it may be impregnated with a compound or be gauged to allow measurements for diagnostic purposes, such as in measuring tear production. The term "strip" should not be used when another term such as "film" is more appropriate.

JP [2] 1-7: Jellies for oral administration

Jellies for Oral Administration are non-flowable gelatinous preparations having a certain shape and size, intended for oral administration.

Tests

JP:
  - □ Uniformity of dosage units: Unless otherwise specified, jellies for oral administration meet the requirements of Uniformity of Dosage Units JP 6.02
  - □ Dissolution: Unless otherwise specified, jellies for oral administration meet the requirements of Dissolution Test JP 6.10 or show an appropriate disintegration

JP [2] 4: Preparation for dialysis

Dialysis agents are liquid or solid preparations that are to be dissolved before use, intended for peritoneal dialysis or hemodialysis. They are classified into peritoneal dialysis agents and hemodialysis agents.

Tests

JP:
  - □ Bacterial Endotoxines/Pyrogens: Unless otherwise specified, dialysis agents meet the requirements of Bacterial Endotoxins Test JP 4.01.
  - □ Uniformity of dosage units: The solid preparations which are to be dissolved before use among Dialysis agents have an appropriate uniformity of dosage units.

- Unless otherwise specified, peritoneal dialysis agents meet the requirements of Sterility Test JP 4.06.
- Extractable volume: Unless otherwise specified, peritoneal dialysis agents meet the requirements for parenteral infusions under Test for Extractable Volume of Parenteral Preparations JP 6.05. The mass of content may convert to the volume by dividing by the density.
- Foreign and particulate matter: Unless otherwise specified, peritoneal dialysis agents meet the requirements of Foreign Insoluble Matter Test for Injections JP 6.06 and of Insoluble Particulate Matter Test for Injections JP 6.07.
- Material of containers: Containers for Injections meet the requirements of Test for Glass Containers for Injections JP 7.01 or the requirements of Test Methods for Plastic Containers JP 7.02.
- Material of closures: Unless otherwise specified, the rubber closures of the containers meet the requirements of Test for Rubber Closure for Aqueous Infusions JP 7.03.

Index

Note: Page numbers in *italic* denote figures, those in **bold** denote tables.

SI Units Used in the Book and Other Relevant Units

Quantity		Unit				
Name	Symbol	Name	Symbol	Expression in SI Units	Expression in Other SI Units	Conversion of Other Units into SI Units
Wave number	ν	Reciprocal meter	1/m	m^{-1}		
Wavelength	λ	Micrometer	μm	10^{-6} m		
		Nanometer	nm	10^{-9} m		
Surface area	A, S	Square meter	m^2	m^2		
Volume	V	Cubic meter	m^3	m^3		$1\ mL = 1\ cm^3 = 10^{-6}\ m^3 = 0.001\ L$
Frequency	ν	Hertz	Hz	s^{-1}		
Density	ρ	Kilograms per cubic meter	kg/m^3	$kg \cdot m^{-3}$		$1\ g \cdot cm^{-3} = 10^{-3}\ kg \cdot m^{-3}$
Velocity	v	Meters per second	m/s	$m \cdot s^{-1}$		
Force	F	Newton	N	$m \cdot kg \cdot s^{-2}$		$1\ dyn = 1\ g \cdot cm \cdot s^{-2} = 10^{-5}\ N$ $1\ kp = 9.80665\ N$
Pressure	p	Pascal	Pa	$m^{-1} \cdot kg \cdot s^{-2}$	$N \cdot m^{-2}$	$1\ dyn \cdot cm^{-2} = 10^{-1}\ Pa = 10^{-1}\ N \cdot m^{-2}$ $1\ atm = 101325\ Pa = 101.325\ kPa$ $1\ bar = 10^5\ Pa = 0.1\ MPa$ $1\ mm\ Hg = 133.322387\ Pa$ $1\ Torr = 133.322368\ Pa$ $1\ psi = 6.894757\ kPa$
Dynamic viscosity	η	Pascal second	Pa·s	$m^{-1} \cdot kg \cdot s^{-1}$	$N \cdot s \cdot m^{-2}$	$1\ P = 10^{-1}\ Pa \cdot s = 10^{-1}\ N \cdot s \cdot m^{-2}$ $1\ cP = 1\ mPa \cdot s$
Kinematic viscosity	ν	Square meters per second	m^2/s	$m^2 \cdot s^{-1}$	$Pa \cdot m^3 \cdot s \cdot kg^{-1}$ $N \cdot m \cdot s \cdot kg^{-1}$	$1\ St = 1\ cm^2 \cdot s^{-1} = 10^{-4}\ m^2 \cdot s^{-1}$
Energy	W	Joule	J	$m^2 \cdot kg \cdot s^{-2}$	$N \cdot m$	$1\ erg = 1\ cm^2 \cdot g \cdot s^{-2} = 1\ dyn \cdot cm = 10^{-7}\ J$ $1\ cal = 4.1868\ J$
Power	P	Watt	W	$m^2 \cdot kg \cdot s^{-3}$	$N \cdot m \cdot s^{-1}$	$1\ erg/s = 1\ dyn \cdot cm \cdot s^{-1} = 10^{-7}\ W = 3.41214\ Btu \cdot h^{-1} = 1\ W$
Absorbed dose	D	Gray	Gy	$m^2 \cdot s^{-2}$	$J \cdot kg^{-1}$	$1\ rad = 10^{-2}\ Gy$
Electric voltage	U	Volt	V	$m^2 \cdot kg \cdot s^{-3} \cdot A^{-1}$	$W \cdot A^{-1}$	
Electrical resistance	R	Ohm	Ω	$m^2 \cdot kg \cdot s^{-3} \cdot A^{-2}$	$V \cdot A^{-1}$	
Electrical charge (amount of electricity)	Q	Coulomb	C	$A \cdot s$		
Activity of a radioactive substance	A	Bq		s^{-1}		$1\ Ci = 37 \cdot 10^9\ Bq = 37 \cdot 10^9\ s^{-1}$
Molarity	C	Moles per cubic meter	mol/m^3	$mol \cdot m^{-3}$		$1\ mol \cdot L^{-1} = 1\ M = 1\ mol \cdot dm^{-3} = 10^3\ mol \cdot m^{-3}$
Mass concentration	ρ	Kilograms per cubic meter	$kg \cdot m^{-3}$			$1\ g \cdot L^{-1} = 1\ g \cdot dm^{-3} = 1\ kg \cdot m^{-3}$